D1687786

International Union Against Cancer

Manual of Clinical Oncology

UICC Manual of Clinical Oncology

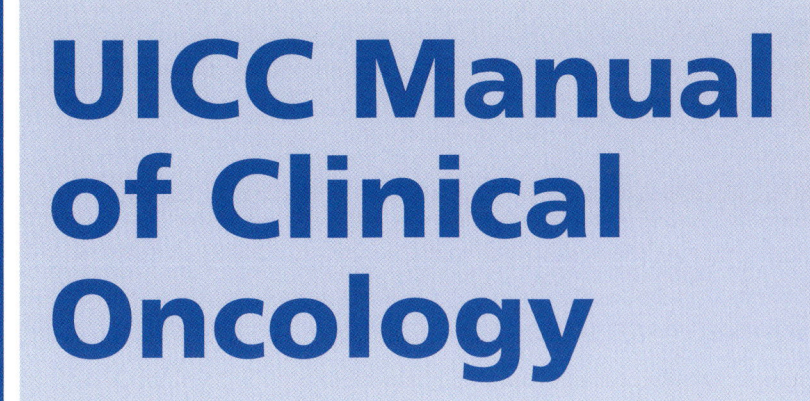

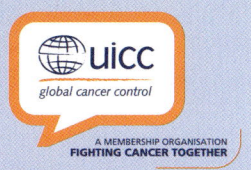

NINTH EDITION

EDITORS

Brian O'Sullivan (Editor in Chief)
MD, FRCPC, FRCPI, FFRRCSI (Hon), FASTRO
Professor, Department of Radiation Oncology
Bartley-Smith / Wharton Chair in Radiation Oncology, The Princess Margaret Cancer Centre / University of Toronto, Toronto, Ontario, Canada

James D. Brierley
BSc, MB, FRCP, FRCR, FRCP(C)
Professor, Department of Radiation Oncology, The Princess Margaret Cancer Centre / University of Toronto, Ontario, Canada

Anil K. D'Cruz
MS, DNB, FRCS
Director, Tata Memorial Hospital, Professor, Department of Head and Neck Surgical Oncology, Mumbai, India

Martin F. Fey
Dr med.
Professor, Department of Medical Oncology, Inselspital and University Hospital, Bern, Switzerland

Raphael Pollock
MD, PhD
Professor, Department of Surgery, Director of the Division of Surgical Oncology, Chief of Surgical Services
The James NCICCC / Ohio State University, Columbus, Ohio, USA

Jan B. Vermorken
MD, PhD
Emeritus Professor, University of Antwerp; Consultant, Department of Medical Oncology, Antwerp University Hospital, Edegem, Belgium

Shao Hui Huang (Editorial Coordinator)
MD, MSc, MRT(T)
Assistant Professor, Department of Radiation Oncology,
The Princess Margaret Cancer Centre / University of Toronto, Toronto, Ontario, Canada

WILEY Blackwell

This edition first published 2015 © 2015 by UICC. Published 2015 by John Wiley & Sons, Ltd

This Work is a co-publication between the UICC and John Wiley & Sons, Ltd.

Registered office: John Wiley & Sons, Ltd, The Atrium, Southern Gate, Chichester, West Sussex, PO19 8SQ, UK

Editorial offices: 9600 Garsington Road, Oxford, OX4 2DQ, UK
The Atrium, Southern Gate, Chichester, West Sussex, PO19 8SQ, UK
111 River Street, Hoboken, NJ 07030–5774, USA

For details of our global editorial offices, for customer services and for information about how to apply for permission to reuse the copyright material in this book please see our website at www.wiley.com/wiley-blackwell

The right of the author to be identified as the author of this work has been asserted in accordance with the UK Copyright, Designs and Patents Act 1988.

All rights reserved. No part of this publication may be reproduced, stored in a retrieval system, or transmitted, in any form or by any means, electronic, mechanical, photocopying, recording or otherwise, except as permitted by the UK Copyright, Designs and Patents Act 1988, without the prior permission of the publisher.

Designations used by companies to distinguish their products are often claimed as trademarks. All brand names and product names used in this book are trade names, service marks, trademarks or registered trademarks of their respective owners. The publisher is not associated with any product or vendor mentioned in this book. It is sold on the understanding that the publisher is not engaged in rendering professional services. If professional advice or other expert assistance is required, the services of a competent professional should be sought.

The contents of this work are intended to further general scientific research, understanding, and discussion only and are not intended and should not be relied upon as recommending or promoting a specific method, diagnosis, or treatment by health science practitioners for any particular patient. The publisher and the author make no representations or warranties with respect to the accuracy or completeness of the contents of this work and specifically disclaim all warranties, including without limitation any implied warranties of fitness for a particular purpose. In view of ongoing research, equipment modifications, changes in governmental regulations, and the constant flow of information relating to the use of medicines, equipment, and devices, the reader is urged to review and evaluate the information provided in the package insert or instructions for each medicine, equipment, or device for, among other things, any changes in the instructions or indication of usage and for added warnings and precautions. Readers should consult with a specialist where appropriate. The fact that an organization or Website is referred to in this work as a citation and/or a potential source of further information does not mean that the author or the publisher endorses the information the organization or Website may provide or recommendations it may make. Further, readers should be aware that Internet Websites listed in this work may have changed or disappeared between when this work was written and when it is read. No warranty may be created or extended by any promotional statements for this work. Neither the publisher nor the author shall be liable for any damages arising herefrom.

Library of Congress Cataloging-in-Publication Data

UICC manual of clinical oncology / editors, Brian O'Sullivan, editor in chief; James Brierley [and five others]. — Ninth edition.
   p. ; cm.
   Manual of clinical oncology
   Preceeded by UICC manual of clinical oncology / editor, Raphael E. Pollock. 8th ed. 2004.
   Includes bibliographical references and index.
   ISBN 978-1-4443-3244-5 (cloth)
   I. O'Sullivan, Brian, 1952– , editor.   II. Brierley, James, editor.   III. International Union against Cancer, issuing body.   IV. Title: Manual of clinical oncology.
   [DNLM: 1. Neoplasms—Handbooks. QZ 39]
   RC262.5
   616.99'4—dc23
                                                                                            2015021962

Wiley also publishes its books in a variety of electronic formats. Some content that appears in print may not be available in electronic books.

Cover image: Photo of banner © UICC.

Set in 9pt/12pt Frutiger Light by Aptara Inc., New Delhi, India
Printed and bound in Singapore by Markono Print Media Pte Ltd

Dedication

This *Manual* is dedicated to Leslie H. Sobin MD, an internationally renowned pathologist and previous long-term Chair of the UICC TNM Prognostic Factor Committee. Les, as he is known to colleagues all over the world, has devoted most of his career to promoting multidisciplinary cancer control in a truly global manner.

Contents

Foreword x
Preface xi
About the Editors xiii
Contributors xvi

PART 1 General principles of cancer diagnosis and management   1

Principles of knowledge generation and translation

1 – Cancer epidemiology   3

2 – Levels of evidence, guidelines and standards   12

3 – Prognosis and classification of cancer   23

4 – Principles of cancer staging   34

5 – Assessment of treatment outcome   40

6 – Cancer informatics   53

Principles of cancer diagnosis

7 – Imaging   63

8 – Pathology   83

Principles of treatment

9 – Principles of surgery   98

10 – Principles of radiotherapy   108

11 – Principles of systemic therapy   124

Special settings, supportive care and survivorship

12 – Treatment in pregnancy   134

13 – Treatment in the elderly   139

14 – Oncology emergencies   145

15 – Supportive care during curative treatment   155

16 – Pain management in cancer   168

17 – Palliative care   174

18 – Survivorship   184

19 – Rehabilitation   194

PART 2 Site-specific multidisciplinary cancer management   203

Thoracic malignancies

20 – Lung   205

Breast

21 – Breast   221

Gastrointestinal malignancies

22 – Liver   241

23 – Biliary tract and pancreas   263
23.1 – Biliary tract   263
23.2 – Pancreas   270

24 – Oesophagus   280

25 – Stomach   297

26 – Colon, rectum and anus   308
26.1 – Colon and rectum   308
26.2 – Anus   327

Genitourinary malignancies

27 – Prostate   333

28 – Bladder and other urothelium   343

29 – Kidney   354

30 – Testicular germ cell tumours   368

31 – Penis   384

Haematological malignancies

32 – Lymphoma   392

33 – Myeloma   415

34 – Leukaemia   427

Gynaecological cancers

35 – Cervix   449

36 – Uterus   467

37 – Ovary and fallopian tube   479

38 – Vulva   495

Head and neck cancer

39 – General principles of head and neck cancer management   503

40 – Nasopharynx   512

41 – Oral cavity   524

42 – Larynx and hypopharynx   542

43 – Oropharynx   559

44 – Major salivary glands   571

45 – Nasal cavity and paranasal sinus   586

46 – Head and neck unknown primary   597

Endocrine tumors

47 – Pituitary   609

48 – Thyroid   626

49 – Adrenal tumours   641

50 – Neuroendocrine tumours   656

Dermatological cancer

51 – Skin: Basal cell carcinoma, squamous cell carcinoma and Merkel cell carcinoma   674

52 – Melanoma   689

Central nervous system and ocular cancers

53 – Central nervous system   706

54 – Eye: Choroidal melanoma, retinoblastoma, ocular adnexal lymphoma and eyelid cancers   726

Sarcoma

55 – Bone (osteosarcoma) 745

56 – Soft tissue 754

Childhood malignancies

57 – Paediatric tumors 768

Specific cancer situations

58 – Cancer of unknown primary (non-head and neck) 788

59 – HIV and transplant-related neoplasms 797

59.1 – HIV-related neoplasms 797

59.2 – Post-transplantation lymphoproliferative disease 809

59.3 – Cancer following solid organ transplantation 812

Index 815

Foreword

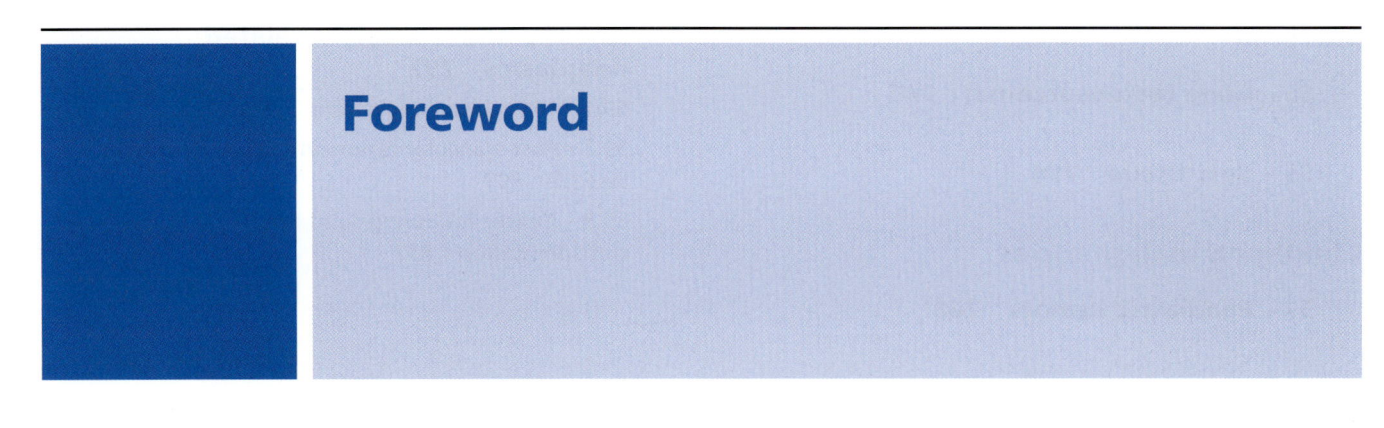

UICC unites the cancer community to reduce the global cancer burden, to promote greater equity and to integrate cancer control into the world health and development agenda with the goal of delivering on the World Cancer Declaration. One of the nine targets of the Declaration that shape the overarching goal of improving cancer survival is the education and training of healthcare professionals. The *UICC Manual of Clinical Oncology* has for many years been part of UICC's educational platform. I have always kept the latest edition of this book as an essential oncology guide in my library since my early years in oncology. By bringing together for the 9th edition a multidisciplinary authorship from across the globe with the purpose of generating an accessible and realistic guide for cancer management in all resource settings, Dr O'Sullivan and the editorial team of the *UICC Manual of Clinical Oncology* have further strengthened UICC's commitment to improve cancer services and patient outcomes.

M. Tezer Kutluk MD, PhD, FAAP
President
Union for International Cancer Control
Geneva

Preface

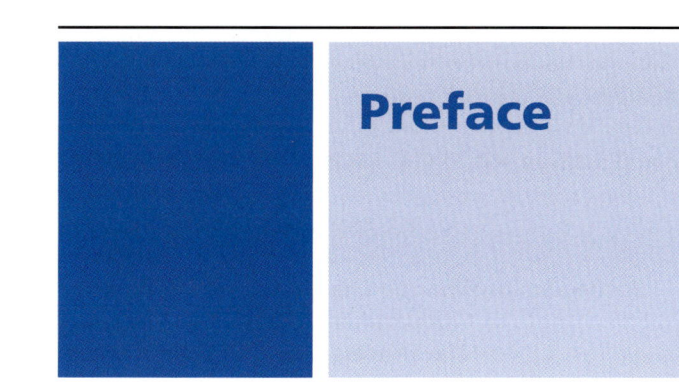

It is with great pride that I introduce the 9th edition of the *UICC Manual of Clinical Oncology*, representing the work of a remarkably diverse international group of colleagues. The *Manual* continues to emphasize a devotion to multidisciplinary assessment and care. Disease-site chapters have been co-authored wherever appropriate by representatives of medical, radiation and surgical oncology in addressing the different fields of cancer management. As well, an international panel of authors has been assembled that strives to emphasize, where relevant, needs in jurisdictions where a disease may be most prevalent. For example, many head and neck cancer chapters are authored from India which sustains an unfair burden of tobacco-related mucosal cancers, but the nasopharyngeal and oropharyngeal chapters are authored by specialists from South East-Asia and the Western World, respectively, in recognition of the unique disease incidence and profile in these locations.

As in previous editions, the target readership comprises oncologists-in-training and the many subspecialty disciplines and allied health practitioners involved with multimodality cancer treatment programmes, as well as practising physicians and others throughout the world who care for cancer patients. Wherever feasible, a succinct style is used and characterized by bullet point displays and tabular depictions instead of the traditional dense text that characterizes many textbooks. In large part this convention is concentrated in the disease-site chapters which form the backbone of the manual and where the hallmark is immediate access to information for readers. The philosophy is particularly mindful of the needs of jurisdictions where information is less available and practitioners may be unusually busy and working in smaller units. For all chapters, references are provided as recommended reading without encumbering the direct narratives of specialists with knowledge and experience of the domain under discussion.

This edition has been completely revised and all chapters rewritten. New chapters address information needs and approaches that highlight areas of contemporary oncology, including, among others, practical understanding and application of evidence-based medicine, cancer informatics, oncology outcome reporting, symptom management, survivorship and end of life needs of cancer patients. Each disease-site chapter also incorporates cancer staging from the *UICC's TNM Classification of Malignant Tumours*, 7th Edition (2009) and a complete chapter is devoted to the history and principles of cancer staging that evolved at the UICC from the time it first introduced TNM more than 60 years ago.

Since publication of the 8th edition in 2004, there has been a necessary need to integrate knowledge about non-anatomical factors with traditional classification of disease extent into prognostic algorithms which also influence cancer diagnosis and therapy. Of particular importance are molecular characteristics, but other very relevant factors pertain to patient issues, such as age, co-morbidity and ability to tolerate treatment, as well as the health service environment, including access to care, education and skill/knowledge of practitioners. For this reason each disease-site chapter employs a standard classification format that identifies prognostic factors according to their current relevance in the clinic. This classifies factors as to whether they are *essential* to guide treatment decision-making, provide *additional* information that may facilitate research, teaching, or cancer programme management, or represent *new and promising* developments in oncology without yet having a firm foothold in overall cancer control. These concepts are emphasized using the UICC's standard tabular format in each anatomical site-specific chapter. The source for *essential* factors is from publicly available guidelines that mandate their requirement for treatment decision-making. They include internationally recognized guidelines such as those of NCCN, ESMO, ASTRO, ESTRO and ASCO, as well as published guidelines from individual cancer institutions or agencies where available. In addition, the cancer incidence and prevalence data are almost entirely from Globocan 2012 (http://globocan.iarc.fr/Default.aspx) and Surveillance, Epidemiology, and End Results Program (SEER) (http://SEER.cancer.gov).

Finally, and most importantly, I would like to thank our readers, whose efforts on behalf of oncology patients worldwide offer the very best hope for a future free of malignant disease. I hope you will enjoy this book as much as we, the editors and authors, enjoyed the global spirit of collaboration and interaction needed to prepare it for you and our patients.

Brian O'Sullivan MD, FRCPC, FRCPI, FFRRCSI (Hon), FASTRO
Editor-in-Chief
UICC Manual of Clinical Oncology
Professor
Bartley-Smith/Wharton Chair in Radiation Oncology
Department of Radiation Oncology
The Princess Margaret Cancer Centre
University of Toronto, Canada

Acknowledgement

I would like to take this opportunity to thank my co-editors and all the authors of the *Manual* for their dedication in volunteering their time on behalf of this project.

Special thanks are also extended to the Editorial Coordinator, Shao Hui (Sophie) Huang, who volunteered tirelessly in supporting the editorial team, and to the staff at UICC and Wiley.

About the Editors

Brian O'Sullivan MD, FRCPC, FRCPI, FFRRCSI (Hon), FASTRO

Brian O'Sullivan is a Professor in the Department of Radiation Oncology at the University of Toronto, Toronto, Ontario, Canada. He also holds the Bartley-Smith/Wharton Distinguished Chair in Radiation Oncology in the Department of Radiation Oncology at The Princess Margaret Cancer Centre, University of Toronto. He is the Head and Neck Oncology Program Chair at The Princess Margaret Cancer Centre, the co-Chair of the US NCI Head and Neck Steering Committee, Coordinating Center for Clinical Trials, CTEP, and a full standing member of the Commission of the International Commission on Radiation Units (ICRU). He is the recipient of numerous international awards, and research grants. He has published almost 300 peer reviewed papers, in excess of 50 book chapters and has written or edited six oncology textbooks. His interests include sarcoma and head and neck cancer, translational research, IMRT delivery and the principles of image-guided radiotherapy, chemoradiotherapy and molecular targeting. He is a member of the TNM Committee of the Union for International Cancer Control (UICC), Chair of the UICC Prognostic Classification Sub-Committee and represents the UICC as liaison in several oncology sites to the American Joint Committee on Cancer (AJCC).

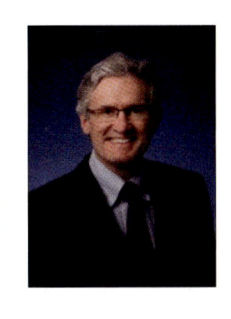

Professor, Department of Radiation Oncology
Bartley-Smith / Wharton Chair in Radiation Oncology
The Princess Margaret Cancer Centre
University of Toronto
Toronto, ON, Canada

James D. Brierley BSc, MB, FRCP, FRCR, FRCP(C)

James Brierley is Professor of Radiation Oncology at the University of Toronto, The Princess Margaret Cancer Centre. He obtained his medical degree from Westminster Medical School, University of London. He initially did postgraduate training in Internal Medicine before transferring to Clinical Oncology. He is interested in and has written extensively on thyroid cancer, the role of radiation in gastrointestinal malignancy, and cancer staging and surveillance, and is actively involved in research into the role of radiation in the management of gastrointestinal and endocrine malignancies and ensuring staging data is collected and used on a population basis. He is the previous head of the Gastrointestinal Site Group at The Princess Margaret Cancer Centre and is currently the Canadian Partnership Against Cancer Expert Lead, Staging and Surveillance. He is a Member of the AJCC Executive and Chair of the AJCC Education and Promotions Working Group, Co-Chair of the UICC TNM Prognostic Factors Core Group and Co-Editor of the UICC 8th edition TNM Classification of Malignant Tumours.

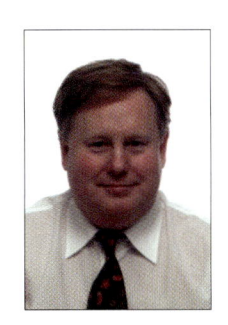

Professor, Department of Radiation Oncology
The Princess Margaret Cancer Centre
University of Toronto
Toronto, ON, Canada

Anil K. D'Cruz MS, DNB, FRCS

Dr D'Cruz is Director at the Tata Memorial Hospital, Mumbai, India as well as Professor & Surgeon, Department of Head & Neck Surgery. He is a distinguished leader in the field of oncology and on the Board of Directors of the Union for International Cancer Control (UICC), Geneva, Foundation of Head Neck Oncology India and the Asian Society of Head Neck Oncology. He has more than 150 peer-reviewed publications and chapters to his name and is also an editor for a two volume text book on head and neck surgery. He is Associate Editor of *Head Neck Oncology Journal* and member of the Editorial Board of many reputed national and international journals. He has delivered more than 250 invited lectures and 50 orations.

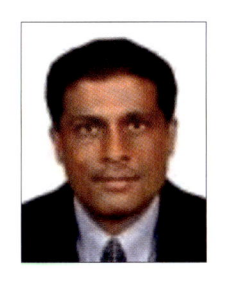

Professor, Department of Head
and Neck Surgical Oncology
Director, Tata Memorial Centre
Mumbai, India

About the Editors

Martin F. Fey MD, Dr. med
Martin Fey is Professor and Head of Department of Medical Oncology at the University of Bern, Switzerland. He is also Head of the Department of Oncology, Laboratory Medicine and Hospital Pharmacy at the Inselspital, Bern. He received his medical degree from the Berne University Medical School. He was the recipient of the Robert-Wenner Award of the Swiss Cancer League and Ellermann Award of the Swiss Society of Haematology. He has more than 250 peer-reviewed publications to his credit, mainly in clinical and experimental haematological oncology. He leads clinical trials in leukaemia, lymphoma, breast cancer and other types of tumours. He was the Chairman of the Leukaemia Group of the Swiss Group for Clinical Cancer Research (SAKK) from 1990 to 1995 and a Principal Investigator of the SAKK and the International Breast Cancer Study Group (IBCSG) from 1993 to 2002. His interests include leukaemia, lymphoma, breast cancer and the design of clinical trials. He is a member of the Cantonal Ethics Committee for Clinical Trials of the Canton of Bern, Switzerland.

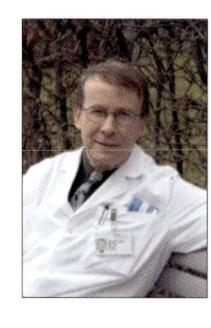

Professor of Medical Oncology
Department of Medical Oncology
Inselspital and University Hospital
Bern, Switzerland

Raphael Pollock MD, PhD
Raphael Pollock was born in Chicago, Illinois and graduated from Oberlin College, Oberlin, Ohio in 1972. This was followed by medical school at the St Louis University School of Medicine, Chicago, IL, residencies in General Surgery at the University of Chicago and Rush Medical College, a fellowship in Surgical Oncology at The University of Texas M. D. Anderson Cancer Center, and a PhD. in Tumor Immunology from the Graduate School of the Biological Sciences at the University of Texas-Houston Health Sciences Center. Dr Pollock joined the Department of Surgical Oncology at The University of Texas M. D. Anderson Cancer Center as a faculty member in 1984. He became Chairman of the Department of Surgical Oncology in 1993 and Head of the Division of Surgery at The University of Texas M. D. Anderson Cancer Center in 1997. In 2006–2007 Dr Pollock served as President of the Society of Surgical Oncology; from 1999-2011 he served as Editor-in-Chief of Cancer. In 2013 Dr Pollock left M. D. Anderson to become Director and Professor, Division of Surgical Oncology and Chief of Surgical Services at The James Comprehensive Cancer Center at The Ohio State University Medical Center, Columbus, Ohio. Dr Pollock serves as Director of the Sarcoma Research Laboratory at The Ohio State University Medical Center and is the Principal Investigator on behalf of the US NIH/NCI SARC Sarcoma SPORE grant program. Dr Pollock is a member of the US NIH/NCI Board of Scientific Counselors.

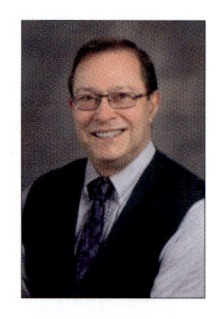

Director of the Division of Surgical Oncology
Chief of Surgical Services
The James NCICCC / Ohio State University
Columbus, OH, USA

Jan B. Vermorken MD, PhD
Jan B. Vermorken was born in 1944, graduated in 1970 from the University of Amsterdam, the Netherlands and became a board-certified specialist in internal medicine in 1975. Since that time he has worked in the field of Medical Oncology and was officially registered as a Medical Oncologist in the Netherlands in 1992. He received his PhD in Medical Sciences in 1986 from the Vrije Universiteit in Amsterdam. From May 1997 until 1 October 2009, he was Professor of Oncology at the University of Antwerp (UA), and head of the Department of Medical Oncology at the University Hospital Antwerp (UZA), in Edegem, Belgium. After his retirement he remains connected to both University (emeritus Professor) and University Hospital. His main fields of interest are gynaecological oncology, and head and neck oncology. He devotes a significant amount of time to teaching, professional training and continuing medical education. Professor Vermorken is member of various scientific societies and of several editorial boards of international journals, reviewer of multiple cancer journals and author or co-author of more than 500 publications in international journals. From 1 January 2009 until 1 January 2014 he was Editor-in-Chief of *Annals of Oncology*, the official journal of the European Society for Medical Oncology and the Japanese Society of Medical Oncology. On 1 March 2013 he received the title of Commander in the Order of Leopold for his contributions to oncology.

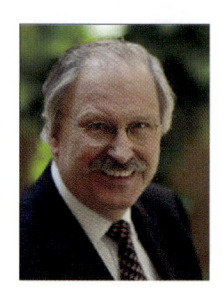

Emeritus Professor of Oncology
Faculty of Medicine and Health Sciences,
University of Antwerp
Antwerp, Belgium
and
Department of Medical Oncology
Antwerp University Hospital
Edegem, Belgium

Shao Hui (Sophie) Huang
MD, MSc, MRT (T)

Shao Hui (Sophie) Huang is an Assistant Professor in the Department of Radiation Oncology at the University of Toronto. She is an MD trained in China, and completed her Hons BSc in Radiation Therapy at the University of Toronto in 2003. Since graduation, she works as a radiation therapist at The Princess Margaret Cancer Centre. Sophie currently divides her time among maintaining the Head-and-Neck Cancer Anthology of Outcomes System at the institution, coordinating the multidisciplinary Head-and-Neck Cancer Conference, clinical and translational research, and delivering radiation treatment for head and neck cancers. She has been the principal investigator and co-investigator in many research projects and has more than 40 peer-reviewed publications. Her major interest is outcome research, especially in HPV-related oropharyngeal cancer. She was the first to describe the unusual distant metastasis pattern in HPV-related oropharyngeal cancer. She has received several awards at international Scientific Meetings.

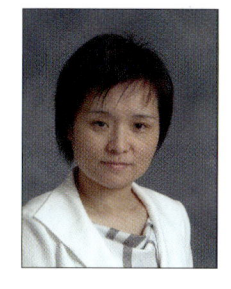

Assistant Professor MRT (T),
Department of Radiation Oncology
The Princess Margaret Cancer Centre
University of Toronto
Toronto, ON, Canada

Contributors

Matti S. Aapro MD
Multidisciplinary Oncology Institute
Clinique de Genolier
Genolier, Switzerland

Eddie K. Abdalla MD
Professor and Chairman
Department of Surgery
Chief of Surgical Oncology
The Lebanese American University
Beirut, Lebanon

Vera M. Abeler MD, PhD (Retired)
Consultant in Pathology
Department of Pathology
Oslo University Hospital
The Norwegian Radium Hospital
Oslo, Norway

Stefan Aebi MD
Head, Cancer Center and Division of
Medical Oncology
Lucerne Cantonal Hospital
Lucerne, Switzerland

Jai Prakash Agarwal MD
Professor
Department of Radiation Oncology
Tata Memorial Centre
Mumbai, India

Peter Albers MD
Professor and Chairman
Department of Urology
University Hospital Dusseldorf
Dusseldorf, Germany

Dawna Allore RN
Symptom Management and Supportive Care
Program
University of Michigan Comprehensive Cancer
Center
Ann Arbor, MI, USA

Maria Almond MD, MPH
PsychOncology Clinic
University of Michigan
Ann Arbor, MI, USA

Supreeta Arya MD, DNB, DMRD
Professor, Department of
Radio-diagnosis
Tata Memorial Centre
Mumbai, India

William F. Auffermann MD, PhD
Department of Radiology
Emory University
Winship Cancer Institute
Atlanta, GA, USA

Hatem A. Azim Jr MD, PhD
Department of Medicine
BrEAST Data Centre
Institut Jules Bordet
Université Libre de Bruxelles
Brussels, Belgium

Sumitra Bakshi MD
Associate Professor, Anesthesiology
Department of Anesthesiology
Critical Care & Pain
Tata Memorial Centre
Mumbai, India

Christopher Baliski MD, FRCSC
Head of Surgical Oncology
University of British Columbia and BC Cancer
Agency
Kelowna, BC, Canada

Brian K. Bednarski MD
Assistant Professor
Department of Surgical Oncology
The University of Texas M. D. Anderson
Cancer Center
Houston, TX, USA

J. Sybil Biermann MD
Professor, Department of
Orthopaedic Surgery
University of Michigan
Ann Arbor, MI, USA

Carsten Bokemeyer MD
Professor, Department of Oncology,
Hematology, BMT with Section Pneumology
University Hospital Hamburg-Eppendorf
Hamburg, Germany

Fabrice Bonnet MD, PhD
Service de Médecine Interne et Maladies
Infectieuses
Hôpital Saint-André, CHU de Bordeaux
INSERM, ISPED, University of Bordeaux
Bordeaux, France

Savtaj S. Brar MD, FRCSC
Surgical Oncologist
Department of Surgery
Mount Sinai Hospital
Toronto, ON, Canada

James D. Brierley BSc, MB, FRCP, FRCR, FRCP(C)
Professor, Department of Radiation Oncology
The Princess Margaret Cancer Centre
University of Toronto, Toronto
ON, Canada

Emile Brihi MD
Associate Professor of Radiation Oncology
Division of Radiation Oncology
The Lebanese American University
Beirut, Lebanon

Melissa C. Brouwers PhD
Department of Oncology
McMaster University
Hamilton, ON, Canada

Gina Brown FRCR
Consultant Radiologist
Department of Radiology
Royal Marsden Hospital
London & Surrey, UK

Claire Casselman LMSW
Clinical Care Coordinator
PsychOncology Clinic
University of Michigan
Ann Arbor, MI, USA

Pamela Catton MD, MHPE, FRCPC
Director, ELLICSR and Medical Director, Patient Education and Survivorship Programs
The Princess Margaret Cancer Centre/
University Health Network
Professor of Radiation Oncology, University of Toronto
Toronto, ON, Canada

Anthony T.C. Chan MD
Department of Clinical Oncology
Chinese University of Hong Kong
Hong Kong, China

Jimmy Y. W. Chan FRCS
Department of Otolaryngology
University of Hong Kong
Hong Kong, China

Joanna S.Y. Chan MD
Department of Pathology, Anatomy, & Cell Biology
Thomas Jefferson University
Philadelphia, PA, USA

Ian Chau FRCP
Consultant Medical Oncologist
Department of Radiology
Royal Marsden Hospital
London & Surrey, UK

Devendra Chaukar MS, DNB
Professor and Head
Department of Head and Neck Surgical Oncology, Tata Memorial Centre
Mumbai, India

Sylvain Choquet MD
Département d'Hématologie Clinique
Hôpital Pitié-Salpêtrière-Charles Foix, APHP
UPMC University of Paris
Paris, France

Rashmi Chugh MD
Associate Professor, Division of Hematology/Oncology
Department of Internal medicine
University of Michigan
Ann Arbor, MI, USA

Caroline Chung MD, FRCPC, CIP
Assistant Professor
Department of Radiation Oncology
The Princess Margaret Cancer Centre
University of Toronto
Toronto, ON, Canada

Dominique Costagliola PhD
Sorbonne Universités,
UPMC University of Paris, IUC
INSERM, Institut Pierre Louis d'Epidémiologie et de Santé Publique
Paris, France

Carien L. Creutzberg MD, PhD
Professor
Department of Radiation Oncology
Leiden University Medical Center
Leiden, The Netherlands

Juanita Crook MD, FRCPC
Professor of Radiation Oncology
British Columbia Cancer Agency
Department of Radiation Oncology and Developmental Radiotherapeutics
Cancer Center for the Southern Interior
Kelowna, BC, Canada

Michael Crump MD, FRCP(C)
Hematologist, Division of Medical Oncology and Hematology
The Princess Margaret Cancer Centre
University of Toronto
Toronto, ON, Canada

Mitali Dandekar MS, DNB
Clinical Fellow, Department of Head and Neck Surgical Oncology
Tata Memorial Centre
Mumbai, India

Elizabeth J. Davis MD
Fellow, Division of Hematology/Oncology
Department of Internal Medicine
University of Michigan
Ann Arbor, MI, USA

Ian D. Davis MBBS, PhD, FRACP, FAChPM
Medical Oncologist
Professor of Medicine, Monash University and Eastern Health
Victoria, Australia

Anil K. D'Cruz MS, DNB, FRCS
Director, Tata Memorial Centre
Professor, Department of Head and Neck Surgical Oncology
Tata Memorial Centre
Mumbai, India

Andre Dekker PhD
Principal Investigator, Department of Radiation Oncology (MAASTRO)
GROW School for Oncology and Developmental Biology
University of Maastricht
Maastricht, The Netherlands

Isabelle Demeestere MD, PhD
Research Laboratory on Human Reproduction
Université Libre de Bruxelles
Brussels, Belgium

Dustin Deming MD
University of Wisconsin
Carbone Cancer Center
Madison, WI, USA

Lynette Denny MBChB (UCT), MMED (O&G), PhD, FCOG (SA)
Head, Department of Obstetrics & Gynaecology
Faculty of Health Sciences
University of Cape Town and Groote Schuur Hospital
Cape Town, South Africa

Colleen Dickie MRT(T)(MR), MSc
Assistant Professor, Department of Radiation Oncology
The Princess Margaret Cancer Centre
University of Toronto
Toronto, ON, Canada

Rajesh Dikshit PhD
Professor – Epidemiology
Tata Memorial Centre Centre for Cancer Epidemiology
Mumbai, India

Rossitza Draganova-Tacheva MD
Department of Pathology, Anatomy, & Cell Biology
Thomas Jefferson University
Philadelphia, PA, USA

Gillian M. Duchesne MS, MD, FRCR, FRANZCR
Professor Radiation Oncology Research
Sir Peter MacCallum Department of Oncology
University of Melbourne
Melbourne, Victoria, Australia

Prateek Dwivedi MSc
Techna Institute/The Princess Margaret Cancer Centre
University Health Network,
University of Toronto
Toronto, ON, Canada

Contributors

Massimo Falconi MD
Professor, Pancreatic Surgery Unit
Salute e Vita
University-San Raffaele Hospital
Milan, Italy

Wentao Fang MD
Professor, Department of Thoracic Surgery
Shanghai Chest Hospital
Jiaotong University Medical School
Shanghai, China

Mary Feng MD
Associate Professor, Department of Radiation Oncology
University of Michigan
Ann Arbor, MI, USA

J.E. Ferguson III MD, PhD
Department of Urology
University of North Carolina School of Medicine
Chapel Hill, NC, USA

Sherise D. Ferguson MD
Department of Neurosurgery
The University of Texas M. D. Anderson Cancer Center
Houston, TX, USA

Felix Fernandez MD
Division of Thoracic Surgery
Department of Surgery
Emory University
Winship Cancer Institute
Atlanta, GA, USA

Martin F. Fey MD, Dr med.
Professor of Medical Oncology
Head of Department of Medical Oncology
Inselspital and University Hospital
Bern, Switzerland

Paul T. Finger MD
Clinical Professor of Ophthalmology
New York University School of Medicine
Director, The Ocular Tumor Services:
The New York Eye Cancer Center
The New York Eye and Ear Infirmary
of Mt. Sinai
Manhattan Eye, Ear and
Throat Hospital
New York, NY, USA

Anna R. Franklin MD
Assistant Professor, Division of Pediatrics
The University of Texas M. D. Anderson Cancer Center
Houston, TX, USA

Oreste Gentilini MD
Department of Breast Surgery
European Institute of Oncology
Milan, Italy

Hady Ghanem MD
Assistant Professor of Medicine
Head of Division of Hematology/Oncology
Division of Medical Oncology
The Lebanese American University
Beirut, Lebanon

Sarbani Ghosh Laskar MD, DNB
Professor
Department of Radiation Oncology
Tata Memorial Centre
Mumbai, India

Bruce J. Giantonio MD, FACP
Abramson Cancer Center
The University of Pennsylvania
Philadelphia, PA, USA

Theresa A. Gillis MD
Medical Director, Oncology Rehabilitation Services
Helen F. Graham Cancer Center
Christiana Care Health System
Wilmington, DE
Clinical Associate Professor
Department of Rehabilitation Medicine
Jefferson Medical College
Philadelphia, PA, USA

Meredith Giuliani MD, Med, FRCPC
Assistant Professor, Department of Radiation Oncology
The Princess Margaret Cancer Centre
University of Toronto
Toronto, ON, Canada

Rob Glynne-Jones FRCP, FRCR
Consultant Radiation Oncologist
Radiotherapy Department
Mount Vernon Centre for Cancer Treatment
Mount Vernon Hospital
Northwood, UK

David P. Goldstein MD, MSc, FRCSC, FACS
Assistant Professor
Head and Neck Surgical Oncology and Reconstructive Microsurgery
Department of Otolaryngology – Head & Neck Surgery
Department of Surgical Oncology
The Princess Margaret Cancer Centre
University of Toronto
Toronto, ON, Canada

Mary Gospodarowicz MD, FRCPC, FRCR (Hon)
Professor
Department of Radiation Oncology
The Princess Margaret Cancer Centre
University of Toronto
Toronto, ON, Canada

Cai Grau MD, PhD
Professor
Department of Oncology
Aarhus University Hospital
Aarhus, Denmark

Vincent Gregoire MD, PhD, Hon FRCR
Professor
Cancer Center and Department of Radiation Oncology
Institut de Recherche Expérimentale et Clinique
Université Catholique de Louvain
Cliniques Universitaires St-Luc
Brussels, Belgium

Xufeng Guo MD
Department of Thoracic Surgery
Shanghai Chest Hospital
Jiaotong University Medical School
Shanghai, China

Abha Gupta MD, MSc, FRCPC
Department of Medical Oncology
The Princess Margaret Cancer Centre
University of Toronto
Toronto, ON, Canada

Tejpal Gupta MD, DNB
Associate Professor, Department of Radiation Oncology
Tata Memorial Centre
Mumbai, India

N. Gutierrez MD
Haematology Department
University Hospital of Salamanca, IBSAL
Salamanca, Spain

Mouhammed Amir Habra MD
Department of Endocrine Neoplasia and Hormonal Disorders
The University of Texas M. D. Anderson Cancer Center
Houston, TX, USA

Christopher L. Hallemeier MD
Radiation Oncology
Mayo Clinic
Rochester, MN, USA

Karin Haustermans MD, PhD
Professor, Department of Radiation Oncology
Leuven Cancer Institute
University Hospital Gasthuisberg
Leuven, Belgium

Kristin A. Higgins MD
Department of Radiation Oncology
Emory University
Winship Cancer Institute
Atlanta, GA, USA

Andrea Hayes-Jordan MD
Associate Professor in Surgical Oncology and Pediatrics, Department of Surgery
The University of Texas M. D. Anderson Cancer Center
Houston, TX, USA

Andrew Hope MD
Assistant Professor, Department of Radiation Oncology
The Princess Margaret Cancer Centre
University of Toronto
Toronto, ON, Canada

Winston W. Huh MD
Associate Professor, Division of Pediatrics
The University of Texas M. D. Anderson Cancer Center
Houston, TX, USA

Shao Hui Huang MD, MSc, MRT(T)
Assistant Professor, Department of Radiation Oncology
The Princess Margaret Cancer Centre
University of Toronto
Toronto, ON, Canada

David A. Jaffray PhD
Professor, Department of Radiation Oncology
Techna Institute/The Princess Margaret Cancer Centre
University of Toronto
Toronto, ON, Canada

P. N. Jain MD, MNAMS, FICA
Professor, Anesthesiology, Critical Care & Pain
Head, Division of Pain
Department of Anesthesiology
Critical Care & Pain
Tata Memorial Centre
Mumbai, India

Robert T. Jensen MD
Chief, Cell Biology Section, Digestive Diseases Branch, National Institute of Diabetes and Digestive and Kidney Diseases (NIDDK),
NIH Bethesda, MD, USA

Wei Jiang MD, PhD
Department of Pathology, Anatomy, & Cell Biology
Thomas Jefferson University
Philadelphia, PA, USA

Jennifer M. Jones PhD
Acting Director, Cancer Survivorship Program
The Princess Margaret Cancer Centre
Associate Professor
Department of Psychiatry
University of Toronto
Toronto, ON, Canada

Robert Jones MBChB, PhD, FRCP (Glas)
Consultant Medical Oncologist
Institute of Cancer Sciences
University of Glasgow
Glasgow, UK

Amit Joshi MD, DM
Associate Professor, Department of Medical Oncology
Tata Memorial Centre
Mumbai, India

Shubhada Kane MD(Path)
Professor & Head, Department of Pathology
Tata Memorial Centre
Mumbai, India

Danielle Karsies MS, RD, CSO, AFFA Group Exercise Certified
Lead Clinical Oncology Dietitian
Cancer Center Nutrition Services
Symptom Management and Supportive Care Program
University of Michigan Comprehensive Cancer Center
Ann Arbor, MI, USA

Matthew H. G. Katz MD
Assistant Professor, Department of Surgical Oncology
The University of Texas M. D. Anderson Cancer Center
Houston, TX, USA

Fadlo R. Khuri MD, FACP
Professor and Chair, Department of Hematology and Medical Oncology
Emory University
Winship Cancer Institute
Atlanta, GA, USA

Jonathan King MD
University of Wisconsin
Carbone Cancer Center
Madison, WI, USA

Henry Kitchener FRCOG, PhD
Professor of Gynaecological Oncology
Faculty Institute for Cancer Sciences
University of Manchester
Manchester Academic Health Science Centre
St Mary's Hospital
Manchester, UK

Felicia Knaul PhD
Director of the Harvard Global Equity Initiative and Harvard Medical School
Associate Professor, Harvard Medical School
Boston, MA
USA
Founder and President, Tómatelo a Pecho A.C
Senior Economist, Mexican Health Foundation
Visiting Professor/Researcher, National Institute Public Health
Mexico

Rahul Krishnatry MD
Senior Registrar, Department of Radiation Oncology
Tata Memorial Centre
Mumbai, India

Gunnar B. Kristensen MD, PhD
Professor in Gynecologic Oncology
Department of Gynecological Oncology and Institute for Cancer Genetics and Informatics
Oslo University Hospital, The Norwegian Radium Hospital
Institute for Clinical Medicine, Oslo University
Oslo, Norway

Monika K. Krzyzanowska MD, MPH, FRCPC
Assistant Professor
Department of Medical Oncology & Hematology
The Princess Margaret Cancer Centre
Department of Medicine
University of Toronto
Toronto, ON, Canada

Dik Kwekkeboom MD
Professor, Department of Nuclear Medicine
Erasmus MC
Rotterdam, The Netherlands

Howard Kynaston MD, FRCS (Urol)
Professor and Consultant Urologist
Institute of Cancer and Genetics
School of Medicine
Cardiff University
Cardiff, UK

Jerome M. Laurence MBChB, FRACS, FRCSC, PhD
Department of Transplantation Surgery
University of Toronto
Multi-Organ Transplant Service
University Health Network
Toronto, ON, Canada

Armelle Lavolé
Service de Pneumologie
Hôpital Tenon, APHP
Equipe de Recherche 2 et GRC-UPMC 04
Theranoscan
Université Pierre et Marie Curie
Paris, France

Quynh-Thu Le MD
Department of Radiation Oncology
Stanford University Medical Center
Stanford, CA, USA

Anne W. M. Lee MD
Center of Clinical Oncology
The University of Hong Kong-Shenzhen Hospital
China

Zhigang Li MD
Department of Cardiothoracic Surgery
Changhai Hospital
Second University of Military Medicine
Shanghai, China

Lisa Licitra MD
Chief of Head and Neck Cancer Medical Oncology Unit
Fondazione IRCCS "Istituto Nazionale dei Tumouri"
Milan, Italy

Kristina Lindemann MD, PhD
Consultant in Gynecologic Oncology
Department of Gynecologic Oncology
Oslo University Hospital, The Norwegian Radium Hospital
Oslo, Norway

Jun Liu MD
Department of Radiation Oncology
Shanghai Chest Hospital
Jiaotong University Medical School
Shanghai, China

Caroline Lohrisch MD, FRCPC
Clinical Associate Professor
Division of Medical Oncology
University of British Columbia and BC Cancer Agency
Vancouver, BC, Canada

Anja Lorch MD
Professor, Department of Urology
University Hospital Dusseldorf
Dusseldorf, Germany

Judith Manola MS
Department of Biostatistics and Computational Biology
Dana-Farber Cancer Institute
Boston, MA, USA

Teng Mao MD
Department of Thoracic Surgery
Shanghai Chest Hospital
Jiaotong University Medical School
Shanghai, China

Kim Margolin MD
Professor, Division of Oncology
Co-director, Pigmented Lesion and Melanoma Program
Stanford University
Stanford, CA, USA

Malcolm Mason MD, FRCP, FRCR, FSB
Professor of Clinical Oncology
Institute of Cancer and Genetics
School of Medicine
Cardiff University
Cardiff, UK

M. V. Matteos MD, PhD
Haematology Department
University Hospital of Salamanca, IBSAL
Salamanca, Spain

Mary Francis McAleer MD, PhD
Associate Professor, Department of Radiation Oncology
The University of Texas M. D. Anderson Cancer Center
Houston, TX, USA

Ian E. McCutcheon MD, FRCS(C)
Department of Neurosurgery
The University of Texas M. D. Anderson Cancer Center
Houston, TX, USA

Robert R. McWilliams MD
Medical Oncology,
Mayo Clinic
Rochester, MN, USA

Hisham Mehanna PhD, BMedSc (Hons), MBChB (Hons), FRCS, FRCS (ORL-HNS)
Professor and Chair of Head and Neck Surgery
Director, Institute of Head and Neck Studies and Education
School of Cancer Sciences
University of Birmingham
Birmingham, UK

Terry Michaelson B.Comm
Radiation Medicine Program/The Princess Margaret Cancer Centre
TECHNA Institute/UHN
Toronto, ON, Canada

Hatel Moonat MD
Pediatric Hematology-Oncology Fellow, Division of Pediatrics
The University of Texas M. D. Anderson Cancer Center
Houston, TX, USA

Brendan J. Moran FRCSI, FRCS
National Clinical Lead for Low Rectal Cancer & Consultant Colorectal Surgeon
Department of Surgery
Hampshire Hospitals Foundation Trust
Basingstoke, Hampshire, UK

Mary Ann Muckaden MD (Radiation Oncology), MSc (Palliative Medicine)
Tata Memorial Centre
Homi Bhabha National University
Mumbai, India

Naveen B. Mummudi MD
Assistant Professor
Department of Radiation Oncology,
Christian Medical College, Vellore,
Tamil Nadu, India

Ludvig Paul Muren MSc, PhD
Assistant Professor
Department of Medical Physics
Aarhus University Hospital
Aarhus, Denmark

Vedang Murthy MD, DNB, DipEpp
Associate Professor, Department of Radiation Oncology
Tata Memorial Centre
Mumbai, India

Do-Hyun Nam MD, PhD
Professor, Department of Neurosurgery
Samsung Medical Center
Sungkyunkwan University School of Medicine, Gangnamgu
Seoul, Republic of Korea

W.T. Ng MD
Department of Clinical Oncology
Pamela Youde Nethersole
Eastern Hospital
Hong Kong, China

Piero Nicolai MD
Professor and Chairman,
Department of Otorhinolaryngology
University of Brescia
Brescia, Italy

E. M. Ocio MD
Haematology Department
University Hospital of
Salamanca
Salamanca, Spain

Ivo A. Olivotto MD, FRCPC
Professor and Head, Division of Radiation Oncology
University of Calgary and Tom Baker Cancer Centre
Calgary, AB, Canada

M. H. M. Oonk MD, PhD
Department of Gynecological Oncology
University Medical Center Groningen
University of Groningen
Groningen, The Netherlands

Brian O'Sullivan MB, FRCPC, FRCPI, FFRRCSI (Hon)
Professor, Department of Radiation Oncology
Bartley-Smith / Wharton Chair in Radiation Oncology
The Princess Margaret Cancer Centre
University of Toronto
Toronto, ON, Canada

Dermot O'Toole MD
Associate Professor and Consultant Physician
Department of Clinical Medicine & Gastroenterology
Trinity Centre for Health Sciences
St James's Hospital & Trinity College
Department of Neuroendocrine Tumours
St Vincent's University Hospital
Dublin, Ireland

Gemma Owens MB BCh BSc (Hons)
Academic Clinical Fellow in Gynaecological Oncology
Faculty Institute for Cancer Sciences
University of Manchester
Manchester Academic Health Science Centre
St Mary's Hospital
Manchester, UK

Lance Pagliaro MD
Department of Genitourinary
Medical Oncology
The University of Texas M. D. Anderson Cancer Center
Houston, TX, USA

Prathamesh S. Pai MS(ENT), DNB, DORL
Professor & Surgeon, Department of Head & Neck Surgical Oncology
Tata Memorial Centre
Mumbai, India

B. Paiva PhD
Clínica Universidad de Navarra
CIMA, IDISNA
Navarra, Spain

Gouri Pantvaidya MS, |DNB, MRCS
Associate Professor, Department of Head & Neck Surgical Oncology
Tata Memorial Centre
Mumbai, India

U.-F. Pape MD
Division of Hepatology and Gastroenterology
Department of Internal Medicine
Campus Virchow-Klinikum
Berlin, Germany

Nicholas Pavlidis MD
Professor of Oncology
Department of Medical Oncology
Medical School
University of Ioannina
Ioannina, Greece

Fedro A. Peccatori MD, PhD
Department of Gynecological Oncology
Fertility and Procreation Unit
European Institute of Oncology
Milan, Italy

Stephen Peiper MD
Department of Pathology, Anatomy, & Cell Biology
Thomas Jefferson University
Philadelphia, PA, USA

George Pentheroudakis MD
Associate Professor of Oncology
Department of Medical Oncology
Medical School
University of Ioannina
Ioannina, Greece

Nancy D. Perrier MD, FACS
Walter and Ruth Sterling Endowed Professor
Professor of Surgery
Associate Director of the Multidisciplinary Endocrine Center
Chief, Section of Surgical Endocrinology
Department of Surgical Oncology, The University of Texas M. D. Anderson Cancer Center
Houston, TX, USA

Curtis Pettaway MD
Department of Urology
The University of Texas M. D. Anderson Cancer Center
Houston, TX, USA

Raphael Pollock MD, PhD
Professor, Department of Surgery
Director of the Division of Surgical Oncology,
Chief of Surgical Services
The James NCICCC / Ohio State University
Columbus, OH, USA

Sandro V. Porceddu BSc, MBBS(Hons), MD, FRANZCR
Princess Alexandra Hospital & School of Medicine
University of Queensland
Brisbane, Queensland, Australia

Kumar Prabhash MD, DM
Professor, Department of Medical Oncology
Tata Memorial Centre
Mumbai, India

E. Pras MD, PhD
Department of Radiotherapy
University Medical Center Groningen
University of Groningen
Groningen, The Netherlands

Nilendu Purandare DMRD, DNB
Associate Professor and Consultant
Radiologist
Department of Nuclear Medicine & Molecular
Imaging
Tata Memorial Centre
Mumbai, India

Laurent Quéro MD, PhD
Service de Cancérologie-Radiothérapie
Hôpital Saint Louis, APHP
INSERM
Université Paris Denis Diderot
Paris, France

Preetha Rajaraman PhD
Professor of Hematology and Medical Oncology
Centre for Global Health; Division of Cancer
Epidemiology and Genetics
U.S. National Cancer Institute
New Delhi, India

Suresh S. Ramalingam MD
Professor of Hematology and
Medical Oncology
Department of Hematology and
Medical Oncology
Emory University
Winship Cancer Institute
Atlanta, GA, USA

Venkatesh Rangarajan DRM, DNB
Professor and Head, Department of
Nuclear Medicine & Molecular Imaging
Tata Memorial Centre
Mumbai, India

W. Kimryn Rathmell
Department of Medicine
Division of Hematology-Oncology
University of North Carolina School of Medicine
Chapel Hill, NC, USA

**K. Thomas Robbins MD
FRCSC FACS**
Professor, Otolaryngology Head and Neck
Surgery
Executive Director, Simmons Cancer
Institute at SIU
Simmons Cancer Institute Endowed
Chair of Excellence in Oncology
Springfield, IL, USA

H. Ian Robins MD, PhD
University of Wisconsin
Carbone Cancer Center
Madison, WI, USA

**Danielle Rodin BA, MD,
MPH Candidate**
Radiation Oncology Residency Program
The Princess Margaret Cancer Centre
University of Toronto
Toronto, ON, Canada

Paula Rodríguez-Otero MD, PhD
Haematology Department
Clínica Universidad de Navarra
CIMA, IDISNA
Navarra, Spain

**Minerva Angélica Romero
Arenas MD, MPH**
Department of Surgical Oncology
Section of Surgical Endocrinology
The University of Texas M. D. Anderson
Cancer Center
Houston, TX, USA

Jacob M. Rowe MD
Department of Hematology and Bone Marrow
Transplantation
Rambam Health Care Campus
Bruce Rappaport Faculty of Medicine
Technion
Israel Institute of Technology
Haifa, Israel
Department of Hematology
Shaare Zedek Medical Center
Jerusalem, Israel

R. Bryan Rumble MSc
American Society of Clinical Oncology
Alexandria, VA, USA

J. San Miguel MD, PhD
Director of Clinical & Translational Medicine
Clínica Universidad de Navarra CIMA, IDISNA
Navarra, Spain

Takeshi Sano MD
Director of Gastroenterological Surgery
Cancer Institute Hospital
Tokyo, Japan

Heinz Schmidberger MD
Professor, Department of Radiation Oncology
University Medical Center Mainz
Mainz, Germany

Shomik Sengupta FRACS, MS, MD
Director of Training & Research, Urology
Department, Austin Health *and*
Clinical Associate Professor
Austin Department of Surgery
University of Melbourne, Heidelberg
Victoria, Australia

Geoffrey Siegel MD
Resident, Department of Orthopaedic
Surgery
Wayne State University School of
Medicine
Oakwood Heritage Hospital
Taylor, MI, USA

Rory L. Smoot MD
Hepatobiliary and Pancreatic Surgery
Mayo Clinic
Rochester, MN, USA

Leslie Sobin MD
Armed Forces Institute of Pathology
Washington, DC, USA

**H. Peter Soyer MD,
FACD**
Dermatology Research Centre
University of Queensland
School of Medicine
Translational Research Institute
Brisbane, Queensland, Australia

**Jean-Philippe Spano
MD, PhD**
Département d'Oncologie Médicale
Hôpital Pitié-Salpêtrière-Charles
Foix, APHP
Sobonne Universités,
UPMC University of Paris
IUC
INSERM, Institut Pierre Louis d'Epidémiologie
et de Santé Publique
Paris, France

Fiona Stewart PhD
Division of Experimental Therapy
Netherlands Cancer Institute
Amsterdam, The Netherlands

Roger Stupp MD
Professor and Chairman, Department of
Oncology and Cancer Center
University Hospital Zurich
Zurich, Switzerland

Henry C. K. Sze FRCR
Department of Clinical Oncology
Chinese University of Hong Kong
Hong Kong, China

Laura H. Tang MD
Professor, Department of Pathology
Memorial Sloan-Kettering Cancer
New York, NY, USA

Kerry Tobias DO
Medical Director, Supportive Care and Survivorship
University of Arizona Cancer Center – Phoenix
Dignity Health
St. Joseph's Hospital and Medical Center
Phoenix, AZ, USA

Mark J. Truty MD, MSc
Section Head – Hepatobiliary and Pancreatic Surgery
Mayo Clinic College of Medicine
Rochester, MD, USA

Richard W. C. Tsang MD, FRCP(C)
Radiation Oncologist
Radiation Medicine Program
The Princess Margaret Cancer Centre
Department of Radiation Oncology
University of Toronto
Toronto, ON, Canada

Susan Urba MD
Professor of Internal Medicine
Division of Hematology/Oncology
Medical Director, Symptom Management and Supportive Care Program
University of Michigan Comprehensive Cancer Center
Ann Arbor, MI, USA

Abhishek D. Vaidya MS, DNB
Former Senior Specialist Registrar
Head Neck Oncology
Department of Head and Neck Surgical Oncology
Tata Memorial Centre
Mumbai
Assistant Professor
Department of Surgical Oncology, DMIMS
Sawangi-Wardha, India

Richa Vaish MS
Senior Resident, Department of Head and Neck Surgical Oncology
Tata Memorial Centre
Mumbai, India

A. G. J. van der Zee MD, PhD
Department of Gynecological Oncology
University Medical Center Groningen
University of Groningen
Groningen, The Netherlands

Michael J. Veness MBBS(Hons), MMed, MD (USYD), MD (UNSW), FRANZCR
Westmead Hospital
University of Sydney
Sydney, New South Wales, Australia

Jan B. Vermorken MD, PhD
Emeritus Professor of Oncology
Department of Medical Oncology
Antwerp University Hospital
Edegem, Belgium

Suzette Walker DNP, FNP-BC, AOCNP
University of Michigan Comprehensive Cancer Center
Adjunct Clinical Professor, University of Michigan School of Nursing
Ann Arbor, MI, USA

Eric M. Wallen MD
Department of Urology
University of North Carolina School of Medicine
Chapel Hill, NC, USA

Rohan Walvekar MD
Associate Professor, Department of Otolaryngology – Head & Neck Surgery
Director, Head & Neck Service
Louisiana State University
New Orleans, LA, USA

Zi-Xuan Wang PhD
Department of Pathology, Anatomy, & Cell Biology
Thomas Jefferson University
Philadelphia, PA, USA

Leon Van Wijk MBChB FFRAD(T) (SA)
Department of Radiation Oncology
Groote Schuur Hospital
Cape Town, South Africa

Christian Winter MD
Department of Urology
Malteser-Hospital St. Josef Hospital
Krefeld-Uerdingen
Germany

Christian Wittekind MD
Institut für Pathologie des Universitätsklinikums
Leipzig, Germany

Wei Xu PhD
Department of Biostatistics
The Princess Margaret Cancer Centre
Toronto, ON, Canada

Tsila Zuckerman MD
Department of Hematology and Bone Marrow Transplantation
Rambam Health Care Campus
Bruce Rappaport Faculty of Medicine
Technion, Israel Institute of Technology
Haifa, Israel

PART 1

General principles of cancer diagnosis and management

1 Cancer epidemiology

Rajesh Dikshit[1] and Preetha Rajaraman[2]

[1]Tata Memorial Centre, Centre for Cancer Epidemiology, Mumbai, India
[2]Centre for Global Health; Division of Cancer Epidemiology and Genetics, U.S. National Cancer Institute, New Delhi, India

Introduction

Epidemiology is the study of the distribution and determinants of disease in specified populations, and the application of this information to the control of health-related problems. Cancer epidemiology thus encompasses understanding the distribution of cancer morbidity and mortality, identifying the causes of cancer and evaluating preventive measures and use of health services.

Distribution of disease refers to the identification, description and interpretation of the patterns of cancer among different populations over different time periods. This branch of cancer epidemiology, often referred to as *descriptive cancer epidemiology*, has provided insights into the disease burden of cancer and trends of cancer over time, and has also helped in generating hypotheses for aetiological research. Key to accurate descriptive cancer epidemiology is the availability of high-quality population-based cancer registries in many areas of the world.

The term *determinant of disease* refers to the study of disease aetiology. Knowledge about the causes and preventive strategies for cancer has largely arisen from carefully conducted epidemiological studies, often referred to as *analytical epidemiology*. The search for causes in an epidemiological setting is not limited to lifestyle factors, but also includes infectious agents and genetic factors. Over the past few decades, the field of epidemiology has evolved with the use of biomarkers, including genetic markers, to deepen our understanding of both exposure and outcome. This particular approach to understanding disease aetiology is often termed *molecular epidemiology*.

Along with the identification of the causes of cancer, epidemiological studies have been used to evaluate the success of primary and secondary prevention strategies in controlling the burden of cancer. These studies are often conducted as *field intervention trials* and assess the feasibility and success of primary preventive measures and screening programmes in different population settings.

Study designs in cancer epidemiology (Box 1.1 and Table 1.1)

Descriptive studies

A well-functioning cancer surveillance system which provides accurate information on cancer incidence, mortality and time trends is a key feature of an effective cancer control programme. The task of cancer surveillance is undertaken by population-based cancer registries (PBCRs). These registries collect cancer data by age, cancer site and date of diagnosis

---

Box 1.1 Introduction to cancer epidemiology

- Descriptive cancer epidemiology is the study of the distribution of cancer in different geographical areas over different time periods. This information is mainly derived from population-based cancer registries (PBCRs)
- Cancer epidemiology is also concerned with identifying the causes of cancer: this is mainly achieved through observational study designs such as case–control and cohort studies
- The branch of epidemiology that uses biomarkers of exposure and disease to understand the aetiology of cancer is referred to as 'molecular epidemiology'
- Since cancer is a relatively rare disease, case–control studies are often the study design of choice. Given the potential for selection and recall bias, these studies should be conducted with utmost care to minimize bias for meaningful interpretation of study results
- Although expensive and requiring longer follow-up, cohort or longitudinal studies are powerful study designs to understand the aetiology of cancer
- Experimental studies which involve randomization of individuals into two or more study groups are commonly used to study treatment efficacy ('clinical trials'). This design can also be used in the field to study the effectiveness of interventions such as vaccination (by randomization of individuals into vaccinated and non-vaccinated groups)

UICC Manual of Clinical Oncology, Ninth Edition. Edited by Brian O'Sullivan, James D. Brierley, Anil K. D'Cruz, Martin F. Fey, Raphael Pollock, Jan B. Vermorken and Shao Hui Huang. © 2015 UICC. Published 2015 by John Wiley & Sons, Ltd.

Table 1.1 Summary of the scope of cancer epidemiology

Main goal	Approach	Statistical measures
Distribution of cancer	Population-based cancer registries (PBCRs)	Incidence rates, mortality rates, cumulative risk
Determinants of cancer (lifestyle, environmental, infection, genetic)	Case–control studies, cohort studies, molecular epidemiology (including genetic markers)	Odds ratio, relative risk, attributable risk
Public health (screening, primary prevention measures)	Field intervention trials	Hazard ratio, mortality ratio

for populations in well-defined geographical areas. PBCRs can also provide data on population-based survival for different cancer sites in different populations. The quality and completeness of the data depends upon the availability and utilization of health services by cancer patients, and proper documentation by various facilities in which cancer is diagnosed and treated. Key requirements for a well-functioning PBCR are: accurate census data for the population covered by the registry by age and gender; access to various sources of cancer diagnosis and treatment; and support from local policy-makers as well as leading cancer diagnostic and treatment centres. While the numbers of high-quality PBCRs have been increasing worldwide, the large majority is still located in high-income countries. In the absence of PBCRs, many countries depend upon data from hospital-based cancer registries (HBCRs) and pathology-based cancer registries to estimate cancer burden. Data from these registries, however, are not suitable for cancer control planning, given the potential biases due to referral patterns and underestimation of incidence for cancer sites where histology is uncommon. In order to promote descriptive epidemiology research and increase the number of cancer registries in low resource settings, the International Agency for Research on Cancer (IARC), in collaboration with a number of global partners, including UICC, the U.S. National Cancer Institute and Centers for Disease Control and Prevention (CDC), has launched the Global Initiative for Cancer Registry Development' (GICR; www.gicr.iarc.fr). The GICR functions with the help of IARC regional hubs which provide assistance in the establishment of cancer registries.

Analytical studies

Analytical studies fall into two main categories: *observational* and *experimental*.

Observational studies

An observational study is a non-interventional investigation of disease causation in a human population. Such studies are based on observing associations between the exposure(s) and disease(s) of interest. Measurement of exposure is usually based on some combination of lifestyle data from questionnaires, external monitoring of exposure (e.g. for air pollutants) and biomarkers of exposure. New advances in microchip technologies and informatics are being used to understand the role of genetics as well as the interaction between environmental exposures and genes. Observational studies yield measures of association between exposure and disease, but interpretation of causality requires further information, including the following considerations:

- *Temporality*. Does exposure precede disease? For a factor to be causal for a disease, it must occur before the disease.
- *Strength* of the association, measured by the relative risk or odds ratio. The stronger the association, the more likely that the relationship is causal.
- Existence of a *dose–response* relationship. If the risk of disease increases with exposure dose, this provides further evidence for causality.
- *Replication* of findings. If an association is observed in various studies and settings, this provides further support for causality.
- *Biological plausibility* of the association. A relationship is more likely to be causal if the existing biological literature supports the finding.
- *Ruling out alternative explanations*. Alternative explanations for the observed results should be considered to rule out the possibility of spurious associations due to confounding or bias (see below).

As individuals are not randomly assigned to exposure groups in observational study settings, these designs can lead to non-causal associations, particularly due to:
- Confounding
- Selection bias
- Misclassification.

Confounding occurs when a variable that is not part of the disease causal pathway is associated with both disease and outcome. Confounding can be addressed by appropriate study design, data collection and analysis. In order to statistically control for confounders during analysis, it is essential to obtain information on potential confounding variables during data collection. For example, in a study measuring the effect of alcohol intake on lung cancer, results could be confounded by smoking, as smoking is associated with both the exposure under investigation (alcohol intake) and is also independently a risk factor for the disease (lung cancer); therefore, the confounding effect of smoking needs to be addressed either at the design stage (e.g. matching for smoking status or restricting the study to non-smokers) or at the analysis stage (by adjusting for smoking information in statistical models).

Most observational studies rely on data collected from accurate reporting of information, e.g. by study participants, physician records or laboratory procedures. Errors in classification of exposure or disease can occur if this information is not properly provided or recorded. This type of bias is called *misclassification bias* or *information bias*. In case–control studies particularly, the exposure or disease frequencies among study participants may not be representative of the target population, resulting in *selection bias*, which can produce inaccurate measures of association.

Careful interpretation of results from observational studies should consider the study design (including selection of cases and controls), potential biases and confounding to rule out alternative explanations. In order to conclude if the observed association is causal, further considerations include the strength of association, temporal relation between exposure and disease, dose–response gradient, biological coherence and consistency of results across studies.

Common study designs for analytical observational studies include *cohort* and *case–control* studies.

Cohort studies

In a cohort study, a group of individuals free of the disease(s) of interest is enrolled and followed up to ascertain different endpoints such as premalignant conditions, occurrence of cancer or death. Exposure measurements are ideally collected at the time of enrolment (prospective cohort study), but can also be collected in subsequent questionnaires or be historically reconstructed (retrospective cohort study). Disease risk is then compared between groups classified based on their exposure. Cohort studies resemble clinical trials in that both study designs compare disease risk between exposure groups. However, since the allotment of exposure is based on natural variation between the groups rather than random allocation by the investigator, more care needs to be taken in interpreting observed associations. Cohort studies allow estimation of the *incidence rate* (the instantaneous rate of occurrence of new disease events) as well as the *cumulative risk* (the cumulative probability of the disease during a given time interval). The ratio of the incidence rates in groups based on different categories of exposure is termed the *relative risk*. While cohort studies are very effective in determining disease aetiology, they can be expensive and difficult to implement logistically as they require long-term follow-up to obtain disease endpoints, particularly for rare diseases like cancer.

Case–control studies

To investigate aetiological factors for relatively rare diseases, the case–control study is often the design of choice for reasons of speed and efficiency. In a study to investigate cancer aetiology, individuals diagnosed with the cancer of interest are recruited from a defined population in a defined time period. A similar group of cancer-free individuals is sampled as a 'control' from the same study base from which the cases arise. The distribution of exposure among cases is then compared with that among controls, and the *odds ratio*, which approximates the relative risk when the disease prevalence is low, is computed as a measure to identify the strength of association between the exposure and disease. Case–control studies appear easy to conduct, but can give misleading results if cases and controls are not properly selected (leading to *selection bias*), or if the information on exposure is not properly collected, e.g. because of poor questionnaire design or administration, or improper collection, storage or analysis of biomarkers (leading to *exposure misclassification*). Additionally, if cases are more likely to report or recall exposure to a given factor than controls, this can lead to spurious results due to *reporting* or *recall* bias.

Experimental studies

In experimental studies, the investigator randomly allocates study subjects to exposure or no exposure. Study subjects are then followed up to observe the outcome(s) of interest. The random allocation makes these studies less susceptible to many of the biases that can be present in observational studies. Nonetheless, experimental studies are susceptible to selection bias if subjects being enrolled in the study are a selective group of individuals (e.g. because of high refusal rates for participation) or if there is considerable drop-out due to incomplete follow-up. Experimental study designs are less commonly used to study disease causation given that it is often unethical and/or logistically difficult to randomize subjects. These designs are thus most commonly used to study the efficacy of treatment, and then are most commonly referred to as 'clinical trials'. Experimental designs are also used in field settings to study the effectiveness of interventions such as the introduction of vaccines or vitamin supplementation, and are commonly known as 'field intervention trials'.

Global burden of cancer (Fig. 1.1)

Cancer is becoming the major cause of death worldwide. The World Health Organization (WHO) statistics for the year 2011 indicate that 7.9 million deaths worldwide were due to cancer (followed by 7 million deaths from ischaemic heart disease and 6.2 million deaths from stroke). An estimated 14.1 million new cases and 8.2 million deaths from cancer (excluding non-melanoma skin cancer) occurred in 2012, with corresponding age standardized incidence and mortality rates of 182 and 102 per 100,000 respectively. More than 60% of the world's cancer cases occur in Africa, Asia and Central and South America. According to GLOBOCAN estimates, the 5-year prevalence of cancer was 32.6 million for both sexes combined in 2012. The numbers of new cancer cases and new cancer deaths were slightly higher in males than females. The five most commonly occurring cancers worldwide among males in 2012 were lung (16.7% of the total), prostate (15.0%), colorectal (10.0%), stomach (8.5%) and liver (7.5%). Among females, the most common sites were breast (25.2% of the total), colorectal (9.2%), lung (8.7%), cervix (7.9%) and stomach (4.8%).

While the above estimates reflect overall global patterns, there are stark differences in cancer patterns across the globe. One way to understand these differences in burden and type of cancer is to classify countries according to their human development

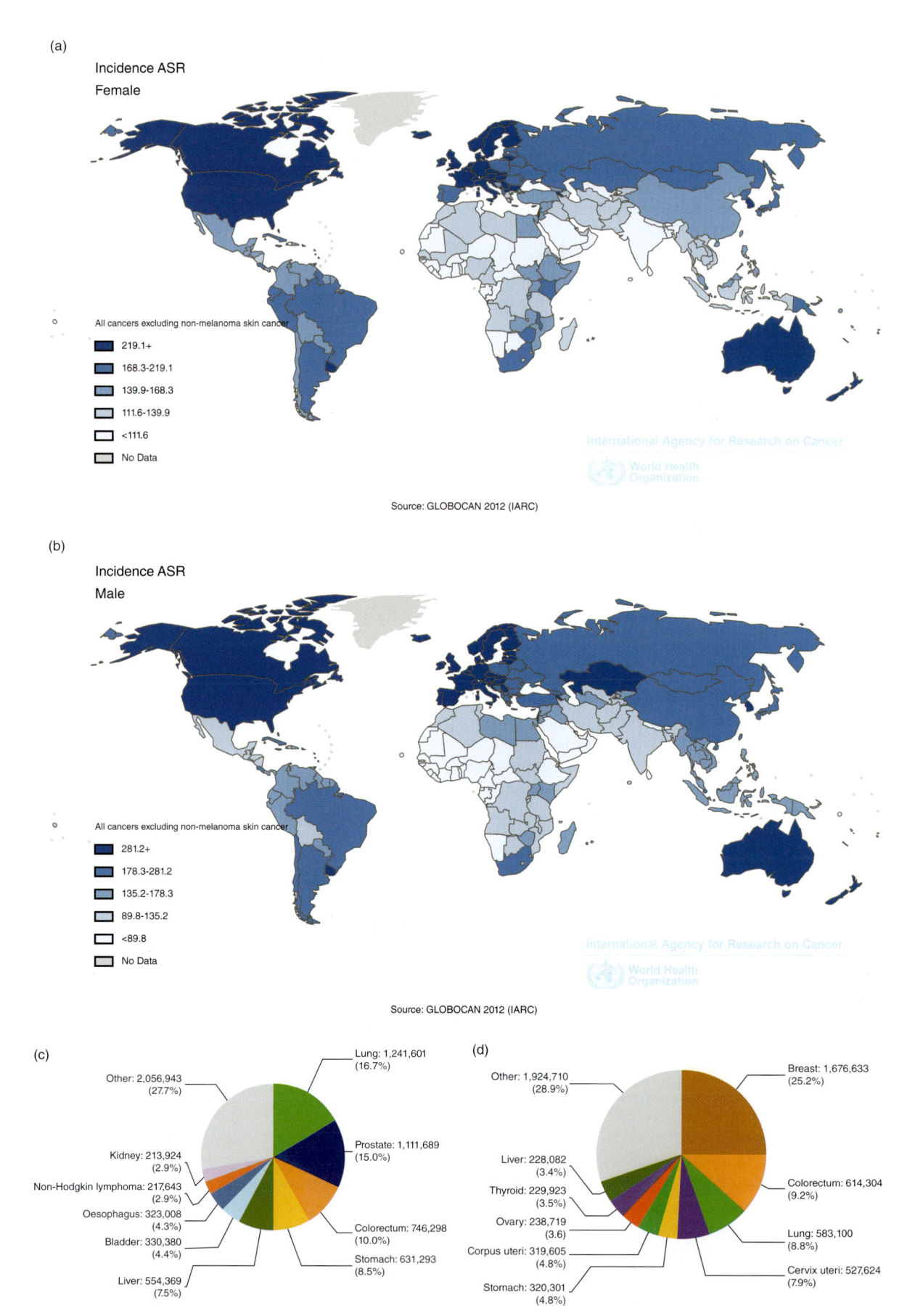

Figure 1.1 (a, b) World Cancer Incidence (WHO 2012) for males and females. (c, d) Percentage distribution of common cancer sites among males and females.
ASR, age-standardized rate. Data source: GLOBOCAN 2012. Reproduced with permission of WHO.

index (HDI). The United Nations Development Programme developed this composite index of three basic dimensions of human development: long and healthy life, level of education and standard of living as measured by gross national income per capita. Lung, breast, prostate and colorectal cancers are the most frequent cancers in countries with high or very high HDIs. On the other hand, countries with low or medium HDIs have a higher burden of infection-related cancers such as stomach, liver and cervical cancers. In recent years, countries with low or medium HDIs have also been witnessing a rise in cancers of the breast, colorectum and lung, indicating that they are undergoing a transition in economy and human development.

It is estimated that there will be >20 million new cancer cases by the year 2025. Countries with medium HDIs will experience the greatest increase in cancer burden, largely due to demographic changes with increases in life expectancy. Adoption of the higher-risk behaviours and lifestyle of more affluent countries (e.g. use of tobacco, higher fat diets) is also responsible for the changing profile of cancer in these settings.

Risk factors for cancer (Table 1.2)

Current knowledge indicates that lifestyle and/or environmental factors are the major contributors to the aetiology of the majority of cancers, although a small proportion can be explained by inherent susceptibility. The *attributable fraction* of a given risk factor is the proportion of the disease of interest that is thought to be due to that risk factor.

Tobacco

Tobacco use in any form (including smoking or chewing) is the single largest cause of cancer worldwide. It has been associated with cancers of the oral cavity, pharynx, oesophagus, stomach, liver, pancreas, nasal cavity, larynx, lung, cervix, ovary, uterus, kidney and bladder, and with myeloid leukaemia. At least 16% of all cancers are estimated to be related to tobacco use, with a higher proportion of tobacco-related cancers among men (25%) than women (4%). In general, the risk of cancer related to smoking and smokeless tobacco use increases with the duration and amount of tobacco smoke/chewed. Even involuntary or passive smoking (the inhalation of second-hand smoke by non-smokers) has been shown to cause cancer, with an estimated 25% increase in lung cancer risk compared to non-smokers. Successful quitting of tobacco smoking has been associated with decreased risk, but risk still remains higher than for never-smokers. Tobacco smoke contains >7000 chemical compounds and smokeless tobacco products >3000, of which many are known carcinogens. Broad classes of carcinogens in tobacco smoke include polycyclic aromatic hydrocarbons, N-nitrosamines and aromatic amines. Similarly, smokeless tobacco products contain at least 28 carcinogens including tobacco-specific nitrosamines, N-nitrosoamino acids and volatile aldehydes such as formaldehyde and acetaldehyde, as well as

Table 1.2 Major risk factors for cancer

Risk factors	Cancer type
Tobacco use (smoking and chewing)	Oral cavity, pharynx, oesophagus, stomach, liver, pancreas, nasal cavity, larynx, lung, cervix, ovary, uterus, kidney, bladder, myeloid leukaemia
Alcohol	Mouth, nasopharynx, oropharynx, oesophagus, colorectum, liver, larynx, female breast
Chronic infection with human papillomavirus (HPV)	Cervix, oropharynx
Chronic infection with hepatitis B and C virus (HBV, HCV)	Liver
Chronic infection with *Helicobacter pylori*	Stomach
Obesity and physical activity	Colon, breast (postmenopausal), kidney, endometrium, oesophagus (adenocarcinoma), pancreas
Diet	Colon, breast, prostate
Reproductive and hormonal factors	Breast, ovary, endometrium
Occupation (exposure to asbestos, heavy metals, diesel exhaust)	Lung, urinary bladder
Pollution (air and indoor)	Lung, bladder, skin
Genetic susceptibility	All
Chemical compounds Aflotoxin (naturally occurring) Aspirin	Liver Protective effect on colon cancer

metals including cadmium, lead, arsenic, nickel and chromium. The major pathways by which tobacco use produces cancer are thought to be DNA binding and consequent mutation, as well as inflammation and epigenetic mechanisms.

Alcohol

Alcohol intake is associated with increased risk for cancers of the oral cavity, hypopharynx, oropharynx, oesophagus, colorectum, liver, larynx and female breast. In addition to these cancer sites, there is some suggestive (but inconclusive) evidence for increased risk of cancers of the stomach, pancreas, prostate, kidney and bladder. There appears to be a positive dose–response relationship with the amount of alcohol consumed. Evidence suggests that the risk of head and neck cancer decreases with time since cessation of drinking. To date, no conclusive differences in carcinogenicity among alcohol beverages have been noted. There does seem to be a synergistic effect between tobacco smoking and alcohol consumption on risk of cancers of the oral cavity, pharynx, larynx and oesophagus, whereby the risk of consuming both tobacco and alcohol is greater than the individual risk of each of these factors. Approximately 4.2% of all cancer deaths have been attributed to alcohol use.

Alcoholic beverages contain several carcinogenic compounds such as ethanol, acetaldehyde, aflatoxin and ethyl carbamate. The main mechanisms by which alcohol is thought to act as a carcinogen include: the genotoxic effect of acetaldehyde; the induction of cytochrome P450 2E1 and associated oxidative stress; increased oestrogen concentration; acting as a solvent for tobacco carcinogens; and altering folate metabolism and DNA repair.

Infections

There is growing epidemiological evidence that chronic infection with viruses, bacteria and macroparasites are strong risk factors for specific cancer sites. Overall, about 2 million (16%) of the total 12.7 million new cancer cases in 2008 are thought to be attributable to infection. The attributable fraction of cancer due to infection varies widely by geographical region, with the lowest rates in North America, Australia and New Zealand (<4%), and highest in sub-Saharan Africa (33%). Table 1.3 lists the infectious agents that have confirmed associations with cancer.

Infection with *Helicobacter pylori* is associated with gastric adenocarcinoma in the non-cardiac part of the stomach. Chronic infection with the hepatitis B (HBV) and/or hepatitis C (HCV) viruses has been consistently associated with hepatocellular carcinoma. Worldwide, the fraction of hepatocellular carcinoma attributable to infection with these viruses is estimated to be 77%. Infection with the human papillomavirus (HPV) is a necessary (but not sufficient) cause of cervical cancer. Generally, 13 high-risk HPV types are classified as carcinogens (HPV 16, 18, 31, 33, 35, 39, 45, 51, 52, 56, 58, 59 and 68). The two most common oncogenic HPV types for cervical cancer are HPV 16 and 18. In addition to cervical cancer, HPV is also related to the risk of anogenital and oropharyngeal cancers. Individuals infected with the human immunodeficiency virus (HIV) have increased risk of acquired immune deficiency syndrome (AIDS)-defining cancers (Kaposi sarcoma, non-Hodgkin lymphoma [NHL] and cervical cancer) and other virus-related cancers. The fact that only a portion of infected individuals develop cancer suggests that infection is not sufficient to produce cancer. Further, there is geographical variation in both infection rates and rates of infection-related cancer, suggesting that much of the infection-related cancer is preventable.

Obesity and physical activity:

Overweight and obesity are associated with increased risk for cancers of the colon, breast (postmenopausal), kidney, endometrium, oesophagus (adenocarcinoma) and pancreas. There is also evidence that obesity increases risk of cancers of the gall bladder (in women), ovary and thyroid, non-Hodgkin lymphoma, multiple myeloma and leukaemia. Overweight and obesity are generally determined from the body mass index (BMI), which is calculated from the weight in kilograms divided by the square of the height in metres. Individuals with a BMI of over 25 kg/m^2 are considered to be overweight, while individuals with a BMI of over 30 kg/m^2 are considered as obese. The association of BMI with cancer risk generally demonstrates a dose–response relationship. However, BMI provides no information about body fat distribution. Other measures of body composition include the waist-to-hip circumference ratio (WHR) and skinfold thickness. Some studies indicate that measures of central adiposity may be better measures of cancer risk in certain populations than overall BMI.

Physical activity contributes to reduction in the risk of all obesity-related cancers, probably at least partially due to protection against weight gain. There is also evidence that physical activity has an independent effect on incidence as well as survival of patients with breast or colon cancers, possibly by acting through hormonal mechanisms.

Diet

There are many methodological challenges in measuring dietary intake, and therefore the exact role of dietary factors in causing human cancers remains unclear. Initial studies on diet and cancer revealed that diets rich in fruits, vegetables and whole grain protect against cancer. However, it is now clear that this protection might not be as strong as previously thought. Similarly, the role of fat in the development of many cancer types was

Table 1.3 Associations between infectious agents and human cancers (World Cancer Report 2014)

Cancer site	Infectious agent
Stomach	*Helicobacter pylori*
Liver	Hepatitis B, C virus, *Opisthorchis viverrini*, *Clonorchis sinensis*
Cervix	Human papillomavirus
Anogenital (penis, vulva, vagina, anus)	Human papillomavirus
Nasopharynx	Epstein–Barr virus
Oropharynx	Human papillomavirus
Non-Hodgkin lymphoma	*Helicobacter pylori*, Epstein–Barr virus, hepatitis C virus, human T-cell lymphotropic virus type 1
Kaposi sarcoma	Herpes virus with or without human immunodeficiency virus (HIV)
Hodgkin lymphoma	Epstein–Barr virus
Bladder	*Schistosoma haematobium*

thought to be important. However, recent prospective studies have demonstrated little or no relationship between fat intake and the risk of breast, colon and prostate cancer.

Higher consumption of meat is associated with increased risk for colon cancer and possibly breast and prostate cancer. In addition to the food itself, the method of food preparation (e.g. grilling) and differences in metabolism are also important. Grilled and barbecued meat and fish contain carcinogenic polycyclic aromatic hydrocarbons and hetrocyclic amines, and high intake of these foods has been associated with increased risk of colorectal and stomach cancer. On the other hand, high intake of calcium, vitamin D and folate has been associated with a reduced risk of colorectal cancer. A Mediterranean-style diet which is high in cereals, fruits and vegetables, and low in animal products has been effective in weight loss (and associated with reduced cancer risk). Similarly, reduced consumption of soda and other sugar-sweetened beverages has resulted in weight loss.

Further research is required to fully understand the role of diet in cancer, including understanding the role of dietary behaviours during childhood and in early adult life.

Reproductive and hormonal factors

Epidemiological evidence for the carcinogenic effect of reproductive and hormonal factors is strongest for breast cancer, and moderately convincing for endometrial and ovarian cancer. Risk of developing breast cancer is almost double in nulliparous women compared to parous women. Women with lower age at first childbirth are at lower risk of developing breast cancer, and the risk increases linearly with later ages at first childbirth. While the protective effect of full-term pregnancy on breast cancer is well established, there is little evidence for the relationship with short-term pregnancies, including miscarriages and abortion. Early age at menarche and late age at menopause are also associated with increased risk of breast cancer. Women with early surgical menopause before the age of 40 years have approximately half of the risk of those who have natural menopause. Uses of hormone replacement therapy (HRT) and oestrogen–progesterone oral contraceptives have been associated with increased risk of breast cancer.

Nulliparity, early age at menarche and late age at menopause also increase the risk of ovarian and endometrial cancer. Use of oral contraceptive is associated with reduced risk of ovarian and postmenopausal endometrial cancer. Prostate and testicular cancer are also linked to hormonal factors; however, further studies are required to fully understand the relationship.

Occupation

The most comprehensive source of occupational exposures associated with cancer is maintained in a series of monographs published by the IARC. According to the IARC monographs, 32 occupational agents and 11 exposure circumstances have been identified as human carcinogens. Some of the identified agents (e.g. mustard gas) are now of only historical interest, while other workplace exposures such as asbestos, polycyclic aromatic hydrocarbons, heavy metals, diesel engine emissions and silica are still widespread. Due to the widespread existence of mixed exposures in the occupational setting, it is sometimes not possible to identify the exact agent responsible for carcinogenesis, and the occupational groups themselves are labelled as carcinogenic (e.g. painters and workers engaged in aluminium production or in rubber manufacture). It is not the occupation itself that confers a risk, rather the exposure or conditions at work that are responsible for the carcinogenic effects. Although the overall burden of occupational cancer is small, this burden may be substantial among the exposed occupational group. Research on exposure biomarkers has substantially contributed to the understanding of occupational cancer aetiology. For example, ethylene oxide was identified as a human carcinogen after the detection of specific protein adducts in exposed workers.

Pollution

Large numbers of people are exposed to environmental pollution from air, water and soil. Many of these pollutants are known or possible carcinogens. Emissions from multiple sources pollute the ambient air, but mainly stem from vehicle emissions, power generation and a range of carcinogenic compounds from industrial waste, including diesel emissions, polycyclic aromatic hydrocarbons and compounds containing asbestos, arsenic and chromium. Complex air pollution mixtures are characterized in terms of summary indicators such as $PM_{2.5}$, which is the mass concentration of fine particulate matter of <2.5 μm in diameter. Ambient $PM_{2.5}$ exposure has been estimated to contribute to 223,000 deaths from lung cancer globally.

In many countries (particularly in East, South and Central Asia), people are exposed to indoor air pollution from the burning of solid fuels such as coal or biomass for household cooking or heating. Exposure to indoor burning of coal has been strongly associated with lung cancer, and indoor burning of biomass may also be responsible for lung cancer.

Another major source of non-occupational carcinogen exposure is asbestos from the installation, degradation and repair of asbestos-containing products during house maintenance. Exposure to asbestos results in an increased risk of mesothelioma and may cause lung cancer, particularly among smokers.

Consumption of drinking water contaminated with arsenic causes cancers of the skin, lung and bladder, and possibly of other organs such as the liver and kidney. Drinking water may also be polluted with carcinogenic organic compounds, e.g. chlorinated solvents and pesticides. High nitrate levels in drinking water have been associated with stomach cancer.

Although the role of pollution in cancer causation is small in terms of attributable risk, pollution presents an important cancer hazard in certain geographical areas, despite the fact that cancer due to pollution is amenable to primary prevention.

Radiation

Exposure to ionizing radiation from both natural and man-made sources has been consistently linked with increased risk of several cancers, including non-chronic lymphocytic leukaemia (CLL) and cancers of the female breast, lung and thyroid. Evidence for increased risk, particularly at moderate-to-high doses, also exists for basal cell carcinoma of the skin, and cancers of the bone, brain, rectum and bladder.

While the main source of exposure to ionizing radiation in the general population remains natural radiation (cosmic rays and radionuclides originating from the Earth's crust), exposure from medical procedures is becoming an increasingly common source in many countries. Exposure to indoor radon is the main source of elevated exposure to natural ionizing radiation, while exposure to man-made ionizing radiation occurs mainly in the course of medical care due to diagnostic procedures (e.g. radiography and computed tomography) or treatment (e.g. radiotherapy). Exposure to ionizing radiation causes multiple types of DNA damage, including single-strand and double-stand breaks. Exposure to non-ionizing radiation in the form of ultraviolet radiation from both the sun and tanning devices causes all types of skin cancer, including melanoma. Exposure to extremely low-frequency magnetic fields has been associated with childhood leukaemia in some studies, but interpretation of this increased risk is difficult given the potential biases. Exposure to a radiofrequency electromagnetic field (including use of mobile phones) has been classified as possibly carcinogenic to humans (group 2B) in the IARC monograph series, largely based on reports of an association between heavy use of mobile phones and risk of glioma and acoustic neuroma. However, due to possible biases such as the self-reporting of mobile phone use, these associations have been difficult to interpret, particularly in the absence of strong supporting biological data. At present, there is insufficient evidence to assess cancer risk due to environmental exposure from transmitters of low-frequency electromagnetic fields, including from television, radio and mobile phone networks.

Genetic susceptibility

Familial aggregation has been shown for many cancers, including those of the breast, colon and prostate. Individuals with high-penetrant gene mutations have greatly increased risk of certain cancers (e.g. *BRCA 1* and *BRCA 2* for breast cancer). However, such high-penetrant mutations are very rare in the general population and likely account for a very small proportion of cancer cases globally.

With advances in microarray technologies it is possible to study more common genetic variants which confer smaller relative risk. Initial studies to identify the risk of common variants in the population using a candidate gene approach (in which variants were selected by investigators based on probable function) were mostly unsuccessful, mainly because the prior probabilities for these candidates was very low.. In the last decade, the genome-wide association study (GWAS) approach (which does not assume prior functionality of any the genotyped variants) has been successfully used to identify risk loci for several cancers. As the effect size for these variants is usually small, very large sample sizes are required to detect true associations. By design, GWAS studies examine a high volume of markers, or 'tag SNPs' (single nucleotide polymorphisms) across the genome, and thus detected associations are not necessarily the 'causal' variant. To correct for multiple comparisons and the associated probability of detecting chance findings, GWAS studies impose a much more stringent threshold for statistical significance ($P = \leq 5 \times 10^{-8}$), and replication of results is essential to establish a conclusive finding. To date, nearly 400 distinct genetic loci have been conclusively identified for common cancer types (breast, colon and prostate), as well as rare cancer type (e.g. Ewing sarcoma, neuroblastoma and paediatric cancers). Notable examples of common variants increasing the risk of cancer include *NAT2* variants with bladder cancer, variants in alcohol dehydrogenase genes with aerodigestive cancers, and *FGFR2* variants with breast cancer. Given the lack of dependence of genetic markers on disease development, the case–control study design is well-suited to identify new genetic loci.

Other factors

Poor oral hygiene, ill-fitting dentures and use of mouth wash with high alcohol content are all factors that have been associated with oral cancer. Additionally, some pharmaceutical drugs used in cancer treatment or as immunosuppressant or hormonal agents have also been associated with cancer development. The *Aristolochia* plant (used in traditional Chinese medicine as an antirheumatic and diuretic) has been associated with increased risk of cancer of the renal pelvis and ureter. Some naturally occurring chemicals from plants, fungi, lichens and bacteria are also carcinogenic (e.g. aflotoxins, ochratoxin or sterigmatocystin are associated with liver cancer). A protective role of aspirin and other non-steroidal anti-inflammatory drugs has been demonstrated for colorectal cancer. Epidemiological studies have indicated that metformin, a widely used oral antidiabetic drug, may reduce the risk of several cancer types; however, this requires further confirmation.

Prevention and cancer control

Prevention of cancer comprises three stages: primary prevention (by avoiding exposure to carcinogenic agents); secondary prevention (by early detection of premalignant or early stage disease); and tertiary prevention (by providing effective treatment). A successful cancer control plan requires the proper integration and implementation of these activities at a population level, as well as continuous surveillance to evaluate the success of these activities.

The knowledge gained regarding modifiable risk factors for cancer has made it possible to achieve primary prevention of cancer by changing lifestyle and avoiding exposure to known carcinogens. The key preventable exposure is to tobacco in its many forms. Tobacco control is not only the top priority for cancer control but also for many other chronic diseases. The WHO launched the Framework Convention on Tobacco Control (FCTC) to stimulate international efforts to reduce tobacco-related harms. There are two main approaches to tobacco control: one is directed towards the tobacco industry (by regulating price, availability and packaging), and the second towards current users or populations vulnerable to initiation of tobacco use (by education and restrictions). Ongoing epidemiological surveillance efforts have been implemented to monitor the progress of the WHO framework convention on tobacco control.

Obesity and physical inactivity are also largely modifiable risk factors for cancer which can be controlled by changing lifestyle behaviours. Behavioural weight loss programmes focusing on reduced caloric intake and participation in moderate-intensity physical activity have been shown to result in weight loss and reduced incidence of diabetes. Ongoing trials are evaluating the benefits of weight loss on reduction in cancer incidence and improvement in cancer survival.

Yet another means for the primary prevention of cancer is vaccination against infections clearly linked to cancer. Thanks to the widespread introduction of HBV vaccination, the incidence of liver cancer has decreased dramatically in the past few decades. Following the recent development of prophylactic vaccines for the control of HPV-related cancer, vaccination of adolescent girls is being recommended and implemented in most parts of the world.

Secondary prevention of cancer can be achieved by implementing population-based early detection programmes for cancers of the cervix, colorectum and breast. These programmes aim to detect premalignant or early-stage disease when effective treatment is available. Common methods of cervical cancer screening include Pap smear testing, testing for HPV DNA and visual inspection of the cervix. For colon cancer, both faecal occult blood testing and faecal immunohistochemical testing have been shown to be effective. Screening with mammography permits detection of early-stage breast cancer. Studies are currently underway to evaluate the effectiveness of clinical breast examination in reducing breast cancer mortality. Population-based screening/early detection programmes require political commitment, engagement of civil society and the ability to mobilize a large number of healthcare professionals. Implementation of primary and secondary prevention measures requires legislative and regulatory initiatives as well as population-wide campaigning. Monitoring and evaluating the success of these efforts using epidemiological study designs is key.

Conclusion

Despite being a relatively young field, cancer epidemiology has successfully quantified patterns of disease and identified several key causes of cancer, thus paving the way for the development of cancer control programmes. Epidemiological surveillance systems have been set up to monitor the burden of cancer and to evaluate the effectiveness of preventive measures. Newer technologies and methodologies are being used to improve the precision of epidemiological studies by improving the classification of exposure and outcome. In addition to traditional data on risk factors from questionnaires, large epidemiological studies are now using complex methods of exposure assessment and collecting various biospecimens (such as blood, tumour tissue and saliva) to examine the role of various biomarkers (e.g. variations in DNA, proteins, metabolites and microbiome) in the hope of gaining a better understanding of the complex aetiological role of the environment and genes in the development of cancer.

More detailed information on the epidemiology of individual cancers is given in the relevant chapters.

Recommended reading

A Catalog of Published Genome-wide Association Studies. Available at http://www.genome.gov.gwastudies

Adami H, Hunter D, Trichopoulos D, eds (2008) *Textbook of Cancer Epidemiology*. New York: Oxford University Press.

Burton PR, Clayton DG, Cardon LR *et al.*; Wellcome Trust Case Control Consortium (2007) Genome-wide association study of 14,000 cases of seven common diseases and 3000 shared controls. *Nature* 447:661–678.

De Martel C, Ferelay J, Franceschi S *et al.* (2012) Global burden of cancers attributable to infection in 2008: a review and synthetic analysis. *Lancet Oncol* 13:607–615.

Ferlay J, Soerjomataram I, Ervik M *et al.* (2013) GLOBOCAN 2012 v1.0, Cancer incidence and mortality worldwide: IARC Cancer Base no. 11. Lyon, IARC.

Global Initiative for Cancer Registry Development in Low and Middle income Countries. Available at http://gicr.iarc.fr/

IARC (2007) Smokeless tobacco and some tobacco specific N-nitorosamines. *IARC Monogr Eval Carcinog Risks Hum* 89:1–592.

IARC (2013) Non-ionizing radiation, part 2: radiofrequency electromagnetic fields. *IARC Monogr Eval Carcinog Risks Hum* 102:1–460.

Pukkala E (2010) Nordic biological specimen bank cohorts as a basis for studies of cancer causes and controls: quality control tools for study cohorts with more than two million samples donors and 130,000 prospective cancers. In: Dillner J, ed. *Methods in Biobanking*. New York: Springer, pp. 61–112.

Renehan AG, Tyson M, Egger M *et al.* (2008) Body mass index and incidence of cancer: a systematic review and meta-analysis of prospective observational studies. *Lancet* 371:569–578.

Stewart BW, Wild C, eds. (2014). *World Cancer Report 2014*. Lyon: IARC.

WHO (2011) *WHO Report on the Global Tobacco Epidemic, 2011. Warning about Dangers of Tobacco*. Geneva: WHO.

World Cancer Research Fund/American Institute for Cancer Research (2007) *Food, Nutrition, Physical Activity, and the Prevention of Cancer; A Global Perspective*. Washington, DC: American Institute for Cancer Research.

2 Level of evidence, guidelines and standards

R. Bryan Rumble[1*] and Melissa C. Brouwers[2]

[1]American Society of Clinical Oncology, Alexandria, VA, USA
[2]Department of Oncology, McMaster University, Hamilton, ON, Canada

Introduction

Clinical practice guidelines (CPGs) and standards documents are decision-making tools that are informed by evidence and consensus of interpretation of this evidence by experts. They are created with the intent of improving patient care and, more recently, have been used to facilitate evidence-informed clinical policy and improvements to health systems. Through their application, patient care can be improved by ensuring the most effective and promising care options are identified, less effective or even harmful care options are abandoned, and undesirable levels of practice variation (that may reflect inequities or varied quality of care) can be mitigated. These tools can help ensure scarce resource dollars are used appropriately; while this may not translate into support for less expensive care options, CPGs and clinical practice standards can assist in identifying care options in which further investments may not be necessary.

In this chapter we will discuss both CPGs and clinical standards documents, and will examine their similarities and differences. The levels of evidence concept will be discussed to explain how these rubrics can be an important methodological component used to develop CPGs and standards. The majority of this chapter will then be dedicated to an in-depth examination of the components of a high-quality CPG – from selecting a topic and forming a development group through to creating recommendations and planning for future updating. The reader will then be directed to additional resources that support the development, evaluation and implementation of guidelines.

The goals of this chapter are two-fold. For readers who would like to know more about guidelines, standards and evidence/evidence quality, we provide an introduction to the core concepts and strategies that will allow them to better incorporate these tools into their clinical practice. For those readers who are more familiar with these concepts, we provide a framework for assessing the quality of any given guideline or standard according to well-accepted criteria, allowing them to focus attention on the best available guidance. We begin with an examination of CPGs and standards documents.

Clinical practice guidelines

High-quality CPGs are systematically developed statements, informed by research evidence, values, and local/regional circumstances to assist patients and clinicians to make decisions. There are key elements to this definition that are worth noting. High-quality CPGs use a synthesis of the research evidence on specific clinical questions and interpretation and consensus of this evidence by experts to inform recommendations for action. The consensus process by experts is important as the evidence alone can never determine what should be done in any given clinical situation; this decision must be made by patients and clinicians with consideration of all relevant factors as part of a considered judgement process.

CPGs are useful in providing options aimed to assist patients and providers of a general operating procedure or practice, but they should be flexible enough that they can be modified to fit specific needs without losing any of their utility. For this reason, they are normative, as they not only include the best evidence on the topic, but they also reflect the values, knowledge and expertise of the creators.

CPGs are used to answer clinical questions and provide guidance on the full spectrum of topics, such as prevention, screening, diagnosis, treatment and follow-up. Within the CPG, users will be advised on what clinical care option is most appropriate for what patient, what are the likely outcomes (both the benefits and risks associated with different options), what might be the barriers to action, and in some cases, what are the costs or

---

* The opinions expressed in this article are those of the authors and do not necessarily represent the views of the American Society of Clinical Oncology.

UICC Manual of Clinical Oncology, Ninth Edition. Edited by Brian O'Sullivan, James D. Brierley, Anil K. D'Cruz, Martin F. Fey, Raphael Pollock, Jan B. Vermorken and Shao Hui Huang. © 2015 UICC. Published 2015 by John Wiley & Sons, Ltd.

resource implications associated with the option. Thus, some of the key issues that are addressed in a CPG are:

- What is the problem (e.g. disease, condition) that needs to be addressed (diagnosis)?
- What is the variation of certain attributes within a population (differential diagnosis/symptom prevalence studies)?
- Which care option should be offered in specific clinical situations and for specific patient subgroups (or what should be done to prevent harm or exposure)?
- What are the likely outcomes if certain treatments are given (prognosis)?
- What are the main resource considerations?
- What is the optimum algorithm, flow chart or other tool to guide practice?

The research question(s) that direct the type of evidence reviewed in a CPG is (are) at least partially determined by the goal of the guideline, e.g. is the CPG intended to provide clinical guidance for practice versus intended to inform policy and adherence philosophy to support the distinction. For example, for CPGs intended to inform practice, the guideline may be more focused on what it is possible to achieve, while considering relevant limitations such as drug/device/technique availability, clinician training and expertise, funding, legislation/legal limitations, and any other considerations that might be nationally, geographically or culturally dependent. CPGs intended to inform practice may more typically answer the question 'what *can* we do?' In contrast, CPGs intended to inform policy may be more focused on what it is possible to achieve in an ideal environment; therefore, these CPGs answer the question 'what *should* we do?' under ideal circumstances. CPGs created to inform policy may result in substantive changes to how health care is practised in the locale in which it is implemented if the recommendations result in an increase in the availability (either via new approval or new funding) of drugs, devices or techniques. Thus, part of the CPG creator's responsibility is to ensure the objectives of the document, its intended purpose and key target users are explicitly articulated.

In summary, high-quality CPGs should provide users with a set of actionable recommendations, an unbiased evidence base to justify the recommendations, the consensus interpretation by credible experts to contextualize the evidence for a given setting, and tools to support the application of recommendations (Box 2.1).

> **Box 2.1** Clinical practice guidelines: Key points
>
> - CPGs are patient-focused actionable recommendations intended to improve care
> - CPGs use evidence and consensus interpretation of this evidence to craft recommendations
> - CPGs are tools designed to assist in decision-making and not formulaic protocols
> - CPGs can answer both 'what should we do?' and 'what can we do?' guideline questions or objectives

Clinical standards

While similar to CPGs in that guidance is given, clinical standards are usually created to serve a different purpose from guidelines: to ensure uniformity in practice patterns or to ensure legal and/or professional obligations are met. As such, standards often go beyond the CPG by identifying which of the recommendations are optional and which are mandatory. Clinical standards may be developed, for example, by institutions or institutional groups, professional organizations, accreditation groups, or as part of a specific quality improvement initiative. Standards may include recommendations that reflect 'expected practice' or 'minimum practice expectations', and they may also be accompanied by benchmarks or performance goals. While they may be similar to CPGs in content, in practice the purpose of the standard may be quite different and may be very jurisdiction specific. For this reason, what a 'standards' document means may be interpreted differently from jurisdiction to jurisdiction, while CPGs are more generalizable across jurisdictions.

Despite the different purposes that standards documents are created for compared with CPGs, the methodology used to create them can be similar: systematic review of the evidence with a consensus process, while taking into account legal and professional needs. Standards documents provide mostly mandatory requirements (i.e. they must be implemented) with few optional components (Box 2.2). This is in contrast to CPGs where most recommendations are considered statements to assist in decision-making processes; in standards documents, all recommendations are considered mandatory and any non-mandatory, discretionary elements are all clearly defined. Examples of standards documents are explicit infection control instructions, patient intake forms, patient release forms, charting protocols, etc., all of which would contain elements that satisfy best practice, as well as any legal requirements and/or professional obligations. Table 2.1 details the similarities and differences between guidelines and standards.

Levels of evidence

In developing a CPG, understanding the quality and quantity of evidence is important in determining the definitiveness of and confidence in the resulting recommendations (Box 2.3). Levels of evidence describe the strength of the evidence according to the study design used, the execution of the study design and

> **Box 2.2** Standards: Key points
>
> - Standards comprise a series of performance expectations
> - Standards often identify minimum acceptable outcomes
> - Standards are useful in ensuring uniformity through regulation

Table 2.1 Guidelines versus standards

	Supported by	Objective	Intended to
Clinical practice guidelines	Evidence Consensus	Recommendations assist in decision-making	Assist in making informed decisions by identifying treatment options
Standards	Evidence Consensus Legal requirements Professional obligations	Recommendations set out expectations of performance	Ensure minimum goals are consistently achieved Ensure uniformity of outcomes

the ability of the study to mitigate bias. It is important to consider the study designs of the included evidence when crafting recommendations, as the level of evidence provides an indirect measure of the reliability of each study to report on what it is intended to. This indirect measure of validity then provides a measure of each study's capacity to inform recommendations; higher level evidence should allow for greater confidence in making definitive recommendations, while lower level evidence would only allow for more conservative recommendations as each study's level of evidence, methodological limitations and quality need to be taken into account. One might expect differing levels of adherence to recommendations as a function of the quality of the evidence base.

A high-quality CPG will use methods that are designed to identify and obtain the best available evidence in order to make the most robust and reliable recommendations. However, what comprises the 'best available evidence' for any given research question is dependent on many factors, including the research question(s) itself, the clinical setting (e.g. therapeutic, prognostic, diagnostic, etc.) and whether the clinical topic is nascent or mature (i.e. for nascent topics, there may be an absence of randomized evidence and systematic reviews compared with mature topics for which high-level evidence should be available). For most clinical questions, the highest level of evidence is provided by a systematic review comprised of homogeneous randomized clinical trials (RCTs) with narrow confidence intervals; for this reason, high-quality CPGs use a systematic review of the literature as the evidence base for their recommendations. However, the evidence included in any systematic review is dependent on the amount and type of evidence available, and could comprise the ideal of homogeneous RCTs with narrow confidence intervals or a series of cohort studies, depending on the research topic and how much evidence is available. Table 2.2 describes the levels of evidence according to study design and clinical situation.

Published study designs

For evidence that is available in the published literature, the two highest levels available for any given topic are (1) a systematic review (with or without meta-analysis) of homogeneous RCTs with narrow confidence intervals; and (2) one or more adequately powered RCTs with narrow confidence intervals. From these two designs, our confidence that each further design is actually measuring what it was intended to measure decreases until we come to the lowest level of evidence available in the published literature, the case report. The reason that such importance is placed on the outcomes of RCTs and systematic reviews of these RCTs is the greater likelihood that these types of studies address bias and reduce or mitigate spurious causality interpretations. Two important aspects of RCTs are the use of randomization (patients are placed into two or more groups using a process intended to ensure each patient has an equal chance of being placed into any of the groups) and blinding (patients should not know which arm they have been placed into, nor should the researchers or the assessors). These attributes of a carefully designed and executed RCT ensure greater internal validity of the study; that the study outcomes are more likely measuring what the study intended to measure, and that the outcomes observed can be attributed to the intervention alone. As it becomes difficult or impossible to randomize patients to different treatment arms, less rigorous designs must be used, and internal validity may also decrease, which reduces confidence in their findings. At the same time, it becomes impossible to blind patients, clinicians and assessors to allocation or condition, reducing confidence further. The lowest level of evidence contains none of the attributes of an RCT, and an RCT or systematic review based on RCTs contains none of the methodological weaknesses of case reports.

> **Box 2.3** Levels of evidence: Key points
>
> - Levels of evidence are a way of describing the strength of the evidence by study design and study quality
> - Levels of evidence provide a measure of confidence in the study findings
> - High-level evidence allows for more definitive recommendations and ones in which there is greater confidence
> - Low-level evidence allows for conservative recommendations only
> - Highest level of published evidence is a high-quality systematic review of homogeneous RCTs with narrow confidence intervals
> - Lowest level of published evidence is a case report
> - There are clinical situations that may explain evidence gaps in the published literature, like all-or-none outcomes and SpPin/SnNout outcomes, but which still represent high-level evidence equivalent to high-level published evidence

Clinical situations

Aside from what is available in the published literature, there are specific clinical situations that must be taken into account when clinical guidance is desired. Often, when reviewing

Table 2.2 Levels of evidence

		Published study designs	Clinical situations
←More reliable Less reliable→	←High quality Modify according to quality assessment Low quality→	Systematic review	
		Randomized controlled trial (RCT)	
			All-or-none outcomes (for therapy/harm or prognosis)* Absolute SpPins/SnNouts (for diagnosis)**
		Quasi-RCT	
		Non-randomized controlled trial	
		Controlled before-and-after study	
		Prospective cohort study	
		Retrospective cohort study	
		Historically controlled trial	
		Nested case–control study	
		Case–control study	
		Cross-sectional study	
		Before-and-after comparison	
		Case reports and case series	
			Expert opinion without explicit critical appraisal, or based on physiology, bench research, or first principles

*An all-or-none outcome is one where *all* patients experienced a negative outcome and/or a negative adverse effect with a previous treatment and now, with a new treatment, *none* or few patients do. The magnitude of benefit can explain the absence of randomized evidence as it would be unethical to allocate patients to a substandard treatment.

**SpPins are where the specificity is so high that a positive result rules in the diagnosis; SnNouts are where the sensitivity is so high that a negative results rules out the diagnosis.

the evidence on a particular clinical situation, appropriate treatment comparisons are missing from the literature as clinicians have moved on to using other treatments or a novel intervention has become standard treatment in the absence of comparative evidence. This situation may result where efficacy has been demonstrated in such a dramatic way that equipoise could no longer be assumed and the intervention was implemented without comparative studies being performed (as it is unethical to allocate patients to receive a substandard treatment or diagnostic test) in any of the following clinical situations: all-or-none outcomes, SpPin/SnNout situations, expert opinion, physiology, bench research and first principles.

Simply stated, an all-or-none outcome is a clinical situation where *all* patients experienced a negative outcome and/or a negative adverse effect with a previous treatment and now, with a new treatment, *none* of them do. If a new treatment shows an all-or-none outcome, randomization of patients into a trial to test its effectiveness becomes unethical and this may be responsible for gaps in the evidence in the published literature. All-or-none outcomes are a factor to examine in CPGs of therapeutic effectiveness where gaps in the comparative literature exist, and the supporting evidence may be found in non-comparative cohort studies or other designs.

Similar to all-or-none outcomes in therapeutic situations, in diagnostic studies there are SpPin and SnNout situations. An SpPin outcome is one where the specificity of a diagnostic test is so high that a positive result always rules the test condition in (e.g. the CAGE questionnaire for determining alcohol dependency – the test is so specific that a positive result always rules alcoholism in). An SnNout outcome is one where the sensitivity of a diagnostic test is so high that a negative test always rules the test condition out (e.g. the loss of retinal vein pulsation in diagnosing high intracranial pressure – the test is so sensitive that a negative result always rules high intracranial pressure out). In cases like these, no further comparative research may be found in the published literature due to the absolute effectiveness of these two index tests, and this may have to be taken into consideration when seeking supporting evidence for CPGs and standards documents.

Both all-or-none outcomes and SpPin/SnNout outcomes are considered high-level evidence, equivalent to the high-level comparative designs found in the published literature. At the low end of the spectrum where there remains an absence of published evidence, recommendations may have to be based on one of the four lowest levels of unpublished evidence: expert opinion without critical appraisal, physiology, bench research or first principles, but none of these will be discussed further in this chapter.

Creating a high-quality CPG

There are many methodological and social components that contribute to a high-quality CPG, starting with topic selection and continuing on through to the drafting of the final recommendations, while also outlining a process for future updating (Box 2.4). Table 2.3 details the components of a quality CPG.

Topic selection

CPG development usually begins with selection of a topic. Selections may be based on interest or need, but it should also consider where the greatest need for guidance is as this will result in the greatest impacts on patient outcomes. Some of the factors that may result in new guideline projects are newly discovered, or new approvals for, drugs, devices or techniques for which clinicians and patients require guidance. New guidelines may also be required to address variations in practice patterns or to implement new policy. Whatever the impetus for topic selection, the project can be guided by coming up with a high-level question which represents the 'what we want to know', i.e. the issue the guideline intends to address. This high-level question is intended to be broad, and is similar to the type of question used in a narrative review. However, because this is being used in a CPG and not a narrative review, the response to this high-level question is a recommendation and not a review.

CPG development group

Either prior to or following the selection of the topic, a guideline development group should be formed. Generally, CPG development groups use a multidisciplinary approach, where a group is formed comprised of representative members from all the relevant stakeholder groups, such as medical/radiation/surgical oncologists, general practice physicians, methodologists, policymakers, nurses, social workers and patients/survivors/other caregivers (equivalent to the Steering Committee of a clinical trial), while a smaller subgroup from that larger group is responsible for the majority of the development, which expedites the process. Using this model, the larger group is approached for input and guidance at key milestones in development only. All members of the CPG development group should be assessed for any existing or potential conflicts of interest, and these should be reported in as transparent a method as possible. From the outset, members should have a clear understanding of the methods being used to create the CPGs and their role(s). In addition, it is advised to have an explicit description of authorship and how participation will be attributed to avoid misunderstandings at the conclusion of the projects.

Box 2.4 Creating a high-quality CGP: Key points

- Topics should be selected based on greatest need, which should result in the greatest impact for patients
- CPG development group should be comprised of all relevant stakeholders, and include members with both clinical and methodological expertise
- A protocol should be created to guide the entire process, and this protocol should be made publicly available for transparency
- Research questions should be created using the PICO(T) elements (or alternatives) to guide the process
- Introduction section should provide background information on the topic and make an argument for why a CPG is the best way to address this research question
- Methods section should be detailed enough to allow for reproducibility, and cover all the necessary components of a high-quality CPG
- Results section should mirror the Methods section, where every item described in the Methods section has a corresponding response in the Results section
- Discussion section should include a considered judgement process where the importance and meaning of the evidence obtained is contextualized in consideration of all other relevant factors determined by the setting in which the recommendations will be implemented and the values of the involved stakeholders
- Conclusion should be limited to what will become the recommendations along with the supporting evidence expressed in narrative form; the original research questions should be answered as explicitly as possible considering the evidence and the considered judgement process
- Recommendations should be worded in a way that makes them as actionable as possible, as determined by the strength and quality of the evidence as well as the factors examined in the considered judgement process
- Before being finalized and made publicly available, the guideline and the drafted recommendations should be distributed for comment in an External Review process
- CPGs should include in their protocol, and in the final published product, a plan for future updating to ensure currency and relevancy
- CPGs should be updated at regular intervals based on need and/or on meeting standards of currency: whatever method of updating is used, it is important that guidelines in use reflect current best practice

---

Protocol development

CPG development should be guided by a protocol, which serves several purposes. As a high-quality CPG uses a systematic review of the published literature as its evidence base, using (and strictly following) a protocol ensures reproducibility. While the recommendations that may emerge from a systematic review may legitimately vary from context to context, the evidence base should be reproducible. A protocol also clearly identifies all components of the research project, helping to reduce or eliminate external demands that could expand the population of interest, inclusion or exclusion criteria, etc. in a process known as scope creep. Keeping the project scope under control and the guideline on track through the use of a protocol facilitates timely development, helping to ensure healthcare resources are used as efficiently as possible.

Like a clinical study protocol, CPG protocols should be made publicly available so that others do not duplicate research efforts by starting similar guideline projects, and so that others can review the methods used and reproduce the guideline where controversy exists. The PROSPERO registry (http://www.crd.york.ac.uk/NIHR_PROSPERO/) hosts information on planned, ongoing and completed systematic reviews. For all guideline projects that use a systematic review as the evidence base for their recommendations, the details of the systematic review portion of the project should be posted to this site for transparency.

Table 2.3 Components of a high-quality CPG

Development stage	Component	Structure
Topic selection	Topic	Topics should be chosen based on where the largest benefit could be attained. This could be determined by considering: • Availability of new drugs/devices/techniques • Unexplained or unwanted variation in practice • Burden of disease • Opportunity for change The topic is what the recommendations are intended to address, and may be stated in the form of a question. This high-level question represents what the guideline is intended to answer (therefore, the answer to this question would be a recommendation)
Determine the CPG development group	Development/writing group	The guideline development group should have representation from all relevant stakeholders, including clinicians (specialists and/or community physicians where appropriate), health research methodologists, public health professionals/policy-makers, patient representatives, implementers, and any other relevant members
Protocol development	Protocol	A protocol should be created to guide the project, and this protocol should be publicly available to ensure: • The project stays on topic • Methods are explicitly determined *a priori* • Reproducibility • Clarity among the group members regarding roles, responsibilities, timelines, governance (i.e. decision-making)
Guideline development and sections	Research question	A CPG is driven by a well-designed research question. Rubrics exist to help structure a question, and the PICO method is a common rubric: P – patient/population I – intervention C – comparison O – outcome(s) Note: Other methods, such as PICOH (where H represents the healthcare setting) and PECO (where E represents exposure) may be used instead of PICO(T) where appropriate. The rubric chosen should be the one best suited to structure the research question in a sensible way A high-quality guideline ensures that: • The (P)atient/population in the obtained evidence is equal to or generalizable to the population of interest (e.g. the population to whom the recommendations will apply) • The (I)ntervention is homogeneous with respect to dose, timing, setting, etc. • The (C)omparison is appropriate, and in most cases, should be the current standard treatment. Where this is not the case, an explanation should be given that is sensible, and would not decrease the strength of any recommendations • The (O)utcomes of interest are the most important ones that should be considered when informing the recommendations Using the PICO elements creates researchable questions that are answered with data, in contrast to the topic question that is answered with a recommendation
	Introduction	The Introduction should introduce the topic, why it is important, and how a CPG could address this. It should also provide basic data to support this by describing incidence, prevalence, and information on burden (e.g. mortality/morbidity) where possible or appropriate

Development stage	Component	Structure

	Methods	The Methods section should give sufficient detail to allow for reproducibility. Ideally, it should include (at a minimum) descriptions of:
		• Literature search:
		  ▪ Inclusion/exclusion criteria (from the protocol)
		  ▪ How the evidence was obtained (what databases were searched, other sources examined, etc.)
		  ▪ How studies were chosen
		  ▪ Which evidence was retained for inclusion
		  ▪ How the data were extracted
		  ▪ The quality assessment
		• Synthesis and consensus:
		  ▪ Any data analysis planned, including pooling
		  ▪ Any formal methods used to reach consensus on the interpretation of the data or crafting of recommendations
		  ▪ Other
		• If costs are included, how these costs will be weighed against evidence of clinical benefit and harm
		• How the values of the group are going to be considered and reflected

	Results	The Results section should report on all of the items covered in the Methods sections, e.g. for each section in the Methods section there should be a response within the Results section. Therefore, the content of the Results section is wholly determined by the content of the Methods section, but should include descriptions of: • Literature search results • Characteristics of the retained evidence • Data extraction results (outcomes) • Study quality results • Any data synthesis, either pooled or narrative summaries
	Discussion	The Discussion section should include a considered judgment process where the evidence in totality (its quality, quantity, consistency, relevance, generalizability, precision) is weighed against all other relevant factors such as: • Potential clinical impact (assessment of the relative benefits and harms) • Values (including patient and other stakeholders) • Costs (where appropriate) • Expert opinion • Patient perspectives • Legal or legislated requirements • Any other relevant factors It is important to take these factors into account in a considered judgment process, as these items may be external to the evidence itself, but may be a modifying factor in recommendation construction At a minimum, the Discussion section should summarize what the importance of the results is as contextualized with all other relevant factors in the considered judgment process, and should lead directly into the Conclusion
	Conclusion	The Conclusion section should follow the Discussion section, and is where all the research questions are definitively answered. As some research questions do not directly lead to a recommendation, it is here that all research questions are answered as informed by both the evidence and the considered judgment process
	Recommendations	Recommendations should be presented according to the following framework: • Should be clear, concise, and actionable (e.g. after reading the recommendation, it should be clear what should be done for whom, who should do it, and when it should be done) • A description of the supporting evidence and its strength should be provided • The expected benefits and harms should be stated • Qualifying statements may be added where appropriate (e.g. to address specific subgroups of patients to whom the recommendations would not apply or would only apply with modifications)
External review	External review	Before being made publicly available, the Recommendations should be sent to a representative body of content experts in an external review process
Updating	Updating	High-quality CPGs should include a plan for updating at regular intervals to maintain currency and clinical relevance

Guideline development
Research question
Where the topic selection process described earlier results in a high-level 'what we want to know' question, the actual research questions are constructed using a rubric, such as the PICO(T) process. There are alternatives to PICO(T), such as PICOH (where H represents the healthcare setting) and PECO (where E represents exposure), and the rubric which best answers the research questions should be chosen. For illustrative purposes, all examples used in this chapter will refer to the PICO(T) method only.

The PICO(T) elements are as follows:

P   Patient or population of interest (to whom the recommendations would apply)
I   Intervention of interest (what is being examined)
C   Comparisons of interest (usually the current standard)
O   Outcomes of interest (the measure examined to determine efficacy)
(T) Time (optional, and only used if there is a temporal outcome related to any of the other elements)

Using this method will help to ensure that researchable CPG questions are constructed, providing the foundation to articulate the specific eligibility criteria that will be used to guide the systematic review. Further, as the response to these targeted research questions are data, focusing the research questions in this way helps to limit the amount of evidence reviewed by decreasing the number of non-relevant papers obtained (increasing the signal-to-noise ratio). This facilitates both timely development and formulation of recommendations as the necessary parameters are documented and well described.

An example of a well-constructed research question created using the PICO(T) elements for a high-level question is given below.

- *High-level question*: What is the most appropriate treatment for premenopausal women with advanced breast cancer?
- *Targeted research question constructed using the PICO(T) elements*: In premenopausal women with advanced (non-resectable locally advanced or metastatic) breast cancer, is there a benefit associated with docetaxel compared with docetaxel + PF-3512676 if 5-year survival is the outcome of interest?

From this targeted research question, the breakdown according to the PICO(T) elements is:

P   Premenopausal women with advanced (non-resectable locally advanced or metastatic) breast cancer
I   Docetaxel + PF-3512676
C   Docetaxel
O   5-year survival
(T) Not relevant in this example

From this example it is clear how a recommendation would address the high-level question, and how data would address the targeted research question, allowing a recommendation to be made.

High-quality CPGs ensure that:
- The patient population identified in the research question is representative of, and generalizable to, the population to whom the recommendations would apply.
- The intervention reported in the acquired evidence is homogeneous with respect to dose, timing, setting, etc., making its comparison against other options appropriate and informative.
- The comparison examined in the CPG is appropriate, and in most cases the appropriate comparator is the current standard. Where the comparator is not the current standard, alternative possibilities such as all-or-none situations should be investigated, and an explanation should be given that is reasonable and supports any recommendations formed.
- The outcomes of interest are the most appropriate outcomes that would determine superiority or equivalency, and are meaningful to both patients and clinicians.

Introduction
The Introduction section should set the stage for the guideline project by introducing the topic: why it is important and why a CPG is the appropriate method to address this gap. A good Introduction will describe the current clinical milieu by providing some historical information on the current state of research on this topic, as well as data on incidence, prevalence, mortality, morbidity, etc. where possible. This section should also clearly state the intended purpose(s) of the document and intended audience(s).

Methods
The Methods section should reflect what was described in the project protocol, and should give enough detail to allow it to be reproduced. The minimum description should include details of:
- Inclusion/exclusion criteria (including information on the appropriate elements: patients/populations, interventions, comparisons, outcomes, years, publication type/study design, language, etc.)
- How the evidence was obtained (what databases were searched, other sources)
- Which evidence was retained for inclusion
- How the data were extracted (manual methods versus electronic tools, validation, auditing, retention, etc.)
- Details of the quality assessment (state which tools are going to be used for which type of evidence, etc.)
- Details of the data analysis, including if pooling is planned or not.

Other details that could be detailed in the Methods section include:
- Topic selection
- How the CPG development group was formed and how members were assessed for conflicts of interest
- Protocol development, including whether it was made publicly available or was posted for public review, and

what changes were made based on that feedback prior to finalization
- How the research question(s) was (were) created, and any changes that occurred between the first drafted questions and the ones that were retained for the CPG
- How consensus is to be achieved
- Any plans for future updating.

Results

As the Results section mirrors the Methods section in the sense that every element described in the Methods section should have an appropriate response in the Results section, the content of the Results section is wholly determined by the content of the Methods section. A high-quality CPG will have the same number of components in the Results section as in the Methods section with no missing sections, and all completed sections should be addressed appropriately. The Results section should not include any interpretation of the evidence reviewed, but should comprise summaries and a synthesis of the evidence obtained and the results of the quality assessment only.

Results of the quality assessment

Quality assessment of the individual studies included in a CPG provides a direct measure of the internal and external validity of the study, and this information provides an indirect measure of the confidence a reviewer can have in the conclusions (in consideration of the study design used). Higher quality evidence allows for greater confidence that the study outcomes were true and reported what they intended to report (internal validity), and that these results would be applicable to the population of interest (external validity). While there are some quality assessment tools that are universal, and that may be applied to many different study designs and publication types (e.g. GRADE, Cochrane risk of bias), many are specific to one publication type or study design only, as each has its own inherent strengths and limitations (Table 2.4). This makes each tool more suitable for use in some specific situations than others. For this reason, the choice of tool used should be decided only after consideration of all applicable instruments.

The quality assessment is used to confirm that the appropriate level of methodological rigour was followed in the execution of the study, and that no flaws were detected that would cause a reviewer to doubt its findings. This is done by examining the methods used according to the stated study design (e.g. higher-level studies like RCTs have more rigorous methodological requirements than cohort studies, and this continues on down through the possible study designs assessed), keeping in mind that quality assessment of methodological rigour is an indirect measure of the internal validity of the study. Following the quality assessment, the evidence from well-performed studies is incorporated into the CPG according to the study design used. In contrast, the evidence from poorly executed studies – those with methodological flaws that would bring the study's conclusions into question – may have the level of evidence associated with its study design or publication type downgraded accordingly. The methodological flaws detected in a study should be fully described, and how they affect clinical interpretation should be discussed as they may impact any recommendations informed by that study.

Table 2.4 Quality appraisal and completeness of reporting tools by study design/publication type

Study design/ publication type	Quality assessment tools
Clinical practice guidelines	Appraisal of Guidelines Research & Evaluation (AGREE II) www.agreetrust.org
	Strength Of Recommendation Taxonomy (SORT) http://www.aafp.org/afp/20040201/548.html
	Scottish Intercollegiate Guideline Network (SIGN) http://www.sign.ac.uk/guidelines/fulltext/50/index.html
Systematic reviews	Assessment for Multiple Systematic Reviews (AMSTAR) http://amstar.ca/Amstar_Checklist.php
Randomized controlled trials	Jadad AR, Moore RA, Carroll D et al. (1996) Assessing the quality of reports of randomized clinical trials: Is blinding necessary? *Control Clin Trials* 17(1):1–12.
	Detsky AS, Naylor CD, O'Rourke K, McGeer AJ, L'Abbe KA. (1992). Incorporating variations in the quality of individual randomized trials into meta-analysis. *J Clin Epidemiol* 45(3):255–265
Diagnostic studies	Diagnostic Accuracy Critical Appraisal Sheet (DACA-CEBM) http://www.cebm.net/index.aspx?o=6913
	Scottish Intercollegiate Guideline Network Diagnostic Studies(SIGN-DS) http://www.sign.ac.uk/guidelines/fulltext/50/checklist5.html
	QUality Assessment of Diagnostic Accuracy Studies (QUADAS-2) www.quadas.org
Other	Cochrane risk of bias www.cochrane-handbook.org
	GRADing quality of Evidence and strength of recommendations (GRADE) http://www.gradeworkinggroup.org/

Discussion

In contrast to the Results section, which should be a summary and synthesis of the obtained evidence only, the Discussion

section should incorporate a considered judgement process where the evidence in totality (as determined by quality, quantity and consistency) is weighed against all other relevant factors. These could include, but are not limited to:
- Potential clinical impact (possible overall benefits versus harms)
- Values (of all relevant stakeholders)
- Costs
- Expert opinion
- Patient perspectives
- Legal, professional or other requirements.

Although external to the evidence itself, these items are important to the process as they may influence the final recommendations, which cannot be made based upon the evidence alone. A properly written Discussion section should summarize the evidence obtained and contextualize that information within the milieu that the recommendations will be applied to. This section should logically follow from the Results and should logically lead into the Conclusion.

Conclusion

The Conclusion section of a CPG should comprise what will become the final recommendations along with the supporting evidence, albeit expressed in narrative form. Here, the research questions should be addressed in as much detail as possible as determined by the evidence and consideration of the other factors included in the considered judgement process. It should follow logically from the Discussion section, and provides the bridge between the considered judgement process that informed the Discussion and the final recommendations.

Recommendations

The Recommendations should be worded to be as actionable as possible as determined by the strength and quality of the evidence reviewed and in consideration of the other relevant factors examined in the considered judgement process. The recommendations should come directly from the Conclusions section, but be translated into statements that makes them actionable – a necessary process that will facilitate the implementation process. Where the evidence obtained was of high quality, high quantity and high consistency, strong recommendations can be offered using language that reflects that strength. Where there are fewer studies and/or studies of poorer quality or with inconsistent results, recommendations can be softened by using language appropriate to that evidence. In situations where harms are possible, contraindications should be given. In consideration of other relevant factors, such as what to do in the presence of co-morbidities, qualifying statements may be given as well to modify recommendations as needed. Table 2.5 shows how the strength of the recommendations mirrors the quality, quantity and consistency of the evidence reviewed. Note that the factors considered in the considered judgement process may further strengthen, weaken or otherwise modify any recommendations beyond the framework described in Table 2.5.

External review

External review of the full draft of a CPG by key stakeholders is an important step in the development process. It serves as a mechanism to make colleagues and peers aware of new evidence and recommendations that will influence their practice, and it also provides a mechanism by which these individuals can shape and inform the recommendations. External review may result in new interpretations of the evidence the CPG group had not previously considered, gauge the general acceptance of the new recommendations and identify potential problem areas which will challenge the implementation of the recommendations. The external review, including a

Table 2.5 Relationship of recommendation strength to evidence reviewed

Recommendation type		Benefits versus Risks/Burdens	Methodological attributes
Strong recommendation	High-quality evidence	Benefits clearly outweigh harms/burdens, or *vice versa*	Homogeneous RCTs or a systematic review of homogeneous RCTs with narrow confidence intervals, or overwhelming evidence from observational studies
	Moderate quality evidence	Benefits clearly outweigh harms/burdens, or *vice versa*	RCTs or a systematic review of RCTs with limitations, or strong evidence from observational studies
	Low- or very low-quality evidence	Benefits clearly outweigh harms/burdens, or *vice versa*	Observational studies or case series
Weak recommendation	High-quality evidence	Close balance between benefits and harms/burdens	RCTs or a systematic review of RCTs with some limitations or overwhelming evidence from observational studies
	Moderate quality evidence	Close balance between benefits and harms/burdens	RCTs or a systematic review of RCTs with major limitations or very strong evidence from observational studies
	Low- or very low-quality evidence	Uncertainty in the relationship between benefits and harms/burdens, or all are closely related	Observational studies or case series

response by the originating CPG group, is an asset to any high-quality CPG.

Updating

CPGs should include a plan for updating in either the protocol or the Methods section of the published product. The trigger for updating a guideline may be based on either need or meeting a standard, or a combination of the two, and this should be detailed in the document. Planned updating based on need ensures that the document remains current and reflects best practice. Some of the reasons to update a guideline based on need would be:

- Changes in the evidence on existing benefits and harms/burdens
- Changes in the values placed on previous or current evidence
- Changes in the availability of resources
- Improvements in current practice.

As an alternative to (or in combination with) a needs-based approach, ensuring that a standard is met may also be used as the trigger for updating. Many entities that aggregate or endorse existing CPGs, including the Institute of Medicine and the National Guidelines Clearinghouse (NGC) (www.guideline.gov), have placed a limit on when a guideline is considered out-of-date at 5 years. Therefore, in order to keep a CPG listed in the NGC database, a guideline topic must be reviewed for relevancy at least every 5 years; otherwise it will be removed and archived. To ensure guidelines reflect best practice, a needs-based approach is likely the best solution, with meeting the standard the alternative option for topics that have not changed based on new research.

Conclusions

CPGs can serve many purposes: they can assist in clinical decision-making, promote development of credible and defensible clinical policies, serve as a key step to an overall quality improvement effort, and serve as a means to create a culture in which participants understand and become receptive to the use of evidence. In the past several decades, considerable advancements have been achieved in the science and practice of CPGs. As such, there are several existing tools and resources to support development and application of CPGs so that new groups are not starting from scratch. A list of some of these key resources is provided in the Recommended reading.

Recommended reading

AGREE Enterprise: www.AGREEtrust.org

CEPGuidelines. http://www.youtube.com/user/CEPguidelines (a series of short practical videos on all the steps related to CPG development).

Guideline International Network: www.g-i-n.net

Guidelines Resource Centre: http://www.cancerview.ca/cv/portal/Home/TreatmentAndSupport/TSProfessionals/ClinicalGuidelines/GRCMain?_afrLoop=1521618018968000&lang=en&_afrWindowMode=0&_adf.ctrl-state=3icw10tkt_328 (one of the most comprehensive sites on practice guidance, tools and resources related to the development, evaluation and application of CPGs).

Institute of Medicine (2011) *Clinical Practice Guidelines We Can Trust*. Washington, DC: The National Academies Press.

Institute of Medicine (2011) *Standards for Systematic Reviews*. Washington, DC: The National Academies Press.

3 Prognosis and classification of cancer

Brian O'Sullivan, James Brierley and Mary Gospodarowicz

Department of Radiation Oncology, The Princess Margaret Cancer Centre, University of Toronto, Toronto, ON, Canada

Introduction

Although cancers share a common characteristic of uncontrolled growth and the ability to form metastases, they present a formidable challenge for classification due to their very heterogeneous nature. Taxonomy is the science or practice of classification. It provides a conceptual framework for discussion, analysis and information retrieval. In oncology, a number of classifications deal with heterogeneity of disease extent and severity, but the taxonomy of cancer is complex and fraught with inconsistencies in application.

The basic elements required to characterize each cancer are well accepted: they include the organ or site of origin, the histological type and the extent of disease at the time of management. However, numerous additional elements influence the outcome of patients and reside in domains generally identified as in the tumour, in the patient and in the environment surrounding the patient. These additional components of the description of the cancer are collectively considered prognostic factors, are important in many aspects of cancer investigation and management, and represent the focus of this chapter. These factors include any measure that, among patients with a given cancer, is associated with a subsequent clinical outcome (i.e. an endpoint of interest). An effective and feasible classification system is needed to address the various dimensions of prognosis and an understanding of the methodological principles should permit such a classification to be implemented and used consistently.

Axes of classification and taxonomy

The World Health Organization (WHO) stewards a classification of diseases (the International Classification of Diseases [ICD]) that is the international standard diagnostic classification to permit systematic recording, analysis, interpretation and comparison of mortality and morbidity data in all jurisdictions. It has also been extended to comprise a WHO 'family' of international classifications (WHO-FIC) that serves as an international framework of building blocks of health information systems. WHO-FIC contains two reference classifications: ICD to capture information on mortality and morbidity, and International Classification of Functioning (ICF) to address the domains of human functioning and disability. Specialty-based adaptations of the ICF and ICD, such as the International Classification of Diseases for Oncology (ICD-O-3), represent a dual axis classification for topography and morphology. Currently, cancer disease extent, an important pillar of cancer description, is not classified, although some approaches in this regard are in development for the forthcoming ICD-11 classification. Largely, this third dimension of the triangle of information needed for oncology practice is provided by the TNM classification of disease extent.

However, beyond these parameters, additional factors and processes exist that impact on the management and understanding of cancer (i.e. prognostic factors), making it important to have an agreed framework for their classification but which is not currently included in WHO-FIC. This chapter will address the approach used in the site-specific chapters of this Manual. Clearly, other classifications that address prognostic factors in cancers that may be used or developed need to be further aligned and maintained in the context of such axes to permit uniform use and interpretation. In addition, certain terms need to be agreed upon by establishing taxonomy and some methodological concepts appreciated to address this field more comprehensively.

The prognostic factor landscape

While prognostic factors are usually described in the context of overall survival, they may also be defined for many relevant oncology outcomes, including local control, organ

---

UICC Manual of Clinical Oncology, Ninth Edition. Edited by Brian O'Sullivan, James D. Brierley, Anil K. D'Cruz, Martin F. Fey, Raphael Pollock, Jan B. Vermorken and Shao Hui Huang. © 2015 UICC. Published 2015 by John Wiley & Sons, Ltd.

preservation, palliative interventions, probability and duration of response to treatment, biochemical response in diseases where this is relevant, quality of life, etc. In addition, the scope of discussion is wide since it applies to many domains of evaluation relevant to the patient, the treatment and the disease. For the latter, an explosion of information is also coming from the evolving interest in the evaluation of molecular biomarkers. The taxonomy of prognostic factors (molecular, genetic, '-omics', etc.) has not been established as the science is in flux and is rapidly changing. We can expect that with progress in our understanding of this field, an accepted taxonomy will evolve to facilitate communication between clinicians and other investigators. Not surprisingly, while biomarker discovery is thriving, incorporation of biomarkers into clinical practice is lagging behind expectations for numerous reasons, many of which will be mentioned.

Many of these concepts require broader discussion than can be accomplished in this chapter, and the reader is referred to the Recommended reading section. Of particular importance are the four publications of the Prognosis Research Strategy (PROGRESS) Group that deal in turn with: (1) frameworks for researching clinical outcomes, (2) prognostic factor research, (3) prognostic model research and (4) stratified medicine research including predicting individual treatment response to foster 'personalized medicine'.

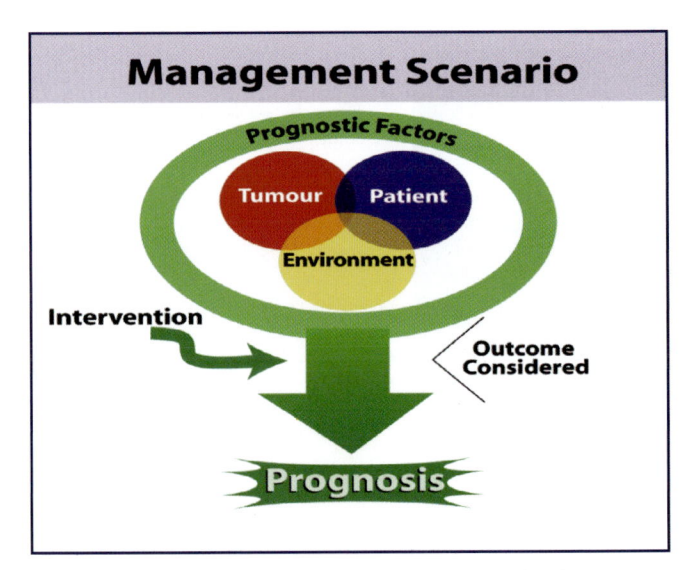

Figure 3.1 Representation of the interaction among the three domains of prognostic factors (tumour, host and environment). The prognostic factors are expressed in the context of the proposed therapeutic intervention and for a given endpoint of interest (e.g. survival, response, local tumour control, organ preservation). In addition, the prognosis itself must be interpreted in the context of both the treatment (because it may change the prognosis) and the endpoint (which must be relevant to the prognosis).
Data source: Gospodarowicz (2006). Reproduced with permission of John Wiley & Sons.

Setting or 'scenario' of the patient with cancer

Prognosis is not static in cancer. The disease itself evolves in a given patient if it is not controlled or if pathways of care change depending on response to earlier interventions; moreover, the tolerance of the patient can change as treatments are deployed, or the patient ages (especially if the patient has a chronic, more indolent disease), and interventions ordinarily available for a given presentation may need to be modified or disqualified because of earlier management. Therefore, when performing prognostic factor studies there is a need to identify and address outcomes pertinent to the individual study at specific intervals and intervention episodes in the evolution of the disease course, while also comparing similar types of patients for these outcomes (see Study population section).

Because of the numerous interacting circumstances impacting on prognostic outcome, it is useful to apply the concept of a 'management scenario', which embargos the prognostic attributes that exist at a given time point, enabling one to then consider how prognosis is influenced by the choice of the planned intervention and the outcome of interest (Fig. 3.1). An application of this concept is illustrated by a patient evaluated following neoadjuvant treatment. In essence this represents a transition to a new state or *scenario* compared to the situation before initiation of treatment. It is especially apparent if new treatment pathways are initiated as a consequence of an intermediate response to neoadjuvant treatments, even though there is no actual disease progression or recurrence. A more overt example is represented by an actual recurrence because the patient generally is now in a more complicated predicament and has clearly entered a new *scenario* with a different prognosis compared to baseline and one that needs to be evaluated in the context of a new treatment.

In summary, prognostic factors must always be considered in context. Only very rarely is it helpful to combine cases in studies that differ with respect to their clinical circumstance (e.g. primary versus recurrent disease, localized versus metastatic disease, curative versus palliative) or their potentially different pathological types within the same anatomical setting (e.g. non-small cell versus small cell lung carcinoma) and management in these settings. The construct extends to prognostic factors for different endpoints as noted earlier, e.g. local control, survival, organ preservation or symptom relief, as prognostic factors may differ depending on the endpoint chosen. However, unless specified, the prognostic factor discussion typically refers to initial diagnosis and survival.

Purpose of prognostic factor analysis

Prognostic factors have important application in different domains of cancer control, including direct *patient care*, *research* and *cancer control programmes* (Table 3.1). They may define important aspects of the disease at diagnosis (e.g. the

Table 3.1 Purpose of prognostic factors

Category	Application of prognostic factor
Patient care	Select appropriate diagnostic tests Select an appropriate treatment plan Predict the outcome for individual patient Establish informed consent through understanding prognosis Assess the outcome of therapeutic intervention Select appropriate follow-up monitoring Provide patient and caregiver education
Research	Improve the efficiency of research design and data analysis Enhance the confidence of prediction Demarcate phenomena for scientific explanation Design future studies Identify subgroups with poor outcomes for experimental therapy Identify groups with excellent outcomes for simplified therapy Identify candidates for organ preservation trials
Cancer control programme	Plan resource requirements Assess the impact of screening programmes Introduce and monitor clinical practice guidelines Monitor results Provide public education Explain variation in the observed outcomes

anatomical extent of disease defined by the TNM classification) in addition to the site of origin (e.g. lung or breast) and morphological type or histology (e.g. adenocarcinoma or squamous cell carcinoma). They are also equally relevant to other settings (e.g. at the time of recurrence) when a patient enters a new treatment 'scenario' (see earlier discussion), although the details may change for different settings and with emphasis on different goals and endpoints.

Guiding individual treatment (patient care)

Generally, prognostic factors guide the treatment that should be used and its degree of intensity; they may form the basis for entry into clinical trials or be incorporated as stratification parameters in randomized clinical trials to ensure balance between different arms of the trial. Prognostic factors may also define subgroups of an apparently similar population that need different treatments: these may also evolve in the course of a given disease as events unfold that may be influenced by clinical, interventional and biological factors that may impact on management decisions. Different approaches are evolving (see later) and include approaches such as the use of nomograms and prognostic groupings to attempt to harness various forms of available data into a coherent means to predict outcome of individuals or groups of patients.

Guiding research

Prognostic factors have applications that involve the different domains of clinical research, laboratory/translational research or health services research. All research areas require these elements, although the focus may differ for different researchers. However, a hallmark is the necessity to group patients (or in some cases tumours) with similar characteristics to guide treatment and/or anticipate outcome or behaviour in a reliable way; alternatively, an important focus is the corollary when outliers emerge who do not conform to such predictions and thereby provide a focus for research into factors underpinning differential outcomes. Addressing the study of these factors is always underpinned by the need for effective study design, analysis, and prediction of outcome, response or tumour behaviour in a manner that is as unambiguous as possible in order to further the goals of research.

Facilitating cancer control

Prognostic factors and prognostic studies are also relevant beyond the individual (i.e. a specific patient or a particular tumour), such as in studies or management pertaining to social deprivation, healthcare access and quality, and the physical environment of the patient. Such factors may significantly impact treatment outcomes and should not be overlooked since they may be as important as novel discoveries emerging from other research areas. Their use can also contribute to the identification of individuals at greater risk of compromised outcome in a healthcare system, or the monitoring of results of interventions including the early results of screening. Programmes such as public education and the implementation and monitoring of clinical practice guidelines at a population level also require an understanding of the clinical cohorts existing in a jurisdiction, as does resource planning to address the needs of specific groups.

Methodological requirements

Study population

Perhaps the most important principle in prognostic factor studies concerns the description of the population being studied and the consequent accrual of a homogeneous case series from which to conduct the study. This usually governs the results of the study and its general applicability to other cohorts.

Cohort assembly

In any study, the cohort for analysis should be assembled properly. In general, this principle commences with achieving an adequate study cohort size (case numbers) to provide sufficient statistical power to support potential conclusions. The well-conducted study is also characterized by the consideration of additional factors with the aim of minimizing confounding effects from other biases that may arise at this phase of the study. These include, where possible, prospective data collection and a hypothesis created for the study prior to patient accrual and data collection. Reasons for exclusion of cases should be identified and where possible eligibility criteria identified from the outset, including criteria for handling patients who may not have completed protocol interventions or assessments (including tumour assays where applicable). There should also be attention to identifying known confounders that may independently alter the prognosis, in the event that such factors are not the primary focus of the study. Factors such as co-morbidities, smoking status, other descriptors of the disease as well as characteristics of the patient (including age, socioeconomic, functional or psychological factors) may all be important as noted later (see Prognosis linked to co-morbidity section).

Inception cohort and establishing 'time-zero'

Defining an inception cohort properly from the outset (i.e. choice of the cohort relevant to time-zero for the study) is an additional critical underlying construct with significant epidemiological implications for any study in this area. Time-zero represents the inception or commencement point for a study; it may be the date of diagnosis, date of recurrence or any other relevant date to mark the start of the situation under study (e.g. initiation of palliative treatment if that is the setting under evaluation in the study), and needs to be consistently applied. It generally identifies the commencement of the intervention and evaluation period and is an important safeguard against combining dissimilar cases where the prognosis can vary greatly for many reasons, thereby confounding the results of the study.

Patients with recurrent or metastatic disease can be expected to have a different prognosis compared to those with primary localized disease, and also have different prognostic factors. Steps must be taken to avoid grouping such cases together. This can pose a problem when a study is structured only from available tissue specimens without reference to accurate accompanying clinical information. Importantly, prognostic factors can be researched, the results of this research can also be applied at any point of the disease, and the context may differ along the history of a patient's disease. This is because the prognosis of a patient evolves when recurrence manifests in the disease trajectory and is also dependent on interventions (usually a specific treatment or alternatively withholding of treatment for entirely appropriate reasons) that may have already taken place for a preceding management scenario.

Challenges in prognostic factor studies
Uncertainties about prognostic attribution among variables

It is important to understand the principles underlying the prognostic factor(s) under evaluation in a study, especially if the goal is to make inference to a different cohort or population of patients presenting at a later time.

Non-baseline factors

A problem is posed by addressing patients defined by parameters that are not available at diagnosis, or even prior to commencement of treatment, especially when inconsistent inclusion criteria prevail and inadequate description of cases exists. In truth this relates to statements about patients who have not yet undergone the treatment or intervention (the latter may include passage of time through surveillance or watchful waiting policies), and the factor of interest may eventually become apparent at a later time but be reported in a manner suggesting it was known from the outset. This is especially a problem of retrospective studies, including planned or unplanned retrospective evaluations in prospective trials.

Examples include statements relating resection margin status to the potential presence of residual disease, since this cannot be attributed until after a tumour resection is attempted. This is important since a tumour that has undergone resection with involved surgical resection margins often has a less favourable prognosis compared to one where no disease remains. However, incomplete disease removal could be multifactorial and likely caused by more invasive unfavourable disease, but could also be consequent to the treatment environment and expertise that resulted in poor planning or execution of the surgery. The fact that the resection status is conditional on the surgery having taken place may also have additional implications. Thus, trials or treatment guidelines requiring exclusion of cases who did not experience complete resection may impact on their general applicability in a disease. Finally, an additional sub-theme is that the consequence on cancer control may vary depending on whether or not adjuvant treatment, such as radiotherapy, is administered at the time.

'Responding'" versus 'non-responding' cases

Similar problems to the 'non-baseline' problem variant may manifest in other guises, characterized by inferring prognosis from parameters that require the treatment to be administered and the response of the disease to be measured. In essence, the original prognostic estimate may be revised with the ensuing passage of time. It may be impossible to separate real 'causality' in the relationship to an intervention since the 'responding' may have fared well with many different potential available treatments. For this reason prognostic factor studies should not compare responding to non-responding cases, irrespective of whether the post-treatment response is measured by objective clinical measurements of gross disease, by measures in the lab on a resected specimen, or potentially by newer imaging techniques such as functional imaging.

Prognosis linked to co-morbidity

It is also important to avoid comparing the outcomes of patient groups assembled according to whether or not a treatment can actually be delivered (e.g. resectable disease versus unresectable tumour). Sometimes this may be less overt, existing under the façade of differences in co-morbidity, performance status or age that may significantly influence the ability to deliver a treatment such as major surgery, or intensive chemotherapy or radiotherapy, with no contribution from the disease itself. This problem is pervasive in retrospective studies and investigators must be vigilant about attributing prognostic outcome to such treatment allocation or to prognostic factors identified in this way as they may be confounded by treatment selection problems of this type. Multivariate analysis is important in attempting to understand these problems (see Statistical techniques section).

Traditional prognostic factors

Although novel investigations and assessments (e.g. new biomarkers) may potentially be subjected to special scrutiny for reliability, traditional parameters also need similar consideration. These need to be considered to avoid spurious and non-relevant associations in the study conclusions. Thus, factors requiring interpretation of medical imaging studies or histological assessment (including diagnosis, but potentially also attributes such as tumour grade) have often been found to be vulnerable to interobserver variability. An example is represented by the assessment of the important prognostic factor for local recurrence, circumferential resection margin (CRM) involvement, in the preoperative evaluation of rectal cancer. This factor is addressed by magnetic resonance imaging (MRI) and requires application of agreed consensus criteria to determine it. Research into and understanding imaging factors of this type are important in any studies that require accurate imaging to be undertaken at baseline, especially where it is the focus of the study.

Biological prognostic factors

Laboratory assays depend on the quality control of specimen procurement, preservation and the process of assay performance if they are to give the best opportunity for evaluation of putative laboratory-based prognostic factors and use in clinical translation. Among other elements, this concerns the need for assay standardization in biomarker-driven trials. A current example is the assessment of persistently elevated post-treatment plasma Epstein–Barr virus (EBV) DNA in nasopharyngeal carcinoma. This assay has been shown to have large variability, even when performed in experienced clinical laboratories, and application of consistent processes are needed if this important prognostic factor is to provide the required value in guiding treatment intensity (see Le et al. in the Recommended reading). The whole area of biomarker exploration has received significant attention in recent years, prompted by the description and observation of significant inadequacies in the quality of publications in the area of biomarker research. Consensus guidelines have been developed, including the Biospecimen Reporting for Improved Study Quality (BRISQ) and the Reporting Recommendations for Tumor Marker Prognostic Studies (REMARK). These timely standards follow a similar approach to that led by some of the same authors for reporting clinical trials (the CONSORT guidelines) and for which many of the significant statistical formalities are similar. Generally, these guidelines emphasize optimal design, conduct and presentation/publication of studies and have been published by several journals simultaneously (including necessity for author adherence to these guidelines as a criterion for review and publication by certain journals) and posted prominently on international oncology-based websites.

Study endpoints

Earlier we discussed the importance of the context of prognosis as relates to the treatment being used and the outcome under assessment (e.g. functional, oncological, survival versus organ preservation, symptom relief versus disease control). Considerable discussion of traditional endpoints and treatment response assessment is provided in Chapter 5. In addition, more recent assessments have also focussed on other important domains that include evaluation of functional status and other patient reported outcome (PRO) measures. An important taxonomy of PROs is available and addresses a wide range of functional attributes and health-related quality of life assessments and how these should be chosen and used (see US Food and Drug Administration (FDA) Guidance for Industry document in the Recommended reading). Chapter 18 on survivorship also considers the important domains that address other endpoints beyond survival and disease control, such as psychosocial, quality of life, cost-effectiveness, return to work, etc. If prognostic factors studies are to be undertaken properly, it is important in all these discussions that the elements and principles underpinning the definition and measurement of endpoints are understood.

Statistical techniques

Frequently, prognostic factor studies require the impact of multiple co-variates to be examined in relation to the chosen clinical endpoints. This involves multivariate analysis to assess the independence of the impact of factors on outcome. Numerous techniques are available but close collaboration is required between a clinical statistician and a clinical researcher to discuss such issues. Among the latter are optimal approaches to address interaction among variables and the development, testing and validation of prognostic models. In general, such techniques can be divided into those that employ mathematical models that assume a linear impact of the baseline factors on the outcome (i.e. logistic regression and Cox proportional hazards regression), decision-rule approaches (i.e. conjunctive consolidation and recursive partitioning) for which linearity is not assumed, and machine-learning techniques that include neural networks. Of importance, the technique should not become the major focus of these analyses but, rather, the output from the data analysis in the way it illustrates the relevance of the prognostic factor and how it can inform the scientific and clinical context.

Some methodological pitfalls in prognostic factor analyses and interpretation are summarized in Table 3.2.

Table 3.2 Some methodological pitfalls in prognostic factor analyses and interpretation

- Insufficient attention to inception cohort description
- Inadequate power in the study cohort
- Insufficient description of study initiation (time-zero) and point of interest in the disease trajectory (e.g. at diagnosis, after neoadjuvant treatment, after surgery, at recurrence, etc.)
- Mixture of dissimilar cases, e.g. primary versus recurrent cases, or patients with or without metastases, or those with or without co-morbidity, etc.
- Non-representativeness of cases to the setting of interest
- Poor analysis and absence of training and validation datasets
- Endpoints not defined adequately, if at all
- Biospecimen robustness and laboratory test validation in the case of biomarkers and molecular assessments
- Inadequate definition of the prognostic factor itself

Taxonomy in prognostic factor discussion

As the prognostic research horizon is wide and varied, there is ample opportunity for inconsistency, discordance and misunderstanding. At the same time, there is a need to integrate prognostic factors in various ways to achieve greater refinement in predictive outcome. An initial simple step would be to agree about terms that represent important cornerstones of models to permit factors to be addressed and integrated cohesively, but still allow their independent roles to be appreciated where these need to be maintained. This is especially important with the introduction of molecular factors and how they can be integrated with more traditional descriptions of disease (i.e. site of origin, histological subtype and TNM stage). This is an evolving area as the scientific community responds to the large body of information that is emerging; a few illustrative examples are given below.

Defining disease type and extent

A starting point will be agreement on essential terms to define these parameters. For example, the UICC and AJCC suggest the following for the upcoming eighth edition of the TNM:
- The terms *stage* (disease extent) and *staging* (investigations that lead to defining disease extent and documentation of disease extent according to an accepted classification system) should be restricted to the description of anatomical disease extent.
- Pathological features of the disease (including molecular characterization) should be termed tumour *profile* or *profiling*.
- Combinations or unions of *stage* with *profile* and with other non-anatomical factors will be compiled into *prognostic groups* (see discussion below), generally using high-quality statistical methods. These may correlate with or be identical to prognostic indices, another term used to combine distinct characteristics about the patient scenario under study. Usually this is for the primary first *scenario* of management with curative outcome as the focus, but it can also be applied to other settings potentially with different outcome goals.

Biomarker terminology

In defining biomarker terminologies a mechanistic focus is probably preferable, especially when addressing molecular test-specific evaluations rather than a technological or modality-specific method governed by the test itself. The latter approach may rely on existing assessment technologies that may evolve with time and become obsolete. This area is beyond the current scope, which is mainly intended to guide the reader in the epidemiological principles underpinning prognostic factor research. However, biomarkers can also be subtyped by the way they are utilized, as indicated in recent guidelines responding to the needs of regulatory requirements: (see Febbo et al. in the Recommended reading).

- *Diagnostic markers* (these are not generally considered prognostic but are included for completeness according to recent guidelines and there is overlap as indicated for 'companion diagnostics'), e.g.:
    - Cytogenics, fluorescent *in situ* hybridization (FISH) or polymerase chain reaction (PCR) for Philadelphia chromosome or *BCR–ABL* rearrangement in chronic myelogenous leukaemia, or
    - Immunohistochemistry for prostate-specific antigen (PSA) in biopsy of bone metastasis.
- *Prognostic markers*: markers associated with reduced (or improved) outcome.
- *Predictive markers*: markers that predict for activity of a therapy.
- *Companion diagnostic markers*: markers that may be diagnostic, prognostic or predictive, but are used to identify a subgroup of patients for whom a therapy has shown benefit. This subtype has been introduced into the regulatory framework largely to address the interests of industry (i.e. for developments in drug, device, biomarker and information technology) in prognosis research, including tests for 'companion diagnostics', sometimes referred to as stratified or 'personalized' medicine.

Some markers may be both prognostic and predictive. For instance, receptor status in breast cancer has both attributes. Some markers may be prognostic in one tumour setting and predictive in another. The recent interest in programmed death 1 (PD-1) pathway inhibitors also highlights this emerging field with tumours (e.g. melanoma, kidney and lung) that express PD-L1 carrying an adverse prognosis but possibly responding with unexpectedly durable responses to targeting of these pathways with immune checkpoint inhibitors and other targeted therapies.

Unions of prognostic factors and combination treatment algorithms

Often the prognostic value of clinical data can be enhanced or more helpfully applied in the clinic if sensible unions of factors are undertaken to create groups of patients who may have different or more robust prognoses for the scenario than are provided by a unidimensional approach based around a single factor or descriptor. For example, a typical outcome for a patient with a given stage of cancer might be significantly altered in the presence of poor performance status. Much effort is ongoing to address this, especially as new molecular discoveries emerge that may modulate the nature of prognosis described in a traditional way. The following sections address several areas of ongoing discussion.

Importance of disease profile and disease extent (stage)

TNM has acquired durable success as the exemplar for characterizing prognosis in cancer over many decades. However, this status is often criticised for an apparent lack of attention to inclusion of all realms of the prognostic problem. Moreover, in the absence of an alternative and widely accepted framework, the medical and scientific communities have at times been tempted to embed other prognostic classifications into TNM, potentially risking abrogating or camouflaging the important impact of anatomical disease extent for some disease subsets. This potentially disregards some of the important rationales behind defining the extent of disease used in other domains, such as those of cancer registry activities and outcomes, health services population-based research as well as evaluating early results of screening programmes. The danger of an approach without broad recognition of the cancer control problem is that neither *tumour profile* nor *disease extent (stage)* will be addressed and acknowledged properly.

A critical need is a framework or repository to classify prognostic factors broadly and, furthermore, bring them to the clinic in a manner that is relevant and augments information from TNM without diminishing the value of any factors for cancer control activities.

At present, in the TNM stage classification the T, N and M categories are combined to create anatomically based *stage* groups (I–IV) that stratify for outcome. The UICC has also introduced separate *prognostic* groups (I–IV) that combine other non-anatomical factors to further differentiate prognosis while maintaining anatomical *stage* groups. So far, such *prognostic* groups are limited to a few diseases (e.g., prostate and oesophagus) in the seventh edition of the TNM classification because of limited available data for other disease. In the future it is anticipated that data will become available to permit other diseases to combine non-anatomical and anatomical factors in the same way and populate the potential third component of TNM for each disease. Some examples are already emerging for the eighth edition, in particular in the viral-related tumours of the head and neck (i.e. almost all nasopharyngeal cancers and many oropharyngeal cancers). This represents a means of addressing the goal of amalgamating *profile* factors and *stage* factors as relevant prognostic groups within TNM.

Treatment decision algorithms and nomograms

More complex decision algorithms have also been created that include nomograms that permit individualized case prognostication, but fall short in the area of aggregate groupings that are needed for comparison of results by institution or by patients subjected to different interventions. These have been widely used for cancer prognostication, primarily because of their ability to reduce statistical predictive models to a single numerical estimate of the probability of an event that is tailored to the profile of an individual patient. Often attractive graphical interfaces, commonly displayed on desktop computers and hand-held devices, facilitate interaction with individual patients about their personal disease situation.

Clearly, it is also appealing to encompass multiple dimensions of prognosis in this way. On the other hand, a limitation is that nomograms largely relate to individual prognosis at this time and additional development will be needed to address groups of patients since one of the goals of the stage classifications is to compare results across groups, in trials and between regions. Another challenge concerns the statistical underpinnings of these models that require careful scrutiny, including the degree of uncertainty surrounding the point estimates, lack of published confidence intervals and limited validation studies. The general tenets embodied in the 'scenario' concept discussed earlier underpin the use of nomograms; these are usually scenario-specific and users should avoid using them outside of the original management context within which they were developed, such as for incorrect subsets of a disease, for endpoints that differ from that for which they were intended, or following interventions that did not underpin their formulation. A recent review (see Iasonos et al. in the Recommended reading) cautions that the methodology underlying the construction of nomograms should be understood by clinical users so that prognostic estimates are appropriately communicated.

Framework for classification of prognostic factors

As mentioned earlier, well-defined and accepted classifications of diseases that include cancer do exist. The best known is the ICD-O-3 classification that is widely used by cancer registries and administrative bodies. The WHO Classification of Tumors forms the basis for the histological classification of cancer. The TNM classification published by the UICC and AJCC is the standard system for recording anatomical disease extent. In contrast to these evidence- and consensus-based agreements, no consensus on an optimal classification for prognostic factors exists.

At the UICC we have previously proposed a framework for describing prognostic factors in cancer and this is used throughout this Manual. It includes a 'subject-based' (i.e. tumour, host and environment) classification developed to highlight the scope of the different sources for potential prognostic factors, and a 'clinical relevance' classification to highlight those factors indispensable for good clinical practice and identify additional factors of interest, or in development, in different cancers.

A description of the 'subject-based' elements is outlined followed by the 'relevance classification' schema. These elements can be presented in the form of a cross-tabulation or prognostic

Table 3.3 Example of the UICC prognostic factors summary 'grid'

Prognostic factors	Tumour related	Host related	Environment related
Essential*	Anatomical disease extent Histological type	Age	Availability of access to a radiotherapy facility
Additional	Tumour bulk Tumour marker level Programmed death 1 (PD-1) receptor and its ligands (PD-L1)	Race Gender Cardiac function	Expertise of a treatment at the specific level (e.g. surgery or radiotherapy)
New and promising	Epidermal growth factor receptor (EGFR) (lung, head and neck) Gene expression patterns	Germline p53	Access to information

*The origin of essential factors as imperatives for treatment decisions is known and available clinical practice guidelines.

Table 3.4 Examples of tumour-related prognostic factors

Category	Examples
Pathology	Molecular tumour characteristics; gene expression patterns Morphological classification, e.g. adenocarcinoma, squamous Histological grade Growth pattern, e.g. papillary vs solid, cribriform vs tubular vs solid Pattern of invasion, e.g. perineural, small vessel invasion
Anatomical tumour extent	TNM categories Tumour bulk Single vs multifocal tumour Number of sites of involvement Tumour markers, e.g. prostate-specific antigen (PSA), alpha-fetoprotein (AFP), carcinoembryonic antigen (CEA)
Tumour biology	Tumour markers, e.g. HER2neu, CD20, programmed death 1 (PD-1) receptor and its ligands (PD-L1) Proliferation indices, e.g. S-phase fraction, MiB-1 Molecular markers e.g. $p53$, Rb, $Bcl-2$
Symptoms related to the presence of tumour	Weight loss Pain Oedema Fever
Performance when related to tumour effect (large size, bleeding, fever)	

factor summary 'grid' (Table 3.3) for a particular cancer type. Generally, they are depicted in each disease-site chapter of this Manual, typically for the overall survival outcome endpoint.

It should be acknowledged that the classification of prognostic factors described below may not always be straightforward. Sometimes, a certain prognostic factor can be considered as a hybrid of two or more categories. Nevertheless, the classification is a starting point for a taxonomy for use in prognostic factor classification.

Subject-based classification (tumour, host and environment)

Tumour-related prognostic factors

Tumour-related factors include those directly related to the presence of the tumour or its effect on the host, and most commonly comprise those that reflect tumour pathology, tumour biology and anatomical disease (Table 3.4).

Tumour profile (qualitative assessment of disease)

Pathological hallmarks of cancer. Histological type has traditionally defined the disease under consideration. While it is of crucial importance, additional factors such as grade, pattern of growth, immunophenotype and, more recently, gene expression patterns also reflect the fundamental type of disease under consideration and, parenthetically, the qualitative character of the tumour and how it may behave irrespective of burden. This is considered the *profile* of the tumour. In contrast, multifocality, presence of lymphatic or vascular invasion, infiltration patterns that also affect the outcome may relate both to type of disease and the extent. Hormone receptors, expression of proliferation-related factors and, increasingly, molecular tumour characteristics that have been shown to affect outcomes for a variety of cancers relate more to the type or *profile* of cancer rather than the disease extent. Generally, the presence of symptoms has been considered a host factor, but may also be a tumour-related factor and one that also influences other parameters such as performance status. A classic example is the presence of B symptoms (night sweats, fever and weight loss) in Hodgkin lymphoma.

Refining 'traditional' versus defining 'new' disease. Most new tumour-related molecular factors, such as gene expression patterns, deal with disease characterization, but a fundamental factor to consider in this milieu is the definition of a particular cancer as a distinct disease entity. While today histology forms the basis of tumour classification, the recent revolution in molecular medicine has challenged this classification and has led to redefinition of many cancers according to molecular and genetic tumour characteristics. These newer criteria have now been accepted in acute leukaemia and some subtypes of lymphoma, and are being considered in other cancers.

Thus, it is important to be vigilant to the possibility that some new discoveries demonstrating differential prognosis within subgroups of an apparently well-defined cancer may actually differentiate entirely different diseases that in the future may not even be considered homogeneous entities. The recently described epidemic of human papillomavirus (HPV)-related oropharyngeal cancer illustrates that the 'biomarker-status' of the HPV virus in conferring a more favourable prognosis within a single disease entity compared to the traditional smoking and alcohol-related version of the disease is potentially overstated. In essence, the disease is caused by this factor (HPV) and, therefore, HPV seems to represent at best a 'diagnostic biomarker' rather than a marker of response within an otherwise consistent disease entity, which is the usual paradigm for 'prognostic' or 'predictive' biomarkers (see Biomarker terminology section). Tumours with and without virus aetiology in this location are entirely different by virtually all available parameters. These include laboratory assessment, patient demographics and aetiology, as well as clinical and outcome assessment. Indeed, the only shared features may be their origin in a similar anatomical region and some superficial similarities in histology, but the latter can usually be readily distinguished by experienced pathologists.

Tumour burden or stage (quantitative measures of disease)

Non-morphological techniques. The second important group of tumour prognostic factors relates to the anatomical extent of disease, the so-called 'stage', and is classified according to the TNM classification. However, in addition to the TNM categories and stage groupings, other factors describing disease extent, including tumour bulk, number of involved sites or involvement of specific organs, and tumour histology may also have an impact on prognosis. Confounding this are additional nuances such as those posed by the presence of tumour deposits (satellites) or isolated tumour cells that are detected by potentially reliable techniques morphologically, or findings suggestive of metastatic tumour cells or their components demonstrated by non-morphological techniques such as flow cytometry or DNA analysis. Many of these concepts are already incorporated into the present TNM system, such as with the use of the abbreviations 'i' and 'mol' for isolated tumour cells and molecular techniques, respectively.

Tumour blood markers as quantitative descriptors. Conflicting opinions may exist between what represents burden of disease characterized by classical staging criteria such as those of TNM (which already captures these quantitative descriptors in certain diseases such as testis and prostate cancer) compared to the true molecular characteristics of the tumour, which are probably best used to define true *qualitative* differences in tumours irrespective of the extent of disease. Tumour markers such as prostate-specific antigen (PSA), α-fetoprotein (AFP) and β-human chorionic gonadotropin (hCG) are used in everyday practice and strongly correlate with tumour burden, but they are not typical biomarkers of qualitatively different behaviour. The same applies to rare cancers such as nasopharyngeal cancer, most typically seen in South-East Asia, where the presence of molecularly determined elevated levels of DNA-defined EBV copy number in the plasma of patients represents a *quantitative* indicator of the burden of disease at diagnosis, or following treatment (see Biological prognostic factors section), but not apparently a *qualitative* descriptor of the disease behaviour.

Host-related prognostic factors

These are factors present in the body of the host (patient) that are not directly related to malignancy, but through interference with the behaviour of the tumour or effect on treatment have the potential to significantly impact the outcome. A history of prior cancer and treatment of that cancer also places survivors at risk for future events. The cancer survivor also has an additional burden to bear in that there is inconsistency in how long-term medical records or treatment are maintained and retained in different jurisdictions, making it difficult to readily advise on additional treatment needed for a new cancer diagnosis in some patients. This problem overlaps with the problems of environment-related factors discussed below.

Host demographics

These are factors that characterize the demography of the patient, such as age, gender, racial origin and inherited conditions (Table 3.5). A hallmark is that almost none of these factors is influenced by treatment intervention, but many can independently influence the outcome of other factors.

Acquired host factors

These comprise acquired factors not directly related to the cancer, but which impact on a patient's ability to tolerate or undergo treatment, such as immunodeficiency, performance status related to co-morbid illness, impact of co-morbidity and

Table 3.5 Examples of host-related prognostic factors

	Definition	Examples
Host demographics	Factors that characterize the demography of the patient and cannot be influenced by medical intervention	Age Gender Race Level of education Socioeconomic status Religion Congenital co-morbidity: • Inherited immune deficiency • von Recklinghausen disease
Acquired host factors	Factors not directly related to the cancer but that impact on ability to tolerate or undergo optimal treatment	Modifiable co-morbidity: • Co-existent illness (e.g. inflammatory bowel disease, collagen vascular disease) • Weight • Cardiac status • Acquired immune deficiency • Infection • Mental health Performance status Compliance: • Social reaction to illness • Influence of habits, drugs, alcohol, smoking, etc. • Belief in alternative therapies • Mental health

co-existent illness themselves, and factors that relate to the host beliefs, attitude and compliance with therapy.

Some factors such as cognitive impairment and psychological problems (both intrinsic or in response to illness) probably reside in between the two host domains.

Environment-related prognostic factors

This area is potentially the least appreciated in circumstances emphasizing research relating to the *tumour* and *host*, and especially the former. Paradoxically, *environment-related factors* often have significantly greater impact on the outcome of patients. They comprise those factors that operate external to the patient and can be specific either to an individual patient or, more frequently, to groups of patients residing in the same geographical area or even undergoing similar treatment protocols that are not applied correctly. Furthermore, they are also the factors that are potentially most readily addressed for the benefit of patients, provided the logistics of delivering care properly can be addressed. Several categories of environmental factors can be considered (Table 3.6).

Treatment and education

These two characteristics are grouped together since they typically influence treatment implementation directly in the clinic. Obviously there is overlap since *education* also influences aspects of the quality measures in place on a broader scale as well. *Treatment*-related issues (e.g. expertise, access, ageism, healthcare delivery processes) and *educational* issues (e.g. participation in continuing education, development of practice guidelines, access to information including the internet) all have direct impact on how care is provided to patients on a day-to-day basis (Table 3.6). There may also be factors related to a society focus, such as a patient's socioeconomic and nutritional status, and the presence and attitude to ageism, which can all influence treatment selection and outcome.

Quality management

Quality issues (e.g. quality of treatment, quality of the healthcare facility, the presence of quality control programmes, access to affordable health insurance) also all serve to impact on outcome, but generally reflect motivations to ensure that resources (time, staff and facilities) and attitudes are in place to deliver treatments by healthcare practitioners in the most desirable way without compromise and in an environment that promotes error elimination and sustainable programmatic delivery. Surprisingly perhaps, the latter are not solely problems of low income countries, as illustrated by recent descriptions of radiotherapy treatment outcome in clinical trials in the developed world (see Recommended reading).

Clinical relevance-based classification

To consider the relevance of prognostic factors in clinical practice, prognostic factors are also considered according to three distinct categories: *essential*, *additional*, and *new and promising factors* that create the stratification within the prognostic factor summary 'grids' (see Table 3.3) used in the disease-site chapters of this Manual.

Table 3.6 Examples of environment-related prognostic factors

		Related to:	
	Treatment	**Education**	**Quality**
Physician	Choice of physician or specialty: • Quality of diagnosis • Accuracy of staging Choice of treatment Expertise of physician: 'narrow experts' Timeliness of treatment Ageism	Ignorance of medical profession Access to internet Knowledge, education of the patient Participation in clinical trials Participation in continuing education	Quality of treatment Skill of the physician Treatment verification
Healthcare system	Access to appropriate diagnostic methods Access to care: • Distance • Waiting lists • Monopoly control of access to care Availability of publicly-funded screening programmes	Continuing medical education Lack of audit of local results Access to internet Development of practice guidelines Dissemination of new knowledge	Quality of equipment Quality management in treatment facility Maintenance of health records Availability of universal health insurance Quality of diagnostic services Implementation of screening programmes Promotion of an error-free environment
Society	Preference for unconventional therapies Socioeconomic status Appropriate geographical distribution of cancer centres Individual payment status Access to transportation, car, etc. Ageism	Literacy Access to information	Access to an affordable health programme Nutritional status of the population

Essential factors

These represent factors fundamental to decisions about the goals and choice of treatment, and include details regarding the selection of treatment modality and specific interventions. *Essential* factors are exclusively those that are required by published clinical practice guidelines (e.g. National Comprehensive Cancer Network [NCCN], European Society for Medical Oncology [ESMO], etc.) and it may be helpful to recognize the source of these recommendations when ordaining their use in tables or other communications.

Additional factors

These factors allow finer prognostication, but are not an absolute requirement for treatment-related decision-making processes. Their role is to communicate prognosis. They are particularly important in areas involving pre-emptive measures to ensure balanced comparisons of different patient groups (e.g. as stratification procedures in clinical trials), but they do not in themselves influence treatment choice.

New and promising factors

These factors are those that shed new light on the biology of disease or the prognosis for patients, but for which currently there is, at best, incomplete evidence of an independent effect on outcome or prognosis.

Conclusion

With progress in treatment and prognostic factor research, and improved outcomes, prognostic factors are becoming more relevant for selection and modification of treatment. These factors are defined as variables that can account for some of the heterogeneity associated with the expected course and outcome of a disease. In addressing this area, there is an important need to encourage optimal research procedures and statistical methods to ensure that these factors can be classified and used for their intended purpose. Consistency in using terminology and processes is needed to enhance communication in this field. Cancer prognosis differs according to specific scenarios, and prognostic factors should be considered within a given context or scenario and for a given outcome, most commonly before a definitive treatment plan is formulated. Since treatment interventions also have a major impact on the outcome, it is important to discuss prognostic factors in the context of a specific treatment plan or therapeutic intervention.

Recommended reading

Altman DG (2006) Studies investigating prognostic factors: conduct and evaluation. In: Gospodarowicz M, B. O'Sullivan B, Sobin L, eds. *Prognostic Factors in Cancer*, 3rd edn. New Jersey: John Wiley & Sons, Inc.:39–54.

Concato J (2001) Challenges in prognostic analysis. *Cancer* 91(8 Suppl):1607–1614.

Febbo PG, Ladanyi M et al. (2011) NCCN Task Force report: Evaluating the clinical utility of tumor markers in oncology. *J Natl Compr Canc Netw* 9(Suppl 5): S1–32; quiz S33.

Gospodarowicz M, O'Sullivan B, et al. (2006). Prognostic factors: principles and applications. In: Gospodarowicz M, O'Sullivan B, Sobin L, eds. *Prognostic Factors in Cancer*, 3rd edn. New Jersey: John Wiley & Sons, Inc.:23–38.

Hanahan D (2014) Rethinking the war on cancer. *Lancet* 383:558–563.

Hanahan D, Weinberg RA (2011) Hallmarks of cancer: the next generation. *Cell* 144(5):646–674.

Hemingway H, Croft P et al. (2013) Prognosis research strategy (PROGRESS) 1: a framework for researching clinical outcomes. *BMJ* 346:e5595.

Hingorani AD, Windt DA et al. (2013) Prognosis research strategy (PROGRESS) 4: stratified medicine research. *BMJ* 346:e5793.

Hodgson D, Tannock I (2013) Guide to studies of diagnositc tests, prognostic factors, and treatments. In: Tannock T, Hill R, Bristow R, Harrington L, eds. *The Basic Science of Oncology*, 5th edn. McGraw-Hill:485–507.

Iasonos A, Schrag D et al. (2008) How to build and interpret a nomogram for cancer prognosis. *J Clin Oncol* 26(8):1364–1370.

Le QT, Zhang Q et al. (2013) An international collaboration to harmonize the quantitative plasma Epstein-Barr virus DNA assay for future biomarker-guided trials in nasopharyngeal carcinoma. *Clin Cancer Res* 19(8):2208–2215.

Ludwig JA, Weinstein JN (2005) Biomarkers in cancer staging, prognosis and treatment selection. *Nat Rev Cancer* 5(11):845–856.

McShane B, Simon F (2001) Statistical methods for the analysis of prognostic factor studies. Gospodarowicz M, Henson D, Hutter R et al., eds. *Prognostic Factors in Cancer*, 2nd edn. Wiley-Liss:37.

McShane LM, Altman DG et al. (2005) REporting recommendations for tumor MARKer prognostic studies (REMARK). *Nat Clin Pract Oncol* 2(8):416–422.

McShane LM, Hayes DF (2012) Publication of tumor marker research results: the necessity for complete and transparent reporting. *J Clin Oncol* 30(34):4223–4232.

Moore HM, Kelly AB et al. (2011) Biospecimen reporting for improved study quality (BRISQ). *Cancer Cytopathol* 119(2):92–101.

O'Sullivan B, Shah J (2011). Head and neck cancer staging and prognosis. Perspectives of the UICC and the AJCC. In: Bernier J, ed. *Head and Neck Cancer – Multimodality Management*. Heidelberg: Springer:135–155.

Peters LJ, O'Sullivan B et al. (2010) Critical impact of radiotherapy protocol compliance and quality in the treatment of advanced head and neck cancer: results from TROG 02.02. *J Clin Oncol* 28(18):2996–3001.

Pollock BH (2009) Cheaper, faster, better: chasing the elusive clinical trial end point. *J Clin Oncol* 27(17):2747–2748.

Riley RD, Hayden JA et al. (2013) Prognosis Research Strategy (PROGRESS) 2: prognostic factor research. *PLoS Med* 10(2):e1001380.

Steyerberg EW, Moons KG et al. (2013) Prognosis Research Strategy (PROGRESS) 3: prognostic model research. *PLoS Med* 10(2):e1001381.

World Health Organization (2011) *International Statistical Classification of Diseases and Related Health Problems (10th revision, edition 2010) (ICD-10)*. Geneva: WHO Press:(2):1–195.

Wuthrick EJ, Zhang Q et al. (2015) Institutional clinical trial accrual volume and survival of patients with head and neck cancer. *J Clin Oncol* 33(2):156–164.

4 Principles of cancer staging*

Leslie Sobin[1], James D. Brierley[2], Mary Gospodarowicz[2], Brian O'Sullivan[2] and Christian Wittekind[3]

[1]Armed Forces Institute of Pathology, Washington, DC, USA
[2]Department of Radiation Oncology, The Princess Margaret Cancer Centre, University of Toronto, Toronto, ON, Canada
[3]Institut für Pathologie des Universitätsklinikums, Leipzig, Germany

History of the TNM system

The TNM System for the classification of malignant tumours was developed by Pierre Denoix (France) between the years 1943 and 1952.

In 1950, the UICC appointed a Committee on Tumour Nomenclature and Statistics and adopted, as a basis for its work on clinical stage classification, the general definitions of local extension of malignant tumours suggested by the World Health Organization (WHO) Sub-Committee on The Registration of Cases of Cancer as well as Their Statistical Presentation.

In 1953, the Committee held a joint meeting with the International Commission on Stage-Grouping in Cancer and Presentation of the Results of Treatment of Cancer appointed by the International Congress of Radiology. Agreement was reached on a general technique for classification by anatomical extent of the disease, using the TNM system.

In 1954, the Research Commission of the UICC set up a special Committee on Clinical Stage Classification and Applied Statistics to "pursue studies in this field and to extend the general technique of classification to cancer at all sites".

In 1958, the Committee published the first recommendations for the clinical stage classification of cancers of the breast and larynx, and for the presentation of results. A second publication in 1959 presented revised proposals for the breast, for clinical use and evaluation over a 5-year period (1960–1964).

Between 1960 and 1967, the Committee published nine brochures describing proposals for the classification of 23 sites. It was recommended that the classification proposals for each site be subjected to prospective or retrospective trial for a 5-year period.

In 1968, these brochures were combined in a booklet, the *Livre de Poche*, and a year later, a complementary booklet was published detailing recommendations for the setting-up of field trials, for the presentation of end results, and for the determination and expression of cancer survival rates. The *Livre de Poche* was subsequently translated into 11 languages.

In 1974 and 1978, second and third editions were published containing new site classifications and amendments to previously published classifications. The third edition was enlarged and revised in 1982. It contained new classifications for selected tumours of childhood. This was carried out in collaboration with La Société Internationale d'Oncologie Pédiatrique (SIOP). A classification of ophthalmic tumours was published separately in 1985.

Over the years some users introduced variations in the rules of classification of certain sites. In order to correct this development, the antithesis of standardization, the national TNM committees in 1982 agreed to formulate a single TNM. A series of meetings was held to unify and update existing classifications as well as to develop new ones. The result was the fourth edition of the TNM.

In 1993, the project published the *TNM Supplement*. The purpose of this work was to promote the uniform use of the TNM by providing detailed explanations of the TNM rules with practical examples. It also included proposals for new classifications and optional expansions of selected categories. Second and third editions appeared in 2001 and 2003, and the fourth in 2012.

In 1995, the project published *Prognostic Factors in Cancer*, a compilation and discussion of prognostic factors in cancer, both anatomical and non-anatomical, at each of the body sites. This was expanded in the second edition in 2001 with emphasis on the relevance of different prognostic factors. The subsequent third edition in 2006 attempted to refine this by providing evidence-based criteria for relevance.

The present seventh edition of *TNM Classification* contains rules of classification and staging that correspond with those appearing in the seventh edition of the *AJCC Cancer Staging Manual* (2009) and have the approval of all national TNM committees. These are listed on pages xv–xvi of the *TNM Classification of Malignant Tumours*, 7th edition, together with the names of the members of the UICC committees who have

*This chapter is reproduced from *TNM Classification of Malignant Tumours* © and published 2010 by Blackwell Publishing, Ltd.

UICC Manual of Clinical Oncology, Ninth Edition. Edited by Brian O'Sullivan, James D. Brierley, Anil K. D'Cruz, Martin F. Fey, Raphael Pollock, Jan B. Vermorken and Shao Hui Huang. © 2015 UICC. Published 2015 by John Wiley & Sons, Ltd.

been associated with the TNM system. The UICC recognizes the need for stability in the TNM classification so that data can be accumulated in an orderly way over reasonable periods of time. Accordingly, it is the intention that the classifications published in this booklet should remain unchanged until some major advance in diagnosis or treatment relevant to a particular site requires reconsideration of the current classification.

To develop and sustain a classification system acceptable to all requires the closest of liaison between national and international committees. Only in this way will all oncologists be able to use a 'common language' when comparing their clinical material and assessing the results of treatment. While the classification is based on published evidence, in controversial areas it is based on international consensus.

The continuing objective of the UICC is to achieve common consent in the classification of the anatomical extent of disease.

The practice of dividing cancer cases into groups according to so-called stages arose from the fact that survival rates were higher for cases in whom the disease was localized than for those in whom the disease had extended beyond the organ of origin. These groups were often referred to as early cases and late cases, respectively, implying some regular progression with time. Actually, the stage of disease at the time of diagnosis may be a reflection not only of the rate of growth and extension of the neoplasm, but also of the type of tumour and of the tumour–host relationship.

The anatomical staging of cancer is hallowed by tradition and for the purpose of analysis of groups of patients, it is often necessary to use such a method. The UICC believes that it is important to reach agreement on the recording of accurate information on the anatomical extent of the disease for each site, because the precise clinical description of malignant neoplasms and histopathological classification may serve a number of related objectives, namely to:
1 Aid the clinician in the planning of treatment
2 Give some indication of prognosis
3 Assist in evaluation of the results of treatment
4 Facilitate the exchange of information between treatment centres
5 Contribute to the continuing investigation of human cancer
6 Support cancer control activities.

The principal purpose to be served by international agreement on the classification of cancer cases by extent of disease is to provide a method of conveying clinical experience to others without ambiguity.

There are many bases or axes of tumour classification, e.g. the anatomical site and the clinical and pathological extent of disease, the reported duration of symptoms or signs, the gender and age of the patient, and the histological type and grade. All of these bases or axes represent variables that are known to have an influence on the outcome of the disease. Classification by anatomical extent of disease as determined clinically and histopathologically is the primary one with which the TNM system deals.

The clinician's immediate task is to make a judgement as to prognosis and a decision as to the most effective course of treatment. This judgement and this decision require, among other things, an objective assessment of the anatomical extent of the disease. In accomplishing this, the trend is away from 'staging' to meaningful description, with or without some form of summarization.

To meet the stated objectives, a system of classification is needed:
1 Whose basic principles are applicable to all sites regardless of treatment, and
2 Which may be supplemented later by information that becomes available from histopathology and/or surgery.
The TNM system meets these requirements.

General rules of the TNM system

The TNM system for describing the anatomical extent of disease is based on the assessment of three components:
 T Extent of the primary tumour
 N Absence or presence and extent of regional lymph node metastasis
 M Absence or presence of distant metastasis
The addition of numbers to these three components indicates the extent of the malignant disease, thus:
 T0, T1, T2, T3, T4
 N0, N1, N2, N3
 M0, M1
In effect, the system is a 'shorthand notation' for describing the extent of a particular malignant tumour. The *general rules* applicable to all sites are as follows:
1 All cases should be confirmed microscopically. Any cases not so proved must be reported separately.
2 Two classifications are described for each site, namely:
 - *Clinical classification:* the pretreatment clinical classification designated TNM (or cTNM) is essential to select and evaluate therapy. This is based on evidence acquired before treatment. Such evidence arises from physical examination, imaging, endoscopy, biopsy, surgical exploration and other relevant examinations.
 - *Pathological classification:* the postsurgical histopathological classification, designated pTNM, is used to guide adjuvant therapy and provides additional data to estimate prognosis and calculate end results. This is based on evidence acquired before treatment, supplemented or modified by additional evidence acquired from surgery and from pathological examination.
   ○ The pathological assessment of the primary tumour (pT) entails a resection of the primary tumour or biopsy adequate to evaluate the highest pT category.
   ○ The pathological assessment of the regional lymph nodes (pN) entails removal of adequate numbers of lymph nodes to validate the absence of regional lymph node metastasis (pN0) or sufficient numbers to evaluate the highest pN category. An excisional biopsy of a lymph node without pathological assessment of the primary is insufficient to fully evaluate the pN category and is a clinical classification.

- The pathological assessment of distant metastasis (pM) entails microscopic examination.
3 After assigning T, N, M and/or pT, pN and pM categories, cases may be grouped into stages. The TNM classification and stage groups, once established, must remain unchanged in the medical records.

    Clinical and pathological data may be combined when only partial information is available either in the pathological classification or the clinical classification.
4 If there is doubt concerning the correct T, N or M category to which a particular case should be allotted, then the lower (i.e. less advanced) category should be chosen. This will also be reflected in the stage grouping.
5 In the case of multiple primary tumours in one organ, the tumour with the highest T category should be classified and the multiplicity or the number of tumours should be indicated in parenthesis, e.g. T2(m) or T2(5). In simultaneous bilateral primary cancers of paired organs, each tumour should be classified independently. In tumours of the liver, ovary and fallopian tube, multiplicity is a criterion of T classification, and in tumours of the lung, multiplicity may be a criterion of the T or M classification.
6 Definitions of TNM categories and stage grouping may be telescoped or expanded for clinical or research purposes as long as the recommended basic definitions are not changed. For instance, any T, N or M classification can be divided into subgroups.

    For more details on classification the reader is referred to the *TNM Supplement*.

Anatomical regions and sites

The sites in the TNM classification are listed according to the code number of the International Classification of Diseases for Oncology. Each region or site is described under the following headings:
- Rules for classification with the procedures for assessing the T, N and M categories
- Anatomical sites, and subsites if appropriate
- Definition of the regional lymph nodes
- TNM: clinical classification
- pTNM: pathological classification
- G: histopathological grading
- Stage grouping
- Summary.

TNM clinical classification

The following general definitions are used throughout:

T: Primary tumour
TX Primary tumour cannot be assessed
T0 No evidence of primary tumour
Tis Carcinoma *in situ*
T1–T4 Increasing size and/or local extent of the primary tumour

N: Regional lymph nodes
NX Regional lymph nodes cannot be assessed
N0 No regional lymph node metastasis
N1–N3 Increasing involvement of regional lymph nodes

M: Distant metastasis
M0 No distant metastasis
M1 Distant metastasis

Note: The MX category is considered to be inappropriate as clinical assessment of metastasis can be based on physical examination alone. (The use of MX may result in exclusion from staging.)

The category M1 may be further specified according to the following notation:

Pulmonary	PUL	Bone marrow	MAR
Osseous	OSS	Pleura	PLE
Hepatic	HEP	Peritoneum	PER
Brain	BRA	Adrenals	ADR
Lymph nodes	LYM	Skin	SKI
Others	OTH		

Subdivisions of TNM

Subdivisions of some of the main categories are available for those who need greater specificity (e.g. T1a, T1b, or N2a, N2b).

The following general definitions are used throughout:

pT: Primary tumour
pTX Primary tumour cannot be assessed histologically
pT0 No histological evidence of primary tumour
pTis Carcinoma *in situ*
pT1–4 Increasing size and/or local extent of the primary tumour histologically

pN: Regional lymph nodes
pNX Regional lymph nodes cannot be assessed histologically
pN0 No regional lymph node metastasis histologically
pN1–3 Increasing involvement of regional lymph nodes histologically

Notes:
1 Direct extension of the primary tumour into lymph nodes is classified as lymph node metastasis.
2 Tumour deposits (satellites), i.e. macro- or micro-scopic nests or nodules, in the lymph drainage area of a primary carcinoma without histological evidence of residual lymph node in the nodule may represent discontinuous spread, venous invasion (V1/2) or a totally replaced lymph node. If a nodule is considered by the pathologist to be a totally replaced lymph

node (generally having a smooth contour), it should be recorded as a positive lymph node, and each such nodule should be counted separately as a lymph node in the final pN determination.
3 Metastasis in a lymph node other than a regional lymph node is classified as a distant metastasis.
4 When size is a criterion for pN classification, the metastasis within the node is measured, not of the entire lymph node.
5 Cases with micrometastasis only, i.e. no metastasis >0.2 cm, can be identified by the addition of (mi), e.g. pN1(mi).
6 The number of resected and positive nodes should be recorded.

Sentinel lymph node

The sentinel lymph node is the first lymph node to receive lymphatic drainage from a primary tumour. If it contains metastatic tumour, this indicates that other lymph nodes may contain tumour. If it does not contain metastatic tumour, other lymph nodes are not likely to contain tumour. Occasionally there is more than one sentinel lymph node.

The following designations are applicable when sentinel lymph node assessment is attempted:
pNX(sn) Sentinel lymph node could not be assessed
pN0(sn) No sentinel lymph node metastasis
pN1(sn) Sentinel lymph node metastasis

Isolated tumour cells

Isolated tumour cells (ITCs) are single tumour cells or small clusters of cells not >0.2 mm in greatest extent that can be detected by routine H&E stains or immunohistochemistry. A proposed additional criterion is a cluster of <200 cells in a single histological cross-section. ITCs do not typically show evidence of metastatic activity (e.g. proliferation or stromal reaction) or penetration of vascular or lymphatic sinus walls. Cases with ITCs in lymph nodes or at distant sites should be classified as N0 or M0, respectively. The same applies to cases with findings suggestive of tumour cells or their components by non-morphological techniques such as flow cytometry or DNA analysis. These cases should be analysed separately. Their classification is as follows:
pN0 No regional lymph node metastasis histologically, no examination for ITCs
pN0(i–) No regional lymph node metastasis histologically, negative morphological findings for ITCs
pN0(i+) No regional lymph node metastasis histologically, positive morphological findings for ITCs
pN0(mol–) No regional lymph node metastasis histologically, negative non-morphological findings for ITCs
pN0(mol+) No regional lymph node metastasis histologically, positive non-morphological findings for ITCs

Cases with or examined for isolated tumour cells can be classified as follows:
pN0(i–)(sn) No sentinel lymph node metastasis histologically, negative morphological findings for ITCs
pN0(i+)(sn) No sentinel lymph node metastasis histologically, positive morphological findings for ITCs
pN0(mol–)(sn) No sentinel lymph node metastasis histologically, negative non-morphological findings for ITCs
pN0(mol+)(sn) No sentinel lymph node metastasis histologically, positive non-morphological findings for ITCs

pM: Distant metastasis
pM1 Distant metastasis microscopically confirmed

Note: pM0 and pMX are not valid categories.
The category pM1 may be further specified in the same way as M1 (see above).
ITCs found in bone marrow with morphological techniques are classified according to the scheme for M, e.g. M0(i+). For non-morphological findings, 'mol' is used in addition to M0, e.g. M0(mol+).

Histopathological grading

In most sites, further information regarding the primary tumour may be recorded under the following heading:

G: Histopathological grading
GX Grade of differentiation cannot be assessed
G1 Well differentiated
G2 Moderately differentiated
G3 Poorly differentiated
G4 Undifferentiated

Notes:
1 Grades 3 and 4 can be combined in some circumstances as 'G3–4, poorly differentiated or undifferentiated'.
2 The bone and soft tissue sarcoma classifications also use 'high grade' and 'low grade'.
3 Special systems of grading are recommended for tumours of breast, corpus uteri, prostate and liver.

Additional descriptors

For identification of special cases in the TNM or pTNM classification, the m, y, r and a symbols may be used. Although they do not affect the stage grouping, they indicate cases needing separate analysis.
m The suffix m, in parentheses, is used to indicate the presence of multiple primary tumours at a single site. See TNM general rule 5 above.
y In those cases in which classification is performed during or following multimodality therapy, the cTNM or pTNM

category is identified by a y prefix. The ycTNM or ypTNM categorizes the tumour extent actually present at the time of that examination. The y categorization is not an estimate of the tumour extent prior to multimodality therapy.

r Recurrent tumours, when classified after a disease-free interval, are identified by the prefix r.

a The prefix a indicates that classification is first determined at autopsy.

Operational descriptors

L: Lymphatic invasion

LX Lymphatic invasion cannot be assessed
L0 No lymphatic invasion
L1 Lymphatic invasion

V: Venous invasion

VX Venous invasion cannot be assessed
V0 No venous invasion
V1 Microscopic venous invasion
V2 Macroscopic venous invasion

Note: Macroscopic involvement of the wall of veins (with no tumour within the veins) is classified as V2.

Pn: Perineural invasion

PnX Perineural invasion cannot be assessed
Pn0 No perineural invasion
Pn1 Perineural invasion

C-factor

The C-factor, or certainty factor, reflects the validity of classification according to the diagnostic methods employed. Its use is optional.

The C-factor definitions are:

C1 Evidence from standard diagnostic means (e.g. inspection, palpation and standard radiography, intraluminal endoscopy for tumours of certain organs)
C2 Evidence obtained by special diagnostic means (e.g. radiographic imaging in special projections, tomography, computed tomography [CT], ultrasonography, lymphography, angiography; scintigraphy; magnetic resonance imaging [MRI]; endoscopy, biopsy and cytology)
C3 Evidence from surgical exploration, including biopsy and cytology
C4 Evidence of the extent of disease following definitive surgery and pathological examination of the resected specimen
C5 Evidence from autopsy

Example: Degrees of C may be applied to the T, N and M categories. A case might be described as T3C2, N2C1, M0C2.

The TNM clinical classification is therefore equivalent to C1, C2 and C3 in varying degrees of certainty, while the pTNM pathological classification generally is equivalent to C4.

Residual tumour (R) classification

The absence or presence of residual tumour after treatment is described by the symbol R. More details can be found in the *TNM Supplement*.

TNM and pTNM describe the anatomical extent of cancer in general without considering treatment. They can be supplemented by the R classification, which deals with tumour status after treatment. The R classification reflects the effects of therapy, influences further therapeutic procedures and is a strong predictor of prognosis.

The R definitions are:
RX Presence of residual tumour cannot be assessed
R0 No residual tumour
R1 Microscopic residual tumour
R2 Macroscopic residual tumour

Note: Some consider the R classification to apply only to the primary tumour and its local or regional extent. Others have applied it more broadly to include distant metastasis. The specific usage should be indicated when the R is used.

Stage grouping

The TNM system is used to describe and record the anatomical extent of disease. For the purposes of tabulation and analysis, it is useful to condense these categories into stage groups. For consistency, in the TNM system, carcinoma *in situ* is categorized Stage 0; in general, tumours localized to the organ of origin as Stages I and II; locally extensive spread, particularly to regional lymph nodes, as Stage III; and those with distant metastasis as Stage IV. The stage adopted ensures, as far as possible, that each group is more or less homogeneous with respect to survival, and that the survival rates of these groups for each cancer site are distinct.

For pathological stage groups, if sufficient tissue has been removed for pathological examination to evaluate the highest T and N categories, M1 may be either clinical (cM1) or pathological (pM1). However, if only a distant metastasis has had microscopic confirmation, the classification is pathological (pM1) and the stage is pathological.

Prognostic grouping

Although the anatomical extent of disease, as categorized by TNM, is a very powerful prognostic indicator in cancer, it is recognized that many factors have a significant impact on predicting outcomes. Some have been incorporated into the stage grouping, e.g. grade in soft tissue sarcoma and age in thyroid cancer. These classifications are unchanged in the seventh edition. In the newly revised classifications for carcinomas of the oesophagus and prostate, *stage grouping* has been maintained as defining the anatomical extent of disease and new *prognostic groupings* that incorporate other prognostic factors have been proposed.

Stage summary

As a means of reference, a simple summary of the chief points that distinguish the most important categories and stage or prognostic grouping has been added to each chapter. These abridged definitions are not completely adequate, and the full definitions should always be consulted.

Related classifications

Since 1958, the WHO has been involved in a programme aimed at providing internationally accepted criteria for the histological diagnosis of tumours. This has resulted in the *International Histological Classification of Tumours,* which contains, in an illustrated multivolume series, definitions of tumour types and a proposed nomenclature. A new series, *WHO Classification of Tumours – Pathology and Genetics of Tumours,* continues this effort. (Information on these publications is available at http://www.iarc.fr)

The *WHO International Classification of Diseases for Oncology (ICD-O)* is a coding system for neoplasms by topography and morphology and for indicating behaviour (e.g. malignant, benign). This coded nomenclature is identical in the morphology field for neoplasms to the *Systematized Nomenclature of Medicine* (SNOMED).

In the interest of promoting national and international collaboration in cancer research and specifically of facilitating cooperation in clinical investigations, it is recommended that the *WHO Classification of Tumours* be used for classification and definition of tumour types, and that the ICD-O code be used for storage and retrieval of data.

Recommended reading

College of American Pathologists. *SNOMED International: The Systematized Nomenclature of Human and Veterinary Medicine.* Northfield: College of American Pathologists. Available at http://www.cap.org

Edge SB, Byrd DR, Compton CC et al., eds. American Joint Committee on Cancer (AJCC) (2009) *AJCC Cancer Staging Manual*, 7th edn. New York: Springer.

Fritz A, Percy C, Jack A et al., eds. (2000) *WHO International Classification of Diseases for Oncology ICD-O*, 3rd edn. Geneva: WHO.

Gospodarowicz MK, O'Sullivan B, Sobin LH, eds. International Union Against Cancer (UICC) (2006) *Prognostic Factors in Cancer*, 3rd edn. New York: Wiley.

Hermanek P, Hutter RVP, Sobin LH, Wittekind Ch (1999) Classification of isolated tumour cells and micrometastasis. *Cancer* 86:2668–2673.

Sobin, LS, Gospodarowicz, MK, Wittekind, Ch (2009) *TNM Classification of Malignant Tumours*, 7th edn. Wiley Blackwell, Oxford.

Wittekind Ch, Compton, CC, Brierley JD, et al., eds. International Union Against Cancer (UICC) (2012) *TNM Supplement. A Commentary on Uniform Use*, 4th edn. Oxford: Wiley Blackwell.

5 Assessment of treatment outcome

Judith Manola[1], Wei Xu[2] and Bruce J. Giantonio[3]

[1]Department of Biostatistics and Computational Biology, Dana-Farber Cancer Institute, Boston, MA, USA
[2]Department of Biostatistics, The Princess Margaret Cancer Centre, Toronto, ON, Canada
[3]Abramson Cancer Center, The University of Pennsylvania, Philadelphia, PA, USA

Outcome reporting: General overview

Clinical endpoints in outcome reporting

Statistical methods are widely used in cancer studies. Their purpose is usually to estimate the treatment effect and its variation, calculate P-values from observed clinical data, apply hypothesis testing and quantify the risk of false-positive conclusions. The most commonly used clinical endpoints in outcome reporting are survival-related time-to-event measures, tumour response, toxicity and quality of life (QoL).

Definitions of commonly used clinical survival-related endpoints are:

- *Overall survival (OS)*: the time from either date of diagnosis or treatment (or randomization/registration date for prospective clinical trials), to the date of death from any cause. Patients alive at the time of the analysis are censored at the date last known to be alive.
- *Cause (or cancer)-specific survival (CSS)*: where events are defined as death due to cancer. Patients who die of other causes or who are still alive are censored at the date of death or date last recorded to be alive.
- *Progression-free survival (PFS)*: where events are defined as the first documented disease (tumour) progression or death due to any cause. Time is censored at the date of last disease evaluation if patients are alive without progression.
- *Disease-free survival (DFS)*: in studies among patients who are rendered free of disease, this is the preferred term, rather than progression-free survival. The treatment of patients who have other intervening endpoints, such as second primary cancers, should be explicit.
- *Other endpoints*:
  - *Local control (LC)*: time to local failure (disease failure at the primary tumour site)
  - *Regional control (RC)*: time to regional failure (disease failure at the adjacent lymph node regions)
  - *Distant control (DC) or distant metastasis-free survival (DMFS)*: time to distant failure (disease spread to remote sites).

These endpoints pose the problem of competing risks, and the statistical analysis must take such competing risks into account.

Measurement of effect size and competing risk

Survival is the most common clinical endpoint used to measure effect size of an intervention. A survival rate is a statistical index of the probable frequency of a specific outcome (death) for a group of cancer patients at a specific time point. The simplest measure for survival is the proportion of surviving patients at the end of the study period (or, conversely, the frequency of death). However, this is only informative if all patients are observed for the same length of time and the vital status is known for every patient in the study. In practice, this is unrealistic because the duration of observation is generally not consistent for each case and for some the vital status may be unknown at the time of analysis.

To address this, an actuarial rate of survival is more appropriate. In actuarial survival analysis, patients who are observed until the event (i.e. death) occurs are termed 'uncensored' cases, while those who survive beyond the end of follow-up or are lost at some point during the study period are termed 'censored' cases. There are two basic methods to determine the actuarial rate of survival:

- *Life table method*:
  - Divides the total period over which a group is observed into fixed intervals
  - For each interval, the proportion surviving to the end of the interval is calculated on the basis of numbers known to have experienced the event (e.g. death) during the interval and the number estimated to have been at risk at the start of the interval
  - May be used by, for example, insurance companies, but is rarely used in clinical trials.

UICC Manual of Clinical Oncology, Ninth Edition. Edited by Brian O'Sullivan, James D. Brierley, Anil K. D'Cruz, Martin F. Fey, Raphael Pollock, Jan B. Vermorken and Shao Hui Huang. © 2015 UICC. Published 2015 by John Wiley & Sons, Ltd.

- *Kaplan–Meier (KM) method:*
  - Uses the exact times that events occurred, rather than the intervals of follow-up (as in the life table method)
  - Calculates the proportion surviving at each point when a death occurs, i.e. a stepwise change in the cumulative survival rate appears to occur independent of the intervals
  - If there are withdrawals before the time of event, they are subtracted from the number at risk
  - Widely used for survival analysis for both clinical trials and retrospective studies, especially when sample size is small and useful fixed intervals cannot be generated.

The actuarial rate of survival estimation is applicable to many clinical endpoints, such as overall survival (OS) and progression-free survival (PFS). Results can be reported either as medians or rates at a specific time point, such as 5 years, along with confidence intervals.

Non-stratified or stratified (if a stratification process is employed in the randomization scheme to balance arms) log-rank tests are frequently applied to compare the treatment effect among various groups.

The Cox proportional hazards regression model is commonly used to estimate the hazard ratio (HR), along with confidence intervals (e.g. 95% CI). Here HR can be interpreted as the chance of an event occurring under one treatment divided by the chance of the event occurring under another treatment in a given study.

Competing risks are present when a patient is at risk for more than one mutually exclusive event, such as death from different causes, and the occurrence of one of these will prevent any other event from ever being observed. In this case, the competing risks method of analysis is recommended:
- More appropriate when event(s) caused by confounding causes (e.g. smoking-related mortalities) other than the cause under investigation (e.g. index cancer death) occur sufficiently frequently that they cannot be ignored.
- Cumulative incidence curves are used for failure types (such as local or regional failure, distant metastases, second primary tumour, death without recurrence) to take into account competing risks. Competing risk regression models are used to assess the treatment effect in such circumstances.

Commonly used conventions, including addressing competing risk issues, for clinical endpoints are summarized in Table 5.1.

Adjustment for the impact of multiple variables

For a cancer patient, multiple factors may affect clinical outcomes. Multivariable analysis models are commonly used to assess and construct prognostic or predictive models with multiple clinical factors. 'Multivariable' means multiple variables measured on the same patient. Stepwise selection algorithms can be used for the model selection process. Multivariable regression analysis can also be used to assess the interaction effect between treatment and other clinical or demographic factors. When conducting multivariable analysis, an approximate rule of thumb is that a minimum of 10 events per predictor variable is needed.

Outcome reporting: Specific issues

Toxicity reporting
- Toxicities are usually evaluated using incidence rates of adverse events based on the National Cancer Institute (NCI) Common Terminology Criteria for Adverse Events (CTCAE).
- Serious adverse events (SAEs) are listed by patient and tabulated by type of adverse event.
- Exact binomial two-sided confidence intervals (CIs) are generated to assess the rates of adverse events of interest. The width of the CI should correspond to the design assumptions of the clinical trial, if applicable.
- For treatment effect assessment, Wilson's score with continuity correction can be used to generate CIs for the difference in adverse event of interest rates between treatment arms.
- KM methods and Cox models can be used to assess the time to development of late toxicity.

Table 5.1 Treatment of first observed events for various common endpoints

First event	OS	CSS	PFS	LC	RC	DC
None (alive, no disease)	Censor	Censor	Censor	Censor	Censor	Censor
Local (primary site) failure	N/A	N/A	Event	Event	N/A	Competing risk
Regional (lymph node) failure	N/A	N/A	Event	N/A	Event	Competing risk
Distant (remote sites) metastasis	N/A	N/A	Event	N/A	N/A	Event
Death due to index cancer	Event	Event	Event	Competing risk	Competing risk	Competing risk
Death due to other causes	Event	Competing risk	Event	Competing risk	Competing risk	Competing risk

CSS, cause (or cancer)-specific survival; PFS, progression-free survival; LC, local control; RC, regional control; DC, distant control; N/A, occurrence of event is ignored in the analysis.

- Ordinal regression models can be applied to assess toxicity based on the CTCAE grade.

Quality of life reporting

Instruments have been developed to assess the QoL of cancer patients for a range of physical and psychological functions. These are usually questionnaires that may combine specific disease- or treatment-related questions as well as general questions. Most score a number of different dimensions, including physical, emotional and social functions, and some provide a total score derived from the individual dimensions.
- Distributions of QoL measures need to be described for each time point in terms of mean, median, standard deviation, minimum, maximum and graphically (i.e. in the form of a histogram, bar plot or series of box plots).
- In some clinical studies, the primary objective of QoL analysis is to assess the change in the pattern of the QoL scores under treatments.
- Linear regression models can be used to assess the difference between the QoL score at each follow-up time point and the baseline measures.
- The change can be defined as an increase by a specific number of points (i.e. a 10-point increase) between baseline and the assessment at specific follow-up time points.
- For more comprehensive evaluation, mixed-effects model regression can be applied to model the repeated measurement of QoL scores over time.

Sample size estimation in clinical trials

Sample size is an important factor in the assessment of treatment effects in clinical studies. Underestimation of sample size may result in the treatment effect being regarded as statistically non-significant even though clinical significance exists. For exploratory and hypothesis-generating studies, the sample sizes can be determined based on feasibility and costs. For well-designed studies such as clinical trials, formal sample size and power analysis need to be conducted. Sample size calculations are conducted with consideration of the following:
- Type of study design
- Analysis method
- Significance level
- Statistical power
- Measurement variability
- Effect size.

Two-sided statistical tests are recommended. For studies with multiple hypotheses, multiple test corrections, such as Bonferroni adjustment, need to be conducted to adjust for inflated false-positive errors.

Interim analysis of clinical trials

Interim analysis can be used to assess the safety and efficacy of clinical studies after partial information has been observed. The investigators are ethically obliged to assess the data at hand and to make a deliberate consideration of terminating the study earlier than planned when a treatment is:
- Overwhelmingly beneficial (efficacy)
- Unlikely to improve upon the control (futility)
- Unacceptably harmful (toxicity) while the study is ongoing.

The stopping boundaries for efficacy can be computed using the Lan–DeMets approximation to the O'Brien–Fleming boundary. Besides the major hypothesis test, sensitivity analyses and subgroup analyses can be performed. Since such analyses are exploratory and hypothesis generating, multiple test correction is not always necessary and $P = <0.05$ can be used to define nominal signals. Such planned analyses should be specified before the study is undertaken.

Adjustment for missing data in outcome reporting

The reliability and interpretability of results from clinical trials can be substantially impaired by missing data. For example, missing data can limit the ability to draw definitive conclusions from studies or lead to biased inferences about drug safety. There are two ways of handling missing data:
- If the missing data can be shown to occur under a missing completely at random (MCAR) mechanism, then they can be ignored and the statistical analysis is performed using only samples with complete data.
- If the missing at random (MAR) assumption can be supported, then imputation methods such as multiple imputation can be applied to impute the missing data based on baseline characteristics, and analyses can be conducted as if all the data were observed. Plans to use multiple imputation should be stated before the study is undertaken.

Assessment of response: General considerations and overview

The efficacy of cancer therapy is most accurately reflected in improved survival and symptom reduction. Yet, intermediary endpoints, such as changes in tumour size, tumour-related chemical markers and tumour metabolism, aid in clinical decision-making and the evaluation of new treatments.

Definition of response evaluation

Response evaluation is defined as a *system* comprising validated techniques for the measurement of tumour burden and criteria for evaluating those measurements. The goal of response evaluation is to detect changes in the disease burden associated with an intervention in a manner that is reliable, valid and practical.
- *Reliable* means that the system can be reproduced across patients, across studies, across disease stages and over time.

- *Valid* means that the system measures and evaluates disease burden in a way that is known to be important to the patient's ultimate outcome.
- *Practical* means that the system is affordable, minimally invasive and 'sensible'.

Applications of tumour response assessment
Clinical research
Clinical trial endpoints that depend on response evaluation include response rate (RR), progression-free survival (PFS) and time to progression (TTP). RR is defined as the proportion of patients who achieve a partial or complete response. Frequently, especially if RR is the study's primary endpoint, the response must be sustained for a minimum time interval and confirmed at a second assessment. PFS is defined as the time from study entry until documentation of disease progression according to the response criteria or death without progression for any cause. TTP is simply the time from study entry until disease progression. Thus, an accurate and reproducible means of assessing response is central to the conduct of clinical research utilizing these endpoints. For patients whose response or progression is not observed, it is important to document the time from study entry to last disease assessment without response or progression.

Clinical decision-making
The current system of defining cancers based on tissue subtypes of the organ of origin ignores the molecular heterogeneity of those cancers, and this in part can explain the variable treatment responsiveness within a particular disease type. Early identification of non-effective treatment in individual patients is critical to prevent unnecessary toxicity and to allow treatment to be changed to a potentially effective one. Historically, identification relies on tumour response assessment obtained through anatomical and metabolic imaging, assessment of markers secreted by tumour cells and at times overall clinical impression.

While much work has been undertaken to establish guidelines of response assessment for clinical research, clinicians are cautioned on applying those guidelines to daily practice. To date, similar systems of response assessment to guide clinical decision-making do not exist.

Response assessment may also provide prognostic information that can be utilized in guiding therapy decisions.

Assessment of response using anatomical methods

Guiding principles for anatomical response evaluation
- The same method of response evaluation must be used over time to ensure accuracy.
- The methods of response evaluation must have well-defined and established procedures to ensure reproducibility.
- Standardized metrics must be used for reporting measurements and the assessment of overall response.
- All anatomical size measurements should be recorded in metric notation (millimetres), using calipers if clinically assessed.
- All baseline evaluations should be performed as close as possible to the start of treatment and never >4 weeks before the beginning of the treatment.
- A target lesion should be selected based on well-defined margins that allow reproducible measurement.

Response evaluation by imaging
- *Computed tomography (CT)*:
  - Commonly used for solid tumours
  - The RECIST 1.1 guidelines define measurability of lesions on CT scan based on the assumption that CT slice thickness is ≤5 mm. When CT scans are of a slice thickness >5 mm, the minimum size for a measurable lesion should be twice the slice thickness
  - Optimal visualization requires administration of intravenous (IV) contrast and adequate coverage of anatomical regions where disease is likely to have metastasized (usually chest/abdomen/pelvis)
  - Results are easily stored for future reference and possible central review
  - Best currently available and reproducible method to measure lesions selected for response assessment.
- *X-ray ('plain films')*:
  - Feasible and widely available, commonly used for chest imaging
  - Not good for identifying new lesions
  - CT is preferred since it is more sensitive than plain X-ray, particularly in identifying new lesions
  - Lesions on chest X-ray may be considered measurable if they are clearly defined and surrounded by aerated lung.
- *Magnetic resonance imaging (MRI)*:
  - Utility for response assessment is similar to that for CT, but requires more precise set-up for the particular type of tumour
  - Not as globally available as CT; more time consuming and costlier
  - Utility limited based on anatomical regions.
- *Ultrasonography*:
  - Not appropriate for assessing solid tumour response
  - Examination is subjective; difficult to make consistent assessments across multiple evaluations
  - Cannot reproduce entire examination for later independent review
  - Can be impeded by gas or other materials in the gastrointestinal tract
  - If new lesions are identified by ultrasound in the course of the study, confirmation by CT or MRI is advised.

Response evaluation by physical examination
- *Palpation*:
  - Used for lesions in the neck, lymph nodes, liver, spleen and prostate (via digital rectal exam)

- Appropriate when lesions are superficial, at least 10 mm in size and can be assessed using calipers
- Difficult to detect small changes objectively. If used in clinical research for response assessment, there should be clear instructions in the protocol about how to perform the measurements
- Assessment should be performed under similar conditions, with the same instrument and by the same person whenever possible
- Difficult to document conditions for possible central review
- Not easy to use in a clinical trial if a central response review is required.
- *Visual assessment*:
  - Used for skin lesions, lesions in the respiratory, female reproductive, urinary and alimentary canals
  - Usually require the use of a 'scope' – microscope or magnifier, endoscopy, colonoscopy, cystoscopy, laparoscopy, colposcopy
  - Not advised for objective evaluation of solid tumours
  - May accompany a procedure for excising visible lesions
  - Can be used to detect recurrence following complete response or surgical resection. While this is a beneficial therapeutic intervention, the excision of lesions makes it impossible to determine treatment effect related to a previously administered intervention, unless there is a pathological complete response
- While video records are possible (such as ultrasonography), it can be difficult to standardize these procedures and readings
- For skin lesions, photographic documentation with a ruler in the field is considered the standard.

RECIST (Response Evaluation Criteria In Solid Tumors), versions 1.0, 1.1

RECIST, since its initial publication in 2000, and subsequent update in 2008, has become the most widely used system for assessing response in cancer clinical trials, and is the preferred and accepted system for use in new drug applications to regulatory agencies. The differences between the two versions are summarized in Table 5.2, and the following discussion will be limited to the specifics and use of version 1.1. Of note, for trials that currently use version 1.0, it is recommended that the studies be completed using that version of the criteria.

In the RECIST system, response assessment is based on the determination of the single largest diameter of the lesion being measured as this measurement directly correlates with volume (this is in contrast to the bi-dimensional measurement used in the WHO criteria, as discussed below).

Lesions to be included in the evaluation are characterized as being either *target* or *non-target* lesions, and assessment

Table 5.2 Comparison of Version 1.0 versus Version 1.1 of the Response Evaluation Criteria in Solid Tumors (RECIST)

	RECIST 1.0	RECIST 1.1
Minimum size of target lesion	≥10 mm on helical CT; ≥20 mm on non-helical CT and MRI	≥10 mm on helical CT or MRI ≥20 mm on chest X-ray
Overall tumour burden	Maximum of ten target lesions total (maximum of five per organ)	Maximum of five target lesions total (maximum of two per organ)
Measurement	One-dimensional (1D) longest diameter of tumour	1D longest diameter of tumour; short axis of lymph nodes
New lesions	None	Clarified
Measurement of cystic and bone lesions	None	Clarified
Lymph node measurement	None	Lymph nodes ≥15 mm are target lesions Lymph nodes <10 mm are non-pathological
Response criteria for PD for target	20% increase over smallest sum on study or new lesions	20% increase over smallest sum on study and at least 5-mm increase or new lesions
Response criteria for PD for non-target	Unequivocal progression considered as PD	More detailed description of 'unequivocal progression'
Confirmation of CR and PR	After at least 28 days	Only required if response is primary endpoint and not randomized
18FDG-PET	None	Used only to support CT if PD or to confirm CR

CR, complete response; PR, partial response; PD, progressive disease.

Source: Yaghmai *et al.* (2011) *AJR* 197:18–27. Reproduced with permission of the *American Journal of Roentgenology*.

of both categories is included in the overall determination of treatment effect. To identify appropriate target lesions, all lesions are initially characterized as measurable and non-measurable based on criteria listed below. Only measureable lesions can be designated as target lesions, whereas non-target lesions can be classified as either measurable or non-measureable. The first step is to identify measureable and non-measureable lesions, and then to assign the required number of target lesions.

Defining measurable and non-measurable lesions in RECIST
Measurable tumour lesions
- Must be readily and accurately measurable in at least one dimension (longest diameter in the plane of measurement is to be recorded) with a minimum size of:
  - 10 mm by CT scan (with CT scan slice thickness no >5 mm)
  - 10-mm caliper measurement by clinical exam (per RECIST 1.1 guidelines, lesions that cannot be accurately measured with calipers should be recorded as non-measurable)
  - 20 mm by chest X-ray.
- Only the soft tissue component of a lytic or a mixed lytic/blastic bone metastasis can be considered as measurable disease if it meets the above criteria.

Measurable lymph nodes
- Unlike tumour lesions, the *shortest* axis of the lymph node in question must meet the following size criterion (by CT imaging with CT scan slice thickness no >5 mm) to be considered a measurable malignant lymph node: measurable (target) ≥15-mm.

Non-measurable lesions
- Any lesion that does not meet the criteria listed for measurable tumour or lymph node lesions (see above)
- Leptomeningeal disease
- Ascites
- Pleural or pericardial effusion
- Inflammatory breast disease
- Lymphangitic involvement of skin or lung
- Abdominal masses/abdominal organomegaly identified by physical exam that is not measurable by reproducible imaging techniques
- Blastic bone lesions
- Lymph node: 10–<15 mm

Tumour lesions situated in a previously irradiated area, or in an area subjected to other locoregional therapy, are usually not considered measurable unless progression of the lesion has been demonstrated.

Bone lesions detected by bone scan, positron emission tomography (PET) scan or plain films are not considered adequate imaging techniques to measure bone lesions. However, these techniques can be used to confirm the presence or disappearance of bone lesions.

Defining 'target' and 'non-target' lesions in RECIST
Target lesions
- Must represent all involved organs. A maximum of five lesions in total (and a maximum of two lesions per organ) are recorded and measured at baseline.
- Should be selected on the basis of their size and the ease of reproducible repeated measurements.
- A sum of the diameters (longest for non-nodal lesions, short axis for nodal lesions) for all target lesions is be calculated and reported as the baseline sum of diameters.

Non-target lesions
- All other lesions, including pathological lymph nodes, should be identified as non-target lesions and should also be recorded at baseline.
- Measurements are not required for non-target lesions, and these lesions should be followed simply as being 'present', 'absent' or demonstrating 'unequivocal progression'.

Response evaluation in RECIST
Target lesions

Complete response (CR)	Disappearance of all target lesions; any pathological lymph nodes must have a short axis of <10 mm
Partial response (PR)	>30% decrease in sum of diameters since baseline; no new lesions
Stable disease (SD)	Neither PR nor PD
Progressive disease (PD)	>20% increase in sum of diameters of target lesions since nadir (absolute increase of >5 mm) or appearance of a new lesion

Non-target lesions

CR	Disappearance of all non-target lesions; all lymph nodes <10 mm (short axis)
Non-CR/Non-PD	Persistence of non-target lesion(s)
PD	Unequivocal progression of existing non-target lesions or new lesion

Evaluation of best overall response in RECIST
The best overall response is defined as the best response recorded from the start of the study treatment until the end of treatment, taking into account any requirement for confirmation. The patient's best overall response assignment will depend on the findings of both target and non-target disease and will also take into consideration the appearance of new lesions.

Confirmation of response
Confirmatory measurement can be protocol specific:
- Non-randomized trials where response is the primary endpoint: confirmation of PR and CR is *required* to ensure responses identified are not the result of measurement error.

- Randomized trials (phase II or III) or studies where stable disease or progression is the primary endpoint: confirmation of response is *not required* since it will not add value to the interpretation of trial results. However, elimination of the requirement for response confirmation may increase the importance of central review to protect against bias, particularly for studies that are not blinded.
- In the case of SD, measurements must have met the SD criteria at least once after study entry at a minimum interval (in general not <6–8 weeks) defined in the study protocol. When SD is believed to be the best response, it must also meet the protocol-specified minimum time from baseline. If the minimum time is not met when SD is otherwise the best time point response, the patient's best response depends on the subsequent assessments.

New lesions
- The appearance of new malignant lesions defines disease progression.
- The finding of a new lesion should be unequivocal, i.e. not attributable to differences in scanning technique, change in imaging modality, or findings thought to represent something other than a tumour.
- A lesion identified on a follow-up study in an anatomical location that was not scanned at baseline is considered a new lesion and will indicate disease progression.

Special considerations for RECIST response evaluation

Response evaluation by pathological determinants of disease
- *Tumour markers*:
  - Tumour markers alone cannot be used to assess objective tumour response. If markers are initially above the upper normal limit, however, they must normalize for a patient to be considered in complete response. Because tumour markers are disease specific, instructions for their measurement should be incorporated into protocols on a disease-specific basis. The disease-specific use of markers is discussed below.
- *Cytology/histology*:
  - These techniques can be used to differentiate between PR and CR in rare cases if required by protocol (e.g. residual lesions in tumour types such as germ cell tumours, where known residual benign tumours can remain).
  - When effusions are known to be a potential adverse effect of treatment (e.g. with certain taxane compounds or angiogenesis inhibitors), cytological confirmation of the neoplastic origin of any effusion that appears or worsens during treatment can be considered if the measurable tumour has met criteria for response or stable disease, in order to differentiate between response (or stable disease) and progressive disease.

Lesions that are too small to measure
- If it is likely the lesion has disappeared, the measurement = 0 mm.
- If the lesion is believed to be present and is faintly seen but too small to measure, a default value of 5 mm should be assigned.
- If the radiologist is able to provide an actual measure, that should be recorded, even if it is <5 mm.

Lesions that split or coalesce on treatment
- Fragmenting of non-nodal lesions:
  - The longest diameters of the fragmented portions should be added together to calculate the target lesion sum.
- Coalescing lesions:
  - If a plane between them is identified, obtain maximal diameter measurements of each individual lesion
  - If the lesions have truly coalesced, the longest diameter in this instance should be the maximal longest diameter for the 'coalesced lesion'.

When the findings for progression of disease are equivocal, treatment may continue until the next scheduled assessment.

New lesions *on the basis of fluorodeoxyglucose (FDG)-PET imaging*
Negative FDG-PET at baseline but a positive FDG-PET at follow-up defines PD based on a new lesion:
- If the positive FDG-PET at follow-up corresponds to a new site of disease confirmed by CT, this is PD.
- If the positive FDG-PET at follow-up is not confirmed as a new site of disease on CT, additional follow-up CT scans are needed to determine if progression is truly occurring at that site (if so, the date of PD will be the date of the initial abnormal FDG-PET scan).
- If the positive FDG-PET at follow-up corresponds to a pre-existing site of disease on CT that is not progressing on the basis of the anatomical images, this is not PD.

Limitations of anatomical response evaluation
- Changes in size may not reflect the activity of agents that are principally cytostatic.
- A dependence on a change in size as the principal measure limits the ability to precisely characterize response in tumours that do not change in size during therapy.
- Construction of continuous plots of fractional shrinkage or growth ('waterfall' plots) may provide a more accurate assessment of treatment effect across a study population.
- There is well-established interobserver variability in CT scan size measurements.
- The degree of response may be under- or over-estimated by CT imaging.

Table 5.3 Standardized response criteria. Descriptions are intended to provide an overview and do not contain all of the nuances of response assessment. Further detail is provided in the cited papers.

Cancer type	System	Year adopted	Response category			Other categories/ remarks	Reference
			CR	PR	PD	SD		
Solid tumours	RECIST	2009 (v 1.1)	Disappearance of target lesions, reduction in short axis of lymph nodes to <10mm	At least a 30% decrease in SLD of target lesions from baseline	At least a 20% increase in SLD of target lesions from smallest sum on study, where increase is at least 5 mm, or appearance of new lesions	Neither PR nor PD	Response confirmation required if response is study's primary endpoint	Eisenhauer et al. (2009) Eur J Cancer 45:228–247
Solid tumours	WHO	1981	Disappearance of all known disease	≥50% decrease in total tumour load (using SPD) with no new lesions and no progression of any existing lesion	≥25% increase in the size of one or more measurable lesions or appearance of new lesions	Neither PR nor PD	Separate criteria for non-measurable, bone lesions	Miller et al. (1981) Cancer 47:207–214
Immune-related response in solid tumours	irRC	2009	Disappearance of all known disease	≥50% decrease in tumour burden compared with baseline in two observations at least 4 weeks apart	At least a 25% increase in tumour burden compared with nadir at any time point in two consecutive observations at least 4 weeks apart	Neither PR nor PD	Index lesions at baseline include up to ten visceral and five cutaneous lesions At each follow-up, up to five new, measurable lesions are added in	Wolchok et al. (2009) Clin Cancer Res 15:7412–7420
Hepatocellular carcinoma	EASL	2001	Response: reduction in viable tumour volume estimated visually as extent of contrast uptake at arterial-phase CT or MRI				Modification of WHO criteria to include assessment of viable enhancing lesions	Bruix et al. (2001) J Hepatol 35:421–430
	mRECIST	2005	Disapearance of any intratumoural arterial enhancement in all target lesions	≥30% decrease in the sum of diameters of *viable* (enhancing) target lesions	At least 20% increase in the sum of diameters of *viable* (enhancing) target lesions	Neither PR nor PD	Modification of RECIST criteria to include assessment of viable enhancing lesions	Llovet et al. (2008) J Natl Cancer Inst 100:698–711
	RECICL	2010	100% tumournecrotizing effect or 100% tumour size reduction	Tumour necrotizing effect or tumour size reduction between 50% and 100%	Tumour growth >25% regardless of necrotizing effect, or emergence of new lesion	Neither PR nor PD	Used in combination with RECIST to evaluate tumour-necrotizing effect after locoregional therapies (presence of non-stained low-density area on dynamic CT)	Kudo et al. (2010) Hepatol Res 40:686–692

(continued)

Table 5.3 (Continued)

Cancer type	System	Year adopted	Response category – CR	Response category – PR	Response category – PD	Response category – SD	Other categories/remarks	Reference
Gastro-intestinal stromal tumour	Choi	2007	Disappearance of all lesions, no new lesions	≥10% decrease in size or ≥15% decrease in tumour density (HU) on CT	≥10% increase in size and does not meet PR criteria by tumour density, new lesions, or new/enlarged intratumoural nodule	Neither PR nor PD		Choi et al. (2007) J Clin Oncol 25:1753–1759
Renal cell carcinoma	MASS	2010	Favourable response: no new lesion and either (1) a decrease in tumour size of ≥20%, or (2) one or more predominantly solid enhancing lesions with marked decreased attenuation (≥40 HU)		Unfavourable response: increase in tumour size of ≥20% in the absence of marked central necrosis or marked decreased attenuation or new metastases, marked central fill-in, or new enhancement of a previously homogeneously hypoattenuating, non-enhancing mass	Neither a favourable nor an unfavourable response		Smith et al. (2010) AJR Am J Roentgenol 194:1470–1478
Prostate cancer PSA	PCWG2	2008	Report percentage change in PSA from baseline to 12 weeks and maximum decline in PSA		≥25% increase and an absolute increase of ≥2 ng/mL from nadir (if decrease observed) or from baseline after 12 weeks	Stable disease not categorized	Specific criteria depend on clinical trial endpoints	Scher et al. (2008) J Clin Oncol 26:1148–1159
Soft tissue			RECIST – record complete elimination of disease at any site separately	RECIST – record changes in nodal and visceral soft tissue sites separately. Only report changes in nodes ≥2 cm at baseline	RECIST – progression at first progression confirmed by a second scan ≥6 weeks later			
Bone			Report outcome of no new lesions		Two or more new lesions			
Glioma	RANO	2013	Disappearance of all enhancing and non-enhancing disease (sustained for ≥4 weeks), no new lesions, no corticosteroids, clinically stable or improved	≥50% decrease of all measurable enhancing lesions (sustained for ≥4 weeks), no progression of non-measurable disease, stable or improved non-enhancing lesions (T2/FLAIR), no new lesions, stable or reduced corticosteroid dose, clinically stable or improved	≥25% increase of enhancing lesions on stable or increasing doses of corticosteroids, significant increase in non-enhancing (T2/FLAIR) lesions, any new lesion	Does not qualify for CR, PR or PD, stable non-enhancing (T2/FLAIR) lesions, stable or reduced corticosteroid dose, clinically stable or improved	Adaptation of MacDonald criteria to incorporate T2-weighted or FLAIR imaging	Chinot et al. (2013) Curr Neurol Neurosci Rep 13:347–357

Cancer type	System	Year adopted	Response category			Other categories/remarks	Reference
			CR	PR	PD	SD		
Lymphoma	IWG/IHP	2007	Disappearance of all detectable clinical evidence of disease and disease-related symptoms. A residual mass that is PET-negative is permitted	>50% decrease in SPD of up to six of the largest dominant nodes or masses, no increase in size of other nodes, liver or spleen, no new sites, or meeting CR criteria but with bone marrow involvement	Appearance of any new lesion of >1.5 cm in any axis, or >50% increase from nadir in SPD of previously involved nodes, or 50% increase in longest diameter of any node	Neither CR, PR nor PD	See Cheson et al. (2007) for details about PET imaging	Cheson et al. (2007) J Clin Oncol 25:579–586
Myeloma	IMWG	2006 (enhanced 2008)	Negative immunofixation of serum and urine, disappearance of any soft tissue plasmacytomas, <5% plasma cells in bone marrow	Generally, ≥50% reduction of serum M protein or in the difference between involved and uninvolved free light chain (FLC) levels, or in bone marrow plasma cells, or in size of soft tissue plasmacytomas	Generally, increase of 25% from lowest response value in serum or urine M-component, FLC levels, bone marrow plasma cells or development of new lesions, or development of hypercalcaemia	Not meeting criteria for CR, VGPR, PR or PD	*Stringent CR*: CR, plus normal FLC ratio and absence of clonal cells in bone marrow. *VGPR*: serum and urine M-component detectable by immunofixation, but not on electropheresis or ≥90% reduction in serum M-component plus urine M-component <100 mg/24 hours	Kyle, Rajkumar (2009) Leukemia 23:3–9
Acute Myeloid Leukemia		2003	Complete Remission: Morphologic leukemia-free state (less than 5% blasts in aspirate, no Auer rods or EMD), platelets > 100 × 10⁹/L, and ANC > 1 × 10⁹/L. Subsets: cytogenetic CR, molecular CR	Partial Remission: Platelets and ANC as for CR, with either decrease in blasts of ≥50% to 5% to 25%, or decrease to <5% blasts with Auer rods present	Recurrence: Reappearance of leukemic blasts in peripheral blood or ≥5% blasts in bone marrow not attributable to other cause	Not defined	Early Treatment Assessment: may be used to guide future treatment. Treatment Failure: failure to achieve a CR on a phase III trial or less than PR on phase I or II trial	Cheson et al (2003) J Clin Oncol 21:4642–4649
Myelodysplastic syndrome		2006	*Bone marrow*: ≤5% myeloblasts with normal maturation of all cell lines. *Peripheral blood*: Hgb ≥11 g/dL, platelets ≥100 × 10⁹/L, neutrophils ≥1 × 10⁹/L, blasts 0%	All CR criteria if abnormal before treatment except bone marrow blasts decreased by ≥50% over pretreatment but still >5%	Increase in % blasts to ≥50% and any of: ≥50% decrement from maximum remission/response in granulocytes or platelets, reduction in Hgb by ≥2 g/dL, transfusion dependence	Neither PR nor PD	Other categories: Marrow CR; Failure; Relapse after CR or PR; Cytogenetic response; Categories for haematological improvement	Cheson et al. (2006) Blood 108:419–425

CR, complete response; PR, partial response; PD, progressive disease; VGPR, very good partial response; FLAIR, fluid-attenuated inversion recovery; PET, positron emission tomography; Hgb, haemoglobin; PSA, prostate-specific antigen; SPD, sum of the greatest perpendicular diameters; SLD, sum of the longest unidimensional diameters, EMD, extramedullary disease.

- With CT imaging there is limited ability to distinguish viable tumour from necrotic or fibrotic tissue.
- RR, TTP and PFS do not necessarily serve as accurate surrogates for overall survival.

Future directions for anatomical response evaluation include three-dimensional measurement of tumour volumes, but the machinery and expertise for this are not widely available and this measurement has yet to be incorporated into guidelines.

Disease-specific response criteria

Table 5.3 summarizes common systems for response evaluation in specific tumour types. While these are primarily anatomical systems, some of them incorporate biomarkers and metabolic systems, as discussed below.

Assessment of response using biochemical markers

Biochemical markers may be substances produced by cancer or other cells in response to cancer, or gene expression patterns in tumour tissue. Caution in interpretation and careful quality control are important in all stages of analysis:

- *Pre-analysis*:
  - Ensure that the correct test is ordered
  - Use the correct type of specimen
  - Assure specimen stability
  - Conduct test at the right point in time; use the right 'baseline'
  - Avoid improper specimen timing (e.g. collect prostate-specific antigen [PSA] before any clinical manipulation of the prostate)
  - Be aware of confounding clinical and lifestyle conditions to ensure proper interpretation.
- *Assay validation, internal quality control (IQC), proficiency testing (PT)*:
  - Use well-characterized methods
  - Assess reproducibility
  - Follow established objective criteria for assay acceptance
  - Include an appropriate number of IQC specimens, using material resembling patient sera, in concentrations appropriate to the clinical application
  - Assess concentrations over the working range for PT
  - Assess assay interferences
  - Evaluate interpretation as well as technical results.
- *Post-analysis*:
  - Obtain brief, relevant clinical information if interpretation is to be made by the lab
  - Provide appropriate reference intervals from a relevant healthy population
  - Document interpretation criteria
  - Define the percentage increase or decrease that constitutes a significant change
  - Ongoing audit of clinical utility of results
  - Document change in methods, implications for interpretation.

Source: http://www.aacc.org/members/nacb/LMPG/Online-Guide/PublishedGuidelines/tumor/Pages/default.aspx

As is true for the anatomical measurements described above, pretreatment assessments can be prognostic (used for staging). Changes from baseline are used to assess response. Table 5.4 shows a subset of markers considered useful for response assessment in particular. (Markers used exclusively for prognosis are not included.)

Assessment of response using methods for metabolic evaluation of tumours

Types of assessments

- *PET (molecular imaging)*:
  - Commonly used in lymphoma, non-small cell lung, breast and colorectal cancers
  - Uses a radiopharmaceutical tracer, commonly ^{18}F-FDG, which is differentially taken up by cancer cells that have abnormally accelerated rates of glycolysis in the presence of oxygen (Warburg effect)
  - Quantified using the maximum standardized uptake value (SUV_{max})
  - Can be used as a complement to CT scanning in the assessment of new lesions
  - FDG uptake period of 60 minutes is required prior to imaging.
- *Combination CT/PET*:
  - Fusion or co-registration of separate CT and PET images taken sequentially in the same scanning session
  - Provides precise localization of regions of interest (ROI) defined by PET imaging agent uptake
  - Variability in the performance of the CT component of the fusion study, including the absence of intravenously administered iodinated contrast material, means it cannot substitute for diagnostic quality CT imaging.

Metabolic imaging using PET with ^{18}F-FDG

In several diseases, PET utilizing ^{18}F-FDG as tracer may be able to identify volumetrically smaller tumours than can be detected by CT imaging. Additionally, in several diseases, a strong relationship between ^{18}F-FDG uptake and cancer cell number has been demonstrated, such that a decline in uptake may closely correlate with a reduction in viable tumour cells (and *vice versa*). This relationship has been demonstrated for oesophageal, lung, head and neck and breast cancer, and lymphoma.

Determination of response using metabolic imaging

Quantitative interpretation

The physical properties of the tracer and its detection allow for a quantitative evaluation of its uptake in tissues. The SUV is by

Table 5.4 Biomarkers of response

Disease	Marker	Remarks	Reference
Breast cancer (metastatic)	CA15-3 CA27.29 Carcinoembryonic antigen (CEA)	Not to be used alone; use only with imaging, history and physical exam Increasing levels may be used to indicate treatment failure Use caution to interpret rising levels during the first 4–6 weeks of treatment; spurious rises may occur	http://www.asco.org/guidelines/breasttm Copyright © 2007 ASCO
Colorectal cancer (metastatic)	CEA	Marker of choice for monitoring during systemic therapy Measure at start of treatment and every 1–3 months during active treatment Restage if levels persistently rise above baseline (rising levels suggest progressive disease even in the absence of corroborating radiographs) Use caution when interpreting a rising CEA level during the first 4–6 weeks of new therapy; spurious rises may occur, especially after oxaliplatin; see guidelines for list of exceptions	http://www.asco.org/guidelines/gitm Copyright © 2006 by ASCO
Pancreatic cancer	CA19-9	Not to be used alone or routinely for monitoring response to treatment Measure at start of treatment and every 1–3 months during active treatment (for locally-advanced metastatic disease) Elevation may be indicative of progressive disease; seek confirmation with other studies	http://www.asco.org/guidelines/gitm Copyright © 2006 by ASCO
Germ cell tumours	Alpha-fetoprotein (AFP) Human chorionic gonadotropin (hCG)	Used to monitor response to treatment and surveillance after treatment for all kinds of NSGCT and for patients with Stage II3c seminoma	http://www.asco.org/guidelines/germcelltm Copyright © 2010 by ASCO
Bladder cancer (superficial)	Nuclear matrix protein (NMP) 22	Two tests available, a qualitative point-of-care assay and a quantitative ELISA assay Approved by the FDA for the detection and monitoring of patients with known bladder cancer	Apolo et al. (2009) Future Oncol 5:977–992
	Bladder tumour antigen (BTA)	BTA-stat is a qualitative point-of-care assay BTA-TRAK is a quantitative ELISA assay Both are FDA approved for monitoring for recurrence	
	Urine cytology	Standard method for detecting tumour cells in urine	
	ImmunoCyt	Based on visualizing CEA and mucin Approved by FDA to aid in management of bladder cancer in conjunction with cytology and cystoscopy	
	UroVysion	Labelled DNA probes using FISH to look for alterations in chromosomes 3, 7, 19 and 9p21 Approved by FDA for use in conjunction with cystoscopy to monitor for recurrence	
Thyroid cancer	Thyroglobulin	Used routinely to monitor for recurrence	

NSGCT, non-seminomatous germ cell tumour; FISH, fluorescence *in situ* hybridization.

far the most commonly used metric for assessing tissue accumulation of tracer. To ensure reproducibility of SUVs, standardization of PET image acquisition is required: this is best achieved by performing scans on the same scanner with comparable doses of FDG and uptake times.

Critical issues that affect the general application of metabolic imaging for assessment of response are:

- Variability in selecting ROI for determination of SUV (i.e. total tumour volume versus maximally active region of tumour)
- Determining which method of SUV normalization to use
- Using standardized criteria for changes in SUV that correlate with response
- Degree of change in SUV may depend on tumour type.

Qualitative interpretation

A qualitative interpretation of metabolic imaging findings is limited to the visual assessment of the distribution and intensity of ^{18}F-FDG uptake by the tumour as compared to normal tissue, and areas of abnormal accumulation are identified. This approach is suboptimal as there are limited data on the reproducibility of qualitative interpretation of PET imaging.

Barriers to the use of metabolic imaging for tumour response assessment are:
- Limited integration and validation in clinical trials
- Variability in test performance
- Lack of uniformly accepted treatment response metrics
- Inability to detect minimal tumour burden versus no tumour burden.

PET may have a prognostic role; the time to normalization of PET may reflect the rate of cell kill and therefore predict likelihood of cure. However, the incorporation of metabolic evaluation of treatment response into the commonly used RECIST version 1.1 is limited due to several issues to be discussed below. Two sets of response criteria for metabolic assessment of tumour response have been developed: the EORTC and the PERCIST criteria (see Wahl et al. (2009) in the Recommended reading).

Assessment of response using patient-reported outcomes

A patient-reported outcome (PRO) is any report of the status of a patient's health condition that comes directly from the patient, without interpretation of the patient's response by a clinician or anyone else.
- Findings measured by a well-defined and reliable PRO instrument can be used to show improvement associated with treatment, if the instrument measures the concept that is improved.
- Typically include patient symptoms, signs or an aspect of functioning directly related to the disease status.
- If the goal of a clinical trial is to test a treatment for disease, PRO assessments are typically secondary.
- If the goal of a clinical trial is to test a treatment for symptoms, PRO assessments may be primary.
  Factors to consider in choosing an instrument are:
- Concepts being measured
- Number of items/response burden
- Context/conceptual framework/cultural suitability
- Medical condition and population for intended use
- Methods of administration, data collection
- Response options and recall period
- Scoring and weighting.

The instrument's development should be well documented and its properties well established:
- Published report of instrument validation
- Validated in population relevant for intended use:
  - Score reliability: extent to which instrument produces same score for same subject under same circumstances
  - Construct validity: extent to which instrument measures what it intends to measure
  - Ability to detect change: sensitivity to clinically meaningful differences over time.

Recommended reading

Altman DG, McShane LM, Sauerbrei W, Taube S (2012) Reporting recommendations for tumor marker prognostic studies (REMARK): explanation and elaboration. *BMC Med* 10:51.

Anderson KC, Kyle RA, Rajkumar SV, Stewart AK, Weber D, Richardson P (2008) Clinically relevant end points and new drug approvals for myeloma. *Leukemia* 22:231–239.

Concato J, Peduzzi P, Holfold TR et al. (1995) Importance of events per independent variable in proportional hazards analysis. I. Background, goals, and general strategy. *J Clin Epidemiol* 48:1495–501.

Dancey JE, Dodd LE, Ford R et al. (2009) Recommendations for the assessment of progression in randomised cancer treatment trials. *Eur J Cancer* 45:281–289.

Gichangi A, Vach W (2005) The analysis of competing risks data: a guided tour. *Stat Med* 132(4):1–41.

Lan KKG, DeMets DL (1983) Discrete sequential boundaries for clinical trials. *Biometrika* 70(3):659–663.

Newcombe RG (1998) Two-sided confidence intervals for the single proportion: comparison of seven methods. *Stat Med* 17(8):857–872.

Nishino M, Giobbie-Hurder A, Gargano M et al. (2013) Developing a common language for tumor response to immunotherapy: immune-related response criteria using unidimensional measurements. *Clin Cancer Res* 19(14):3936–3943.

Sargent DJ, Rubinstein L, Schwartz L et al. (2009) Validation of novel imaging methodologies for use as cancer clinical trial end-points. *Eur J Cancer* 45:290–299.

U.S. Department of Health and Human Services, Food and Drug Administration (2009) *Guidance for Industry: Patient-Reported Outcome Measures: Use in Medical Product Development to Support Labeling Claims.* Available at www.fda.gov/RegulatoryInformation/Guidances/ucm122046.htm

Wahl RL, Jacene H, Kasamon Y, Lodge MA (2009) From RECIST to PERCIST: Evolving considerations for PET response criteria in solid tumors. *J Nucl Med* 50 (Suppl 1):122S–150S.

6 Cancer informatics

David A. Jaffray[1,2], Andrew Hope[1,2], Prateek Dwivedi[1,3], Terry Michaelson[1,3], and Andre Dekker[4]

[1]Techna Institute/The Princess Margaret Cancer Centre, Toronto, ON, Canada
[2]Department of Radiation Oncology, University of Toronto, Toronto, ON, Canada
[3]University Health Network, University of Toronto, Toronto, ON, Canada
[4]Department of Radiation Oncology (MAASTRO), GROW School for Oncology and Developmental Biology, University of Maastricht, Maastricht, The Netherlands

Introduction

While the term 'informatics' was first coined in 1966 by Mikhailov, the science of information is age-old. The academic field of informatics involves the practice of information processing and the engineering of information systems, including studies of the structure, algorithms, behaviour, and interactions of natural and artificial systems which store, process, access, and communicate information. The field of informatics is very broad, considering the interaction between humans and information systems, the construction of computer interfaces, and the development of conceptual and theoretical foundations for describing information. According to Greenes *et al.*, the term medical informatics includes "the cognitive, information processing, and communication tasks of medical practice, education, and research, including information science and the technology to support these tasks".

Arguably, cancer care is one of the most complex processes in medicine, with remarkable levels of intricacy in the underlying biology of the disease (site, morphology, histology, genomics, microenvironment), the disposition of the patient (genetics, co-morbidities, psychosocial and economic factors), and the interaction with the process of cancer care (clinicians, interventions, outcomes, support). While modern science is rapidly revealing the true complexity of cancer, this complexity is further escalated in the clinical context by the interplay between the disease, the patient, and the interventions we currently deliver. Patients with the same general type of cancer and a similar genetic profile exhibit a wide variation in the speed and extent of disease pathogenesis, degree of malignancy, and response to treatment both with respect to control and toxicity. Within a given tumour, there are differences in somatic mutations, gene expression, and microenvironmental factors (e.g. hypoxia).

The term 'panomics' is used by the American Society of Clinical Oncology (ASCO) as an umbrella term for molecular level signatures, such as genomics, proteomics, metabolomics and transcriptomics, which combine with factors in the tumour's environment to drive tumour development and behaviour. Understanding cancer and advancing more personalized cancer treatment regimens requires access to the full spectrum of bio-clinical data for the individual and for large cohorts. Regardless of whether these data are being used in mechanistic research or in the pursuit of biomarker-based clinical decision strategies, we need to integrate diverse, multimodal information (clinical-, imaging-, treatment-, tissue-derived data) in a quantitative manner to generate biological insight and provide specific clinical predictions and decision support that has clinical relevance.

The adoption of informatics methods and frameworks to document the state of the host and his/her disease, understand the underlying nature and guide the application and development of novel interventions is the field of 'cancer informatics'. While the concepts motivating the definition and development of the field of cancer informatics are not novel, the recent and rapid development of new methods of characterizing the patient and his/her disease requires oncology to embrace the field of cancer informatics if this new information is to be used to its fullest extent to *guide decisions for the individual patient* and to advance our *understanding of the disease.*

The linkage between high-quality clinical care and the development of important insights that drive cancer research is becoming ever more evident. This perspective dissolves the traditional boundaries between 'clinical' and 'research' informatics activities and is pushing academic cancer centres to adopt a more integrative approach to their informatics strategy (Fig. 6.1). This holistic approach sees the clinical and research records as part of a continuum, with appropriate mechanisms

---

UICC Manual of Clinical Oncology, Ninth Edition. Edited by Brian O'Sullivan, James D. Brierley, Anil K. D'Cruz, Martin F. Fey, Raphael Pollock, Jan B. Vermorken and Shao Hui Huang. © 2015 UICC. Published 2015 by John Wiley & Sons, Ltd.

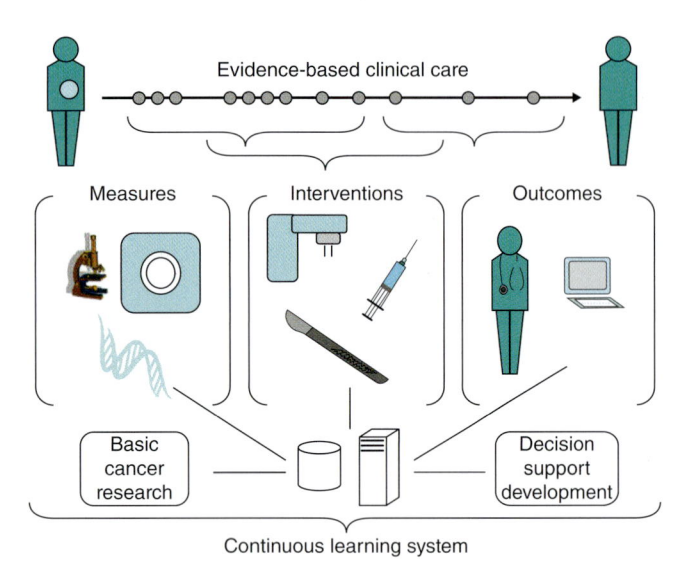

Figure 6.1 Delivery of patient-centred cancer care is one of the most intense, extended interactions a person has with the healthcare system. The quantity and variety of data, criticality of decision-making and extended time course from diagnosis through treatment and on to follow-up define one of the most complex informatics problems in health care. Progressive cancer care organizations are positioning informatics to enable the data associated with the delivery of evidence-based clinical care to drive the basic cancer research agenda, as well as create decision-support systems that fully enable personalized cancer care.

in place to assure data security, patient consent, and data governance. This concept is highlighted by the gradual emergence of clinically viable decision-support systems (e.g. IBM Watson) that facilitate interpretation of new data sources (e.g. genomics data) which lie in the hinterland between routine clinical practice and research. The electronic medical record and wealth of data sources distributed in the various health information subsystems of a modern cancer centre (e.g. radiology, pathology, anaesthesia, radiation and medical oncology) become important components of the cancer informatics system that, when brought together, offer the potential both to improve the quality of care and to advance our understanding of cancer.

In this chapter, the various informatics elements and processes associated with a cancer care and research facility of the future are described as a primer. The depth of presentation should provide the reader with a foundation that motivates the need for an informatics strategy in cancer care and research, describes the structural and technical elements of an informatics architecture, highlights some of the important operational components, and stimulates further reading on this critical part of a comprehensive cancer programme.

Infrastructure and elements

Electronic medical record

The technology of a modern electronic medical record (EMR) includes many components, starting with an underlying secure physical network, an operations architecture for enabling secure access control, defined policies and procedures for information system use, large-scale storage subsystems (including redundancy, back-up and archival, local or cloud), numerous vendor-provided data generation and processing systems (computed tomography [CT] scanners, Picture Archival and Communication System (PACS), digital pathology), desktop functionality (administrative, email), all in addition to several 'central' medical record systems. These central systems are used for all patients, regardless of their specific interaction within the hospital and include patient registration, primary medical record keeping, dictation, scheduling and billing systems. These systems have become critical to clinical operations and require uptime performance in excess of 99.9%. The elimination of the traditional 'paper chart' largely prevents clinical operations from continuing when the EMR is inaccessible. This is particularly the case in cancer care, wherein the patient's diagnosis and treatment history is integral to assessment and decision-making. In addition to the internal systems, there is also a highly regulated interface (e.g. firewall) between the EMR systems and the Internet. This interface is selectively bidirectional to facilitate staff and system access to external sources (e.g. PubMed, www), while simultaneously restricting access by external entities to specific systems or applications (e.g. remote servicing of technologies). An example that is particularly relevant in cancer care is the development of a 'patient portal' to allow patients to gain secure access to their test results, schedule appointments and/or participate in self-reporting of outcomes or levels of distress. In general, hospital EMR systems do not provide comprehensive oncology solutions. This reflects the fact that cancer care has evolved into a highly specialized practice within modern medicine that does not readily fit within the functionality of the hospital's EMR: as a result, dedicated EMRs for the needs of oncology have also been developed. While the EMR provides a partial health record and is typically associated with a specific healthcare provider, the electronic health record (EHR) refers to a complete health record under the custodianship of a healthcare provider(s). This record holds all relevant health information about a person over their lifetime and is often described as a person-centric record, which can be used by many approved healthcare providers or healthcare organizations. In the context of cancer, the EHR opens the opportunity for rapid referral, coordinated care and patient follow-up. The distribution of patient care into the community offers significant quality and economic benefits for both effective palliation as well as survivorship.

Dedicated computer-assisted intervention and information technology for cancer care

Cancer interventions are complex procedures that are derived from immediate, patient-specific information, including specialized histological assays, detailed medical imaging studies (magnetic resonance imaging [MRI], fluorodeoxyglucose [FDG]-positron emission tomography [PET]), as well as genetic sequencing results, all integrated to determine the appropriate therapy. As a result, dedicated oncology information systems that are distinct from the hospital's EMR have been developed. These comprehensive systems support the prescription of complex drug and radiation treatment schedules. In the context of medical oncology, these systems provide internal safety systems for selection of preapproved drug protocols, as well as robotic dispensation of drugs. In radiation treatments, these same systems are used to control the actions of the radiation treatment units and assure the prescribed radiation dose is accurately delivered by the treatment machine. These systems have also been extended to manage more complex treatments using image guidance to target the tumour and intensity modulation of the radiation beams to sculpt the radiation dose and avoid normal tissues. It can be expected that the development of image-guided, robotic surgery will also drive the development of dedicated oncology informatics tools into surgery, thereby providing the potential for coordination across the continuum of cancer interventions. While these systems allow controlled, protocol-defined delivery of care, they also provide detailed records of the treatment for each patient and have significant value for retrospective analyses. The quantity of data collected in the oncology EMR is staggering and continues to expand with the adoption of daily imaging during radiation delivery, the development of image-based assessments of response to therapy (e.g. RECIST) and the continued growth in panomics (e.g. genetics, radiomics, immunohistochemical scores). Of course, these oncology-specific systems are connected to the central EMR to assure exchange of scheduling, billing, current status of cancer therapy and other safety-related information (e.g. known allergies). In addition to keeping the details of the cancer treatment record, these oncology EMRs are also serving as repositories of outcomes collection. This combination is very powerful as it can provide the clinician with an accurate patient-specific context during patient interaction and in-clinic outcomes collection.

Point-of-care technology

Collecting cancer outcomes, adverse events and level of patient distress is considered best practice for delivering high-quality cancer care and a means to increase expertise development in the clinical staff. There is more and more evidence that outcomes, including outcomes related to quality of life, should not only be reported by the physician but also by the patient. While clearly a long-standing tradition in world-leading cancer centres, the value of outcomes collection as a means for system level learning, facilitating basic research and supporting expertise development by the clinician is becoming more widely recognized. This recognition is putting greater emphasis on the need for effective data collection at the 'point of care'. Point-of-care interactions are complex and the methods of collection need to be tuned to the specific task if they are to be successful in terms of (1) enabling high-quality data collection (e.g. patient understanding the query), (2) assuring a context for the data that are being collected (e.g. query appropriate for patient) and (3) respecting the time and effort constraints of the participants (e.g. time spent by both clinician and patient). Since conventional EMR systems are designed for interactions during treatment delivery, they are rarely designed to support the workflow and needs of the clinician or patient to facilitate reporting or outcomes collection. As a result, dedicated software (or paper-based) tools (e.g. Cancer Care Ontario and the Princess Margaret's Formatted Anthology Synoptic Tick [FAST] Sheet) are often used as an extension to conventional EMR systems. These systems range from dedicated 'apps' through to the use of survey-type technologies to determine outcomes or assess patient distress (e.g. Cancer Care Ontario's DART initiative). Well-engineered implementations leverage other data sources in the EMR to make these tools more effective, including the provision of key information for the clinician to utilize in the clinical interaction, or the routing of patient-reported distress symptoms (e.g. DART) to the appropriate clinical support team. The emergence of point-of-care technologies highlights the tight interplay between effective informatics strategies and clinic operations – a concept that cannot be over emphasized. Current thinking supports an integrated approach wherein the value of high-quality outcomes collection is worth significant organizational, cultural and financial investment.

Cancer research data infrastructure

Cancer care and research requires integration of diverse, multimodal information (clinical-, imaging-, treatment-, tissue-derived data, outcomes). From an informatics perspective the challenges are that this information has very different scales (from the genome to society), very different dimensions (from a full DNA sequence and multiple time-point 3D image sets to age and marital status), and comes from different sources (biobanks, electronic hospital records, PACS, pathology slides, socioeconomic databases). The integration into well-curated and linked datastores, so that cancer research can take the required holistic approach, is an active area of research, sometimes called 'clinical research informatics' or 'translational bioinformatics'. Two main approaches can be taken to build these clinical research databases: *centralized* and *federated*. In the *centralized* approach, there exist one or more central databases where investigators can store and access the information. This access is usually limited to investigators during the course of the study. As a rule, cancer information is rarely completely contained in a single *centralized* system. As described above, oncology practice requires both hospital-level and oncology-level systems to co-exist. The addition of research databases and point-of-care data collection systems requires cancer informatics systems to function through *federation* with the use of 'global identifiers' to enable records to be linked and associated with a specific patient.

This concept is being extended to reach beyond the clinical setting. Upon publication of study results, more and more scientific journals, especially in the cancer biology domain, are requesting or requiring research data to be shared in the form of supplementary material or in publicly accessible archives, both to demonstrate scientific integrity of the published results as well as to enable reuse of the data for other research questions. Examples of widely used data stores are The Cancer Imaging Archive (TCIA; http://cancerimagingarchive.net/), which allows researchers to share de-identified image collections for open science, the Gene Expression Omnibus for gene expression data and Cancer Data (https://www.cancerdata.org/) for clinical cancer data. The integration of these rather monolithic archives was the admirable founding principle of the cancer Biomedical Informatics Grid (caBIG), although it proved to be too ambitious. Examples with similar aims albeit on a smaller scale and more community driven include the Dutch Translational Research IT project (TraIT; http://www.ctmm-trait.nl/) and the USA National Cancer Informatics Program (http://cbiit.nci.nih.gov/ncip).

While attractive, these centralized approaches suffer from the requirement that the information is disclosed by the institute where it was captured. This can be problematic from a practical point of view (the volume of data may be too large to share and it takes a lot of time to curate the data for others to reuse) and has ethical/privacy concerns (see below). Also, the data shared through these libraries or through publications are often limited because much of the health information collected in everyday patient care is not necessarily available for research. This has led to a *federated data sharing* approach where either the data remain permanently inside the hospital with the analysis of data done locally, or metadata are made available in public catalogues but the underlying data only disclosed to specific users asking a specific research question. Examples of the federated approach are the EU Biobanking and Biomolecular Resources Research Infrastructure (BBMRI; http://bbmri.eu/), which maintains a European-wide catalogue of biobanks, and BioMedBridges (http://www.biomedbridges.eu/), which aims to provide informatics tools to link research databases. The promise of these approaches and the need for large data pools has stimulated the development of global initiatives to facilitate sharing of genomic and clinical data. The Global Alliance for Genomics and Health (Global Alliance) was launched in 2014 to create a broad community as represented by over 200 entities that work together to create interoperable approaches to enable the sharing of genomic and clinical data. The development of these 'open science' models that link academics, providers, industry, technology and patient organizations is a trend that is likely to continue.

Multi-institutional data sharing is not a new concept. The earliest form of large-scale, multi-institutional cancer research databases is the *cancer registry*. Cancer registries are the most widespread cancer informatics activity in the world. They are fundamental building blocks for the establishment of cancer control programmes and illustrate the benefit of investing in cancer informatics at the most basic level. These systems are now being linked to socioeconomic and geospatial data sources to better understand the causes, progression, required services and survival at a comprehensive health systems scale.

Data models and interoperability

Data collection protocols

Data modelling starts with a definition of the data elements that need to be collected. This often takes the form of a data dictionary document that describes terms, formats, etc. of the data to be collected. The step beyond the data dictionary is the process and protocol for data collection that describes not only which data elements to collect, but also how they should be collected, and can include standard operating procedures (e.g. for tissue collection). For technology-based data collection such as radiology or radiotherapy, these would typically also include quality assurance guidelines and standardized image acquisition and/or calculation parameters. The development of a standardized set of data to be collected for cancer care and research is not a trivial task. There are nominally 15 major categories of cancer (e.g. head and neck, lung, genitourinary) and each of these can have dramatically different sets of information that are believed to be relevant for care and for subsequent research. For example, the importance of a patient's smoking history is clearly relevant in lung and head and neck cancer; however, one would not expect marital status to be a prognostic factor, yet there is emerging data that demonstrates its role in predicting survival. A few organizations, e.g. the Moffitt Cancer Center's Total Cancer Care Protocol, have been quite successful in building standardized data collection protocols for cancer with 100–200 'standardized elements'; however, extending this protocol to operate across multiple institutions is complicated by the local variations in research ethics approval for the consenting and data collection process. A framework to accomplish this begins by defining a common set of data for all cancer patients, recognizing the differences for each disease site and cohorts within each disease site. To be successful in this endeavour, a flexible data model is imperative as the 'standardized elements' emerge and the protocols change. The definition of a data model and the data collection protocol are key starting points in the establishment of an effective cancer informatics system.

Databases, data warehouses and beyond

The most common architecture to organize and store structured data is the relational database, sometimes referred to as an SQL database (SQL refers to 'structured query language', which is a common interface to such databases). A relational database is a collection of tables with relationships defined between the columns of the tables. Typically, a database diagram is available that shows all tables and their relations. Non-relational databases (NoSQLs) are also often used in cancer research to support simple data elements (e.g. spreadsheets, text files and collection of documents on a file system), as well as more comprehensive 'Big Data' type stores. Although a full discussion of the pros and cons are beyond the scope here, SQL databases are in general more structured and can handle more complex queries easier, but are less flexible than NoSQL databases. This flexibility is an important distinction in cancer informatics because of the changes in care and data collection protocols driven by advancement in research and the speed of these innovations reaching the bedside. As a result, the supporting data models continue to evolve and change, thereby continuing to emphasize the need for the flexibility of NoSQL databases. Due to the nature of technology deployment, cancer centres have a collection of relational and non-relational databases associated with a variety of vendors and products. A major issue with these distributed databases is that their data model is defined locally, inside the application, such that the query language is not well-standardized across vendors and such that the technical application interfaces to the databases also vary between vendors. To address this, it is very common to establish a 'data warehouse' that copies and combines these multiple data sources into a central data repository and relies on the global identifier concept. This allows the organization to define one entry point for clinical, managerial, financial and research data. Maintaining these links is not straightforward due to the ongoing upgrades and enhancements of the individual products, and these warehouses can easily become out of date if the links are not maintained and new data are stored in adjacent systems. In general, there is no simple solution to this problem and, as a result, cancer centres require a level of dedicated information technology expertise to maintain operability. There are efforts underway to allow systems to automatically create associations between data and what they mean. The concept of a 'semantic' web has been proposed and is being advanced by a World Wide Web consortium (W3C) effort to standardize and promote common data formats using 'machine readable' extensions to the principle of the World Wide Web. There is evidence that a semantic architecture for clinical research environments is starting to emerge, but more work will be needed to ensure that there is scalability in the architecture as complexity of the data and volume of records increases.

Pursuing data interoperability

Closely linked to the data model is the ability of data to be shared with others, such as between vendors' products inside the hospital, or between different hospitals' EMR systems, or between hospitals and outside systems such as registries, clinical trial systems, etc. Interoperability can be defined at multiple levels (Table 6.1). Technical and syntactic interopability is the minimal requirement for any data sharing, which means it has to be agreed which (technical) protocol is used to transfer data; implying that data representation should be equal among participating sites. Emerging standards such as HL7 FHIR (Fast Healthcare Interoperability Resource) not only simplify technical interoperability, but also allow for more flexible workflows,

Table 6.1 Levels of system interoperability

Level 0	No interoperability at all
Level 1	Technical and syntactical interoperability (no semantic interoperability)
Level 2	Two orthogonal levels of partial semantic interoperability *Level 2a*: Unidirectional semantic interoperability *Level 2b*: Bidirectional semantic interoperability
Level 3	Full semantic interoperability, sharable context, seamless cooperability

Source: Stroetman 2009. Reproduced with permission of European Union.

medical device integration and support for mobile and cloud deployments. Semantic interoperability goes further. It is defined as: "The ability of any communicating entity (not only computers) to share unambiguous meaning. For computers, this is the ability to exchange information and have that information properly interpreted by the receiving system in the same sense as intended by the transmitting system". For semantic interoperability, one needs to use terminological systems (which are here loosely defined as a thesaurus, classification, vocabulary, nomenclature or coding system) which are known by both sender and receiver, e.g. SNOMED-CT, ICD-10, CTCAE and the NCI Thesaurus. An ontology is one or a combination of terminology systems specific to a certain domain: it provides the consensus on the meaning of concepts and the relations between the concepts. The US National Center for Biomedical Ontology hosts the broadest collection of ontologies via the Bioportal (http://bioportal.bioontology.org/). Ontologies represent an important investment that needs to be made to enable sharing of data without the loss of meaning of those data. Such investments are long term and require forethought. Unfortunately, it has taken a long time to convince people that such approaches are the only way that we can learn from the masses of clinical and research data that are constantly being generated across the clinical and research enterprises of cancer centres.

Informatics: From data to knowledge

Informatics for medical and scientific objectives

In terms of research, there are many topics at the crossroads of informatics and medicine, but *clinical informatics* and *bioinformatics* are often seen as the two major disciplines. Clinical (also referred to as medical) informatics is focused on using informatics approaches to deliver patient care. Some examples of research in this field include data sharing/standards between hospitals; electronic hospital record development; clinical decision-support systems; informatics-supported evidence-based medicine; and computer-aided diagnoses. In contrast, bioinformatics is focused on panomics data. The volume and complexity of these data have made bioinformatics a separate scientific discipline with topics such as ontologies, machine learning, data mining and high-performance computing. Perhaps the main distinction from a research perspective is that in *bioinformatics* one often deals with an extremely high volume of relatively homogeneous (in terms of syntax and semantics) data on a limited set of patients or animals. In *clinical informatics*, a smaller volume of very heterogeneous data on a high number of patients needs to be analysed. With the entry of biological analysis into the clinical domain and the predictive and prognostic ability of panomic data sources, the domains of bioinformatics and clinical informatics are starting to merge, hence the now commonly-used term *translational bioinformatics*.

Informatics for operational issues

Cancer care is highly multidisciplinary and requires continuous coordination between caregivers often from disparate departments and institutions. Ensuring a smooth patient flow, i.e. that the care path of each cancer patient leads to a correct and timely cancer diagnosis and treatment, is a constant worry for cancer centres and health systems. This is especially the case in specific cancers, such as head and neck and lung cancer, which are known to have a tumour doubling time in the order of weeks, which means waiting causes a noticeable growth in the tumour and subsequent lower chance of achieving control. Such worries have led to waiting time norms being formulated by governments, care payers and/or professional bodies. The evaluation of cancer patient flow and throughput and analysing decisions to optimize these is part of a field called *operations research*. This informatics-heavy discipline not only needs the aforementioned clinical databases to group patients in relevant care paths, but also needs information on available financial and human resources, medical equipment utilization, as well as detailed timing information on the care path (e.g. dates of diagnosis, multidisciplinary team meeting, surgery, first fraction of radiotherapy). Operations researchers can then analyse where bottlenecks occur and simulate whether resource or process changes affect the waiting times in a positive manner. It is expected that such a data-driven operations research approach becomes an increasing part of cancer informatics as limits on healthcare resources, more personalized approaches and higher demands on patient throughput require well-informed and thoughtful management decisions in cancer programmes.

Accessing health information

Privacy and disclosures

There is worldwide consensus that health information is very personal and needs to be protected from disclosure. Although regulatory frameworks vary widely between countries and even between institutions, there is generally a distinction between the following disclosures:
1 *Disclosures between healthcare professionals in individual health care*. An example is the exchange of patient information between a general practitioner and a hospital. The regulatory framework for such disclosures is often based on an 'opt-out' mechanism, meaning the professionals can assume they have the patient's permission to exchange all health information they think the other healthcare professional needs to care for that individual patient. In an 'opt-out' system, the patient needs to actively object to some or all of his/her health information being exchanged, a request that generally has to be adhered to.
2 *Disclosure in the process of conducting a clinical trial*. An example is the entry of information in a trial database hosted by the pharmaceutical company that sponsors the trial. The regulatory framework for clinical trials is almost invariably based on the Declaration of Helsinki principle of informed consent, meaning the trial subject has specifically given permission to disclose his/her health information within the context of the clinical trial. Such consent can be withdrawn at any time before, during or after the clinical trial, with a subsequent mandatory purging of the information from the trial database.
3 *Disclosure by reusing existing information from individual healthcare or clinical trials*. An example is storing health information in a national cancer registry. The reuse of information is where regulatory approaches differ considerably. Some require informed consent similar to that for clinical trials, but most regulatory frameworks have an opt-out–based exemption that allows the reuse of health information for public health and/or research purposes unless patients specifically object to such a disclosure. Often such an exemption is coupled to the obligation to remove identifying information as much as possible before disclosing information (see Data anonymization below).

The above categorization is quite broad and it should be noted that many exceptions exist. Examples are the disclosure of health information to employers and insurance companies or from people who are not (legally) able to consent, and of health information that may be of direct benefit to those other than the individual patient (e.g. knowledge of a genetic disposition may be beneficial to family members). As regulations vary and are dependent on the type of disclosure, it is strongly recommended to seek legal advice on all matters of health information disclosures and/or to appoint a health information privacy officer who specializes in the field. Informatics developments to support legal frameworks focus on using newer technologies to engage patients in the disclosure process, e.g. by making informed consent open, more dynamic, portable and under the control of patients themselves. This would enable disclosures of health information to be made on the basis of consent rather than having to revert to the less ideal opt-out solutions.

Data anonymization

A topic related to privacy of personal health information is the definition of 'personal' and the ways to make health information no longer relatable to a person, i.e. the creation of anonymized data. Generally speaking, anonymized data are no longer considered to be personal health information and can thus be disclosed. Data are anonymized if "all identifying elements have been eliminated from a set of personal data. No element may be left in the information which could, by exercising reasonable effort, serve to re-identify the person(s) concerned". Note that pseudonymized data (where identifiers are replaced with pseudonyms which are reversible) might still be defined as personal health information, such as in the European Union. Some countries have defined in some detail what are considered to be identifying elements, e.g. the US Health Insurance Portability and Accountability Act (HIPAA) has defined a list of elements considered to be identifying. Other guidance is being offered by standard bodies such as the National Electrical Manufacturers Association (NEMA) that has defined confidentiality profiles for medical images in Annex E of Part 15 of the Digital Imaging and Communications in Medicine (DICOM) standard. DICOM de-identification tools such as the Clinical Trial Processor have implemented these parts of the standards. Guidance on standardized methods for anonymization of genomic data has yet to emerge, as the very nature of the data is identifying. Various encryption schemes or limiting the amount of genomic data that are available are helpful, but the limits of anonymization should be addressed during the consent process.

After identifying and removing or replacing these obvious identifiers, a risk analysis is often undertaken by healthcare organizations to estimate if indeed re-identification takes more than a 'reasonable effort'. Typically such a risk analysis would involve three questions:
- Is it possible to isolate some or all records which identify an individual in the dataset? (e.g. are there possible identifiers left, such as very rare diseases, extreme body height or weight, sparsely populated regions, possible face reconstruction from images?)
- Is it possible to link two or more records concerning the same individual across two or multiple databases? (e.g. if information on the patient has been shared before in another project, can these be linked and does this link provide a risk?)
- Is it possible to infer identifiable elements from a combination of non-identifiable elements? (e.g. from multiple statements of age at specific dates, the exact birth date may be derived)

Governance of access to patient data

Large databases are essential for cancer informatics research and efforts should be taken to implement data governance and maximize appropriate access. Most critically, all data, especially clinical data, require context. Clinical data (especially outcomes or toxicity) are always interpreted through the lens of the observer and often require consideration of the clinical state of a patient. Even patient-reported outcomes can be misinterpreted if the status of treatment, disease progression or other co-morbid conditions are not considered. As such, the ultimate interpretation of research results should involve the individuals collecting the data as well as clinical experts functioning as part of the research team. Similarly, applications to access informatics data should be reviewed by a team including clinical experts to ensure that the data being accessed will address the research question. However, clinical data and the resulting databases are (in most jurisdictions) 'owned' by the institution rather than by individual clinicians or researchers. As such, institutions should take care to ensure that collaborative informatics data can be appropriately accessed by interested researchers and clinicians.

The establishment of a Data Governance Committee to broker and monitor appropriate access to patient-related data is recommended. This committee should ideally include representation from all contributing sources, including oncology specialties (radiation, medical and surgical), radiology, pathology and ancillary services (nursing, speech language pathology, nutrition, etc.). This committee ensures that the people making the decision regarding access are not conflicted in their decision. It also ensures that researchers are paired with clinical counterparts to ensure proper understanding of the data. In cancer, this committee considers both access to data and access to banked tissue, and should ensure tumour site experts are appropriately involved. In some environments, the committee can also maintain the link between the clinical identifiers and the research identifiers, so that updates to the anonymized dataset can be provided. To be clear, the Data Governance Committee does not take the place of the ethics board, but is a critical addition to ensure that privacy policies are being met and that data are being appropriately accessed and interpreted.

Future horizons

Patient- and caregiver-managed medical data

The development of advanced EMR capabilities, the liberation of data sharing through the Internet and the release of low-cost, patient-supported health measurement tools (e.g. blood glucose monitors) is precipitating greater awareness by individuals of their medical data and their capacity to collect and manage these data. As a result, the separation between 'institutional' medical and 'personal' health records is becoming blurred. This transition allows the development of 'learning systems' that are not part of the medical establishment at all, but rather systems that provide individuals with assistance in managing their own cancer care decisions, as well as being able to broker datasets to organizations that need specific questions answered. CancerCommons, Sage Bionetworks' BRIDGE project and the Patient-Centered Outcomes Research network are examples of patient-driven data sharing and research entities. The role of these systems and their interface with conventional clinical care are evolving and this evolution is likely to accelerate as relevant health-related measurements ranging from gene sequencing through to lifestyle monitoring technologies become less and less expensive.

Decision support and learning engines

A potential benefit of investing in cancer informatics is to deliver clinical decision support systems (CDSs) for cancer treatment. The Healthcare Information and Management Systems Society (HIMSS) defines these as systems that "enhance health-related decisions and actions with pertinent, organized clinical knowledge and patient information to improve health and healthcare delivery. Information recipients can include patients, clinicians and others involved in patient care delivery; information delivered can include general clinical knowledge and guidance, intelligently processed patient data, or a mixture of both; and information delivery formats can be drawn from a rich palette of options that includes data and order entry facilitators, filtered data displays, reference information, alerts, and others". Two main categories of CDS are identified by Gartner, Inc.: those with and those without a knowledge base. A CDS with a knowledge base relies on a 'database' of knowledge to which the patient's data are matched to provide a suggested best decision. The knowledge base can consist of guidelines and data-based prediction models such as nomograms and/or mathematical models. The development of such systems requires structured data and a clearly defined methodological process (Fig. 6.2). In contrast, a CDS without a knowledge base analyses historical clinical data and tries to find patterns of interest that might support a decision for a new patient. The latter approach reuses historical data for decision support, has been named 'rapid learning' and is being pursued in the form of systems such ASCO's CancerLinq and IBM's Watson health initiative.

Real world learning versus randomized clinical trials

The development of comprehensive, integrated electronic medical records that focus on outcomes has always held the promise of increasing the performance of the healthcare system through both the delivery of care to the individual patient, as well as the capacity to learn from a broad cohort of patients as they interact with the healthcare system. This concept is highlighted in the Institute of Medicine's Characteristics of a Learning Health Care System (Table 6.2) This approach requires multiple components to be present, including the integration of science and informatics, establishment of patient–clinician partnerships, incentives and a culture of learning. This is consistent with McDonald's 1997 review 'Barriers to electronic medical record systems', in which he argues that the technical issues are not the issue, rather two "grand challenges" need to be solved: "the efficient capture of physician gathered information, and the identification of a minimum but affordable set of variables needed to assess quality and outcomes of care".

An interesting example of this development comes from the Intermountain Health Care Corporation's Latter-Day Saints (LDS) Hospital. This organization has been the leader in the development of EMRs for more than 25 years and is also leading the development of real world learning (RWL) approaches. Intermountain has recently partnered with Deloitte to create PopulationMiner to

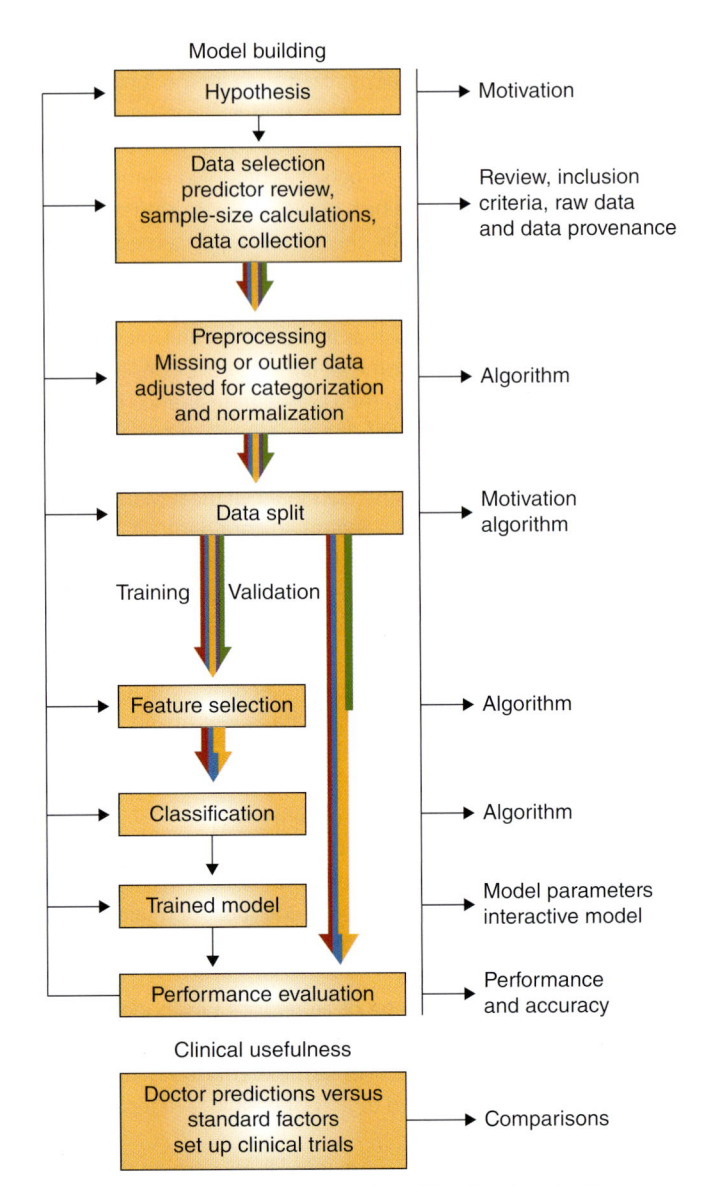

Figure 6.2 Model development and machine learning pipeline employed in cancer informatics research.
Source: Lambin P, van Stiphout RG, Starmans MH, et al: Predicting outcomes in radiation oncology-multifactorial decision support systems. *Nat Rev Clin Oncol* 10:27-40, 2013. Reproduced with permission of Nature Publishing Group.

provide insights from millions of patients, allowing rapid hypothesis generation and validation across a range of traditionally isolated business functions, including drug development, drug safety, pharmacoepidemiology, and health economics and outcomes research. The potential for highly integrated, reduced bias data collection to contribute to building robust evidence-based medicine cannot be ignored. A future in which randomized controlled trials (RCTs) and real-world approaches are applied in a coordinated approach to assure RCT outcomes are realized in the non-trial clinical setting and cancer care is advanced in a rapid and robust fashion. Not only are these approaches potentially powerful, but they may also be cost-effective. Walters et al. in 2014 demonstrated that retrospective analyses of outcomes in

Table 6.2 Characteristics of a learning healthcare system. These must all be present for a system to function as an effective learning system. It is clear that the technological issues are not the greatest challenge

Science and informatics	*Real-time access to knowledge*: A learning healthcare system continuously and reliably captures, curates and delivers the best available evidence to guide, support, tailor and improve clinical decision-making and care safety and quality
	Digital capture of the care experience: A learning healthcare system captures the care experience on digital platforms for real-time generation and application of knowledge for care improvement
Patient–clinician partnership	*Engaged, empowered patients*: A learning healthcare system is anchored in patient needs and perspectives, and promotes the inclusion of patients, families and other caregivers as vital members of the continuously learing care team
Incentives	*Incentives aligned for value*: In a learning healthcare system, incentives are actively aligned to encourage continuous improvement, identify and reduce waste, and reward high-value care
	Full transparency: A learning healthcare system systematically monitors the safety, quality, processes, prices, costs and outcomes of care, and makes information available for care improvement, informed choices and decision-making by clinicians, patients and their families
Culture	*Leadership-instilled culture of learning*: A learning healthcare system is stewarded by leadership committed to a culture of teamwork, collaboration and adaptability in support of continuous learning as a core aim
	Supportive system competencies: In a learning healthcare system, complex care operations and processes are constantly refined through ongoing team training and skill building, systems analysis and information development, and creation of the feedback loops for continuous learning and system development

Source: Institute of Medicine (2013). Reproduced with permission of The National Academies Press.

head and neck cancer can prove to be costly, and advise the collection of data meaningful to patients, providers and payers throughout the patient's entire treatment cycle.

Summary

Classical motivation for the adoption of EMR systems was focused on pragmatic issues related to eliminating the inefficiencies associated with searching for a patient chart in a busy clinic or delivering effective care using only a subset of the patient's medical record available to the clinician. While these are strong motivators, they pale in comparison to the needs and promises that have emerged as the quantity and complexity of healthcare data have exploded over the past two decades. In many ways, cancer has been at the epicentre of this explosion with massive expansions in genomic, medical imaging, pathology and treatment-related records. An informatics-powered cancer care and research paradigm has grown from these early efforts and this paradigm promises not only to address the pragmatic issues of having the right information at the right location and the right time, but also to create a *system* of data collection and learning that improves the quality of care, allows a remarkable degree of personalization in the delivery of therapy and enables learning (both human and machine) about the practice of medicine and the nature of cancer.

Recommended reading

Abernethy AP, Etheredge LM, Ganz PA *et al.* (2010) Rapid-learning system for cancer care. *J Clin Oncol* 28:4268–4274.

caBIG Strategic Planning Workspace (2007). The Cancer Biomedical Informatics Grid (caBIG): infrastructure and applications for a worldwide research community. *Stud Health Technol Inform* 129:330–334.

Clark K, Vendt B, Smith K *et al.* (2013) The Cancer Imaging Archive (TCIA): maintaining and operating a public information repository. *J Digit Imaging* 26:1045–1057.

Cruz JA, Wishart DA (2006) Applications of machine learning in cancer prediction and prognosis. *Cancer Inform* 2:59–77.

Edgar R., Domrachev M, Lash AE (2002) Gene Expression Omnibus: NCBI gene expression and hybridization array data repository. *Nucleic Acids Res* 30:207–210.

Edwards C. (2014) Using patient data for personalized cancer treatments. *Commun ACM* 57:13–15.

European Union Agency for Fundamental Rights & Council of Europe (2013) *Handbook on European Data Protection Law*. Available at http://www.coe.int/t/dghl/standardsetting/dataprotection/TPD_documents/Handbook.pdf

Friend SH, Norman TC (2013) Metcalfe's law and the biology information commons. *Nat Biotechnol* 31:297–303.

Fleurence RL, Curtis LH, Califf RM, Platt R, Selby JV, Brown JS (2014). Launching PCORnet, a national patient-centered clinical research network. *J Am Med Inform Assoc* 21(4):578–582.

Freymann JB, Kirby JS, Perry JH, Clunie DA, Jaffe CC (2012) Image data sharing for biomedical research–meeting HIPAA requirements for De-identification. *J Digit Imaging Off J Soc Comput Appl Radiol* 25, 14–24.

Kaye J, Whitley EA, Lund D, Morrison M, Teare H, Melham K (2014) Dynamic consent: a patient interface for twenty-first century research networks. *Eur J Hum Genet* [Epub ahead of print].

Lambin P, Roelofs E, Reymen B *et al.* (2013) Rapid Learning health care in oncology' – an approach towards decision support systems enabling customised radiotherapy. *Radiother Oncol* 109:159–164.

Lambin P, Rios-Velazquez E, Leijenaar R *et al.* (2012) Radiomics: extracting more information from medical images using advanced feature analysis. *Eur J Cancer* 48(4):441–446.

Lunshof JE, Chadwick R, Vorhaus DB, Church GM (2008) From genetic privacy to open consent. *Nat Rev Genet* 9:406–411.

Meldolesi E, van Soest J, Dinapoli N et al. (2014) An umbrella protocol for standardized data collection (SDC) in rectal cancer: A prospective uniform naming and procedure convention to support personalized medicine. *Radiother Oncol* 112:59–62.

Pierce CD, Booth D, Ogbuji C et al. (2012) SemanticDB: Semantic Web Infrastructure for Clinical Research and Quality Reporting. *Curr Bioinform* 7.

Shrager J, Tenenbaum JM, Travers M (2011) Cancer Commons: Biomedicine in the internet age. Elkin S, ed. *Collab Comput Technol Biomed Res* 161–177.

Stroetman V et al. (2009) *Semantic Interoperability For Better Health And Safer Healthcare*. Available at http://eprints.ucl.ac.uk/66190/

Veer LJ, Bernards R (2008) Enabling personalized cancer medicine through analysis of gene-expression patterns. *Nature* 452:564–570.

Walters RS, Albright HW, Weber RS et al. (2014) Developing a system to track meaningful outcome measures in head and neck cancer treatment. *Head Neck* 36:226–230.

7 Imaging

Supreeta Arya[1], Venkatesh Rangarajan[2] and Nilendu Purandare[2]

[1]Department of Radio-diagnosis, Tata Memorial Centre, Mumbai, India
[2]Department of Nuclear Medicine & Molecular Imaging, Tata Memorial Centre, Mumbai, India

General principles

Imaging plays a vital role in cancer diagnosis (including guided biopsy), staging, assessment of treatment response, detection of recurrence and identification of post-treatment normal tissue changes. Imaging can be morphological (providing anatomical information) or functional (yielding physiological information).

Morphological imaging

Computed tomography (CT) and magnetic resonance imaging (MRI) are the most commonly used morphological imaging methods. Ultrasound (US) as well as plain radiography, such as chest X-ray (CXR), skeletal radiography (for bone tumours), panoramic radiography (for the mandible in oral cancers), mammography (a type of soft tissue radiography) and occasionally barium studies are also useful in certain situations. Features including the strengths and limitations of the various morphological imaging studies are shown in Table 7.1.

Computed tomography

Conventional CT acquired images via section by section scanning; this was succeeded by helical CT (volumetric scanning). Recently, multidetector CT (MDCT) has widely replaced helical CT and revolutionized CT imaging. MDCT enables:

- Faster scanning
- Increased volume coverage in a single breath-hold
- High-resolution multiplanar reformations (with 16 and higher row detector scanners, which are ideal for oncological imaging)
- Increased lesion detection
- Increased accuracy of anatomical (T and M) staging.

Contrast-enhanced CT (CE-CT) is performed after intravenous administration of a non-ionic, low osmolar, iodinated contrast agent. This opacifies vasculature, increases soft tissue contrast and helps in the characterization of pathology. However it should be cautiously administered in patients with renal impairment (i.e. creatinine >1.5 mg/dL, glomerular filtration rate [GFR] <60 mL/min), weighing risks against benefits.

Magnetic resonance imaging

MRI is another widely used imaging method in oncology owing to its superior soft tissue contrast. Advanced MRI can also provide functional information. The morphological and functional information is obtained by studying various MRI sequences, as shown in Table 7.2. Various tissues display differing signal intensity (SI) on different MRI sequences (Table 7.3).

Table 7.1 Morphological imaging

CT	MRI	Ultrasound	Radiography
Cross-sectional imaging with a wide field of view Inferior soft tissue contrast compared to MRI	Cross-sectional imaging with wide field of view; with limitations due to movement Exquisite soft tissue characterization	Cross-sectional imaging with limited field of view Bone and bowel gas interfere with visibility Operator dependent	Planar imaging with no soft tissue characterization
Employs intravenous and oral contrast (in abdomen and pelvis)	Uses intravenous gadolinium, but not mandatory for all regions	Routinely no contrast; contrast-enhanced ultrasound has been used for detection and characterization of focal lesions (mostly liver)	Barium studies with oral contrast and angiography with intravenous contrast

UICC Manual of Clinical Oncology, Ninth Edition. Edited by Brian O'Sullivan, James D. Brierley, Anil K. D'Cruz, Martin F. Fey, Raphael Pollock, Jan B. Vermorken and Shao Hui Huang. © 2015 UICC. Published 2015 by John Wiley & Sons, Ltd.

Table 7.2 Information from MRI

Sequences for morphological information	Sequences for functional information
T1W T2W and fat-suppressed T2W Gadolinium-enhanced T1W FLAIR (brain) STIR (head and neck) FIESTA/TRUFISP (abdomen and pelvis) Gradient echo (GRE) and susceptibility-weighted imaging (SWI): for blood products and calcification (brain, musculoskeletal) Chemical shift imaging (adrenal, liver)	*Dynamic contrast-enhanced (DCE) perfusion MRI using T1W sequences*: malignant tumours show rapid early enhancement; benign tumours show slow gradual enhancement *Dynamic susceptibility contrast (DSC) perfusion MR imaging using T2*-weighted sequences* *Diffusion-weighted imaging (DWI) with apparent diffusion co-efficient (ADC) maps*: highly cellular tissues (malignant tumours) show restricted diffusion (high signal on the b-value image with low signal on the ADC map) *Spectroscopy*: characterizes tissues according to metabolite level *Diffusion tensor tractography*: demonstrates orientation and integrity of white matter fibres *in vivo*

Table 7.4 shows some advantages and disadvantages of CT and MRI.

Ultrasound

US is performed through various routes:
- Abdominal
- Endoscopic
- Transvaginal (TVS)
- Transrectal: to evaluate the cervix and prostate
- Endorectal: to evaluate the layers of the rectal wall
- Soft parts: for thyroid, superficial nodes, breast, testes.

US is useful for:
- Differentiating solid versus cystic lesions
- Differentiating liver metastases versus haemangiomas

Table 7.3 MRI signal intensity in various tissues on different sequences

	T1W	T2W	Post-gadolinium enhancement	STIR (short tau inversion recovery)
Fat (including yellow bone marrow)	High (bright)	High	No	Low (dark)
Water	Low	Very high	No	Very high
Tumour (*exceptions: melanomas have high T1W signal intensity [SI]; meningiomas can have low T2W SI)	Low*	Intermediate to high* (depending on grade and water content) Necrotic foci have SI similar to water	Homogeneous or heterogeneous enhancement No	High Very high
Inflammation (in laryngeal cartilages and sinonasal mucosa)	Low	Very high (>adjacent tumour)	Homogenous enhancement (> adjacent tumour)	Very high
Oedematous paranasal sinus mucosa	Low	Very high	Does not enhance	Very high
Fibrosis	Low	Very Low (dark signal)	Absent in mature fibrosis, mild enhancement in early stages	Low
Tumour-invaded marrow	Low (compared to normal marrow)	Variable	Enhancement	High
Blood	High in subacute stage (weeks–months) Low in hyperacute/acute stages (hours–days) or in chronic stage (years)	Low or high (depends on stage)	No	**GRE/SWI** Blooms (appears very dark)

Table 7.4 CT versus MRI

	CT	MRI
Scanning speed	(+) Very fast (most with MDCT) (+) Less susceptible to motion artefact	(−) Long scan duration (−) Sensitive to coughing, breathing, swallowing, peristalsis, blood flow and patient movement
Ionizing radiation	(−) Yes	(+) No
Dental amalgam artefact	(+) Yes; may be minimized by gantry angulation	(−) Less
Reaction to contrast	(−) More frequent, including anaphylaxis	(+) Less frequent (−) Occasionally nephrogenic systemic fibrosis (in GFR <30 mL/min/1.73m^2)
Multiplanar reformations	(+) By indirect reconstruction (only with 16- and higher row MDCT)	(+) By direct multiplanar imaging
Depiction of bone and calcification	(+) Superior (most specific for demonstration of cortical erosion)	(+) Very sensitive for marrow and skull base invasion (−) Can overestimate cortical erosion in the mandible (chemical shift artefacts) (−) Decreased specificity for marrow (tumour versus inflammation)
Soft tissue contrast	(−) Inferior	(+) Superior for: • Tumour versus inflammation • Recurrence versus fibrosis • Invasion of muscles, cavernous sinus, dura and perineural spread

+, advantage; −, disadvantage.

- Characterizing ovarian masses (by TVS)
- Guided fine needle aspiration (FNA)/biopsy
- Selecting thyroid nodules and superficial nodes for guided FNA
- Detecting tumour thrombus and assessing lesion vascularity with colour and power Doppler.

Functional imaging

The commonly used functional imaging methods are positron emission tomography (PET), bone scintigraphy and single photon emission computed tomography (SPECT).

PET and PET-CT

Images are acquired by external detection on a PET scanner of decaying positrons emitted by a radiotracer injected into the human body. The commonly used radiotracer in clinical practice is ^{18}F-fluorodeoxyglucose (^{18}FDG).

The principles of PET scanning are:
- Cancer cells have increased glucose metabolism
- Increased uptake of ^{18}FDG by tumour occurs due to up-regulation of glucose transporters
- Reduced hexokinase levels limit further metabolism of ^{18}FDG, leading to radiotracer accumulation and reflecting as areas of hypermetabolism.

Several non-FDG tracers used to study various biological processes are:
- ^{18}F-fluorothymidine(FLT): proliferation
- ^{18}F-fluoromisonidazole: hypoxia
- Somatostatin receptor expression: ^{68}Ga-DOTATOC/TATE.

PET alone lacks spatial resolution, but when combined with CT/MRI it provides anatomical and functional information.

Bone scinitigraphy/bone scan

This method commonly uses ^{99m}Tc-methylene diphosphonate (MDP) to assess bone metastases; however, it lacks specificity in accurately differentiating benign processes from malignant involvement.

SPECT and SPECT-CT

This imaging method gives accurate spatial localization of an uptake seen on a planar (two-dimensional) scan; by obtaining tomographic sections of the abnormality. When CT is combined with SPECT, precise anatomical overlay can be combined with functional information.

Site-specific imaging studies

Central nervous system
Contrast-enhanced MRI (CE-MRI)
- Gold standard for brain and spine: for medulloblastoma, germ cell tumours, leptomeningeal metastases, primary central nervous system (CNS) lymphomas, intracranial and spinal ependymomas
- Ideal for tumour definition

- Enhancement present in high-grade tumours and absent in low-grade tumours

MRI schedule
- Pretherapy
- Postoperative/post biopsy: within 24–48 hours; no later than 72 hours
- For response assessment (post-adjuvant treatment): 4 weeks in high-grade tumours and 8 weeks in low-grade tumours
- Follow-up

MRI studies
- *Ideal*: Multiplanar MRI with T1 weighted (T1W) and T2 weighted (T2W), fluid-attenuated inversion recovery (FLAIR), gradient recalled echo (GRE)/susceptibility-weighted imaging (SWI), post-gadolinium T1W sequences, MR spectroscopy, perfusion and diffusion-weighted imaging (DWI)
- *Minimal*: T1W and T2W/FLAIR with post-gadolinium T1W sequences in axial and coronal/sagittal planes; 4-mm slice thickness; no gap
- MR spectroscopy:
  - Shows metabolites: choline, creatinine, N-acetyl aspartate (NAA), lipid and lactate in normal and tumour tissue:
    - Choline peaks with elevated choline-to-NAA ratios seen in tumours; lipid and lactate peaks in necrosis
  - Evolving role in grading gliomas, distinguishing gliomas and metastases, and differentiating recurrence versus pseudoprogression
- MR perfusion: dynamic susceptibility CE-MRI (DSC MRI):
  - Compares cerebral blood volume (rCBV) values in tumour and normal brain parenchyma to:
    - Distinguish tumour from radiation injury (increased rCBV in tumour; decreased in pseudoprogression after radiation and temozolomide)
    - Grade tumours (higher perfusion in high grade). Figure 7.1 shows hyperperfusion in a right frontoparietal lobe tumour, suggesting a high-grade tumour
    - Guide biopsy
- DWI-MRI:
  - Can differentiate between abscess (restricted diffusion) and metastases (no restriction)
  - In immediate postoperative period (<72 hours) may distinguish ischaemic foci (with restricted diffusion) from residual tumour, both of which can enhance
  - Evolving role in evaluating pseudoprogression

Computed tomography
- If MRI cannot be performed (patients with claustrophobia/implants)
- In the immediate postoperative setting

FDG-PET-CT
- Not routinely used as accuracy is questionable in recurrent glioma

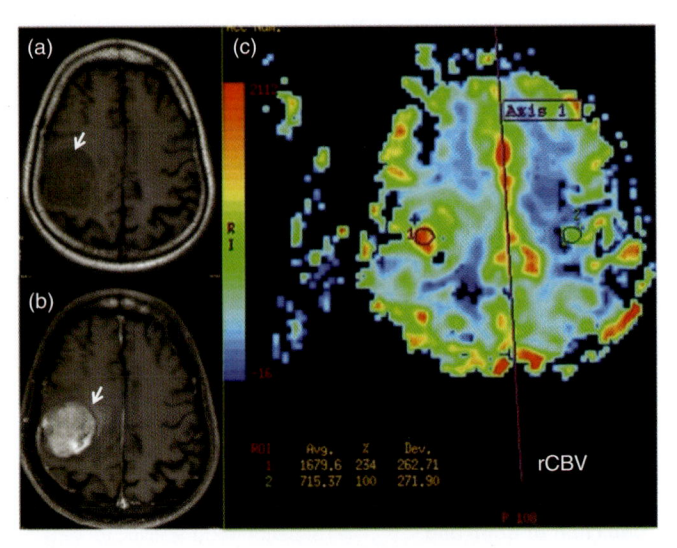

Figure 7.1 (a) T1W non-contrast axial MRI shows a hypointense mass (arrow) in the right frontoparietal lobe. (b) Contrast-enhanced T1W MRI shows enhancement (arrow). (c) Perfusion map showing the focus of hyperperfusion as a red zone, suggesting a high-grade tumor. Note rCBV in ROI 1 (in red zone) = 234%; standard value in contralateral brain parenchyma ROI 2 = 100%.

PET with other tracers:
- ^{11}C-methionine-PET has very high sensitivity and specificity for detection of recurrent glioma (requires on-site cyclotron due to the short half-life of the radiotracer)
- ^{18}F-fluorothymidine (FLT) and ^{18}F-fluoroethyl L-tyrosine (FET) are promising non-FDG glioma radiotracers. Figure 7.2 shows the value of FLT-PET in detecting a recurrent glioma of the left cerebral hemisphere
- SPECT agents like ^{99m}Tc-sestamibi, ^{99m}Tc-tetrofosmin and ^{99m}Tc-glucoheptonate have been used for the detection of recurrent glioma

Response assessment (high-grade gliomas)
Table 7.5 describes the McDonald & RANO criteria to assess response to surgery and adjuvant therapy.

Criteria for pseudoprogression on conventional MRI
1. ≥25% enlargement of enhancing lesions; unequivocal increase in T2/FLAIR lesions
2. No new lesion outside radiation field
3. No clinical worsening
4. Decreased corticosteroid dose

Confirmed only on next MRI exam:
- If stable/decreased with no clinical worsening: *'pseudoprogression'*
- If increased/new lesion outside radiation field; clinical worsening on stable/increased corticosteroid dose: *'progression'*

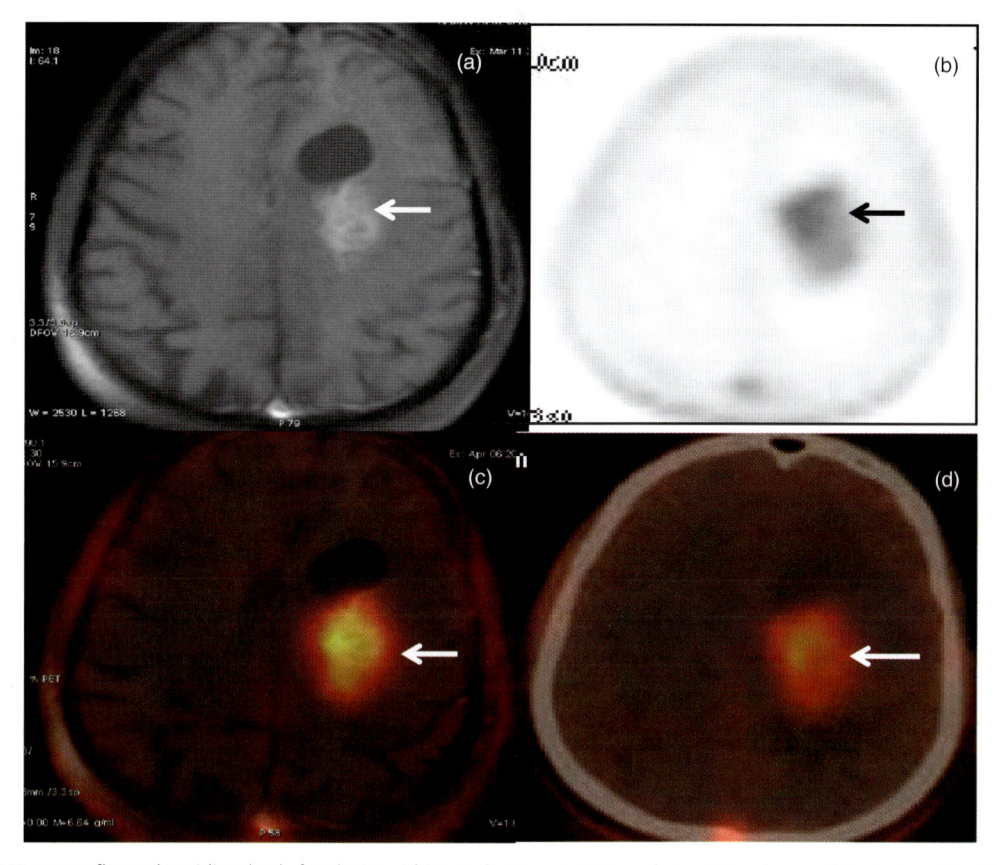

Figure 7.2 New PET tracer, fluorothymidine (FLT), for distinguishing radiation necrosis and recurrent glioma of the left cerebral hemisphere. (a) Contrast-enhanced T1W MRI shows irregular enhancement in the left frontal lobe (arrow) associated with the resection cyst (seen just anterior to the enhancing area). (b) FLT-PET image shows increased tracer concentration in the left cerebral hemisphere (arrow). (c) Fused PET-MRI. (d) PET-CT showing FLT uptake correlating with the morphological abnormality (arrow); histopathology confirmed recurrence.

Table 7.5 Response assessment guidelines for gliomas

Criteria	Features	Comments
McDonald*	Relies on increased gadolinium enhancement for tumour recurrence	Limitations: • Increased enhancement can be due to pseudoprogression (early), radiation necrosis (late), seizure, inflammation or tumour • Lack of enhancement with antiangiogenic therapy (pseudoresponse)
RANO (Response Assessment in Neuro-oncology)* for high grade gliomas	Relies on T2/FLAIR hyperintensity + gadolinium-enhanced T1 lesions	More reliable to distinguish: • Pseudoresponse (decreased enhancement; increased FLAIR hyperintensity) from • True response (decrease in both enhancement and FLAIR hyperintensity)

*Both criteria incorporate clinical assessment and corticosteroid dose.

Thyroid cancers
- US is the modality of choice for thyroid nodule detection and characterization
- Scintigraphy (^{99m}TcO4/^{123}I/^{131}I) used for:
  - Detection/ablation of residual disease
  - Evaluation of nodule function (only when thyroid-stimulating hormone [TSH] low)
- CT/MRI for evaluating extent in advanced disease; in goitre with substernal extension
- PET-CT for post-treatment follow-up (select cases, e.g. those with high thyroglobulin and normal scintigraphy; or to identify metastases in anaplastic thyroid cancer)

Approach to thyroid nodule
TSH is measured in an enlarged thyroid/suspected nodules to decide further evaluation (Table 7.6).
- If multiple nodules are seen on US, the nodule(s) with suspicious features is (are) needled (which need not be the largest nodule)
- US-guided FNA with 23–27-gauge needles; on-site cytology exam under light microscopy increases yield

Table 7.6 Thyroid stimulating hormone (TSH) levels and imaging

TSH level	Imaging	Result	Implication
Low	Scintigraphy	Hyperfunctioning	Hyperthyroidism
Normal/ high	Ultrasound	Diffuse heterogeneous non-nodular gland; no nodes	Probably benign
		Solitary nodule (defined as discrete lesion within gland distinct from surrounding parenchyma) or multinodular thyroid	Study nodule features to decide FNA

- One to three aspirations usually give adequate yield
- US thyroid incomplete without evaluation of nodes; if nodes suspicious or abnormal on US, any sized thyroid nodule/even diffusely heterogeneous gland/alternately the node needs FNA
- Preoperative US needed prior to thyroidectomy for status of contralateral lobe and both sides of neck for nodes
- Extracapsular spread with adjacent deep structure invasion/mediastinal extension requires further staging with CT/MRI
- Thyroid US is very sensitive, but non-specific; hence FNA is widely indicated (Table 7.7)
- Implications of FNA results are discussed in Chapter 48

Post-therapy imaging in papillary thyroid cancers
See Table 7.8.

Medullary thyroid cancers
If medullary thyroid cancer is detected on US-guided FNA, preoperative work-up with CE-CT neck, chest and abdomen is indicated for bulky cervical nodal metastases and/or serum calcitonin of >400 pg/mL.

Follow-up imaging after surgery
- US of neck
- If serum calcitonin is >150 pg/mL above baseline level, metastatic work-up is recommended, including CE-CT neck, chest, abdomen, pelvis ± MRI spine, bone scan and/or FDG-PET-CT

Head and neck cancers
Pretreatment imaging
Standard diagnostic and staging studies include:
- *CE-CT head and neck*: to assess size and extent of primary tumour and extent of neck disease

Table 7.7 Ultrasound features of thyroid nodule and guided fine needle aspiration (FNA)

Features		Implication	FNA
Solid nodule	Microcalcification	Most specific feature for malignancy	Yes if ≥1 cm
	Coarse calcification	Seen in multinodular goitre/medullary/ papillary cancers Ominous in solitary nodules	Yes if ≥1.5 cm
	Iso-hyperechoic	Follicular neoplasm	Yes if ≥1.5 cm
	Darkly hypoechoic	Favours malignancy	Yes if ≥1 cm
	• Increased vascularity, ill-defined margins and a taller than wide nodule are other ominous features • Complete uniform hypoechoic halo specific for benignancy		
High risk history* and small nodule with suspicious features		Suspect malignancy	Yes if >5 mm
Purely cystic		Benign	No
Solid cystic nodule		Ominous if solid parts have suspicious features	Yes if ≥2.0 cm
Spongiform nodule		Nodular hyperplasia (99.7–100% specificity for benignancy)	No

*High-risk history: history of thyroid cancer in one or more first-degree relatives; history of external beam radiation as a child; exposure to ionizing radiation in childhood or adolescence; prior hemithyroidectomy with discovery of thyroid cancer, ^{18}FDG avidity on PET scanning; calcitonin >100 pg/mL, multiple endocrine neoplasia; familial medullary thyroid cancer (FMTC). Adapted from ATA Guidelines 2009.

- *CE-MRI*: preferred for:
  - Assessing tumour extent in nasopharyngeal cancer and other skull base tumours
  - Paranasal sinus cancers complicated by oedema
  - Oropharyngeal cancer if the tongue base is involved
  - Salivary gland tumours with suspected perineural spread (Fig. 7.3)
  - Oral tongue cancers and if patient has dental artefact
- *In general, CT is preferred in the infrahyoid neck and MRI is preferred in the suprahyoid neck*
- CT is also preferred in gingival, buccal and retromolar trigone cancers for assessing mandibular invasion as it has high specificity for bone erosion and because the incidence of bone erosion is high in these cancers (Fig. 7.4)
- *FDG-PET-CT*: useful for patients with an initial 'unknown primary' presentation to identify the potential mucosal primary;

Table 7.8 Post-therapy imaging (papillary thyroid cancers)

Clinical situation	Imaging strategy
Post thyroidectomy (surgical details not available or residual thyroid suspected)	US (thyroid bed and nodes) (not specific in the thyroid bed up to 3 months after total thyroidectomy) Scintigraphy if US negative or small residual thyroid suitable for ablation
Post-total thyroidectomy (no macroscopic tumour)	Consider diagnostic ^{131}I scan after thyroid stimulating hormone (TSH) stimulation for planning radioiodine ablation
Post-therapeutic ^{131}I administration	Whole body scanning with ^{131}I to look for residual disease and metastases if re-ablation planned
6 months/1 year post ^{131}I therapy	US and serum thyroglobulin (Tg) If US negative and raised Tg → high-dose whole body ^{131}I scan (after TSH stimulation) to identify residual thyroid suitable for ablation
Rising Tg levels and absent ^{131}I uptake	^{18}FDG-PET-CT
High-risk patients with poorly differentiated thyroid cancers unlikely to concentrate ^{131}I, Hurthle cell carcinoma and tall cell variant	^{18}FDG-PET-CT

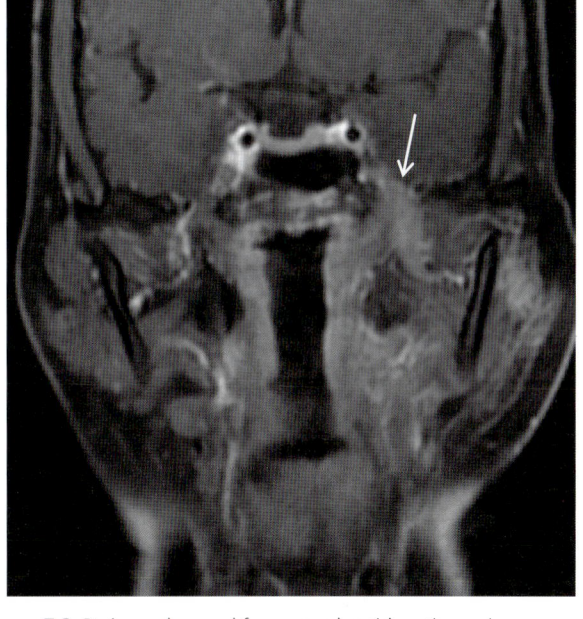

Figure 7.3 Perineural spread from an adenoid cystic carcinoma of the parotid. Contrast-enhanced, fat-suppressed coronal T1W MRI shows perineural spread along the mandibular nerve, seen as enhancement along the left foramen ovale (arrow). Note the absence of enhancement on the contralateral side.

identifying distant metastases (in those with Stage III or IV cancers) and occasionally to assess extent of neck disease
- *CXR*: in all
- *CT chest*: in advanced disease for lung metastases and baseline imaging of thorax if PET-CT is not done
- *Bone scan*: in advanced disease if PET is not available
- CT, MRI, US and PET-CT offer similar accuracy for neck nodes in clinically negative neck (Fig. 7.5); FDG-PET-CT is of no additional value in the N0 neck
- *Panoramic radiography*: useful for planning dental treatment prior to radiotherapy.

Table 7.9 describes the role of imaging in the various head and neck regions

Figure 7.4 Multidetector CT (MDCT) using multiplanar reformation and a bone algorithm for assessing the mandible. Oblique reformations of the mandible (a, b) on a 16-slice MDCT scanner depict the entire alveolar crest of the retromolar trigone in a case of squamous cell cancer demonstrating cortical erosion (arrows). (a) Bone window image (obtained with a soft tissue algorithm image). (b) Bone algorithm image (reconstructed with same dataset) shows higher image resolution. Adapted from Arya 2013. Reproduced with permission of Elsevier.

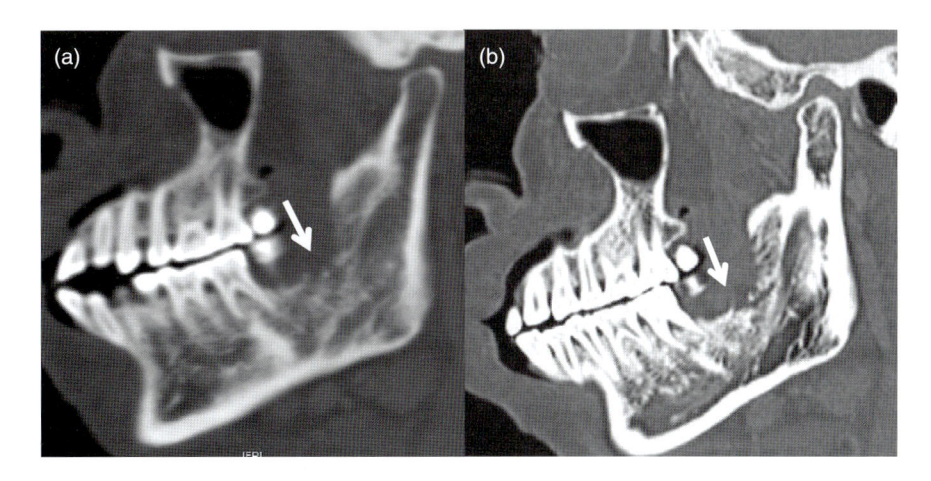

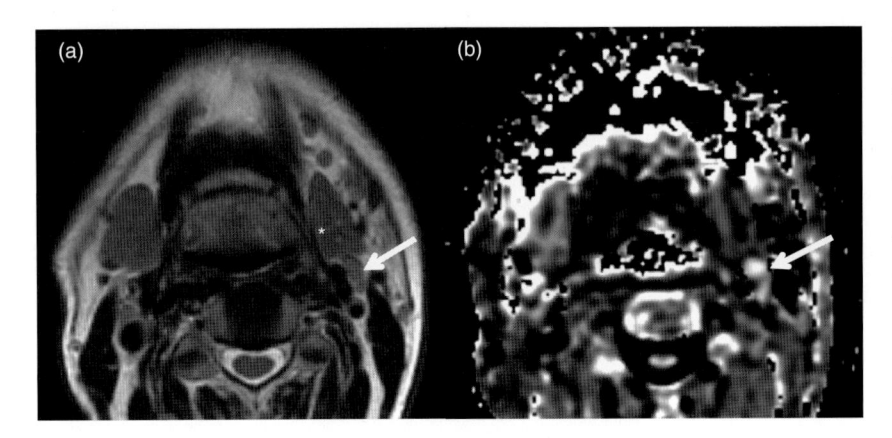

Figure 7.5 Diffusion-weighted imaging (DWI) for sub-centimetre neck nodes. Known case of oral tongue squamous cancer along the left lateral border. (a) T2W axial MR image shows an unremarkable sub-centimetre node at left level II (arrow); * shows the submandibular gland (b) DWI (b = 1000 image). Arrow shows the node with restricted diffusion (bright), which showed a low value on the ADC map (not shown). Histopathology confirmed metastasis. However, it is reported in the recent literature that DWI is highly sensitive for detecting nodes, but cannot reliably distinguish between a benign or metastatic aetiology.

Table 7.9 Imaging in various head and neck regions

Region	Imaging
Oral tongue, floor of mouth	CE-MRI is optimal; can show: • Extrinsic muscle invasion • Posterior and inferior soft tissue extent • Perineural spread • Bone invasion* (seen in <10% cases in tongue cancers) MDCT alternate method, but with inferior soft tissue characterization *MRI highly accurate for marrow invasion; but can overestimate mandibular cortical erosion and inferior alveolar canal involvement. CT can be problem solving for bone erosion as it has the highest specificity (87%) for mandibular invasion.
Gingiva, buccal mucosa, lips, retromolar trigone	MDCT with puffed cheek technique; can demonstrate: • Bone erosion (with high positive predictive value) • Posterior soft tissue extent to decide resectability
Hard palate	CE-MRI (for perineural spread) and MDCT (for bone erosion) are complementary
Oropharynx	CE-MRI better depicts: • Skull base invasion • Perineural spread • Prevertebral fascial invasion • Retropharyngeal adenopathy MDCT is a close second alternative
Nasopharynx	CE-MRI as compared to MDCT is superior in showing: • Local extent • Marrow invasion • Perineural spread PET-CT (optional): more useful for metastatic work-up and mapping extent of nodal disease
Larynx/hypopharynx	MDCT preferred due to fast speed of scanning; complements endoscopy with information on: • Laryngeal cartilages • Pre-epiglottic and paraglottic spaces *Laryngeal cartilage invasion*: • CT has 95% negative predictive value (NPV) • Lower positive predictive value: 　▪ 15–40% for thyroid cartilage sclerosis 　▪ 74% for cartilage destruction 　▪ 81% for extralaryngeal spread • MRI has high NPV (95%) and overall specificity of 82% for all cartilages and 75% for thyroid cartilage using revised criteria • *When CT equivocal/positive → MRI (problem solving)→ if negative → no cartilage invasion*

Region	Imaging
Salivary glands	CE-MRI best for differentiating benign and malignant, and for perineural spread MDCT alternate method
Nasal cavity and paranasal sinuses	CE-MRI: for perineural spread, soft tissue extent and addressing secretions MDCT for bone erosion is complementary
Parapharyngeal masses	Dynamic* CE-MRI/MDCT MR angiography for demonstrating multiple paragangliomas *Notes*: 1. Imaging diagnosis of paragangliomas may obviate need for biopsy 2. Paragangliomas may not always show characteristic flow-voids on T1/T2W MRI sequences; hence dynamic imaging to resolve. 3. *Paragangliomas show early enhancement (<1 minute) with rapid washout, while schwannomas and pleomorphic adenomas show delayed enhancement
Neck nodes	Both CT and MRI may show: • Enlarged necrotic nodes • Perinodal spread and adjacent muscle invasion • Invasion of carotid artery (circumferential contact ≥270) In non-necrotic sub-centimetre nodes, MRI features of internal heterogeneity and irregular margins may help characterize nodes as metastatic nodes

Imaging to evaluate radiotherapy response and for surveillance

- In patients who have been treated with primary radiotherapy, CT/MRI head and neck is generally performed at 8–12 weeks after radiotherapy to assess treatment response
- FDG-PET-CT may be used in addition to CT/MRI head and neck for suspected residual disease and assessment of metastatic disease if salvage treatment is planned
- CT thorax may be indicated if there is abnormality on baseline CT or prior to salvage surgery for residual disease if PET-CT is not done
- FDG-PET-CT done ≥ 12 weeks has a high negative predictive value of 95% for locoregional disease in treated head and neck squamous cancer; those with a negative 3-month PET-CT gain limited benefit from further PET-CT surveillance

Post-treatment changes on imaging

- *Expected postoperative changes:*
  - Asymmetry
  - Loss of bulk
  - Soft tissue surrounding carotid sheath
  - Myocutaneous flap with sharp interfaces
- *Expected post-radiotherapy changes:*
  - Skin and platysmal thickening
  - Subcutaneous fat reticulation
  - Thickened endolaryngeal structures and pharyngeal walls
  - Atrophied salivary glands
- *Abnormal post-treatment changes: see Table 7.10*

Table 7.10 Abnormal post-treatment changes

Postoperative	Fluid collection	Serous retention cyst, haematoma, abscess
	Fluid collection with air locules and enhancing walls	Abscess
6–12 months post radiation	Non-enhancing mucosal thickening with air locules	Mucosal necrosis
1–3 years post treatment	Enhancing mass (expanding contours) with restricted diffusion (low apparent diffusion co-efficient [ADC] values)	Recurrence
1–3 years post radiation	Bone/cartilage: • Destruction with sclerosis and sequestra *without soft tissue mass* • *Stable uptake on PET*	Osteo/chondroradionecrosis
	Ring-enhancing lesion in the brain parenchyma with surrounding oedema Raised lactate on spectroscopy High ADC values on DWI No uptake on PET scanning	Temporal lobe necrosis

Breast cancer
Screening
The role of mammography for breast cancer screening is debated. It is generally recommended to perform 2-yearly screening from 50 to 74 years of age for average-risk population, and annually (with breast MRI) starting at an earlier age for high-risk population (see Chapter 21).

Diagnosis
- For any palpable lump/single duct spontaneous nipple discharge/breast asymmetry with *clinical suspicion of malignancy, bilateral mammography is required at any age* with US for problem solving
- For a palpable lump without high suspicion of malignancy:
  - Mammography required in patients aged >30 years ± US
  - US in patients aged <30 years ± mammography.
- Well-accepted indications for MRI breast are:
  - High-risk history with *BRCA* mutation
  - Evaluation of implants
  - Axillary nodes with occult primary and dense breasts on mammography

Table 7.11 describes the BIRADS system for mammography reporting. Figure 7.6 illustrates a BIRADS 5 lesion.

Work-up in proven breast cancer (BIRADS category 6)
- *Clinical Stage I–IIB:*
  - Bilateral mammograms ± US
  - MRI breast (optional)
- *Clinical Stage IIIA and above:*
  - Mammography
  - CT chest, abdomen and pelvis + bone scan
  - FDG-PET-CT (optional)

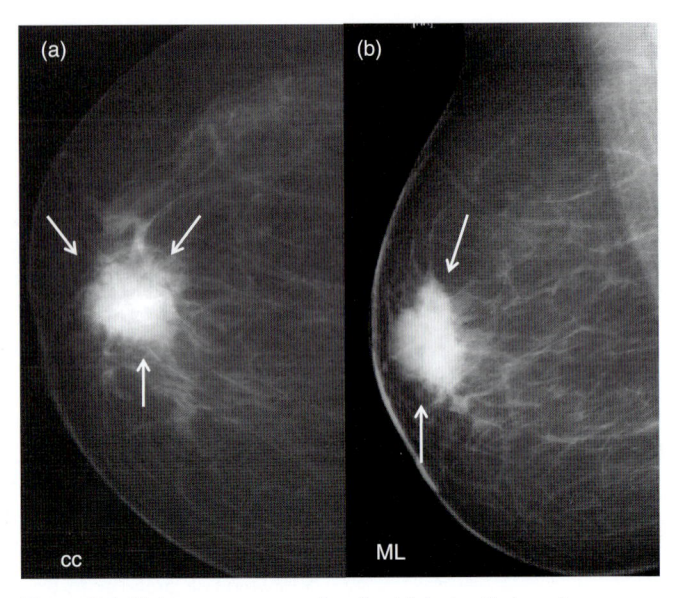

Figure 7.6 Right mammogram showing high-density breast mass with spiculated margins (arrows). (a) Craniocaudal view (CC); (b) mediolateral view (ML). BIRADS category 5. Subsequent histopathology showed an infiltrating duct carcinoma.

Response assessment (locally advanced/metastatic)
- CT chest, abdomen and pelvis + bone scan
- FDG-PET-CT (optional)

Follow-up (in treated cases)
- Clinical and mammography (at 18 months)
- Metastatic work-up if symptomatic

Thoracic cancers
Non-small cell lung cancer (NSCLC) or small cell lung cancer (SCLC)
Screening
- Screening with low-dose CT chest resulted in a 20% reduction in disease-specific mortality from lung cancer (National Lung Screening Trial 2011)
- In high-risk heavy smokers (≥30 pack years) aged 55–74 years, screening with annual low-dose CT scan is indicated if facilities to provide comprehensive care to screen positives are available

Detection
Lung nodules are detected commonly on CT scanning.
- Solitary pulmonary nodule (SPN) refers to a focal intraparenchymal lung lesion of ≤3 cm without atelectasis, pleural effusion or adenopathy
- A lesion >3 cm is defined as a lung mass

Image-guided transthoracic needle biopsy is dependent on the nodule size and location, and the skill of the operator. The

Table 7.11 Mammography: BIRADS system

Category 0:	Additional evaluation required
Category 1:	Negative
Category 2:	Benign (definite)
Category 3:	Probably benign (<2% probability of malignancy)
Category 4:	Suspicious (3–94% probability of malignancy); merits biopsy
4A:	Low suspicion (2–10% probability of malignancy)
4B:	Intermediate suspicion (11–50% probability of malignancy)
4C:	Moderate suspicion (51–94% probability of malignancy)
Category 5:	Highly suggestive of malignancy (≥95%)
Category 6:	Biopsy-proven malignancy

goal of imaging is to non-invasively differentiate benignity from malignancy. Comparison of current and previous imaging is essential to see nodule growth rate.
- Absence of growth over a 2-year period is considered a reliable sign of benignity, requiring no further evaluation
- An SPN visible on CXR with benign central calcification does not require further evaluation

No single imaging algorithm is uniformly accepted for imaging SPNs (practices vary amongst institutions). Table 7.12 shows the features of SPNs seen on various imaging studies.

Staging
Imaging helps stratify proven NSCLC into early operable and advanced stages.
- CT chest and abdomen is often the initial investigation (information about tumour size, mediastinal and chest wall invasion; metastatic disease)
- MRI thorax can be helpful in superior sulcus tumours (extension to spinal canal, neural foraminae and brachial plexus)
- *All operable NSCLCs with curative intent are also ideally imaged with FDG-PET-CT and MRI brain* (latter is mandatory even with a negative PET)
- Adding PET-CT to the conventional work-up can prevent futile thoracotomies in up to 20% of cases (Fig. 7.7)
- Integrated PET-CT outperforms CT for mediastinal nodal staging (sensitivity and specificity for CT: 53% and 73%; for PET-CT: 72% and 93%)
- CT brain, chest and abdomen with bone scintigraphy may be used for staging if PET and MRI are not available
- Bone scintigraphy: has lower sensitivity (86%) and specificity (87%) than PET (93% and 98%, respectively) for skeletal metastases
- Histopathological nodal staging is a prerequisite for operable NSCLCs:
  - Can be initially done by endobronchial US-guided FNA followed by mediastinoscopy (gold standard) if negative
  - Positive nodes on PET-CT/CT have to be confirmed by histopathology
  - High negative predictive value (NPV) of PET can obviate need for invasive mediastinoscopy in peripheral T1aN0 tumours

Response assessment (to neoadjuvant treatment)
- CT chest and abdomen
- FDG-PET-CT (optional)
- Metabolic responders on PET have a better prognosis than non-responders

Gastrointestinal and hepatobiliary cancers
Oesophageal cancer
Staging
- Initial staging includes CT lower neck, chest and abdomen; MDCT is preferred if available

Table 7.12 Solitary pulmonary nodule (SPN) features

Imaging method	Criteria	Features favouring	
		Benign nodule	Malignant nodule
CXR	Margins	Well-defined smooth	Lobulated Irregular Spiculated
	Calcification	Central nodular Pop-corn Diffuse Laminated	Eccentric Stippled
CT	Margins	Well-defined smooth	Irregular, spiculated
	Calcification	Same as on CXR	Same as on CXR
	Density	Ground glass <5 mm	Mixed partially ground glass/solid and >10 mm
	Contrast enhancement	Absent or <15 HU	20–60 HU (this criterion has 99% sensitivity, 54% specificity)
PET-CT	Uptake	Low/no uptake	High uptake
	• PET sensitivity (96.8%), specificity (77.8%) for detecting malignant nodules (meta-analysis) • False-negative PET results have been found with bronchioloalveolar carcinomas and small lesions <1.0 cm; false-positive results with infectious and granulomatous conditions		

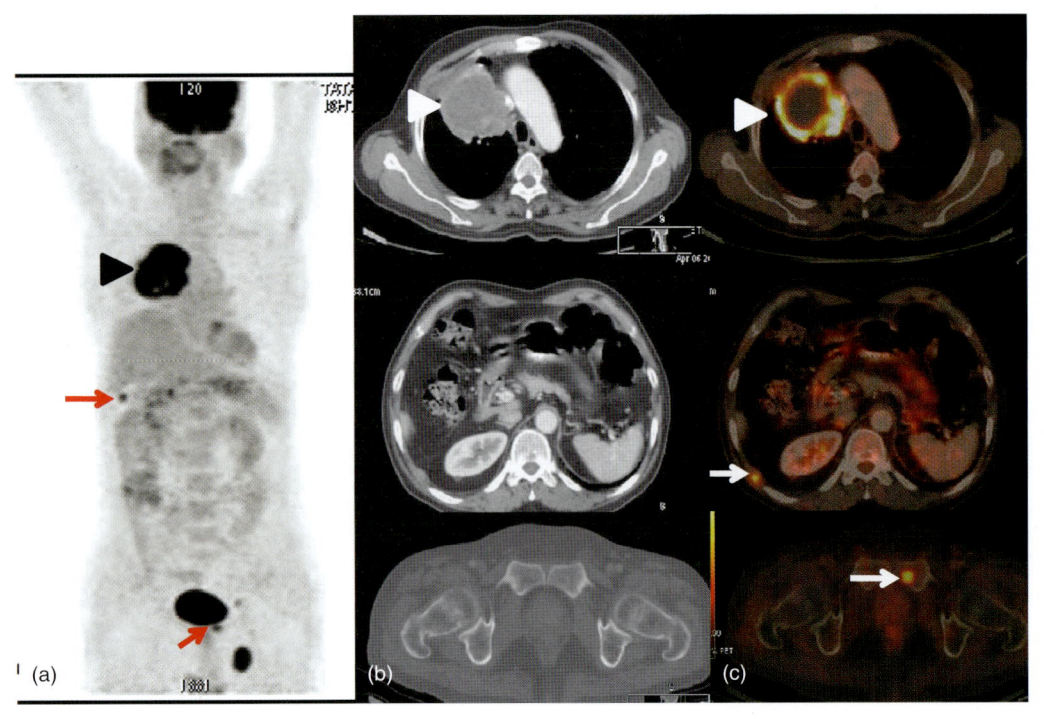

Figure 7.7 Upstaging by PET-CT in non-small cell lung cancer. (a) Coronal PET MIP image. (b) Axial CT images and (c) fused PET-CT images show the right upper lobe mass (arrowheads). Arrows in (a) and (c) show occult metastases in the abdominal wall and the pubic bone, not obvious in (b).

- If CT does not reveal metastases, FDG-PET-CT (if available) can prevent futile surgeries in 10–20% of cases
- CT has reliable sensitivity of 80–85% for T4 disease (to predict infiltration of the aorta and bronchus):
  - *Aorta*: circumferential contact (CC) of oesophagus with aorta is measured:
    - Aorta free if CC <45°; invaded if CC >90°; borderline if CC 45–90°
  - *Bronchial/tracheal invasion*: predicted if tumour deeply indents the posterior wall of left main bronchus/reaches along the left posterolateral tracheal wall
- CT sensitivity to differentiate T1, T2 and T3 categories is limited
- Endoscopic US (EUS) is superior to CT for T categories, particularly for early stages
- EUS-guided FNA is more sensitive for regional nodes, while CT is more specific for metastatic abdominal nodes (low false positives)
- *Hence, EUS ± guided FNA is indicated only in select cases to differentiate between T1–2N0* (which are treated with upfront surgery) *from T3N+* (which require neoadjuvant chemotherapy)

Response assessment (to neoadjuvant therapy)
- CT chest and abdomen, but morphological imaging has limitations in assessing therapeutic response
- FDG-PET has been used as a surrogate marker to predict early response to neoadjuvant treatment and to definitive chemoradiation therapy

Gastric cancer
Staging
- MDCT chest, abdomen and pelvis is a single comprehensive method for staging
- EUS, MRI and PET-CT are other methods
- The overall accuracies of MDCT, EUS and MRI are equivalent for T staging and serosal involvement, but EUS is more accurate in *proximal early gastric cancers* (89% accuracy) and is a must before planning endoscopic resections
- MDCT is more accurate than helical CT for T staging (overall accuracy of 89% and 73%, respectively); a 16-row or higher detector scanner provides optimal high-resolution multiplanar reformations
- MDCT, EUS and MRI are all equivalent and unreliable for nodal staging (sensitivity 70–80%)
- PET-CT has lower median sensitivity of 55% for lymph node metastases
- MDCT, MRI and PET-CT have high (and equivalent) sensitivity and specificity for hepatic metastases, but with poor sensitivity for peritoneal metastases
- PET-CT can be negative in one-third of gastric cancers; in mucinous and diffuse tumours
- EUS has a role in proximal tumours to confirm T1–2N0 status, where upfront surgery is contemplated, as T3–4N+ tumours require neoadjuvant therapy prior to restaging
- *Suggested work-up*:
  - MDCT chest, abdomen and pelvis→ EUS in select cases (see immediately above)
  - Helical CT to be used if MDCT not available

Table 7.13 Imaging in hepatocellular carcinoma (HCC)

	Recommended imaging	Criteria	Implication of imaging findings	Guideline body
Surveillance	*Abdominal* US every 6 months; 4 months if new nodule detected	In cirrhotic patients *or* Non-cirrhotic HBV carriers with high viral load or HCV positives	Size of nodule to be monitored – growing/ stable Growing nodule → investigate Stable → US follow-up	EASL-EORTC
Diagnosis	*4D CT and/or Dynamic multiphase CE-MRI*	*Lesion >2 cm*: one imaging method *Lesion 1–2 cm*: one method in centres of excellence; two methods in others	Arterial phase hypervascularity and portal venous or delayed-phase washout indicates HCC	EASL-EORTC
Staging	1. *4D CT/dynamic CE-MRI and* 2. *CT thorax + bone scan for* resectability assessment	Number and size of nodules Vascular invasion Extrahepatic spread	*Stage 0*: single nodule <2 cm *Stage A*: single or up to three nodules ≤3 cm *Stage B*: multinodular *Stage C*: portal vein invasion and extrahepatic spread	Barcelona Clinic Liver Cancer (BCLC) system
Response assessment (within 2 years)	*Dynamic CE-CT or dynamic CE-MRI* 1 month after any therapy; every 3 months in first year; every 6 months up to 2 years	Modified RECIST (m-RECIST)	Target lesions: • *Complete response*: disappearance of intratumoural arterial enhancement in all target lesions • *Partial response*: 30% decrease in the sum of diameters of viable enhancing target lesions with respect to baseline sum of diameters of target lesions	EASL-EORTC
Response assessment after 2 years	*Ultrasound every 6 months*	Appearance of new nodule	Monitor nodule growth as for Surveillance	EASL-EORTC

HBV, hepatitis B virus; HCV, hepatitis C virus.

Response assessment (post neoadjuvant therapy)
• CT chest, abdomen and pelvis

Hepatocellular carcinoma
Present guidelines recommend non-invasive methods for diagnosis and staging of hepatocellular carcinoma (Table 7.13) as needle tract seeding with biopsy has been known.

Biliary cancers
The role of imaging in biliary cancers is described in Table 7.14.

Pancreatic adenocarcinoma
Diagnosis, staging and assessment of resectability
• With contrast-enhanced pancreatic protocol, CT abdomen or pancreas protocol, MRI abdomen with MRCP for: diagnosis, T staging, vascular relations, adenopathy and hepatic metastases
• Tumour–vascular relationship is the most important factor in assessing resectability. The five important vessels are the coeliac artery (CA), hepatic artery (HA), main portal vein (MPV), superior mesenteric vein (SMV) and superior mesenteric artery (SMA)

Table 7.14 Imaging in biliary cancers

Issue	Imaging methods
Diagnosis (by imaging and histopathology with FNA/biopsy/biliary brush cytology)	Abdominal US (first line) MDCT/CT abdomen *or* MRI abdomen with MRCP
Staging and assessing resectability	MDCT/CT abdomen with delayed phase imaging *or* MRI abdomen with MRCP (preferred over PTC) *and* CXR/CT chest PTC (*if therapeutic intervention planned*; performed in gall bladder cancer only if MRCP not available) PET-CT (optional if suspected metastases)

MRCP, magnetic resonance cholangiopancreatography; PTC, percutaneous transhepatic cholangiopancreatography.

- Optimal CT study requires thin sections (≤3 mm) in the non-contrast, arterial and/or pancreatic parenchymal phase and portal venous phases
- 16 or higher-slice MDCT affords thin sections with high-quality multiplanar reformations to study vascular relations
- EUS is complementary; can provide information on vessels and nodes
- EUS-guided FNA is safer and with better yield than CT-guided FNA
- CT chest/CXR needed for pulmonary metastases
- No evidence for PET-CT in preoperative staging
- Pancreatic adenocarcinoma is divided into:
  - Resectable
  - Borderline resectable (BR)
  - Locally-advanced unresectable
  - Metastatic
- BR tumours may be down-staged with neoadjuvant chemotherapy/radiotherapy and restaged to assess resectability; hence the need for stratification as described in Table 7.15

Colon cancer (sporadic)
Staging
- MDCT abdomen and pelvis is more reliable than helical CT for T staging; both are less reliable for N staging

Table 7.15 Imaging criteria for resectability in pancreatic head adenocarcinoma

Resectable	Borderline resectable	Unresectable
No distant metastases	No distant metastases	Distant metastases Nodal metastases beyond the field of resection
Clear fat planes around CA, HA and SMA	1 Tumour: SMA contact ≤180° 2 Gastroduodenal artery encasement up to HA with direct abutment* or short segment encasement** of HA without extension to the coeliac axis	Tumour:-SMA circumferential contact >180° CA abutment Aortic encasement
No radiographic evidence of SMV/MPV distortion	1 Short segment safely reconstructible occlusion of SMV or MPV due to thrombus or encasement 2 Involvement of SMV/MPV with distortion or luminal narrowing	SMV/MPV occlusion which is non-reconstructible (no suitable vessel above or below for reconstruction)

*Abutment = tumour vessel contact of ≤180°.
**Encasement = tumour vessel contact >180°.
CA, coeliac artery; HA, hepatic artery; MPV, main portal vein; SMV, superior mesenteric vein; SMA, superior mesenteric artery.

- CT chest/CXR is to be added for metastatic work-up (there is no consensus on optimal chest strategy in colorectal cancers, but CT is superior to CXR)
- MRI can be problem solving for hepatic metastases; adding DWI improves accuracy (meta-analysis)
- PET-CT is not recommended in the initial staging except when CT reveals curable M1 disease
- *Suggested work-up*: MDCT abdomen and pelvis (helical CT if MDCT is not available) + CT chest/CXR

Response assessment (with neoadjuvant and palliative therapy)
- CT abdomen and pelvis

Follow-up
- CT abdomen and chest (in Stage II–III disease)
  or
- Abdominal US liver and CXR
- Small debated role for PET-CT when carcionoembryonic antigen (CEA) rising and CT negative

Rectal cancer
Staging
Issues in rectal cancer staging are:
- Circumferential resection margin (CRM), which is the distance from the tumour/perirectal node to the mesorectal fascia (MRF):
  - CRM is positive when node/tumour/peritumoural fat stranding is <1 mm from MRF
  - CRM is threatened if tumour/node is 1–2 mm from the MRF
  - CRM is negative if >2 mm from the MRF
- T, N and M categories

- Imaging in rectal cancer can be used to determine which patients are appropriately treated with upfront surgery or who benefit from preoperative chemoradiation (Fig. 7.8)
- Locoregional disease extent seen on imaging can influence radiotherapy planning
- Specific imaging methods for the issues:
  - High-resolution external MRI pelvis (HR-MRI) using external coil:
    - Multiplanar T2W sequences are sufficient
    - Post-gadolinium images are not required (ESGAR 2013 recommendation)
    - Minimum magnet field strength is 1.0 T; 1.5-T magnet is optimal
  - MDCT/CT
  - Endorectal US (ERUS)
- MRI with endorectal coil (ER-MRI) is not required (failed insertions in stenosing tumours, cannot demonstrate the MRF and hence the CRM status)
- PET is not recommended for initial staging.
- *CRM + T category*:
  - ERUS is highly accurate for T category, but may not display MRF (for CRM status); also unsuitable for obstructing tumours

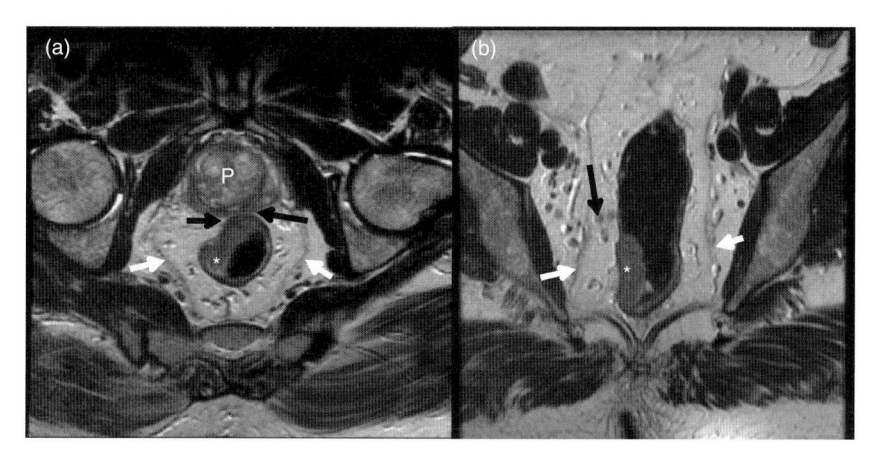

Figure 7.8 MRI in rectal cancer. (a) Axial and (b) coronal T2W images (post-gadolinium sequences are not mandated). The tumour (*) is located along the right lateral rectal wall without extension into the perirectal fat. Black arrows in (a) show the intact fat plane with the prostate (P): category T2. The black arrow in (b) shows tiny perirectal deposits (<3 mm in size): N1c category. White arrows show the mesorectal fascia (MRF), which is free (hence the circumferential resection margin is negative). MRI staging justifies surgery (upfront) without preoperative chemoradiation.

- Hence, ERUS is recommended only for specific differentiation between T1 and T2 tumours
- HR-MRI is the modality of choice for T category and CRM status (meta-analysis)
- HR-MRI also provides information on sphincter complex and extramural venous invasion
- MDCT is suboptimal for prediction of CRM in low anterior tumours; has lower accuracy for T category, cannot predict sphincter status; hence, cannot ideally replace MRI in local staging of rectal cancer
- *Nodal status*:
  - ERUS and HR-MRI have similar sensitivity and specificity for regional nodes (but greater than CT)
  - However, both ERUS and HR-MRI have lower sensitivity for N category than for T category (66% and 67% versus 94% and 94%, respectively)
  - Advantage of HR-MRI/CT over ERUS is the iliac and retroperitoneal node visualization
- *M category*:
  - MDCT chest, abdomen and pelvis is commonly employed
  - MRI is slightly superior for hepatic metastases and could be a problem-solving method
- *Suggested work-up*:
  - HR-MRI pelvis (add ERUS in T1 tumours) + MDCT chest abdomen and pelvis

  or
  - MDCT/CT pelvis and abdomen (if MRI not available) + CT chest/CXR

Response assessment
- HR-MRI pelvis is commonly used for local restaging (preferred to MDCT)
- CT thorax, abdomen and pelvis is optional for metastatic work-up (<7% change in management)
- Conflicting reports exist about the role of MRI in local restaging following preoperative chemoradiation
- Prediction of T category, nodal status and complete response was poor in a multicentre study
- DW-MRI and PET-CT are investigational

Follow-up
- CT abdomen, pelvis and chest (in Stage II and III disease)

  or
- Abdominal US liver and CXR
- Small debated role for PET-CT when CEA rising and CT negative

Anal cancer
Staging
- *Local staging*: MRI pelvis or MDCT/CT pelvis
- *Metastatic work-up*: CT abdomen + CT chest/CXR

Response assessment
- MRI can complement clinical examination

Follow-up
- No imaging if complete response
- For slow responders or initial node-positive disease → similar to rectal cancer

Gastrointestinal stromal tumours
Tumours of ≤2 cm are benign/low risk, with malignant potential related to tumour size (5 cm) and location. Rectal/oesophageal gastrointestinal stromal tumours (GISTs) are more likely to be malignant.
- *Small gastric GIST* (detection and follow-up):
  - EUS
- *Large GIST* (detection and staging; and follow-up in high risk):
  - Biphasic CE-CT abdomen (in gastric/colonic GIST); *MRI pelvis* (in rectal GIST)
  - *CXR/CT chest* for lung metastases
  - Percutaneous biopsy of large non-metastatic GIST to be planned with care, particularly in cystic tumours to prevent rupture and spillage
  - PET-CT as baseline investigation only if subsequent response assessment with imatinib therapy is needed

Response assessment (to imatinib therapy in inoperable/metastatic GIST)
- With CE-CT or PETCT
- For assessment of response, Choi criteria are preferred to RECIST (described below):
  - On CE-CT, 10% decrease in size *or* 15% decrease in density indicates partial response
  - PET criteria: >70% decrease in maximum standard uptake value (SUVmax) as compared to pretreatment value *or* an absolute (SUVmax) of <2.5 indicates partial response (Fig. 7.9)

Musculoskeletal tumours
Bone tumours
Diagnosis
Imaging has an important role in assisting diagnosis of bone tumours.
- *Plain radiograph of bone* in two planes including both joints is the initial method:
  - Lesion characteristics that along with age narrow differential diagnoses prior to biopsy are location, matrix, zone of transition, periosteal reaction and soft tissue component
- *CT* can be problem solving:
  - For radiographically occult bone destruction in complex anatomical regions (pelvis, ribs, sacrum, sacroiliac joint, skull base)
  - To show nidus in osteoid osteoma (with thin sections)
  - To depict subtle mineralization in lytic tumours

Staging
- *Local staging:*
  - MRI whole bone with adjacent joints is best method for studying marrow, skip lesions, soft tissue, joint and neurovascular bundle; also guides biopsy
- *Distant work-up:*
  - Non-contrast CT chest +
  - Bone scan/FDG-PET-CT(if available); PET-CT is superior to bone scan for marrow metastases in Ewing sarcoma

Response assessment
- MRI + radiographs
- *Optional*:
  - Early post-chemotherapy response predicted by dynamic contrast-enhanced (DCE)-MRI and DWI-MRI correlates well with histological necrosis
  - FDG-PET-CT useful as early surrogate marker for response prediction
  - In Ewing sarcoma and osteosarcoma, strong correlation exists between FDG uptake and degree of post-chemotherapy histological tumour necrosis
  - DCE-MRI can distinguish scar from residual tumour
  - DWI-MRI is useful to differentiate viable tumour and necrotic tissue during treatment of metastases

Follow-up
- Local imaging + non-contrast CT chest/CXR + bone scan (for Ewing sarcoma)

Soft tissue sarcomas (limb and retroperitoneal)
Detection, characterization and local staging
- *MRI limb*
- For retroperitoneal sarcomas, *CT/MRI abdomen* is equivalent
- Limb radiographs may help by depicting phleboliths, calcification, myositis ossificans and bone erosion. CT may be problem solving in these cases
- Imaging can be used to plan and guide core biopsy performed by an experienced surgeon/radiologist
- Biopsy pathway should be through a single muscle and compartment; should avoid intermuscular plane and neurovascular bundle; such that the path of biopsy and scar are removed at surgery
- Peritoneal approach for biopsy is contraindicated for retroperitoneal sarcomas

Distant work-up
- *Non-contrast CT chest*

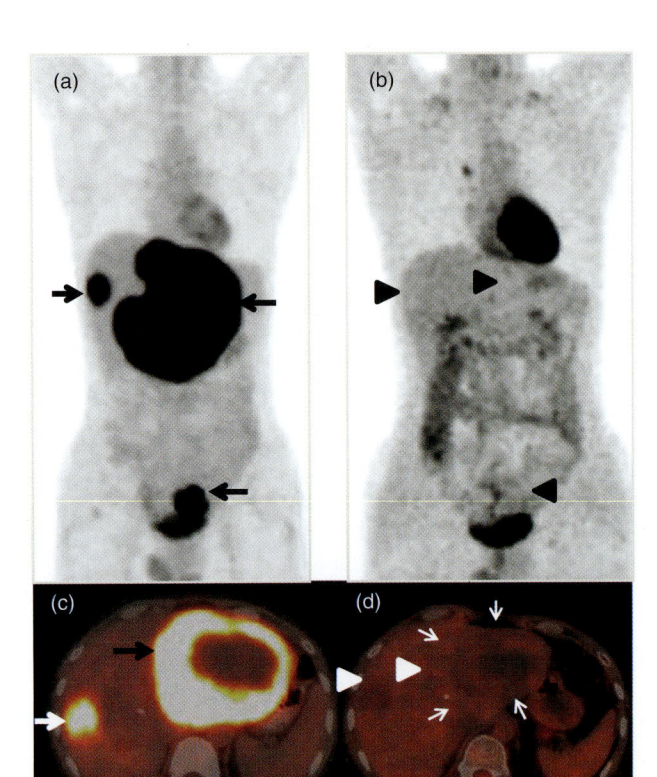

Figure 7.9 PET predicting response to imatinib in metastatic gastrointestinal stromal tumour (GIST). (a, b) Coronal PET MIP images. (c, d) Fused PET-CT images. (a) and (c) show intense FDG uptake in the lesions (arrows). (b) and (d) show complete metabolic response (arrowheads). Note the absence of significant change in the size of the lesions in (d) (arrows).

- *Consider CT/MRI brain* in alveolar soft part sarcoma, angiosarcoma, clear cell sarcoma
- *Consider CT abdomen* in extremity myxoid liposarcomas; regional node evaluation for epitheloid sarcomas

Follow-up
- US/MRI (limb) and CT/US abdomen for retroperitoneal sarcomas
- CXR (in low-grade sarcomas)
- Non-contrast CT chest in intermediate- and high-grade tumours (latter require closer follow-up)

Paediatric solid abdominal tumours

Table 7.16 describes imaging for common abdominal tumours in children.

Lymphomas and multiple myeloma

- Staging and response evaluation of Hodgkin and non-Hodgkin lymphomas with imaging is mandatory; commonly with *CT neck, thorax, abdomen and pelvis*
- *FDG-PET-CT* used alternately if available
- Interim response evaluation is mandatory in adult Hodgkin disease; early response to therapy seen on FDG-PET-CT is of prognostic significance
- In multiple myeloma:
  - Skeletal survey is recommended
  - MRI recommended if symptoms of cord compression
  - Bone scan is of limited value and not recommended

Gynaecological cancers
Cervical cancers
Pretreatment evaluation
- With the exception of CXR, imaging is not mandated, although it is encouraged in the revised International Federation of Gynecology and Obstetrics (FIGO) clinical staging
- In practice, cross-sectional imaging is often employed to plan treatment, but imaging is optional in tumours of Stage ≤IB
- Imaging can assist evaluation by demonstrating disease extent
- Intravenous pyelogram (IVP) and barium enema are no longer necessary
- CT abdomen and pelvis commonly used; as effective as MRI for nodal disease
- MRI is more accurate than CT for primary disease evaluation (tumour volume, invasion of cervical stroma, parametria, vagina, uterine corpus, bladder and rectum); the negative predictive value of MRI to rule out parametrial invasion is very high (Fig. 7.10); addition of DWI-MRI improves staging
- PET-CT shows superior performance in nodal staging of advanced disease when CT is negative (evolving evidence)
- Sentinel node biopsy is under evaluation
- *Suggested work-up*: CXR + MRI/CT pelvis + CT/US abdomen

Follow-up
- Imaging is required if clinically indicated (CT abdomen and pelvis + CXR/CT chest)
- DWI-MRI and DCE-MRI can help differentiate recurrence from radiation fibrosis

Endometrial cancers
Detection
- Transvaginal sonography (TVS) is indicated in postmenopausal bleeding
- Endometrial biopsy is recommended if endometrial thickness is >4 mm in postmenopausal bleeding
- *Disease extent*:
  - MRI pelvis preferred to CT for local extent
  - MRI demonstrates depth of myometrial invasion, cervical and adnexal invasion, tumour volume and nodes
  - Addition of DCE-MRI and DWI improves accuracy of staging
- *Suggested work-up*: MRI/CT pelvis + MRI/CT abdomen + CT chest/CXR

Table 7.16 Imaging in paediatric solid tumours

Tumour	Imaging			
	Local	Lung	Bone	Follow-up*
Neuroblastoma	CT/MRI of local part: can show *image-defined risk factors (IDRFs)*	–	MIBG scintigraphy + bone scan	MIBG scintigraphy + CT/MRI abdomen
Wilms tumour	CT/MRI	CXR or CT chest	–	CXR + CT/MRI abdomen
Rhabdomyosarcoma	MRI in limb tumours CT/MRI (abdominal or pelvic tumours)	Non-contrast CT chest	Bone scan Whole body MRI: investigational	CXR + CT/MRI (local)
Hepatoblastoma	CT/MRI: *pretreatment imaging stratifies patients to monitor chemotherapy response and assess resectability (PRETEXT staging)*	Non-contrast CT chest	–	CXR + CT/MRI abdomen

*Alternative to CT/MRI: ultrasonography of local part until higher imaging indicated.

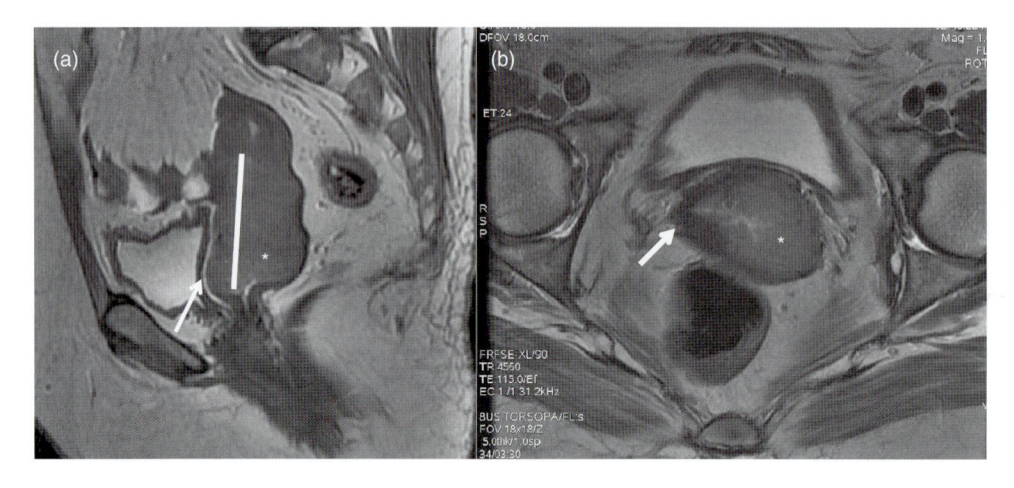

Figure 7.10 MRI in staging carcinoma of the cervix. (a) Axial T2W MRI shows a hyperintense mass in the cervix (*) extending into the lower uterine corpus. Fat plane with the bladder is preserved (arrow). (b) Preservation of the darkly hypointense stromal stripe on the right (arrow) is 95% specific for the absence of parametrial invasion.

Follow-up
- Imaging used if clinically indicated (CT abdomen and pelvis + CXR/CT chest)

Ovarian cancers
Screening
- Not recommended, as it does not reduce mortality

Detection
- Abdominal US and TVS are common first-line diagnostic investigations
- TVS helps differentiate between benign and malignant ovarian neoplasms
- Guided FNA is contraindicated in early ovarian lesions to prevent cyst rupture and peritoneal spillage
- MRI may be an optional imaging method for lesions indeterminate on US; addition of DWI and DCE-MRI improves characterization

Disease extent and response assessment
- CT abdomen and pelvis + CT chest/CXR

Follow-up
- In epithelial ovarian cancers, imaging is indicated only if clinical examination/tumour markers indicate disease recurrence
- CT abdomen and pelvis + CXR/ CT chest are then recommended
- PET-CT is as yet investigational

Urogenital cancers
Renal cancers
Detection and staging
- Most renal neoplasms are incidentally detected on US/CT abdomen; US has lower accuracy for detecting lesions of <2.0 cm (58%) than CT (100%)
- US, CT and MRI can distinguish solid from cystic masses
- Bosniak CT/MRI classification categorizes renal cysts into five types to predict malignancy; MRI may upgrade the Bosniak classification:
  - Bosniak type I and II cysts are benign and require no intervention/follow-up
  - Type III and above require investigation
- CT and MRI abdomen and pelvis are used to characterize renal masses; can show ominous features requiring surgery without need for FNA/biopsy
- MDCT is the mainstay for staging:
  - For predicting invasion of renal sinus fat, perinephric region and adrenals (85–98% specificity)
  - For assessing renal vein and inferior vena cava (IVC) for thrombus (specificity 97%; sensitivity 84%)
- MRI is equally accurate for staging, but is used as a problem-solving modality
- CT angiography is indicated for *preoperative renal vascular anatomy*
- Both CT and MRI have lower accuracy for nodal staging
- CT chest (preferred)/CXR is added for metastatic work-up
- Bone scan and CT/MRI brain are required only if clinically indicated
- FDG-PET has no established role in initial staging, but has a role in evaluating recurrence

Suggested follow-up
- US abdomen and CXR
- Annual CT chest and abdomen is advised in high-risk cases

Prostate cancer
Imaging for staging is currently recommended only in intermediate- and high-risk cancers.

Detection
- TRUS-guided needle biopsy of the prostate (with periprostatic local anaesthetic) is the test of choice for diagnosis; minimum ten cores, ideally 12 cores, obtained with a

18-gauge needle. TRUS without biopsy has limited role in detection
- Need for TRUS-guided biopsy is decided by serial prostate-specific antigen (PSA), DRE and clinical parameters
- Indication for MR-guided biopsy is high suspicion of cancer despite negative result on TRUS-guided biopsy
- Transperineal US-guided extended prostate biopsy has been proven to be as effective as TRUS-guided biopsy

Staging
- Accuracy of TRUS for local staging is 37–80% and can be used if MRI is not available
- Colour Doppler US can improve detection but does not improve staging accuracy
- *MRI pelvis is the most accurate and complete method for local staging.* MRI using endorectal coil and T2W sequences achieves high spatial resolution; it is the best technique for *extracapsular extension*, *seminal vesicle* and *neurovascular bundle invasion*
  - A 6–8-week delay is recommended between a biopsy and a staging MRI examination
- Addition of MR spectroscopy, DWI-MRI and DCE-MRI improves detection and staging accuracy (85–90%); can guide biopsy
- CT abdomen and pelvis is used for evaluation of abdominal and pelvic adenopathy in locally-advanced cases; equivalent to MRI for lymph node staging
- ^{99m}Tc-MDP bone scan *is usually performed for skeletal metastases* in high Gleason score and locally-advanced tumours
- ^{18}F-PET-CT (if available) has superior sensitivity and specificity to ^{99}Tc-MDP bone scan for skeletal metastases
- ^{18}FDG-PET-CT has no established role in routine staging
- PET-CT with new tracers such as ^{11}C-choline, ^{11}C-acetate and ^{18}F-choline is promising for detecting nodal and metastatic disease in high-risk cases

Follow-up
- TRUS/MRI pelvis may be used if clinically indicated
- ^{18}FDG-PET-CT has a potential role in the detection of recurrence in poorly differentiated cancers and/or rising PSA levels

Bladder cancer
Only *muscle invasive* bladder cancers (that comprise 20–30%) require imaging to evaluate disease extent.

Detection
- CT is the modality of choice for investigating haematuria
- CT has a sensitivity of 79–89% and specificity of 91–94% in diagnosing bladder cancers
- Conventional US has a limited role in assessing bladder tumours; presence of hydronephrosis suggests muscle-invasive bladder cancer

Staging
- *CT chest, abdomen and pelvis* for local staging and distant disease (for liver, abdominopelvic nodes, distant metastases)
- *CT urography* for information about upper urinary tracts
- CT pelvis can show extravesical local disease (T3b) with a high negative predictive value, but has limitations in demonstrating exact locoregional spread
- MRI pelvis is superior for local staging, particularly for extravesical disease
- CT/MRI should ideally precede or follow cystoscopy/transurethral resection of bladder tumour (TURBT) by 2 weeks
- Bone scan is required if clinically indicated
- FDG-PET-CT is not routinely recommended in staging, but has an evolving role

Testicular tumours (non-seminomatous germ cell tumours and seminoma)
Diagnosis
- High-resolution bilateral testicular US is essential; it can confirm a solid mass and display the size and status of the contralateral testis
- *Trans-scrotal testicular biopsy is contraindicated and condemned*

Staging
- CT abdomen and pelvis is commonly used, particularly to show retroperitoneal adenopathy; alternately; MRI can be used
- Chest can be imaged with CXR; CT chest is mandatory when CT abdomen reveals retroperitoneal adenopathy
- Bone scan or brain imaging is required only if clinically indicated
- PET-CT is *not* recommended in routine initial staging

Response assessment
- CT abdomen with CXR/CT chest
- PET-CT has no role in routine practice

Follow-up
- CXR + CT abdomen; CT pelvis in Stages II and III
- PET-CT has an optional role only in the follow-up of Stage II and III seminomas

Recommended reading

Beets-Tan RG, Lambregts DM, Maas M et al. (2013) Magnetic resonance imaging for the clinical management of rectal cancer patients: recommendations from the 2012 European Society of Gastrointestinal and Abdominal Radiology (ESGAR) consensus meeting. *Eur Radiol* 23(9):2522–2531.

Beitler JJ, Muller S, Grist WJ et al. (2010) Prognostic accuracy of computed tomography findings for patients with laryngeal cancer undergoing laryngectomy. *J Clin Oncol* 28(14):2318–2322.

Callery MP, Chang KJ, Fishman EK, Talamonti MS, William Traverso L, Linehan DC (2009). Pretreatment assessment of resectable and borderline resectable pancreatic cancer: expert consensus statement. *Ann Surg Oncol* 16(7):1727–1733.

Chinot OL, Macdonald DR, Abrey LE, Zahlmann G, Kerloëguen Y, Cloughesy TF (2013) Response assessment criteria for glioblastoma: practical adaptation and implementation in clinical trials of antiangiogenic therapy. *Curr Neurol Neurosci Rep* 13(5):347.

European Association for the Study of the Liver; European Organization for Research and Treatment of Cancer (2012) EASL-EORTC clinical practice guidelines: management of hepatocellular carcinoma. *J Hepatol* 56(4):908–943.

Gotzsche PC, Nielsen M (2011) Screening for breast cancer with mammography. *Cochrane Database Syst Rev* (1):CD001877.

Hanly AM, Ryan EM, Rogers AC, McNamara DA, Madoff RD, Winter DC; MERRION Study Group (2014) Multicenter Evaluation of Rectal cancer Re-imaging post Neoadjuvant (MERRION) therapy. *Ann Surg* 259(4):723–727.

Hricak H, Choyke PL, Eberhardt SC, Leibel SA, Scardino PT (2007). Imaging prostate cancer: a multidisciplinary perspective. *Radiology* 243(1):28–53.

Liao LJ, Lo WC, Hsu WL, Wang CT, Lai MS (2012) Detection of cervical lymph node metastasis in head and neck cancer patients with clinically N0 neck – a meta-analysis comparing different imaging modalities. *BMC Cancer* 12:236.

Oka K, Yakushiji T, Sato H, Hirai T, Yamashita Y, Mizuta H (2010) The value of diffusion-weighted imaging for monitoring the chemotherapeutic response of osteosarcoma: a comparison between average apparent diffusion coefficient and minimum apparent diffusion coefficient. *Skeletal Radiol* 39(2):141–146.

Wu Y, Li P, Zhang H *et al.* (2013) Diagnostic value of fluorine 18 fluorodeoxyglucose positron emission tomography/computed tomography for the detection of metastases in non-small-cell lung cancer patients. *Int J Cancer* 132(2):E37–47.

8 Pathology

Joanna S.Y. Chan, Rossitza Draganova-Tacheva, Wei Jiang, Zi-Xuan Wang and Stephen Peiper

Department of Pathology, Anatomy, & Cell Biology, Thomas Jefferson University, Philadelphia, PA, USA

Anatomical pathology is made up of several fields, most notably surgical pathology, cytology, haematopathology and molecular pathology, each of which will be discussed separately. In conjunction with the presenting clinical manifestations, the anatomical pathologist is able to make a tissue diagnosis, which will guide the best possible patient care.

Surgical pathology

Surgical pathology is the practice of establishing disease diagnosis on the basis of patient tissue obtained by biopsy or resection performed by clinicians and surgeons. The gross anatomy of the specimen is evaluated with attention to the size, appearance and architecture expected for a given tissue type. The specimen is then triaged for appropriate processing. For the majority of diagnoses, the tissue is fixed (usually in formalin), dissected and then stained for evaluation by light microscopy (Fig. 8.1).

Clinical information

Before a tissue diagnosis of any type can be rendered, a certain amount of clinical information must accompany the specimen to facilitate safe and accurate specimen handling. In particular, demographic material must be specified as required by the Joint Commission on Accreditation of Healthcare Organizations (JCAHO). All patient specimens must be submitted with at least two patient identifiers, the name of the requesting physician, date and time of procedure when the patient specimen was acquired, and specimen identification. The clinical request must also include relevant history. In addition, a specific clinical request or question from the providing physician can be very helpful both in the proper handling of the specimen and in generating an accurate and germane pathological diagnosis.

Clinician requests may include specific specimen handling designations, such as 'intraoperative diagnosis', 'rush', 'routine' or 'gross only'. Such designations, along with the clinical history, facilitate appropriate handling of specimens in a timely manner.

Specimen handling

It is important that after being appropriately labelled, pathology specimens are transported as quickly as possible to pathology laboratories to prevent autolysis, which can significantly limit their diagnostic quality. Autolysis refers to the self-destruction of a cell through the action of its own enzymes, and takes place as soon as tissue is removed from its blood supply. A variety of factors affect autolysis rate:
- Increase in temperature: can occur during sample mishandling; will frequently accelerate autolysis
- Particular tissue types, such as pancreatic tissue, are more susceptible to autolysis as a function of their inherent enzymatic composition.

The loss of histological features, which occurs as a consequence of autolysis, increases the difficulty of making a microscopic diagnosis. To maximize the diagnostic potential of a specimen, autolysis is retarded by refrigeration, frequently at temperatures just above the freezing point of water. Additionally, particular attention should be directed at the rapid transport and processing of specimens with increased risk of autolysis. Autolysis is arrested by the process of fixation of the specimen, which is discussed below.

Fixation

In addition to arresting autolysis, fixation allows tissue to be thinly sectioned, inactivates infectious agents, stabilizes tissue components and allows proper staining with various agents. The standard fixative solution for most tissues is 10% phosphate-buffered formalin. In addition, a number

---

UICC Manual of Clinical Oncology, Ninth Edition. Edited by Brian O'Sullivan, James D. Brierley, Anil K. D'Cruz, Martin F. Fey, Raphael Pollock, Jan B. Vermorken and Shao Hui Huang. © 2015 UICC. Published 2015 by John Wiley & Sons, Ltd.

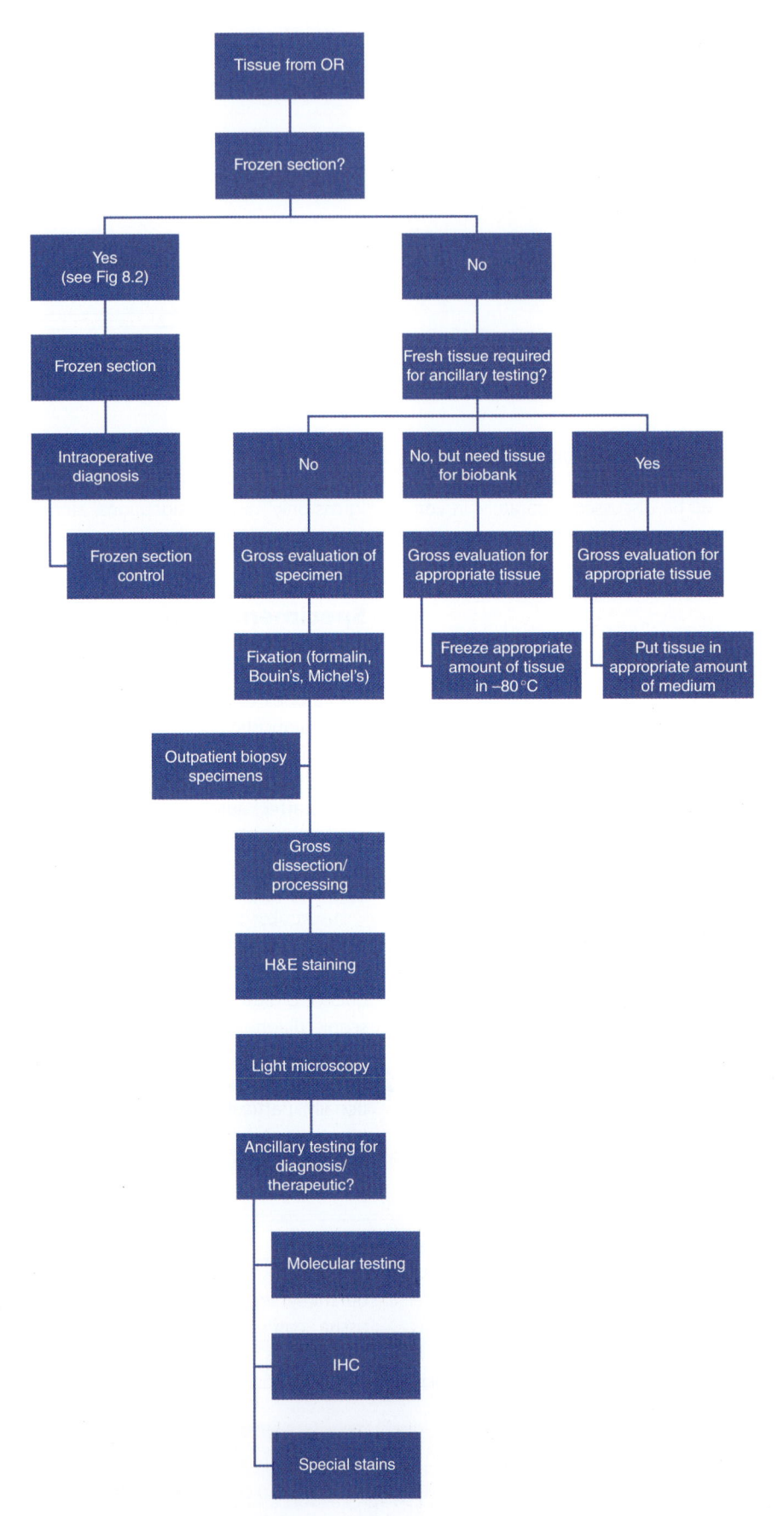

Figure 8.1 Typical work flow of specimen in surgical pathology.

of less commonly used fixative agents are available depending on the presenting diagnostic question and specific specimen type, such as glutaraldehyde for specimens that require electron microscopy. As discussed below, the initial fixative strategy can be critical to the resulting histological and molecular characterization of the specimen. Pre- or peri-procedural consultation with the anatomical pathologist regarding the appropriate specimen handling is recommended in the case of ambiguity.

The process of fixation irrevocably alters protein structure, solubilizes certain tissue components, shrinks tissue and degrades nucleic acids. These alterations can limit the type of examination done, particularly certain molecular and immunohistochemical (IHC) tests. Tissue fixation precludes intraoperative diagnosis, i.e. frozen section analysis. Rapid transport of these specimens in the 'fresh' state, without application of formalin fixative, is essential.

In some specific instances, the length of time of formalin fixation should be noted, as it may affect outcomes in later ancillary testing, such as hormone receptor testing in breast carcinoma. Consultation with the anatomical pathologist regarding the most appropriate fixative agent and time of fixation may be of great value to the clinician. This is particularly true when multiple modalities of diagnostic testing are required, such as in the case of haematological malignancies.

Intraoperative consultation

Intraoperative consultation, also commonly called 'frozen sections', is a service provided by pathologists where rapid diagnosis is given to guide intra- and peri-operative treatment. In an intraoperative consultation, unfixed tissue is sent to the pathology laboratory directly from the operating room. The specimen is then grossly evaluated, before being processed for immediate histological evaluation, as outlined in Fig. 8.2.

In the case of intraoperative consultation, clinical history and a direct clinical question are critical in guiding the diagnostic approach. It is helpful if the submitting physician indicates the reason for the consultation. There are a few common reasons:

- *Guide surgical plan*. This is one of the most frequent indications for intraoperative consultation, as clinicians frequently alter their surgical plan based on multiple staging factors, such as depth of invasion or presence of metastasis. Two such examples are:
  - *Depth of invasion*. In endometrial adenocarcinoma, a Stage 1A tumour with depth of invasion of <50% of the myometrial wall only requires a total hysterectomy and salpingo-oophorectomy. Tumours with myometrial invasion of deeper than 50%, requires pelvic lymph node and peritoneal sampling in addition to total hysterectomy and salpingo-oophorectomy.
  - *Presence of metastasis*. In pancreatic adenocarcinoma, a single neoplastic lesion within the head of pancreas mass can be resected in a Whipple procedure. If metastatic disease is present at the time of laparotomy, however, surgical resection would not be considered standard of care.
- *Evaluate surgical margins*. In cases where limited resection is required because of critical or limited adjacent anatomy, evaluation of the surgical margins for neoplastic cells is required to limit excessively large *en bloc* resections.
- *Confirmation of lesional tissue*. Occasionally the tissue necessary for histological diagnosis is difficult to obtain, e.g. in the case of highly necrotic tumours. These lesions are frequently difficult to confidently sample for viable and diagnostically adequate tissue at the time of biopsy or resection. The periprocedural pathological consultation may prevent the need for repeat biopsy or resection.
- *Guide pathology processing*. Some tissues require specific handling that differs from routine pathology, particularly specimens that require multiple or more advanced diagnostic pathological

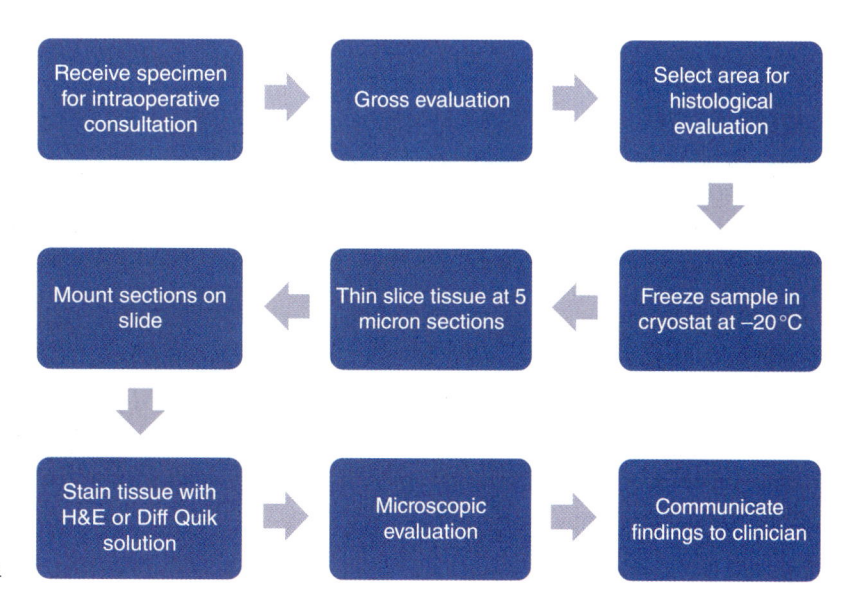

Figure 8.2 Intraoperative consultation work flow.

modalities. For example, lymphoid tissue submitted for a haematopoietic diagnosis is often partitioned into fixed tissue for histological diagnosis and unfixed tissue for flow cytometry.

- *To identify the presence of tissue or the organ of origin of the specimen*. Occasionally, it can be difficult to grossly distinguish tissue type or viability in the operating room or procedure suite, such as during parathyroidectomy, when it may be grossly difficult to identify a discrete parathyroid gland in the background of thyroid tissue. Histological confirmation of parathyroid tissue is frequently required via an intraoperative consultation to confirm an adequate resection.

While intraoperative diagnosis via frozen section can be useful to clinicians, there are also several limitations:

- *Limited sampling*. While every effort is made to freeze the area that best answers the clinical question, only a small piece of tissue can be microscopically evaluated. In heterogeneous lesions, the frozen section may not adequately represent the entire specimen. In the case of mucinous ovarian tumours, adenocarcinoma may arise in the background of otherwise benign cystadenoma.
- *Frozen artefact*. Unlike routine histological sections, tissue sampled for intraoperative consultations are frozen in a −20 °C cryostat to allow the thin sections necessary for microscopic evaluation to be cut. The process of freezing can create artificial changes that can obscure cytological features necessary for diagnosis. One such artefact is nuclear clearing, which can look similar to some histological features of papillary thyroid carcinoma.
- *Lack of special studies*. Making the correct pathological diagnosis often requires the use of special studies such as IHC or special stains. As these stains may take 24 hours to process, they cannot be used in rapid intraoperative consultation. Micrometastasis to axillary lymph nodes for metastatic breast carcinoma, particularly lobular type, can be virtually impossible to diagnose without immunohistochemical staining (Fig. 8.3). Diagnosis of such subtle pathology can be limited during rapid intraoperative consultation.
- *Tissue- and neoplastic-specific limitations*. Inherent limitations of the frozen technique preclude diagnosis of haematological malignancy. In addition, particular tissue types, such as adipose and bony tissue, are not amenable to evaluation by frozen sample processing. In these instances, diagnosis must be deferred to permanent processing.

The consulting physician must keep in mind that these limitations may result in apparent discrepancy between an intraoperative diagnosis and a final diagnosis. Currently, a 3% major discrepancy rate is reported by the College of American Pathologists (CAP). These discrepancies are divided into four major categories:

- *Sampling error*. As discussed previously, only a small piece of tissue can be frozen for evaluation. Even when the entire tissue is submitted for freezing, only a small percentage of tissue is available on the slide for microscopic examination, and deeper sections may reveal a different diagnosis.
- *Interpretive error*. The combination of freezing artefact, lack of special studies and lack of consultation may lead to an interpretive error by the pathologist.
- *Technical error*. A poor frozen section technique can lead to interpretation errors. Sections that are cut too thick or poorly mounted on the slide can obscure important histological features. Certain types of tissue can be difficult to evaluate on frozen section, and frozen section analysis should be avoided if possible for these.
- *Incorrect/incomplete clinical history*. Clinical history is necessary to place histological features into diagnostic context. One example is a history of radiation or prior procedures, which can cause cytological atypia that can easily be mistaken for dysplasia. A history of malignancy can also contextualize dysplastic cells.

Intraoperative consultations are a collaborative process between the clinician and pathologist. A specimen clearly designated as requiring an intraoperative consultation with appropriate clinical history will generally lead to a diagnosis that can allow the clinician or surgeon to direct patient care. However, given the limitations of intraoperative diagnosis, the results of these consultations should be considered more as an immediate director of care. The final diagnosis should only be considered following evaluation of the permanent sections.

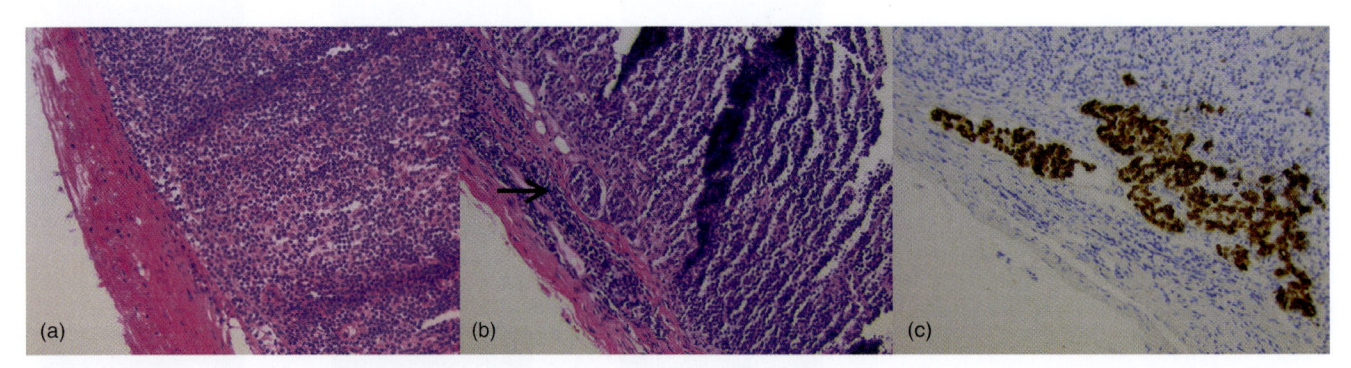

Figure 8.3 Three images of the same area of a sentinel axillary lymph node sent for intraoperative consultation for metastatic poorly differentiated breast carcinoma. (a) Intraoperative diagnosis slide. (b) Permanent section of same tissue, with micrometastasis (arrow). (c) Immunohistochemistry for pan-cytokeratin of same tissue highlighting metastatic cells. H&E, 20×; IHC, 20×.

Gross evaluation

All specimens received in pathology require a gross evaluation. Even small biopsy specimens must be described and measured to ensure appropriate histological evaluation. Large resection specimens need to be oriented, measured and evaluated for gross abnormalities prior to dissection. Accurate gross characterization along with clinical information typically guides later orientation and dissection. The components of gross evaluation and dissections are:

- *Orientation*. While most specimens can be oriented by anatomical landmark, complex specimens may require additional orientation by the surgeon, such as a neck dissection or partial breast resection. This orientation can be done in *in situ* or immediately *ex vivo*, often with sutures, ink or clips.
- *Description*. All gross features and lesions are measured and described, including size, colour and texture.
- *Dissection*. Hollow organs are opened and solid organs are serially sectioned at 5–10-mm intervals to identify pathological processes. The specimen sampling should not only allow for identification of a lesion, but also identify prognostic features, such as stage, presence of lymphovascular invasion and margin status.

Entire specimens are rarely submitted for microscopic evaluation. Instead, specific areas are sampled to render a complete diagnosis. Many lesions have a characteristic gross appearance, underscoring the importance of accurate clinical history and conscientious gross characterization.

An example of typical tissue processing can be considered for a mixed germ cell tumour of the testis. These tumours are often made up of various tissue types, each with its own specific gross appearance, histology and prognostic significance. In general, histological evaluation is performed for every 1–2 cm of lesion. The interface between lesion and uninvolved tissue is sampled as well to evaluate their relationship. Besides sampling representative areas of all identified lesions, representative sections of all anatomical organs included in the specimen are also submitted.

Surgical resections for malignancy often include lymphadenectomy as part of the staging procedure. For some procedures to be considered an adequate staging resection, a minimum number of lymph nodes needs to be evaluated, such as at least 12 lymph nodes in colon cancer. Therefore, all lymph nodes must be identified and evaluated microscopically for metastasis. The same degree of meticulous analysis is performed for each lymph node sampled. In addition, any remaining remnants of tissue used for intraoperative consultation are submitted for permanent sectioning to create a frozen section control.

Processing and mounting

After the specimen is dissected and tissue is selected for histological diagnosis, it is submitted for processing. Processing allows the tissue to be infiltrated with paraffin, which provides a structural framework with a density similar to that of tissue. The similar density of the tissue and paraffin allows the thinnest possible sections to be cut.

The tissue is dehydrated, cleared and infiltrated with paraffin. This process may take several hours. The processed tissue is then oriented and embedded in a paraffin block so that it can be sectioned such that the orientation of a three-dimensional object is apparent on a two-dimensional slide. In certain situations, such as margins or hollow pieces of tissue, appropriate orientation is critical. Once the tissue is embedded, it is thinly sectioned at 4-μm intervals to be mounted on a glass slide. For biopsy material (gastrointestinal, gynaecological, skin, etc.), multiple slides are prepared from a single block in order to provide maximal sampling of the tissue. Some practices prepare an unstained slide in between two different levels (e.g. prostate biopsies) to minimize the loss of small areas of interest on deeper sections.

Histological evaluation

Once the tissue section is mounted on a glass slide, it is stained for routine histological evaluation by light microscopy. The most common stain is haematoxylin and eosin (H&E). Haematoxylin, a natural dye that is extracted from the Logwood tree, is an aromatic carbon molecule which is electron rich and has an affinity for nucleic acids, but can also non-specifically stain mucin and calcium. As a result, the nuclei of cells, calcific atheromatous plaques and mucinous materials within tumours or extracellular matrix stain an avid blue when evaluated on typical light microscopy. Eosin is a negatively charged synthetic dye that binds to positively charged proteins and carbohydrates in the cytoplasm and connective tissue. These structures typically stain a light to avid pink.

While H&E may be sufficient in most routine pathology, special studies are often utilized for a definitive diagnosis. These include special histochemical stains, IHC studies and molecular analyses, including *in situ* hybridization and applied genomic techniques.

Special histochemical stains

In contrast to many molecular assays, most histochemical stains can be performed on formalin-fixed tissues. The most commonly used stains in the laboratory are listed in Table 8.1. These special stains can be useful in determining cell type, identifying microorganisms and highlighting tissue structures.

The use of special stains in cancer diagnosis is, however, somewhat limited. A reticulin stain may be useful in differentiating a regenerative nodule from a well-differentiated hepatocellular carcinoma. Mucin stains are most commonly used in the differential diagnosis of carcinoma to confirm the presence of glandular differentiation seen in adenocarcinoma. An elastin stain can help highlight the elastic lamina of arteries and veins to aid in the diagnosis of lymphovascular invasion. Special stains for microorganisms sometimes help to distinguish an infectious/pseudotumour process from a neoplastic process. Examples of these stains are shown in Fig. 8.4.

Table 8.1 Commonly used histochemical stains

Stain	Targets	Comment
Mucin		
Alcian blue	Acid mucin: blue (normal intestinal epithelium)	
Periodic acid-Schiff (PAS)-alcian blue	Intestinal metaplasia: purple Normal gastric epithelium: pink	
Mucicarmine	Mucin: deep rose to red *Cryptococcus*: capsule stains deep rose to red	Confirms adenocarcinoma differentiation
Connective tissue		
Trichrome (Masson)	Collagen: blue Nuclei: black Cytoplasm, keratin, muscle: red	Liver (assess fibrosis)
Reticulin (Gomori, Snook)	Reticulin: black	Organ architecture (liver, spleen)
Elastic stain (van Gieson)	Elastic fibres: blue-black to black	Identification of arteries and veins in vasculitis and tumour lymphovascular invasion
Pigments, minerals and cytoplasmic granules		
Fontana–Masson	Melanin: black	Melanoma
Iron (Perl's)	Iron: blue	
Calcium (von Kossa)	Calcium: black	
Microorganisms		
Gram (Brown Hopps, Brown Brenn)	Gram-positive bacteria: blue Gram-negative bacteria: red	
Gomori-methenamine silver (GMS)	Fungi: black *Pneumocystis jirovecii*: black	Bacteria will also stain black There may be considerable background staining
PAS	Fungi: red	Stains glycogen, mucin, mucoprotein, glycoprotein, and fungi.
Acid fast bacilli (AFB) (Ziehl–Neelsen, Kinyoun, Fite)	*Mycobacteria*: bright red *Nocardia*: pink	Acid-fast: high lipid content of the cell wall of mycobacteria causes them to bind and retain the basic carbol-fuchsin dye even after strong decolourization with acid-alcohol Also stains *Cryptosporidium parvum*, *Isospora* and *Cyclospora* cysts and hooklets of cysticerci Fite stain is used to identify *Mycobacterium leprae*
Warthin starry	Spirochetes: black *Helicobacter pylori*: black *Bartonella henselae*: black	Silver nitrate-based method
Others		
Congo red	Amyloid: apple-green birefringence during polarization	
Oil red O	Fat: red	Frozen tissue needed (lipids removed by most fixatives or tissue processing)

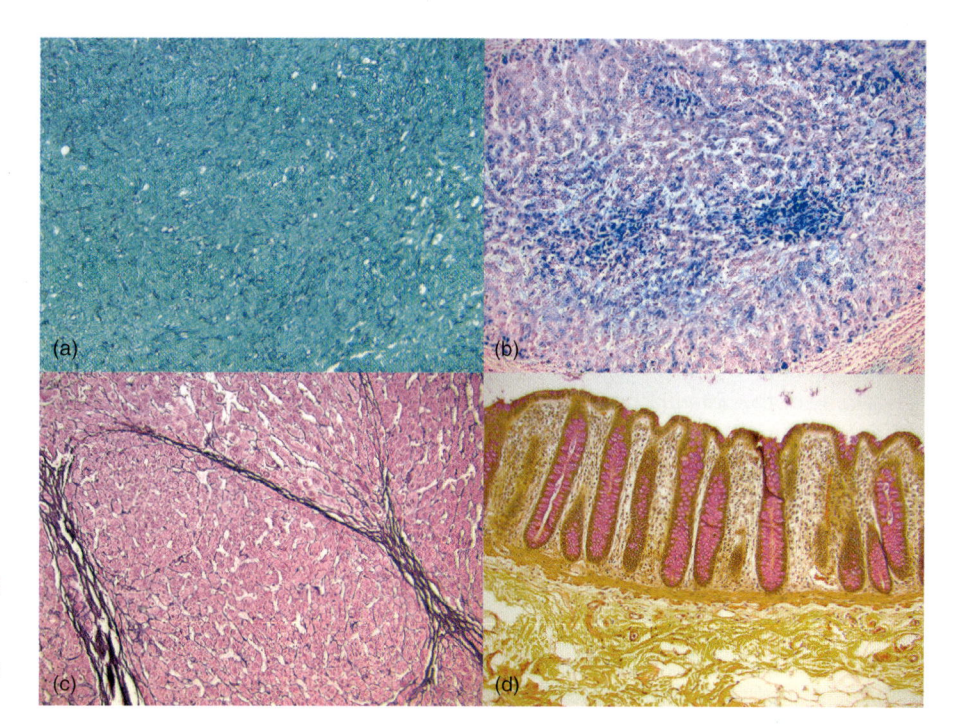

Figure 8.4 Special histochemical stains. (a) Gomori-methanamine stain highlighting fungal organisms. (b) Iron stain in liver. (c) Reticulin stain in a cirrhotic liver. (d) Mucicarmine stain highlighting mucin in colonic mucosa.

Immunohistochemistry

After examination of the H&E slides, additional information about the lesional tissue may be necessary to provide the most correct diagnosis. IHC compliments light microscopy by providing information at a cellular level.

IHC is based on the specific binding between antigen and antibody. Two antibodies are used in tandem in order to maximize the conspicuity of the antibody–antigen interaction with a technique similar to the commonly performed enzyme-linked immunosorbant assay (ELISA) technique frequently performed in biochemistry laboratories. The principle aim of the antigen-primary antibody-secondary antibody IHC technique is to have the highest signal-to-noise ratio. Several more advanced methods such as signal amplification, blocking non-specific background staining and antigen retrieval are often employed to optimize visualization of the specific reaction products.

The most common indications for IHC use include:
- *Diagnosis and classification of tumours.* A fairly exhaustive list is provided in Table 8.2 for common cell lineage markers.
- *Carcinoma of unknown primary.* A wide variety of somewhat specific IHC markers for different cell types are available. By using the available IHC stains (Tables 8.2 and 8.3), the primary lineage of a neoplastic cell can frequently be determined by a reductive process using multiple stains. This is particularly useful in the setting of metastatic disease in which the selection of treatment modality is dependent on the underlying primary cell type. Unfortunately, no single immunostain is entirely specific, and a diagnosis should be based on histomorphological findings, clinical history and multiple IHC stains with a selected panel of antibodies. The aggregate pathological

Table 8.2 Common immunohistochemistry lineage markers

Epithelial markers	AE1/AE3, Cam5.2, CK7, CK20, CK5/6, EMA, CEA
Vascular markers	CD31, CD34, ERG
Melanocytic markers	Melan A/Mart1, HMB45, tyrosinase, S100
Lymphoid markers	CD3 (T cells), CD20 (B cells), CD15, CD30, Pax5, others
Histiocytic markers	CD68, CD163
Neuroendocrine markers	Synaptophysin, chromogranin, CD56
Muscle markers	Smooth muscle actin, desmin, caldesmon (smooth muscle), myogenin (skeletal muscle), MyoD1 (skeletal muscle)

Table 8.3 CK7/CK20 immunohistochemistry expression patterns in common epithelial cancers

CK7/CK20 expression pattern	Common cancers
CK7+/CK20+	Pancreas, bile duct, stomach
CK7+/CK20−	Lung, breast, endometrium, ovary
CK7−/CK20+	Colon
CK7−/CK20−	Kidney, liver, adrenal, prostate

information will contribute to the decision-making process for determining the most accurate diagnosis.
- *Prognostic and predictive markers, particularly in the evaluation of breast carcinoma.* For breast carcinomas, the current guidelines published by the American Society of Clinical Oncology(ASCO)/CAP recommend that oestrogen receptor (ER) and progesterone receptor (PR) status be determined on all invasive breast cancers and breast cancer recurrences, and human epidermal growth factor receptor 2 (*HER2*) or *ERBB2* status be determined in all invasive breast cancers.

  The ER and PR biomarkers provide an indication of prognosis and of the potential benefit of hormonal therapy. Generally, ER/PR-positive tumours are more likely to respond to endocrine therapy and have a better prognosis, stage-for-stage, than receptor-negative tumours.

  The tumour marker, *HER2*, is an oncogene on the long arm of chromosome 17 that is amplified in approximately 20% of breast cancers. Amplification is associated with a worse prognosis (higher rate of recurrence and mortality) in patients with newly diagnosed breast cancer who do not receive any adjuvant systemic therapy. Interestingly, *HER2* status also appears to be predictive for response to different chemotherapeutic agents. Herceptin (trastuzumab) is the first molecularly targeted drug. Currently, there are multiple FDA-approved companion diagnostic tests which determine eligibility for treatment with Herceptin (trastuzumab) based on the presence of *HER2* amplification.

  The guidelines for analysis of these biomarkers propose detailed testing algorithms that rely on accuracy and reproducibility of the assay performance. Specimen selection criteria, fixation time in formalin and interpretation criteria have all been specified. In the presence of appropriate internal and external controls, ER and PR assays are considered positive if at least 1% of the tumour nuclei have positive staining. For *HER2* analysis, either IHC or fluorescence *in situ* hybridization (FISH) assay may be performed. A positive *HER2* result is an IHC staining of 3+ (uniform, intense membrane staining of >30% of invasive tumour cells), a FISH result of >6 *HER2* gene copies per nucleus or a FISH ratio (*HER2* gene signals to chromosome 17 signals) of >2.2; a negative result is an IHC staining of 0 or 1+, a FISH result of <4.0 *HER2* gene copies per nucleus or a FISH ratio of <1.8. Equivocal results require additional action for final determination.
- *Screening for familial cancer syndromes.* Approximately 2–7% of colorectal carcinomas are attributed to an aetiology of Lynch syndrome, or hereditary non-polyposis colorectal cancer (HNPCC). Individuals with Lynch syndrome have a germline mutation in one of several genes encoding proteins involved in DNA mismatch repair, including *MLH1*, *MSH2*, *MSH6* and *PMS2*. Either IHC or microsatellite instability IHC testing may be performed on tumour tissue as a screening test for this syndrome (see also Molecular pathology). If the result is positive, additional genetic testing should be performed on blood cells to determine a germline mutation.
- *Identification of microinvasion and micrometastasis.* For breast carcinoma, sometimes it is difficult to distinguish between *in situ* lesions and microinvasive cancer on H&E sections. As a result, IHC evaluation for antigens of myoepithelial markers such as p63, calponin, smooth muscle actin and smooth muscle myosin heavy chain can be used for evaluation. IHC is also particularly useful in sentinel lymph node biopsy for breast cancer and melanoma. Lymph nodes that may appear negative on H&E sections now require analysis by IHC to rule out the presence of isolated tumour cells or micrometastasis in the lymph nodes provided during these oncological resections.

Pathology reporting

Once a diagnosis is finalized, the results need to be made available to the clinicians in a timely fashion. For routine pathology in which there are no special requirements, such as a biopsy, a final report can usually be issued in 2 working days, as recommended in CAP guidelines. The final pathological report should contain the following demographic and clinical information: institution identifiers, patient identifiers, name of the pathologist responsible for the report, submitting physician, date of procedure and date the specimen was received. Essential pathological information to be conveyed to the ordering physician in the report includes the intraoperative diagnosis, gross description, final diagnosis and synoptic report (see CAP guidelines) for malignant tumours. An example of a CAP-approved synoptic is shown in Fig. 8.5. The synoptic reports contain all the relevant information for prognosis as well as pathological staging.

The final diagnoses can often be broadly classified as one of four categories: benign, premalignant, malignant and, rarely, lesions of uncertain malignant potential. Figure 8.6 is an example of a premalignant lesion compared to an invasive carcinoma of the cervix. The definition of terms commonly seen in pathology reports is given in Table 8.4.

Occasionally, an addendum report is issued to report additional findings which do not change the final diagnosis. Rarely, a final diagnosis may be revised for various reasons, including intra- or extra-departmental review requested by the clinician or pathologist, or additional clinical information or ancillary testing become available. In these instances, an amendment report is issued and, more importantly, there is direct discussion with the clinician or surgeon.

Communication between pathologist and clinician

Effective communication between pathologist and clinician is critical to ensuring correct diagnosis and an appropriate patient treatment plan. The pathologist requires germane clinical, radiological and prior treatment information in order to establish the correct pathological diagnosis. The anatomical pathologist makes every attempt to communicate critical values in a timely manner to clinicians. A critical value is a pathologic diagnosis that may require the clinician's immediate attention. Such diagnoses include fat in endometrial curettage specimen, malignancy in superior vena cava syndrome, or transplant rejection.

> **Synoptic Report Example**
> **CARCINOMA OF THE LUNG**
>
> Specimen type: Lung, left upper lobe
> Procedure: Lobectomy
> Specimen integrity: Intact
>
> Tumor site: Upper lobe
> Tumor size: 1.7 x 1.5 x 1.2 cm
> Tumor focality: Unifocal
> Histologic type: Squamous cell carcinoma
> Visceral pleural invasion: Not identified
> Direct tumor extension into extrapulmonary structures: Not applicable
> Bronchial margin: Uninvolved by invasive carcinoma
> Vascular margin: Uninvolved by invasive carcinoma
> Parenchymal (stapled) margin: Not applicable
> Parietal pleural margin: Not applicable
> Chest wall margin: Not applicable
> Other attached tissue margin: Not applicable
> Distance to closest margin: 4.2 cm from vascular margin
> Neoadjuvant treatment effect: Not applicable
> Lymph-vascular invasion: Not identified
>
> Pathologic staging (pTNM):
> Primary tumor: pT1a
> Regional lymph nodes: pN0
> Number examined: 5
> Number involved: 0

Figure 8.5 Example of CAP-approved synoptic report for lung adenocarcinoma.

The pathologist also needs to communicate with the clinicians when an urgent or unexpected diagnosis is reached, such as unsuspected malignancy in a fracture site or unrecognized infection, which may result in a rapid change in the plan of care. As stated above, a change in diagnosis should always prompt direct communication with the clinician.

Cytopathology

Cytopathology is a branch of anatomical pathology that utilizes evaluation of morphology of single cells or small cell clusters. It is becoming increasingly important for detection, screening and follow-up of benign and malignant neoplasms. Cytopathology is reliable and cost-effective, and usually employs simple and non-invasive patient techniques to obtain specimens.

The most common types of non-gynaecological specimens received in cytology laboratories are:

- Fine needle aspiration (FNA) biopsy: solid or cystic lesions
- Body fluids: urine, cerebrospinal fluid, pleural, pericardial and peritoneal fluids
- Washings: most commonly bronchial and peritoneal
- Scrapes or brushings: respiratory and gastrointestinal tracts
- Bronchoalveolar lavage (BAL)
- Direct smears: secretions, sputum, mucosal and skin lesions.

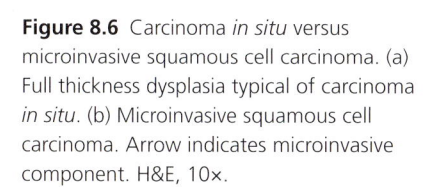

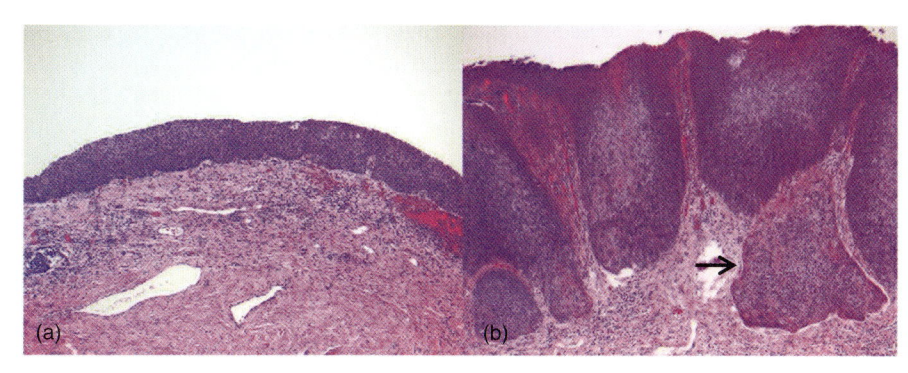

Figure 8.6 Carcinoma *in situ* versus microinvasive squamous cell carcinoma. (a) Full thickness dysplasia typical of carcinoma *in situ*. (b) Microinvasive squamous cell carcinoma. Arrow indicates microinvasive component. H&E, 10×.

Table 8.4 Terms commonly used in pathology diagnoses

Neoplasm	Abnormal mass of tissue, growth of which exceeds and persists in the same excessive manner after cessation of the stimuli which evoked the change
Adenoma	Epithelial neoplasm that forms glandular patterns. Depending on context, may imply low-grade dysplasia, i.e. tubular adenoma of the colon
Sarcoma	Malignant tumour arising from mesenchymal tissue
Carcinoma	Malignant neoplasm of epithelial cell origin. May be further subclassified based on histology, i.e. *adenocarcinoma* (glandular growth pattern)
Carcinoma in situ	Dysplastic changes involving the entire thickness, but confined to the epithelium with no mesenchymal invasion; usually considered a premalignant condition
Dysplasia	Disordered epithelial growth, characterized by a loss of uniformity in individual cells as well as loss of architectural orientation
Metaplasia	Transformation of one cell type to another; does not necessarily denote malignancy
Pleomorphism	Variation in size and shape; usually referring to nuclei or individual cells

Gynaecological specimens include:
- Conventional Papanicolaou (Pap) cervical smears
- Liquid-based cervical preparations: ThinPrep, SurePath and others.

Collection and processing of specimens

Proper collection and fixation of the specimens is of paramount importance for an optimal diagnostic cell sample. The majority of false-negative and false-positive diagnoses arise from problems with collection and fixation of specimens. Different methods are employed in the collection of specimens depending on the type of specimen and laboratory. The individual obtaining the specimen should be familiar with the techniques and be aware that the sample should be fixed as soon as possible after collection to minimize artefacts. Some special diagnostic tests such as molecular, cytogenetic, IHC and flow cytometry may require collecting the specimen in a specific media or fixative.

Laboratories create protocols that include guidance for specimen collection, processing and recording of the specimens. Similar to surgical pathology, the specimens must be identified with the patient's name and a unique identifier, such as a birth date, and must be accompanied by a requisition form with the requesting physician's name, date of specimen collection, specimen source and appropriate clinical information.

After processing and staining, the samples are examined by light microscopy. Most laboratories use a combination of Diff Quik stain for air-dried slides and Papanicolaou stain for alcohol-fixed smears. Cell blocks can be created by centrifuging cytology specimens and concentrating the cells into a pellet. These cells are then fixed in formalin and then processed in a manner similar to tissue samples in surgical pathology. This allows the cells to be stained with H&E, as well as be used for IHC and special staining for characterization of unknown tumours and molecular studies.

Screening, reporting and quality control

The majority of cytology volume is gynaecological specimens. The screening of slides prior to final diagnosis is performed by certified cytotechnologists or pathologists. Although a cytology technologist may issue final diagnoses for normal cervical cytology specimens, a pathologist performs final interpretation of all non-gynaecological and abnormal gynaecological specimens. A random review of 10% of normal cervical cytology specimens is required for quality assurance. The cytology report should use a nomenclature of which all involved in the patient's care are fully aware. To make the cervical terminology uniform, reproducible and unambiguous to clinicians, most laboratories use the Bethesda System for Reporting Cervical Cytology 2001. Thyroid cytology reports are also being standardized using the Bethesda System for Reporting Thyroid Cytopathology. For non-thyroid, non-gynaecological specimens, narrative reports are used.

Laboratories must have mechanisms for internal and external quality control with the objective of avoiding false-negative and false-positive tests. These mechanisms should include measures relating to the screening and final interpretation of the specimens. This includes correlating cytology to relevant surgical pathology specimens as well as the previously mentioned random review of normal cervical cytology.

Cytological methods and types of specimens

The *Papanicolaou (Pap) test* for uterine cervix cancer screening was the first cancer screening test and is the most successful. Because the Pap smear is easily obtained and highly sensitive for premalignant disease, it is a good screening tool for cervical carcinoma. Screening programmes in developed countries have led to a large decline in cervical cancer incidence and mortality. About 80% of new cases occur in developing countries, which lack well-established screening programmes. In order for Pap smears to be effective in preventing squamous cell carcinoma, guidelines for follow-up and management of patients with pre-invasive lesions are critical.

Fine needle aspiration (FNA) biopsy of solid or cystic lesions uses a thin (22–25 G) needle to apply suction under negative pressure. For masses that are superficial and easily palpable, FNA may be performed by palpation without image guidance. For small, deeper lesions, image-guided FNA can be done in conjunction with a radiologist and interventionalist. Very small lesions, several millimetres in greatest dimension, can be successfully targeted using multiple imaging modalities, including ultrasound (US), computed tomography (CT), magnetic resonance imaging (MRI) or endoscopic ultrasound procedures. This has become an effective diagnostic tool that can establish a diagnosis without a more invasive biopsy. Image-guided FNA biopsy can be quickly accomplished in most body sites with minimal risk and discomfort, avoiding more invasive, risky and costly procedures. The active participation of a cytopathologist or cytotechnologist in the evaluation of the adequacy of specimens assures that sufficient cells for diagnosis are obtained with a minimum number of samples, thereby reducing patient risk and discomfort and the inconvenience of returning for additional samples if the initial material obtained is insufficient. The most common body sites biopsied using FNA are thyroid, lung, liver, breast, pancreas, salivary glands and other head & neck lesions, lymph nodes, mediastinum and retroperitoneal lesions including of the kidney and adrenal glands.

Thyroid FNA biopsy is the standard method for diagnosis of thyroid lesions. It is a common cytology specimen. Based on cytological diagnosis and in some cases in conjunction with molecular tests (*BRAF*, *NRAS* and analysis of other mutations), patients are appropriately triaged for timely clinical management or surgical intervention. Examples of thyroid cytopathology are shown in Figs. 8.7 and 8.8.

Endobronchial ultrasound-guided fine needle aspiration (EBUS-FNA) biopsy is a novel technique for initial lung cancer diagnosis and staging, and evaluation of unexplained mediastinal/hilar lymphadenopathy. It is a reliable, minimally invasive alternative to mediastinoscopy for the detection of nodal disease, reducing the need for surgical staging in up to two-thirds of patients.

Due to its anatomical location, the pancreas is relatively inaccessible to conventional methods of study. Taking a wedge biopsy or large-bore needle biopsy often leads to serious complications. With the introduction of modern endoscopic and imaging techniques, *endoscopic ultrasound-guided fine needle aspiration (EUS-FNA) biopsy* is rapidly gaining recognition as an excellent method of obtaining a pathological diagnosis among patients with benign and malignant lesions of the pancreas.

Urine cytology is a good example of a test used for the diagnosis of symptomatic patients and follow-up of patients with a history of urinary tract neoplasia. Voided urine specimens are easily obtained and do not require a specially equipped laboratory. To increase the specificity and sensitivity of the test, urine cytology can be combined with FISH to detect chromosomal aberrations. The UroVysion test was approved by the FDA for monitoring patients with known histories of carcinoma of the urinary bladder after initial diagnosis.

The *cytopathological analysis of body cavity fluids* has an important role in the diagnosis and staging of various neoplasms. The finding of malignant cells in serous effusions or washings implies an advanced stage cancer. Serous effusions may be removed at the time of surgical exploration or sampled by inserting a wide-bore needle through the body wall into the fluid-containing cavity. Peritoneal fluid is removed by abdominal paracentesis, pleural fluid by thoracentesis and pericardial fluid by pericardiocentesis. Most neoplasms in serous effusions are readily classifiable in terms of the primary neoplasm. Metastatic adenocarcinomas are by far the most common type of neoplasm to be found in serous effusions. Most adenocarcinoma cells in serous effusions originate from breast, lung or ovary. Other common tumour types are small cell carcinoma, squamous cell carcinoma, melanomas, lymphomas and malignant mesothelioma.

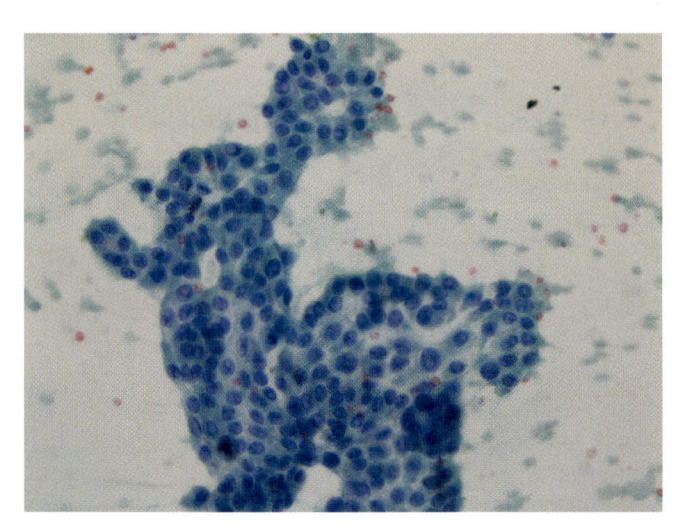

Figure 8.7 Papillary thyroid carcinoma. Papillary fragment showing enlarged ovoid nuclei with fine granular chromatin, nuclear grooves and many intranuclear pseudoinclusions. Papanicolaou, 40×.

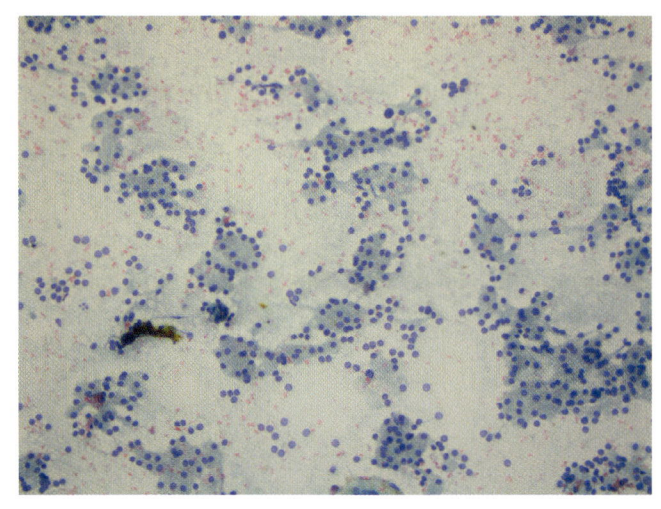

Figure 8.8 Follicular neoplasm. Cellular smear showing follicular cells arranged in microfollicles and small crowded groups. No colloid is present in the background. Papanicolaou, 20×.

Diagnostic haematopathology

The logistics for handling and processing specimens for the diagnosis of haematological malignancies have extensive overlap with those for other neoplastic disorders (i.e. solid tumours), but multiple additional analyses may be performed to enhance diagnostic accuracy. This section focuses on the specific measures that differ from those in the handling of non-haematological disorders and discusses the specialized studies that can enhance the diagnosis of lymphomas and leukaemias. These studies include:

- Cytogenomic analysis, including karyotyping and *in situ* hybridization with probes for the diagnosis of numerical, i.e. aneuploidy, and structural, i.e. translocations, rearrangements
- Immunophenotype analysis by flow cytometry
- Molecular genetic analysis.

The primary specimens for the diagnosis of lymphomas and leukaemias are lymph node and bone marrow biopsies and aspirates, respectively. For the diagnosis of lymphomas, an excisional biopsy of an intact lymph node is strongly preferred over aspirations or core needle biopsies for proper classification. The major reason for this requirement is the importance of overall nodal morphology in establishment of accurate diagnosis. The pattern of effacement of nodal architecture and the distribution of the neoplastic lymphoid infiltrate are part of the diagnostic criteria for lymphoma. In addition, in optimal practice, it is desirable to submit unfixed tissue for cytogenomic and immunophenotype studies, microbiological culture in some instances and the preparation of imprints ('touch preps'). Currently, most relevant molecular studies, notably analysis of immunoglobulin heavy chain (*IGH@* gene) rearrangement, can be performed on routinely processed tissues that have been fixed in formalin and embedded in paraffin (FFPE).

Optimal processing of lymph node biopsies requires coordinating tissue handling with the surgeon performing the lymph node biopsy. Typically, members of the haematopathology service obtain the biopsied lymph node fresh (without fixation) and divide the lymph node by sectioning (coronally) through the hilus. A common transport medium for haematopathology specimens is RPMI culture medium, which preserves cellular viability and does not preclude ancillary testing. Representative tissue from one side of the node should be submitted for cytogenetics and flow cytometry, and microbiological culture if clinically indicated. Imprints may be prepared before fixing the tissue in neutral buffered formalin. After fixation of the other side of the lymph node (as well as the remaining tissue from the side used for cytogenomics and flow cytometry) for several hours, multiple 3-mm sections should be submitted for histopathology. Cytogenomic analysis for chromosomal translocations and rearrangements (including *BCL6* and *IGH@* rearrangement using break-apart probes) can be performed on the imprints, cell suspensions or FFPE sections. However, for karyotype analysis, it is necessary to make suspensions of single cells. The karyotype has the advantage of detecting numerical and major structural abnormalities that are not included in the usual sets of probes used to identify known translocations that are diagnostic of specific lymphoma subtypes. Similarly, flow cytometric analysis is performed on single cell suspensions of live cells. It is an important diagnostic test because it is the only method to detect expression of immunoglobulin proteins on the cell surface, and thus, is fundamental to identifying monoclonal (i.e. clonally-restricted exclusive kappa or lambda) cell surface immunoglobulin light chain expression, as well as other diagnostic signatures defined by cell surface antigens, such as co-expression of cell surface CD5 and pan B-lymphocyte antigens (such as CD19 and CD20) in chronic lymphocytic leukaemia/small lymphocytic lymphoma.

The analysis of bone marrow pathology involves the interpretation of multiple types of processed specimens, including smears and sections of the clotted bone marrow aspirate, sections of the (decalcified) bone marrow biopsy and peripheral blood:

- *Bone marrow aspirate analysis.* The bone marrow aspirate smear provides insight into the dynamic status of haematopoiesis based on Wright-Giemsa staining, including the differentiation and maturation of myeloid, erythroid, and megakaryocytic precursors. This preparation may be used for establishing a differential count, which enables the calculation of the ratio of myeloid to erythroid precursors (M:E ratio) and blast percentages.
- *Bone marrow clot analysis.* Analysis of sections of the bone marrow clot shows the cellularity of bone marrow spicules and the morphology of bone marrow cells and infiltrates, if present. In addition, the bone marrow biopsy sections demonstrate the intact relationships of bone marrow cells with medullary bone, which is of particular importance for identifying paratrabecular lymphomatous infiltrates. Decalcified specimens cannot be used for molecular genetic studies; therefore the bone marrow biopsy is excluded from this analysis. The primary material for this type of study is from the bone marrow aspirate smears or the bone marrow clot section.
- *Peripheral blood.* Peripheral blood obtained through a minimally invasive venepuncture can be used to both quantitatively and qualitatively evaluate the functional status of bone marrow. A differential count of haematopoietic cell types can be determined through either manual or automated methods. Blood cell morphology can also be determined through microscopic evaluation of a peripheral smear.

In situ hybridization, typically detected using fluorescent probes, is routinely used for the detection of reciprocal translocations that are diagnostic of a specific malignancy, with the classic example being the Philadelphia chromosome, t(9; 22) in chronic myelogenous leukaemia. Translocations may also define subtypes of a specific malignancy, illustrated by the numerous translocations and rearrangements, beyond the scope of this chapter, used in the diagnosis of leukaemias and lymphomas. In addition, multiple solid tumours, sarcomas in particular, have specific translocations. In general, the translocations have a driver gene, which imparts the oncogenic mechanism through unscheduled and/or high level expression of the encoded protein, which may be altered to confer oncogenic activity. The fusion gene partner may contribute to structural alteration/stabilization of the encoded oncoprotein, confer a hybrid function or upregulate the expression of a wild-type protein. Translocations can be detected with fusion probes from each of the two genes involved in the translocations. The normal pattern is two copies of each gene, typically shown in FISH as two green and two red signals. In the case of translocations, both sides of the reciprocal translocation are shown as a fusion of a green and red signal, totalling two, and a normal green and red signal that are separate. In addition, break-apart probes can be used to detect translocations for which the 'driver' gene is known, but the partner is either variable or unknown. In this case, probes from contiguous regions of a gene known to be involved in the rearrangement are labelled with green and red, which gives a normal pattern of two green–red fusions. In the case of a translocation or rearrangement, such as occurs in the retinoic acid receptor gene in acute promyelocytic leukaemia, the *IGH@* gene in various B-lineage lymphomas, and the *ALK* gene in adenocarcinoma of the lung, the rearranged gene will separate into green and red signals and the uninvolved gene will retain the green–red fusion signal. *In situ* hybridization for RNA in FFPE sections has been shown to be of clinical utility for the detection of Epstein–Barr virus short small nuclear RNAs (EBER) and for kappa and lambda light chain mRNA transcripts to demonstrate clonal expression of immunoglobulin light chains.

Molecular pathology

The approach described in previous sections provides a comprehensive perspective for the pathological analysis of tissues to establish a diagnosis, as well as the stage and grade of a malignancy. In many instances this information is sufficient to finalize the diagnosis. Molecular pathology is an additional diagnostic method that can enhance clinical understanding of a patient's disease process. For solid tumours, the detection of specific gene mutations is currently being used as a 'companion diagnostic' to predict the responsiveness of a tumour for targeted therapies or as an aid in diagnosis, as briefly explained in the examples provided below. For haematological malignancies, current classification systems heavily rely on specific gene abnormalities detected by FISH, as described in Diagnostic haematopathology section.

DNA sequencing techniques

The point mutations and small deletions/insertions harboured in tumour cells, but not present in the germline, are called somatic mutations. Since somatic mutations in cellular oncogenes are typically heterozygous, 50% of abnormal sequences could be detected if the tissue examined contained 100% tumour cells.

The crucial first step for any mutation detection is professional examination of FFPE tumour tissues by a pathologist to determine areas that contain specific malignant cell types and sufficient tumour load for optimal analysis. Real-time polymerase chain reaction (RT-PCR)-based methods are commonly used for detection of specific mutations with a sensitivity of 5–10% of tumour cells in the population. Sanger DNA sequencing is another widely used method in clinical molecular laboratories that can detect any mutations in a targeted genomic region flanked by primers, with a sensitivity of about 25% malignant cells. False-negative results for mutation detection can occur from a dilutional effect of normal and reactive cells that can render the mutation load below the limits of resolution of molecular testing. For any solid tumour case that needs a molecular assay, it is necessary for a pathologist to review all H&E slides to determine the best tissue block and then to select regions of the tumour from the H&E slide of the chosen block by circling the areas that contain a sufficient number of tumour cells for optimal analysis. Six unstained sections with a thickness of 10 μm and one slide stained with H&E are requested for any DNA-based molecular assays performed in our molecular pathology laboratory. Microdissection is performed under a microscope by matching tissues from unstained slides to the marked areas on the H&E-stained slide for DNA extraction. An area of tumour as small as 1 cm × 1 cm often has a yield of several micrograms of DNA when this is extracted from two to three slides.

Predictive and prognostic significance

The most commonly used predictive analyses currently include the detection of (1) mutations in *KRAS* codons 12 and 13 and *BRAF* codon 600 which are associated with resistance of metastatic colorectal adenocarcinoma to therapy with monoclonal antibodies to the epidermal growth factor receptor (EGFR); (2) mutations or in-frame microdeletions in exons 18–21 of EGFR for sensitivity of adenocarcinoma of the lung to therapy with EGFR tyrosine kinase inhibitor (TKI); and (3) detection of the *BRAF V600* mutations that provide eligibility for treatment of advanced melanoma with vemurafenib, a *BRAF* mutation-specific kinase inhibitor. The detection of mutations in cytopathology specimens may also be of clinical utility. We routinely test all thyroid FNA specimens that show significant atypia for the presence of *BRAF* and *NRAS* mutations, which are associated with papillary and follicular carcinomas, respectively, to provide insight for further clinical management of these patients. Sufficient DNA for a sequencing analysis can be derived from cells from one aspiration of an FNA.

In situ hybridization, which was described in the Diagnostic haematopathology section, may also be used to detect gene copy number abnormalities in non-haematological malignancy. The *HER2* gene was the first to be found to be amplified in an adult human tumour, breast cancer, resulting in increased expression of the product, a cell surface tyrosine kinase. As previously mentioned, the HER2 protein was the first molecular target for directed therapy, trastuzumab. Since *HER2* gene amplification and overexpression is present in approximately 25% of cases of mammary carcinoma, eligibility for the targeted therapy is dependent upon the verification of *HER2* gene amplification or protein overexpression, the first companion diagnostic laboratory study. Since patients with tumours having HER2 protein overexpression in the absence of gene amplification may not show a clinical response to trastuzumab, *in situ* hybridization appears to be the most effective technique, which has also been found to have greater overall cost effectiveness. A set of comprehensive guidelines have been established for HER2 testing, including fixation from 6 to 48 hours in neutral buffered formalin for both IHC and *in situ* hybridization. Recently, a chromogenic *in situ* hybridization test for *HER2* gene amplification has been approved by the FDA in the USA. Examples of these detection methods are shown in Fig. 8.9. This approach allows for simultaneous visualization of histopathology and gene copy number, which facilitates the requirement for analysis of 20 cells in two independent areas of invasive carcinoma.

Future molecular techniques

At this time, the number of FDA-approved targeted therapies is limited and the associated companion diagnostic tests are performed on an individual basis. It is anticipated that the number of antagonists for oncological targets will continue to increase. It is currently estimated that approximately 80% of the pipeline of late-stage oncology therapies are directed against molecular targets. Over 500 compounds are under study and about 140 targets are in development. In this context, it will be critical to have an efficient method for mutational analysis of multiple exons/genes. Desktop next-generation sequencing (NGS), which has the ability to easily sequence several hundred exons simultaneously with a mutation detection sensitivity for specimens that contain only 10% tumour cells, represents an ideal technology to analyse a wide spectrum of candidate genes for eligibility for therapy with targeted agents.

Multiple databases are available to assist in the identification of clinical trials that employ targeted antagonists and the corresponding genes. The "My Cancer Genome" database (www.mycancergenome.org) provides a catalogue of mutated genes in specific tumours and clinical trials with targeted therapies. The COSMIC (Catalog of Somatic Mutations In Cancer; http://cancer.sanger.ac.uk/cancergenome/projects/cosmic/) database provides a listing of mutations that occur in specific malignancies and their relative frequency.

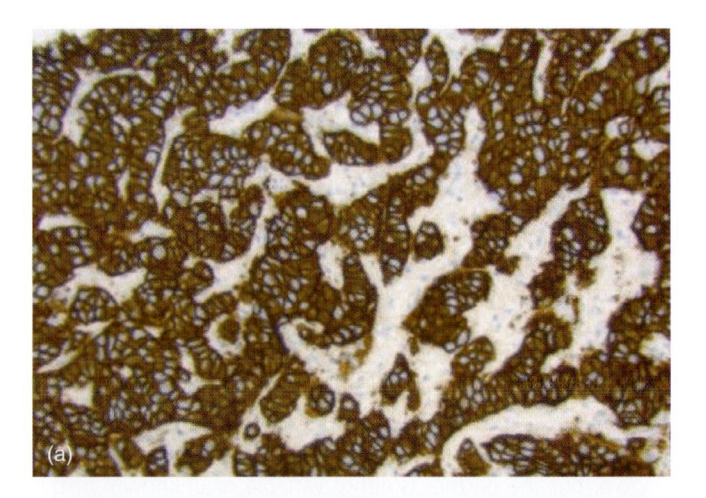

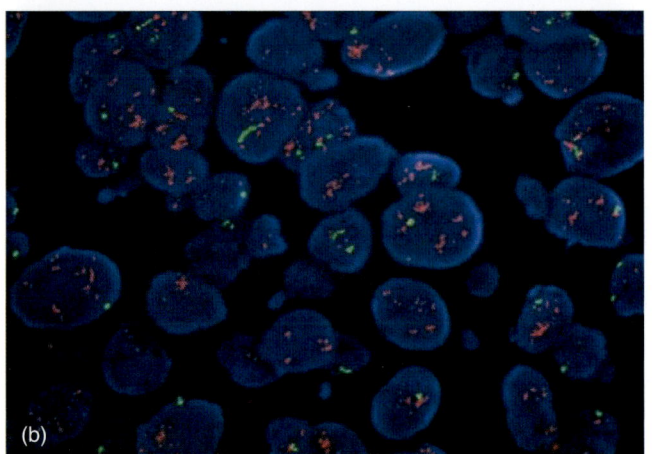

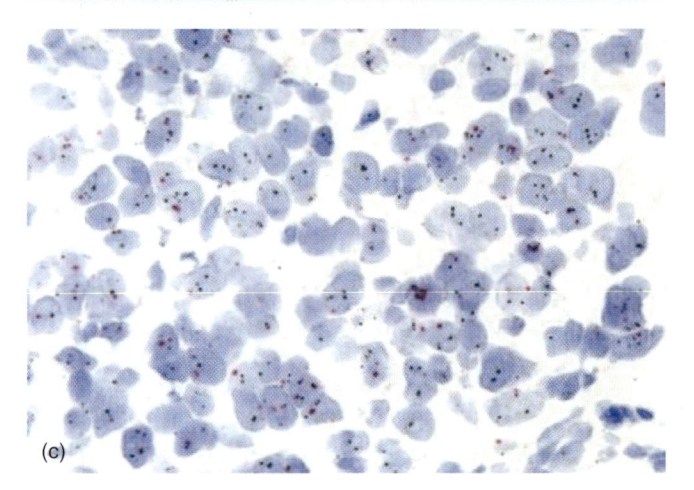

Figure 8.9 Detection methods for *HER2* gene amplification.
(a) Immunohistochemical staining for HER2 showing 3+ amplification.
(b) *HER2* amplification by fluorescent *in situ* hybridization (FISH).
(c) *HER2* amplification by chromogenic *in situ* hybridization (CISH).

Conclusion

Anatomical pathology is a tissue-based diagnostic specialty that uses multiple modalities to provide the most accurate diagnoses. The pathological examination of tissues represents a critical milestone in the diagnostic process and a key component of the infrastructure for clinical and translational research. Under the guidance of experienced pathologists, traditional pathological studies provide strong insights into disease processes, such as tumour type, grade and stage for malignancies, and represent one of the most cost-effective diagnostic analyses in modern medicine. However, further interrogation of routinely processed tissues using contemporary genomic methods, including Next Generation Sequencing, will enhance the classification and stratification of diseases in patients. In conjunction with clinical context, modern pathology incorporates standard diagnostic techniques with cutting-edge molecular methods to generate diagnoses that can best guide patient care.

Recommended reading

Surgical pathology

College of American Pathologists Accreditation Checklists (2013) Available at www.cap.org

Kumar V, Abbas A, Fausto N (2005) *Robbins and Cotran Pathologic Basis of Disease*, 7th edn. Philadelphia: Elsevier.

Lester, SC (2005) *Manual of Surgical Pathology*, 2nd edn. Philadelphia: Elsevier.

Rosai J (2004) *Rosai and Ackerman's Surgical Pathology*, 9th edn. Philadelphia: Elsevier.

Westra WH, Hruban RH, Phelps TH *et al*. (2009) *Surgical Pathology Dissection: An Illustrated Guide*, 2nd edn. Springer.

Wolff AC, Hammond EH, Schwartz JN *et al*. (2007) American Society of Clinical Oncology/College of American Pathologists guideline recommendations for human epidermal growth factor receptor 2 testing in breast cancer. *J Clin Oncol* 25(1):118–145.

Cytopathology

Ali SZ, Cibas ES (2009) *The Bethesda System for Reporting Thyroid Cytopathology: Definitions, Criteria, and Explanatory Notes*. New York, NY: Springer.

Bibbo M, Wilbur D (2009) *Comprehensive Cytopathology: Expert Consult*, 3rd edn. Philadelphia: Elsevier.

Solomon D, Nayar R, Davey D, Wilbur D (2004) *The Bethesda System for Reporting Cervical Cytology: Definitions Criteria, and Explanatory Notes*. New York, NY: Springer.

Molecular pathology

Vanderbilt-Ingram Cancer Center www.mycancergenome.org

Wellcome Trust Sanger Institute, Genome Research Limited cancer.sanger.ac.uk/cancergenome/projects/cosmic/

9 Principles of surgery

Matthew H.G. Katz and Brian K. Bednarski

Department of Surgical Oncology, The University of Texas M.D. Anderson Cancer Center, Houston, TX, USA

Introduction

In the clinical management of patients with solid tumours, pattern recognition by surgeons skilled in the timely and appropriate application of operative procedures for cancer is invaluable. Indeed, surgeons often represent the nucleus of the multidisciplinary cancer care team. A complete understanding of the common patterns of presentation of solid tumours, patterns of their response to treatment, and patterns of spread and recurrence is therefore of utmost importance to the surgical oncologist. This knowledge provides a guide for diagnostic interventions and pretreatment staging; influences the use, timing and extent of surgical operations; allows proper incorporation of interventions into the overall multimodality care plan; and permits the development of rational and cost-effective postoperative surveillance strategies.

Patterns of tumour spread

The hallmark of malignancy is the presence of abnormal cells that have the ability and potential to invade locally and disseminate both regionally and to distant sites of the body. Cancer cells within the primary tumour may infiltrate through their tissues of origin directly into adjacent organs, exfoliate and implant directly onto the surface of nearby structures, or access the blood or lymphatic system through which they may circulate to distant locations. Cancer cells may disseminate from the primary tumour using one of these routes primarily, or using more than one simultaneously. Often, cancer types are associated with a characteristic route of metastasis. Ovarian cancer cells, for example, commonly dislodge from the primary tumour and exfoliate into the peritoneal cavity. Basal cell carcinomas and bladder cancers tend to invade locoregionally. Follicular thyroid cancer favours metastasis through the bloodstream, while papillary thyroid cancer characteristically spreads primarily through the lymphatic system.

Combined with the anatomical relationships of its primary tumour, the common method(s) of metastasis associated with a cancer may suggest a characteristic pattern of metastatic disease. For example, gastric adenocarcinoma, which disseminates through both the circulatory and lymphatic systems, is often associated with metastases in the regional lymph nodes along the foregut vasculature and the liver due to the flow of venous blood from the colon into the portal circulation. Metastatic disease may also be noted as drop metastases in the ovary or as tumour implants elsewhere in the peritoneal cavity when the primary invades through the stomach wall. In contrast, because soft tissue sarcomas primarily metastasize through the bloodstream but not the lymphatic system, metastases from these tumours are often found in the liver and lung, but are rarely identified in regional lymph nodes. Some cancers have a particularly marked preference for organ-specific metastasis, e.g. choroidal melanoma almost exclusively seeds to the liver.

A complete understanding of the metastatic patterns associated with each cancer subtype is critically important to the design and performance of effective cancer operations. Regional lymphadenectomy is not routinely advocated as part of curative operations for soft tissue sarcoma, for example; because sarcomas do not generally spread via lymphatic channels, cancer cells are rarely identified in the regional lymph node basins draining these tumours. Resection of regional lymphatics would therefore add to technical complexity and risk, but add little to the oncological efficacy of the procedure. On the other hand, lymphatic dissemination is commonly observed in association with carcinoid tumours of the midgut, often even when the primary tumour itself is very small. An aggressive lymphatic resection is therefore recommended as part of curative resection of these cancers to prevent complications associated with locoregional recurrence.

Although the likelihood of lymphatic involvement by cancer is to some extent disease specific, it can also be predicted on the basis of disease stage and other histopathological factors

---

UICC Manual of Clinical Oncology, Ninth Edition. Edited by Brian O'Sullivan, James D. Brierley, Anil K. D'Cruz, Martin F. Fey, Raphael Pollock, Jan B. Vermorken and Shao Hui Huang. © 2015 UICC. Published 2015 by John Wiley & Sons, Ltd.

associated with the primary tumour. Adenocarcinoma of the stomach limited to the mucosa and submucosa is associated with lymphatic metastases in only 10–15% of cases, and thus local endoscopic mucosal resection may be appropriate for many patients with this stage of disease; those most appropriate might be selected on the basis of favourable prognostic features such as small tumour size, well-differentiated histology and the absence of lymphovascular invasion. Similarly, superficial cancers of the rectum, which are properly selected on the basis of size and histological grade, may be safely resected with local operations which are associated with less morbidity than radical resections. More advanced disease associated with a higher likelihood of lymphatic involvement would mandate a more comprehensive resection designed to clear both the local disease as well as the regional lymphatic vessels and lymph nodes, such as low anterior resection with total mesorectal excision.

It should be emphasized that in many cancers that spread to the lymphatics (e.g. adenocarcinomas of the pancreas and stomach), a direct influence of the extent of radical lymphadenectomy on recurrence or survival has not been clearly demonstrated, but lymphadenectomy is still recommended as it provides comprehensive staging and prognostic information that may be used to determine the need for and to individualize postoperative therapies. Indeed, the adverse effects of 'stage migration' may occur when patients who undergo an inadequate lymphadenectomy and are falsely declared to have no lymphatic involvement, do not receive postoperative therapies that would otherwise be mandated if a thorough sampling of the regional lymph nodes had identified existing metastatic disease.

Resectability and operability

The role of surgery in the care of patients with solid cancer depends in large part on the extent to which a tumour is surgically 'resectable'. Although the term 'resectable' implies an emphasis upon the anatomical and technical features of the tumour that place constraints upon its complete extirpation, determination of the role of surgery is complex and must be individualized to each clinical scenario. Indeed, it requires evaluation of tumour anatomy in the context of anticipated morbidity, associated risk and tumour behaviour. Surgical operations should be performed only when the benefit expected from surgery is favourable relative to the risks and potential morbidity associated with it. From a pragmatic standpoint, it may therefore be more appropriate to make decisions based upon 'operability', which takes into account features of both tumour and host.

Surgical margin (R–) status

The completeness – or radicality – of a surgical resection for cancer is routinely measured by a clinical assessment of the margins of resection. The extent of residual cancer left in the body following surgical resection is described by the symbol R: R2 indicates an incomplete gross resection and the presence of macroscopic disease following resection; R1 indicates resection of all gross disease but the presence of residual microscopic tumour cells; and R0 indicates resection of all macroscopic and microscopic cancer. Because the presence of residual disease following surgery has profound prognostic importance and clinical relevance, R status must be accurately assessed and recorded following all cancer operations.

The surgeon makes the distinction between an R0/R1 and R2 resection intraoperatively by examining the tumour bed following extirpation. In contrast, the pathologist makes the distinction between an R0 and R1 resection following a thorough microscopic examination of the surgical margins in the pathology suite. For such assessments to be meaningful, the margins examined should be thoroughly described and labelled, and, ideally, evaluated using an identical histopathological protocol. Typically, the histopathological status of the surgical margins is evaluated using stained, permanent samples of tissue at the margins of resection. However, intraoperative assessment of surgical margins may be useful in some cases. Using frozen section analysis, the tissue margins are inked, frozen and sectioned, followed by thawing, fixation and staining. Alternatively, the tumour can be pressed onto glass slides to make an imprint, followed by fixation and staining. Using either method, examination by the pathologist can be performed while the patient is still under anaesthesia. In the event cancer cells are identified at the margin, additional tissue can be re-resected. Although false-negative results can occur due to processing, and thus definitive analysis of the margins must await final evaluation, the use of these rapid assessments can improve rates of margin-negative resection. Patients with breast cancer treated with breast conservation surgery who undergo intraoperative margin assessment, for example, have a lower rate of reoperation and re-resection than patients who do not undergo these evaluations.

Although the status of surgical margins can only be definitively assessed following removal of the specimen, the likelihood of achieving negative margins should be predicted prior to surgery based on the results of a clinical work-up that includes a physical examination and radiographic studies, as the identification of anatomical limitations that prohibit R0 resection (e.g. size of the tumour, its location, or the relationships between it and vital structures) will most certainly influence the therapeutic plan. Palliative therapies, for example, would be more appropriate than attempted curative resection of a painful abdominal tumour for which margin-positive resection (or inability to resect at all) could have been predicted preoperatively.

Anticipated operative morbidity

Although resectable from a purely technical standpoint, some tumours may be considered unresectable because extirpation of the tumour to negative margins would require sacrifice of normal, unreconstructable anatomical structures to a degree incompatible with maintenance of quality or even quantity of life. For example, resection of soft tissue sarcomas of the extremities may require neurovascular disruption leading to loss of function or even amputation. In such cases, the anticipated morbidity associated with such sacrifice must be balanced with the desire to achieve clear margins.

Perioperative risk

The risk of the operation is associated with multiple factors, including the type of operation performed, the clinical context in which it is performed, and the age and pre-existing co-morbidities of the patient.

Certain operations are associated with greater technical complexity than others. Addition of secondary procedures may further increase technical complexity. Pancreaticoduodenectomy with *en bloc* resection and reconstruction of the portal vein, for example, is more complex than standard pancreaticoduodenectomy, which is more complex than segmental mastectomy. The difficulties associated with precisely measuring and categorizing surgical complexity notwithstanding, an increase in surgical complexity is generally associated with an increase in perioperative risk and surgical complications.

The clinical context within which a surgical procedure is performed is also an important factor associated with perioperative risk. Cancer operations generally carry a higher level of risk than similar operations performed for benign disease due to the effects of multiple factors, including pre-existing co-morbidity, circulating catabolic mediators and cancer cachexia, and cytotoxic therapies delivered in the preoperative period. Surgical risk may be further modulated by the acuity with which the operation is performed. Hemicolectomy for colon cancer performed emergently in the setting of an obstructing tumour of the sigmoid may be accompanied by an unprepared bowel, dehydration and electrolyte imbalances, cachexia and malnutrition that are not associated with elective colectomy.

Patient characteristics also contribute significantly to perioperative risk, and critical emphasis must be placed on the identification and optimization of reversible physiological risk factors. Performance status, a crude measure of the effects of cancer on a patient's activities of daily living, is routinely measured using the Eastern Cooperative Oncology Group (ECOG) or Karnovsky system, and is graded simply with physical exam and historical data from complete disablement (cannot carry out any self-care, totally confined to bed or chair) to full activity (able to carry out all predisease performance without restriction). The extent of a patient's pre-existing co-morbidities can be calculated using tools such as the Adult Comorbidity Index-27 (ACE-27) or the Charlson Score, both of which have been shown to be predictors of postoperative complications and poor overall surgical outcomes. A related but distinct clinical entity, frailty, is also being increasingly recognized as a measurable predictor of surgical risk. Clinically, frailty is characterized by progressive loss of function, malnutrition, sarcopenia, osteopenia and impaired cognition. It can be clinically identified according to objective clinical criteria: exhaustion, weak grip strength, weight loss, slow walking speed and low physical activity. The prevalence of frailty among the elderly is significant, and may be particularly pervasive among older patients with cancer. Because performance status, co-morbidity, frailty, malnutrition and other related constructs can contribute to a poor functional reserve in times of stress, each must be carefully evaluated prior to surgical intervention. Preoperative medical assessment with additional input from medical subspecialties such as cardiology, nephrology and geriatrics may be helpful in many elective circumstances.

Tumour behaviour

An evaluation of a tumour's behaviour (its 'tumour biology') is essential to determining the role and predicting the efficacy of surgical care. Occasionally, the behaviour of a cancer is such that the results of surgery will be inadequate despite the apparent resectability of the solid tumour from a technical perspective. For example, pancreatic adenocarcinoma may present with small volume, oligometastatic disease in the liver. Despite the technical resectability of both the primary tumour and the liver disease, the use of surgery in this circumstance has historically been associated with poor outcomes due to the presence of occult metastatic disease that manifests as early postoperative cancer 'recurrence' and early death.

Although tumour behaviour is most routinely estimated on the basis of the natural history of a given tumour type (i.e. anaplastic thyroid cancer has historically behaved more aggressively than papillary thyroid cancer), other clinical clues may provide additional insight into the behaviour of a particular tumour. Serological tumour markers, such as the cancer antigens CA125 and carcinoembryonic antigen (CEA), may be used to assess the extent of many cancers, and may be particularly valuable in the evaluation of cancers commonly associated with micrometastatic, radiographically-occult disease. Other clues, such as Ki-67, tumour grade and mitotic index, may be determined by analysis of a tumour biopsy and may provide further insight into the potential natural history of a given tumour. Important clinical markers can also be obtained by history and physical examination. A recent onset of cachexia and pain, for example, may indicate aggressive and/or advanced cancer not amenable to curative surgery even in the presence of radiographic findings that suggest more limited disease.

Incorporation of surgery into multimodality treatment plans

As the science of medicine has advanced, so too has the care of cancer patients. With advances in chemotherapy, biological therapy, radiation, endoscopic therapies, interventional radiology applications and surgical techniques, the need for a multidisciplinary approach to the treatment of cancer has become more important than ever before. The integration of these multiple therapies into a cohesive treatment plan requires surgeons providing oncological care to be knowledgeable of the benefits of non-operative therapies as well as the impact of those therapies on surgical outcomes. This enables the surgeon to be an active participant in the development of the treatment plan.

The sequence in which therapies are administered may impact – positively and negatively – both perioperative outcomes and long-term oncological results. Furthermore, the decision to administer radiation, chemotherapy or other non-operative treatments in either the preoperative or postoperative setting may influence the surgical plan and intraoperative events. For instance, as is seen in the treatment of soft tissue sarcomas of the extremity, the administration of external beam radiation prior to surgery may reduce the extent of resection necessary to completely extirpate the tumour. However, preoperative radiation may also increase the potential for postoperative wound complications. These potential effects must be thoughtfully considered to appropriately design the resection, to plan the reconstruction and to anticipate events in the postoperative period.

Although surgical resection is a local therapeutic modality that has historically been applied primarily in the setting of localized disease, improvements in medical therapies have also resulted in prolonged survival of patients with many metastatic cancers. This has led to the need to critically re-evaluate the role for surgery – both with palliative and curative intent – in some patients with systemic disease. For example, an ongoing debate centres on the role for resection of the primary tumour in patients with metastatic colorectal cancer. In complex scenarios like this one, the surgeon must evaluate the risk of morbidity from surgical resection of the primary tumour in the context of the potential for the success of novel systemic therapies in prolonging survival through the control of systemic disease. Concerns to be addressed include the potential for local complications due to obstruction, bleeding or perforation from the primary tumour. In addition to the effects of systemic therapy, the other concepts to incorporate into the decision-making process are the availability of other non-surgical treatment options such as endoscopic therapies, including endoluminal stents and ablation, as well as external beam radiation. These situations are very challenging for the patient, the surgeon, the medical oncologist and all other participating specialties.

Given the complexities associated with oncological decision-making and the innumerable treatment modalities available for each clinical scenario, the benefit of a cohesive, multidisciplinary treatment plan cannot be overstated. This plan can be generated through regular multidisciplinary conferences (e.g. 'tumour boards'), which facilitate a comprehensive review of all pertinent data and a frank discussion regarding the risks and benefits associated with each treatment modality. The result is an agreement on a treatment approach that can be communicated to the patient with the confidence that all options have been reviewed. The role and utility of each treatment may be re-evaluated on the basis of physical exam, history and restaging studies at subsequent meetings. Real-time multidisciplinary evaluation may be further facilitated by evaluation and treatment in dedicated disease-specific or disease site-specific clinics that bring medical oncologists, pathologists, radiation oncologists, radiologists and surgeons together. Whatever the strategy employed, it is important for surgeons to avoid being labelled as technicians by actively participating in discussions and sharing their unique perspective on balancing benefits and risk of surgical intervention, and to involve other specialties appropriately in order to mitigate any associated surgical morbidity.

Curative surgical therapy and treatment sequencing

Surgery

Margin-negative resection of the primary tumour is the cornerstone of definitive surgical therapy for most solid cancers. Such a resection involves removal of the cancer along with a margin of normal tissue. When performed with intent to cure, surgical dissection is conducted through normal tissues surrounding the tumour; dissection directly upon the tumour is avoided to prevent neglecting infiltrating tumour cells or contamination of non-cancerous tissues. Indeed, although a zone of compressed reactive tissue may be observed around the tumour, tumour cells frequently infiltrate through this pseudocapsule. Organs or structures in contact with the tumour should therefore be resected – completely or partially – en bloc with the cancer.

The extent of normal tissue surrounding the tumour that is resected as part of curative resection varies by tumour type, location and anatomical relationships between the tumour and adjacent structures. The risk for local recurrence following an inadequate local resection must be balanced with the increase in morbidity that may be associated with larger operations. For example, although all melanomas were once resected with wide margins (3–5 cm of normal tissue surrounding the lesion), those aggressive resections carried significant morbidity and, it is now recognized, were not associated with a lower rate of local recurrence than resections with narrower margins. Indeed, curative resections of melanomas measuring <1 mm in thickness are performed with margins only 1 cm wide. Thicker melanomas should be resected with 2-cm margins, as the rate of local recurrence following resection with less aggressive operations is unacceptable. Margins of 2 cm are also the objective in curative resections for soft tissue sarcomas, but narrower margins may be accepted in certain cases if vital structures can be preserved.

In some anatomical areas, resection with a substantial margin of soft tissue may not be attainable due to the proximity of vital structures. For example, the margin most commonly found to be positive for residual cancer cells following pancreaticoduodenectomy is that adjacent to the superior mesenteric artery, a structure that cannot be removed without significant morbidity. The free margin of tissue removed at this margin is routinely measured in millimetres. In other cases, a more significant resection of soft tissue or organs than would otherwise appear necessary may be mandated by the anatomy of the tumour and its relationship with adjacent structures. For example, resection of the duodenum – even when not directly involved by cancer – is required as part of pancreaticoduodenectomy because the duodenum shares its blood supply with the pancreatic head, and this blood supply is sacrificed as part of tumour resection.

Given these anatomical relationships and limitations, the extent of the resection may be modulated, particularly in the context of available adjuvant and neoadjuvant therapies. In curative operations for patients with rectal cancer, division of the mesorectum 2–5 cm distal to the most distal aspect of the tumour is associated with the most favourable local recurrence rates. Prior to the use of neoadjuvant chemoradiation, the surgical management of rectal cancer mandated a 5-cm distal margin to ensure adequate removal of all submucosal spread of the tumour. This had greatest impact upon patients with low rectal cancers who could not undergo sphincter-preserving surgery and were instead relegated to permanent colostomy. However, as knowledge of rectal cancer biology grew, techniques of surgical resection changed and the concept of preoperative treatment with chemoradiation became standard of care, the 5-cm rule began to be challenged in this unique subset of patients and subsequently has been rewritten. The key realization was that a universal rule is inappropriate. For upper and middle rectal tumours where the complete excision of the mesorectum may not be required to adequately excise the tumour, the 5-cm rule for the distal margin remains the goal secondary to the potential for tumour deposits and lymph nodes to be involved distal to the tumour within the mesorectum. On the other hand, for low rectal tumours where the mesorectum is completely excised, a goal of 2 cm is adequate to safely guard against microscopically positive margins secondary to submucosal spread of tumour cells. These limits continue to be re-evaluated to determine if even narrower margins could be utilized without compromising the risk of microscopically positive margins or local recurrence. This has led to further efforts to identify criteria to determine which patients would be best suited for an oncologically sound narrow margin excision of a low rectal cancer. The result of these advances has been a change from assigning all patients to the morbidity of an abdominoperineal resection and permanent colostomy, to increasing the rate of sphincter preservation in appropriately selected patients.

Although the efforts in rectal cancer have primarily focused on the oncological validity of a narrower margin of excision, a current debate regarding the surgical management of retroperitoneal sarcomas is whether appropriate management of surgical margins requires the pre-emptive resection of all adjacent organs potentially at risk for involvement. This concept of a more radical approach to the resection of retroperitoneal sarcomas is based on the theory that residual microscopic disease may be left *in situ*, despite gross macroscopic resection of clearly affected organs and structures, secondary to the complex anatomical relationships of these retroperitoneal tumours. The concern for an inadequate R1 resection notwithstanding, the decision to remove macroscopically uninvolved organs must be balanced with the morbidity and loss of function that would be expected following extirpation. The results of retrospective studies suggest that the more aggressive surgical approach can improve local recurrence rates. In order to get a definitive answer as to best approach, a formal prospective study would be necessary, which is challenging when working with such rare diseases.

Some low-grade or early-stage cancers may be cured with resection of the primary tumour alone. However, dissemination through the lymphatic vessels and microscopic and macroscopic involvement of regional lymph nodes is common and may also lead to locoregional recurrence and considerable morbidity. Regional lymphadenectomy is therefore routinely performed as part of curative operations for many solid malignancies that tend to metastasize through the lymphatic system. Indeed, a thorough lymphatic resection may be the primary determinant of the anatomical extent of the operation. For example, cancers in the caecum are resected with right hemicolectomy, an operation that involves resection of the entire mesocolon to the right of the superior mesenteric vessels up to and including the right branch of the middle colic artery. The extensive colonic resection is performed not for issues relating to margins on the colon, but instead because thorough lymphadenectomy of the nodes along the ileocolic and right colic vessels requires sacrifice of those vessels which supply the right colon.

Adjuvant therapy

With respect to surgical oncology, adjuvant therapy refers to the administration of non-operative treatments following potentially curative surgery for cancer. The goal of those treatments, which may include systemic chemotherapy, radiation therapy, immunotherapy, hormone therapy or others, is to prolong survival and to enhance the likelihood of cure through the eradication of residual microscopic disease that may be located at locoregional and/or distant sites. Postoperative therapies delivered in the adjuvant mode must be distinguished from palliative therapies, as might be administered following a non-curative, margin-positive operation.

Adjuvant therapy is effective for some cancers but not for others. For example, systemic chemotherapy administered following pancreaticoduodenectomy prolongs both the disease-free survival and the overall survival of patients with localized pancreatic adenocarcinoma. The role of radiation therapy in this context is not as clearly defined, and it may in fact be harmful. Patients with localized neuroendocrine tumours, in contrast, do not benefit from the administration of systemic chemotherapy in the postoperative setting, even though systemic chemotherapy may prolong the survival of patients with unresectable neuroendocrine tumours. The efficacy of adjuvant therapies may also vary on the basis of disease stage. Although patients with node-positive colon cancer clearly benefit from the administration of systemic chemotherapy following colectomy, patients with superficial, node-negative tumours do not. Some (but not all) patients with deeply invasive, node-negative cancers may benefit; treatment is often offered to those with adverse prognostic features, such as lymphovascular invasion or poor differentiation.

The administration of adjuvant therapies following curative resection may be delayed or even abandoned in those patients who develop perioperative complications or those who do not recuperate from surgery expeditiously. It is therefore of utmost importance that surgical operations for cancer be performed with low complication rates. Furthermore, the likelihood of a patient receiving adjuvant therapy in the postoperative period (e.g. the prospect of expeditious perioperative recovery to an extent sufficient to initiate postoperative therapy) must be estimated *prior to surgery*. In some cases, alternative treatment strategies may need to be pursued based on the results of that assessment.

Neoadjuvant therapy

In contrast to adjuvant therapy, neoadjuvant therapy is administered prior to surgical resection. Neoadjuvant therapies, like those administered in the postoperative setting, may be used in an attempt to eradicate micrometastatic disease that might serve as a source of postoperative recurrence. Neoadjuvant therapy can also be used to facilitate margin-negative resection by reducing either the size or anatomical extent of a cancer; this 'down-staging' effect may either allow resection of previously unresectable cancers or may reduce the scope of a planned operation. For example, preoperative radiotherapy administered to patients with distal rectal cancer, who would otherwise require *de novo* abdominoperineal resection with removal of the anal sphincter, may often lead to successful sphincter preservation procedures associated with similar survival but superior quality of life. Preoperative chemotherapy is often administered to women with locally advanced breast cancers and may allow breast conservation surgery in some women with advanced disease.

The delivery of non-operative therapies prior to surgery has several potential advantages over the delivery of those same therapies following surgery. External beam radiation with concurrent sensitizing chemotherapy is more effective and less toxic than postoperative chemoradiation when delivered to periampullary cancers because the intact blood supply and well-oxygenated cancer cells are more susceptible to injury. Following surgery, the cells in the tumour bed may be hypoxic and more radioresistant. Furthermore, following surgery the small bowel used in gastrointestinal reconstruction is radiated, increasing the risk of strictures and gastrointestinal toxicity. Among patients with rectal cancer, preoperative chemoradiation is associated with better local tumour control and lower short- and long-term toxicity rates. To the extent that evolving micrometastases distant from the primary tumour may confound attempts at surgical cure, the delivery of preoperative therapy may address this disease early and select patients with a tumour load most appropriate for subsequent resection. Finally, the efficacy of neoadjuvant therapies can be monitored by observation of the cancer *in situ*; effective therapies may then be delivered in the postoperative setting or in the event of tumour recurrence.

The potential disadvantages of preoperative therapy must also be considered. The application of non-surgical strategies delays definitive local control. To the extent that many operations are designed to both cure and palliate symptoms of cancer, such delays in surgical therapy may mandate that alternative palliative strategies be considered. For example, the administration of neoadjuvant therapy to patients with pancreatic cancer who have biliary obstruction due to tumour requires endoscopic or percutaneous drainage of the biliary tree prior to the administration of non-operative treatments. The potential complication rates and costs associated with these temporary palliative manoeuvers must be thoughtfully considered.

Intraoperative therapies

For some cancers, adjunctive therapies may also be delivered during the surgical procedure itself and the surgeon should be aware of the role, advantages, and limitations of such therapies. Instillation of heated mitomycin C into the peritoneum, for example, is an important component of cytoreductive surgical procedures performed for peritoneal surface malignancies. Administration of chemotherapy directly into the abdominal cavity exposes the tumours to higher concentrations of drug than in other tissues, thus enhancing efficacy and reducing systemic toxicity. Radiation therapy may also be delivered intraoperatively directly to an exposed tumour, using either external beams or locally-implanted radioactive devices and catheters. Radioactive brachytherapy catheters can be loaded with radioactive wires and left in the surgical bed for days. When used for soft tissue sarcomas, such treatments may cut the treatment time from weeks down to days.

Non-curative surgery for cancer

The goals of non-curative surgical therapy must be clearly defined, and must be extraordinarily well communicated to both the patient and family. Most non-curative surgical procedures fit broadly into one of the following categories.

Cancer screening and surveillance

Screening and surveillance is not appropriate for all cancers. Cancers for which screening is particularly effective are those associated with a high-risk population, those that are treatable, and those for which effective, low-cost screening tests exist. Because such tests are performed for asymptomatic individuals, it is critical that they are non-invasive, are associated with minimal risk and have little effect on either short- or long-term quality of life. For this reason, invasive surgical procedures are rarely performed for these purposes.

Important examples of screening and surveillance procedures that lie within the purview of the surgical oncologist, however, do exist. Sigmoidoscopy and colonoscopy, for example, are often recommended for asymptomatic individuals >50 years of age to screen for colorectal cancer, as screening for colorectal cancer has been well-documented to reduce cancer-related mortality. Colonoscopy is a useful test in this scenario as the study itself is associated with low morbidity, the incidence of occult malignancy is high among older individuals, premalignant tumours (adenoma) with a well-defined risk for conversion to malignancy can be identified endoscopically with high sensitivity, and a curative treatment for such tumours is readily available. Similarly, periodic surveillance for recurrent colorectal cancer with endoscopy is appropriate following a potentially curative operation for colorectal cancer as metachronous tumours may develop in the remnant colorectum even in the absence of symptoms, and such disease is often curable. Screening endoscopy for pancreatic cancer in asymptomatic individuals, in contrast, is not generally advocated due in large part to an absence of a well-defined group at high risk for the disease, and its role following curative resection of pancreatic cancer is also unclear as no curative treatment option exists for patients in whom recurrent disease is identified.

Diagnosis

Appropriate treatment of cancer is dependent upon acquisition and evaluation of abnormal tissue. For this reason, the surgical oncologist is often called upon to perform surgical procedures and other interventions to acquire tissue sufficient for cytopathological or histopathological analysis. Although the primary goal of those procedures may be to secure a diagnosis of cancer, additional pathological information can often be gleaned from tissue biopsy that may have important clinical implications with regard to both treatment and prognosis. Close cooperation between the surgeon performing the biopsy and the pathologist evaluating the specimen is therefore of utmost importance.

Several technical methods exist for biopsy of solid tumours. The technique selected depends on factors associated with both the tumour and patient; in general, the least invasive intervention that can reliably obtain the necessary pathological data should be selected. Superficial tumours which are either visible to the eye (e.g. skin nevi) or are clinically palpable (e.g. breast or rectal nodules and tumours) may often be biopsied under direct visualization. In contrast, tumours which cannot be readily identified due to their size or anatomical location (e.g. retroperitoneal sarcomas, colon polyps or adrenal tumours) may require biopsy under ultrasonographic, computed tomography (CT)/magnetic resonance imaging (MRI) or endoscopic guidance. Occasionally, surgical exploration and exposure may be required for adequate acquisition of tumour tissue. In such cases, minimally invasive laparoscopic approaches are often used.

Needles can be used to acquire either cytological (fine needle aspiration [FNA]) or histological (core biopsy) samples for analysis. Cellular samples are often adequate to determine the presence or absence of malignancy, are inexpensive, and are relatively simple to acquire using a small (22 or 25 gauge) needle and syringe. The technique leads to little tissue destruction. Furthermore, the cytological specimens, albeit small, may be used for research applications ranging from immunocytochemistry to sequencing. However, FNA biopsy has important disadvantages. First, examination of disaggregated cells may not be sufficient to precisely determine cancer histotype, and the samples give no indication of the cytoarchitecture of the tumour. FNA therefore cannot precisely distinguish premalignant lesions from invasive cancer. Tissue samples large enough to provide histopathological information can be secured using larger-diameter 'core' needles. However, these needles can cause greater tissue injury and are associated with a more significant potential for complications in certain clinical scenarios. For example, FNA biopsy has historically been preferred to core needle biopsy for tumours of the pancreas due to concerns over the potential for bleeding or pancreatitis following instrumentation with large-core needles. Recently, however, the development of smaller-diameter core needles has allayed these concerns to some degree.

Both of these biopsy instruments have additional potential disadvantages. First, because they only sample a small portion of a lesion, false-negative FNA or core biopsies may occur in the setting of histopathological heterogeneity. Second, 'seeding' of tumour cells along needle tracks has been (albeit infrequently) reported. These disadvantages notwithstanding, needle biopsy is now routinely performed to interrogate abnormalities of the breast, thyroid, lung and other organs.

Surgical excisional and incisional biopsies may be performed for a variety of indications. Skin nevi and other skin lesions are highly appropriate for this approach. Whenever possible, skin lesions are completely excised using a full-thickness, excisional biopsy to clear margins as this technique reduces the potential for a 'false-negative' result due to sampling error. Excisional biopsy is also appropriate for relatively small tumours that can be palpated, visualized or located endoscopically. Incisional biopsy, or surgical removal of a portion of the tumour, may be more appropriate for larger tumours or for lesions in cosmetically challenging areas (e.g. the face). Proper planning of incision should be performed to minimize the tissue loss that may subsequently occur as part of curative resection of the tumour. It is important to emphasize that excisional or incisional biopsies are preferable to shave biopsies for skin lesions, particularly for the evaluation of pigmented lesions presumed to be melanoma, as the depth of invasion of such tumours has important clinical relevance.

In many cases, histopathological diagnosis can be determined on the basis of simple haematoxylin and eosin (H&E) slide preparations. In others, a precise diagnosis may require immunohistochemical studies or flow cytometry. The surgeon should understand the differential diagnoses of a tumour and be alert to the requirements of the pathologist in discriminating between them. A discussion with the pathologist prior to and following the acquisition of tissue is good practice.

Cancer staging

Staging is the clinical process whereby the extent of a cancer is determined. Cancer stage can be used to help estimate the prognosis of an individual patient based upon the natural history of prior patients with a similar extent of disease. The cancer stage designation may also be used to determine treatment and facilitate research. Although the specifics vary by tumour type, the stage of each cancer is determined primarily by the anatomical extent of its primary tumour (T, e.g. maximum tumour diameter or tumour depth of invasion); the degree to which regional lymph nodes are involved by cancer (N); and the presence or absence of metastases (M). The American Joint Committee on Cancer (AJCC) and UICC share a standardized TNM system on this basis. Additional non-anatomical data may be used in the staging process for some solid cancers, such as the presence of ulceration (e.g. melanoma, breast). Stage can be determined clinically (cTNM) on the basis of results of the physical examination and radiographic studies, or with greater precision pathologically (pTNM) using results of microscopic examination of biopsy or other surgical specimens. Stage may also be assessed following non-operative therapies either clinically or pathologically (ycTNM or ypTNM), at the time of recurrence (rTNM) or at autopsy (aTNM).

The presence of tumour within regional lymph nodes can be estimated radiographically or definitively detected pathologically using any of the biopsy techniques previously described. For many cancers treated surgically, selective or complete regional lymphadenectomies performed as part of curative operations provide the most accurate data with regard to the oncological status of regional lymph nodes. The extent of cancer within regional lymph nodes associated with melanoma and cancers of the breast (among, potentially, others), can also be estimated using a sentinel lymph node technique. Using this technique, the lymph nodes most likely to harbour cancer cells are identified intraoperatively following injection of dye and/or nuclear material into the primary tumour and evaluation of the regional lymphatic basins visually and/or with a nuclear detection counter. The status of all remaining lymphatics in the basin is then established based upon the status of the 'sentinel' nodes; patients with negative sentinel nodes are presumed to have no additional disease in the other lymphatics, and are spared the potential morbidities of a more complete lymphatic dissection. In contrast, patients with positive sentinel lymph nodes are presumed to have additional disease elsewhere in the regional lymph node basin. A formal lymphadenectomy is routinely performed in such cases.

The diagnosis of cancer at metastatic sites distant to the primary tumour is often performed radiographically, but occasionally pathological diagnosis may require needle, endoscopic or even surgical biopsy.

Palliation

Palliative surgical procedures are performed either to relieve or to prevent the symptoms and suffering associated with cancer. No attempt at cure is made, although certain palliative operations may involve resection of all gross disease. Palliative operations can be performed either electively or emergently for symptoms such as pain (e.g. splanchnic block for pancreatic cancer), perforation (e.g., emergent diverting colostomy for perforated colon cancer), haemorrhage (e.g. partial gastrectomy for bleeding secondary to gastric cancer), obstruction (e.g. diverting colostomy for obstructing colon cancer) or infection (e.g. soft tissue resection, mastectomy or even amputation for infected soft tissue tumours) associated with solid cancers. Often, palliative operations are less 'radical' than operations performed with curative intent. For example, palliative gastrectomy performed to remove an intractably bleeding malignant ulcer would be performed without significant dissection of the regional lymphatics; such a limited operation would be considered insufficient in the elective, curative setting.

Patients may be selected for palliative operations instead of surgical ones on the basis of both patient- and tumour-associated factors. Cancer patients may be poor candidates for radical curative procedures secondary to cancer-related cachexia, malnutrition, frailty or pre-existing co-morbidities even in the presence of a technically resectable primary tumour that might be resected for cure in others. In other cases, the anatomical relationship between the cancer and adjacent organs or vital structures may preclude curative resection of a localized tumour without significant morbidity or mortality. Alternatively, the presence of distant metastatic disease may preclude the resection of some cancers for cure, even when both the primary and metastatic disease is technically resectable. In such cases, palliative operations may be a useful adjunct to non-surgical palliative therapies to improve quality of life.

The application of palliative surgery, particularly in the emergent setting, requires thoughtful consideration by the surgeon, multidisciplinary consultation and thorough discussion with the patient and his/her family. Palliative operations are often performed for less-than-optimal surgical candidates and under extreme conditions (such as operation for bleeding or obstruction) that preclude preoperative optimization of the patient's physiology. Complication rates associated with such procedures are therefore often high, even when compared to those associated with more extensive curative operations that may also be used for the same cancer. For example, gastrojejunostomy performed for palliation of gastric outlet obstruction by cancer has a mortality rate as high as one-third in some series; curative pancreaticoduodenectomy for cancer has a mortality rate of 1–5% in optimized patients. For these reasons, the risk-to-benefit profile of a palliative operation must be thoroughly considered. Less invasive methods of palliation (e.g. endoscopic drainage of the biliary tree, stenting of the duodenum or colon to prevent impending instruction) should always be considered, especially when risk is high or anticipated postoperative survival is low.

Reconstruction

Reconstructive surgical operations are often required to repair the soft tissue defects created by primary resection of sarcomas, and cancers of the breast and skin. Complex reconstructive procedures may also be employed to re-establish continuity of the gastrointestinal or aerodigestive tracts following extirpative operations. The complexity of reconstructions may range from simple incisional closures to complex tissue transfer procedures requiring microvascular anastomoses. The importance of these procedures cannot be emphasized enough as their quality can contribute significantly to both quantity and quality of life following cancer surgery.

Prevention

As high-risk groups for solid tumours are being increasingly defined, surgery is increasingly being used in cancer prevention. The goal of such operations is to reduce or eliminate the possibility of cancer developing in patients at high risk for the disease. For example, patients with a genetic predisposition for breast cancer, such as patients who test positive for mutations in the BRCA 1 or BRCA 2 gene, may be offered bilateral prophylactic mastectomy. Similarly, patients with familial adenomatous polyposis due to a germline mutation in the adenomatous polyposis coli (APC) gene may benefit from proctocolectomy or total colectomy prior to a diagnosis of cancer.

Surgical complications

Surgical complications may have profound effects upon the treatment and outcome of the patient with cancer. Indeed, an adverse association between complications and long-term survival in surgical patients in general, and cancer patients specifically, has been well documented. This may in part be related to the long-term sequelae of inflammation and immunosuppression associated with some complications; in cancer patients it may also reflect the inability of patients who suffer from complications to receive all intended oncology therapy. Attention should therefore be given to both prospectively documenting and minimizing complications. Several standardized tools are available for this purpose.

Quality of surgical care

Given the increasing complexity of cancer management, including the variety of anatomical, strategic and multispecialty variables that impact surgical resection, the issue of providing quality surgical cancer care has become an important topic of discussion. This is further affected by the increase in surgical specialization and the increased interest in centralization of complex medical care. Significant research effort has focused on the impact of both hospital and surgeon volume upon outcomes following complex cancer operations. Evidence suggests an association exists between hospital volume and perioperative mortality and overall survival in pancreatic cancer, rectal cancer and oesophageal cancer, among others. A similar association may exist between surgeon volume and surgical and oncological outcomes. These results support the concept of surgeons dedicated to cancer care. However, with the increasing age of the global population, the corresponding increase in incidence of cancer and the impending effects of surgeon shortage, the ability to truly centralize complex oncological surgical care is a formidable challenge.

Postoperative surveillance

Despite potentially curative operations for cancer and treatment using advanced multimodality treatment protocols, recurrence following surgical therapy may occur. In some patients, postoperative recurrence may develop from residual microscopic (or macroscopic) locoregional disease that was not completely addressed surgically in an R1 or R2 operation. In others, postoperative recurrence may develop at distant sites years following an apparently complete R0 procedure. In such cases, recurrence is presumed to arise from dormant micrometastatic tumour cells that were present at the time of the initial operation.

The primary goal of postoperative surveillance programmes is to detect recurrent disease prior to the onset of symptoms, when both the cancer and patient may be most amenable to therapy. Surveillance may involve scheduled clinical evaluations, tumour marker assays and radiographic imaging studies. The use of routine postoperative surveillance following resection of colorectal cancer has been associated with improved overall survival rates. However, surveillance following curative resection of other cancer types (e.g. small cell lung cancer, pancreatic cancer) has not been definitively shown to translate into an improvement in survival. This is significant, because postoperative surveillance programmes are associated with significant costs, such as fear and anxiety, financial costs associated with the studies employed and opportunity costs such as transportation, lost wages and time away from family.

New technologies

Following the rapid introduction of laparoscopic cholecystectomy and the unsystematic and often chaotic dissemination of early 'minimally invasive' surgical technologies, surgeons learned important lessons regarding the potential hazards associated with new technologies and the need for rigorous evaluation of and training in the application of such technologies to minimize perioperative morbidity. In the application of new surgical technologies into operations for cancer, additional challenges exist. Perhaps the biggest of these is the need to understand the interplay between new technologies and the wide variety of biological cancer behaviours that exist among tumour types, and the effect of new technologies on these behaviours. Specifically, in addition to their potential impact upon short-term perioperative metrics (e.g. complication rates, intensity and/or duration of postoperative pain), the potential impact of new technologies on tumour growth, metastasis and recurrence needs to be fully and completely explored in a systematic manner.

Within the context of an understanding of and respect for cancer biology, surgical oncologists have therefore begun to systematically evaluate the role of minimally invasive procedures in the treatment of cancer. Indeed, surgeons have taken leadership roles in designing and implementing clinical trials evaluating the use of laparoscopic surgery for solid tumours. For instance, the treatment of colon cancer using laparoscopic surgery has been well studied in both the USA and in Europe. Randomized prospective trials have demonstrated several important short-term perioperative benefits of laparoscopy, such as shorter hospital stays and decreased narcotic use. More importantly, however, the trials have confirmed that a laparoscopic approach to the treatment of colorectal cancer is safe and similar to an open approach with regard to both perioperative oncological metrics (e.g. rates of negative margins and lymph node retrieval) and long-term oncological metrics such as median duration of disease-free survival. These studies have revolutionized the treatment of primary colorectal cancer and have set the standard for evaluation of new surgical technologies in surgical cancer care.

Although oncological equipoise has been demonstrated between laparoscopic and open resection for colon cancer, it is critical to recognize that some tumours exhibit biological behaviours that might be less compatible with existing minimally invasive technologies. For example, The abdominal insufflation associated with laparoscopy has been suggested to lead to an increase in peritoneal dissemination in patients with adrenal cortical carcinoma and gall bladder cancer. Given the rarity of these diseases, conduct of prospective clinical trials like the ones performed to evaluate laparoscopy for colon cancer is unrealistic. However, given the concerns raised and the ambiguity in the literature, it is incumbent upon the surgical oncologist to utilize these techniques cautiously.

The most recent tool brought to the forefront of cancer therapy is the surgical robot. The surgical robot (e.g. DaVinci system) provides several technical advantages over standard laparoscopy. First, it improves surgical dexterity over that associated with unwristed laparoscopic instrumentation by providing six degrees of freedom (forward/backward, up/down, left/right, pitch, yaw, roll). The surgical robot thereby facilitates movements and manoeuvers essentially identical to those of the human hand and wrist. The robot also reduces the effect of tremor and allows for scalable surgeon–robot motion. These features are important to the conduct of delicate operations that require a high level of precision, such as microsurgical anastomoses and lymphadenectomies. The robot also provides high-definition, three-dimensional optics that allow enhanced visualization, and the ability to operate in a comfortable, ergonomic environment. However, the robot also has disadvantages, such as its limited field of view that precludes the ability to operate in multiple quadrants without being redocked. Use of robotic surgery has been well established in the treatment of prostate cancer and recently has been implemented in the treatment of other solid tumours. From a technical standpoint, the robot may be most appropriate for operations confined to small spaces such as the pelvis, and may be less appropriate for operations that require sweeping, broad fields of view, such as pancreatectomy.

As technology continues to evolve, the scope of applications in surgical oncology will continue to grow. For instance, in the age of video-conferencing via tablet computers and cell phones, the concept of 'telesurgery' has been introduced. Together with robotics, telesurgery applications now allow off-site mentoring of another surgeon, or even operation of surgical robots from a distance. These technologies and their appropriate implementation into the field of oncology are understandably areas of great interest and study. The use of telesurgical systems could enhance access to oncology care in underdeveloped geographical areas, improve dissemination of surgical expertise from high-volume centres to satellite clinics, or even permit the primary conduct of cancer operations in remote locations. Certainly, as this technology continues to be incorporated into medical practice, it will certainly require extensive safeguards for privacy protection and critical evaluation of the patient–doctor relationship in these settings to assure fully informed consent and appropriate intraoperative use.

Technology is a powerful tool and as oncological surgery continues to grow and evolve in the 21st century, active participation of surgeons in the development, use and study of these concepts is required to ensure enhancement of oncological care while simultaneously furthering the understanding of appropriate applications of the technology. The oncological surgeon as an endproduct consumer of technology products is in a unique position to help guide the development of the technology and needs to be an active participant as an advocate for cancer patients.

Recommended reading

Bagaria SP, Faries MB, Morton DL (2010) Sentinel node biopsy in melanoma: technical considerations of the procedure as performed at the John Wayne Cancer Institute. *J Surg Oncol* 101:669–676.

Gardner TB, Barth RJ, Zaki BI et al. (2010) Effect of initiating a multidisciplinary care clinic on access and time to treatment in patients with pancreatic adenocarcinoma. *J Oncol Pract* 6:288–292.

Khuri SF, Henderson WG, DePalma RG et al. (2005) Determinants of long-term survival after major surgery and the adverse effect of postoperative complications. *Ann Surg* 242:326–341; discussion 341–323.

Kuhry E, Schwenk W, Gaupset R et al. (2008) Long-term outcome of laparoscopic surgery for colorectal cancer: a cochrane systematic review of randomised controlled trials. *Cancer Treat Rev* 34:498–504.

Lamb BW, Brown KF, Nagpal K et al. (2011) Quality of care management decisions by multidisciplinary cancer teams: a systematic review. *Ann Surg Oncol* 18:2116–2125.

Matsuda A, Matsumoto S, Seya T et al. (2013) Does postoperative complication have a negative impact on long-term outcomes following hepatic resection for colorectal liver metastasis?: a meta-analysis. *Ann Surg Oncol* 20:2485–2492.

Merkow RP, Bentrem DJ, Cohen ME et al. (2013) Effect of cancer surgery complexity on short-term outcomes, risk predictions, and hospital comparisons. *J Am Coll Surg* 217(4):685–693.

Saxton A, Velanovich V. (2011) Preoperative frailty and quality of life as predictors of postoperative complications. *Ann Surg* 253:1223–1229.

10 Principles of radiotherapy

Vincent Gregoire[1], Cai Grau[2], Karin Haustermans[3], Ludvig Paul Muren[4] and Fiona Stewart[5]

[1]Cancer Center and Department of Radiation Oncology, Institut de Recherche Expérimentale et Clinique, Université Catholique de Louvain, Cliniques Universitaires St-Luc, Brussels, Belgium
[2]Department of Oncology, Aarhus University Hospital, Aarhus, Denmark
[3]Department of Radiation Oncology, Leuven Cancer Institute, University Hospital Gasthuisberg, Leuven, Belgium
[4]Department of Medical Physics, Aarhus University Hospital, Aarhus, Denmark
[5]Division of Experimental Therapy, Netherlands Cancer Institute, Amsterdam, The Netherlands

Introduction: Radiation oncology and radiation biology in the global picture of oncology

Radiation therapy represents one of the main treatment modalities for solid malignant tumours. It is estimated that more than one in two cancer patients will benefit from radiotherapy during the course of their disease. Similar to surgery, the primary objective of radiotherapy is to achieve local tumour control, which is an essential prerequisite for cancer cure. Radiotherapy can be delivered as the only therapeutic intervention for patients for whom a non-surgical approach is preferred to maintain a better organ function (e.g. head and neck carcinoma, anal carcinoma, prostate carcinoma), for locally advanced non-resectable tumours (e.g. non-small cell lung carcinoma, cervical carcinoma, oesophageal carcinoma), for highly radiosensitive tumours (e.g. Hodgkin lymphoma) or for non-operable patients for medical reasons. For small tumours, radiotherapy is typically delivered as a single modality, whereas for locally advanced stages, it is most frequently delivered in association with radiosensitizing agents such as chemotherapy, targeted agents or hypoxic cell sensitizers. Radiotherapy (or concomitant chemoradiation) can also be delivered in association with surgery, either as a preoperative modality (neoadjuvant radiotherapy) to improve resection with free margins (e.g. rectal carcinoma) or as a postoperative modality (adjuvant radiotherapy) to improve local and/or regional control (e.g. breast carcinoma, head and neck carcinoma), and thus the overall therapeutic outcome. Radiotherapy can also be delivered as a palliative option to alleviate pain not controlled by drugs (e.g. bone metastasis), to re-establish continuity in an organ (e.g. airway obstruction), to control bleeding or to decompress a critical organ (e.g. brain or spinal metastasis). In these circumstances, lower total doses and a higher dose per fraction are typically delivered to maximize the cost-effectiveness ratio.

During the second half of the last century, key technological innovations in radiotherapy technology, diagnostic imaging and computer science greatly modified the routine practice of radiotherapy, leading to substantial improvements in treatment delivery and outcome. The introduction of deeply penetrating external photon beams, initially from ^{60}Co in the 1950s, and those from high-energy electron linear accelerators (linacs) in the 1960s, allowed the target dose to be increased without increasing normal tissue morbidity. During the 1970s and 1980s, treatment planning based on the use of planar diagnostic X-rays was widely implemented. The increasing use of X-ray computed tomography (CT) in the 1980s and magnetic resonance imaging (MRI) in the 1990s enabled much more reliable three-dimensional assessment of the location and extent of the disease. With these imaging improvements and advances in treatment planning techniques, it became practical to design treatment fields that conformed more closely to the target volume. This technique is usually referred to as conformal radiotherapy (CRT) or three-dimensional conformal therapy (3D-CRT).

The concept of intensity-modulated radiation therapy (IMRT) arose in the 1980s because radiotherapy treatment planning optimization algorithms predicted that the optimal radiation pattern from any single direction was typically non-uniform. It was shown that a collective set of intensity-modulated beams from multiple directions could be designed to produce dose homogeneity similar to conventional radiotherapy within the tumour but with superior conformality, especially for concave or other complex-shaped target volumes, thereby sparing nearby normal tissues.

UICC Manual of Clinical Oncology, Ninth Edition. Edited by Brian O'Sullivan, James D. Brierley, Anil K. D'Cruz, Martin F. Fey, Raphael Pollock, Jan B. Vermorken and Shao Hui Huang. © 2015 UICC. Published 2015 by John Wiley & Sons, Ltd.

The use of IMRT has grown rapidly. In a survey performed in 2003 in the USA, one-third of radiation oncologists were using IMRT. In 2005, a similar US survey showed that more than two-thirds of radiation oncologists were using some form of IMRT, mainly for increased normal tissue sparing or target dose escalation. In other countries, and especially in those countries lacking the financial incentive, IMRT tends to be used in much more selected cases. Among the sites treated by IMRT, head and neck malignancies and prostate cancers are by far the most common, followed by central nervous system, lung, breast and gastrointestinal tumours. However, thus far, only a few prospective randomized trials have reported superiority of IMRT over conventional treatments, either in terms of efficacy or morbidity reduction. These studies were for head and neck, breast and prostate cancers.

Alongside these improvements in dose delivery, numerous studies in radiation biology have been conducted, and have also complementarily contributed to the development of radiotherapy over the last few decades. In a nutshell, radiation biology aims at individualizing the various molecular, cellular and tissue pathways involved after radiation exposure, at highlighting the differences in response between normal tissue and cancer cells, and finally at proposing strategies to selectively improve the therapeutic ratio of radiotherapy (Fig. 10.1). There are many examples illustrating how knowledge of radiation biology has translated into improved efficacy of radiotherapy. One of the first examples is probably the demonstration of differences in cell proliferation and cell recovery after fractionated irradiations between normal and cancer cells, which have led to the clinical validation of accelerated fractionation and hyperfractionated regimens in various tumour types such as head and neck and lung. The study of tumour microenvironment and the demonstration that tumours are typically more hypoxic than the surrounding normal tissues have led to the development of hypoxic sensitizers (e.g. nimorazole), which have been shown to improve locoregional tumour control probability in cervical, lung and head and neck tumours. More recently, the individualization of cancer selective molecular pathways involved in early response after ionizing radiation has led to the introduction of protocols combining radiation with specific targeted agents. The story of the epidermal growth factor receptor (EGFR) pathways and the inhibitory antibody C225 (cetuximab) is probably one of the most recent examples illustrating how the discovery of a key molecular determinant of cancer cell phenotype have led to significant improvement in cancer cure.

In the following sections, the concepts briefly outlined above will be elaborated with special emphasis on how improved dose delivery and a better understanding of radiation biology can lead to the development of more effective treatment protocols.

Biological basis of radiation oncology

Molecular and cellular radiation biology
DNA damage and repair

As indicated by its name, the principal damaging effects of ionizing radiation arise from its ability to ionize, or eject, electrons from molecules within cells. Almost all the photons produced by linear accelerators have sufficient energy to cause such ionizations. Most biological damage, however, is caused by the ejected electrons themselves, which ionize the molecules they collide with, progressively slowing down with each collision. At the end of electron tracks, interactions with other molecules become more frequent, giving rise to clusters of ionizations. The clusters are such that many ionizations occur within a few base pairs of the DNA. These clusters are a unique characteristic of ionizing radiation, in contrast to other forms of radiation such as ultraviolet (UV) or DNA-damaging drugs such as topoisomerase inhibitors. Only a small amount of the damage is clustered, but when these clusters occur in DNA, the cell has particular difficulty coping with the damage.

Ionized molecules are highly reactive and undergo a rapid cascade of chemical changes, which can lead to the breaking of chemical bonds. This can disrupt the structure of macromolecules such as DNA, leading to severe consequences if not repaired adequately or in time. Ionizing radiation deposits its energy randomly, thus causing damage to all molecules in the cell. As DNA is present in only two copies, has very limited turnover, is the largest molecule and thus the biggest target, and is central to all cellular functions, the consequence of permanent damage to DNA can therefore be serious and often lethal to the cell.

There is also compelling experimental evidence that the DNA is the principal target for radiation-induced cell killing. Elegant experiments have been carried out irradiating individual

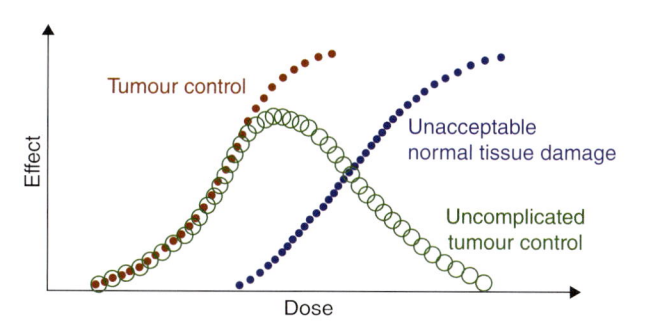

Figure 10.1 Therapeutic ratio is defined by the comparison of dose–response relationships between tumours and normal tissues. The greater the separation between curves, the higher is the therapeutic ratio. There are situations where the tumours (e.g. lymphomas, seminomas) are so radiosensitive (tumour response curve on the left) that irradiation can be done with no or minimal dose delivered to normal tissues, thus creating a high therapeutic ratio; there are situations where the tumours (e.g. glioblastoma, melanoma) are so radioresistant (tumour response curve similar to the normal tissue response curve but displaced to the right) that irradiation also delivers a high dose to normal tissues, thus creating a low therapeutic ratio. Strategies for improving the therapeutic ratio typically aim to displace the tumour response curve to the left.

cells with small polonium needles producing short-range α-particles. High doses could be given to plasma membranes and cytoplasm without causing cell death. However, as soon as the needle was placed so that the nucleus received even one or two α-particles, cell death resulted. Other experiments have used radioactively-labelled compounds to irradiate principally the plasma membrane (^{125}I-concanavalin) or principally the DNA (^{3}H-labelled thymidine), and compared this with homogeneous cell irradiation with X-rays. Cell death closely correlated only with dose to the nucleus, and not with either the plasma membrane or the cytoplasm.

Owing to the importance of DNA, cells and organisms have developed a complex series of processes and pathways for ensuring that the DNA remains intact and unaltered in the face of continuous attack from within (e.g. oxidation and alkylation owing to metabolism) and from the outside (e.g. ingested chemicals, UV and ionizing radiation). These include different forms of DNA repair to cope with the different forms of DNA damage induced by different agents. Specialized repair systems have therefore evolved for detecting and repairing damage to bases (base excision repair [BER]), single-strand breaks (single-strand break repair [SSBR], closely related to BER) and double-strand breaks (homologous recombination [HR] and non-homologous end-joining [NHEJ]). There are also other DNA repair pathways, such as those for correcting the mismatches of bases in DNA which can occur during replication, such as mismatch repair (MMR), and for repairing bulky lesions or DNA adducts such as those caused by UV light and some drugs such as cisplatin (nucleotide excision repair [NER]). However, neither MMR nor NER appears to be important for ionizing radiation, since cells with mutations or deletions in genes on these pathways are not more sensitive to ionizing radiation. In contrast, mutations or deletions in genes involved in BER, SSBR, HR or NHEJ can all, under certain circumstances, lead to increased radiosensitivity.

To give an idea of the scale of damage, 1 Gy of irradiation will cause in each cell approximately 10^5 ionizations, >1000 damaged DNA bases, around 1000 single-strand DNA breaks (SSBs) and around 20–40 double-strand DNA breaks (DSBs). To put this into further perspective, 1 Gy will kill only about 30% of cells of a typical mammalian cell line, including human. This relatively limited cytotoxicity, despite the large numbers of induced lesions per cell, is the consequence of efficient DNA repair.

Cellular DNA comprises two opposing strands linked by hydrogen bonds and forming a double helical structure. Each strand is a linear chain of the four bases – adenine (A), cytosine (C), guanine (G) and thymine (T) – connected by sugar molecules and a phosphate group, the so-called sugar–phosphate backbone. The order of the bases is the code determining not only which protein is made but also whether a gene is active (transcribed) or not. In turn, this double helix is wound at regular intervals around a complex of a specific class of proteins (histones), forming nucleosomes, resembling beads on a string. Many other proteins are also associated with the DNA; these control DNA metabolism, including transcription, replication and repair. The DNA plus its associated proteins is called chromatin. There are further levels of folding and looping, finally making up the compact structure of the chromosomes.

This structure poses various challenges to the cell for repairing DNA damage. First, specialized proteins have to be sufficiently abundant and mobile to detect damage within seconds or minutes of it occurring. Second, the chromatin usually needs to be remodelled (e.g. the structure opened up) to allow access of repair proteins. This may entail removal of nucleosomes close to the break, among other changes. The correct repair, accessory and signalling proteins then need to be recruited, often mediated by histone modifications, and tightly coordinated. This includes stopping various processes such as transcription and cell cycle progression to allow the concentration on repair. Repair progress needs to be continually monitored so that the chromatin will be reset to its original state after completion of repair, and then normal cellular processes resumed.

Cell survival curve and dose–response relationship

When a tumour regrows after non-curative dose of radiotherapy, it does so because some neoplastic cells, called stem cells, were not killed. Radiobiologists have therefore recognized that the key to understanding tumour response is to ask how many stem cells are left. It is almost impossible to recognize tumour stem cells *in situ*, and therefore assays have been developed to detect stem cells by their ability to form a colony within some growth environment. These are therefore called 'clonogenic' or "colony-forming" cells – cells that form colonies exceeding about 50 cells within a defined growth environment. The number 50 represents approximately five or six generations of proliferation.

In this context, a cell survival curve is a plot of the surviving fraction against dose (of radiation, cytotoxic drug or other cell-killing agent). As cell kill is a random process after ionizing radiation, survival is an exponential function of dose and thereby cell survival curves are typically depicted on a linear logarithmic scale (Fig. 10.2). Several models have been proposed to fit the cell survival curves, and the linear quadratic (LQ) model has been widely adopted as it gives a better description of the dose–response relationship in the dose range of 1–3 Gy, which more closely relates to the dose per fraction of 2 Gy typically used in daily clinical radiotherapy.

According to the LQ model, the formula for the cell survival curve is $S = \exp\text{-}(\alpha D + \beta D^2)$ where S is the surviving fraction and α and β parameters with dimension of Gy^{-1} and Gy^{-2}, respectively. According to this LQ model, the $\alpha{:}\beta$ ratio (in Gy) expresses the shape (or 'bendiness') of the curve, a low ratio indicating a more "bendy" curve. Typically, tumours and early reacting normal tissues (see next section) have higher $\alpha{:}\beta$ ratios (>10) compared to late reacting normal tissues (around 2–3).

Empirical attempts to establish dose–response relationships in the clinic date back to the first decade of radiotherapy. In 1936 the clinical scientist Holthusen was the first to present a theoretical analysis of dose–response relationships, and this has

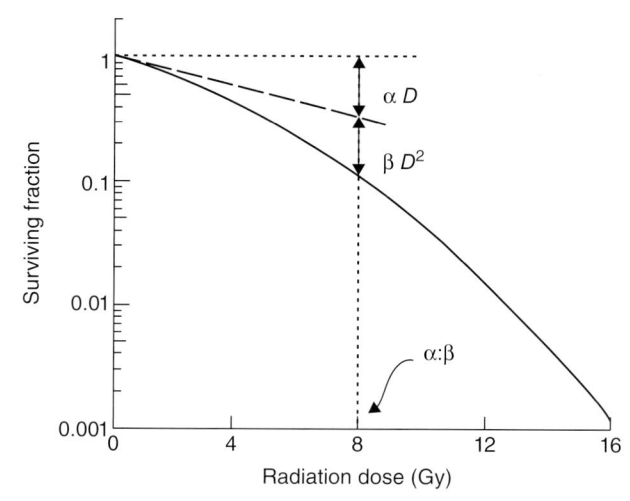

Figure 10.2 A typical cell survival curve for cells irradiated in tissue culture, plotted on a logarithmic scale. The parameter α corresponds to the slope of the initial part of the curve, whereas the ratio α:β depicts the curvature or 'bendiness' of the curve. D is the total dose and d the fraction size.

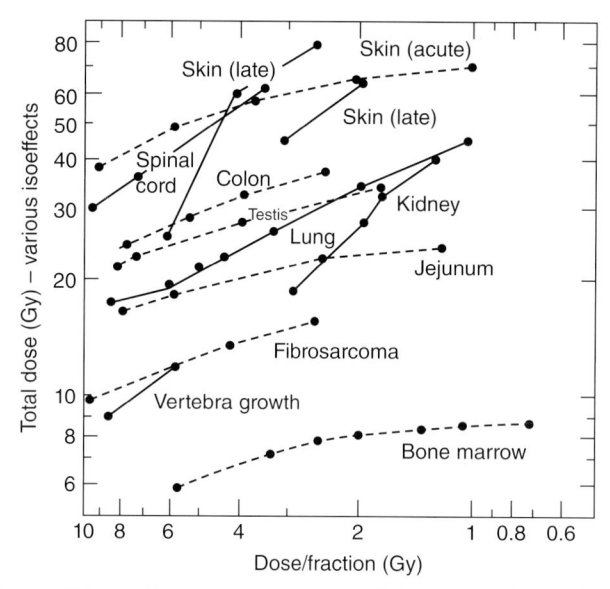

Figure 10.3 Relationship between the total dose required to produce a given biological effect and the dose per fraction in various normal tissues and tumours in experimental animals. The curves for late-responding tissues (unbroken line) are typically steeper than for early-responding tissues and tumour (broken lines).

had a major impact on the conceptual development of radiotherapy optimization. Holthusen demonstrated the sigmoid shape of dose–response curves both for normal tissue reactions (i.e. skin telangiectasia) and local control of skin cancer (see Fig. 10.1). He noted the resemblance between these curves and the cumulative distribution functions known from statistics, and this led him to the idea that the dose–response curve simply reflects the variability in clinical radio-responsiveness of individual patients. This remains one of the main hypotheses for the origin of the dose–response relationships and has had a renaissance in recent years with the growing interest in interpatient variability in response to radiotherapy.

Fractionation sensitivity

The relationships between total dose and dose per fraction for tumours, late responding tissues and acutely responding tissues provide the basic information required to optimize radiotherapy according to the dose per fraction and number of fractions. A milestone in this subject was the publication by Thames in 1982 of an overview of isoeffect curves for various normal tissues and tumours, mainly in mice (Fig. 10.3). These curves showed the relationship between the total radiation dose required to produce a given biological effect and the dose per fraction: the lower the dose per fraction the higher the total dose required to produce a given effect. This survey showed that the isoeffective total dose increases more rapidly with decreasing dose per fraction for late effects (tissues with a low α:β ratio) than for acute effects and tumour response (tissues with a higher α:β ratio). It can be deduced immediately from this plot that use of lower doses per fraction will tend to spare late reactions if the total dose is adjusted to keep the acute reactions constant. This is the radiobiological basis of using hyperfractionated radiotherapy which allows an increase in the total dose delivered to the tumour while keeping a similar level of late normal tissue toxicity.

The LQ cell survival model can be used to describe this relationship between total isoeffective dose and the dose per fraction in fractionated radiotherapy. The LQ model can thus form a robust quantitative environment for considering the balance between acute and late reactions (and effect on the tumour) as dose per fraction and total dose are changed. This is one of the most important developments in radiobiology applied to therapy.

The LQ approach leads to various formulae for calculating isoeffect relationships for radiotherapy, all based on similar underlying assumptions. These formulae seek to describe a range of fractionation schedules that are isoeffective. The simplest method of comparing the effectiveness of schedules consisting of different total doses and doses per fraction is to convert each schedule into an equivalent schedule in 2-Gy fractions that would produce the same biological effect. This is the recommended approach:

$$EQD_2 = D \cdot [d + (\alpha/\beta)]/[2 + (\alpha/\beta)]$$

where EQD_2 is the dose in 2-Gy fractions that is biologically equivalent to a total dose D given with a fraction size of d Gy. Values of EQD_2 can be numerically added for separate parts of a treatment schedule. They have the advantage that since 2 Gy is a commonly used dose per fraction clinically, EQD_2 values will be recognized by radiation oncologists as being of a familiar size. However, it should be stressed that this model should only be used within a range of dose per fraction of 1 and 6–8 Gy as it overestimates the tolerance dose for lower and for higher doses per fraction.

Tumour and normal cell repopulation

Each fraction during a course of fractionated radiotherapy reduces the total population of clonogenic cells in a tumour, leading to progressive tumour shrinkage. In general, clonogenic cells that survive radiation can repopulate the tumour by proliferation and/or reduced cell loss. Repopulation of clonogenic tumour cells might occur during the course of fractionated radiotherapy and thereby reduce the efficacy of treatment. If a tumour has the capacity to repopulate, any prolongation of the overall treatment time results in a higher number of clonogenic tumour cells that need to be inactivated and thereby requires a higher radiation dose to achieve local tumour control. The so-called time factor of fractionated radiotherapy has been largely attributed to repopulation of clonogenic tumour cells during treatment. Repopulation of clonogenic tumour cells during fractionated radiotherapy has been shown in a large variety of different experimental and clinical studies. The results are most consistent for squamous cell carcinomas (e.g. head and neck, lung, cervix), but for other tumour types evidence for a time factor is also accumulating. The rate, kinetics and underlying radiobiological mechanisms of repopulation vary substantially between tumour types as well as between different tumour lines of the same tumour type.

The possible existence of a tumour time factor in clinical radiotherapy became more widely acknowledged following a publication by Withers in 1988 entitled 'The hazard of accelerated tumour clonogen repopulation during radiotherapy'. This review examined the correlation between tumour control and overall treatment time for squamous cell carcinomas of the head and neck and led to the graph showing that as overall time increases, a greater total radiation dose has been required to control these tumours. The other important conclusion was that there seemed to be an initial flat portion to this relationship (the so-called 'dog leg'). This implied that, for treatment times shorter than 3–4 weeks, tumour proliferation may have little effect and that, as shown for experimental tumours, it also takes time for accelerated repopulation to be 'switched on' in human tumours. For treatment times longer than 4 weeks, the effect of proliferation was equivalent to a loss of radiation dose of about 0.6 Gy/day. Thus, accelerated fractionation, which uses an overall treatment time shorter than the conventional 6–7 weeks, should increase tumour cure rates by restricting the time available for tumour cell proliferation. For example, the dose in a 5-week schedule would be effectively larger than that in a 7-week schedule by a factor 0.6 Gy/day – (49–35 days) = 8.4 Gy, or slightly above 10% of a 70-Gy treatment. Since this publication, the effect of cell proliferation on tumour control has also been reported for lung and cervix tumours.

The kinetics and radiobiological mechanisms of repopulation have been studied in an extensive series of experiments in which fractionated irradiation was given to human tumour xenografts under various experimental conditions. A switch to rapid repopulation was observed after about 3 weeks of fractionated irradiation, with the clonogen doubling time decreasing from 9.8 days during the first 3 weeks to 3.4 days thereafter. In this study, acceleration of repopulation was preceded by a decrease in tumour hypoxia after 2 weeks of fractionated irradiation, suggesting that improved tumour oxygenation might trigger repopulation in tumours either by facilitating more proliferation and/or by reducing cell loss. Increased labelling indices for BrdUrd (S-phase fraction) and Ki67 (growth fraction) during fractionated irradiation indicate that increased proliferation contributes directly to repopulation.

In contrast to this concept, it has been suggested, particularly for well-differentiated tumours, that an actively regulated regenerative response of surviving clonogens, reminiscent of a normal epithelium, represents the major mechanism of clonogen repopulation. Signalling via the EGFR has been proposed as a potential molecular mechanism of this regulated regenerative response underlying repopulation.

Tumour microenvironment

Tumours can only grow when they receive sufficient oxygen and nutrients. In order to obtain a sufficient supply of both, new vessels sprout from the existing normal vasculature. This process is referred to as angiogenesis. However, very frequently the tumours outgrow their blood supply. The vasculature that is formed is also very primitive with tortuous and often non-functional vessels. The combination of these two phenomena leads to the development of areas within a tumour that are hypoxic and acidic. Hypoxic cells in these areas might still be viable, but the partial pressure of oxygen (PO_2) can typically reach very low level below 1 mmHg. Classically, two types of hypoxia are recognized: chronic or diffusion limited hypoxia, and acute or perfusion limited hypoxia. In the former, areas of necrosis are frequently observed. These are typically located at 100–180 μm from the blood vessels, which corresponds to the diffusion distance of oxygen from vessels. More recently, acute hypoxia has been described, resulting from the periodic opening and closing of immature blood vessels under high interstitial pressure.

Direct measurements of PO_2 with the Eppendorf electrode in patients have shown a large range of oxygen concentrations in human tumours. Although there is a wide variation both in space and time of hypoxia within a tumour, the variability in hypoxic fractions between tumours is even greater. Because of this large intertumour variability, it becomes possible to stratify tumours according to their hypoxic fraction into different prognostic subgroups that may receive different treatments. In head and neck cancer, a multicentre meta-analysis identified the hypoxic fraction measured by the Eppendorf electrode as the most significant negative prognostic factor in patients treated with radiotherapy. Also, it has been shown that hypoxia is an important prognostic factor in patients treated with surgery. Hoeckel et al. showed that poorly oxygenated cervical tumours treated with surgery alone had a significantly poorer disease-free survival and overall survival. This is indirect evidence that hypoxia causes a more malignant phenotype. Several pathways are activated by hypoxia and these are the basis for both hypoxia tolerance and malignancy. Understanding these pathways will lead to the development of biomarkers for hypoxia and ultimately to new molecular targeting agents.

Oxygen is also a key player in the response of tumour cells to ionizing radiation. When radiation is absorbed in the tumour, free radicals are formed. These radicals are highly reactive and can break chemical bonds. They initiate the chain of events that leads to biological damage. These radicals also interact with water to produce peroxy radicals, RO_2*, which then undergoes further reaction to form organic peroxides, ROOH. This leads to a stable change in the chemical composition of the target, and the damage is said to be chemically 'fixed' by oxygen. In the absence of oxygen, the free radicals can react with H^+, thus chemically restoring their original form without causing any damage. To quantitate the enhanced efficacy of ionizing radiation by oxygen, the 'oxygen enhancement ratio (OER)"', which is the ratio of radiation doses to induce a given biological effect under hypoxic and normoxic conditions, has been defined. For low linear energy transfer (LET) radiation, such as X-rays, typical OER values reach a factor of 2.8 under very low oxygen concentration. In fractionated radiotherapy, every fraction preferentially kills the well-oxygenated cells. The remaining hypoxic cells will then get access to oxygen. This phenomenon is called reoxygenation, and it is one of the reasons fractionation is used in the clinic.

Several therapeutic approaches have been tested to overcome the problem of hypoxia resistance. A first approach is to raise the oxygen content of the inspired air. This can be done with hyperbaric oxygen. As an alternative, carbogen (95% oxygen combined with 5% carbon dioxide) was used in the ARCON (accelerated radiotherapy with carbogen and nicotinamide) trial. Both measures mainly overcome diffusion-limited hypoxia. ARCON is a therapeutic strategy that combines radiation treatment modifications, with the aim of counteracting various resistance mechanisms. To limit clonogenic repopulation during therapy, the overall duration of the radiotherapy is reduced, generally by delivering several fractions per day. This accelerated radiotherapy is combined with inhalation of carbogen to decrease diffusion-limited hypoxia, and with oral intake of nicotinamide, a vasoactive agent, to decrease perfusion-limited hypoxia. In 345 patients with advanced laryngeal cancer, the 5-year regional control was significantly improved with ARCON (93%) compared with standard radiotherapy (86%; $P = 0.04$) with equal levels of toxicity. The improvement in regional control was specifically observed in patients with hypoxic tumours and not in patients with well-oxygenated tumours (100% versus 55%, respectively; $P = 0.01$). Also, in muscle invasive bladder cancer, 323 patients were randomized to radiation alone or to radiation with carbogen and nicotinamide (CON). Radiation plus CON produced a small but non-significant improvement in cystoscopic control. Differences in overall survival, risk of death and local relapse were significantly in favour of CON. Late morbidity was similar in both trial arms.

A second approach to overcome tumour hypoxia is the use of hypoxic cell radiosensitizers. These compounds mimic oxygen.

One of the agents widely tested in the clinic is nimorazole. In the DAHANCA 5 study (a Danish study group of head and neck cancer), a highly significant improvement in locoregional control was observed when nimorazole was combined with radiation in the treatment of supraglottic and pharyngeal carcinomas.

A third approach is the use of bioreductive drugs acting as selective hypoxic cell cytotoxins. These compounds undergo intracellular reduction to form active cytotoxic species under low oxygen tension. Tirapazamine is an example of such a drug. It has been tested in a phase III randomized trial in patients with previously untreated Stage III or IV squamous cell carcinoma of the oral cavity, oropharynx, hypopharynx or larynx. Eight hundred and sixty-one patients were randomly assigned to receive definitive radiotherapy concurrently with either cisplatin or cisplatin plus tirapazamine. There were no significant differences in failure-free survival, time to locoregional failure or quality of life. But retrospective analysis of the data has shown that a significant proportion of patients did not receive appropriate radiotherapy. When these patients were excluded from the data analysis, a borderline improvement of efficacy was observed in favour of the tirapazamine group.

Acute and late reactions in irradiate normal tissues

There is increasing awareness that radiotherapy, although a very effective form of cancer therapy, is associated with a range of both acute and long-term side effects, some of which may seriously impair quality of life or be life threatening. These side effects are caused by a combination of cell killing and stimulation of inflammatory, thrombotic and fibrogenic processes. Side effects may develop during the course of radiotherapy (acute reactions) or be delayed for months or years after treatment (late reactions). The time of onset of damage and recovery potential depend on the proliferative and cellular organization of the tissue, as well as on the radiation dose, fractionation schedule and the volume of tissue irradiated.

Acute reactions
General principles
Acute radiation injury is mainly seen in mucosal tissues (e.g. skin, oral mucosa, intestine) and the haematopoietic system, which have rapid natural cell turnover rates. Such tissues have what has been described as a 'hierarchical' structure, in that there are distinct populations of stem cells (capable of unlimited division), transit cells (capable of limited proliferation) and post-mitotic, fully differentiated, functional cells. The cell killing effects of radiation are mediated mainly by DNA damage, leading to either rapid apoptotic cell loss (in a few cell types such as lymphocytes and salivary gland acinar cells) or reproductive failure of stem and transit cells at subsequent mitoses, in the majority of cell types. Tissue damage occurs when the rate of cell depletion exceeds the proliferative capacity of the remaining cells.

Time of expression of acute reactions
Mature functional cells in hierarchical tissues generally die from natural senescence rather than from irradiation. The time of onset of acute damage is therefore dependent on the natural lifespan of these functional cells; this may be <1 week for the small intestine or 3–4 weeks for bone marrow. The maximum extent of damage is determined by the proportion of stem cells that have been killed, which depends on dose and on the radiation sensitivity of the tissue stem cells. The rate of tissue healing depends on the extent of cell depletion and the proliferative capacity of the surviving cells. Providing that sufficient stem cells survived, proliferative regeneration will usually give rise to complete healing of acute normal tissue damage. Since all tissues and organs have more mature differentiated cells than are required for adequate function, there may be significant cell killing without any observable tissue damage. Conversely, proliferative regeneration to fully restore the original cell numbers in a tissue will take longer than the time to observable healing.

Consequential tissue damage
In normal tissues that have an important barrier function against mechanical or chemical insult (e.g. oral, intestinal and bladder mucosa), high doses causing severe acute damage may disrupt this barrier function and lead to secondary infections. This initiates a chronic phase of inflammation and abnormal tissue remodelling, fibrosis and secondary processes like strictures or obstructions, which have been termed 'consequential late effects'. In these situations there is no complete healing after the acute phase of damage, despite ongoing proliferative regeneration.

Manifestation of acute reactions
Acute mucosal reactions manifest as erythema and oedema (caused by early vascular damage), parenchymal cell death and hypoplasia, leading to desquamation and ulceration, followed by re-epithelialization. In the oral mucosa, the hypoplastic phase is associated with patchy or confluent mucositis (depending on dose); in the intestine, hypoplasia gives rise to malabsorption, electrolyte loss and diarrhoea, with the risk of ulceration and sepsis.

In the salivary glands, hypoplasia causes a reduction in the production of saliva from the parotid glands and mucin from the submandibular glands, resulting in xerostomia. The stem cells in the salivary glands are particularly radiosensitive and if the entire gland is exposed to doses commonly used to treat head and neck cancers, there will be insufficient surviving stem cells to repopulate the gland and the resulting xerostomia is likely to be permanent.

In the urinary bladder, increased urination frequency and urgency occur during fractionated radiotherapy, but this acute response is due to changes in prostaglandin metabolism and decreased urothelial barrier function, resulting in oedema and alterations in bladder tone, rather than cell loss. There is no urothelial cell depletion in the acute phase of bladder damage, since these cells have a very long cell turnover time and cell loss consequently does not occur until many months after irradiation (unless bladder infection precipitates early desquamation).

Late tissue reactions
General principles
Late radiation damage is the result of complex biological responses at both the cell and tissue levels. In contrast to hierarchical tissues, many organs have slow turnover rates and they do not have well-defined stem cell populations with separate functional cells tissues (e.g. heart, lung, kidney, liver, brain). These slow turnover tissues have been termed 'flexible' in that their differentiated, functional cells are normally in G0 phase, although they can be recruited into the cell cycle in response to injury. Since radiation cell death in parenchymal cells is mostly expressed when cells attempt to go through mitosis, the onset of cell death is delayed in tissues with a slow turnover rate.

Time of expression of late reactions
There is an inverse correlation between time of expression of late radiation injury and the basal cell turnover rate of tissues (damage is expressed earlier in lung than in heart or brain). The time of onset and rate of progression of late radiation injury are also dependent on the radiation dose, in contrast to acute radiation injury. This is because cell killing of functional cells stimulates compensatory proliferation in other functional cells, which then express their radiation damage as they attempt to go through mitosis. This sets up an avalanche effect, where higher doses cause more cell death and compensatory proliferation, precipitating more damage and shortening the latent time for expression of tissue injury. A major contrast between acute and late damage is that compensatory proliferation in hierarchical tissues leads to tissue recovery, whereas in slow turnover flexible tissues it is associated with further progression of damage. This is illustrated by the development of telangiectasia (dilated, fragile capillaries with reduced functionality) in irradiated skin of breast cancer patients, where both the incidence and severity of telangiectasia increase, in proportion to dose, from about 6 months to >10 years after treatment. Most types of late radiation damage are progressive and irreversible, despite the stimulated proliferation in parenchymal cells, although some specific inflammatory and immune pathologies, e.g. pneumonitis, do resolve in time.

Manifestation of late radiation damage
Cell loss, vascular damage, inflammation and fibrosis are the underlying mechanisms of late radiation damage, but the influence these changes have on organ function varies. Microvascular damage causes telangiectasia and visible haemorrhage in skin and mucosal tissues (e.g. rectum, bladder), but telangiectasia also develops in the central nervous system (CNS), kidney and other internal organs, where the resulting haemorrhages may initially go undetected. Microvascular damage may lead to secondary necrosis and parenchymal cell loss, e.g. white matter necrosis in the irradiated spinal cord with resulting paralysis,

congestive heart failure in the irradiated heart and bone necrosis in the irradiated jaw. The consequences of fibrosis also vary according to tissue type. In skin this may lead to symptoms such as 'frozen shoulder', in bladder to a permanent reduction in bladder capacity with resulting increased frequency and nocturia, and in tube-like structures fibrosis may lead to strictures and stenosis (e.g. intestine, oesophagus). In other organs, fibrosis is associated with a general reduction in function or organ failure, depending on dose (lungs, kidney, heart). In many tissues, e.g. lungs, there may be distinct waves of damage, with an early vascular and inflammatory phase (pneumonitis), followed by a later fibrotic phase of damage.

Influence of fractionation on tissue tolerance

The biological effects of radiation depend strongly on how the total dose is delivered in time. The main factors involved are: (1) repair of sublethal damage, which occurs within minutes to hours and is influenced by the size of the dose per fraction; and (2) tissue regeneration by proliferation of surviving cells, which occurs within days to weeks and is influenced by overall treatment time.

Influence of the dose per fraction

Clinical radiotherapy is generally given as a series of fractionated doses over a period of several weeks. The rationale for this is that repair of sublethal damage takes place after each fractionated dose and that this will increase the tissue tolerance to radiation. Of course, this is based on the premise that repair during fractionated schedules is greater in normal tissues than in tumours! The relationship between total tolerance dose and the size of the dose per fraction varies according to tissue type, and can be described by the LQ model and $\alpha:\beta$ ratio of the tissue, as discussed earlier. The lower the $\alpha:\beta$ ratio of a tissue, the greater will be its sensitivity to changes in the dose per fraction, with high doses per fraction causing more tissue damage than low doses per fraction, for the same total dose. Acute radiation damage in rapidly dividing tissues is described by high $\alpha:\beta$ ratios, e.g. 8–12 Gy for oral mucositis. Late radiation damage is described by much lower $\alpha:\beta$ ratios, e.g. 2–4 Gy for fibrosis. Late radiation effects are therefore more sensitive to changes in dose per fraction than acute effects. There are many clinical examples demonstrating that doses per fraction of >3 Gy cause more late complications than conventional doses of 2 Gy per fraction, unless the total dose is reduced. Conversely, hyperfractionation with doses per fraction of <2 Gy leads to relative sparing of late normal tissue injury.

In order to exploit the sparing effects of fractionated radiotherapy, there must be sufficient time between fractions for complete repair of sublethal damage. The estimated half-times for repair vary among tissues, e.g. 30–45 minutes for the intestine and oral mucosa, and >1.5 hours for the kidney and spinal cord. Intervals of <6 hours between fractions are likely to be associated with incomplete repair in slow turnover tissues. Indeed, there are several clinical examples where multiple fractions per day were given with 2–4.5 hours between fractions and this led to very severe late complications.

Influence of overall treatment time

Proliferative regeneration of rapid turnover tissues results in increased acute radiation tolerance for longer overall treatment times. This is a homeostatic, compensatory response to cell loss, whereby the cell cycle time of surviving stem cells decreases. There is also a temporary loss of asymmetric cell division, in that both daughter cells remain as stem cells rather than one cell entering the transit cell/differentiated cell lineage. These mechanisms allow the tissue to repopulate to normal levels quickly and efficiently. In rapidly proliferating tissues, like oral and intestinal mucosa, compensatory proliferation starts early in a course of fractionated radiotherapy (1–2 weeks) and at its maximum may completely counteract the cell killing induced by 2 Gy per day. The effects of this can be seen clinically, where oral mucositis actually starts to heal during the last weeks of radiotherapy, despite continued irradiation. Shortened overall treatment times will lead to an increased incidence of acute reactions as there is less time for compensatory proliferation to regenerate the tissue.

Since compensatory proliferation is triggered by cell loss, this will not normally occur in slowly proliferating tissues during a 6–7-week course of radiotherapy. Stimulated proliferation does occur in these slow turnover tissues, but this usually starts several months after radiotherapy and, as explained above, it may precipitate further damage rather than tissue recovery. There is therefore little or no influence of modest changes in overall treatment time (e.g. 3–8 weeks) on late radiation damage.

Re-irradiation of previously treated tissue

Re-irradiation of previously treated areas may become necessary for recurrent cancer, new primary tumours (common in head and neck cancer patients) or nodal and metastatic disease. Factors that need to be taken into account include: (1) previous dose and extent of field overlap; (2) whether there are additional treatments proposed, e.g. chemotherapy; (3) the critical organs and tissues at risk; (4) how much time has elapsed since the initial treatment; and (5) whether there are any practical alternatives to re-irradiation?

Rapidly proliferating tissues generally recover well from the acute radiation injury and will tolerate re-irradiation to full doses after an interval of a few months. Retreatment tolerance depends on the level of cell killing from the first treatment and on the extent of compensatory proliferation that has occurred before re-irradiation; recovery of the stem cell compartment may take longer than apparent functional recovery of the tissue. Clinical experience is generally consistent with animal studies in that there is little increase in acute toxicity for re-irradiation schedules, providing that tolerance is not exceeded in the first treatment.

Some slowly proliferating tissues are capable of partial proliferative and functional recovery, although this takes several months and some residual damage remains. Preclinical data show that there is good recovery in the lung from the pneumonitis phase of damage after initial treatments of <50% full tolerance, and partial recovery after higher doses. The re-irradiation tolerance for the fibrotic phase of lung injury is, however, less than for pneumonitis. Clinical data also indicate good tolerance for palliative re-irradiation (with low doses) and selected patients can be re-irradiated with higher doses, with some increase in incidence of pneumonitis. The spinal cord is another example of a slowly proliferating normal tissue that has substantial long-term recovery after initial doses equivalent to 50–60% full tolerance, with greater recovery at longer intervals (2–3 years) than at 6 months.

Other slowly proliferating tissues (e.g. kidney and heart) do not show long-term recovery and retreatment tolerance. In these tissues, the damage is progressive, even after subthreshold doses, and retreatment tolerance actually decreases with time from first treatment.

The clinical re-irradiation data indicate that for the majority of late effects there is some long-term recovery and re-irradiation can be considered if other options are not available. The largest clinical experience is for head and neck cancers, which demonstrates that long-term tumour control can be achieved in selected patients at the price of some increased late toxicity. Late effects are generally more severe in re-irradiated patients, especially when re-irradiation is combined with chemotherapy, but toxicity is less than would be predicted based on total initial and re-treatment doses (i.e. there is some long-term recovery). Because of the increased toxicity risk, these patients should receive the best available treatment planning and more limited radiotherapy fields. If possible, concurrent chemotherapy should be avoided. Hyperfractionated schedules with low doses per fraction can also reduce the risk of late toxicity.

Partial organ irradiation

Structural tissue tolerance (damage per unit area) depends on radiation sensitivity and there is little evidence that this varies with the volume irradiated, although it can be altered by patient-related factors, e.g. diabetes, and the addition of chemotherapy. By contrast, the ability of an irradiated tissue to maintain its function can vary considerably according to the irradiated volume and tissue architecture.

Paired organs, like kidneys or salivary glands, and organs in which the functional subunits are arranged in parallel, e.g. lung and liver, have low tolerance to whole organ irradiation, but small volumes can be irradiated to much higher doses without compromising organ function. This is due to the functional reserve capacity, where <50% of the organ is required to maintain adequate function under normal physiological conditions. In such tissues, the risk of complication depends on the distribution of the dose in the whole organ, with a threshold volume below which functional damage will not develop, even after high doses. Above this threshold, there will be increasingly severe functional organ impairment with increasing dose, as well as a substantial volume effect for a given dose.

By contrast, organs like the spinal cord and oesophagus have a more serial organization where the inactivation of one critical subunit may cause loss of function in the whole organ. Radiation damage in such tissues is binary, with a threshold dose below which there is normal function and above which there is loss of function, e.g. radiation induced myelopathy or oesophageal obstruction. For these tissues, the risk of complication is strongly influenced by high-dose regions, even small hot spots of dose inhomogeneity. The probability of complications for a given dose increases with the length of the organ irradiated, but the magnitude of the volume effect is generally smaller than for parallel and paired organs.

Several theoretical models have been developed to estimate normal tissue complication probability (NTCP) for partial volume irradiations and inhomogeneous dose distributions. However, these models cannot properly account for all biological variables, like regional differences in tissue sensitivity, the functional status of non-irradiated tissue, microvascular damage underlying late tissue effects, co-morbidity factors, etc. Therefore, models should be treated with caution and constantly re-evaluated using new clinical data. Clinical data on partial organ irradiation have been extensively reviewed within the QUANTEC (quantitative normal tissue effects in the clinic) program, which gives guidelines for normal tissue tolerance after both whole- and partial-organ irradiation with fractionated radiotherapy. This review includes dose/volume data on each organ system and summarizes recommended dose constraints (published in a special issue of *Int J Radiation Oncol Biol Phys* 2010;76(3)).

Combination with chemotherapy and targeted agents

For many tumour sites, radiotherapy is more and more often combined with some form of systemic treatment – cytostatic drugs, hormonal treatment or more recently molecular targeting agents. Depending on the goal of the combination, the drugs can be given in a sequential or in a concomitant way. When given sequentially, the full dose of the drugs can be administered with the aim of eradicating systemic disease. The sequential sequence only makes sense when the tumour is drug and radiation sensitive, such as Hodgkin lymphoma. Drugs are given concomitantly when the interaction with radiation enhances the effect. However, for toxicity reasons, the dose of the drugs usually needs to be lowered, which decreases their systemic effect. The main aim of concomitant treatment is to further improve locoregional control. Examples of combined modality treatments are those for glioblastoma where radiation is combined with temozolomide, head and neck cancer and cervical cancer where radiation is combined with cisplatin, and non-small cell lung cancer and small cell lung cancer where the combination of radiation and chemotherapy is superior to radiation alone. Also, in rectal cancer as well as in anal cancer, it has been shown that the addition of 5-fluorouracil (5-FU)-based chemotherapy improves locoregional control. In all these studies the addition of chemotherapy comes at the price of increased acute toxicity. The underlying mechanisms of the improved efficacy of combined chemoradiation are not fully understood. Some of the drugs used, such as cisplatin, have been shown to cause DNA damage in the form of DNA adducts, breaks and intercalation. During the repair of the DNA adducts, radiation-induced single-strand breaks might be converted to double-strand breaks. Through this mechanism cisplatin inhibits the repair process and in this way also contributes to the enhanced effect of radiation. Usually, chemotherapy is most effective on cycling cells as most of these drugs are inhibitors of cell division. Due to their selective effect in certain phases of the cell cycle, the remaining cells will be synchronized. Depending on the phase of the cell cycle they are synchronized in, they might be more sensitive to radiation. Although this phenomenon has been illustrated in preclinical research, it is hard to demonstrate it in the clinic. Some of the drugs cause an increase in apoptosis. However, they can only do so after incorporation into the DNA, which could be facilitated by the DNA breaks caused by radiation. Tumour reoxygenation resulting from tumour cell kill induced by chemotherapy decreasing the distance between the remaining cells and blood vessels is another potential mechanism for an increased effect of the radiation when combined with chemotherapy.

In daily clinical circumstances, however, it is very difficult to optimally sequence the administration of the drug and radiotherapy to try to fully benefit from the possible interaction mechanisms with ionizing radiation. The fact that the combination works so well is then probably more related to the inhibition of proliferation by chemotherapy rather than to the mechanisms mentioned above. The drugs counteract the repopulation triggered by radiation.

In recent years, the so-called molecular targeting agents became progressively available. They are mainly used in combination with classical cytotoxic drugs, but they have also been tested in combination with radiotherapy. These small molecules or antibodies to surface receptors interact with the molecular pathways linked to radioresistance, such as the EGFR pathway. The expression of specific genes involved in radioresistance can also be altered using short antisense RNA, short interference RNA or aptamers. Theoretically, these compounds are more tumour specific as they target pathways involved in radiation response that are often differentially expressed in tumours and normal tissues. Combining these compounds with radiation however, requires thorough knowledge of the molecular pathways in the tumour cells that lead to radioresistance. These molecular mechanisms are increasingly understood, which makes it possible to identify potential targets. As intertumour variability is very important, these highly specific drugs require treatment to be tailored to the individual tumour, maximizing tumour cell kill and minimizing normal tissue damage. The largest clinical experience on the inhibition of the EGFR pathway comes from head and neck tumours, where high EGFR expression has been shown to be an independent prognostic factor for overall and disease-free survival. When combined with radiotherapy, cetuximab, a monoclonal antibody against EGFR, has been shown to significantly improve overall survival in patients with Stage III and IV squamous cell carcinoma of the oropharynx, hypopharynx and larynx. Unfortunately, subsequent trials looking at the combination of various EGFR inhibitors with standard chemoradiation were negative. Also, in rectal cancer and lung cancer the combination of EGFR inhibitors with standard chemoradiation led to disappointing results. A possible explanation could be that the addition of EGFR inhibition to chemoradiation leads to inhibition of proliferation and thus to less efficient tumour cell kill by the chemotherapy. These findings clearly illustrate that preclinical research on how to sequence or combine these different agents is essential.

Several studies have also looked at combining vascular endothelial growth factor (VEGF) targeting with radiation. The VEGF receptor is mainly expressed on endothelial cells and its activation leads to endothelial cell proliferation, migration and survival. High levels of VEGF are typically associated with poor prognosis. Antiangiogenic treatments have been proposed to transiently normalize the tumour vasculature by pruning the immature vessels, resulting in a transient increase in oxygenation, and thereby creating a window of opportunity for enhanced radioresponse. Such combination treatment with an antiangiogenic agent and irradiation could be superior to individual treatment alone. Direct evidence was obtained in rectal cancer patients for the antivascular effect of bevacizumab (Avastin®), a humanized monoclonal antibody to VEGF that was the first angiogenesis inhibitor to be approved for cancer treatment. However, at present many obstacles still have to be conquered to use this combination in daily clinical routine. The molecular interactions between the angiogenesis inhibitor and radiotherapy still need to be unravelled to be able to optimize this treatment combination. Another important hurdle to overcome is the development of resistance or tumour escape to antiangiogenic agents, caused by the up-regulation of compensatory proangiogenic signalling or pre-existing multiplicity of redundant proangiogenic signals, which can compensate for loss of VEGF signalling. Also, the combination of these drugs with radiation leads to unexpected side effects, such as in-field intestinal toxicity or cartilage necrosis with fistulization.

General principles of radiation oncology

Role of radiotherapy in the management of cancer

Radiotherapy is one of the most effective treatment modalities to cure cancer. It has been estimated that radiotherapy used alone or in combination with other modalities was responsible for almost 40% of cancer cures, whereas almost 50% were attributable to surgery and 11% to systemic treatments alone. The development of new radiation techniques such as IMRT together with a more accurate selection and delineation of target volumes, and the concomitant use of biological modifiers (e.g. chemotherapy, targeted agents, hypoxic cell sensitizers) are likely to further increase the beneficial use of radiotherapy.

Curative radiotherapy

A planning study performed in the mid-2000s in Australia concluded that following available evidence-based guidelines for radiotherapy indications, overall a little >50% of cancer patients benefited from radiotherapy. These figures ranged from just a few percent for patients with haematological diseases such as leukaemia, to close to 90% for patients with cancers of the CNS. When expressed as a percentage of the total number of cancers, patients with breast, lung, prostate, rectum and head and neck carcinoma accounted for almost two-thirds of the indications. These estimates are probably conservative as indications for radiotherapy for skin cancers and benign diseases were not taken into account. Also, this study focused on external beam radiotherapy and did not consider brachytherapy, which is a key component of the treatment for some tumours such as cervical cancers. Furthermore, more recent randomized studies in head and neck, prostate and breast cancers have further validated the use of radiotherapy as the primary modality or as an adjuvant postoperative treatment, which will likely impact on the utilization rate of radiotherapy. One also needs to consider a retreatment rate of around 20–25%, either for recurrent disease or metastatic evolution (see Palliative radiotherapy below). Although performed in Australia, this study is likely to be also valid for other parts of the world such as Europe and North America.

For the great majority of the radiotherapy indications, a conventional fractionation (dose of 2 Gy per fraction) is advised, although the use of non-conventional fractionation regimens such as hyperfractionation or hypofractionation has been validated, for example, for some stages of head and neck squamous cell carcinoma and non-small cell lung cancer, respectively. For all of these indications, the overall treatment time should be maintained as scheduled without introduction of any treatment break. This is especially true for squamous cell carcinoma (e.g. head and neck, lung, cervix) where any treatment prolongation has been associated with a lower probability of cure. For these indications, all measures should be taken (e.g. to treat more than five times a week) to recuperate the lost fractions in the event of patient no-show or machine breakdown.. In case of severe acute toxicity, all supportive care measures (e.g. feeding tube, use of narcotics in case of severe pain) should be utilized in order to minimize the potential length of the treatment interruption. In this context also, when radiotherapy is associated with concomitant chemotherapy, if treatment de-escalation is deemed necessary, chemotherapy could be omitted, but in any case, radiotherapy should be maintained with the total dose and overall treatment time as prescribed.

Palliative radiotherapy

The goals of palliative radiotherapy are to relieve pain and/or other symptoms and thus to improve quality of life. It is mainly used for bone and brain metastasis, but irradiation of the primary tumour site and/or the regional lymph nodes may also be required to alleviate local symptoms when no other options are possible or effective. It has been estimated that at least 14% of patients will require palliative radiotherapy as their first entry into the disease. In addition, additional patients may require palliative radiotherapy later in their disease history for locoregional recurrence after initial successful locoregional treatment and/or for distant metastasis. Altogether, around 25–30% of patients may benefit from palliative radiotherapy at some point during their disease history. This percentage is likely to vary from country to country depending on the typical pattern of patient referral to the various oncological specialties and the lack of financial incentive for physicians to refer patients to radiation oncologists, and the availability of radiotherapy centres. For palliative radiotherapy, specific regimens typically using lower total dose and fewer fractions with higher doses (e.g. 8-Gy single fraction for bone metastasis) have been validated to be extremely cost-effective. Such short courses can be repeated if necessary.

Radiation dose prescription, reporting and recording in external beam delivery: the ICRU concepts

To be cost-effective, radiotherapy requires that a given dose is delivered accurately and homogeneously to precisely selected and delineated tumour volumes with no or minimal dose delivered to the surrounding normal tissues. Such objectives are facilitated by the use of a set of recommendations aimed at homogenizing the delivery of radiotherapy across centres. In this context, the International Commission on Radiation Units and Measurements (ICRU) has developed guidelines (ICRU reports #29, #50, #62, #83) for prescribing, recording and reporting the dose of the radiation therapy.

Definition of target volumes

Selection and delineation of target volumes is the first obligatory step in the planning process, as dose cannot be prescribed, recorded and reported without specification of tumour volumes and volumes of normal tissue at risk.

The *gross tumour volume* (GTV) is the gross demonstrable extent and location of the tumour. It consists of the primary tumour, the regional lymph nodes or the distant metastases according to the clinical situation. The GTV can be delineated on anatomical (e.g. CT or MRI) or functional (e.g. positron emission tomography [PET] with various tracers) imaging modalities; it can be delineated before the start of treatment and subsequently during treatment to capture a change in tumour volume.

It is known that tumours have the potential to microscopically infiltrate into the surrounding normal tissues and/or disseminate through the lymphatic network to reach the regional lymph node stations. In this framework, the *clinical target volume* (CTV) is the volume that contains a demonstrable GTV and/or subclinical malignant disease that must be eliminated. Data on the incidence of regional tumour and lymph node involvement have been accumulated for various primary tumour sites and based on these data, recommendations for the identification and delineation of CTVs have been proposed. There may be more than one specified GTV and corresponding CTV. It should be emphasized that both the GTV and the CTV are oncological concepts requiring a sound clinical knowledge for their optimal definition.

Before starting the dose optimization process, because of tumour motion (e.g. lung tumour), variation in organ filling (e.g. of the rectum) and variation in patient positioning, additional geometric margins need to be added to the CTV. The *planning target volume* (PTV) is thus a geometric concept used for treatment planning that ensures that the prescribed dose is actually delivered to the CTV with a clinically acceptable probability. Each CTV should have a corresponding PTV. Recommendations have been published on how to calculate margins to determine the PTVs.

The *organs at risk* (OAR) are tissues which if irradiated above tolerance could suffer significant morbidity, and thus influence the treatment planning and/or the dose prescription. Care has to be when delineating OARs. For example, for 'hollow' organs (e.g. the rectum, orbit), the wall and not the full organ including the content needs to be contoured; also for finite normal tissues (e.g. the parotids, lungs), the full organ has to be contoured as the measurements to evaluate radiation toxicity in these organs (e.g. mean parotid dose, V_{20Gy} for the lung) are related to the entire volume. Recent publications (QUANTEC) have summarized normal tissue tolerances to fractionated irradiation.

Uncertainties and variations in the position of the OARs during treatment must also be considered before dose optimization. Thus, margins have to be added to the OARs using principles similar to those for the PTV, leading to the concept of *planning organ at risk volume* (PRV). The selection of the margin will however depend on the structure of the OAR, being more critical for organs such as the spinal cord or nerves (i.e. serial-like organs) than for organs such as the parotid glands or the lungs (i.e. parallel-like organs) . In practice, for these latter organs, an OAR–PRV margin of 0 mm could be used.

Planning aims and treatment optimization

In IMRT, the distribution of dose to multiple volumes is prioritized and tailored through an iterative process, referred to as 'optimization'. This process consists of three major components: (1) the definition of the 'planning aim(s)' using image-based information from which the desired absorbed dose levels are specified for all the PTVs and PRVs; (2) a complex beam delivery 'optimization' process to achieve and, if needed, modify the initial 'planning aim(s)'; and (3) a complete set of accepted final values, which becomes the 'treatment prescription' and, together with the required 'technical data,' represent the 'accepted treatment plan'. The prescription is a description of the volumes of interest, the dose and/or dose–volume requirements for the PTV, the fractionation scheme, the normal tissue constraints and the dose distribution(s) that have been planned. This final process is the responsibility of the treating physician.

Dose–volume prescription, reporting and recording

In 3D-CRT and in IMRT, dose prescription, reporting and recording in the PTV and PRV is done on a volumetric basis, as the dose distribution can be explicitly visualized on a dose–volume histogram (DVH). Prescription should be based on dose–volume specifications, and the use of an ICRU reference point dose is no longer recommended. Whatever dose–volume prescription value is chosen, the median dose ($D_{50\%}$) should be reported and recorded as it represents a typical dose within the PTV, and is usually closest to the dose value of the more traditional ICRU reference point. The radiation oncologist should not rely solely on the DVH for treatment evaluation, but should also carefully inspect the absorbed dose distributions slice-by-slice (or in three dimensions) to ensure that the PTV is being adequately irradiated and normal sensitive tissues avoided as far as possible, and to verify the absence of hot spots outside of delineated structures. Treatment plan evaluation should also include verification of dose homogeneity, which characterizes the uniformity of dose distribution within the target volume, and dose conformity, which characterizes the degree to which the high-dose region conforms to the PTV. An acceptable plan should be both highly conformed and highly homogeneous.

As mentioned above, the functional arrangement of normal tissue cells has been typically described as parallel or parallel-like (e.g. lung, parotid), or serial or serial-like (e.g. spinal cord, nerve). For parallel-like structures, the mean absorbed dose can be a useful measure of absorbed dose, as commonly done for parotid glands. For lungs, dose–volume reporting specifying V_D, which is the volume that receives at least the absorbed dose D specified in Gy, is a concept that has been commonly used and can also be easily obtained from a DVH. For serial-like structures, the maximum absorbed dose as specified by a single calculation point (D_{max}) has often been reported, but this is based on a single point and has great delineation uncertainty. Instead, it is recommended to report the near-maximum dose, e.g. $D_{2\%}$. To obtain a true value of $D_{2\%}$, the entire organ should be contoured. When this is not possible (e.g. for the spinal cord), the anatomical description of the delineated regions should be described when reporting the $D_{2\%}$. When organs are not clearly classified as a serial-like or parallel-like structure, such as the kidney, it is recommended to report and record at least three dose–volume specifications. These would include D_{mean}, $D_{2\%}$ and a third specification, V_D, which correlates well with an absorbed dose D and if exceeded within some volume has a known high probability of causing a serious complication. Other specifications of risk, as deemed to be relevant by the radiation oncologist, may also be reported and recorded.

The reported and recorded dose prescriptions and technical data defining the accepted plan are only meaningful if there is adequate quality control in the whole process to ensure that the doses are being delivered as accurately as planned. This is particularly relevant in IMRT as sharp dose gradients are typically generated. It is beyond the scope of this chapter to give an in-depth review of the quality assurance (QA) programmes required, but it should be clearly understood that both machine-specific and patient-specific QA should be performed.

Dose distributions of different radiotherapy modalities

Today radiotherapy is offered with a range of different planning and delivery solutions, of varying complexity. The dose distributions resulting from each approach have certain characteristics, in particular with respect to the achievable conformity, i.e. the ability to shape the dose distribution to individual patients.

A milestone achievement in radiotherapy was the introduction in the 1970s and 1980s of medical linear accelerators that could deliver high-energy (MV) photon and electron beams. Using such beams, deep-seated tumours could for the first time be reached without giving considerably higher doses to the tissues located in front of the tumour. In what is usually referred to as two-dimensional radiotherapy (2D-RT), beam portals were defined in the X-ray simulation process, involving standardized set-ups both in terms of field configurations (one to four beam directions) and the anatomical boundaries. The use of two opposing fields or four-field box techniques allowed the delivery of relatively homogenous dose distributions to the whole irradiated volume, or the volume (the 'box') located in the intersection of the four beams, respectively.

While the first breakthrough in radiotherapy delivery was a result of the development of accelerator physics, the next paradigm shift came as a result of advances in imaging physics and in computer science. The advent of CT and its later introduction as a tool for radiotherapy planning, combined with the development of computerized treatment planning and dose calculation algorithms, led to what is usually referred to as 3D-CRT. These components form the basis for all contemporary radiotherapy planning and delivery.

The concept of 3D-CRT soon developed. In the planning phase of 3D-CRT, beams from different directions are directed towards the PTV, with the selection of beams based on a 3D representation of the patient created from a CT image series. Using the same 3D patient model, the resulting dose distribution throughout the patient volume is estimated using dose calculation algorithms of different physical sophistication and hence accuracy. The term conformal arises from the introduction of beam shaping devices – originally customized blocks, later multileaf collimators (MLCs) – that during radiotherapy delivery effectively shape the beam portals to the projections of the PTV, leading to dose distributions conforming to the shape of the PTV and sparing large parts of normal tissues from receiving doses in the prescription dose range.

Beginning in the mid-1990s, the field of linac-based stereotactic radiotherapy also developed. Stereotactic radiotherapy was originally developed as an alternative to surgery in the management of intracranial lesions, delivered using dedicated radiation devices such as the Gammaknife. Using the beam-shaping possibilities of 3D-CRT, highly conformal dose distributions can be achieved by irradiating the target from a large number of directions. Today, this modality is also used to treat small, well-localized tumours outside the skull, such as in the lungs and liver, in what was first referred to as stereotactic body radiotherapy (SBRT) and more recently as stereotactic ablative radiotherapy (SABR).

The introduction of MLCs also enabled a further development towards what is current state-of-the-art photon-based radiotherapy, so-called intensity-modulated radiotherapy (IMRT). The term intensity modulation refers to the use of radiation beams with a non-uniform intensity across the beam port, realized through computer-controlled movement of the MLC. IMRT is tightly connected with the term inverse planning, which refers to a radiotherapy planning process where the intensity patterns of the beams are iteratively optimized to achieve the initially defined treatment goals, formulated in so-called DVH constraints. With IMRT, concavely shaped dose distributions could be obtained, giving the possibility of sparing normal tissues in very close vicinity of the PTV, such as the rectum in radiotherapy for prostate cancer, and the spinal cord, brainstem and salivary glands in radiotherapy for head and neck tumours. Figure 10.4 compares a box technique and IMRT (tomotherapy or volumetric-modulated arc therapy [VMAT]).

With time, different IMRT solutions have been developed. The main MLC-based solutions are referred to as step-and-shoot

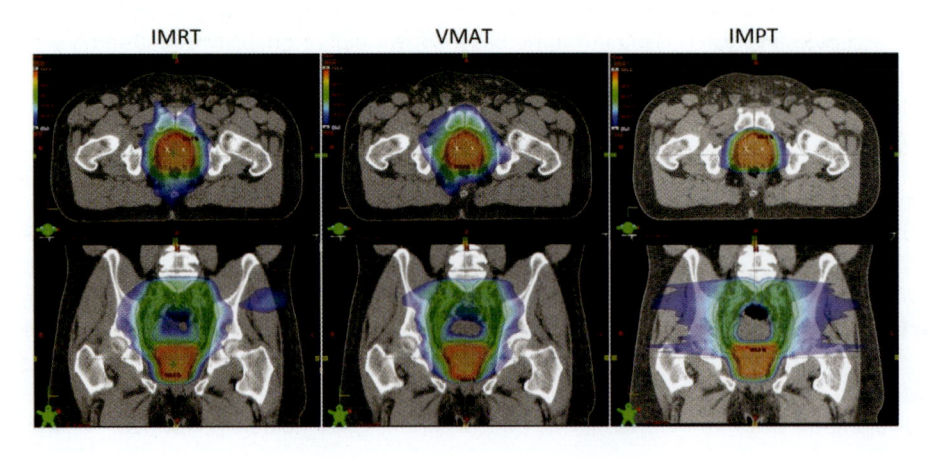

Figure 10.4 Comparison of dose distributions for simultaneously integrated treatment of a patient with locally-advanced prostate cancer irradiated with intensity-modulated radiotherapy (IMRT), volumetric-modulated radiotherapy (VMAT) and intensity-modulated proton therapy (IMPT). Source: Sara Thörnqvist, Aarhus University (2013). Reproduced with permission..

IMRT and dynamic IMRT, which differ in the way the beam modulation is achieved with the MLC movements. In step-and-shoot delivery, the intensity patterns are built up through a number of beam segments where the MLC is stationary, while in dynamic delivery, the MLC is moving during beam-on.

More recently, a new variation of IMRT has been developed, often referred to as rotational IMRT. This can be seen as a development of what was known as arc therapy, a rotational form of 3D-CRT where the target was continuously irradiated during gantry rotation, and where mechanical shaping devices were used in a dynamic way. Today, the term rotational IMRT covers treatment with tomotherapy, where the patient is treated using rotational delivery of a narrow fan beam similar to the principle of imaging tomography, and of VMAT, which can be considered as a combination of arc therapy and dynamic IMRT. VMAT is achieved using conventional linacs equipped with MLCs, offers better conformity than conventional IMRT and is therefore to a large extent now replacing conventional IMRT in many institutions.

In parallel with the considerable development and refinement of photon-based external beam radiotherapy, the use of heavy charged particles, including protons and other nuclei such as carbon ions, has also been explored. All photon-based radiotherapy is limited by the physical properties of photons, as the maximum dose of a photon beam is found at a relatively limited depth, with significant dose deposition beyond the target. This makes it difficult to fully protect neighbouring healthy normal tissues during radiotherapy. Radiotherapy with charged particles exploits the fundamentally different physical properties of these particles. In particle therapy, a term that covers radiotherapy with both protons and carbon ions, most of the energy is deposited at the end of the particle range, at the so-called Bragg peak (BP), sparing healthy tissue both in the path to the target volume as well as beyond the target. Radiotherapy with protons was initially proposed in 1946, but it has taken a long time to mature technologically. The technological development of this modality has been substantial during in the past 5–10 years, and is now used in a rapidly increasing number of facilities worldwide. Proton and particle therapy is currently used for only 1% of all radiotherapy courses, but it has been estimated that it could be more widely used. With the installation of new particle therapy facilities, evidence will need to be generated to demonstrate the utility of such treatment.

Brachytherapy

In contrast to external beam radiotherapy, brachytherapy involves placing short-range radioactive material or sources in or near the tumour. The source is usually enclosed in a protective capsule or wire, and the irradiation only affects a localized area around the radiation sources, allowing a very conformal plan and low volume of exposed normal tissue. It is commonly used to treat cervical, uterine and prostate cancers and less frequently to treat head and neck, eye, lung and gastrointestinal tumours. It can be combined with external beam radiation.

Brachytherapy can be given over a short overall treatment time such as 5–7 days compared to several weeks for external beam radiotherapy. There are radiobiological advantages for this in that interstitial brachytherapy reduces the risks of prolonged treatment and repopulation in the management of squamous cell carcinomas by enabling the radiation to be given over a short treatment time. Repopulation is not a concern for tumours such as prostate cancer in which permanent brachytherapy is used. In high dose rate (HDR) brachytherapy, the higher dose rate may result in less repair of sublethally damaged cells and the increased risk of normal tissue toxicity. Pulse dose rate (PDR) brachytherapy allows the use of HDR, but by increasing the overall treatment time it reduces the risk of normal tissue toxicity. Reoxygenation is also more likely in low dose rate (LDR) and PDR than HDR brachytherapy.

A more detailed description of technique and results is given elsewhere in the relevant disease-site chapters as necessary. Definitions used in brachytherapy are given in Table 9.1.

Individualized radiotherapy: Adaptive and tailored

Contemporary high-precision radiotherapy techniques like IMRT and stereotactic radiotherapy have enabled highly conformal and individualized dose distributions, delivering high doses to the target and lower doses to the surrounding healthy tissue. However, the consequence of the increasingly conformal dose distributions is a higher sensitivity to modifications in dose distribution from planning to treatment, and during the course of fractionated radiotherapy. Set-up errors and anatomical changes may cause deviations between planned and delivered dose distribution, which can lead to under-dosage of tumour

Table 10.1 Definitions of terminology used in brachytherapy

Interstitial	Radiation source placed within the tumour (e.g. prostate and head and neck cancers)
Intracavity	Radiation source placed within an organ cavity (e.g. uterine and oesophageal cancers)
Temporary	Radiation source removed after the prescribed dose has been administered
Permanent	Radiation source left in place and decays over time
Low dose rate (LDR)	Radiation source left in place and decays over time at 0.4–2 Gy/h. All permanent (usually <0.4 Gy/h) and some temporary brachytherapy
High dose rate (HDR)	>12 Gy/h
Pulse dose rate (PDR)	Usually uses HDR but pulsed through an applicator over a large number of fractions to simulate LDR

volume and/or over-dosage of normal tissue if not properly corrected for. The soft tissue deformations occurring during the treatment course due to weight loss, tissue shrinkage, breathing motion or deformation of tumour/normal tissues need to be monitored by frequent (daily or weekly) volumetric imaging. Complete 3D volumetric information on soft tissue can be obtained in the treatment room using either ultrasound, CT or MRI. Cone-beam CT (CBCT) using kilovolt or megavolt X-ray equipment mounted on the treatment gantry is a versatile imaging method where 3D volumetric images are constructed from 2D projections, and thus providing both set-up and anatomical information of the patient on the couch prior to treatment. The linear accelerator-based CBCT has thus made repeated imaging and adaptive radiotherapy feasible. Especially for critical normal tissues like the spinal cord, optic nerves, salivary glands, heart, kidneys or rectum in close proximity to the high-dose tumour volume, significant anatomical changes will require adaptive planning to fulfil the desired treatment goal. Anatomical studies during IMRT suggest that up to 25% of patients treated with curative radiotherapy experience changes, which have dosimetric consequences. However, it is also clear from the published data that a large heterogeneity exists among patients with respect to the size and consequences of the changes observed in these relatively small cohorts.

Adaptive strategies involve developing a new treatment plan on the basis of the new anatomical information. Currently, two basic strategies are emerging: *plan selection* and *replanning*. In plan selection, the best dose plan for the anatomy on the day is selected from a library of three to five prefabricated plans. Such a strategy is useful for large daily variations in, for example, bladder or rectal filling, and can lead to significant reduction of the irradiated volume of normal tissues. Replanning is a more tedious process, which involves recontouring, reoptimization, plan evaluation, dose reconstruction and dose accumulation. Since the temporal anatomical changes often evolve smoothly, these cases might be well suited for creating computational algorithms for automatic segmentation, based on the original organ contouring.

A logical next step in adaptive radiotherapy is to incorporate more biological features into the initial treatment planning (dose painting) and systematically adapt the treatment as both the anatomical and biological features change during the course of treatment. This emerging concept is called biology-guided adaptive radiotherapy (BiGART). Relevant biological features for BiGART include hypoxia, proliferation, cell density and intrinsic radioresistance. The principle in dose painting is redistribution and escalation of the radiation dose to these radioresistant parts of the tumour. A biologically more effective dose distribution might be achieved while simultaneously sparing normal tissues. Functional imaging modalities for BiGART include dynamic CT with contrast, diffusion-weighted MRI, dynamic contrast-enhanced MRI and PET/CT with various tracers. A number of studies have shown that functional imaging information on, for example, hypoxia is prognostic for the outcome of radiotherapy.

The main challenges in BiGART are resolution and dynamics: the biological features are likely to be more heterogeneous at a microscopic level than can be picked up with current imaging. If so, current imaging and delivery techniques are probably too coarse to fully address the biological distribution. The dynamics of the biological features of interest determine how frequently the patient needs to be subjected to repetitive imaging during radiotherapy. A few early studies have shown that dose painting and BiGART in principle is possible, although not yet practical nor cost-effective on a daily or even weekly basis.

Organization of a radiation oncology department

It is obvious from the above that modern radiotherapy is a highly specialized treatment, for which patients need to be selected properly based on guidelines and evidence, by medical experts working in a broad multidisciplinary oncology team. Planning and delivering radiation therapy is a complex process (Fig. 10.5), based on high-tech software and hardware, and involving a

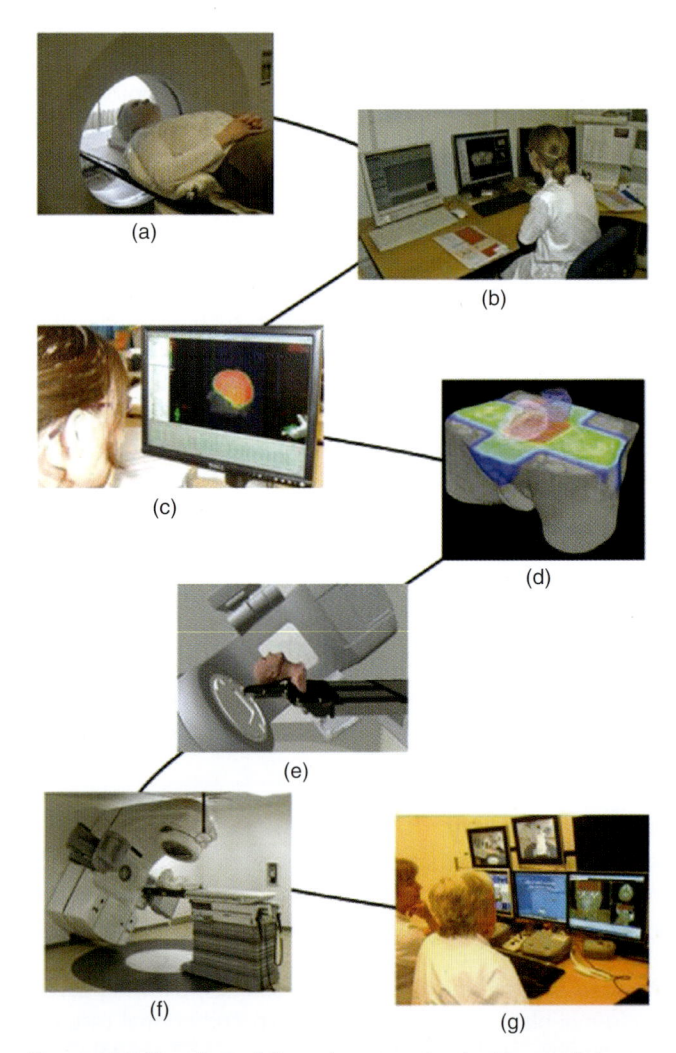

Figure 10.5 Flowchart of the various steps involved in a typical radiotherapy treatment. (a) Planning CT scan; (b) contouring; (c) dose planning; (d) plan evaluation; (e) quality assurance; (f) set-up; (g) image guidance and delivery.

wide range of staffs, e.g. physicians, physicists, radiographers and radiation therapists/nurses. Due to the high risks involved in radiotherapy, training to a high skill level is crucial.

Planning of radiotherapy starts with a CT scan of the patient immobilized in the treatment position on a flatbed couch. The GTV, CTVs and OARs are then outlined on each CT slice with the aid of multimodality imaging (MRI/PET/SPECT). Margins for uncertainties (biological, organ motion, patient positioning) are added. The fully segmented CT scanning forms the basis for computer-aided dose planning. Beam orientations delivering high doses to the tumour while avoiding as much critical tissue as possible are chosen. The resulting accumulated radiation dose distribution is calculated, and one or more plans are produced. Evaluation of treatment plans at the planning review involves careful assessment of the doses that will be given to the target volumes as well as the organs at risk. The dose distributions superimposed on the CT slices is visually inspected, ensuring an accurate representation of the spatial relationships in the patient. The best treatment plan is chosen. Since the gantry of the linear accelerator can rotate 360° around the patient, there is a risk of collision of the gantry with the treatment couch or the patient. Any plan should be tested for the risk of collision before the first treatment of the patient. When the dose plan is evaluated, accepted and quality checked, the patient is brought to the linear accelerator and placed on the treatment couch, assisted by radiation therapists/nurses. Laser beams in the room guide the position of the patient relative to the isocentre of the machine. In recent years, set-up using external laser-guided markers has been gradually replaced by image-guided set-up: imaging devices on the accelerator are used for online daily imaging and matching of internal markers (bony anatomy, gold markers) or even soft tissue (cone-beam CT).

During the course of radiotherapy, patients are monitored for side effects by the staff, and appropriate supportive care is delivered. Most patients remain ambulatory and can complete the treatment as outpatients, but hospitalization may be needed, especially if the patient is also receiving concurrent medical treatments (e.g. chemotherapy or targeted biotherapy).

Long-term follow-up after curative radiotherapy is important in order to monitor the effect and sequelae of the radiotherapy. Late chronic side effects occur months or years after treatment, and are generally progressive, so a rehabilitation and surveillance programme is important. Early detection of recurrence may enable salvage treatment, and long-term cancer survivors are also at a high risk of developing new secondary tumours, which should also be detected early.

Recommended reading

Ahn GO, Brown M. (2007) Targeting tumors with hypoxia-activated cytotoxins. *Front Biosci* 12:3483–3501.

Bentzen SM (2006) Preventing or reducing late side effects of radiation therapy: radiobiology meets molecular pathology. *Nat Rev Cancer* 6:702–713.

Bentzen SM, Constine LS, Deasy JO *et al.* (2010) Quantitative Analyses of Normal Tissue Effects in the Clinic (QUANTEC): an introduction to the scientific issues. *Int J Radiat Oncol Biol Phys* 76(3 Suppl):S3–9.

Bernier J, Hall EJ, Giaccia A (2004) Radiation oncology: a century of achievements. *Nat Rev Cancer* 4(9):737–747.

Brown JM (2002) Tumor microenvironment and the response to anticancer therapy. *Cancer Biol Ther* 1(5):453–458.

Brush J, Lipnick SL, Phillips T *et al.* (2007) Molecular mechanisms of late normal tissue injury. *Semin Radiat Oncol* 17:121–130.

Choy H, Kim DW (2003) Chemotherapy and irradiation interaction. *Semin Oncol* 30(4 Suppl 9):3–10.

Delaney G, Jacob S, Featherstone C, Barton M (2005) The role of radiotherapy in cancer treatment: estimating optimal utilization from a review of evidence-based clinical guidelines. *Cancer* 104(6):1129–1137. Erratum in *Cancer* 2006;107(3):660.

Grau C, Høyer M, Alber M, Overgaard J, Muren LP (2013) Biology-Guided Adaptive Radiotherapy (BiGART) – more than a vision? *Acta Oncolog* 52(7):1243–1247.

Gregoire V, Jeraj R, Lee JA *et al.* (2012) Radiotherapy for head and neck tumours in 2012 and beyond: conformal, tailored, and adaptive? *Lancet Oncol* 13:E292–300.

International Commission on Radiation Units and Measurements (ICRU) (2010) Prescribing, Recording, and Reporting Photon-Beam Intensity-Modulated Radiation Therapy (IMRT). ICRU Report 83. *J ICRU* 10(1).

Jacob S, Wong K, Delaney GP, Adams P, Barton MB (2010) Estimation of an optimal utilisation rate for palliative radiotherapy in newly diagnosed cancer patients. *Clin Oncol* 22(1):56–64.

Jeggo P, Löbrich M (2006) Radiation-induced DNA damage responses. *Radiat Prot Dosimetry* 122(1–4):124–127.

Jeggo P, Lavin MF (2009) Cellular radiosensitivity: how much better do we understand it? *Int J Radiat Biol* 85(12):1061–1081.

Joiner M, van der Kogel A, eds (2009) *Basic Clinical Radiobiology*, 4th edn. London: Hodder Arnold.

Marks LB, Yorke ED, Jackson A *et al.* (2010) Use of normal tissue complication probability models in the clinic. *Int J Radiat Oncol Biol Phys* 76:S10–19.

Nieder C, Milas L, Ang KK (2000) Tissue tolerance to re-irradiation. *Semin Radiat Oncol* 10:200–209.

Overgaard J (2007) Hypoxic radiosensitization: adored and ignored. *J Clin Oncol* 25(26):4066–4074.

Niyazi M, Maihoefer C, Krause M, Rödel C, Budach W, Belka C (2011) Radiotherapy and "new" drugs-new side effects? *Radiat Oncol* 6:177.

Overgaard J (2011) Hypoxic modification of radiotherapy in squamous cell carcinoma of the head and neck–a systematic review and meta-analysis. *Radiother Oncol* 100(1):22–32.

Peng F, Chen M (2010) Antiangiogenic therapy: a novel approach to overcome tumor hypoxia. *Chin J Cancer* 29(8):715–720.

Smith RP, Heron DE, Huq S, Yue NJ (2006) Modern radiation treatment planning and delivery – from Röntgen to real time. *Hematol Oncol Clin North Am* 20:45–62.

Tanderup K, Georg D, Pötter R, Kirisits C, Grau C, Lindegaard JC (2010) Adaptive management of cervical cancer radiotherapy. *Semin Radiat Oncol* 20:121–129.

Thames HD Jr, Withers HR, Peters LJ, Fletcher GH (1982) Changes in early and late radiation responses with altered dose fractionation: implications for dose-survival relationships. *Int J Radiat Oncol Biol Phys* 8(2):219–226.

Wilson GD, Bentzen SM, Harari PM (2006) Biologic basis for combining drugs with radiation. *Semin Radiat Oncol* 16(1):2–9.

Withers HR, Taylor JM, Maciejewski B (1988) The hazard of accelerated tumor clonogen repopulation during radiotherapy. *Acta Oncol* 27(2):131–146.

11 Principles of systemic therapy

Martin F. Fey[1] and Stefan Aebi[2]

[1]Department of Medical Oncology, Inselspital and University Hospital, Bern, Switzerland
[2]Cancer Center and Division of Medical Oncology, Lucerne Cantonal Hospital, Lucerne, Switzerland

Types of anticancer drugs

If cancer were a strictly localized type of disease, local therapy, notably surgery and/or radiotherapy, would be appropriate, with little need for systemic treatment, i.e. cancer drugs. However, one of the hallmarks of many cancers is their propensity to invade or infiltrate neighbouring tissue and anatomical structures, and to spread via the bloodstream or the lymphatic channels. Haematological cancers, particularly the leukaemias, disseminate early in their natural history and must be viewed as systemic disorders from diagnosis. Successful treatment of cancer must, therefore, account for this fundamental biological feature, and drugs have become one of the most important tools to improve outcome in cancer medicine. Systemic therapy was until recently often termed cancer 'chemotherapy', but in view of the developments in this field, particularly with the advent of therapeutic monoclonal antibodies and small molecules (mostly '-nibs', a suffix indicating an iNhIBitor), the more general term 'systemic' treatment seems appropriate.

Cytotoxic chemotherapy

In the early days of cancer treatment, drugs acting against cancer cells came to be labelled as *chemotherapy*, a term coined by Paul Ehrlich, a German physician who developed the first 'chemical' treatment, not against cancer but for syphilis. Based on the 'cytotoxic' or 'cytostatic' action of chemotherapy, it was hoped that these drugs would kill cancer cells more efficiently than normal cells, and eventually 'cure the disease'. Empirically it was found that normal cells, e.g. bone marrow or mucosal stem cells, although susceptible to damage from chemotherapy, recovered more quickly than the cancer cells. The successful cure of testicular cancer and some types of leukaemias and lymphomas by chemotherapy fostered the pioneers' view that eventually cytostatic or cytotoxic drugs would 'solve' the cancer problem. It was, hence, sobering to realize over time that many common metastatic cancers, notably lung, breast and gastrointestinal carcinomas, were much less susceptible to chemotherapy and treatment results were often unsatisfactory. To add insult to injury, the toxicity of chemotherapy to normal tissues often tipped the balance towards more harm than benefit, at times damaging the reputation of medical oncology in its early days.

Several generations of carefully designed clinical trials eventually made it possible to appraise the true value and place of time-honoured cytostatic drugs such as alkylating agents (e.g. cyclophosphamide), anthracyclines (e.g. adriamycin, so named at a conference held near the Adria, a region of Italy close to the Mediterranean Sea), mitotic spindle poisons (e.g. vincristine), topoisomerase inhibitors (e.g. etoposide) and many others. It also became clear that cytotoxic agents often work best in combination rather than as single drugs, whereby care must be taken to combine drugs with similar anticancer efficacy, yet distinct mechanisms of action and resistance and different toxicity profiles. For example, cisplatin and etoposide used in combination in small cell lung cancer have different toxicities: cisplatin chiefly displays renal and ototoxicity, whilst etoposide mainly suppresses the bone marrow; both, however, require potent antiemetics.

Hormone therapy

Some human cancers are *endocrine responsive*, the prime examples being breast and prostate cancer. It is therefore logical that additive or ablative hormonal therapy should be effective in such cancer types. The finding that orchiectomy yielded valuable responses in metastatic prostate cancer was rewarded

---

UICC Manual of Clinical Oncology, Ninth Edition. Edited by Brian O'Sullivan, James D. Brierley, Anil K. D'Cruz, Martin F. Fey, Raphael Pollock, Jan B. Vermorken and Shao Hui Huang. © 2015 UICC. Published 2015 by John Wiley & Sons, Ltd.

with the Nobel prize, and hormone therapy of breast cancer is now firmly established in the adjuvant and palliative treatment of this group of cancers. Breast cancer is a model disease in this respect as it was arguably the first tumour type for which assessment of a predictive marker, the detection of oestrogen and progesterone receptors on cancer cells, was introduced into routine pathology work-up.

Molecularly targeted therapy

Over the past decades great advances were made to clarify the principles of the molecular and cellular pathology of cancer. It has become clear that cancer mostly arises due to the stepwise acquisition in cancer stem cells and their progeny of somatic mutations in key genes critical for the governance of normal cellular homeostasis and the control of mitotic proliferation, cellular differentiation, cell survival (including programmed cell death, or apoptosis) and perhaps autophagy. In patients with a hereditary cancer predisposition, crucial gene alterations may be present in the germline, but additional somatic mutations are still required to elicit full-blown clinical cancer. These important advances fostered the notion that chemotherapy would eventually be replaced by drugs providing hits against *cancer-cell specific molecular targets*, i.e. altered genes or their protein products (Table 11.1).

The discovery that the protein product of the leukaemogenic *BCR-ABL* fusion oncogene, an activated tyrosine kinase created by the chromosomal translocation t(9; 22) in chronic myelogenous leukaemia (CML), was blocked by a small molecule, imatinib, suggested a new era of cancer therapy. However, the success of this approach with CML, although quoted as a prime example of molecularly targeted cancer therapy, is unfortunately not representative for many other cancer types, particularly solid tumours. The unique feature of CML is that its pathology is governed almost entirely by one single mutation, a major 'driver' of leukaemic transformation and behaviour. In contrast, many cancers, notably solid tumours, display much more complicated patterns of molecular aberrations, including activating mutations of proto-oncogenes and inactivating mutations or deletions of tumour suppressor genes. For example, complete genome sequencing of a lung cancer from a heavy smoker showed that the cancer cells had acquired one mutation per three cigarettes smoked by the patient during his 40 or so pack years, i.e. a myriad of gene alterations instead of a single one. The molecular pathology of colorectal cancer is a model for stepwise accumulation of many diverse, yet important, somatic mutations governing the hyperplasia–adenoma carcinoma pathway known to pathologists. It is hence essential to single out major 'driver' mutations from such a large mutational gene pool, as only these may represent targets for drugs.

Table 11.1 Therapeutic molecular targeting of cancer cells

Cancer type	Target in tumour cells	Drug
Monoclonal antibodies		
B-cell lymphoma	CD20 antigen	Rituximab
Colorectal cancer and head and neck cancer	EGFR	Cetuximab
HER2-positive breast cancer and gastric cancer	*HER2* gene (amplification)	Trastuzumab
Diverse cancers	VEGF/VEGFR	Bevacizumab
Small molecules (mostly tyrosine kinase inhibitors)		
CML	BCR-ABL fusion protein	Imatinib (and newer inhibitors)
Non-small cell lung cancer	EGFR	Erlotinib and gefitinib
Non-small cell lung cancer	ELM–ALK fusion protein	Crizotinib
Melanoma	*BRAF V600E* mutation	Vemurafenib
Diverse cancers	VEGF/VEGFR and other targets	Sunitinib and sorafenib

As a corollary, the detection of cancer gene alterations has led to the development of many new drugs targeting such molecules. Most of them are either small compounds inhibiting tyrosine kinase-dependent pathways (e.g. erlotinib blocks the epidermal growth factor receptor [EGFR] pathway in non-small cell lung cancer) or monoclonal antibodies binding to proteins on the cancer cell surface (e.g. CD20 in B-cell non-Hodgkin lymphomas, EGFR in squamous cell carcinoma of the head and neck, or HER2 in *HER2*-positive breast cancer). Ideally, targeted therapy should hit an abnormal gene product specific to the cancer cell and absent from normal cells, particularly from those derived from the same tissue of origin. This is indeed the case in CML as the BCR-ABL fusion protein is never found in normal haematopoietic cells, or in melanoma with the *BRAF V600E* mutation in the *BRAF* oncogene. Lung cancer agents that target the EGFR pathway work best if an activating *EGFR* gene mutation is present, whereas in colon cancer antibody-mediated anti-EGFR therapy is much less effective when a constitutively active mutated *RAS* oncogene is present in the down-stream section of this pathway.

Agents operating against vascular endothelial growth factor (VEGF) or its receptor (VEGFR) still face the problem of limited efficacy in many cancers, possibly because no established predictive factors can be detected in tumour tissue or patient serum to assess the chances of whether or not this treatment modality will work.

Other molecular abnormalities often seen in cancer have so far largely eluded therapeutic targeting. Examples include the replacement of inactivated or otherwise defective tumour suppressor genes or altered transcription factors, with the notable exception of the *PML-RARA* translocation, t(15; 17) (q24; q21), in acute promyelocytic leukaemia that can be targeted with all-*trans* retinoic acid.

Immune therapy

A fourth avenue with therapeutic potential is *cancer immunology*. Several clinical observations underpin the view that disturbances of immune regulation play a pivotal role in cancer pathology. The 'immune system', whatever it is, may indeed have anticancer cell mechanisms, mostly T-cell mediated. Specific types of cancer may be particularly frequent in immunosuppressed hosts, such as patients with uncontrolled human immunodeficiency virus (HIV)-mediated disease or immunosuppressed organ transplant recipients. A well-established form of 'immune therapy' against cancer is allogeneic stem cell transplantation where an immune response mediated by donor lymphoid cells, the graft-versus-leukaemia/lymphoma effect, is thought to be important in producing the favourable results of allogeneic transplantation in a number of haematological cancers. Recently, novel antibody-mediated approaches to modulate T-cell response to cancer cells have been shown to be of value, notably in metastatic melanoma. However, many attempts at vaccinating cancer patients against cancer-specific antigens have so far failed in the sense that none of these trials produced new therapy standards applicable in routine practice. Interferon- and interleukin-2-based treatments may be mentioned in a somewhat loose connection with 'immunotherapy", but both agents, whilst much hyped when introduced, have lost ground in clinical practice.

Cancer gene therapy

Cancer gene therapy in the strict sense of the term was eagerly tested for some time, and initially expectations were high. It was hoped that genes or gene sequences could be introduced into human cancer cells *in vivo* via suitable gene transfer vectors to rescue defective genes (e.g. an inactivated *p53* tumour suppressor gene), or into immune competent cells *ex vivo*. Such gene-manipulated cells would then be readministered to the patient to foster an immunological cellular anticancer response. However, this field has somewhat run out of clinical steam during the last decade, as initial hopes and concepts have not been realized. Today no 'gene therapy' protocols are available for routine practice, and research focuses instead on the other areas outlined above.

Strategies of systemic cancer treatment

Regardless of the drugs used, systemic anticancer treatment must follow some important basic principles or therapeutic strategies (Table 11.2).

Table 11.2 Strategies of systemic therapy and selected examples of neoplasms

Primary systemic therapy	Leukaemias, lymphomas, advanced germ cell cancers, small cell lung cancer (extensive disease), some sarcomas
Preoperative/ neoadjuvant systemic therapy	Gastric cancer, locally advanced urothelial bladder cancer, osteogenic sarcoma, locally advanced breast cancer, selected cases of ovarian cancer
Adjuvant/ postoperative systemic therapy after radical surgery	Breast cancer, node-positive colorectal cancer, pancreatic cancer, malignant gliomas, non-small cell lung cancer
Palliative systemic therapy	Many metastatic solid tumours, indolent B-cell lymphomas

Adjuvant cancer therapy

Adjuvant systemic cancer therapy represents a treatment given to reduce risk of relapse and improve the chances of cure, when other modalities (mostly surgery) have removed all detectable cancer. 'Radical' cancer surgery as such does not imply that a cancer patient is necessarily cured by local therapy. Depending on its biological and molecular characteristics (reflected by assessable risk factors), a cancer may have spread before diagnosis and local treatment, with an ensuing relapse risk at local and distant sites over time. Based on this definition, adjuvant systemic therapy is mostly considered in solid cancers, including carcinomas and some sarcomas. Examples are lymph node-positive colon cancer or certain types of breast cancer. It is important to understand that postoperative systemic adjuvant treatment is offered in such cases to reduce the risk of later relapse, possibly derived from small populations of residual cancer cells undetectable by current imaging and other diagnostic techniques. Patients (and their physicians) must understand that pre- and postoperative staging with imaging techniques operates at the level of macroscopic tumour detection. In solid tumours, no validated laboratory tests are available to detect residual small cancer cell populations in clinical practice, and thus selection of candidate patients for adjuvant systemic therapy must rely on clinical and pathological risk factors predicting an appreciable risk of unfavourable outcome with local therapy alone. It follows from these arguments that there is no way to assess efficacy of adjuvant therapy in an individual patient. The value of adjuvant systemic treatment can only be assessed by randomized phase III trials with appropriate primary endpoints (ideally overall survival, or disease-free survival if assessment of survival is confounded by treatment effects seen in relapsing patients).

Neoadjuvant or preoperative systemic treatment

This strategy applies to cancers, mostly locally advanced carcinomas or some sarcomas, where sooner or later radical surgery is planned, mostly with curative intent. The goal of pretreatment with systemic therapy (or a combination of systemic treatment and radiotherapy) is to improve the chances of radical tumour surgery, to ensure a possibility of less mutilating surgery or to improve outcome with a 'package deal' of multidisciplinary treatment. Well-founded examples are preoperative treatment of locally-advanced breast cancer to improve the chances of breast-conserving surgery, or of colorectal cancer metastatic to the liver to improve the options of metastasectomy, or pretreatment of the primary tumour in rectal cancer with radiochemotherapy prior to removal of the tumour.

In some instances it is difficult to ensure adequate administration of adjuvant treatment in a demanding postoperative rehabilitation phase, and therefore chemotherapy may more easily be given prior to surgery. Preoperative chemotherapy in operable gastric cancer is a good example in this setting, as the feasibility of giving an appropriate chemotherapy regimen postoperatively after radical gastrectomy and lymphadenectomy is often jeopardized in a prolonged recovery phase. Preoperative chemotherapy may also help to identify patients with a relatively favourable prognosis in whom surgery is worthwhile, such as patients with Stage IIIA non-small cell lung cancer. On the other hand, preoperative therapy might jeopardize the outcome of subsequent surgery, increasing its complication rates, and it may worsen the postoperative course. Therefore, such decisions must be taken in interdisciplinary conferences. If planned outside clinical trials, the respective evidence available in the scientific literature must be respected just as it is in many other situations in cancer medicine.

Treatment of disseminated and/or metastatic cancer

Drug therapy given to cancer patients with advanced disease is sometimes called 'primary' chemotherapy, or 'induction' chemotherapy in specific settings. In some metastatic cancers and in primary systemic disorders, such as the leukaemias, systemic treatment can be given with a *curative intent*. Success of chemotherapy in this setting is seen in inherently chemosensitive cancers, e.g. testicular cancer, or some aggressive lymphomas or acute leukaemias. Treatment of CML with imatinib obviated the need for allogeneic stem cell transplantation, and long-term results suggest that patients with CML adhering to therapy with this targeted agent enjoy a high likelihood of long-term remission, possibly cure (the optimal duration of imatinib treatment in this setting is, however, not firmly established).

However, most solid tumours, and thus many carcinomas, become incurable once disseminated disease is present. In these cases, *palliative treatment* is warranted, provided clinical benefit is proven. In patients with symptomatic metastatic cancers, treatment is warranted to improve quality of life. In patients presenting with metastatic incurable disease, yet without symptoms, the decision of when to start treatment is often less easy. Taking into consideration that side effects of systemic treatment (both from old and new drugs) may be debilitating, the definition of a clear and evidence-based treatment goal in such patients is particularly important. Clinicians should remember that it may be difficult to improve quality of life with palliative chemotherapy in asymptomatic cancer patients. Postponement of symptoms may be a worthwhile goal, as would be the prolongation of life, even in patients who eventually succumb to their cancer. These decisions must be taken based on available trial data suggesting that such goals can indeed be reached. Decision-making may become more and more difficult along the clinical course of disease, there being little evidence to support late lines of treatment in patients who have failed first- and second-line therapies. These principles largely apply to both chemotherapy and the newer 'targeted' drugs.

The literature providing evidence to support palliative systemic treatment in advanced cancers is fraught with a number of problems that should be recognized. In many trials, objective response and/or duration of response, or progression-free survival (PFS) are accepted endpoints. None of these, however, implies true clinical benefit, as they do not always reflect the impact of an objective response assessed by imaging and serum tumour marker assays on clinical symptom control and drug side effects. To label improvement of response rates or duration of response *per se* as 'clinical benefit' may be misleading, unless it is proven that a particular regimen improves the patient's well-being. The term 'clinical benefit' was introduced in a seminal paper describing the beneficial effects of gemcitabine in metastatic pancreatic cancer on pain scores and weight loss, and ideally it should be used in this strict sense in other cancers. Objective response, e.g. as shown by a regression of an asymptomatic lung metastasis on a computed tomography (CT) scan, in the face of considerable toxicity from chemotherapy, would be labelled as 'success' by RECIST criteria or PFS, but as failure when quality of life scores are taken into account. Important measures of success in palliative systemic treatment would thus be improvement of quality of life, reduction of the use of analgesics given to control cancer pain, weight gain and other clinical parameters indicating patient well-being, rather than improvement of imaging parameters *per se*.

Selection of drugs, dosage and dose intervals

The choice of cytostatic or cytotoxic drugs in cancer is largely based on empirical findings that indicate that a given drug may work rather well in one cancer but much less well in another. As mentioned above, it was recognized in the early days of chemotherapy development that in most settings, drug combinations are better than single agent chemotherapy, mainly because of resistance to drugs. A number of principles guide the selection of drug combinations in cancer medicine:

- Only drugs known to be at least partially effective against a given tumour type should be combined.
- Ideally drugs from different classes with different modes of action and distinct mechanisms of resistance should be combined. An example is the CHOP regimen for lymphoma, where cyclophosphamide (an alkylating agent), doxorubicin (an anthracycline acting on topoisomerase and gene transcription), vincristine (a spindle poison) and steroids are combined.
- Drugs with overlapping toxicity should be avoided.
- Dosing of drugs should avoid overdosing with excess toxicity and under-dosing with lack of effect. Ideally, the necessary concentrations of drugs should be achieved at their cellular target structure, or elicit a certain pharmacodynamic effect. In cancer pharmacology, the target concentrations and the cellular effects in tumour tissue are largely unknown; hence, drugs are often given at the maximum tolerated dose as assessed clinically or through routine laboratory parameters. This approach has been criticised in recent years, in particular in the context of molecularly targeted agents.

A paradigm shift from the chemotherapy-type trial-and-error approach of cancer candidate drug selection was introduced when agents became available which were designed to interfere with molecular pathways or specific proteins with an important role in the molecular pathology of a given cancer. These agents chiefly include monoclonal antibodies and small molecules blocking important proteins in the cancer cell, mostly activated tyrosine kinases.

A number of principles dictate the mode by which specific cancer drugs are given, i.e. the strategy of chemotherapy, and other drug regimens. Well-tolerated compounds such as hormones in breast cancer and some of the tyrosine kinase inhibitors are often given continuously, perhaps with interruptions dictated by toxicity. Continuous dosage is, however, rarely possible with cytostatic agents as normal cells need time to recover from the toxicity, notably the mucosa and bone marrow. Recovery from such toxicity typically determines the therapy cycle duration and thus treatment-free intervals. In many instances, the duration of treatment 'cycles' is built around bone marrow toxicity, specifically neutrophil and platelet recovery. Deliberate shortening of the cycle intervals predictably increases toxicity, and is only warranted if a tighter interval provides a clear-cut clinical benefit. This concept of 'dose density' is used with the intention of impeding regrowth of cancer cells in chemotherapy-free intervals. In high-grade lymphoma, for example, CHOP was originally given on Day 1 of a 21-day cycle (CHOP-21); attempts to give it every 2 weeks (CHOP-14) seemed to show promising treatment results, but also more toxicity. In daily practice, however, the term 'dose dense' is often used to denote frequent, short intervals with reduced doses of chemotherapy. Drug dosage should be maintained at the levels published to obtain an optimal result, but often toxicity, e.g. leukopenia, will demand dose reductions. Dose intensity refers to the amount of cytostatic drugs given at defined dosage over time and is expressed in milligrams per square metre per week. Lengthening the cycle interval or dose reductions whilst maintaining the treatment interval both lower dose intensity, but may thus jeopardize outcome. Maintaining dose intensity is of paramount importance in situations where chemotherapy is given with curative intent, e.g. in testicular germ cell cancer. In the palliative setting, great care must be taken to adjust therapy in a way which ensures best symptom control with acceptable toxicity.

Dose intensity may be increased in two ways. First, in chemotherapy regimens with a predominantly myeloid toxicity, leading to neutropenia, neutrophil recovery may be hastened through administration of haematopoietic growth factors or colony-stimulating factors (CSFs), particularly granulocyte CSF (G-CSF). The dose intensity gained is moderate. The chief aim of administering G-CSF is a reduction in the risk of febrile neutropenia rather than improvement of chemotherapy results.

Second, dose escalation is much more marked in high-dose chemotherapy regimens supported by autologous haematopoietic stem cells. By retransfusing the patient's own stem cells harvested prior to high-dose chemotherapy, this modality exploits the possibility of administering particularly high dosages of drugs with explicit bone marrow toxicity. It is obvious that such high-dose regimens must be based on drugs for which the chief dose-limiting feature is bone marrow toxicity. Dose escalation of, for example, anthracyclines, must respect their potential for cardiotoxicity, and the therapeutic margins for vincristine, taxanes and platinum are very narrow because of concern for irreversible neurotoxicity, nephrotoxicity and ototoxicity, respectively. Dose escalation in high-dose chemotherapy regimens is only possible with the adjunct of haematopoietic growth factors to ensure rapid bone marrow reconstitution from retransfused stem cells. This concept is nowadays best used in the treatment of multiple myeloma, relapsed high-grade lymphoma, Hodgkin lymphoma and, perhaps, prognostically adverse cases of testicular cancer. The results of high-dose chemotherapy with autologous stem cell transplantation have been disappointing for solid tumours such as breast, ovarian and small cell lung cancers.

Duration of systemic therapy

The optimal duration of systemic therapy in cancer is in most instances ill defined, surprising as this may sound. Most curative regimens, e.g. R-CHOP in B-cell lymphoma or BEP (bleomycin + etoposide + cisplatin) in testicular cancer, stem from pioneer trials where an arbitrary number of treatment cycles were given; subsequent trials respected these landmarks for fear of jeopardizing the results. It is hence difficult to assess the optimal number of cycles that should be given to an individual patient, as some patients may need the full programme for a successful outcome whereas others may be cured with fewer cycles. Newer trial data studying the optimal number of ABVD (doxorubicin + bleomycin + vinblastine + darcarbacine) cycles given to treat Hodgkin lymphoma suggest that treatment duration and cycle number may be adjusted to clinical risk patterns, or perhaps to the interim assessment of tumour response to treatment. In the adjuvant therapy of breast cancer, six courses of CMF (cyclophosphamide + methotrexate + fluorouracil) have been shown to be as effective as 12 courses, and six cycles of AC (cyclophosphamide + doxorubicin) were equivalent to four cycles. Similarly, 1 year of fluorouracil-based chemotherapy was no more effective than 6 months of adjuvant therapy for colorectal cancer.

In palliative systemic therapy, a given treatment regimen should obviously be ended or changed if unacceptable toxicity occurs, or if there is clear-cut evidence of tumour progression under therapy. Progression should be assessed by objective, clinically-relevant criteria. Changing a treatment regimen simply because a tumour marker rises or because size of a metastasis on a CT scan appears somewhat increased with respect to a previous reference image, may not always be clinically appropriate. Decisions on whether or not to continue treatment once a response is noted are, however, often difficult. In metastatic colorectal or breast cancer, several trials have compared a stop-and-go policy of palliative treatment versus continuous treatment (to maintain remission) and results are somewhat controversial. Individual decisions, largely resting on the patient's self-assessment and attitude, are therefore often warranted. Some patients might prefer a 'break' from treatment once response and clinical benefit have been obtained, whilst others cling to continuing therapy out of fear of impending tumour progression. The same principles largely apply to new targeted agents, e.g. the treatment of metastatic lung cancer with EGFR inhibitors.

Maintenance therapy refers to a strategy where systemic treatment is given to maintain a tumour response that has mostly been obtained with more intense treatment. The aim is to prolong a progression-free interval, and possibly overall survival. Maintenance regimens typically show a restricted toxicity to increase their feasibility and patient acceptance. Examples are the use of rituximab maintenance therapy, given at 2–3-months intervals, for patients with previously untreated follicular CD20-positive B-cell non-Hodgkin lymphoma who achieve a response to rituxumab in combination with chemotherapy, or pemetrexed maintenance in patients with lung adenocarcinoma who have responded to combination chemotherapy. Lenalidomide maintenance is increasingly used to maintain treatment response in myeloma after induction therapy and consolidation with high-dose chemotherapy and autologous stem cell retransfusion.

Refractory or relapsing cancer

Failure of particular cancers to respond to therapy is still one of the greatest problems in clinical oncology. Resistance to drugs may be present from the beginning of treatment, resulting in cancer progression during the respective line of therapy. Often it may evolve in a cancer initially responsive to treatment, possibly through the selection of drug-resistant subclones. In practice, drug resistance of cancer is still the major obstacle to therapeutic success, and this is true for chemotherapy as well as the newer agents. Unfortunately, few predictive *in vitro* tests are available in routine practice to predict whether particular chemotherapy agents will or will not work in a given case. In a number of cancers, predictive factors can be assessed to judge the *a priori* likelihood of treatment success or failure. The absence of oestrogen receptors predicts the failure of a hormonal agent in patients with breast cancer. CML cells with the *BCR-ABL T315I* mutation are resistant to imatinib. Patients with colon cancer are unlikely to benefit from cetuximab, an antibody targeting EGFR, when the constitutively activated mutant *KRAS* is incorporated in a down-stream position. On the other hand, metastatic melanoma harbouring the *BRAF V600E* mutation frequently responds to therapy with vemurafenib.

In cancers that fail to respond to a selected line of therapy, several aspects should be considered. The diagnosis of the cancer type should perhaps be rechecked by an experienced pathologist, as an erroneous diagnosis of the cancer type in question would obviously lead to an incorrect choice of drug regimens. In oral cancer therapies, care should be taken to assess patient compliance with drug intake. For instance, only 50% of patients with early breast cancer complete a 5-year course of adjuvant hormonal therapy. Non-compliance may not always be easy to spot, but a careful history on this topic (whilst avoiding reproachful remarks to the patient) should be taken. If the cancer diagnosis is correct, and non-compliance ruled out with any certainty, drugs should be changed as soon as refractory cancer behaviour is documented. In the next line of treatment, drugs should be selected from a different class of agents with different modes of action to overcome molecular resistance mechanisms. Some localized cancers with an unsatisfactory treatment response may react favourably to involved-site radiotherapy. Truly refractory cancers often have a dismal prognosis even after a change of treatment.

Cancer relapses, as a rule of thumb, may be retreated with the same regimen that was initially successful, provided there has been a sufficiently long treatment-free interval before relapse. It is often assumed that progression- and hence treatment-free intervals of about 1 year or more warrant reuse of the previous line of therapy, with careful monitoring of response. Early relapse after a transient and short treatment-free interval warrants a next-line choice of drugs from a different type or class than used in the previous line. These principles apply equally to regimens used for metastatic cancer or in an adjuvant setting.

When selecting a subsequent line of therapy, long-term toxicity as a result of previous regimens must be considered. The cumulative dose of anthracyclines must be calculated, as a previously accumulated 'anthracycline burden' limits the future use of this drug. Drug-induced polyneuropathy may often persist and worsen under re-exposure to neurotoxic drugs such as lenalidomide, vincristine or the taxanes. Impaired bone marrow reserves may be due to previous exposure to marrow-suppressive drugs and to irradiation of bone segments with active haematopoiesis.

In some patients, relapse may occur in 'chemotherapy sanctuaries' such as the central nervous system (CNS) or the testicles which many cytotoxic agents fail to penetrate. Relapses of acute lymphoblastic leukaemia in the testicles or meninges are examples. If possible, care must be taken to employ preventive measures, such as intrathecal therapy or prophylactic brain irradiation, to overcome this problem.

Monitoring systemic therapy over time

Follow-up of cancer patients under systemic treatment must ensure that acceptable responses and clinical benefit (in the true sense of the term) are obtained, with acceptable toxicity. Assessment of tumour responses in metastatic or disseminated cancers with measurable tumour parameters are discussed in the respective chapters of this book. As a general rule, it must be stressed that systemic cancer therapy should *not* be given over prolonged periods of time without such assessments, as clinicians must ensure that the balance between effect and side effects eventually tips in favour of benefit. In treatment given with curative intent, considerable short-term toxicity may be acceptable in view of a later sustained beneficial result, i.e. cure, e.g. as in when acute leukaemias are treated with intensive chemotherapy and transplantation. The benefit of adjuvant therapy cannot by definition be assessed in individual patients, but monitoring of these patients for toxicity is still of paramount importance.

Toxicity monitoring must respect the expected side effects of the drugs used. Serial peripheral blood counts to identify therapy-induced neutropenia or thrombocytopenia must take into account the expected period when a cell count nadir (i.e. the point in time with the lowest respective cell count) is most likely. A finding of neutropenia should elicit a clinical search for mucosal toxicity, as both often run in parallel, and *vice versa*. Patients receiving anthracyclines must be checked prior to therapy and when approaching the critical cumulative dose by echocardiography or multigated acquisition (MUGA) scan, which provide objective measures of left ventricular ejection fraction. In younger cancer patients who still might wish to father offspring or to become pregnant, gonadal toxicity potentially leading to infertility must be considered before therapy is started. In men, sperm can be banked and stocked in liquid nitrogen after harvest for later attempts at *in vitro* fertilization and in women, oocytes can be harvested and kept, albeit with much greater complexity in terms of time and effort. It is compulsory to inform patients about such options before intensive therapy (including haematopoietic stem cell transplantation programmes which almost always result in sterility).

In contrast to other clinical settings, assessment of therapeutic drug levels plays virtually no role in cancer treatment, except for methotrexate and some newer drugs such as imatinib. Methotrexate is eliminated via the kidneys, and accumulation of this compound or sustained serum and tissue levels may elicit considerable, potentially fatal, mucosal toxicity. In patients who receive medium-to-high doses of methotrexate and hence need normal tissue rescue with leucovorin (folinic acid), serial assessment of methotrexate serum levels is therefore mandatory to ensure proper elimination of the drug and to prompt administration of high doses of leucovorin in case of unexpectedly slow elimination.

Route of administration of systemic therapy

Systemic cancer medicine may be administered via several routes. Although this issue may sound trivial, selecting the best route of administration of anticancer drugs may be crucial to obtaining best results. In drugs where both intravenous and oral routes are available, the choice may depend on several aspects. The oral route poses a problem in terms of patient compliance, which may not always be immediately apparent on follow-up visits. The intravenous route, if feasible, eliminates this problem, but it may be more complicated as each dose requires that the patient travels to the outpatient clinic. Routes of application may have an impact not only on patient compliance, but also on therapy results. For example, the CMF regimen in breast cancer shows a better performance if cyclophosphamide is given orally over 2 weeks instead of parenterally on Days 1 and 8, as in an intravenous CMF regimen. In colorectal cancer, bolus intravenous 5-fluorouracil has been shown to be inferior to continuous intravenous application of the drug around the clock with portable pump systems. Bortezomib used in myeloma yields similar antitumour results but less neurotoxicity when given subcutaneously rather than intravenously.

Treatment of tumour lesions in the CNS requires that intravenous drugs penetrate the blood–brain barrier. This may depend on drug dosage. For example, successful treatment of CNS lymphoma requires high doses of intravenous methotrexate with or without high doses of intravenous cytarabine to ensure sufficient tissue levels of the drug in the CNS. Alternatively, drugs may be given intrathecally into the spinal fluid through a lumbar puncture or – preferentially – a suitable reservoir permitting access to the brain's ventricles. Few drugs are suitable for intrathecal administration, among them methotrexate, cytarabine and glucocorticosteroids.

Drugs given intravenously require a safe and reliable venous access. If peripheral veins are unsuitable, placement of an intravenous access device system may be mandatory. Given the inconvenience of repeated venepunctures when giving serial cycles of intravenous chemotherapy or antibodies, the option of implanting a permanent intravenous catheter system should be widely offered. Some drugs, notably anthracyclines and vincristine, may produce debilitating tissue toxicity if injected accidentally into paravenous tissue, and this must be prevented at all cost. If there is any doubt, the clinician should never hesitate to recommend the implantation of a port-a-cath system.

Some drugs require premedication to prevent or alleviate allergic reactions, e.g. paclitaxel and some monoclonal antibodies, mostly the chimaeric ones consisting of mixed human and mouse moieties (rituximab being the best known example of that kind). Other supportive measures such as antiemetics are discussed in the respective chapter of this book.

Patient co-morbidities

When planning systemic cancer treatment, pre-existing medical conditions, i.e. co-morbidities, must be taken into account. This may pose special problems in an elderly population where a cancer diagnosis must be seen in the context of multiple pre-existing conditions. Table 11.3 gives a few frequent examples to be considered when planning and starting systemic cancer treatment.

Table 11.3 Non-neoplastic co-morbidities and related problems of systemic cancer treatment

Pre-existing medical condition	Cancer drug	Problem
Diabetes mellitus	Steroids	Impaired blood glucose control
Kidney failure	Methotrexate (and other drugs chiefly eliminated via the kidneys)	Tissue toxicity through drug accumulation and/or prolonged drug serum and tissue levels
Labyrinthine hearing impairment	Cisplatin	Exacerbation of hearing loss potentially leading to severe impairment or deafness

(continued)

Table 11.3 Non-neoplastic co-morbidities and related problems of systemic cancer treatment (Continued)

Pre-existing medical condition	Cancer drug	Problem
Peripheral polyneuropathy	Vincristine, lenalidomide, taxanes, oxaliplatin, bortezomib	Worsening of peripheral nerve damage, potentially irreversible
Myelodysplastic syndrome	Any drug with marked bone marrow toxicity	Pancytopenia due to drug-induced suppression of haematopoiesis
Heart failure (coronary or valvular heart disease)	Anthracyclines	Additional impairment of ventricular function
Ascites and/or pleural effusion	Methotrexate	'Third space' with drug accumulation, protracted release, and hence increased tissue toxicity
Hepatic cholestasis	Anthracyclines and other drugs eliminated through bile	Retention of active drug or metabolites thereof with increased toxicity
Multiple pre-existing conditions (diabetes, arterial hypertension, etc.) requiring several drugs, particularly those given orally	Particularly oral cancer drugs	Compliance with taking 'yet another pill' added to an already longish list of drugs for various conditions
History of or active thrombosis	Drugs increasing the risk of thrombosis or thromboembolism, e.g. lenalidomide or bevacizumab	Additional drug-induced risk of thromboembolic events, at times despite anticoagulants or other preventive measures

Pricing of cancer drugs and affordability of systemic therapy

The price of cancer drugs has been spiralling over the past decade, whilst therapeutic advances have often been modest. Patent protection of new drugs ensures that often there is little or no competition for a given compound. For example, a potential gain of life span in metastatic melanoma treated with the anti-CTL4 antibody ipilimumab will cost US$100,000 or more if the costs of treating complications are also considered. Drug prices seem not to reflect the clinical benefit, and may exceed the financial levels stipulated by a number of government bodies, such as the National Institute for Health and Clinical Excellence (NICE) in the UK. NICE arbitrarily suggested that the cost for a life year saved through treatment should not surpass a limit of £30,000 (US$50,000), possibly using the cost of 1 year's treatment with haemodialysis as a yardstick. In many affluent countries, such discussions have as yet had little influence on pricing of newly marketed drugs, and society still shies away from taking up this delicate issue. The principle that 'life is priceless' still seems to prevail over economically oriented discussions, whilst health costs continue to rise to levels that may become unacceptable even in high human development index countries. Solutions to the problem of the rising costs of drugs should be explored through collaboration between governments, the pharmaceutical industry and the medical profession to enable improved access to drugs of clinical benefit.

Recommended reading

Amir E, Seruga B, Martinez-Lopez J et al. (2011) Oncogenic targets, magnitude of benefit, and market pricing of antineoplastic drugs. *J Clin Oncol* 29:2543–2549.

Bamias A, Pignata S, Pujade-Lauraine E (2012) Angiogenesis: a promising therapeutic target for ovarian cancer. *Crit Rev Oncol Hematol* 84:314–326.

Blumenthal GM, Scher NS, Cortazar P et al. (2013). First FDA approval of dual anti-her2 regimen: pertuzumab in combination with trastuzumab and docetaxel for HER2-positive metastatic breast cancer. *Clin Cancer Res* 19(18):4911–4916.

Burris HA, Moore MJ, Andersen J et al. (1997) Improvements in survival and clinical benefit with gemcitabine as first-line therapy for patients with advanced pancreas cancer: a randomized trial. *J Clin Oncol* 15:2403–2413.

Cabanillas F (2010) Front-line management of diffuse large B cell lymphoma. *Curr Opin Oncol* 22:642–645.

Experts in Chronic Myeloid Leukaemia (2013) The price of drugs for chronic myeloid leukemia (CML) is a reflection of the unsustainable prices of cancer drugs: from the perspective of a large group of CML experts. *Blood* 121:4439–4442.

Ocaña A, Amir E, Vera F, Eisenhauer EA, Tannock IF (2011) Addition of bevacizumab to chemotherapy for treatment of solid tumors: similar results but different conclusions. *J Clin Oncol* 29:254–256.

Ou SH, Bartlett CH, Mino-Kenudson M, Cui J, Iafrate AJ (2012) Crizotinib for the treatment of ALK-rearranged non-small cell lung cancer: a success story to usher in the second decade of molecular targeted therapy in oncology. *Oncologist* 17:1351–1375.

12 Treatment in pregnancy

Hatem A. Azim, Jr[1], Fedro A. Peccatori[2], Isabelle Demeestere[3], Oreste Gentilini[4] and Nicholas Pavlidis[5]

[1]Department of Medicine, BrEAST Data Centre, Institut Jules Bordet, Université Libre de Bruxelles, Brussels, Belgium
[2]Department of Gynecological Oncology, Fertility and Procreation Unit, European Institute of Oncology, Milan, Italy
[3]Research Laboratory on Human Reproduction, Université Libre de Bruxelles, Brussels, Belgium
[4]Department of Breast Surgery, European Institute of Oncology, Milan, Italy
[5]Department of Medical Oncology, Medical School, University of Ioannina, Ioannina, Greece

Introduction

The diagnosis of cancer during pregnancy is relatively uncommon. The exact incidence is unknown, although it is estimated that around 1 in 1000 pregnancies is complicated by cancer. Given the relative rarity of this condition, pregnant patients are frequently misdiagnosed with other benign conditions and hence cancer is often diagnosed at relatively late clinical stages. This means therapy cannot be delayed until delivery in the majority of cases. Induction of abortion can be proposed; however, there is no evidence supporting a therapeutic role for this approach. In addition, abortion is considered ethically unacceptable by some individuals and cultural groups. Thus, it is important to provide guidance and clear recommendations on how to manage and counsel women diagnosed with cancer during the course of gestation. Tables 12.1 and 12.2 summarize the general obstetrical and oncological considerations that should be taken into account in managing pregnant cancer patients.

Breast cancer during pregnancy

Epidemiology

Several studies have found that breast cancer is the most common malignant tumour diagnosed during pregnancy. It is estimated that around 1 in 3000 pregnancies is complicated by breast cancer. There has been controversy regarding the prognosis of these patients. Nevertheless, they appear to exhibit an aggressive tumour phenotype mimicking that of

Table 12.1 General obstetric considerations in managing pregnant women with cancer

	Obstetric considerations
Fetal monitoring during pregnancy	Pregnancies should be considered as high obstetrical risk and hence should be closely monitored Monthly monitoring of fetal development and amniotic fluid volume by ultrasound is encouraged
Time of delivery	Target full-term delivery as possible If not possible, late preterm delivery can be considered (i.e. weeks 34–37) Induction of labour on reaching viability (i.e. early preterm) is a discouraged approach as it can have significant short- and long-term sequelae on the newborn. This should be considered only in cases of severe fetal or maternal complications
Mode of delivery	Vaginal delivery allows faster postnatal recovery compared to caesarean section and hence is preferred if treatment needs to be started shortly following delivery
Placenta evaluation	Placental metastasis is rare and most commonly reported with melanoma. However, it is recommended to send the placenta for histological examination
Neonatal care and follow-up	Apgar score, weight, height and blood counts should be measured for the neonate at delivery It is encouraged to join active registries on long-term surveillance of babies born to pregnant cancer patients (www.cancerinpregnancy.org or www.pregnantwithcancer.org)

UICC Manual of Clinical Oncology, Ninth Edition. Edited by Brian O'Sullivan, James D. Brierley, Anil K. D'Cruz, Martin F. Fey, Raphael Pollock, Jan B. Vermorken and Shao Hui Huang. © 2015 UICC. Published 2015 by John Wiley & Sons, Ltd.

Table 12.2 General oncological considerations in managing pregnant women with cancer

	Oncological considerations
Multidisciplinary approach	Whenever possible, pregnant patients with cancer should be treated within institutions with known expertise in managing such cases and within a multidisciplinary team including an oncologist, obstetrician, neonatologist and also a psychologist
Diagnostic radiology and radiotherapy	Radiation doses >100 mGy may result in a risk of childhood cancer and fetal malformations. Staging procedures that involve radiation exposure are usually below this dose. Nevertheless, it is preferred to strictly limit their use during pregnancy Risk of radiation to the fetus is also highly dependent on gestational age Radiation therapy is better postponed until after delivery When radiotherapy is unavoidable due to rapid tumour progression, effort should be made to minimize fetal radiation exposure by optimizing field size, shape and beam energy, as per the American Association of Physicists in Medicine guidelines Estimation of fetal size and position, as well as projected growth over the duration of treatment, is essential in radiotherapy planning in order to minimize the fetal radiation exposure. Patients with brain metastasis often require immediate palliative radiotherapy, and this can be performed during pregnancy provided adequate shielding is established Palliative radiotherapy to the cervical spine, upper thoracic vertebrae and shoulders is also possible as the radiation fields are rather far from the uterus Radiation to the pelvis and lumbar area should be avoided during the course of gestation. If there is an urgent need for such treatment, abortion should be considered
Chemotherapy	Should be avoided during the first trimester Actual weight should be used for dose calculation acknowledging that pharmacokinetics can be relatively altered during pregnancy Should be stopped before week 34 of gestation to avoid delivery during nadir periods Weekly scheduling is an attractive approach as it is associated with shorter nadir periods. In addition it allows close patient monitoring and easy interruption of therapy in case of complications.

breast cancer diagnosed in young women, and hence active and immediate initiation of therapy is warranted in the vast majority of cases.

Diagnosis and staging

- *Breast ultrasound and mammogram*: suspicious breast lumps should be subjected to an ultrasound. A mammogram can be performed during pregnancy provided there is adequate uterine shielding to avoid potential fetal exposure to ionizing radiation.
- *Pathological evaluation*: a core biopsy of suspicious breast lesions should be performed. Fine needle aspirates are not recommended in these cases. Pathological evaluation should be the same as in the non-pregnant setting, including the determination of histological type and grade, oestrogen receptor (ER), progesterone receptor (PgR) and HER2 status, and when feasible a proliferation marker like Ki-67.
- *Abdominal ultrasound*: can be performed any time during pregnancy.
- *Chest X-ray*: can be performed provided there is adequate uterine shielding. It is best avoided during the third trimester due to the abdominal localization of the uterus.
- *Other radiological exams*: bone scan and positron emission tomography (PET) should be avoided during pregnancy. In case of suspicion of bone metastasis, magnetic resonance imaging (MRI) without gadolinium can be performed.

Treatment
Local treatment
- Patients with localized disease in the breast should be considered for surgical resection during pregnancy.
- Surgery, whether mastectomy or breast conserving surgery, should follow the standard indications for outside the pregnancy setting.
- Surgery can be performed any time during pregnancy, even during the first trimester.
- The experience with sentinel node biopsy using technetium-99 during pregnancy remains limited. However, available data are rather reassuring. Hence, it can be considered in centres in which sentinel node biopsy is standard in routine practice. However, the use of blue dye during pregnancy is discouraged as it is associated with a 2% risk of allergic reaction, which can be life-threatening.
- Radiotherapy is better postponed until after delivery. Careful evaluation should be performed for patients considered for breast conserving surgery early during the first trimester as this may delay the initiation of adjuvant radiotherapy.

Systemic treatment
- The decision to offer adjuvant or neoadjuvant chemotherapy should follow the same indications as for outside the pregnancy setting.
- Anthracyclines-based regimens are the most commonly used regimens in the adjuvant/neoadjuvant setting. They are the most tested regimens during pregnancy and appear to have an acceptable safety profile when administered during the course of gestation, starting in the second trimester.
- There is no particular preference for one anthracycline-based regimen over any other.
- Data on taxanes are also reassuring, yet they are more limited compared to those for anthracyclines. Hence, in metastatic patients who have previously been exposed to anthracyclines, taxanes remain the first choice during pregnancy. Weekly paclitaxel may be favoured given its relatively better tolerance compared to docetaxel and its weekly application, which allows close monitoring of pregnancy.
- Tamoxifen is contraindicated during pregnancy as it has been shown to be associated with congenital malformation both in preclinical models and in sporadic clinical reports.
- Trastuzumab should be avoided during pregnancy as it is associated with a high risk of oligohydramnios, which predispose to preterm labour, fetal morbidity and mortality.

Cervical cancer during pregnancy

Epidemiology
The rate of cervical cancer during pregnancy ranges from 1 to –12 per 100,000 pregnancies. The prognosis of cervical cancer diagnosed during pregnancy appears to be comparable to that diagnosed in the non-pregnancy setting.

Diagnosis and staging
- It is generally recommended that all pregnant women undergo a Pap smear and/or HPV typing as a part of their initial prenatal examination.
- Colposcopy can be performed with relatively high sensitivity ranging from 75% to 95%.
- Endocervical curettage should be avoided during pregnancy.
- Pelvic MRI can be considered for adequate staging of nodal involvement.

Treatment
- Radical hysterectomy and/or pelvic radiotherapy with or without cisplatin are the main modalities used in managing cervical cancer. Radical surgery and pelvic radiation would result in pregnancy termination and fetal death. Hence, patients who wish to preserve their pregnancy should be informed that management will require modification of standard local treatment. Whether this potentially has detrimental effects on patient outcome remains unknown.
- Treatment depends on stage and gestational age. In early-stage cervical cancer, definitive treatment can be postponed until after delivery, with close monitoring during pregnancy.
- For more advanced cases (Stage IB1, IB2, IIA) who wish to preserve their pregnancy, a thorough radiological and surgical staging is needed to identify patients who require immediate initiation of therapy.
- Lymphadenectomy can be safely performed during pregnancy. Laparoscopic lymphadenectomy can also be considered in some cases, even if the risk of bleeding or complications may be higher than in non-pregnant cases.
- If the patient needs treatment for a locally advanced or high-risk tumour, platinum-based chemotherapy with or without paclitaxel can be proposed, with a local response rate similar to that in non-pregnant cases.
- Radical surgery can be offered concomitantly with caesarean section in qualified centres.

Lymphomas during pregnancy

Epidemiology
Lymphoma is diagnosed in around 1 in every 6000 pregnancies. The presenting manifestations are similar to those for classical lymphoma, but can be confused with symptoms accompanying the normal pregnancy, such as shortness of breath and fatigue. Prognosis appears comparable to that in the non-pregnancy setting.

Diagnosis and staging
- Patients with palpable lymph nodes should undergo lymph node biopsy.
- Pathological evaluation should follow the same standard procedures as outside the pregnancy setting, including bone marrow biopsy.
- Staging work-up with computed tomography (CT) and PET scan should be avoided during pregnancy. Staging with MRI remains the preferred option with fewest potential fetal adverse effects.

Treatment
- Low-grade lymphomas should be kept under surveillance until delivery. In symptomatic cases in which active treatment is required, a CHOP (cyclophosphamide + doxorubidin + vincristine + prednisolone)-like regimen could be considered.
- Standard chemotherapy (i.e. CHOP for non-Hodgkin lymphoma; and ABVD [Adriamycin + bleomycin + vinblastine + dacarbazine] for Hodgkin lymphoma) can be given at standard doses starting the second trimester

- Rituximab administration is not associated with congenital malformations; however, it has been shown to cause neonatal B-cell depletion, which is generally reversible. Hence, in cases in which postponement of rituximab is regarded to compromise patient prognosis, rituximab can be given during pregnancy provided close monitoring of fetal blood count.

Leukaemia during pregnancy

Epidemiology

Relative to lymphomas, leukaemias are less commonly diagnosed during pregnancy, with an estimated incidence of 1 in 75,000–100,000 pregnancies. Leukaemias diagnosed during pregnancy are mainly acute, more commonly myeloid than lymphoid.

Diagnosis and staging

- Bone marrow examination can be performed as in non-pregnant patients and evaluation should follow the same standard procedures as outside the pregnancy setting.

Treatment

- Patients diagnosed with acute leukaemias should initiate chemotherapy as soon as possible. Hence, women diagnosed early during the first trimester should be considered for an abortion, as initiation of chemotherapy carries a significant high risk of fetal congenital malformations.
- Leukapheresis in the presence of a very high white blood count and leucostasis-related symptoms can be safely performed during pregnancy.
- Treatment with idarubicin and daunorubicin should be avoided during pregnancy even during the second and third trimesters. These are highly lipophilic and have been shown to be associated with high fetal complications. Doxorubicin can be used as an alternative in these cases.
- Patients with chronic myeloid leukaemia can be kept on observation until delivery in the absence of symptoms or significantly deteriorating blood counts. In situations in which active treatment is required, imatinib can be considered after the first trimester, acknowledging that safety data are limited and first trimester exposure is associated with a high rate of congenital malformations. Interferon can be considered as an alternative or if treatment is required during the first trimester

Malignant melanoma during pregnancy

Epidemiology

Melanoma is one of the most common tumours diagnosed during pregnancy, with an incidence higher than that of breast cancer in some studies. Prognosis appears comparable to age- and stage-matched non-pregnant cases.

Diagnosis

- Patients may present with thicker melanoma during pregnancy.
- Sentinel lymph node biopsy can be offered during pregnancy as a part of the staging procedure. The same precautions should be considered as mentioned earlier for breast cancer staging.

Treatment

- Surgical management should follow the same standard procedures as for outside pregnancy.
- In pregnant patients with metastatic melanoma requiring the initiation of systemic therapy, interferon-alpha remains the first option. No safety data are available for ipilimumab or vemurafenib during pregnancy, and hence their use during pregnancy is discouraged. If the relative inferiority of interferon is deemed to significantly affect patient outcome, pregnancy termination should be discussed with the patient.

Other rare malignancies in pregnancy

Ovarian cancer

Epithelial ovarian cancer is a disease of the elderly and hence is rarely diagnosed during pregnancy. Germ cell tumours are more common in young patient; however, reports are limited to a few cases in the literature. Treatment of both should be with chemotherapy, starting in the second trimester with a platinum-based regimen. The preferred partner is paclitaxel, even for germ cell tumours, given the toxicity profile of etoposide during pregnancy even when administered after the first trimester.

Lung cancer

Several reports point to a potential increase of diagnosing lung cancer in young women and during pregnancy, given the increase in cigarette smoking among young females. Staging follow-up should be performed by MRI instead of CT scan. Platinum agents can be administered during pregnancy. Carboplatin has an overall milder toxicity profile compared to cisplatin and hence is relatively favoured during pregnancy. Paclitaxel is the preferred partner given its activity in lung cancer and safety data in managing breast and ovarian cancer, and also few cases of non-small cell lung cancer. Until further safety data are available, the use of epidermal growth factor receptor tyrosine kinase inhibitors during pregnancy should be restricted.

Soft tissue sarcoma

Current data in the literature are restricted to few cases. Patients requiring active treatment during pregnancy should be offered single agent doxorubicin. Given the lack of superiority of doxorubicin combined with ifosfamide on overall survival, avoidance of the administration of ifosfamide is preferred during pregnancy given its toxicity profile and limited information on its safety during pregnancy.

Supportive care

Nausea and vomiting

Treatment with metoclopramide, domperidone or ondansteron is possible throughout pregnancy. Prednisone can also be used, but preferably during the second trimester.

Analgesia

The analgesic of choice is paracetamol. Non-steroidal anti-inflammatory drugs should be avoided, as they are associated with fetal defects, risk of miscarriage and oligohydramnios. Opiates can be used, but they are best avoided close to delivery, as they can be associated with neonatal withdrawal effects.

Infections

Metronidazole, cephalosporins and clarithromycin can be used during pregnancy. More limited data are available for imipenem and meropenem. It is best to avoid quinolones and aminoglycosides because of their potential for fetal adverse effects.

Anaemia and leucopenia

Erythropoietin and granulocyte colony-stimulating factor (G-CSF) should not be used unless there is an urgent need for them, given the limited safety data on their use during pregnancy.

Bone metastases

Bisphosphonates were shown to cause fetal skeletal defects in animal models. They also cause maternal hypocalcaemia that can affect uterine contractions and hence should be avoided in pregnancy.

Conclusions

Cancer during pregnancy should be managed in experienced centres. These cases should be discussed by a multidisciplinary team involving the obstetrical, neonatal and oncological teams to allow adequate counselling of these highly challenging cases. These situations are often emotionally stressful for the patient, her partner and also her family. Hence, an individualized approach should be considered, taking into account cancer prognosis, fetal well-being and the patient's preferences.

Recommended reading

Amant F, Van Calsteren K, Halaska MJ et al. (2012) Long-term cognitive and cardiac outcomes after prenatal exposure to chemotherapy in children aged 18 months or older: an observational study. *Lancet Oncol* 13:256–264.

Azim HA Jr, Peccatori FA, Pavlidis N (2010) Treatment of the pregnant mother with cancer: a systematic review on the use of cytotoxic, endocrine, targeted agents and immunotherapy during pregnancy. Part I: Solid tumors. *Cancer Treat Rev* 36:101–109.

Azim HA Jr, Pavlidis N, Peccatori FA (2010) Treatment of the pregnant mother with cancer: a systematic review on the use of cytotoxic, endocrine, targeted agents and immunotherapy during pregnancy. Part II: Hematological tumors. *Cancer Treat Rev* 36:110–121.

Cardonick E, Usmani A, Ghaffar S. (2010) Perinatal outcomes of a pregnancy complicated by cancer, including neonatal follow-up after in utero exposure to chemotherapy: results of an international registry. *Am J Clin Oncol* 33:221–228.

Loibl, S., Han, S.N., von Minckwitz, G et al. (2012) Treatment of breast cancer during pregnancy: an observational study. *Lancet Oncol* 13:887–896.

Luis SA, Christie DR, Kaminski A, Kenny L, Peres MH (2009) Pregnancy and radiotherapy: management options for minimising risk, case series and comprehensive literature review. *J Med Imaging Radiat Oncol* 53(6):559–568.

Martin DD (2011) Review of radiation therapy in the pregnant cancer patient. *Clin Obstet Gynecol* 54(4):591–601.

Morice P, Uzan C, Gouy S, Verschraegen C, Haie-Meder C (2012) Gynaecological cancers in pregnancy. *Lancet* 379:558–569.

Peccatori FA, Azim HA Jr, Orecchia R et al. (2013) Cancer, pregnancy and fertility: ESMO Clinical Practice Guidelines for diagnosis, treatment and follow-up. *Ann Oncol* 24 Suppl 6:vi160–170.

Van Calsteren K, Heyns L, De Smet F et al. (2010) Cancer during pregnancy: an analysis of 215 patients emphasizing the obstetrical and the neonatal outcomes. *J Clin Oncol* 28:683–689.

Van Calsteren K, Verbesselt R, Ottevanger N et al. (2010) Pharmacokinetics of chemotherapeutic agents in pregnancy: a preclinical and clinical study. *Acta Obstet Gynecol Scand* 89:1338–1345.

13 Treatment in the elderly

Matti S. Aapro

Multidisciplinary Oncology Institute, Clinique de Genolier, Genolier, Switzerland

Introduction

The world's population is ageing with one in five individuals projected to be over the age of 65 years by 2020, and most individuals aged 65 years and above will be in developing countries, even if they represent a smaller proportion of the populations of these countries. Cancer incidence increases with age; thus, the number of older cancer patients will increase significantly. In order to adequately address patients' needs, it is important to understand the specificities of ageing and their implication on the cancer and its treatment.

Definition of elderly and geriatric assessment

There is no age cut-off defining 'elderly', but 70 years is becoming the most commonly used age limit for defining patients as elderly within the field of geriatric oncology. However, the most important factors are the physiological decline of organ reserves and co-morbidities which accelerate this decline and reduce the ability to cope with stress. There is no simple way to assess these processes and little evidence to suggest the superiority of one approach compared to any other. They are however important for many decisions; the type of adjuvant treatment suggested for a patient with a life expectancy of 3 years will differ from that for a patient with a 12-year life expectancy.

The International Society for Geriatric Oncology (SIOG) has recently looked at the rationale for performing a comprehensive geriatric assessment (GA); findings from a GA performed in geriatric oncology patients; the ability of GA to predict oncology treatment-related complications; association between GA findings and overall survival (OS); impact of GA findings on oncology treatment decisions; composition of a GA, including domains and tools; and methods for implementing GA in clinical care. It concluded that GA can be valuable in oncology practice for detection of impairment not identified in routine history or physical examination; prediction of severe treatment-related toxicity; prediction of OS for a variety of tumours and treatment settings; and ability to influence treatment choice and intensity.

The SIOG panel recommended that the following domains be evaluated in a GA: functional status, co-morbidity, cognition, mental health status, fatigue, social status and support, nutrition and presence of geriatric syndromes.

Recognition of cognitive dysfunction may require formal cognitive testing, especially if the patient has preserved language function or if the caregiver does most of the talking. For surgical procedures, the risk of postoperative acute confusional state (known as delirium) is markedly increased in the presence of pre-operative cognitive dysfunction. According to the World Health Organization (WHO), a diagnosis of dementia must include impairment of memory affecting the person's daily functioning and at least one other cognitive dysfunction (e.g. language, visual–spatial function or logical reasoning). There must also be impairment of mental functions such as emotional control, motivation or social behaviour. The duration of the symptoms must be at least 6 months and consciousness must be normal.

The risk of falls is multifactorial and includes muscle weakness, gait deficits and balance deficits. Medications that may increase the fall risk include benzodiazepines, opioid analgesics, sleeping medication and antidepressants.

Although several combinations of tools and various models are available for implementation of GA in oncology practice, the SIOG expert panel could not endorse one over another. One of the issues is also the complexity of these instruments and the time needed to implement them. Thus, various screening instruments have been suggested (Table 13.1) which can indicate if a patient has a short life expectancy. The G-8 instrument (Table 13.2) is now suggested to be incorporated in all EORTC trials.

UICC Manual of Clinical Oncology, Ninth Edition. Edited by Brian O'Sullivan, James D. Brierley, Anil K. D'Cruz, Martin F. Fey, Raphael Pollock, Jan B. Vermorken and Shao Hui Huang. © 2015 UICC. Published 2015 by John Wiley & Sons, Ltd.

Table 13.1 Screening tools

Tool	Components	Data in geriatric studies	Data in oncology patients
VES-13	Age, self-rated health, functional capacity and physical performance	Score predictive of increased risk of death or functional decline over 2 years	Mixed results for identifying CGA impairment in different populations
Groningen Frailty Indicator	Mobility/physical fitness, vision, hearing, nutrition, co-morbidity, cognition, psychosocial	Correlation between the GI score and CGA	Predicts mortality in older cancer patients receiving chemotherapy
G-8	Nutrition, mobility, cognitive defect, polypharmacy, age, self-perceived health status	Derived from MNA	Sensitive for predicting deficits on CGA

CGA, Comprehensive Geriatric Assessment; GI, Groningen Inventory; MNA, Mini-Nutritional Assessment

Table 13.2 G-8 geriatric screening tool

A.	Has food intake declined over the past 3 months due to loss of appetite, digestive problems, chewing or swallowing difficulties?	0 = severe decrease 1 = moderate decrease 2 = no decrease
B.	Weight loss during the past 3 months?	0 = >3 kg 1 = does not know 2 = between 1 and 3 kg 3 = none
C.	Mobility?	0 = bed or chair bound 1 = able to get out of bed/chair but does not go out 2 = goes out
D.	Neuropsychological problems?	0 = severe dementia or depression 1 = mild dementia 2 = no psychological problems
E.	BMI (weight in kg/height in m^2)	0 = BMI <19 1 = BMI 19–<21 2 = BMI 21–<23 3 = BMI ≥23
F.	Takes more than three prescription drugs per day?	0 = yes 1 = no
G.	In comparison with people of the same age, how does the patient consider his/her health status?	0.0 = not as good 0.5 = does not know 1.0 = as good 2.0 = better
H.	Age	0 = >85 years 1 = 80–85 years 2 = <80 years
Total score		0–17

Surgery and the elderly

There is continued debate about the increased risk of acute and delayed complications after surgery in the elderly. Present evidence shows that older cancer patients treated under elective conditions have less operative morbidity and mortality. Self-expanding metallic stents are worth considering in acute decompression of colonic obstruction. Bone lesions, if not amenable to cementoplasty, are frequently considered for fixation and consolidation.

While the American Society of Anesthesiologists (ASA) score is helpful in predicting mortality in the general population, the Physiological and Operative Severity Score for Enumeration of Mortality and Morbidity (POSSUM) and its modification P-POSSUM have been prospectively validated, with the P-POSSUM formula designed to better predict operative mortality in cases where POSSUM overstated the observed mortality. POSSUM and P-POSSUM were also developed to predict outcomes; regrettably, their reliability is poor in the elderly subgroup and most importantly, some information can only be retrieved perioperatively rather than before the decision is made to undergo surgery or consider medical palliation.

The geriatric assessment domains can also be helpful. Thirty-day morbidity is principally related to instrumental activities of daily living (IADL) and brief fatigue inventory (BFI), whereas the postoperative hospital stay correlates with activities of daily living (ADL).

Radiotherapy and the older cancer patient

As for all areas of oncology dealing with the elderly patient, there is a dramatic lack of level I evidence. The SIOG has established a task force to make recommendations for curative radiotherapy in older patients (Table 13.3) and to identify future research priorities. Recent advances in radiation planning and delivery have improved the efficacy of radiotherapy, while reducing its toxicity.

Implications of the ageing process for tolerance to chemotherapy

Decreased organ function complicates treatment: the most frequent issues are impairments in renal function which increase drug toxicity. Liver reserves are not decreased significantly by

Table 13.3 SIOG recommendations for standard radiotherapy in the elderly

Breast cancer	• Fit older patients are candidates for postoperative whole breast radiotherapy (WBRT) after breast conserving therapy (BCS) for invasive cancer and for higher-risk ductal carcinoma *in situ* (DCIS) • WBRT with a boost to the site of excision is appropriate for all older patients with invasive breast cancer. There is no specific subgroup from whom WBRT can be systematically omitted • Patients ≥50 years of age are candidates for shortened treatment schedules when they do not need any lymph node irradiation • Partial breast irradiation should be considered investigational as there in insufficient evidence to support it in the elderly • Post-mastectomy irradiation should be considered for older patients with pT3–4 tumours or those with ≥4 axillary nodes • Axillary irradiation is recommended for macrometastases on sentinel node biopsy or axillary node sampling • 3D CT-based planning is advised to minimize cardiac and lung irradiation, as are alternative techniques such as treatment in the prone or lateral position
Lung cancer	• While surgery remains the standard of care in early-stage non-small cell lung cancer (NSCLC) in the elderly, stereotactic body radiation therapy (SBRT) is a reasonable option in early-stage NSCLC when surgery is contraindicated • For inoperable locoregionally-advanced NSCLC, concomitant chemoradiation is appropriate in fit elderly patients • For operable locoregionally-advanced NSCLC, no elderly-specific recommendations can be made concerning postoperative indications, and decisions should be individualized • In limited-disease SCLC, chemoradiation in the fit elderly is appropriate, with adapted regimens where necessary
Lymphoma	• For early-stage Hodgkin lymphoma, involved-field radiotherapy (IFRT) after short-course chemotherapy is appropriate for elderly patients • For elderly patients with more advanced Hodgkin lymphoma and stage I–II non-Hodgkin lymphoma, IFRT is an option in cases of symptomatic recurrence and in all patients with low-grade lymphoma • In some cases of localized disease, involved-node radiotherapy (INRT) can be considered, using new techniques such as intensity-modulated radiation therapy (IMRT) or 3D conformal radiotherapy (3D-CRT) to decrease the toxicity
Prostate cancer (PC)	*Patients with low-risk PC* • Management selection (hormonal therapy, watchful waiting, external beam radiation therapy (EBRT), brachytherapy or surgery) should be based on geriatric assessment • Significant co-morbidity should be a strong relative contraindication to aggressive treatment *Patients with intermediate or high-risk PC* • Patients with no or mild co-morbidity have a significant overall survival benefit from short-course androgen deprivation therapy (ADT) added to EBRT. In men without moderate or severe co-morbidity, 6 months of hormones added to EBRT should be proposed • For high-risk PC, chemotherapy with EBRT and long-term ADT should be indicated after selection based on geriatric evaluation and treatment tolerance *EBRT technique in the elderly* • 3D-CRT is recommended for all patients. IMRT is generally associated with less grade 3 proctitis, compared with 3D-CRT • Shortened, hypofractionated radiotherapy may be a more convenient alternative in elderly patients • Role of brachytherapy in elderly patients with low-risk PC should be defined in prospective studies taking into account life expectancy and geriatric evaluation
Endometrial cancer	• In low-risk patients, no adjuvant treatment is required • In high-to-intermediate risk patients, vaginal brachytherapy (VBT) alone is the adjuvant treatment of choice • In high-risk patients, no standard optimal treatment is defined. EBRT ± VBT is a reasonable option for this group
Rectal cancer	• Elderly patients with locally advanced rectal cancer can safely receive preoperative long-course chemoradiation with 5-fluorouracil (5-FU) chemotherapy or a 1-week short course of pelvic radiation alone • For elderly patients with early rectal cancer who are medically inoperable, endorectal contact X-ray treatment offers the potential for local control without significant toxicity • Tailored strategies for those elderly patients who receive preoperative treatment with a complete clinical response, such as surveillance or transanal endoscopic microsurgery (TEMS), may be appropriate if there are contraindications to radical surgery, which remains the standard of care • Colorectal cancer oligometastases to the lung and liver can be treated with stereotactic ablative radiotherapy in elderly patients not eligible for surgery, with minimal morbidity and a high likelihood of local control

(continued)

Table 13.3 (Continued)

Central nervous system	• Conformal short-course radiotherapy with or without concomitant temozolomide can be advised for elderly patients with malignant glioma. For elderly patients whose tumour shows *MGMT* methylation it is reasonable to treat initially with temozolomide alone, reserving radiotherapy for patients with progressive disease • For elderly patients with limited brain metastases, stereotactic radiosurgery (SRS) is appropriate
Head and neck cancer	• Radical radiotherapy using IMRT or other highly conformal techniques to reduce acute and late toxicity is appropriate in elderly patients without severe co-morbidities • Aggressive combined modality treatment is appropriate where co-morbidities permit

Source: Kunkler (2014). Reproduced with permission of Oxford University Press.

ageing. Cardiac issues can complicate many treatments and pulmonary issues are limiting factors for surgery and, rarely, for chemotherapy (with the notable exception of bleomycin). Several groups have suggested scores that may help predict the toxicity related to chemotherapy and adapt the doses used in the elderly. These scores are important but complex to use, and are not proven prospectively to improve clinical outcome for patients (Tables 13.4).

Renal function needs to be carefully assessed in order to adapt drug dosage. The probable age-related decrease in renal function is probably best evaluated with an aMDRD formula, rather than the commonly used Cockcroft–Gault one. The level of serum creatinine should not be relied upon to assess renal function as it may appear normal but actually is already indicative of reduced renal clearance of drugs. Many websites allow the calculation of revised drug dosages.

Cardiac function declines are observed in many elderly patients. These patients are at higher risk of complications in the short and longer term, and thus when possible a less cardiotoxic choice of drugs is preferable. Although some guidelines suggest that follow-up of troponin levels after administration of cardiotoxic agents may be of value, there is no substantial evidence for this. Particular attention should be paid to the QTc interval on the electrocardiogram: a prolonged QTc puts the patient at risk of major rhythm disturbances and many drugs should be avoided in such situations.

Specific issues related to cancer treatment and its side effects in the elderly

Febrile neutropenia

Febrile neutropenia, defined as an oral temperature of >38.5 °C or two consecutive readings of >38.0 °C for 2 hours and an absolute neutrophil count of <0.5 × 10^9/L, or expected to fall below 0.5 × 10^9/L, is a major risk factor for infection-related morbidity and mortality and also a significant dose-limiting toxicity in cancer treatment. The importance of the risk is dependent on the number of co-morbidities in any given patient.

Prophylactic granulocyte colony-stimulating factor (G-CSF) is recommended in various evidence-based guidelines which indicate that a risk of >20% of febrile neutropenia is a reason to use primary prophylaxis. A predicted risk of 10–20% is actually probably higher among patients above the age of 65 years. Different forms of G-CSF are available: originators and biosimilars, from short acting like filgrastim or lenograstim (not available in the USA) to longer acting (needing only one injection) like pegfilgrastim and lipegfilgrastim (not available in the USA). The most important factor for their efficacy is use as per EMA or FDA approved labelling. They have no contraindications related to patient age. The European Organization for Research and Treatment of Cancer (EORTC) guidelines and others do not recommend the use of antibiotic prophylaxis (fluoroquinolones), but the UK National Institute for Health and Clinical Excellence (NICE) has issued a position statement which considers this as an alternative to G-CSF usage.

Nausea and vomiting

Elderly patients have a decreased risk of developing nausea and vomiting, but are at a higher risk of complications related to chemotherapy-induced nausea and vomiting (CINV) like dehydration and its consequences on blood pressure and renal function. Current guidelines for CINV prevention (see Chapter 15) are applicable to the elderly patient. Guidelines indicate the preferential use of palonosetron. This is important for elderly patients (who often have cardiac disease) because several 5-hydroxytryptamine 3 (5-HT3)-receptor antagonists carry

Table 13.4 Predictors of toxicity

Laboratory	Clinical
Haemoglobin	Eastern Cooperative Oncology Group performance status (ECOG PS)
Albumin	Diastolic blood pressure
LDH	Mini-Mental Examination
Creatinine clearance	Self-rated health
	Mini-Nutritional Assessment
	Cumulative. Illness Rating Scale for Geriatrics (CIRS-G) co-morbidity
	Instrumental activities of daily living (IADL)

Source: Extermann et al. (2011). Reproduced with permission of Wiley & Sons Ltd.

warnings about potential prolongation of the QTc electrocardiographic interval, which can lead to arrhythmias. As many elderly patients have diabetes, caution is needed when corticosteroids are used. Neurokinin 1 (NK1)-receptor antagonists interact with agents metabolized through the 3A4 pathway, and many are used by elderly patients with co-morbidities.

Drug–drug interactions

Many drugs can interact with each other and it is estimated that if more than six agents are used daily, there is a risk of one significant interaction. As an example of potential interactions, those for agents metabolized through the 3A4 pathway are shown in Table 13.5.

Bone health

Bone loss (osteoporosis) and associated fractures increase with age in both men and women. The WHO has thus identified the following risk factors (other than low bone mineral density) for bone loss: age, gender (female), smoking, personal history of fracture after 50+ years, parental history of hip fracture, low body mass index (<20 kg/m^2), consumption of >3 units of alcohol per day, corticosteroid use and having other diseases (such as rheumatoid arthritis or vitamin D deficiency). Aromatase inhibitors in females with breast cancer and androgen deprivation therapy (ADT) in males accelerate bone loss and significantly increase the risks of fracture. In addition, when metastases in the bone are present, there is a further risk of fractures.

Exercise, smoking cessation, reduction of alcohol consumption and vitamin D and calcium supplements are important in preventing bone loss in patients with cancer. Bisphosphonates such as zoledronic acid or denosumab are recommended for the prevention of fractures in patients with bone metastases, and denosumab is also indicated in the prevention of bone loss-related to adjuvant treatment with aromatase inhibitors. A recent meta-analysis has shown that among postmenopausal women, the rate of breast cancer mortality was 15.2% for those treated with bisphosphonates versus 18.3% for those not receiving bisphosphonates ($P = .004$).

Anaemia

Anaemia is not a normal consequence of ageing and >50% of cases the cause is treatable, which may include iron and vitamin B12 deficiency. It may be a sign of early myelodysplasia or renal insufficiency.

Cobalamin deficiency is related to atrophic gastritis and medications (proton pump inhibitors and metformin). The diagnosis of iron deficiency in the presence of inflammation may represent a challenge. Patients with iron deficiency may need intravenous iron as they may not be able to absorb iron normally.

The use of blood transfusions and erythropoietin-stimulating agents should follow guidelines.

Table 13.5 Drug interactions for a drug metabolized via the 3A4 pathway

	Reason for interaction
Increased drug concentration	
Ketoconazole, itraconazole, voriconazole	Strong CYP3A4 inhibitor[a]
Clarithromycin, telithromycin	Strong CYP3A4 inhibitor[a]
Atazanavir, saquinavir, ritonavir, indinavir, nelfinavir	Strong CYP3A4 inhibitor[a]
Nefazodone	Strong CYP3A4 inhibitor[a]
Fluconazole	Moderate CYP3A4 inhibitor and/or P-glycoprotein (P-GP) inhibitor[b]
Erythromycin	Moderate CYP3A4 inhibitor and/or P-GP inhibitor[b]
Amprenavir, fosamprenavir	Moderate CYP3A4 inhibitor and/or P-GP inhibitor[b]
Verapamil	Moderate CYP3A4 inhibitor and/or P-GP inhibitor[b]
Aprepitant	Moderate CYP3A4 inhibitor and/or P-GP inhibitor[b]
Diltiazem	Moderate CYP3A4 inhibitor and/or P-GP inhibitor[b]
Decreased drug concentration	
Rifampin	Strong CYP3A4 inducer[c]
Rifabutin, rifapentine	Strong CYP3A4 inducer[c]
Phenytoin	Strong CYP3A4 inducer[c]
Phenobarbital	Strong CYP3A4 inducer[c]
Carbamazepine	Strong CYP3A4 inducer[c]
Increased drug concentration	
Midazolam	Sensitive CYP3A4 substrate

[a]Concomitant strong inhibitors of CYP3A4 should not be used.
[b]If alternative treatment cannot be administered, reduce the drug dose.
[c]If alternative treatment cannot be administered, increase the drug dose.

General principles of treatment of cancer in the elderly

The recommendations based on level I evidence available for younger patients are often suggested as being valid for the 'fit' elderly. This is probably correct, provided renal function is taken into account. There is however evidence that even these patients are at risk of increased toxicity and, for example, use of preventative G-CSF is suggested by guidelines in elderly patients even if the risk of febrile neutropenia is only between 10% and 20% as determined in studies in younger patients. The present recommendations of guideline committees are given in the Recommended reading. As for all patients, careful attention to co-morbidities is needed and will decrease the potential problems. A past history of repeated infections and even 'mild' diabetes can be the cause of major toxicities.

Conclusion

Management of the elderly cancer patient requires careful and continuous assessment of all aspects of the individual. Important outcomes in the treatment plan include quality of life and performance status maintenance, not only progression-free survival or overall survival. Best management recognizes and prevents geriatric issues. There is a great need and opportunity for specific care trials in older cancer patients, including studies that look at treating older frail patients.

Recommended reading

Aapro M, Bernard-Marty C, Brain EG et al. (2011) Anthracycline cardiotoxicity in the elderly cancer patient: a SIOG expert position paper. Ann Oncol 22:257–67.

Biganzoli L, Wildiers H, Oakman C et al. (2012) Management of elderly patients with breast cancer: updated recommendations of the International Society of Geriatric Oncology (SIOG) and European Society of Breast Cancer Specialists (EUSOMA). Lancet Oncol 13:148–160.

Decoster L, Van Puyvelde K, Mohile S et al. (2014) Screening tools for multidimensional health problems warranting a geriatric assessment in older cancer patients: an update on SIOG recommendations. Ann Oncol [Epub ahead of print].

Droz JP, Aapro M, Balducci L et al. (2014) Management of prostate cancer in older patients: updated recommendations of a working group of the International Society of Geriatric Oncology. Lancet Oncol 15:e404–e414.

Extermann M, Boler I, Reich RR et al. (2012) Predicting the risk of chemotherapy toxicity in older patients: the Chemotherapy Risk Assessment Scale for High-Age Patients (CRASH) score. Cancer 118:3377–3386.

Falandry C, Bonnefoy M, Freyer G, Gilson E (2014) Biology of cancer and aging: a complex association with cellular senescence. J Clin Oncol 32:2604–2610.

Hurria A, Togawa K, Mohile SG et al. (2011) Predicting chemotherapy toxicity in older adults with cancer: a prospective multicenter study. J Clin Oncol 29:3457–3465.

Kunkler IH, Audisio R, Belkacemi Y et al.; on behalf of the SIOG Radiotherapy Task Force (2014) Review of current best practice and priorities for research in radiation oncology for elderly patients with cancer: the International Society of Geriatric Oncology (SIOG) task force. Ann Oncol 25(11):2134–2146.

Launay-Vacher V (2013) Cancer and the kidney: individualizing dosage according to renal function. Ann Oncol 24:2713–2714

Mathoulin-Pélissier S, Bellera C, Rainfray M, Soubeyran P (2013) Screening methods for geriatric frailty. Lancet Oncol 14:e1–2.

Naeim A, Aapro M, Subbarao R, Balducci L (2014) Supportive care considerations for older adults with cancer. J Clin Oncol 32:2627–2634

Pallis AG, Gridelli C, Wedding U et al. (2014) Management of elderly patients with NSCLC; updated expert's opinion paper: EORTC Elderly Task Force, Lung Cancer Group and International Society for Geriatric Oncology. Ann Oncol 25:1270–1283.

Papamichael D, Audisio RA, Glimelius B et al. (2014) Treatment of colorectal cancer in older patients. International Society of Geriatric Oncology (SIOG) consensus recommendations 2013. Ann Oncol [Epub ahead of print]

Popa MA, Wallace KJ, Brunello A et al. (2014) Potential drug interactions and chemotoxicity in older patients with cancer receiving chemotherapy. J Geriatr Oncol 5:307–314

van Leeuwen BL, Huisman MG, Audisio RA (2013) Surgery in older cancer patients – recent results and new techniques: worth the investment? Interdiscip Top Gerontol 38:124–131.

Wildiers H, Mauer M, Pallis A et al. (2013) End points and trial design in geriatric oncology research: a joint European organisation for research and treatment of cancer–Alliance for Clinical Trials in Oncology–International Society Of Geriatric Oncology position article. J Clin Oncol 31:3711–3718.

14 Oncology emergencies

Jonathan King, Dustin Deming and H. Ian Robins

University of Wisconsin, Carbone Cancer Center, Madison, WI, USA

Superior vena cava syndrome

Superior vena cava syndrome (SVCS) is the clinical manifestation of blood flow obstruction to the superior vena cava (SVC). This was a more common occurrence in the distant past, when syphilitic aortitis and tuberculous mediastinitis were more prevalent. Currently, >95% of cases of SVCS are due to malignancy; 75% of these are of lung origin. Of course, this means that not all cases of SVCS are malignant. Thus, establishing a diagnosis is of prime importance (Table 14.1).

Presenting symptoms
- Syndrome usually evolves insidiously
- Dyspnoea (63%)
- Facial swelling/fullness (50%)
- Cough (24%)
- Arm swelling (18%)
- Chest pain (15%)
- Dysphagia (9%)

Physical examination findings
- Neck vein distention (66%)
- Chest wall venous distension (54%)
- Facial oedema (46%)
- Cyanosis (20%)
- Plethora (19%)
- Arm oedema (14%)
- Other associated symptoms can include hoarseness, syncope and dizziness
- Patients may also describe that the plethora or facial oedema worsens with bending forward or lying down

Diagnostics
It is extremely important to establish that the SVC blood flow is being severely limited and the underlying aetiology for the SVCS, as treatment can differ substantially.

Work-up of SCVs typically begins with a chest X-ray. More often than not, this will be abnormal, thus setting the stage for computed tomography (CT) and magnetic resonance imaging (MRI) scans, bronchoscopy, thoracoscopy, venograms and possibly limited thoracotomy. Given the increased central venous pressure, the risk of bleeding during biopsy can be substantial.

Treatment
In the past, SVCS was considered a medical emergency for which immediate treatment was often given even before a pathological diagnosis had been established. This led to difficulty in accurately diagnosing 50% of patients, which complicated follow-up treatment. We now recognize that the treatment of SVCS is often not medically urgent, as the process has generally been present for weeks.

Treatment for SVCS can consist of chemotherapy, radiation therapy, thrombolytics or anticoagulation, expandable stents, balloon angioplasty, surgical bypass, steroids and/or diuretics. In malignancy-associated SVCS, the choice of treatment depends on the tumour type. For example, lymphomas and small cell lung cancers can respond rapidly to chemotherapy alone, whereas other malignancies will likely require radiotherapy. One may elect to use combination chemoradiotherapy for small cell lung cancer or lymphoma, given the improved survival advantage and locoregional control seen in several studies.

In general, 75% of patients with malignancy-associated SVCS will show improvement in 3–4 days, with 90% having major improvements within 1 week. Patients who do not improve during that first week may have developed a central

Table 14.1 Malignant and non-malignant causes of superior vena cava syndrome

Malignant (95%)	Non-malignant (5%)
Lung cancer (75%)	Granulomatous disease
Small cell cancer (50%)	Tuberculosis
Squamous cell cancer (26%)	Syphilis
Adenocarcinoma (14%)	Histoplasmosis
Large cell carcinoma (10%)	Sarcoidosis
Lymphoma (15%)	Silicosis
Others (primary or metastatic) (10%)	Goitre
	Aortic aneurysm
	Thrombosis
	Thymoma
	Teratoma
	Dennoid cyst
	Fibrosing mediastinitis

vein thrombus; this requires fibrinolytic or antithrombotic therapy. Given the increased central venous pressure and the fact that certain tumours are more friable, caution must be followed before anticoagulants are instituted. For this reason, prophylactic anticoagulation is not standard practice.

Occasionally, steroids can improve symptoms, particularly if the aetiology of the SVCS is lymphoma. They can also decrease swelling while the patient is receiving radiation treatments for the SVCS. Benefits are usually minimal; however, if severe respiratory compromise is present, steroid use would be reasonable.

Diuretics can provide symptomatic relief initially, but caution with regard to fluid status should be observed.

Metastasis to brain

Brain metastasis occurs in 25–35% of patients with systemic cancer, most commonly in those with cancers of the lung or breast, and in malignant melanoma. In general, brain metastases portend a poor prognosis with median survival ranging between 3 and 6 months with whole-brain radiation alone. Now, with neurosurgical resection and stereotactic radiosurgery, survival has improved in selected patients. Generally, with current treatment strategies, median survival has increased to 6 months to 1 year from the onset of central nervous system (CNS) disease.

Presenting symptoms
- Seizure
- Headache
- Cranial nerve deficits
- Incoordination
- Muscle weakness
- Nausea
- Mental status changes.

Physical examination findings
- Thorough cranial nerve and neurological assessment needs to be documented
- Papilloedema is uncommonly seen and reflects increased intracranial pressure

Diagnostics
- MRI or CT scan (with and without contrast):
  - MRI is far preferable (especially if cranial nerve findings suggest a brainstem lesion or exam is suspicious for posterior fossa pathology)

Treatment
Treatment typically begins with corticosteroids (e.g. dexamethasone 10 mg bolus intravenously [IV] or orally [PO], followed by 4 mg IV/PO every 6 hours) to decrease cerebral oedema if present on radiological evaluation. This can result in improvements in symptoms within hours and prevent worsening of symptoms once more definitive treatment is performed.

At the time steroids are introduced, consideration should be given to:
- Checking blood sugars for glucose intolerance
- Ulcer prophylaxis, e.g. with an H2 blocker, proton pump inhibitor or sucralfate
- Thrush prophylaxis, e.g. with nystatin swish and swallow suspension, or clotrimozole troches.

Depending on the patient's functional status, number and location of metastatic lesion(s) in the CNS, and other end-organ involvement, neurosurgical resection or stereotactic radiosurgery can be considered.

Whether or not the lesion is resectable, whole-brain radiation should be considered as the number of future neurological events has been shown to be substantially decreased with radiotherapy. (In some cases localized radiation, i.e. radiosurgery can be considered for lesions <3 cm.) In such patients many radiation oncologists delay whole-brain radiotherapy until the time of recurrence. The initiation or radiation therapy typically is not emergent. Patients can typically be stabilized with the use of steroids.

Spinal cord compression

Spinal cord metastasis with cord compression is a true oncological emergency in that delays in treatment can result in high morbidity with significant neurological deficits. The natural history of disease is toward progressive pain, paralysis, sensory loss and sphincter incontinence. Spinal cord compression is common. In general, 3–7.4% of patients with breast, prostate or lung cancer will present to their physician with metastatic cord compression. In patients with advanced cancer, 5–10% of all patients will have evidence of cord compression at autopsy. Yet, despite its common occurrence, current treatment recommendations are largely empiric.

Presenting symptoms
- Typically back pain as the periosteum is invaded:
  - Pain can be present for weeks to months before evidence of neurological compromise
- Other symptoms can include:
  - Radicular pain or referred pain (e.g. sacroiliac pain with L1 compression)
  - Weakness
  - Sensory loss
  - Urinary retention
  - Rectal sphincter dysfunction

Physical examination findings
A thorough neurological assessment needs to be documented.

Diagnostics
An MRI (with and without contrast) is optimal for confirming the diagnosis; however, a CT scan with contrast can also be used.

Typically, the aetiology is already known, but if the patient has no known diagnosis of cancer, appropriate work-up for a histological diagnosis should be done. If tissue cannot be obtained in an appropriate time frame, and if neurological compromise is already present, treatment should be initiated immediately as delays in therapy can substantially reduce the chance of full neurological recovery and increase morbidity.

Treatment
Treatment typically begins with corticosteroids (e.g., dexamethasone 10 mg bolus IV, followed by 4 mg IV/PO every 6 hours).

At the time steroids are introduced, consideration should be given to:
- Checking blood sugars for glucose intolerance
- Ulcer prophylaxis, e.g. with an H2 blocker, proton pump inhibitor or sucralfate
- Thrush prophylaxis, e.g. with nystatin swish and swallow suspension, or clotrimozole trouches.

To relieve the cord compression, radiotherapy and/or surgical options need to be investigated, taking into account the number of lesions, spine stability, life expectancy and radiosensitivity of the primary tumour.

Historically, laminectomy was the treatment of choice for malignant cord compression. With the advent of radiotherapy, improved local control rates became possible with less spinal instability, as seen with laminectomy. With surgical improvements, vertebral body resection then became favoured as spinal integrity was maintained. In general, radiation therapy is the treatment of choice as it has less treatment-associated morbidity. It should be noted, however, that a phase III clinical study suggested better preservation of neurological function with surgery and radiotherapy. One caveat to performing a surgical intervention (in the face of neurological deterioration) is the need for surgery to be performed emergently. The patients in this study, however, were generally far more advanced clinically in their neurological deterioration than patients seen at our more urban centre. Specific indications for surgical intervention include evidence of bony compression (typically a compression fracture of >50%), spinal instability or progression of symptoms despite radiotherapy.

One concern in a patient with malignant cord compression at a site that was previously irradiated is the development of radiation myelopathy if repeat radiotherapy is employed. It should be noted that if radiation myelopathy were to occur, it would typically present approximately 1 year after therapy. As most such patients have a prognosis of <1 year, and progression of neurological symptoms will inevitably occur without intervention, when considering the alternative (i.e. surgery or progressive cord compression), strong consideration for repeat radiation should be given.

Steroids can usually be tapered off over 2 weeks if symptoms are improving. Appropriate antifungal and antiulcer prophylaxis should always be provided as high-dose steroids can cause thrush, gastritis or a gastrointestinal bleed. Also, monitoring of blood glucose is important as steroids can lead to a hyperglycaemic response.

Neutropenic fever

Antineoplastic therapy affects the cell-mediated and humoral immune systems, predisposing patients to infections. In addition, myelosuppression and mucositis from chemotherapy are both substantial risk factors for developing a life-threatening infection. In immunocompromised hosts, infections can disseminate rapidly, leading to shock and death, so it is important to educate patients to be vigilant for fever or other signs of infection. In general, a single oral temperature of >38.3 °C or of >38.0 °C for at least 1 hour should be considered a fever in a neutropenic patient. Although certain tumours (such as lymphomas, hepatic metastases and tumour necrosis) can cause fevers, tumour fever is a diagnosis of exclusion, and appropriate evaluation for an occult infection needs to be performed.

Neutropenia is defined as an absolute neutrophil count of <1000/mm^3. Once the neutrophil count falls below 500/mm^3, the chance of infection increases significantly. It is estimated that 50–60% of neutropenic patients will develop an established or an occult fever. The typical organisms responsible for neutropenic infection are most commonly bacteria that normally colonize individuals, including aerobic Gram-positive cocci (viridans group streptococci, coagulase-negative staphylococcus, *Enterococcus* spp., *Streptococcus pneumonia*, *Streptococcus pyogenes* or *Staphylococcus aureus*) and aerobic Gram-negative bacilli (especially *Escherichia coli*, *Klebsiella pneumoniae* or *Pseudomonas aeruginosa*).

Presenting symptoms

Clinical signs or symptoms that may suggest infection can be subtle in a neutropenic host. This is likely related to the decreased inflammatory response in the setting of neutropenia.

In general, patients may only complain of fevers or rigors. Other typical clinical signs such as erythema, swelling, purulent drainage and pain may be absent.

Physical examination findings

Primary sites usually include the gastrointestinal tract (secondary to bacterial translocation from chemotherapy-damaged mucosa), skin (from vascular access devices) and possibly periodontal, rectal or respiratory infections (typically in more prolonged neutropenia).

Therefore, examination should give careful attention to the skin and venous access sites to look for erythema, tenderness and discharge, the perianal region to look for a perirectal abscess or cellulitis, and the oropharynx to evaluate for leukoplakia, dental abscess and stomatitis. Internal rectal examinations are avoided in the neutropenic patient to prevent gut flora from entering the surrounding tissue and bloodstream.

Diagnostics

- Initial work-up:
  - Two sets of blood cultures (one from each lumen of the vascular access device if present plus a peripheral blood culture) prior to initiation of antibiotics
  - Chest X-ray
  - Urine culture
  - Other clinically indicated studies or procedures
- Routine cerebrospinal fluid (CSF) examination is *not* recommended, but should be performed if CNS infection is suspected
- Complete blood count is important as it quantifies the degree of neutropenia, and can allow the physician to estimate the time of neutropenia based on the patient's previous response and type of chemotherapy used
- Evaluation of other chemistries (e.g. liver function tests, creatinine, electrolytes) is important as it allows appropriate dosing of antibiotics and monitoring for potential drug toxicity

Treatment

Prompt empiric administration of antibiotics is necessary, as current diagnostic tests cannot rapidly exclude a microbial source of infection.

Initial antibiotic therapy should be broad in spectrum and cover the common pathogens previously mentioned. Also, the initial selection should account for the local antibiotic resistance, patient drug allergies and organ dysfunction that may limit the use of certain antibiotics. Drug interactions should also be considered as patients treated with potentially nephrotoxic chemotherapy (such as cisplatin) may receive added toxicity from the use of aminoglycosides. That said, a standard regimen for empiric antibiotic selection should be followed.

We generally use regimens similar to the guidelines recommended by the Infectious Disease Society of America (2010). High-risk patients require IV antibiotic monotherapy and hospitalization. Monotherapy options include carbapenems (meropenem or imipenum) or piperazillin–tazobactam, or antipseudomonal β-lactam third-generation cephalosporins (like ceftazidime; not ceftriaxone secondary to inferior antipseudomonal efficacy). At our centre, we typically use a fourth-generation cephalosporin (cefepime) at a dose of 2 g IV every 8 hours when given as monotherapy (versus every 12 hours if used in combination with another antibiotic). Typical combinations of empiric therapy in severely ill patients (e.g. those with pneumonia or hypotension) or in cases of suspected antimicrobial resistance can include monotherapy plus the addition of an aminoglycoside or fluroquinolone, and/or vancomycin. Vancomycin is added only if the risk for a Gram-positive *Staphylococcus* infection is considered to be high (indwelling venous access device, severe mucositis, colonized with methicillin-resistant *S. aureus* [MRSA], history of MRSA or haemodynamic instability) and is discontinued after 3–4 days if cultures are negative or susceptibility results are available.

Length of therapy depends mainly on the neutrophil count, response to therapy and pathogen isolated. In general, if the patient remains afebrile and the neutrophil count exceeds 500/mm^3, we typically stop the antibiotic by Day 7. If the patient becomes afebrile and the neutrophil count remains low, depending on the length of anticipated neutropenia, one can either continue the antibiotics until the neutropenia resolves or discontinue the antibiotics after 7 days with close observation. If an infection source is identified (typically <50% of the time), longer antibiotic regimens (typically 10–14 days) are used. The initial broad-spectrum antibiotic can then be adjusted to cover the isolated pathogen based on susceptibility data.

Fevers that persist after 3–4 days on initial broad-spectrum antibiotics implies either a non-bacterial infection, new infection, improper clearance of the initial infection (such as an abscess or infected vascular access device), inadequate antibiotic levels, drug fever or tumour fever. A repeat search for the aetiology of the fever should be done with a focus on these possible causes. Changing antibiotics would not be unreasonable, as well as adding antifungal therapy (e.g. fluconazole or an echinocandin).

Particular concern should be exercised in neutropenic patients who have abdominal pain or nausea. These patients can have typhilitis (necrotizing colitis of the caecum) and require anaerobic coverage and possibly a surgical consultation. Additionally, patients with prolonged neutropenia (such as those undergoing induction chemotherapy for leukaemia or bone marrow transplantation) or on chronic steroids (such as brain cancer patients) can develop *Pneumocystis jiroveci* pneumonia if not on prophylactic therapy (e.g., trimethoprim–sulfamethoxazole [preferred], atovoquone, dapsone or aerosolized pentamidine), particularly if lymphocyte counts are below 400/mm^3.

Currently, the use of colony-stimulating factors prophylactically has reduced the incidence and duration of neutropenia. Routine use of colony-stimulating factors for the febrile neutropenic patient is not necessary, but should be considered in patients at high risk for prolonged neutropenia or infectious complications, and can shorten duration of neutropenia by days.

Hypercalcaemia

Hypercalcaemia can be a potentially life-threatening complication of several cancers. It is most often seen in breast, myeloma, lymphoma, lung, renal cell, head and neck and prostate cancer. Hypercalcaemia can be secondary to destructive bony lesions as well as the release of parathyroid hormone-related peptide (PTHrP), prostaglandins and various osteoclast-activating factors.

Presenting symptoms
- Typically weakness, lethargy and fatigue
- Patients may also have nausea and vomiting, constipation, polyuria, anorexia and dehydration
- Less commonly, patients may present with confusion, seizures or coma

Physical examination findings
- Examination may reveal mental status changes, dry mucous membranes and muscle weakness
- Deep tendon reflexes may be decreased or absent

Diagnostics
- Serum calcium (corrected for hypoalbuminemia) or ionized calcium level confirms the diagnosis
- Electrocardiogram may reveal a shortened QT segment or, less commonly, a first-degree atrioventricluar block or intraventricular block

Treatment
Aggressive hydration with normal saline is the single most important step in treating hypercalcaemia. This is because these patients are almost always dehydrated. Immediate improvements in symptoms can be seen with a decrease in serum calcium within 12–24 hours.

Bisphosphonates (zoledronic acid and pamidronate) have now evolved as the primary agents used in treating and preventing malignancy-associated hypercalcaemia. They bind to bone minerals and help the bones resist breakdown by phosphatases from activated osteoclasts. Almost all patients with tumour-induced hypercalcaemia with calcium of >12 mg/dL should receive a bisphosphonate. Patients with calcium of <12 mg/dL should also be treated with a bisphosphonate if symptomatic. Care must be taken in patients who are in need of impending dental extraction as they will be at risk for osteonecrosis of the jaw if treated with bisphosphonates.

We generally use zolidronate at a dose of 4 mg IV, as studies have shown that this dose can achieve normocalcaemia in >90% patients. Also, this dose appears necessary for humoral hypercalcaemia (versus bone metastases-induced hypercalcaemia).

Loop diuretics (furosemide) are often employed in the treatment of hypercalcaemia as they enhance sodium excretion and, therefore, calciuresis. Again, the key is to correct the fluid deficit first. Once that is done, a loop diuretic can be added, if necessary, with doses adjusted to maintain euvolaemia.

Other treatment options for hypercalcaemia include steroids (useful in hypercalcaemia secondary to lymphoma, myeloma or breast cancer) as well as calcitonin. Although calcitonin can decrease the serum calcium rapidly (within 2–4 hours), the peak effect is small and transient.

Syndrome of inappropriate antidiuretic hormone secretion

Syndrome of inappropriate antidiuretic hormone secretion (SIADH) has a variety of non-malignant aetiologies, but is most commonly associated with small cell lung cancer in the malignant setting. The tumour releases antidiuretic hormone, inappropriately resulting in hyponatraemia and water retention, and associated serum hypo-osmolarity.

Presenting symptoms
- Nausea, vomiting and anorexia
- Patients can be confused, lethargic or weak, and can also present with a seizure

Physical examination findings
Patients should appear euvolaemic without evidence of volume overload or dehydration.

Diagnostics
- Serum osmolarity and sodium are reduced due to a relative volume excess

- Urine sodium in general should be >20 mOsm/kg and urine osmolarity <100 mOsm/kg
- Thyroid stimulating hormone (TSH) and morning cortisol level should be measured to evaluate for other aetiologies of euvolaemic hyponatraemia

Treatment

In general, treatment involves correcting the underlying cause, which in the case of malignancy is the underlying cancer.

Free water restriction can improve the sodium concentration, although this is usually difficult to achieve in an uncontrolled setting.

Demeclocycline (300–600 mg twice a day) or lithium carbonate can improve symptoms by counteracting the effect of antidiuretic hormone by causing nephrogenic diabetes insipidus. These drugs can be especially useful in patients who cannot follow or tolerate a fluid-restriction programme, or in patients whose underlying malignancy is refractory to antineoplastic therapy.

Two aquaretics have recently been approved by the FDA. Conivaptan is a parenteral non-peptide dual AVP V1a- and V2-receptor antagonist. It is approved for use in hospitalized patients with euvolaemic (dilutional) and hypervolaemic hyponatraemia. The drug is given as a 20-mg loading dose followed by a continuous infusion or as intermittent boluses. It should not be used for >4 days. Tolvaptan is a selective oral V2-receptor antagonist also approved for use in hospitalized patients for hypervolaemia and euvolaemic hyponatraemia. The drug is started at a dose of 15 mg once daily and titrated up to 60 mg daily as required; it is best to avoid fluid restriction during the dose-finding phase.

As a cautionary note, both extreme hyponatraemia and an inappropriate approach to its treatment can have disastrous consequences. Consultation with a nephrologist should be sought early in difficult cases. Rapid correction can result in central pontine myelinolysis (CPM) with permanent neurological deficits.

Tumour lysis syndrome

Tumour lysis syndrome (hyperuricaemia, hyperkalaemia, hyperphosphataemia and hypocalcaemia) can develop in patients with leukaemia, lymphomas or bulky small cell carcinomas upon treatment with chemotherapy. This is due to the breakdown of cells with therapy and the release of a large amount of purine precursors into the circulation. The hyperuricaemia can cause urate crystal precipitation in the kidney tubules leading to acute renal failure, and the electrolyte and metabolite abnormalities can lead to cardiac irritability and even sudden death.

Presenting symptoms

- Decreased urine output
- Fatigue
- Change in mental status

Diagnostics

- Hyperuricaemia, hyperkalaemia, hyperphosphataemia, hypocalcaemia
- Oliguric renal failure
- Arrhythmia on electrocardiogram (ECG)

Treatment

- To prevent complications, patients should be well hydrated and started on allopurinol before systemic treatment is begun
- Urine alkalization with sodium bicarbonate (to keep urine pH >7.0) can decrease urate crystal precipitation in the kidney tubules
- Monitoring serum electrolytes and early treatment of electrolyte abnormalities are important during the first few days of therapy to prevent potential cardiac complications
- Rasburicase is a recombinant urate oxidase indicated for the treatment of hyperuricaemia secondary to tumour lysis syndrome

Adrenal insufficiency

Although metastatic involvement of the adrenals is not uncommon, particularly with breast and lung cancer, the development of adrenal insufficiency is rare. Clinical symptoms may include nausea, vomiting, apathy, abdominal pain and hypotension (possibly severe). If suspected, steroid replacement should be started and appropriate work-up initiated. Laboratory analysis, including cortisol and adrenocorticotropic hormone (ACTH) levels and ACTH stimulation tests are often adequate to verify clinical suspicions. Administration of dexamethasone (e.g. 4 mg) is the preferred initial steroid as it is not measured in serum cortisol assays. One common situation is the patient on chronic steroids with a suppressed adrenal gland secondary to negative feedback on the pituitary axis. These patients, when faced with a stressful event (such as infection or surgery), may develop symptoms of adrenal insufficiency because their adrenal gland cannot compensate for the added stressors to the body. In these cases, additional 'stress-dose' steroids (i.e. hydrocortisone 50–100 mg every 6 hours) should be provided until the inciting event resolves.

Thrombosis and hypercoagulability

Laboratory evidence for coagulation abnormalities in cancer patients can be a common finding (up to 90% of cases). This can result in a hypercoagulable state as the various pathological processes disturb the normal haemostatic balance. Typical processes can include thrombocytosis with increase in vascular reactivity, fibrin/fibrinogen degradation products and tissue factor, and also hyperfibrinogenaemia. Hypercoagulability may present as migratory thrombophlebitis, disseminated intravascular coagulation (DIC), marantic endocarditis or a deep venous thrombosis (DVT).

Classically, mucin-containing gastrointestinal malignancies and gliomas are associated with migratory thrombophlebitis, whereas DIC is associated with acute promyelocytic leukaemia. It is reported that 1–15% of patients with cancer will develop a clinically significant thrombosis during the course of their disease. Interestingly, up to 38% of patients with an idiopathic DVT were later found to have an occult malignancy in some cohort studies, suggesting that a work-up for malignancy should be performed in patients with unexplained thrombosis. Occasionally, the risk of thrombosis is increased secondary to treatment (e.g. hormone therapy in breast cancer), but the cause can be difficult to identify in many cases. Initial therapy in the past has been parenteral heparin, followed by oral warfarin. This however has changed with the advent of low molecular weight heparins (LMWHs), which have an improved safety profile and proven efficacy without need for frequent dose titration. It provides physicians with an alternative to intravenous heparin and has allowed treatment in an outpatient setting that was previously not possible. In fact, some data exist to suggest that LMWH may be more efficacious in malignancy-related thrombosis and that extended therapy with LMWH instead of warfarin may be better and safer.

There are various FDA-approved LMWHs commercially available which are produced by chemical or enzymatic depolymerization of unfractionated heparin (UFH). The fragmented LMWHs are approximately one-third the size of UFH and range from 4000 to 6500 Da with a chain length of 12–22 polysaccharides. The anticoagulant activity of LMWHs is similar to that of UFH; however, a shortened polysaccharide chain allows for more specific binding to inhibit factor Xa. UFH binds to antithrombin III, initiating inhibition of several serine proteases in the coagulation cascade, including factors IIa and Xa. The polysaccharide chain is truncated in LMWHs while retaining the high affinity pentasaccharide binding sites. This results in inhibition of factor Xa, but the shortened polysaccharide chain is relatively ineffective at binding factor IIa, resulting in loss of inhibition of factor IIa. In terms of anticoagulation, this results in a reduced anti-IIa activity relative to factor Xa and improved pharmacokinetics.

UFH is given intravenously (if used therapeutically) and requires close monitoring of activated partial thromboplastin time (APTT) with frequent dose adjustments. In contrast, LMWHs are injected subcutaneously once or twice daily and do not typically require routine monitoring. Special considerations for monitoring should be given for patients with renal failure and obesity. LMWHs are cleared by the kidneys and dosing is weight based. The biological half-life is prolonged in patients with renal failure. Dosing in renal failure and weight-adjusted dosing were not addressed in original clinical trials, but monitoring of anti-Xa levels is now recommended. Monitoring in pregnancy may also be considered given the relative increase in renal clearance. Anti-Xa levels can be monitored in serum 4 hours following subcutaneous administration. Various tests are available for monitoring anti-Xa levels and the target therapeutic range is 0.6–1.0 IU/mL.

Thus, as alluded to above, many consider LMWH as the agent of choice for the initial and long-term treatment of venous thromboembolism (VTE) in patients with neoplastic disease, based on randomized clinical studies In 2003, Lee et al. conducted a randomized study of cancer patients with VTE: 336 patients received dalteparin at 200 IU/kg daily for 5–7 days followed by a vitamin K antagonist for 6 months with a target international normalized ratio (INR) of 2–3, whereas the other 336 patients received dalteparin at 200 IU/kg daily for 1 month followed by 150 IU/kg daily for 5 months. It should be noted that the concept of a 25% dose reduction after initial therapy was an arbitrary choice and was not evaluated in comparison to other possibilities. Many will reduce the dose by 50%, and after another few months by an additional 25% to reach a convenient maintenance dose. In the Lee study, the cumulative risk of symptomatic and recurrent VTE during 6 months of anticoagulation was 17% for patients treated with a vitamin K antagonist, compared with 9% for patients treated with dalteparin, a LMWH. The relative risk reduction of 52% was statistically significant (hazard ratio 0.48; $P = 0.002$). One episode of recurrent VTE was prevented for every 13 patients treated with dalteparin. In terms of side effects, no difference in major or minor bleeding was detected between the groups, with 6% of dalteparin-treated patients and 4% of control patients having major bleeding episodes.

Malignant effusions

Malignant effusions can cause significant discomfort to the patient as well as increased morbidity. Potential anatomical sites (pericardium, pleural space, peritoneum) should be evaluated if the patient complains of chest pain, shortness of breath, cough, shoulder pain, nausea or abdominal distension, as removing the fluid can improve symptoms immediately. Unfortunately, malignant effusions portend a poor prognosis, but early treatment can improve survival and quality of life in many cases.

Pericardial effusion/pericardial tamponade

A malignant pericardial effusion develops in 5–15% of patients with cancer (typically leukaemias, lymphomas or breast cancer). This can be a true oncological emergency if tamponade physiology develops.

Presenting symptoms
- Dyspnoea, chest pain, cough, and/or
- Light headedness

Physical examination findings
- Distant heart sounds and jugular venous distension
- Pulsus paradoxus >10 mmHg

Diagnostics
- Widened mediastinum on chest X-ray
- Low voltage and/or electrical alternans on ECG
- Echocardiography, CT or MRI can confirm the diagnosis

Treatment
- Urgent drainage of the fluid through pericardiocentesis will relieve symptoms and tamponade physiology
- Pericardiodesis, placement of a surgical pericardial window or systemic chemotherapy may be used to prevent pericardial effusion reaccumulation

Pleural effusions

Malignant pleural effusions are common in advanced cancers. All new effusions should be sampled to exclude infection.

Presenting symptoms
- Dyspnoea, chest pain, cough, orthopnoea, hiccups

Physical examination findings
- Dullness in the lung bases on auscultation and percussion
- Crackles in the lung fields

Diagnostics
- Fluid in lung bases on chest X-ray
- May be better visualized on CT scan of the chest
- Lateral plain films may be beneficial to estimate the size of the effusion and to determine if it is free flowing
- Thoracentesis with standard studies, including cell count and differential, lactate dehydrogenase, glucose, protein, pH, Gram stain and culture, should be obtained
- Sample for cytology should also be sent, but a negative cytology does not exclude a malignant aetiology:
  - Only about one-third of malignant effusions will yield a positive cytology
- In general, an exudative effusion with negative cultures in a patient with known cancer is a malignant effusion until proven otherwise

Treatment
- Thoracentesis can be both diagnostic and therapeutic
- Controlling the underlying cancer with systemic therapy may reduce the risk of effusion recurrence
- Pleurodesis or chest tube placement can be helpful for recurrent pleural effusions

Malignant ascites

Malignant ascites are seen commonly in gynaecological cancers, gastrointestinal cancers and occasionally breast cancer. Many of these patients will have evidence for carcinomatosis on imaging or previous surgical staging.

Presenting symptoms
- Anorexia
- Dyspnoea with shallow breaths
- Nausea
- Sbdominal pain, abdominal distension, constipation/diarrhoea

Physical examination findings
- Abdominal distension
- Fluid wave
- Shifting dullness on percussion

Diagnostics
- Ultrasound, CT or MRI of the abdomen can confirm the presence of ascitic fluid
- Diagnostic paracentesis should be performed to rule out other aetiologies, with specimens sent for albumin, protein, cell count, culture and cytology
- Serum albumin should be used at the same time to calculate the serum ascites albumin gradient (SAAG): <1.1 g/dL indicates a non-portal hypertension-related aetiology
- Negative cytology does not rule out malignancy as the cause for the ascites

Treatment
- Therapeutic paracentesis to alleviate symptoms:
  - Repeat paracentesis is often necessary
  - Indwelling catheters are sometimes used in some patients for palliation
  - Unfortunately, frequent taps can result in peritonitis, protein depletion and electrolyte disturbances
- Systemic therapy may improve the rate of fluid reaccumulation
- Medical management with diuretics is typically unsuccessful as these patients typically have low serum oncotic pressure and are generally not volume overloaded
- Occasionally, intraperitoneal chemotherapy has been used with some limited success
- More rarely, peritoneal–venous shunting has been performed

Refractory nausea and vomiting

Patients consider chemotherapy- and radiotherapy-induced nausea and vomiting as among the most unpleasant of the acute side effects of their therapies. The significance of such symptoms should not be minimized. It is a tragic situation when a patient quits therapy due to inadequate supportive care. Patients sometimes develop anticipatory nausea and vomiting, which may require time-consuming interventions like hypnosis or behaviour modification and premedication with benzodiazepines. Overall, these symptoms can be so profound that discontinuation of cancer treatment is requested.

The development of new, more effective antiemetics has allowed oncologists to administer more chemotherapy in an outpatient setting than was previously possible. Antiserotonin agents (odansetron, granisetron, palonosetron, dolasetron) are typically the cornerstone of treatment and prevention. A newer compound, aprepitant, belongs to a class of drugs called substance P antagonists. It mediates its effect by blocking the neurokinin 1 (NK1) receptor. This drug is helpful for both acute and late nausea/vomiting. Other older and sometimes useful drugs include: tranquilizers (e.g. haloperidol), benzodiazepines (e.g. lorazepam), antihistamines (e.g. hydroxyzine), phenothiazines (e.g. prochlorperazine), corticosteroids (e.g. dexamethasone) and dopamine antagonists (e.g. metoclopramide). Rehydration of patients with nausea and vomiting is not only sound medical practice, but can help prevent post-therapy emetogenesis. When using highly emetogenic agents, the addition of steroids to an antiserotonin agent (and aprepitant if used) has been shown to have a potentiating effect.

Occasionally the symptoms of nausea and vomiting can be secondary to progressive cancer, with obstruction of a hollow viscous (bowel or ureteral obstruction, constipation), decreased bowel motility (from tense ascites or peritoneal carcinomatosis), metabolic disruption (hypercalcaemia) or CNS disease (brain metastasis). In these cases, antiemetics can help control symptoms, but the underlying aetiology should be corrected if possible.

Use of transfusions and cytokines

Anaemia
Anaemia is often a result of antineoplastic therapy, but factors such as chronic disease, blood loss with iron deficiency, and marrow replacement by tumour can be important factors as well. In general, patients should be considered for blood transfusions if symptomatic or if their haematocrit drops below 24% (haemoglobin <8 g/dL). Higher cut-off values should be allowed for patients with heart disease and/or pulmonary disease. The use of erythropoietin agents can decrease the need for blood transfusions in cancer patients if they develop chemotherapy-induced anaemia. However, recent data suggest these drugs may compromise survival. Thus, their use has sharply been reduced and should be restricted to patients receiving palliative therapy.

Thrombocytopenia
The pathophysiology of thrombocytopenia is similar to that of anaemia. Occasionally, it may be the result of thrombosis, DIC or splenic sequestration. In general, severe bleeding is uncommon if the patient's platelet count exceeds 20,000/mm^3, but easy bruising or petechiae can still be seen. The risk for severe bleeding (intracranial haemorrhage) increases dramatically once the platelet count falls below 10,000/mm^3, so empiric transfusions are recommended when the platelet count falls below 20,000/mm^3 Patients with uraemia, brain tumour or metastases, or uncontrolled hypertension may require prophylactic transfusions at a higher cut-off threshold. In addition, a threshold of at least 50,000/mm^3 is usually necessary for any surgical interventions and at least 100,000/mm^3 for neurosurgical or ophthalmological surgeries. New platelet growth factors are under development, but more studies are needed to determine their efficacy.

Neutropenia
Although the technology for white blood cell transfusion was developed long ago, it has limited practical use in neutropenic patients today. Thus, it is not considered standard practice. However, the use of granulocyte-colony stimulating factor (G-CSF) and granulocyte-macrophage colony stimulating factor (GM-CSF) have found a significant role in the prevention chemotherapy-induced neutropenia. They have been shown to decrease treatment-associated morbidity and are helpful in preventing the number of episodes of neutropenic fevers and infections. In chemotherapy regimens with a high risk of neutropenia (>20%), prophylactic CSFs are appropriate and supported by high levels of evidence, especially in the adjuvant and curative setting. In a high-risk patient with documented febrile neutropenia in the past, CSF use should be considered.

Conclusion

Complications of cancer and its associated therapies can present in numerous ways to any physician in practice today. Given that these presentations can be the first sign of a malignancy, all physicians (not just oncologists) should be aware of how to manage these life-threatening problems. Prompt recognition and treatment cannot be overemphasized, as delay in therapy can result in significant morbidity and mortality. Oncological emergencies are also often a sign of progression of the patient's cancer. These situations can thus also be emotionally stressful for patients and their families. The physician's approach to patient care therefore needs to be thoughtful, compassionate and individualized, not only to the patient's histological disease type and stage, but also according to the patient's preferences, comfort and emotional well-being.

Recommended reading

Altman A (2001) Acute tumor lysis syndrome. *Semin Oncol* 28(2 Suppl 5):3.

Chao B, Lepeak L, Leal T, Robins I (2011) Clinical use of the low molecular weight heparins in cancer patients – focus on the improved patient outcomes. *Thrombosis* 2011:530183.

Ellison DH, Berl T (2007) Syndrome of inappropriate antidiuresis. *N Engl J Med* 366:2064–2072.

Freifeld AG, Bow EJ, Sepkowitz KA *et al.* clinical practice guideline for the use of antimicrobial agents in neutropenic patients with cancer: 2010 Update by the Infectious Disease Society of America." *Clin Infect Dis* 52:e56–e93

Galter-Gvilli A, Fraser A, Paul M, Leibovici L (2005) Meta-analysis: antibiotic prophylaxis reduces mortality in neutropenic patients. *Ann Intern Med* 142:979.

Hirsh J, Bauer KA, Donati MB *et al.* (2008) Parenteral anticoagulants: American College of Chest Physicians Evidence-Based Clinical Practice Guidelines, 8th edn). *Chest* 133(6 Suppl):141S–59S.

Klastersky J, Paesmans M, Rubenstein EB *et al.* (2000) The Multinational Association for Supportive Care in Cancer risk index: a multinational scoring system for identifying low-risk febrile neutropenic cancer patients. *J Clin Oncol* 18:3038–3051.

Lee Y, Levine MN, Baker RI *et al.* (2003) Low-molecular-weight heparin versus a coumarin for the prevention of recurrent venous thromboembolism in patients with cancer. *N Engl J Med* 349:146–153.

Levack P, Graham], Collie D *et al.* (2002) Don't wait for a sensory level- listen to the symptoms: a prospective audit of the delays in diagnosis of malignant cord compression. *Clin Oncol* 14:472.

Lyman GH, Khorana AA, Falanga A *et al.* (2007) American Society of Clinical Oncology guideline: recommendations for venous thromboembolism prophylaxis and treatment in patients with cancer. *J Clin Oncol* 25:5490–5505.

National Comprehensive Cancer Network Clinical Practice Guidelines in Oncology. Myeloid growth factors (v.l.2012). Available at http://www.nccn.org/professionals/physician_gls/PDF/myeloid_growth.pdf [accessed 29 January 2013].

National Comprehensive Cancer Network Clinical Practice Guidelines in Oncology. Prevention and treatment of cancer-related infections (version 1.2012). Available at http://www.nccn.org/professionals/physician_gls/PDF/infections.pdf [Accessed 28 January 2013].

Patchel RA, Tibbs PA, Regine WF *et al.* (2005) Direct decompressive surgical resection in the treatment of spinal cord compression caused by metastatic cancer: a randomized trial. *Lancet* 36:2436–2448.

Sung L, Nathan PC, Alibhai SM, Tomlinson GA, Beyene J (2007) Meta-analysis: effect of prophylactic hematopoietic colony-stimulating factors on mortality and outcomes of infection. *Ann Intern Med* 147:400–411.

Walji N, Chan AK, Peake DR. (2008) Common acute oncological emergencies: diagnosis, investigation, and management. *Postgrad Med J* 84:418–427.

Wilson LD, Detterbeck Fe, Yahalom J (2007) Superior vena cava syndrome with malignant causes. *N Engl Med* 356:1862.

15 Supportive care during curative treatment

Susan Urba[1], Suzette Walker[1], Danielle Karsies[1], Dawna Allore[1], Claire Casselman[2] and Maria Almond[2]

[1]Symptom Management and Supportive Care Program, University of Michigan Comprehensive Cancer Center, Ann Arbor, MI, USA
[2]PsychOncology Clinic, University of Michigan, Ann Arbor, MI, USA

Introduction

The National Cancer Institute in the USA describes 'supportive care' as the care given to improve the quality of life of patients who have a serious or life-threatening disease. The goal of supportive care is to prevent or treat as early as possible the symptoms of a disease, side effects caused by treatment, and psychological, social and spiritual problems related to the disease or its treatment. Many patients who go through chemotherapy, radiation and/or surgery for potentially curative treatment of their cancer may endure frequent and severe toxicities and stress during this period of time. It is incumbent upon the clinician treating the patient to provide proficient support of the patient to maximize quality of life. Some of the most frequent issues encountered are fatigue, diarrhoea, constipation, nausea, pain and psychological distress.

Fatigue

Fatigue is one of the most common symptoms reported in cancer patients. Almost 100% of patients will report fatigue throughout the cancer trajectory. Cancer-related fatigue is distressing and affects the physical, psychosocial and economic status of patients and their caregivers. Fatigue affects the patient's social activities, cognitive performance, relationships, employment and overall sense of well-being. Fatigue affects every component of a patient's life.

Cancer-related fatigue has been formally defined by the National Comprehensive Cancer Network (NCCN) as a distressing, persistent, subjective sense of physical, emotional and/or cognitive tiredness or exhaustion related to cancer or cancer treatment that is not proportional to recent activity and interferes with usual functioning.

Screening and assessment

Fatigue assessment and management should be included in clinical health outcome studies as well as in quality improvement projects. Fatigue is rarely an isolated symptom and often occurs with other issues such as pain and sleep disturbances.

- *Screening*:
  - Initial visit
  - Regular intervals during treatment and following treatment
  - As clinically indicated
  - Screen every patient for fatigue as a vital sign
  - Severity 0–10 scale: (0 = no fatigue, 10 = worst fatigue imaginable), or descriptors (none, mild, moderate, severe)
- *Focused history*:
  - Disease status (rule out recurrence or progression)
  - Review of systems:
    - Onset, pattern, duration
    - Change over time
    - Associated or alleviating factors
    - Interference with function (how is fatigue interfering with your ability to function?)
    - Associated distress
  - Social support status/availability of caregivers
- *Assessment of treatable conditions* that may contribute to fatigue:
  - Medications/side effects
  - Pain
  - Emotional distress (depression, anxiety)
  - Anaemia
  - Sleep disturbances
  - Nutritional deficits (weight loss, dehydration, electrolyte imbalance)
  - Decreased performance status (decreased physical activity)

- Co-morbidities:
  - Alcohol/substance abuse
  - Cardiac dysfunction
  - Pulmonary dysfunction
  - Pulmonary embolism
  - Endocrine dysfunction (hot flushes, thyroid deficiency, adrenal insufficiency, hypogonadism)
  - Gastrointestinal dysfunction
  - Liver dysfunction
  - Infection
  - Neurological dysfunction
  - Renal dysfunction

Treatment
Underlying causes should be corrected if possible.

Anaemia
Check complete blood count (CBC) and iron studies.
- If anaemia is related to low iron intake, increase iron-rich foods such as leafy greens, dried beans such as lima beans and green peas, dried apricots and figs, prunes, nuts and seeds, and iron-fortified foods such as cereals, bread and pasta
- If anaemia is related to disease or treatment, encourage adequate nutrition to support weight maintenance
- Oral or intravenous (IV) iron supplementation. Recheck labs in recommended time frame
- Transfusion:
  - Recheck labs in recommended time frame
  - Educate patient/family on signs and symptoms of low haemoglobin

Electrolyte depletion
Check full profile including potassium, magnesium, calcium and vitamin D.
- Replete as needed
- Vitamin D: check 25-hydroxyvitamin D level:
  - <30 ng/dL: ergocalciferol 50,000 units every week for 8 weeks
  - <15 ng/dLl: ergocalciferol 50,000 units twice a week for 8 weeks
- Recheck labs in recommended time frame

Endocrine disorders
Check for low testosterone and abnormal thyroid function, and consider a cortrosyn stimulation test if appropriate.
- Replace as necessary
- If patient has low testosterone and replacement is necessary, educate patient on medication, side effects and precautions for family members
- Follow-up with patient to see if improvement of symptoms has occurred 1–2 weeks after medication therapy has started:
  - Recheck labs in recommended time frame

Depression
- Psycho/social intervention:
  - Evaluate to determine if depression predates cancer diagnosis and if interventions have been used in the past
  - What was successful?
- Antidepressant therapy:
  - Citalopram: 10–20 mg/day; also helps with anxiety
  - Fluoxetine: 20 mg, up to 60 mg/day
  - Mirtazapine: also may stimulate appetite and help with sleep
  - Bupropion: stimulating effect, less interference with sexual function
- Increase physical activity:
  - Give handouts on walking, stretching and ambulation exercises for patients to start at home

Weight loss and dehydration
- Consider an *appetite stimulant*:
  - Megestrol acetate suspension: 800 mg/day orally
  - Mirtazapine: 15 mg orally at night
  - Dronabinol: 2.5–5 mg orally t.i.d..
- *Diet*:
  - Encourage patients to eat regular meals:
    - Meal skipping can result in low blood glucose levels
  - Counsel the patient to eat at set times during the day and not to wait until they feel hungry or have a desire to eat:
    - Smaller, more frequent meals may be easier to cope with
  - Encourage complex carbohydrates as tolerated for steadier blood glucose levels
  - Ensure the patient is consuming adequate protein to support preservation of lean body mass:
    - Patients undergoing treatment may need up to 1.2–1.5 g of protein/kg/day or more
  - Check for vitamin and mineral deficiencies and treat accordingly:
    - Prescribe a general multivitamin with minerals daily if the patient has a poor diet
- *Hydration*:
  - Decreased blood volume from dehydration requires the heart to pump harder, which can contribute to fatigue
  - Review fluid intake for adequacy (30–35 mL/kg/day) and counsel patients to increase fluid intake as indicated

Strategies for sleep
- Patients and families should be taught to decrease activity close to bed time
- Set a standard time to go to bed and a standard time for awakening
- Avoid long afternoon naps
- Avoid afternoon caffeine
- Make the bedroom quiet and dark
- Combine sleep hygiene with a complimentary therapy such as breathing control, guided imagery or music therapy
- Sleep aids such as diphenhydramine 50 mg orally or zolpidem 5–10 mg orally may be helpful

- Obtain history if insomnia predates cancer diagnosis:
  - Evaluate what strategies the patient has used in the past
- Has patient had a sleep study?:
  - If not, consider ordering one
  - If the patient has had a sleep study, is he/she following the recommended plan of care, such as use of a continuous positive airway pressure (CPAP) machine?

Exercise

Exercise has been shown to decrease fatigue in patients. Many studies in the breast cancer population have demonstrated that patients who exercise on a routine basis have lower fatigue scores then those who do not exercise.
- Referral to physical therapy
- Exercise: 40–50% of cancer patients who exercised regularly during and after treatment had less fatigue and depression, and slept better:
  - Most research on cancer-related fatigue and exercise is in patients with breast and prostate cancer
    - A 2012 meta-analysis of 56 articles showed a positive association between aerobic exercise and relief of fatigue
    - Duration, intensity and frequency varied significantly
    - One study in patients with pancreatic cancer also showed positive effects from aerobic exercise
  - Resistance training is a form of exercise in which muscles contract against external resistance, such as lifting weights:
    - This type of exercise should not be discounted just because research in this area is more limited.
    - Movement of any kind (aerobic, resistance or combination) and for any duration based on patient's ability likely will aid in cancer-related fatigue
  - Extended periods of sedentary behaviour should be avoided:
    - Patient should get up and/or be moving every 2 hours
    - Recommendations should be adjusted based on patient abilities, e.g. a bed-bound patient should try to sit up for 10 minutes every 2 hours, whereas a more mobile patient should take short walks to the kitchen, postbox or longer distances as tolerated every 2 hours

Energy conservation

Energy conservation is defined as the deliberate, planned management of personal energy resources to prevent depletion.
- Alternate periods of rest and planned activity
- Plan activities

Heart and pulmonary issues
- If there are known cardiac and pulmonary issues, optimize medications
- Shortness of breath can be confused with fatigue:
  - Monitor for pulmonary embolism
  - Monitor oxygen level and give oxygen as needed
  - An albuterol inhaler is useful for shortness of breath

Medication management
- Discontinue any non-essential medications
- Methylphenidate 5–10 mg orally up to t.i.d.
- Medication review

Diarrhoea

Diarrhoea may be acute or chronic. It is described as loose and watery bowel movements. Most people experience diarrhoea at least two times a year. Often diarrhoea can be treated with over-the-counter medications. Diarrhoea can lead to dehydration, hypotension, weakness, electrolyte depletion, acute renal failure or, in extreme cases, cardiac arrhythmias, even resulting in death.

Diarrhoea can be classified as:
- *Osmotic diarrhoea* (water is drawn from the body into the bowel)
  - Malabsorption syndromes
  - Maldigestion syndromes
- *Secretory diarrhoea*:
  - Infections
  - Medications
  - Cancer
- *Exudative diarrhoea* (blood or pus in the stool):
  - Inflammatory bowel disease such as Crohn or ulcerative colitis or infections
  - Previous radiation

Common causes of diarrhoea include:
- Infection (bacterial and or viral)
- Foods (see Table 15.2)
- Allergies
- Medications
- Radiation and chemotherapy
- Diseases such as Crohn, inflammatory bowel disease (IBS), ulcerative colitis
- Malabsorption and pancreatic exocrine insufficiency
- Hyperthyroidism
- Alcohol abuse
- Diabetes
- Digestive tract surgery

Assessment
This is described in Table 15.1.

Treatment
Goals of therapy
- Prevent diarrhoea
- Enhance recovery of intestinal mucosa
- Restore normal bowel function
- Maintain nutrition and fluid status
- Correct electrolytes
- Protect skin integrity

Table 15.1 Diarrhoea assessment

Complete history
- Onset
- History of irritable bowel syndrome or other gastrointestinal diagnosis
- Symptoms: abdominal cramps, pain, fever, stool incontinence, nausea/vomiting
- Anyone else in the household with same symptoms?
- Number of stools in 24 hours
- Colour and consistency of stools
- Diet
- Medications
- Treatments including past surgery

Physical exam
- Vital signs including weight

Laboratory studies
- Complete blood count
- Chemistries
- Stool samples
- *Clostridium difficile*
- Ova and parasites
- Bacteria
- Fungus

Box 15.1 Oral rehydration recipe

½ teaspoon of table salt
½ teaspoon of potassium chloride
8 teaspoons (2 tablespoon + 2 teaspoons) of granulated sugar
½ teaspoon of sodium bicarbonate (baking soda)
1 L of water (4 ½ cups)
Combine and stir until well mixed and dissolved
Mix with juice for taste

Nutritional management of diarrhoea
- For patients with chronic diarrhoea, schedule antidiarrhoea medications before all meals
- Consider use of oral rehydration solution such as Pedialyte®, Ceralyte® or homemade oral rehydration recipe (Box 15.1)
- Smaller more frequent meals (5–6 mini-meals/day) are recommended
- Patients with severe malabsorption may need significantly higher intake of calories and protein, as well as vitamin and mineral supplementation:
  - Water-soluble vitamins A, D, E and K may be beneficial if fat malabsorption is suspected
- Avoid blanket dietary restrictions as these can further contribute to malnutrition:
- Patient should keep a food diary to record symptoms or should trial removal of the 'foods to avoid' listed in Table 15.2 one at a time to test for effect, while including more foods from the 'foods to include' listed in Table 15.2

Non-pharmacological management of diarrhoea
- Discontinue all medications that may contribute to diarrhoea if medically possible:
  - Antihypertensives
  - Retrovirals
  - Cholinergic agents
  - Laxatives
  - Magnesium-containing agents
  - Non-steroidal anti-inflammatory drugs (NSAIDs)
  - Medications containing sorbital/mannitol (sugar alcohols)
  - Caffeine-containing medications
- Clean the perianal area frequently to prevent skin breakdown and apply skin protectant after passage of each stool

Pharmacological management of diarrhoea
- Hydrate if needed
- Replace electrolytes as needed (Table 15.3)
- Treat as needed for infectious diarrhoea
- Replace pancreatic enzyme as needed
- Psyllium, guar gum or inulin fibre supplements:
  - Encourage 8 oz of fluid with each dose
- Probiotic rich foods or supplements

Table 15.2 Diarrhoea: Foods to avoid and include

Foods to avoid		Foods to include	
Insoluble fibre	Whole grain breads and cereals, brown rice, wild rice, nuts, seeds, beans, lentils	Soluble fibre	Banana, oatmeal, white rice, white toast, mashed potatoes
Fatty or greasy foods	Fried foods, bacon, sausage, doughnuts, rich desserts and gravies	Potassium- and sodium-rich foods	Broth-based soups, pretzels, saltines, canned apricots, bananas, fruit nectars, sports drinks
Caffeine	Dark colas, coffee, tea, chocolate, energy drinks	Probiotics	Yoghurt, kefir, miso, tempeh
Sugar-free foods (sugar alcohols)	Sugar-free puddings, cookies, gelatine, gum	Dry, salty foods	Saltines or other crackers, toast
Lactose-containing foods	Only avoid if intake of dairy results in increased diarrhoea	Fluids	Drink at least eight cups per day plus one cup of fluid for each loose stool. Avoid large amounts at one time and fluids at room temperature may be better tolerated

Table 15.3 Electrolyte replacement

	Clinical levels	IV replacement dosing[a,b]	Rate of infusion
Hypophosphataemia	2.3–2.7 mg/dL	0.08–0.16 mmol/kg	
	1.5–2.2 mg/dL	0.16–0.32 mmol/kg	
	<1.5 mg/dL	0.32–0.64 mmol/kg	
Hypokalaemia	2.5–3.4 mEq/L, asymptomatic	20–40 mEq	10–20 mEq of K$^+$/h; maximum of 40 mEq of K$^+$/h
	<2.5 mEq/L	40–80 mEq	
Hypomagnesaemia	1–1.5 mg/dL	1–4 g of magnesium sulphate (8–32 mEq), up to 1 mEq/kg	
	<1 mg/dL	4–8 g of magnesium sulphate (32–64 mEq), up to 1.5 mEq/kg	

[a]In patients with normal renal function.
[b]Adjusted body weight is suggested in patients who are significantly obese.

- Prostaglandin inhibitor/serotonin antagonist:
  - Bismuth subsalicylate 15–30 mL every 6 hours
  - Octreotide subcutaneously
  - Cyproheptadine 4 mg tablets t.i.d. to q.i.d.
  - Mesalamine (ulcerative colitis)
- Adsorbent:
  - Kaolin/pectin suspension 30–60 mL every 4 hours
- Bile acid sequestrate:
  - Cholestyramine powder 4–12 g t.i.d.
- Opioid agonist:
  - Codeine 15–60 mg every 4–6 hours
  - Diphenoxylate/atropine 2.5–5 mg every 4–6 hours
  - Loperamide 2–4 mg every 4–6 hours
  - Opium tincture 0.6–1.2 mL every 4–6 hours
- Pancreatic enzyme:
  - Lipase 45,000 units, protease 25,000 units, amylase 20,000 units, one to six capsules with each meal and snack

Table 15.4 Patient education for diarrhoea

Signs and symptoms	Action
Grossly bloody stool Severe lethargy or weakness Signs of dehydration: decreased urine output, sunken eyes, pinched skin does not spring back	Seek emergency care
Excessive thirst and dry mouth Persistent fever Diarrhoea for >2 days 5–7 stools in 24 hours with severe cramps	Seek urgent care within 24 hours
Chronic diarrhoea Recent travel to a foreign country New prescription	Notify healthcare provider

Patient education

Patient education for diarrhoea is described in Table 15.4.

Constipation

Constipation can be a troubling symptom for patients. It occurs in approximately 50% of patients and 85% of patients treated with opioids. Constipation is defined as either reduced frequency or increased difficulty of defaecation. Frequency of defaecation varies among individuals, with a range of three times a day to three times a week. Constipation is often associated with other symptoms such as abdominal pain, bloating, flatulence, malaise and nausea. In severe cases, vomiting may result.

All patients should be monitored for alteration in bowel habit at each clinical encounter. If constipation is present, the cause and severity should be assessed. The patient should be examined to rule out impaction and obstruction. Treatable causes should be identified and treated. Common causes are:
- Drug induced
- Hypercalcaemia
- Hypokalaemia
- Hypothyroidism
- Diabetes
- Gastroparesis
- Dehydration
- Anorexia
- Decreased physical activity
- Depression
- Tumour in the bowel wall or compressing the bowel
  Several drugs classes can cause constipation:
- Opioids
- Antidepressants

Table 15.5 Constipation assessment

History and physical exam
- Date of last bowel movement
- Stool size, colour, consistency, difficult to pass
- Has patient had diarrhoea recently?
- Flatulence
- What has patient tried for relief?
- Abdominal X-ray if needed
- Medication review

Laboratory test
- Chemistries
- Complete blood count
- Thyroid function
- Assess for dehydration
- Assess for depression

- Antispasmodics
- Phenothiazines
- Antiemetics
- Antacids
- Diuretics
- Iron supplements

Assessment

This is described in Table 15.5.
- Evaluate for obstruction:
  - Clinical exam
  - Abdominal X-ray
- If the patient is impacted consider:
  - Glycerine suppository and/or
  - Mineral oil retention enema
  - Perform manual disimpaction if needed

Treatment

The treatment of constipation should include the implementation of preventive measures with the start of opioids. Treatment focuses on increasing fluids, dietary management and physical activity.

Non-pharmacological management of constipation

- *Diet*:
  - Promote adequate fluid intake (30–35 mL/kg/day):
    - Hot liquids may be beneficial
  - Encourage regular meals and snacks to increase episodes of peristalsis to promote gut motility
  - Addition of soluble fibre such as oatmeal, apple sauce, bananas, lentils, pears and white rice
  - Addition of insoluble fibre such as whole wheat and bran, nuts, seeds, fruit and vegetables:
    - Avoid these foods if symptoms of gas, nausea or history of bowel obstructions noted

Box 15.2 Fruit paste recipe

Recipe yields 16: 1-tbsp servings
Calories per serving: 10
⅓ cup of bran
⅓ cup of apple sauce
⅓ cup of mashed stewed prunes

- 1–2 tablespoons of fruit paste recipe before bed followed by 8 oz of water (Box 15.2)
- *Physical activity*:
  - Activity recommendations must be tailored to the individual's physical abilities and health condition
  - Regular physical activity per patient tolerances:
    - Avoid >2 hours of sedentary behaviour, encourage sitting up or additional movement every 2 hours if possible
    - Walking for 15–20 minutes once or twice a day.
- *Toileting*:
  - Ignoring or suppressing the urge to have a bowel movement contributes to constipation:
    - Establishing a routine toileting regimen is helpful
    - Toileting for 5–15 minutes after meals, especially after breakfast

Pharmacological management of constipation

Pharmacological therapy is indicated if symptoms of constipation do not resolve with lifestyle changes. Selection of an agent should be based on the characteristics of the patient, such as contraindications to a specific class, previous laxative use and personal preference. In a randomized study of a laxative combined with a stool softener there was no added benefit from the addition of a stool softener. The pharmacological agents used can be classified into several categories. The goal of treatment is to return the patient to normal bowel function, and for the patient to have at least one bowel movement every 24–48 hours. Care must be taken in patients who take opioids for the abdominal pain often associated with constipation.

- Bulk-forming laxatives (must be taken with plenty of water):
  - Citrucel
  - Fibercon
  - Metamucil
- Emollients:
  - Docusate sodium
- Lubricants:
  - Mineral oil
- Osmotic laxatives:
  - Lactulose (titrate to desired results)
  - Polyethylene glycol
- Stimulants:
  - Senna (up to 8 tablets a day)
  - Bisacodyl (10–15 mg as needed to reach goal)

Table 15.6 Patient education for constipation

Signs and symptoms	Action
Severe abdominal pain, swelling, or vomiting Vomiting brown, yellow or green emesis Rectal bleeding with no history of haemorrhoids or bleeding with constipation	Seek emergency care
No bowel movement in 5–7 days Fever of unknown origin for 24–48 hours Inability to pass gas	Seek urgent care within 24 hours
Dry hard stools Pain with bowel movement	Notify healthcare provider

- Chloride-channel stimulators:
  - Lubiprostone
- Metoclopramide 10 mg orally t.i.d
- Methylnatrexone can be considered in severe opioid-induced constipation

Patient education

Patient education for constipation is described in Table 15.6.

Nausea

Nausea and vomiting is a common side effect of patients who are undergoing chemotherapy or radiation therapy for their cancer treatment. Luckily, today there are numerous categories of medications available to attenuate that feared side effect, and several sets of guidelines to assist the clinician with decision-making. The three sets of antiemetic guidelines probably most widely used worldwide are those from the Multinational Association of Supportive Care in Cancer (MASCC), the National Comprehensive Cancer Network (NCCN) in the USA and the American Society of Clinical Oncology (ASCO). The guidelines are readily available online from those organizations, and while there are some small differences in the recommendations, they are remarkably similar in their general principles. The major take-home points are briefly summarized here. For specific information regarding the names of the agents and dosing, the full set of guidelines should be referred to.

Pharmacological management of nausea

Antiemetic therapy for chemotherapy should be administered prophylactically and in most cases, coverage should be continued for 2–4 days afterwards to prevent delayed nausea and emesis. While there are risk factors for nausea associated with the patient (female gender, low alcohol consumption, age <50 years), the major risk is the emetogenicity of the chemotherapy agent itself.
- *Highly emetogenic chemotherapy* requires a three-drug regimen:
  - Serotonin receptor antagonist
  - Neurokinin 1 (NK1) receptor antagonist
  - Corticosteroid
- *Moderately emetogenic chemotherapy*:
  - Serotonin receptor antagonist
  - Corticosteroid
  - ± NK1 receptor antagonist
- *Low emetogenic chemotherapy*:
  - Single-agent coverage:
    - Corticosteroid
    - Prochlorperazine
    - Dopamine receptor antagonist
    - Serotonin receptor antagonist.
- Minimal emetogenic chemotherapy:
  - No routine prophylaxis

Despite receiving treatment, according to antiemetic guidelines, some patients have persistent nausea that can greatly impact their quality of life.
- The first step a clinician should take is to review the antiemetics that were prescribed, and to make sure that they were administered or taken correctly.
  - Do the antiemetics written on the chemotherapy orders include all the appropriate classes of medication?
    - In recent years, many institutions have initiated standard preprinted orders to be used for the various levels of emetogenicity (high, moderate and low), and this helps to limits errors or omissions on a daily basis
  - If the chemotherapy had moderate emetogenicity, was an NK1 receptor antagonist given?
    - If not, it should be added to the next cycle of chemotherapy
  - Was a corticosteroid given?
    - In one survey to determine the most common deviation from national antiemetic guidelines, the most frequent error was the omission of corticosteroids from the regimen
  - If any of the medications were given orally, did the patient file the prescription and actually take the medication?
    - Poor insurance coverage and the high cost of the medications may preclude a patient from actually filing the prescription.
    - The patient may have misunderstood that the medication should be taken prophylactically at home for 3 days following the chemotherapy to avoid delayed nausea
    - Patients often decide that if they do not have nausea, they do not need to take the medication
    - However, if nausea then occurs, it may be more difficult control it
    - Prevention is typically easier than treatment
- If the medications were correctly ordered and taken, but the patient still suffers nausea, then additional interventions are needed:
  - Medication from another category of antiemetic agents not already administered should be considered (to be added to the current regimen). Examples include:
    - Benzodiazepines
    - Cannabinoids
    - Phenothiazine
    - Dopamine antagonists

Table 15.7 Foods to eat or avoid during nausea

	Recommended foods	Foods that may cause distress
High-protein group	Broiled or baked meat, fish and poultry; cold meat or tuna fish salad; eggs; cream soups made with low-fat milk; lean meats; non-fat yoghurt; skimmed or low-fat milk, mild cheese	Fatty and fried meats; fried eggs; sausage, bacon, milkshakes (unless made with low-fat milk and reduced fat ice cream or frozen yoghurt)
Breads, cereals and rice	Saltines, soda crackers, bread, toast, cold cereal, English muffins, bagels, plain noodles, rice, low-fat or baked corn and potato chips, pretzels, unbuttered popcorn, dry cereals	Doughnuts, pastries, waffles, pancakes, muffins, regular potato chips, French fries, hash browns
Fruits and vegetables	Potatoes (baked, boiled, or mashed), juices, canned or fresh fruits, vegetables if tolerated	Breaded, fried or creamed vegetables, or vegetables with a strong odour, such as broccoli or cauliflower
Beverages, desserts and snacks	Cold fruit-ades, decaffeinated sodas and iced teas, sports drinks, sherbet, fruit-flavoured gelatine, angel food cake, sponge cake, vanilla wafers, pudding made with low-fat milk, popsicles, juice bars, fruit ice, butter or margarine in small amounts, fat-skimmed gravy, salt, cinnamon, spices as tolerated	Alcohol, coffee, pies, ice cream, rich cakes, spicy salad dressings, olives, cream, pepper, chili powder, onion, hot sauce, some seasoning mixtures

Nutritional management of nausea

- Encourage ginger ales, teas, candies or fresh ginger root or consider use of medicinal ginger (0.75 g daily)
- Encourage patients to consume protein-rich foods (eggs, dairy, meat or poultry) with each meal or snack:
  - Some research has shown that a higher protein diet can aid the management of delayed nausea
- Recommend small, frequent meals (five to six meals/day) to aid digestion
- Drink liquids between meals:
  - Avoid large amounts at one time and drink slowly but constantly throughout the day
- Remain upright after meals:
  - Avoid reclining or lying down within 1 hour of eating
- If nausea is triggered by aromas, choose room temperature or cold foods such as cottage cheese, cold sandwiches and yoghurt:
  - Have others cook
- Foods to eat or avoid during nausea are listed in Table 15.7.

Pain (see also Chapter 16)

Pain is a major problem for patients with cancer undergoing therapy. Approximately two-thirds of patients with advanced or metastatic cancer will report pain, and approximately one-third of them will rate it as moderate or severe. The pain may be a result of the cancer itself, or a side effect of the chemotherapy, radiation or surgery used in treatment. It may be acute in duration, occurring primarily during the period of the treatment, or it may be a long-lasting sequela.

In the 1960s, Dame Cicely Saunders introduced the concept of 'total' pain often experienced by cancer patients:
- Physical pain
- Spiritual pain
- Emotional pain
- Social or interpersonal pain

While this section will focus primarily on physical pain, it is crucial for health practitioners to keep in mind the complex interplay of physical and non-physical factors that may affect a patient's experience of pain and response to its treatment.

Assessment of pain

The key to accurate assessment of pain is to ask about it at every patient visit. If the patient has no pain, then the clinician can move on to other enquiries. However, if the patient does have pain, it needs to be assessed both quantitatively and qualitatively.
- Quantitative pain intensity:
  - Visual analogue scale for adults:
    - Simple assessment tool consisting of a 10-cm line with 0 at one end, representing no pain, and 10 at the other end, representing the worst pain ever experienced
  - Visual analogue scale for children:
    - Most typical type of assessment scale for children includes a series of faces that range from smiling (no pain) to crying (severe pain)
- Qualitative pain assessment: descriptors of pain are extremely important, primarily because of the need to differentiate nociceptive pain from neuropathic pain, which can lead to different treatment decisions:
  - *Nociceptive pain* (typical descriptors):
    - Aching
    - Throbbing
    - Stabbing
    - Pressure
  - *Neuropathic pain* (typical descriptors)
    - Burning
    - Tingling

- Shooting
- Electrical sensation
- Hot/cold

Pain syndromes
- *Radiation-induced pain*:
  - Head and neck cancer: oral mucositis, resulting in impaired eating
  - Oesophageal cancer: oesophagitis, resulting in impaired eating
  - Abdominal radiation: abdominal pain and cramping, often with diarrhoea
  - Rectal cancer: proctitis, leading to painful defaecation
  - Skin breakdown: a site of intense radiation can react like a burn, with skin breakdown and oozing, tenderness and burning
- *Chemotherapy-induced pain*:
  - Oral mucositis
  - Neuropathy
  - Cold intolerance
  - Tumour pain
  - Pain at the site of the intravenous catheter if extravasation occurs
- *Surgery-induced pain*:
  - Acute postoperative wound healing
  - Long-term scar formation, particularly in the abdomen
  - Neuropathy at site of surgical incision

Treatment of pain
For the most part, many clinicians follow the general approach described by the World Health Organization (WHO): the three-step analgesic Ladder.
- Non-opioids:
  - Acetaminophen
  - Anti-inflammatory medications
  - Medications should be taken on a scheduled basis, *around the clock*, for best efficacy (check anamnesis)
- Opioids for mild-to-moderate pain
- Opioids for moderate-to-severe pain

Patients may have already tried non-opioids before they even start reporting their pain to their doctor. If so, it should be determined if those medications were taken routinely around the clock. If they were, cancer pain uncontrolled with non-opioids requires the initiation of opioid analgesics.

Opioids for mild-to-moderate pain
- Hydrocodone/acetaminophen combinations:
  - Maximal total dose of acetaminophen should ideally be limited to 3000 mg/day
  - It is important to take a thorough medication history because patients frequently take a hydrocodone/acetaminophen product for pain, as well as over-the-counter supplemental acetaminophen tablets without realizing that they are inadvertently doubling the dosage and increasing their risk for liver toxicity
- Codeine:
  - Available as a single agent, which is most commonly used for coughs:
    - More commonly prescribed in combination with acetaminophen.
- Tramadol:
  - A centrally-acting opioid analgesic, which is also a weak inhibitor of reuptake of norepinephrine and serotonin
  - Indicated for moderate-to-moderately severe chronic pain
- Tapentadol:
  - A centrally-acting analgesic that is a mu-opioid receptor agonist and a norepinephrine reuptake inhibitor
  - Indicated for moderate-to-severe chronic pain and neuropathic pain associated with diabetic peripheral neuropathy:
    - Anecdotally, some practitioners have also used it for patients with peripheral neuropathy associated with chemotherapy, with some success.

Opioids for moderate-to-severe pain
- Morphine:
  - Mainstay of the treatment of most cancer pain, because it is often readily available, cheaper than the other opioid medications and available in multiple forms:
    - Oral tablets, both short- and long-acting
    - Oral liquid formulation for those who cannot swallow tablets; concentrations vary from 1 to 20 mg/mL; higher concentrations for those who need a relatively high dose but cannot swallow a large volume
    - Parenteral formulation which can be given IV, subcutaneously or infused into the epidural or intrathecal space
- Oxycodone:
  - Similar efficacy to morphine, with immediate-release and extended-release tablets available
  - Does not have an IV form and, while an oral liquid formulation exists, it is not readily available at many pharmacies
- Fentanyl:
  - One of the few medications available as a transdermal patch, which gives it an advantage for use in the following patients with:
    - Tumours involving the head and neck or oesophagus, which thus interfere with swallowing tablets
    - Painful mucositis from chemotherapy or radiation
    - Severe nausea during chemotherapy who cannot reliably keep down their pain medications
    - Poor compliance for taking their medications
  - Relatively expensive and some insurance companies require that the patient try oral, less expensive formulations first
- Methadone:
  - Relatively available and inexpensive:
    - Long half-life means it is more difficult to use in elderly patients who may have some renal insufficiency

Treatment of neuropathic pain

In 2011, the International Association for the Study of Pain undertook a systematic review of 22 studies that included 13,683 patients with active cancer who reported pain. It calculated the prevalence of patients with neuropathic pain to be as high as 39%. This determination is important because neuropathic pain requires specific prescribing strategies, in addition to or instead of opioids. Even when patients have completed their anticancer treatment and are considered to be cured, some continue a long battle with residual side effects, such as persistent neuropathic pain from some of the commonly used chemotherapy agents. Because many of these patients have a long projected survival, they require ongoing supportive care and medication adjustments to try to minimize pain and maximize function. Patients may complain of numbness or burning pain, or both. The numbness is typically not very responsive to medications, but may gradually partially resolve the longer the time from chemotherapy. Medication may help the pain, but the patient should be advised that the medications are usually started low and slowly titrated upward over a period of weeks. Therefore, maximal relief may take some time to achieve.

- *Anticonvulsants*:
    - Gabapentin:
        - Official indications are for post-herpetic neuralgia and seizures
        - One of the most commonly used medications for neuropathy associated with cancer and its treatment
        - Wide range of dosing, starting at 100 mg t.i.d. up to 1200 mg t.i.d.; patients often experience relief of the pain at medium doses (300–600 mg t.i.d.)
        - Can be used in combination with tricyclic antidepressants. One study compared single-agent gabapentin to single-agent nortriptyline, and to the two agents in combination. Both single drugs resulted in some pain relief, but the pain with the combination treatment was significantly lower than with either agent alone
    - Pregabalin: official indications are:
        - Neuropathic pain associated with diabetic peripheral neuropathy or spinal cord injury
        - Postherpetic neuralgia
        - Fibromyalgia
        - Adjunct therapy for partial-onset seizures
    - Carbamazepine:
        - Indicated for trigeminal neuralgia
        - Some small studies suggest it may be useful for neuropathic pain
- *Antidepressants*:
    - Tricyclic antidepressants:
        - Amitriptyline, nortriptyline, desipramine: depression and neuropathic pain
            These older medications are nowadays not as commonly used for depression as some of the newer agents, such as selective serotonin reuptake inhibitors (SSRIs) and selective serotonin norepinephrine reuptake inhibitors (SSNRIs). However, they can be particularly helpful in patients who have both depression and neuropathic pain.
            When used to treat depression, the dose is often titrated up to 150 mg/day. However, when used primarily for neuropathy, lower doses of 50–75 mg/day may suffice.
            Side effects include dry mouth, urinary hesitancy and sedation, so the medication should be administered at night time. Nortriptyline has lower anticholinergic effects compared to amitriptyline. The potential for cardiac conduction abnormalities warrants a baseline electrocardiogram (ECG) in patients with a history of heart trouble.
    - SSNRIs:
        - Duloxetine, venlafaxine
        - Major depressive disorder
        - Generalized anxiety disorder
        - Diabetic peripheral neuropathy pain, fibromyalgia, chronic musculoskeletal pain
- *Topical analgesics*:
    - Lidocaine patches 5%: most effective in post-herpetic neuralgia:
        - Patch can be applied directly over the painful area, and covers a surface area of 10 × 14 cm
        - Up to a maximum of three patches can be applied at a time and can be left on for 12 hours
        - Then, they should be removed for a period of 12 hours
        - Patch can be cut into smaller pieces
        - Typically, a relatively low amount of the lidocaine is absorbed, which is insufficient to cause numbness or systemic effects
    - Compounded creams including such agents as ketamine, amitriptyline or lidocaine
    - Capsaicin:
        - Topical cream: 0.025%, 0.075% and 0.1%, applied t.i.d. or q.i.d.
        - Should not be used on open wounds, near the eyes or on the face: can cause local erythema, burning or stinging

Treatment of mucositis

Mucositis is inflammation of the oral mucosa. It can result from chemotherapy or from radiation therapy. In a systematic review of >6000 patients with head and neck cancer receiving radiation therapy, 56% of those receiving altered fractionation developed grade 3 or 4 mucositis. Up to 30% of these patients may be hospitalized for complications of severe mucositis, including pain and dehydration. The National Cancer Institute recommends using a stepped approach:

- Good oral hygiene with a soft toothbrush
- Bland rinses:
    - Salt and soda: ½ teaspoon of salt and 2 tablespoons of baking soda in 32 oz of warm water
    - Patient should swish this around in his/her mouth and then spit it out
    - Can help to keep the mucosa clean and soothed

- Topical anaesthetics:
  - Irrigate mouth before applying topical medication
  - Lidocaine: viscous solution, sprays
  - Benzocaine: sprays, gels
  - Diphenhydramine solution, swish and spit
- Mucosal coating agents:
  - Amphogel
  - Kaopectate
  - Methylcellulose film-forming agents: apply with a Q-tip; can last for 6 hours
  - Gelclair (approved by the US FDA as a device):
    - Adheres to and coats the inside of the mouth
    - Does not cause numbing, stinging or drying
    - Pour packet into glass of water, rinse mouth for 1 minute, gargle, spit out, t.i.d.; patient should not eat or drink for 1 hour
  - MuGard: mucoadhesive oral wound rinse; patient swirls it around his/her mouth and it forms a protective coating
- Analgesics: opioid medications are most typically used
- Growth factor (keratinocyte growth factor-1):
  - Decreases the incidence and duration of severe oral mucositis in patients undergoing high-dose chemotherapy with or without radiation therapy followed by bone marrow transplant for haematological cancers

Nutritional management of mucositis
- Careful adjustment of the diet, in addition to good oral care, can decrease the pain associated with eating
- Choose soft foods that require minimal chewing and are easy to swallow:
  - Yoghurt, cottage cheese
  - Macaroni cheese
  - Mashed potatoes
  - Custards and puddings
  - Scrambled eggs
  - Canned fruits, bananas and apple sauce
  - Soft meats such as meatloaf, hamburger and tender meats in soups
- Avoid foods and liquids that can irritate the mouth:
  - Acidic foods such as oranges, tomatoes, lemons or their juices
  - Spicy or salty foods or condiments
  - Crunchy or coarse foods such as granola, toast, chips and raw vegetables
- Dunk or moisten dry foods with liquid, such as letting cereal set in milk before eating it or pour extra sauce or gravy on meat, pasta or potatoes
- Cook foods until they are soft and tender
- Cut foods into small pieces
- Use a blender or food processor to purée food
- Include milkshakes and/or nutrient-dense oral nutritional supplements.
- Try foods cold or at room temperature as hot foods may be irritating
- Try sucking on ice chips
- If swallowing is hard, tilting the head backward or leaning forward when swallowing may help
- Use a bicarbonate rinse (½ teaspoon of baking soda dissolved in two cups of water) before and after meals

Psychosocial care

A cancer diagnosis and subsequent treatment is disruptive to the lives of patients and families. For many, the experience is traumatic, threatening their quality of life as well as their life expectancy. Attention to the psychological and social (psychosocial) aspects of cancer care may provide opportunities to maximize treatment adherence and outcomes for persons with cancer. Each person's situation will vary depending upon a number of factors (such as age, socioeconomic status, access to support and resources, co-morbidities). This section is intended to suggest approaches to identify persons in need of psychosocial services/resources; types of services/resources; and means to deliver the services/resources.

Communication

Effective communication is the bedrock of delivering skilled and compassionate care to patients and their families. A substantial body of evidence indicates that effective physician–patient communication is positively related to a patient's health outcomes.

Two questions from the provider early in the relationship can help facilitate clear communication and treatment planning:
- What style of communication do you prefer?
  - Some people cope most effectively when given a lot of data and a list of possible scenarios/outcomes/prognosis. ('big picture' communication)
  - Others find this approach to be anxiety-provoking and prefer to be given small amounts of information regarding prognosis and 'next steps'. ('just in time' communication)
  - Does the patient prefer to include family/friends in communication?
- What matters most to you in the experience of illness and treatment?
  - Intended to obtain a picture of the person's values/fears/primary concerns, which can provide an effective touchstone for further communication/clarification

Communication among the treatment team members and regular communication with the patient's primary care physician are essential to success.

Screening for psychosocial needs
- Provided for all patients:
  - Helps to identify patients with unmet psychosocial needs and to focus resources
- Screening is comprehensive: ask about physical, emotional, spiritual, social and practical/tangible needs that contribute to distress from cancer and its treatment

- Screening tools should be brief, easy to complete and review, and sensitive to literacy

Assessment
- Provided for patients identified through screening
- Detailed exploration of domains known to impact patient access to care, mental health, coping abilities and outcomes
- Domains:
  - Physical (always rule out pain/organic causes as source for symptoms related to mood/anxiety)
  - Psychosocial
  - Spiritual
  - Practical/barriers to care (financial, lack of social support, poor access to transportation)
- Include family members when possible in order to better understand the impact of illness on the patient's role in the family

Development and implementation of a plan
Cultural norms and community standards influence the availability of psychosocial services and resources, and influence a person's receptivity to psychosocial care:
- Educational/informational needs
- Crisis intervention as indicated
- Problem-solving for addressing barriers to care
- Education: normalizing reactions, explaining biochemical aspects of anxiety/mood
- Engaging family/social supports as available
- Engaging spiritual care resources as indicated
- Access to mental health services as indicated
- Access to practical/financial resources/services as indicated

Follow-up and re-evaluation
- Scheduled/periodic follow-up is most effective
- Key events when re-evaluation should be considered:
  - Completion of planned chemo/radiation
  - Time of surveillance scans/tests/evaluation
  - Recurrence/progression of disease
  - In anticipation of transition to palliative/hospice care
  - Patient/family reported 'crisis'

Adjustment reactions
- Remember that 'normal' reactions to cancer diagnosis include:
  - Sadness
  - Anxiety/panic attacks
  - Mood swings
  - Depressed mood
  - Irritability
  - Problems with sleep and appetite
- Symptoms often improve with development of the cancer treatment plan, support and time (usually within days/weeks)
- Persistent symptoms (weeks/months) that impair functionality physically/socially and are not adaptive would suggest further assessment/treatment

Depression
- 25% of people with cancer are likely depressed enough at some point in the course of their illness to warrant mental health evaluation and treatment:
  - Advanced disease is correlated with a higher prevalence of depression
- Treatment typically includes a combination of psychological counselling and medication
- Psychotherapeutic interventions:
  - Supportive psychotherapy
  - Cognitive behavioural therapy
- Medications:
  - Choice of medication is dependent on the presenting symptoms and side effect profiles of medications
  - Onset of therapeutic actions often takes 4–6 weeks
  - SSRIs:
    - Citalopram: 20–40 mg/day orally (limited upwards dosing due to evidence of QTc prolongation)
    - Escitalopram: 10–20 mg/day orally
    - Paroxetine: 20–60 mg/day orally (high incidence of discontinuation symptoms)
    - Sertraline: 50–200 mg/day orally
    - Fluoxetine: 20–80 mg/day orally (long half-life).
  - SNRIs:
    - Venlafaxine: 75–300 mg/day orally (noted effectiveness with hot flashes)
    - Duloxetine: 40–60 mg orally daily (may be given in divided doses b.i.d.; effective for neuropathic pain)
  - Tricyclic antidepressants (TCAs):
    - Effective for neuropathic pain and headaches, but increased anticholinergic side effects
    - May cause substantial fatigue, so is best dosed at bedtime
    - Amitriptyline: 50–150 mg/day orally
    - Nortriptyline: 50–150 mg/day orally
  - Aminoketone:
    - Bupropion: 150–450 mg/day orally (stimulating effect).
  - Tetracyclics:
    - Mirtazapine: 15–45 mg orally every night at bedtime (assists with insomnia, particularly at lower doses, and can stimulate appetite).

Anxiety
Patients with cancer who are undergoing anticancer treatment and experience anxiety may benefit from medication or behavioural therapy, or both.
- Cognitive behavioural therapy, including use of relaxation techniques, is a first-line treatment.

- Medications are frequently used as an adjuvant to enable patients to better access appropriate behavioural coping tools:
  - Antidepressants (see above)
  - Buspirone: 15–60 mg total daily (often administered in divided b.i.d. dosing)
  - Benzodiazepines:
    - In some circumstances may be a helpful supplement to antidepressant medications
    - Longer-acting agents, such as clonazepam or lorazepam, are usually preferable to a shorter-acting agent, such as alprazolam, in order to avoid rebound anxiety
    - Short periods of scheduled dosing are preferable to indeterminate periods of intermittent use only as needed

Suicide risk

Patients often express a desire to 'have this all be over', to 'quit' or to 'just end it all'. Careful assessment is needed to determine risk of suicidal intent.

- All patients should receive a standardized suicide screening:
  - Screening can be performed by any member of the treatment team.
- Screening questions are often most effective when prefaced with an explanation that all patients in the treatment setting are asked about any thoughts they have had regarding ending their life:
  - "Some people who are dealing with the stress and difficulties of cancer have told us that they sometimes have thoughts of harming themselves or ending their life. Have you ever had thoughts of ending your life?"
    - If "yes", ask: "How recent were these thoughts?" and "Do you currently have a plan to take your life?"
    - If "yes", ask: "How likely do you think you are to follow through with the plan?" and "Have you ever attempted to take your life?"
    - Patients who respond "yes" to thoughts of ending their life should be referred to a mental health provider
    - Patients who indicate they have a plan should be urgently referred
    - If the patient indicates he/she has a plan and contact with a mental health provider is not possible before the patient leaves the clinic, close follow-up is indicated until a more thorough assessment can be made

- Suicide risk factors may include:
  - Depression and hopelessness
  - Uncontrolled pain
  - Previous suicide attempts
  - Substance abuse
  - Poor social support
  - Family history of suicide

Recommended reading

Adler NE, Page A (2008) *Cancer Care for the Whole Patient: Meeting Psychosocial Health Needs.* Washington, D.C.: National Academies Press, Chapters 1–4.

Berger A (2013) *Principles and Practice of Palliative Care and Supportive Oncology*, 4th edn. Philadelphia: Wolters Kluwer Health/Lippincott Williams & Wilkins, Chapters 40 and 72.

Cancer Care for the Whole Patient: Meeting Psychosocial Health Needs. Available at http://www.nap.edu/catalog/11993.html

Cramp F, Byron-Daniel J (2012) Exercise for the management of cancer-related fatigue in adults. *Cochrane Database Syst Rev* (11):CD006145.

Goldstein N, Morrison RS (2013) What is Neuropathic Pain? How do opioids and nonopioids compare for neuropathic pain management? In: *Evidence-Based Practice of Palliative Medicine*. Philadelphia: Elsevier Saunders:54–59.

Hickey M, Newton S (2012) *Telephone Triage for Oncology Nurses.* Oncology Nursing Society.

Lussier D, Portenoy RK (2010) Adjuvant analgesics in pain management. In: Hanks G, Cherny N, Christakis N, Kaasa S, Fallon M, Portenoy RK, eds. *Oxford Textbook of Palliative Medicine*, 4th edn. Oxford, Oxford University Press:706–733.

Minton O, Richardson A, Sharpe M, Hotopf M, Stone P (2010) Drug therapy for the management of cancer-related fatigue. *Cochrane Database Syst Rev* (7):CD006704.

Mustian KM, Morrow GR, Carroll JK et al (2007) Integrative nonpharmacologic behavioral interventions for the management of cancer-related fatigue. *Oncologist* 12(Suppl 1):52–67.

National Comprehensive Cancer Center (NCCN) Guidelines. Available at http://www.nccn.org/professionals/physician_gls/f_guidelines.asp

Oncology Nutrition Practice Group, Elliot L et al. (2006) *The Clinical Guide to Oncology Nutrition*, 2nd edn. The American Dietetic Association.

Schiller LR (2006) Nutrition management of chronic diarrhea and malabsorption. *Nutr Clin Prac* 21(1):34–39.

16 Pain management in cancer

P. N. Jain and Sumitra Bakshi

Department of Anesthesiology, Critical Care & Pain, Tata Memorial Centre, Mumbai, India

Introduction

Cancer pain is a universal phenomenon affecting the rich as well as poor around the globe. Unfortunately, it is an often neglected symptom and inadequately controlled in the majority of cases. This is despite the fact that, as stated by many international bodies, 80% of patients with cancer pain can be successfully treated. Pain in cancer can be a persistent sequala of the disease process, the cancer treatment or both. Recently, extraordinary breakthroughs in our understanding of cancer pain have opened newer treatment options. Neurobiology of bone pain has changed the management of primary and metastatic bone lesions.

Epidemiology

Pain is experienced by one-third of all cancer patients during the course of disease despite the availability of efficacious analgesics. Pain is the first symptom in 20–50% of all cancer patients. Approximately 30–50% patients on active cancer treatment and 75–95% with advanced disease suffer with pain. This can be associated with the primary cancer, tumour progression or treatment related. Direct involvement by tumour is the commonest cause of pain. Patients with cancer often have multiple causes of pain and multiple sites of pain.

Pain in advanced cancer is described as moderate to severe in approximately 40–50% and excruciating in 25–30% patients. Pain limits daily activity in 41% patients who are in mild-to-moderate pain, and in 94% who are in severe pain. About 33% of cancer survivors also suffer pain, e.g. post mastectomy or post thoracotomy.

The commonest tumour sites associated with pain are:
- Head and neck (67–91%)
- Prostate (56–94%)
- Uterine (30–90%)
- Genitourinary (58–90%)
- Breast (40–89%)
- Pancreatic (72–85%).

Definition of pain and types of pain

The International Association for the Study of Pain (1986) has defined pain as "an unpleasant sensory and emotional experience associated with actual or potential tissue damage or described in terms of such damage".

The types of pain in cancer patients are:
- *Direct effect of the tumour*: related to the cancer spread and involvement of soft tissue and bones, surrounding nerves, obstruction of organs and stretching of capsule of organs
- *Effect of cancer therapy*: post-surgical pain, chemotherapy- and radiotherapy-associated neuropathy and mucositis
- *Unrelated to cancer*: diabetic neuropathy, post-herpetic migraine, muscle spasm and decubitus ulcer.

Pathophysiology

Pain is classified as somatic, visceral or neuropathic depending on the origin of the pain signals. Pathophysiology of cancer pain is often complex with more than one component often present.
- *Somatic pain:*
  - Well-localized pain due to activation of nociceptors in cutaneous or deep tissue, e.g. metastatic bone pain, musculoskeletal pain and post-surgical incision pain
- *Visceral pain*:
  - Deep, squeezing and pressure-like pain that is poorly localized
  - May be referred to cutaneous sites remote from the lesion

---

UICC Manual of Clinical Oncology, Ninth Edition. Edited by Brian O'Sullivan, James D. Brierley, Anil K. D'Cruz, Martin F. Fey, Raphael Pollock, Jan B. Vermorken and Shao Hui Huang. © 2015 UICC. Published 2015 by John Wiley & Sons, Ltd.

- May result from activation of nociceptors form infiltration, compression, extension or stretching of the thoracic, abdominal or pelvic viscera
- *Neuropathic pain*:
  - Often severe; described as burning or of dysaesthetic quality
  - Most common in areas of sensory loss and may be associated with hypersensitivity to noxious and non-noxious stimuli
  - Results from injury to the peripheral or central nervous system (CNS) as a result of tumour compression or infiltration of peripheral nerves or the spinal cord
  - Surgery, radiation therapy or chemotherapy may also cause neural injury

Pain may also be classified according to its temporal distribution:
- *Acute pain*:
  - Associated with subjective and objective physical signs and with hyperactivity of the autonomic nervous system; characterized by a well-defined temporal pattern of pain onset
  - Usually self-limiting and responds to analgesics
  - Can be subacute or episodic
- *Chronic pain*:
  - Persistent pain for >3 months with a less well-defined temporal onset
  - Associated with significant changes in personality, lifestyle and functional ability
- *Breakthrough pain*:
  - Transient flare of pain over and above a controlled baseline pain
  - Often referred to as incident pain

Clinical assessment of pain

Adequate clinical assessment of pain is critical in defining the appropriate therapeutic strategy for each individual patient. The key points are:
- Believe the patient's complaint
- Take a careful clinical history, including:
  - Location(s):
    - Intensity
  - Quality:
    - Nociceptive: aching, throbbing
    - Visceral: squeezing, cramping
    - Neuropathic: burning, tingling, electrical, painful numbness
  - Temporal patterns:
    - Aggravating and alleviating factors
- Perform a careful medical and neurological examination defining the degree of motor or sensory changes to diagnose the involvement of the nervous system:
  - In patients with sensory loss, the presence of allodynia and hyperaesthesia can further define the nature of the sensory problem
- Review appropriate diagnostic studies:
  - Imaging (computed tomography [CT] scan, magnetic resonance imaging [MRI], bone scan) and tumour markers
  - Differentiate between a primary or metastatic site of the tumour
- Evaluate the patient's psychological state: 25% of patients may suffer from depression
- Individualize the therapeutic approach and discuss advance directives with the patient and family

Measurement of pain

Pain is a subjective experience. Various pain scales are available for assessing the intensity of pain, including the verbal rating scale, visual analogue scale and numerical rating scale. Pain is commonly rated on a scale of 0 to 10, where 0 indicates no pain and 10 indicates severe, intolerable pain. The Wong Baker face scale is used for children or the elderly. These scales help to quantify pain and understand the response to pain therapy.

Many validated scales are available for multidimensional pain assessment including:
- *Brief Pain Inventory*: the Wisconsin Brief Pain Questionnaire (BPI) is a self-administered, easily understood method to assess pain. The short version is most commonly used.
- *McGill Pain Questionnaire (MPQ)*: the MPQ is an extensively used pain assessment tool that produces scores for four empirically derived dimensions, as well as several summary scores. The MPQ offers a methodological approach to assess the sensory, affective and evaluative component of pain.
- *Memorial Pain Assessment Card*: this scale was devised by the Analgesic Study section of the Memorial Sloan-Kettering Cancer Center to assess the relative potency of analgesic drugs. It consists of three visual analogue scales that measure pain intensity, pain relief and mood.

Management of cancer pain

The management of cancer pain requires a multidisciplinary approach.

The European Organization for Research and Treatment of Cancer (EORTC) has suggested a three-dimensional pyramid approach. This involves four basic approaches to cancer pain control: surgery and physical methods, psychological and behavioural methods, analgesics and anticancer therapies.

The treatment must be tailored to suit the individual and should be titrated to achieve effective pain relief.

The use of drug therapy should be within the armamentarium of any physician or nurse who cares for the patient with cancer pain. The use of specific interventional blocks often requires trained medical personnel who have clinical experience in managing cancer pain. Such approaches may require referral to specialist centres.

Table 16.1 Commonly available NSAIDs

NSAID	Half-life (hours)	Dosing interval	Adult daily dose	Usual 24-hour adult dose range
Acetaminophen	2	Every 4 hours	325, 650, 1 g	2–4 g
Aspirin	2–3	q.i.d.	600–1500 mg	2.4–6 g
Ibuprofen	6	Every 4–8 hours	200–400 mg	1.2–2.4 g
Naproxen sodium	14	b.i.d.	250, 375, 500 mg	750–1 g
Ketoprofen	2–4	t.i.d.	75 mg	225 mg
Indomethacin	2–4.5	t.i.d or q.i.d.	25–50 mg	<200 mg
Diclofenac	1–2	t.i.d.	50 mg	200 mg
Piroxicam	40–50	Once daily	10, 20 mg	20 mg
Celecoxib	6–12	Once to twice daily	100–200 mg	200 mg

Principles
- Use oral analgesics or other non-invasive routes of administration whenever possible
- Administer in accordance with principles in the World Health Organization (WHO) analgesic ladder

WHO three-step analgesic ladder
The WHO analgesic ladder is a conceptual approach widely used as a clinical and educational tool for recommending type of oral analgesic vis-à-vis intensity of pain.

The key principles include:
- *By the mouth:*
  - Use oral analgesics whenever possible
  - An alternative route can be used in patients with dysphagia, uncontrolled vomiting and gastrointestinal obstruction
- *By the clock:*
  - Patients with pain should take medications at regular, pre-defined intervals
- *By the ladder:*
  - Idea is to escalate analgesics from non-opioid to weak opioid to strong opioid depending upon the pain severity and response
  - Opioid dosing is combined with adjuvant analgesics
  - Adjuvant drugs are prescribed at all stages of the ladder
- *For the individual:*
  - Individualize the dose which provides a satisfactory pain relief with minimum side effects
- *With attention to detail:*
  - Monitor adherence, side effects and adverse effects

Analgesic drug therapy
Mainly classified as:
- Non-opioid analgesics
- Opioid analgesics
- Adjuvant analgesics

Non-opioid analgesics
- Includes acetaminophen and the non-steroidal anti-inflammatory drugs (NSAIDs; Table 16.1)
- NSAIDs are believed to provide analgesia through a peripheral mechanism related to inhibition of the enzyme cyclooxygenase, thereby reducing inflammatory mediators
- These drugs are most commonly used orally and their analgesia is limited by a ceiling effect
- Increasing the dose beyond a certain level provides no increase in pain relief but a proportionate increase in side effects
- Commonest toxicities associated with the use of NSAIDs are gastrointestinal, platelet dysfunction and renal toxicity

Opioid analgesics (Tables 16.2 and 16.3)
- Produce their analgesic effects by binding to discrete opiate receptors in the peripheral and central nervous system
- Do not appear to have a ceiling effect (pure agonists), i.e. as the dose is escalated, the increment in analgesic effect is linear to the point of loss of consciousness
- Effective use requires the balancing of the most desirable effects of pain relief with the undesirable effects of nausea, vomiting, mental clouding, constipation, tolerance and physical dependence
- Selection is based on the need to treat moderate-to-severe pain:
  - Weak opioids are to be used only in moderate pain as they have a maximum recommended dose, e.g. tramadol
- About 10% of patients are unable to metabolize opioids to the active form, e.g. codeine:
  - In case of inadequate pain relief, the opioid needs to be changed
- Strong opioids like morphine, oxycodone, hydromorphone, fentanyl and methadone have a broader dose range
- Long-acting opioids (controlled release or slow release) are used for stable or baseline pain

Table 16.2 Long-acting oral and transdermal opioid preparations

Opioid	Dosing	Pharmacokinetics	Common adverse effects
Morphine IR	Every 4 hours	Tmax = 1.3 hours	Constipation, nausea, giddiness
Morphine ER	Every 12 hours	T½ = 2–4 hours	Constipation, nausea, giddiness
Hydrocodone IR	Every 4–6 hours	Tmax = 1.3 hours	Light headedness, dizziness, sedation, nausea
Oxycodone IR	Every 6 hours	Tmax = 1.6 hours T½ = 3.5 hours	Drowsiness, light headiness, nausea
Oxycodone CR	Every 12 hours	T½ = 4.5 h	Constipation, nausea, somnolence
Oxymorphone IR	Every 4–6 hours	Tmax = 0.5 hours	Nausea, dizziness
Oxymorphone ER	Every 12 hours	Tmax = 5 hours T½ = 9–10 hours	Nausea, dizziness
Fentanyl patch	One patch for 72 hours	Tmax = 34–38 hours	Nausea, vomiting
Buprenorphine patch	One patch for 7 days	Tmax = 24–72 hours	Constipation

IR, immediate release; ER, extended release; CR, controlled release.

- Fast- and shorter-acting opioids are used for breakthrough or incident pain as and when needed via novel routes, e.g. transmucosal, transnasal fentanyl:
  - Traditionally, immediate-release oral morphine is used to control breakthrough pain episodes; however, it far from ideal.

Anticipation and treatment of side effects
The side effects of the opioid analgesics often limit their effective use. The most common side effects are:
- Nausea and vomiting: an antiemetic should be taken along with the opioid, or the opioid should be switched
- Constipation: results from the actions of these drugs at multiple sites:
  - When opioid analgesics are prescribed, a regular bowel regimen including stool softeners with peristalsis enhancer should be started
  - Opioid antagonists (e.g. methylnaltrexone) that do not penetrate the blood–brain barrier are a new effective treatment for opioid-induced constipation
- Sedation and drowsiness: vary with the drug and dose

Table 16.3 Opioid analgesics commonly used for cancer pain management

Drug	Equianalgesic (mg)	Starting oral dose (mg)	Duration of action (hours)
Morphine	10	30–60	4
Codeine	67	200	2–4
Hydrocodone	10	5–10	4–6
Oxymorphone	3.3	10–20	4–6
Oxycodone	6.7	5–15	4–6

- Respiratory depression: rarely a problem because pain stimulates the respiratory centre and tolerance develops to this adverse effect
- Multifocal myoclonus: can occur and is treated by adding clonazepam:
  - Dose reduction of the opioid and opioid rotation also helps

Availability of opioids is a serious issue in the Eastern world. Morphine is often substituted by weaker opioids; hence, it is necessary to know the equianalgesic dose of commonly available preparations.

Adjuvant analgesics
These are not analgesics but act as analgesics. In cancer pain, steroids, anticonvulsants and antidepressants are commonly used as adjuvant analgesics.
- *Antidepressants*: the tricyclic antidepressants (TCAs):
  - Most useful group of psychotropic drugs in the management of cancer pain
  - Analgesic effects are mediated by enhancement of serotonin activity
  - Starting dose of amitriptyline is 10–25 mg at night, increasing gradually in 2–4-weeks periods
  - First-line therapeutic approach for neuropathic pain and should be tried for several weeks before discontinuing it
- *Anticonvulsants*:
  - Stabilize the membrane, suppress the paroxysmal discharge and reduce neuronal hyperexcitability
  - Most commonly used drugs are gabapentin and pregabalin
- *Corticosteroids*:
  - Major indications include refractory neuropathic pain, bone pain and headache due to raised intracranial tension, acute spinal cord compression, superior vena cava syndrome, symptomatic lymphoedema, hepatic capsular distension

- Effective in patients with tumour infiltration in brachial and lumbosacral plexopathy
- Loading dose of 16 mg and maintenance with 4 mg/day of dexamethasone is effective in advanced cancer patients
- *Other adjuvant drugs:*
  - A wide variety of other adjuvant drugs, such as clonidine, benzodiazepine, neuroptics and NMDA antagonists, are used in the management of neuropathic pain
  - Use of ketamine infusion has been found to be effective in certain cases of refractory neuropathic pain
  - Metastatic disease to bone is the most common cause of pain in patients with advanced cancers of the breast, lung and prostrate
  - Bisphosphonates (zoledronic acid and ibandronate) and radionucleotides (strontium-89 and samarium-153) have been found to be effective in the treatment pain with multifocal metastatic bone disease.

Interventional approaches

Around 10% of patients may require interventional techniques for pain relief. Consideration for intervention is indicated when:
- Symptoms cannot be controlled adequately with medications
- Patient cannot tolerate medications
- Non-availability of opioid drugs

Interventions should be initiated at an early stage to have maximal advantage and give a better quality of life:
- A diagnostic block should always precede a therapeutic block
- *Peripheral nerve block:*
  - Definite, although limited, role in the management of pain mapping to single or multiple peripheral nerves
- *Cranial nerve blocks:*
  - Pain caused by head and neck malignancies is often the most challenging management problem for the pain specialist
  - Lasting pain relief is difficult to achieve with discrete nerve blocks because of sensory overlap
  - Technical difficulties may also be encountered because of the tendency for tumours in these regions to erode and destroy the surrounding tissue
- *Intraspinal analgesia:*
  - A good option for spinal or radicular pain caused by primary or metastatic lesions
  - A single injection of steroid or local anaesthetic can be used
  - A permanent intraspinal catheter and implanted subcutaneous pump may be tried if the patient's life expectancy is >3 months
- *Epidural and intrathecal neurolysis:*
  - Alcohol or phenol have been used primarily to manage patients with advanced disease whose pain is either unilateral in the chest or abdomen or midline in the perineum
  - Advantages of neurolysis are the high success rates in appropriately selected patients, ease of performance, adequate and durable pain relief, and ease of repetition when necessary
- *Sympathetic nerve block:*
  - Effective in conditions with vasomotor or viscera-motor hyperactivity:
    - Stellate ganglion block (cervicothoracic ganglion block): useful for pain in the face, upper neck and hemicranium
    - Lumbar sympathetic block: may provide significant relief from intractable pain of urogenital origin; pain due to carcinomatous invasion of local nerves and the plexus in the perineum and lower extremity
    - Coeliac plexus block: widely used as has excellent potential to relieve upper abdominal and referred back pain caused by malignancy involving the upper abdominal structures (pancreas, stomach, duodenum, liver and gall bladder)
    - Superior hypogastric plexus block: can be used to relieve pelvic pain due to malignancy of the rectum, vagina, cervix and other pelvic organs
- *Spinal cord stimulation:*
  - Useful in chronic neuropathic pain in the setting of chemotherapy-induced peripheral neuropathy, and post-radiation nerve injury

Cancer pain syndromes

Post-chemotherapy pain syndromes

Chemotherapy drugs are neurotoxic and cause cellular damage, which may be in the form of neuronal apoptosis and induction of lysosomal storage defects (platinum agents) or microtubular aggregation (taxanes). The drugs associated with neurotoxicity are the vinca alkaloids (vincristine, vindesine, vinblastine), platinum agents (cisplatin), taxanes (paclitaxel, docetaxel) and other non-cytostatic drugs like interferon, thalidomide and amphotericin B.

Treatment includes adjuvant analgesics such as TCAs and anticonvulsant drugs.

Cancer-related bone pain

Bone pain most commonly arises from metastasis from cancers of the breast, prostate and lung, but also from cancers of the kidney and thyroid, and lymphoma and multiple myeloma. Both osteolytic and osteoblastic changes in bone occur from metastasis of tumours of the lung, breast and kidney; osteolysis from multiple myeloma and sarcomas; and osteoblastic lesions commonly from metastatic prostate cancer.

The periosteum is richly innervated by both sympathetic and sensory nerve fibres. In the osteoblastic lesions there is evidence of destructive injury and an increase in density of sensory fibres compared to normal bone. Changes in pH play a role in osteoclastic lesions. Up-regulation of nerve growth factor following nerve injury is responsible for hyperalgesia which is often associated with these lesions.

Treatment:
- Conventional opioids or NSAIDs may not produce adequate analgesia because of the incidental and intermittent nature of the pain and dose-limiting side effects
- Targeted pharmacotherapeutic and interventional approaches are used alone or in combination with traditional analgesics
- Corticosteroids cause pain relief by blocking the cytokine synthesis that contributes to inflammation and nociception
- Bisphosphonates are used for metastatic bone pain and also for correction of hypercalcaemia and prevention of cancer treatment-induced bone loss
- The hormone calcitonin is used for treatment of bone metastasis because of its potential to relieve pain and retain bone density
- Radionucleotides, including phosphorus-32, strontium-89, yttrium-90, samarium-153, are of maximum benefit in multifocal oesteoblastic lesions as they inhibit pain mediators from normal cells
- External beam radiotherapy for localized bone pain

Neuropathic cancer pain

Tumour infiltration into surrounding nerves (e.g. intercostal nerve infiltration secondary to rib metastasis, radiculopathy due to epidural or leptomeningeal spread) can lead to severe neuropathy.

Neuropathies can also be treatment related; post-mastectomy pain, phantom pain and post-thoracotomy pain are common example of postoperative neuropathic pain. Radiation therapy causes pain by damaging peripheral nerves, the spinal cord or brain. It alters the microvascular connective tissues surrounding peripheral nerves, via fibrosis and chronic inflammation in connective tissues, or leads to demyelination and focal necrosis of white and grey matter in the spinal cord.

Treatment of neuropathic pain includes adjuvant drugs like TCAs and anticonvulsant drugs.

Cancer pain emergencies

- Defined as severe or excruciating pain, e.g. 8 out of 10 on a numerical scale (0–10) for >6 hours
- Common causes are pathological fracture, epidural spinal cord compression and severe headache due to raised intracranial pressure
- Rapid titration with IV opioids is the mainstay of treatment:
  - Rarely leads to serious toxicity and pain can be controlled in the emergency room, with admission rarely warranted

Recommended reading

Bruera E, Roca E (1985) Action of oral methylprenisolne in terminal cancer patients. A prospective randomized double blind study. *Cancer Treat Rep* 69:751.

Caraceni A, Portenoy RK, from Working Group of the IASP Task Force on Cancer Pain (1999) An international survey of cancer pain characteristics and syndromes. *Pain* 82:263–274.

Daut RL, Cleeland CS, Flanery RS (1983) The development of the Wisconsin Brief Pain Questionnaire to assess pain in cancer and other diseases. *Pain* 17:197.

De'Courcy JG (2011) Interventional pain management in cancer. *Clin Oncol* 23:407–417.

Eisenberg E, Carr DB, Chalmers TC (1995) Neurolytic celiac plexus block for treatment of cancer pain: A meta-analysis. *Anesth Analg* 80:290–295.

Fishman B, Pasternak S, Wallerstein SL et al. (1986) The Memorial Pain Assessment of cancer pain. *Cancer* 60:1151.

Foley KM (1997) Supportive care and quality of life. In: Devita VT, Hellman S, Rosenberg SA, eds. *Cancer: Principles and Practice of Oncology*, 5th edn. Philadelphia: Lippincott-Raven:2807–2841.

Greenbery HS, Kim JH (1980) Epiduro-spinal cord compression from metastatic lesions, results with new treatment protocol. *Ann Neurol* 8:361.

Graham C, Bond SS, Gretrovitch MM, Cook MR (1980) Use of the McGill Pain Questionnaire in the management of cancer pain: replicability and consistency. *Pain* 8:377.

IASP Subcommittee on Taxonomy (1980) Pain terms: a List with definitions and notes on usage. *Pain* 8:249.

Mercandante S, Antonino G (2013) The long winding road of non steroidal anti-inflammatory drugs and paracetamol in cancer pain treatment: a critical review. *Crit Rev Oncol Hematol* 2013:1701.

Negels W, Pease N, Bekkering G, Dobbels P (2013) Celiac plexus neurolysis for abdominal cancer pain: A systematic review. *Pain Med* 14(8):1140–1163.

Plancarte R, Amescua C, Patt RB et al. (1990) Superior hypogastric plexus block for pelvic cancer pain. *Anaesthesiology* 73:236.

Portenoy RK, Hagen NA (1990) Breakthrough pain: definition, prevalence and characteristics. *Pain* 41:273–282.

World Health Organization (1990) *Cancer Pain relief and Palliative Care*. Report of WHO expert Committee. *WHO Tech Rep* 804:1–73.

Zech DL, Grond S, Lynch J et al. (1995) Validation of World Health Organization guidelines for cancer pain relief: a 10 year prospective study. *Pain* 63:65.

17 Palliative care

Mary Ann Muckaden

Tata Memorial Centre, Homi Bhabha National University, Mumbai, India

Introduction

Worldwide, management strategies for cancer include maximum resource utilization towards prevention, early detection and treatment. GLOBOCAN 2012 data shows cancer as a leading cause of death worldwide, accounting for 8.2 million deaths (around 13% of all deaths), with 48% occurring in the less developed regions. Deaths from cancer worldwide are projected to rise to over 13.1 million by 2030. Life-threatening or advanced disease is a crisis that affects patient and family alike.

Palliative care is defined by the World Health Organization (WHO) as 'an approach that improves the quality of life of patients and their families facing the problems associated with life-threatening illness, through the prevention and relief of suffering by means of early identification and impeccable assessment and treatment of pain and other problems, physical, psychosocial and spiritual'. It is treatment to 'relieve, rather than cure, symptoms' and allow patients to live more comfortably with their disease. It is an urgent humanitarian need for those with cancer and other chronic fatal diseases, particularly in patients with advanced stages of disease for whom there is little chance of cure. Palliative care provided at the appropriate time, i.e. early within the disease course, can even improve survival, as demonstrated in a trial in patients with lung cancer. It improves 'quality of life' while the patient is undergoing disease-modifying therapy (Fig. 17.1).

Thus, palliative care:
- Provides relief from pain and other distressing symptoms
- Affirms life and regards dying as a normal process
- Intends neither to hasten nor postpone death
- Integrates the psychological and spiritual aspects of patient care
- Offers a support system to help patients live as actively as possible until death
- Offers a support system to help the family cope during the patient's illness and in their own bereavement
- Uses a team approach to address the needs of patients and their families, including bereavement counselling, if indicated
- Enhances quality of life and may also positively influence the course of illness
- Is applicable early in the course of illness, in conjunction with other therapies that are intended to prolong life, such as chemotherapy or radiation therapy, and includes those investigations needed to better understand and manage distressing clinical complications.

WHO strategies include:
- Effective public health strategies, comprising community- and home-based care, are essential to provide pain relief and palliative care for patients and their families in low-resource settings
- Improved access to oral morphine is mandatory for the treatment of moderate-to-severe cancer pain, suffered by >80% of cancer patients in the terminal phase
- When disease is progressing, palliative anticancer therapy is part of the armamentarium.

Principles of management

As stated by Dr Robert Twycross 'care of the dying goes far beyond pain and symptom management'. Also, support is not only for the patient but also for families; 'one of the most rewarding of their doctors, nurses and other carers responsibilities'.

Good symptom control is an essential component of effective palliative care and is based on the five principles (EEMMA):
- **E**valuation: diagnosis of each symptom before treatment
- **E**xplanation: to the patient before treatment
- **M**anagement: individualized treatment
- **M**onitoring: continuing review of the impact of treatment
- **A**ttention to detail: no unwarranted assumptions.

UICC Manual of Clinical Oncology, Ninth Edition. Edited by Brian O'Sullivan, James D. Brierley, Anil K. D'Cruz, Martin F. Fey, Raphael Pollock, Jan B. Vermorken and Shao Hui Huang. © 2015 UICC. Published 2015 by John Wiley & Sons, Ltd.

Palliative care

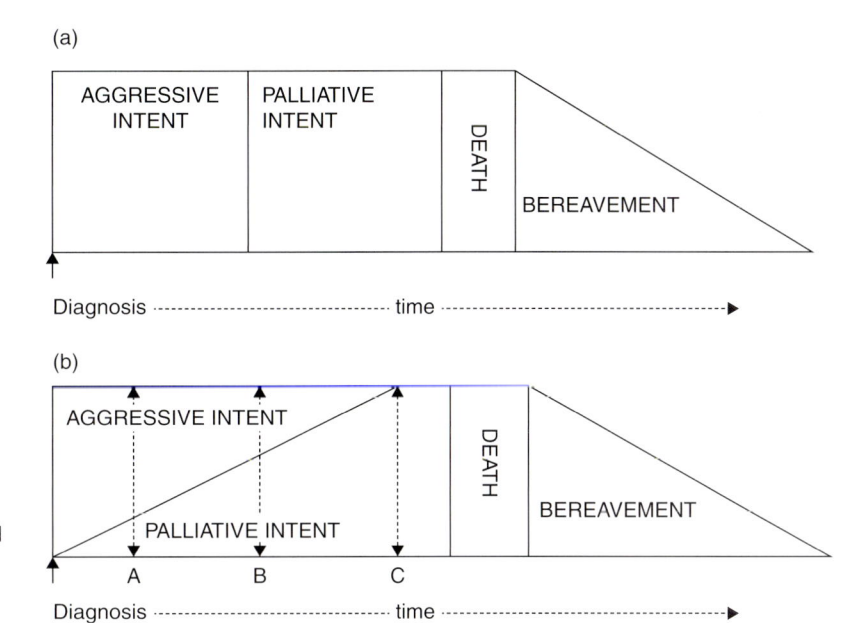

Figure 17.1 (a) Traditional and (b) modern integrated palliative care services model.
Source: Meiring 2011. Reproduced with permission of Health & Medical Publishing Group.

Disease-modifying treatment

The aim of palliative disease-modifying treatment is to reduce tumour size, thus reducing symptoms and improving quality of life:
- Radiation: short term, high daily dose fractionation schedules
- Chemotherapy: for sensitive tumours – simple schedules, easy to administer, often oral, administered at home
- Surgery: amputations, diversion, stents.

Treatment options using anticancer therapy should be continued only until such time as toxicities out way the benefits.

National Comprehensive Cancer Network (NCCN) guidelines consider:
- Shared care between the oncologist, palliative care teams and other professionals like mental health specialists, social services and community services
- Respect for and the need to ascertain patient/family needs, values, beliefs and cultures
- Ongoing communication between all professionals involved in the care pathway, the patient and family, with ongoing review of care at every step
- Discussions of 'advanced care planning' as soon as feasible.

Common symptoms and their control

Nausea and vomiting
Aetiology
The pathophysiology of vomiting is illustrated in Fig. 17.2 and the specific receptors and triggers are listed in Table 17.1.

Management
- *General:*
  - Check plasma levels of creatinine, digoxin and calcium
  - Consider stopping gastric irritant drugs, e.g. antibiotics, corticosteroids, non-steroidal anti-inflammatory drugs (NSAIDs)
  - Reverse cause where feasible, e.g. bisphosphonates for hypercalcaemia
  - May need to start with subcutaneous route and switch to oral route as soon as possible
  - Where the intravenous (IV) route is available, this should be used, followed by the oral route
  - Rectal route is efficacious and should be used where indicated
  - Maintain hydration (subcutaneous route is a good alternative to the intravenous route)
- *Specific:*
  - Appropriate drug depends on receptor stimulation (Table 17.2)

Stimulation of receptors (see Table 17.1) sends message to the vomiting centre (located in brainstem but across the blood–brain barrier)

⇩

Gastric atony, retroperistalsis, thoracic and abdominal muscle contractions

⇩

Vomiting

Figure 17.2 Mechanism of vomiting.

Table 17.1 Receptors and triggers in the vomiting stimulus

	Area	Receptor	Trigger
Chemoreceptor trigger zone (CTZ)	Postrema (base of fourth ventricle)	Dopamine (D_2) 5-Hydroxytryptamine type 3 (5-HT_3) Substance P	Drugs (morphine, digoxin) Hypercalcaemia Uraemia
Cerebral cortex	Higher centre	Gamma-aminobutyric acid (GABA) 5-Hydroxytryptamine (5-HT) Neurokinin 1 (NK1)	Anxiety Raised intracranial pressure (ICP) Hyponatraemia
Vestibular system	Inner ear	Muscarinic cholinergic (ACh_m) Histamine type 1 (H_1) receptors	Movement Vertigo
Gut and serosal surfaces in the viscera	Gastrointestinal tract	5-HT_3 receptors	Radiotherapy Chemotherapy Intestinal distension

Table 17.2 Drugs for nausea and vomiting

Drug	Dose	D_2	H_1	ACh_m	$5HT_2$	$5HT_3$	$5HT_4$
Metoclopromide	10–20 mg every 4–6 hours PO/SC/IV	++	–	–	–	+	++
Domperidone	10–20 mg every 4–8 hours PO	++	–	–	–	–	–
Haloperidol	0.5–2 mg every 6–12 hours PO/SC/IV	+++	–	–	–	–	–
Ondansetron	4–8 mg every 8–12 hours	–	–	–	–	+++	–
Chlorpromazine	25–50 mg every 6–8 hours PO/IV	++	++	+	–	–	–
Diphenhydramine	50–100 mg PO/IV every 4–6 hours	–	++	++	–	–	–
Prochlorperazine	10–20 mg PO/IV every 6 hours or 25 mg PR every 6 hours	++	+	–	–	–	–
Olanzapine	1.25–2.5 mg once daily PO	+	++	++	++	+	–
Dexamethasone	4–20 mg every morning PO/IV/SC	–	–	–	–	?	–

D_2, dopamine type 2; H_1, histamine type 1; ACh_m, muscarinic cholinergic; $5HT_2$, $5HT_3$, $5HT_4$, 5-hydroxytryptamine (serotonin) types 2, 3 and 4.

Constipation
Aetiology
- *Related to cancer/immobility:*
  - Inactivity
  - Lack of exercise
  - Diet low in fibre
  - Low fluid intake
  - Fever
  - Weakness
  - Inability to visit toilet
- *Related to drugs:*
  - Morphine
  - NSAIDs
  - 5-HT3 antagonists, e.g. odansetron
  - Vincristine: paralytic ileus

Management
- *General:*
  - Increase oral intake
  - Encourage fluid intake
  - Mobilize patient where feasible
  - Provide privacy and access to toilet
- *Specific:*
  - Rotate/stop drugs where feasible
  - Laxatives: combine bulking and motility agents (Table 17.3)
  - Use suppository where needed
  - Faecal impaction, see Fig. 17.3

Diarrhoea
Diarrhoea is uncommon. Spurious diarrhoea, caused by sub-acute intestinal obstruction leading to bacterial putrefaction, needs to be ruled out.

Table 17.3 Drugs for constipation

Predominantly softening	Predominantly peristalsis stimulating
Surface wetting agents sodium docusate, poloxamer	Anthracenes: senna, danthron
Osmotic laxatives: lactulose, sorbitol	Polyphenolics: bisacodyl, sodium picosulphate
Bulking agents: ispaghula, methyl cellulose	
Saline laxatives: magnesium sulphate	
Lubricants: liquid paraffin	

Management
- Antibiotics where appropriate
- Antimotility drugs: loperamide for symptomatic relief
- Hydration is essential but should be oral or subcutaneous (1 L can be given per day by hypodermoclysis at home; no need for intravenous hydration)

Bowel obstruction
Bowel obstruction is common. It is a very distressing feature of advanced abdominopelvic cancer and is more common in patients who have undergone previous surgery and/or radiation.

The pathophysiology should be well understood before management is decided:
- Constipation ruled out by per rectum examination:
  - If rectum full: management as for constipation
  - Rectum empty: manage as for bowel obstruction
- Role for surgery is confined to single sites of obstruction and if survival is anticipated to be weeks to months
- Evidence indicates that decision-making should be based on time to relapse, performance status, advanced age and low albumin levels
- Poor prognostic factors include radiologically evident disease sites, carcinomatosis/sarcomatosis and ascites

Management
- Traditionally managed with Ryle's tube aspiration with IV fluids to keep the gut quiescent (drip & suck)
- An alternative approach is conservative management by the subcutaneous route; results are as effective

Subacute obstruction
- Small passage in the obstructed gut, allowing liquid bowel contents to pass
- History: colicky pain, passage of small quantities of stool and flatus
- Physical exam: increased bowel sounds

Management (Table 17.4)
- Corticosteroids (subcutaneous): dexamethasone 4–8 mg every 8 hours for 3–4 days

---

With severe constipation of 5–7 days' duration: Manual evaluation is necessary
⇩
Softening of stool with arachis oil or glycerine overnight
⇩
Gentle manual evacuation
⇩
High phosphate enema (a plain soap water enema will not be effective due to the impaction and can damage the mucosa)
⇩
Continue laxatives

Figure 17.3 Management of faecal impaction.

- Prokinetic drugs: metaclopramide 10 mg every 8 hours (watch for increasing bowel sounds which herald perforation)
- Buscopan: 10 mg for colicky pain if indicated
- Small frequent liquid feeds

There may be reversal for a period of days after which symptoms will recur and obstruction may become complete.

Complete obstruction
- No propulsion of gastric or intestinal contents
- Usually heralds terminal phase
- History: absence of flatus or stool passage, pain due to stretching of the capsule of distended organs and copremesis
- Physical exam: distended abdomen, mild tenderness, absent bowel sounds

Management
- Pain is managed as per the WHO ladder:
  - Step 3 drugs like morphine cause gastric and intestinal stasis:
    - May be indirectly beneficial by causing relaxation of the distended bowel, thus relieving non-colicky pain and reducing vomiting
  - The subcutaneous route is best, using a syringe driver or the Edmonton injector
- Gastric and intestinal secretions are reduced with octreotide, somatostatin or glycopyrolates subcutaneously
- Small sips of water or any other fluid are administered if desired:
  - Ice cubes, if sucked, keep thirst away
- Small quantities of fluids up to 1 L can be transfused (dermoclysis) through the subcutaneous route
- Patient can be cared for at home in the terminal phase

Anorexia and cachexia syndrome
- Weight loss of >5% over the last 6 months:
  - Weight loss should have been ongoing over the last 1–2 months

Table 17.4 Medications for treatment of malignant intestinal obstruction

Drug category	Medication	Dosage
Analgesic drugs	Opioids (SC or transdermal)	As needed to control symptoms
	Steroids (e.g. dexamethasone)	See below
	Antispasmodic/anticholinergics	See below
Antisecretory agents	Dexamethasone	6–20 mg/day SC; trial for 3–5 days
	Octreotide	100–1500 µg/day SC
	Antispasmodic/anticholinergics	
	Hyoscine butylbromide	40–120 mg/day SC
	Glycopyrrolate	0.1–0.4 mg/day SC
	Scopolamine	0.2–2 mg/day SC or 1–2 transdermal patches of 1.5 mg every 3 days
	H_2-receptor antagonists (e.g. famotidine, ranitidine)	As needed to control symptoms
	Proton pump inhibitors	As needed to control symptoms
Antiemetic drugs	Metoclopramide (if no colicky pain)	40–240 mg/day SC
	Haloperidol	5–15 mg/day SC
	Olanzapine	2.5–20 mg/day SL
	Phenothiazines (sedation)	
	Chlorpromazine	50–100 mg rectally or IM every 8 hours
	Prochlorperazine	25 mg rectally every 8 hours
	Methotrimeprazine	6.25–50 mg/day SC
	Dimenhydrinate	50–100 mg/day SC, IV or rectally
	Ondansetron	4–8 mg twice daily IV
Other	Laxative suppositories, enemas	As needed to control symptoms
	Amidotrizoate	Single 50-mL oral dose with metoclopramide, octreotide, dexamethasone SC in partial obstruction

SC, subcutaneously; SL, sublingually; IM, intramuscularly; IV, intravenously.
Source: Tradounsky 2012. Reproduced with permission from College of Family Physicians of Canada.

- In patients with significant fluid retention, large tumour mass or obesity, significant muscle wasting may occur in the absence of weight loss

Management
- *Corticosteroids:*
  - To improve appetite, feeling of well-being, performance status
  - Effect is limited to 4 weeks
  - Dose is between 4 and 16 mg/day
  - Side-effects: fluid retention, candidiasis, myopathy, insomnia, gastritis
- *Progestational drugs:*
  - Improve appetite and increase weight in patients with cancer
  - Take up to 2 weeks to take effect but benefit is more prolonged than with steroids
  - Most appropriate for patients with a longer prognosis
  - Dose 160–800 mg
  - Side effects: nausea, fluid retention, increased risk of thromboembolism
- *Prokinetics:* metoclopramide 10 mg or domperidone 10–20 mg (fewer long-term side effects) t.i.d. half an hour before meals
- *Other medications:*
  - NSAIDs: alone seem to offer little benefit, but may be more effective as part of a multimodal intervention
  - Thalidomide: an anti-inflammatory, antiangiogenic and anticytokine agent that is known to increase fat-free mass as well as appetite

- Investigational drugs: ghrelin, olanzapine (anti-interleukin [IL]-6 antibodies), creatine, myostatin antagonists, gluconeogensis inhibitor (metformin), selective androgen receptor modulator (ostarine)

Parenteral nutrition
- Role in patients with limited life span is controversial:
  - NCCN guidelines do not find adequate evidence for use in patients with <3 months estimated survival
- Hypoproteinaemia will be present in the majority of patients who have undergone extensive anticancer therapies, but the side effects associated with parenteral nutrition would adversely affect quality of life for this group of patients
- Options should be discussed with patient and family

Fatigue and asthenia
Aetiology
Multiple factors interact with each other and contribute to fatigue:
- Direct effects: lipolytic factors, tumour degradation factors, proteolytic factors, invasion of brain or pituitary gland by tumour
- Induced host factors: IL-1, IL-6, tumour necrosis factor (TNF)
- Accompanying factors: psychological issues, anaemia, cachexia, infection, metabolic disorders, endocrine disorders, paraneoplastic syndrome

Management
- Non-pharmacological: counselling, physiotherapy, occupational therapy
- Pharmacological:
  - Corticosteroids
  - Megesterol acetate
  - Other management as described for cachexia
  - Psychostimulants:
    - Methylphenidate and modafinil are known to promote a sense of well-being, reduce fatigue and alleviate depression
    - Methylphenidate is also known to reverse opioid-induced fatigue and sedation
- Specific measures:
  - Correction of anaemia
  - Counselling and antidepressants for major depression
  - Correction of metabolic disorders like hyponatraemia, hypercalcaemia, hypokalaemia, hypoxia, dehydration

Dyspnoea
Where life expectancy is weeks or months, any anticancer intervention is appropriate where symptom benefits outweigh burdens. For dyspnoea, interventions to reduce symptom burden include tapping of pleural effusion and, pericardial drainage (pig tail or window).

Management
- *Dyspnoea on exertion:*
  - Bronchodilators oral or inhaled and low-dose steroids where appropriate
  - Modify lifestyle to space periods of exertion with rest
  - Positioning in sleep (sitting up with support), relaxation therapy, breathing techniques
- *Dyspnoea at rest* (usually heralds terminal phase):
  - Low-dose morphine (2.5–5 mg every 4 hours for opioid-naïve patients or 50% escalation for those already on morphine for pain) reduces awareness of dyspnoea in the terminal phase
  - Benzodiazepines reduce anxiety:
    - Lorazepam 0.5–1 mg orally every 8 hours and when necessary
  - Oxygen therapy using face mask is controversial as it prevents communication between the patient and family:
    - Useful only where measurable PO_2 levels are very low
  - Positioning (as above)
  - Psychological support for patient and family

Delirium
Delirium is common when entering terminal phase, and is very distressing for both the patient and family.

Management
- Reverse cause: dehydration, hypercalcaemia, bladder or bowel distension
- Maximize non-pharmacological interventions: safe familiar environment, quiet room, close family members and known professionals
- Haloperidol: 0.5 mg orally every 4–24 hours (increase dose as required; intravenous infusion if agitated and until controlled)
- Olanzepine: 2.5–7.5 mg orally every 4–8 hours (maximum 30 mg/day)
- When severe, add lorazepam 0.5–2 mg every 4 hours subcutaneously or intravenously
- Support relatives

Bleeding
- May be from surface wound or body cavity
- Usually capillary in origin; rarely erosion can affect veins or even arteries
- If in stool, the colour of stool can guide origin of bleeding: black stools indicate gastric bleed

Management
- External bleed:
  - Local sustained pressure, local application of ethamsylate or tranexemic acid 500-mg tablets crushed and mixed in xylocaine jelly; change every 24 hours
  - Gauze soaked in noradrenaline (1:1000)

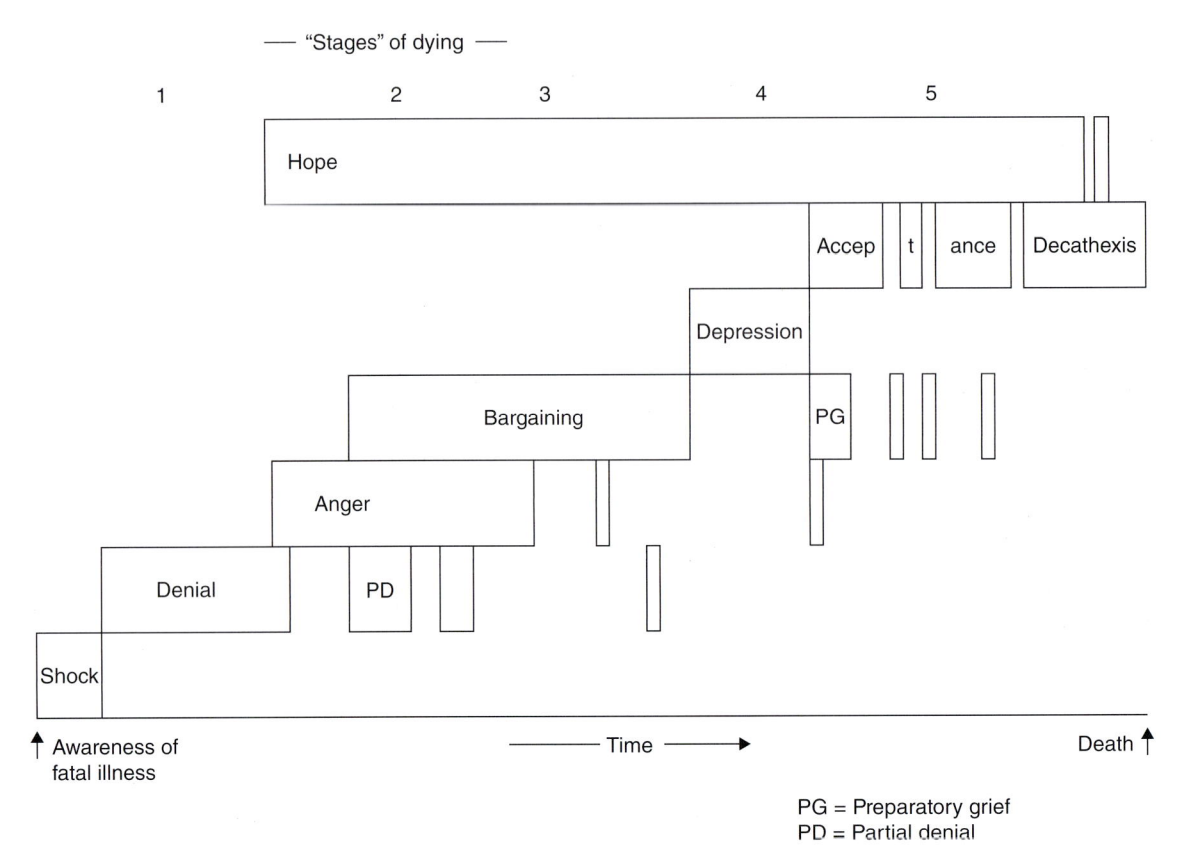

Figure 17.4 Stages of grief.
Source: Kubler-Ross (2011) Reproduced with permission of Taylor & Francis Group.

PG = Preparatory grief
PD = Partial denial

- When severe, consider oral ethamsylate or tranexemic acid 500-mg every 8 hours for 3–5 days until bleeding stops
- Vaginal bleeding: pack using diluted noradrenaline (1:1000), change every 24 hours:
  - Where local management is inadequate to stop bleeding, systemic therapy, as above, should be added to local packing
- Laser therapy, cryotherapy or brachytherapy where appropriate
- Gastroscopy or colonoscopy may be helpful
- Artery embolization, ligation, amputation, if justified, where benefit outweighs morbidity
- Massive bleeds from major vessels are life threatening:
  - Moving the patient is futile, as collapse is imminent
  - Preparation with availability of dark towels, sedation for patient and preparation of the family are essential

Psychological reactions to advanced cancer

Feelings of loss/grief are part of living with advanced cancer. The stages of grief have been described by Kubler Ross (Fig. 17.4), and newer models have been suggested.
- Anticipatory loss/grief recognized
- Most common psychological distress includes depression and anxiety
- More severe distress is manifested by feelings of helplessness, worthlessness and lack of role in family and society
- In severe cases, this may lead to suicidal tendencies, a trait oncologists need to recognize when dealing with patients whose cancer is incurable

Psychological care

- Personalized medical care contributes to maintenance of psychological balance and quality of life in patients suffering from chronic conditions; consistently proven in literature
- Psychological support is provided for every patient and his/her family by the palliative care team at first referral
- Early care can help in coping with grief/loss
- Routine care ranges from active listening and general counselling to prognosis explanations by trained personnel
- Good communication skills are essential:
  - Open communication between the patient and family is facilitated by a multidisciplinary team in atmosphere of confidentiality, trust and privacy, and with appropriate time given to it
- Problem-solving through self-help should be encouraged, with active support from the team for both psychological and financial problems:
  - This continues through the entire disease course and into the bereavement process.

- Support groups have a proven benefit in coping with loss
- Collusion among family members, where present, should be handled with culture-specific skills:
  - Where signs are evident that the patient is interested in his/her prognosis, the family should be counselled to be open with the patient
- 'Breaking bad news' both to the patient and family are important components of palliative care counselling (Table 17.5)
- Where grief is complicated, the patient/family should be referred to a clinical psychologist or psychiatrist for specialized care
- Hypnosis, imagery and other behaviour modifying therapies should be used along with counselling
- Staff should regularly attend training and refresher courses

Social issues and their relevance to palliative care

- Very culture specific
- Rehabilitation of the patient to live as normal a life as possible
- In developing countries, help with social issues can include financial help for devices, a place for temporary stay near to the treatment centre, medications etc.
- Create a network of care as close to the patient's home as feasible
- Use existing resources, adding to them where necessary
- Government and non-governmental organization cooperation

Table 17.5 10 Steps to breaking bad news

1	Preparation: know all the facts before the meeting. Find out who the patient wants present, and ensure privacy and chairs to sit on
2	What does the patient know? Ask for a narrative of events from the patient
3	Is more information wanted? Test the waters, but be aware that it can be very frightening to ask for more information
4	Give a warning shot, e.g. "I'm afraid it looks rather serious" – then allow a pause for the patient to respond
5	Allow denial: denial is a defence mechanism and a way of coping. Allow the patient to control the amount of information he/she receives
6	Explain: increase the patient's information to match the professional's to the appropriate level
7	Listen to concerns: ask "What are your main concerns at the moment?" and then allow space for expression of feelings
8	Encourage ventilation of feelings: this is the *key* phase in terms of patient satisfaction with the interview, because it conveys empathy
9	Summary and plan: summarize concerns, plan treatment, foster appropriate hope
10	Offer availability: most patients need further explanation and support and may benefit greatly from a family meeting

Source: Kaye (1996).

- Families given aid when required to achieve normalcy
- Education for children and empowerment of women after bereavement

Spiritual care

- One of the difficult, yet imperative, areas of care
- Important to distinguish between religion and spirituality
- In Western countries, chaplains care for spiritual distress
- In countries where religion is a way of life, religion and spirituality may be more intertwined and interdependent
- Care for spiritual distress falls upon the palliative care teams
- Wright expands on the role of spiritual and palliative care as:
  - 'Spirituality has come to be regarded as an essential feature of hospice and palliative care.
  - While only 20% of people in Western Europe and 14% in Eastern Europe claimed to attend a religious service on a weekly basis, beliefs had not been discarded: seven of ten adults still claimed to believe in God.
  - Paradoxically, the journey into death is sometimes considered to be the ultimate vehicle for spiritual discovery'
- Narayanasamy states: 'Empirical evidence suggests that spiritual support may act as an adjunct to the palliative care of those facing advanced diseases and end of life'
- A Consensus Conference in 2009, led by Puchalski and Farrell, was based on the belief that spiritual care was a fundamental component of quality palliative care:
  - One prominent finding was 'Spiritual care models offer a framework for health care professionals to connect with their patients; listen to their fears, dreams, and pain; collaborate with their patients as partners in their care; and provide, through the therapeutic relationship, an opportunity for healing'

Ethics and palliative care

A compilation of views from all over the world has brought out the following issues as relevant to ethics in palliative care:
- A duty to alleviate suffering
- Respect for persons
- Autonomy
- Non-maleficence
- Beneficence
- Utility
- Justice
- Human rights

These concepts are crucial to decision-making. Patients need to trust their doctors and all decisions must be made in the best interest of patients. This trust can only be developed over time, with adequate communication skills. Palliative care thus needs to be introduced as early in the course of the illness as possible if optimum benefits are to be achieved. Evidenced-based treatment options should guide decision-making.

End of life care

The WHO (1998) defines end of life care as 'the active, total care of patients whose disease is not responsive to curative treatment' and the National Institute of Health (2004) as 'the underlying disease process should be irreversible, and that the symptoms or impairments resulting from it, require either professional, or informal family/volunteer care in the time leading up to death'.

Features of the patient nearing the end of life include:
- Becomes increasingly weary, weak and sleepy
- Becomes less interested in getting out of bed or receiving visitors
- Becomes less interested in things happening around him/her
- Often becomes confused, occasionally with features of agitated anguish
  Care at this time is challenging, yet rewarding.
- Patient and family preference should be respected
- Advance care planning is essential
- Advance directive documentation is to be encouraged wherever feasible
- Determination of medical futility is part of decision-making
- Decisions regarding interventions, e.g. stents for symptom control, nasogastric feeding and medication versus parenteral nutrition, should be made jointly by the patient and family, supported by professionals. NCCN guidelines indicate a lack of benefit of such interventions when death is estimated to be in weeks
- Route of medication is important:
  - Some drugs are absorbed sublingually, e.g. morphine, buprenorphine hyoscine and lorazepam
  - Subcutaneous route allows ease of administration at home (a cocktail can be prepared for the following 24 hours and administered by the patient or relatives)
  - Rectal and transdermal routes are also preferred at this stage
- Only essential medications should be continued and reviewed regularly

Ethics in end of life care
- Decisions for interventions are based on the 'total clinical goal' for every patient and not just on immediate consequence
- Quality of life is paramount; based on joint decisions between physician and family
- Determination of 'medical futility' extends to decision-making regarding 'withholding and withdrawing' unnecessary interventions, e.g. vasopressors, dialysis, ventilator support, assisted nutrition and hydration
- Advance care directives, written in advance, help in decision-making during the terminal phase:
  - One copy should be held in the patient's medical record and another with treating institution records
  - These are followed in many developed countries
- Advance care directive should include instructions on resuscitation, i.e. 'Do not resuscitate', indicating withholding CPR
- Where decision-making is in conflict, physicians should seek guidance and collaboration from colleagues, higher authorities and the court
- Place of death should be where the patient and family are best supported
- Euthanasia is defined as 'the deliberate and painless termination of life of a person afflicted with an incurable and progressive disease leading inexorably to death':
  - Not to be confused with cessation of futile treatment

Place of care

Hospital versus home care versus hospice care should be the choice of the patient and family, and their decision may change many times over the course of the disease.

Home care
- Adequate support can be provided by home care teams; cost effective; saves unnecessary admissions
- Effective if home care teams can provide adequate holistic care:
  - Training and availability are essential
- Studies have shown the importance of family physicians or hospice rapid response teams for provision of 'out of hours care'

Hospice care
- Hospices can care for patients when symptom control is difficult at home or adequate family support is not available:
  - While patients like to be surrounded by their family, caregivers also need to care for the rest of their family
- In a country like India, this option is not often exercised; family units are strong and are able to provide sufficient care with the help of professionals

Bereavement support

This is an integral component of palliative care.
- Should be offered by all palliative care teams until such time as the next of kin are able to move on in life
- Normal grief is experienced by 90% of families
- Prolonged, delayed or excessive depression can be life threatening and prolonged intervention may be necessary
- Studies have shown that intervention too soon by palliative care teams can be detrimental; early intervention should be reserved for those families showing abnormal grief
- Optimum timing of a bereavement visit is a topic of research and there are currently conflicting reports in literature

Research and palliative care

As in any other branch of clinical medicine, there is a need for evidence-based research. Traditionally, the palliative care of patients at home or in a hospice made research efforts very difficult. However, in the past 10 years there has been a great increase in research, though few studies are at level I or II. It is interesting to note that there as much research is being undertaken by nurses as by doctors.

Paediatric palliative care

As examples from the Western literature, the incidence of children needing palliative care in children in Canada was 14.7 per 10,000 between 1984 and 1994, and in Australia, the crude average incidence is 13.8 per 10,000 for those under the age of 15 years. There are no accurate estimates for developing countries, including India, where childhood death from acute conditions and malnutrition is far higher than from cancer.

- Hynson speculates that the spectre of death is ever present in the cancer disease course as a consequence of infection or any other complication
- The presence of the palliative care physician from the inception of therapy has been referred to as 'upstream palliative care', where the seriousness of the situation is revisited at regular intervals
- In the disease course, transition to palliative care may come after years of treatment, e.g. for acute lymphatic leukaemia; the spectre of sudden death is a reality
- The presence of the palliative care team provides supportive or holistic care, looking after physical symptoms while providing psychological and social support to the family
- The child and family become familiar with the palliative care team who assist in taking care of every need
- As the disease progresses, the involvement of the palliative care team increases
- A good strategy is for the palliative care team to be present at every tumour board meeting
- Children often enter the palliative care pathway while continuing with some form of palliative chemotherapy; this helps the family come to terms with the situation, with the palliative care team supporting them through the whole process
- When chemotherapy is no longer beneficial, family support continues, enabling a smooth transition into palliative care only

Recommended reading

Artherholt SB, Fann JR (2012) Psychosocial care in cancer. *Curr Psychiatry Rep* 14(1):23–29.

Baines M, Oliver DJ, Carter RL (1985) Medical management of intestinal obstruction in patients with advanced malignant disease. *Lancet* 2:990–993.

Butler C, Holdsworth LM, Coulton S, Gage H (2012) Evaluation of a hospice rapid response community service: a controlled evaluation. *BMC Palliat Care* 30:11.

Cairns R (2011) Advance care planning: thinking ahead to achieve our patients' goals. *Br J Commun Nurs* 427:16.

Dennis K, Librach SL, Chow E (2011) Palliative care and oncology: integration leads to better care. *Oncology* 25(13):1271–1275.

Dickman A (2010) *Drugs in Palliative Care*. Oxford: Oxford University Press.

Ferrell BR, Coyle N, eds. (2010) *Oxford Textbook of Palliative Nursing*, 3rd edn. Oxford: Oxford University Press.

Geppert CM, Andrews MR, Druyan ME (2010) Ethical issues in artificial nutrition and hydration: a review. *J Parenter Enteral Nutr* 34(1):79–88.

Hanks G, Cherny NI, Christakis NA, Fallon M, Kaasa S, Portenoy RK, eds. (2009) *Oxford Textbook of Palliative Medicine*, 4th edn. Oxford: Oxford University Press.

Harman SM, Braun UK, Howie LI, Harris PF, Jayes RL (2012) To stent or not to stent: an evidence based approach to palliative procedures at the end of life. *J Pain Symptom Manage* 43(4):795–801.

Holland JC, Breitbart WS, Jacobsen PB, Lederberg MS, Loscalzo MJ, McCorkle R, eds. (2007) *Psycho-Oncology*, 2nd edn. Oxford: Oxford University Press.

Hoskin P, Makin W, eds. (2009) *Oncology for Palliative Medicine*, 2nd edn. Oxford: Oxford University Press.

Hudson P (2003) Home-based support for palliative care families: challenges and recommendations. *Med J Aust* 179(6 Suppl):S35–57.

Jox RJ, Schaider A, Marckmann G, Borasio GD (2012) Medical futility at the end of life: the perspectives of intensive care and palliative care clinicians. *J Med Ethics* 38(9):540–545.

Kaye P (1996) *Breaking Bad News: Ten Step Approach*. Northampton: EPL Publications.

Kissane D, Bultz B, Butow P, Finlay I, eds. (2010) *Handbook of Communication in Oncology and Palliative Care*. Oxford: Oxford University Press.

Jox RJ, Schaider A, Marckmann G, Borasio GD (2012) Medical futility at the end of life: the perspectives of intensive care and palliative care clinicians. *J Med Ethics* 38(9):540–545.

Lorenz KA, Lynn J, Dy SM et al. (2008) Evidence for improving palliative care at the end of life: a systematic review. *Ann Intern Med* 148(2):147–159.

Lloyd-Williams M, Reeve J, Kissane D (2008) Distress in palliative care patients: developing patient-centred approaches to clinical management. *Eur J Cancer* 44(8):1133–1138.

Narayanasamy A (2007) Palliative care and spirituality. *Indian J Palliat Care* 13:32–41.

NCCN Clinical Practical Guidelines in Oncology (NCCN Guidelines). (2012) Version 2.2012 04/23/12 National Comprehensive Cancer Network Inc.

Puchalski C, Ferrell B, Virani R et al. (2009) Improving the quality of spiritual care as a dimension of palliative care: The Report of the Consensus Conference. *J Palliat Med* 12(10):885–904.

Rocque GB, Cleary JF (2012) Palliative care reduces morbidity and mortality in cancer. *Nat Rev Clin Oncol* 10(2):80–89.

Schut H, Stroebe MS (2005) Interventions to enhance adaptation to bereavement. *J Palliat Med* 8(Suppl 1):S140–147.

Sepúlveda C, Marlin A, Yoshida T, Ullrich V (2002) Palliative Care: The World Health Organization's Global Perspective. *J Pain Symptom Manage* 24(2):91–96.

Twycross RG, Wilcock A, Stark Toller C, eds. (2009) *Symptom Management in Advanced Cancer*, 4th edn. Palliative Drugs.com Ltd.

Volker DL, Wu HL (2011) Cancer patients' preferences for control at the end of life. *Qual Health Res* 21(12):1618–1631.

Wright M (2004) Hospice care and models of spirituality. *Eur J Palliat Care* 11(2):75–78.

18 Survivorship

Jennifer M. Jones[1], Felicia Knaul[2], Meredith Giuliani[3], Danielle Rodin[1] and Pamela Catton[1]

[1]The Princess Margaret Cancer Centre/University Health Network, University of Toronto, Toronto, ON, Canada
[2]Harvard Global Equity Initiative, Boston, MA, USA
[3]Department of Radiation Oncology, The Princess Margaret Cancer Centre, University of Toronto, Toronto, ON, Canada

Introduction: Why survivorship?

The issues of living well, with and beyond cancer, begin at diagnosis, continue throughout life and present diverse and unexpected challenges. They are influenced by many factors including: age and developmental phase at diagnosis, type and stage of cancer, complexity of treatment and duration of post-treatment survival. Other factors that impact the survivorship experience include: financial and geographical access to necessary follow-up care and community resources, information and unmet supportive care needs, literacy and level of education, employment status, levels of gender and other types of discrimination, availability of patient protection legislation, and health insurance or financial protection. The impact and interplay of these factors are magnified in low- and middle-income countries (LMICs).

The number of cancer survivors worldwide is significant and projected to grow. According to the World Health Organization (WHO), the incidence of cancer in 2030 will be 21.3 million, up from 13.3 million in 2010. This is primarily due to population ageing and better screening methods. Current estimates are that 25 million people are living post a cancer diagnosis worldwide. In North America, advances in early detection and treatment have resulted in an overall 5-year relative cancer survival rate of 68% though this ranges widely with rates as high as 96% for prostate cancer and as low as 17% for lung cancer. While based on older treatment regimens, North American SEER statistics demonstrate 20-year relative survival in over 50% of patients diagnosed with the following cancers: thyroid (95%), testis (88%), melanoma (83%), prostate (81%), uterus (79%), bladder (68%), non-Hodgkin lymphoma (67%), breast (65%), cervix (60%) and colon (52%). Survivors who are 19 years of age or younger comprise only 1% of prevalent cases, young adults (20–39 years) make up 5%, and those aged 40–59 years account for 24%. The largest subgroup of survivors is those over 60 years of age (70%).

The growing numbers of cancer survivors pose numerous challenges to our healthcare systems. Long-term cancer survivors now present with a range of persistent and late-onset side effects and the evidence base to guide the identification and management of these problems is lacking. Existing cancer care delivery systems have limited capacity to accommodate the growing number of cancer survivors and provide them with access to quality, long-term health care. The combination of these factors is driving innovations in cancer care delivery, a research and education agenda to fill gaps in our knowledge base and skills, and a consumer survivorship advocacy movement to direct individual, organizational and systems change.

Definitions of survivor and survivorship

Cancer survivorship is a relatively new and uncharted area of health care that has still not been adequately defined and researched. Since the concept was first brought forward in the mid-1980s, there has been conflict about its definition, but most institutions have opted for an inclusive approach and this is what is applied in this chapter: cancer survivorship applied to anyone with a personal history of cancer, including caregivers, family members and friends, who have also been affected by the diagnosis (Box 18.1).

The lack of clarity surrounding various definitions should not take away from the very real issues facing cancer patients, cancer care organizations and healthcare delivery systems

---

Dr Pamela Catton passed away on December 23rd 2014. She was a skilled and compassionate clinician, and a creative and driving force in education and cancer survivorship. A true visionary, Dr Catton has left an important and impactful legacy and has been a pathfinder for what we now know as patient-centred care. She is a true example of one person making an important difference in this world.

UICC Manual of Clinical Oncology, Ninth Edition. Edited by Brian O'Sullivan, James D. Brierley, Anil K. D'Cruz, Martin F. Fey, Raphael Pollock, Jan B. Vermorken and Shao Hui Huang. © 2015 UICC. Published 2015 by John Wiley & Sons, Ltd.

> **Box 18.1** Evolving definition of survivor and survivorship
>
> 1985 Dr Fitzhugh Mullan wrote an article in the *New England Journal of Medicine* describing his personal experience of cancer as three seasons of survival. He felt the medical approach was lacking when dealing with his post-treatment supportive care needs.
>
> 1986 Mullan co-founded the National Coalition for Cancer Survivorship (www.canceradvocacy.org), the first community advocacy and support organization to offer a definition of a 'cancer survivor': anyone with a personal history of cancer and those family members and friends who have also been affected by the diagnosis.
>
> 1990 The US National Cancer Institute (NCI) Office of Cancer Survivorship Research was established and adopted this very inclusive definition.
>
> 2006 A report by the Institute of Medicine (IOM), entitled Lost in Transition, made 10 recommendations to improve the quality of cancer care in the USA, particularly directed at the post-treatment, or survivorship, phase of the cancer control continuum.
>
> The survivorship phase has in turn been divided for research purposes into two parts: early post treatment or re-entry (12–60 months post treatment) and extended survivorship, thereafter.
>
> The term 'survivor' continues to generate confusion, discussion and heated debate among cancer patients and healthcare practitioners as to its appropriateness and acceptability in many countries.

Table 18.1 Components of survivorship health care

> - Surveillance for cancer and persistent and late physical and psychological effects
> - Managing persistent and late physical and psychosocial effects
> - Prevention and health promotion
> - Surveillance and co-morbid illness
> - Healthcare coordination to ensure that all long-term health and wellness needs are met

providing cancer care following treatment in variably resourced settings. This chapter highlights opportunities to build quality survivorship care around the world. It addresses the priorities and challenges of clinical care, research, education and advocacy for post-treatment adult survivorship, i.e. individuals who develop cancer aged 18 or older, at any point along the care trajectory following treatment. Beyond the scope of this chapter are the very important issues of survivorship for children living with cancer, and adult survivors of paediatric cancer. The Childhood Cancer Survivor Study has produced a number of review articles (https://ccss.stjude.org/published-research/reviews) that address a variety of outcomes in this population.

Survivorship clinical priorities and challenges

Essential elements of survivorship care

Patients moving out of active treatment have particular requirements for health care that should be oriented to maintain or improve their overall health and wellness. Health in this context reflects the ability to successfully adapt to physical, emotional and social challenges; wellness reflects the ability to proactively achieve a state of positive well-being. Ideally, the goals of post-treatment cancer care should align with this patient-centred wellness approach, and shift away from a disease orientation.

Survivorship health care should include the following components (Table 18.1):

1 Risk-informed surveillance for active cancer, including locoregional recurrence, metastatic spread, treatment-induced second primary cancers and the appearance of new related and unrelated primary cancers
2 Detection and treatment of persistent and late-onset effects of the cancer treatment
3 Routine health checks for common non-cancer health problems
4 Health promotion activities to:
   - Reduce the risk of cancer recurrence or new primaries
   - Mitigate the risk of late effects
   - Ameliorate the symptoms of persistent and late side effects
   - Improve overall wellbeing and quality of life.

These are complex goals and require the involvement of many different healthcare providers. The greater the number of people involved, the greater the need for a coordinated systems of care with excellent team communication. At present, there is substantial variability in the approach taken to and overall quality of care received by survivors.

Surveillance

Ongoing surveillance is an essential component of survivorship care to ensure that new or recurrent cancers are detected at a time when treatment may be most effective. While close surveillance in high-risk periods can result in effective locoregional salvage treatment for many types of cancer, early detection of distant recurrence rarely results in improved outcomes. Evidence from randomized trials of common malignancies, including breast, prostate and gynaecological cancers, have shown that intensive follow-up, comprised of frequent visits with routine blood work, tumour markers and cross-sectional imaging, does not prolong survival. As a result, follow-up guidelines generally recommend against the use of routine tumour markers or imaging. Exceptions include situations where early treatment has been shown to result in long-term survival, such as in the resection of oligometastases of the liver in colorectal cancer. With this evidence, there are ongoing efforts to stem the extensive overuse of imaging to detect metastases in various jurisdictions. Evidence-based guidelines and consensus statements are increasing in number and have been released and updated by the American Society of Clinical Oncology (ASCO) for breast and colorectal cancer follow-up. In addition, the National Comprehensive Cancer Network (NCCN), which has developed over 100 clinical guidelines for cancer, has also incorporated limited consensus-based recommendation for surveillance and management of common problems faced by cancer survivors. The National Guidelines Clearinghouse (www.guideline.gov) and the Cochrane Collaboration (www.thecochranelibrary.com) are searchable databases for guidelines that include what is currently available for cancer patient follow-up. However, guidelines are not available for all cancer types and vary considerably in their comprehensiveness. Many of the guidelines provide inconsistent recommendations regarding the frequency, duration and type of follow-up that is required for different survivor groups. The issue is compounded by the limited uptake of guidelines into clinical practice, and their relevance in LMICs.

It should be noted that surveillance visits also provide an opportunity to screen for persistent and late-onset physical side effects, psychosocial concerns and general health issues. Individuals aged over 70 years represent a major proportion of incident cases, and elderly cancer survivors report poorer quality of life and more chronic conditions, psychological and functional problems, and are at higher risk of functional decline compared to age-matched controls. The frequency and nature of follow-up visits for persistent and late effects should also be tailored to the risk profile of the survivor. An increasing number of clinical practice guidelines are also being developed to assist practitioners in this regard, but much more research is needed to build knowledge in this area.

Managing persistent and late side effects

Significant improvements in long-term survival have come about because of the increasing complexity of cancer treatments over the past three decades, i.e. new chemotherapeutic and biological agents, multiagent chemotherapy protocols with dose intensification, more radical surgeries with improved reconstruction strategies, and high precision, dose escalating, altered fractionation radiation therapy regimens. Combinations of these modalities are usually the norm, and treatment is associated with a wide range of previously undocumented side effects that persist beyond the conclusion of therapy (persistent), or may appear after a latent period of months to years (late onset). These toxicities can be further complicated by pre-existing risk factors such as age, co-morbidities, genetic profile, as well as behavioural and lifestyle factors. They can impact survivors physically, emotionally, practically and spiritually. While there is a growing appreciation of the extent to which cancer survivors must manage persistent and late-onset side effects, knowledge regarding the exact incidence, prevalence and risk is limited, and effective approaches to mitigate many of these side effects are lacking.

Most of the physical side effects tend to be specific to the type of cancer and treatment, and can affect all body systems. The more intensive the treatment, the more likely the symptoms will persist. Although patients are warned of the acute effects of treatment, they are often unprepared for their persistence and slow resolution after treatment. Clinical assessment systems need to be modified to identify late-onset side effects, such as fertility challenges in patients of reproductive age; treatment-induced menopausal symptoms; bone loss in women on aromatase inhibitors or following treatment-induced ovarian failure and in men on antiandrogen therapy; patients at risk for lymphoedema; sexual health issues in both genders; cardiotoxicity; digestive problems; and organ functional loss such as faecal and urinary incontinence.

Cancer survivors can also experience a variety of interrelated side effects that can vary in frequency, intensity and level of perceived distress, and which have been shown to influence functional status, quality of life, cancer recurrence rates and even survival. Fatigue, sleep disturbances, chronic pain, cancer-related cognitive dysfunction, depression and anxiety often cluster together.

Cancer-related fatigue

Cancer-related fatigue (CRF) and related sleep–wake disturbances are among the most commonly reported (up to 50% of survivors) and distressing side effects that can persist for years after successful completion of cancer therapy. This can result in adverse mood changes, emotional distress and amplification of concurrent symptoms, leading to reduced physical, psychosocial and cognitive functioning and interfering with the resumption of normal daily activities, including precancer roles at home and at work. CRF persists even after correction of anaemia or endocrine abnormalities. It is a subjective sense of exhaustion not proportional to recent activity. Survivors describe themselves as being 'bone weary', in spite of adequate amounts of rest and sleep. The aetiology is likely multifactorial. Patients should be routinely screened for CRF after cancer treatment. There is strong and consistent evidence supporting the effectiveness of exercise, education and support, and information addressing sleep hygiene and energy conservation strategies.

Pain

Pain is another very common symptom associated with cancer and its treatment. Over 50% of patients experience pain at some point in the disease process, and up to 75% in the advanced stages of cancer. Pain may be acute or chronic and can fluctuate throughout the course of the disease and into the survivorship phase, thereby reducing quality of life. In a recent US survey, over one-third of cancer survivors reported ongoing pain. Pain may represent recurrent disease, chronic post-treatment pain syndromes or other non-cancer related co-morbidities. Patients should be counselled to report pain promptly, and should be routinely screened for pain during and after cancer treatment. Early identification and effective interdisciplinary management is imperative. Clinicians should also address the related physical and psychosocial concerns.

Cancer-related cognitive dysfunction
Cancer-related cognitive dysfunction (CRCD), otherwise known as chemo-brain and cancer-related brain-fog, is also commonly reported in cancer survivors. In cancers directly involving the brain, the location of the brain tumour or metastasis dictates which cognitive abilities are impacted. In cancers outside of the brain, deficits are less focal but are also commonly reported. Estimates of the frequency of CRCD are as high as 75% during therapy. While most survivors notice symptoms during treatment, some start experiencing symptoms at the time of diagnosis. Cognitive functioning often improves after treatment, but for one in three, symptoms persist for months to years. The precise causes of CRCD are poorly understood, are likely multifactorial and may change over time. They include the cancer diagnosis, surgery, chemotherapy, radiation therapy, and/or other therapy (e.g. stem cell transplant, endocrine treatment), anaemia, hormone changes (e.g. menopause), infection, stress, depression and/or anxiety, fatigue, lack of sleep, lack of proper nutrition, and pain and/or pain medications. There is no agreed upon neurocognitive clinical assessment strategy, and most screening tests do not pick up subtle changes induced by treatment. However, even subtle changes in cognitive functioning may be problematic for those with high cognitive demands. They report changes in attention, concentration, working memory and executive function, and note they have to work harder to achieve pretreatment levels of mental functioning. It is important to rule out other medical conditions that can cause cognitive dysfunction to avoid misdiagnosis. While there are no currently available pharmacological treatments that will eliminate symptoms, dealing with other contributing conditions such as sleep disturbances, depression, anxiety, fatigue and anaemia are beneficial. Cognitive rehabilitation approaches which include information about cognitive problems and validation of experiences, education regarding possible compensatory strategies (e.g. memory aids), and stress reduction (e.g. relaxation training) may contribute to improved functioning, coping and adjustment.

Psychosocial distress
The psychological burden of cancer includes anxiety (particularly fear of recurrence or disease progression), feelings of helplessness and hopelessness, depression and problems due to changes in body image, self-concept, self-esteem and identity. The experience of anxiety may be precipitated by known or unknown stimuli, and can range from normal feelings of vulnerability to disabling problems such as depression, panic and social isolation. While the prevalence of anxiety and/or depression in the first year post diagnosis may be as high as 30–50% and may persist up to 5 years post treatment, there is evidence that long-term survivors do adapt positively and over time successfully resolve many psychological challenges. Incorporating routine screening into surveillance visits is the best method to ensure that psychological issues are consistently addressed. A number of symptom screening tools, such as the Distress Thermometer or the Edmonton Symptom Assessment System (ESAS), are often used to identify distress at regular surveillance visits. Many cancer control jurisdictions have implemented routine distress screening during the treatment phase and are considering modifications to these clinical assessment tools to embed questions related to long-term survivorship issues. When concerns develop into significant distress that affects functioning and quality of life, further assessment and interventions are required. Treatments for psychological distress range from non-pharmacological interventions, such as counselling, cognitive behavioural therapy and support groups, to medications and complementary therapy.

Prevention and health promotion
The aetiology of cancer is a multifactorial interaction of genetic, environmental and lifestyle factors. There is increasing evidence that physical activity, dietary choices, maintaining a healthy weight and smoking cessation may prevent secondary or recurrent cancers, and reduce many of the physical and psychological consequences of cancer treatment. Cancer survivors can be empowered to reduce their risk through health promotion strategies and may be more inclined to make lifestyle changes and adopt more healthy behaviours following the conclusion of cancer treatment to improve their situation.

Exercise
Physical activity, with or without dietary changes, can improve general health and reduce the incidence of breast, colon, endometrial and prostate cancers. There are numerous studies in breast and colon cancer populations which suggest a risk reduction of 25–30%. In breast cancer studies, risk reduction is associated with volume of exercise. The greatest benefit of exercise may in fact be following a cancer diagnosis. An impressive and growing body of literature describes the benefits for the cancer survivor during and after treatment. These benefits include improvements in fatigue, functional capacity, mood, appetite, sleep quality, body composition, treatment tolerance and overall quality of life. Furthermore, there is mounting evidence that physical activity can also reduce cancer recurrence and mortality rates in breast, colorectal and prostate cancer. The physiological benefits of exercise for the cancer survivor are now starting to be revealed and likely occur via several biological mechanisms, including sex hormones, stress and inflammatory cytokines, and adipokine regulatory pathways.

Diet
Dietary factors are linked to the development of one-third of cancers in industrialized countries. Eating fruits and non-starchy vegetables is associated with a decreased risk of upper aerodigestive cancers. Intake of fibre-rich foods is associated with a reduced incidence of colorectal cancer. Dietary behavioural modification interventions have effectively modified the intake of fruit, vegetables, fibre and dietary fat, and resulted in improved weight and body composition. However, the data are inconclusive on whether diet alone can reduce cancer recurrence rates and impact survival. Vitamins and dietary supplements have not been shown to prevent cancer.

Obesity

Obesity is an important cancer risk factor linked convincingly to an increased risk of postmenopausal breast, oesophageal, pancreatic, colorectal, endometrial and kidney cancers. The link between cancer recurrence and obesity is less well defined, but evidence is mounting in postmenopausal breast cancer that it is a poor prognostic factor.

Alcohol and tobacco use

Excessive alcohol consumption increases the risk of developing breast, oropharyngeal, laryngeal, oesophageal, colorectal and liver cancer. The relative risk increases with the amount consumed. When combined with tobacco use, it accounts for over three-quarters of the cancers of the mouth, pharynx, larynx and oesophagus.

Tobacco use alone is strongly linked to an increased risk for numerous cancers. Substantial evidence has shown that continued smoking may reduce the effectiveness of treatment, worsen the side effects and increase the likelihood of a second primary cancer. Smoking cessation has been shown specifically to improve the outcomes of patients with lung and head and neck cancers, in addition to its many other health benefits.

It is reasonable to offer exercise, dietary or smoking cessation programmes to survivors on the basis of improved outcomes. Programmes should be tailored to meet individual survivor goals, ability level and available community resources.

Health promotion aims to create the social, environmental, structural and individual requirements for a health-promoting lifestyle. Patient education and health promotion are usually based on manualized training and treatment programmes that focus on typical problems (i.e. fatigue, cognitive dysfunction, anxiety, fear of recurrence, dietary changes, exercise programmes and smoking cessation). Key components of health promotion programs are to:
- Increase knowledge and confidence
- Apply an effective behaviour change model (such as the transtheoretical model of change, social cognitive theory or cognitive behavioural theory)
- Improve the acquisition of self-management skills and social skills to mobilize support.

Unfortunately adherence and sustainability are big challenges, particularly in certain subgroups like the elderly.

Controlled studies have shown that over time cancer survivors are more likely than population-based controls to adopt multiple healthy behaviours. Follow-up visits provide the clinician with the opportunity to routinely evaluate current behaviours and encourage cancer survivors to maintain a healthy weight and be physically active, and to counsel on alcohol and tobacco use.

Healthcare delivery and coordination

Strategies for the delivery of post-treatment survivorship care are under development in many cancer control jurisdictions, organizations and care settings. Barriers to organizing quality survivorship care include, but are not limited to:
- An acute care orientation that is reactive rather than proactive
- Fragmented and poorly coordinated cancer care system
- Absence of a locus of responsibility for follow-up care among, at times, a group of oncology specialists and the primary care provider
- Poor mechanisms for communication among the many members of the healthcare team
- Lack of guidance about the specific tests, examinations, advice and treatment that make up survivorship care
- Lack of focus on health promotion and chronic disease prevention
- Healthcare providers who are ill prepared to provide comprehensive survivorship care, by virtue of their lack of awareness, knowledge or skill.

The components of high quality care are listed in Table 18.2.

The ultimate objective of good quality cancer care is to achieve desired outcomes for survivors, who want not only to survive the cancer but also to live well. Functional status, quality of life and the experience of cancer care are important outcomes, often overshadowed by the emphasis on reducing recurrence rates and improving survival. Along with individual patient characteristics, the processes and structure of care are important contributors to these outcomes. Process is the set of activities that goes on between the patient and the provider, and includes both the technical and interpersonal quality of care. Structural dimensions of healthcare quality include the resources needed to provide medical care, such as the availability of imaging, specialized services, and even the professional education and competence of the provider.

A number of reports and publications have recommended various service delivery processes and structures for patients following the end of treatment. Several models of follow-up care have been identified, including the interdisciplinary survivorship clinic, with access to specialized services to meet a wide range of needs; nurse-led, family physician-led, specialist or oncologist-led follow-up care; and shared-care models. More recently, survivor-initiated models of care have been identified

Table 18.2 Components of high-quality survivorship care

- Comprehensive, multidisciplinary and accessible
- Tailored to meet individual needs
- Encompasses preventive as well as reactive health management
- Includes specialized rehabilitation services for physical and psychosocial issues
- Empowers survivors to take a role in their own health management to the extent that they wish
- Uses effective communication strategies to promote planned and coordinated follow-up
- Is evidence based and supported by appropriate guidelines, policies and research to ensure that care is outcomes focused, cost-effective and sustainable

Adapted from Lotfi-Jam K, Schofield P, Jefford M (2009). What constitutes ideal survivorship care? *Cancer Forum* 33(3):179–182.

as a possible approach in the UK, with telehealth and ehealth strategies under investigation. Currently, across cancer organizations, the various models of follow-up care have emerged based on local health policy, or by default due to lack of consensus on the most effective approach. Systematic review on survivorship models of care have been performed and, in general, the current evidence is rated as low quality, being based predominantly on consensus guidelines and a limited number of randomized studies in breast, prostate, lung and colorectal cancer patients. The data suggest that nurse-led and family physician models of follow-up care in certain low-risk populations, mostly breast cancer patients, were equivalent for detecting recurrence.

These guidelines reflect a global consensus that the traditional model of oncologist and cancer centre follow-up for the growing number of cancer survivors is not sustainable. There is a movement to increase system capacity by exploring risk-based models, where primary care practitioners (PCPs) take over care of patients in low-risk and low-complexity situations, such as in post-surgical colorectal and prostate cancer patients, and post-adjuvant treatment of breast cancer patients. In patients with persistent ongoing post-treatment issues at a higher risk of recurrence or who need specialized examinations to detect recurrence, e.g. gynaecological and head & neck cancer patients, a shared care model may be more appropriate. This system has a number of strengths with cancer surveillance and side effect management being the focus of the oncologist, and preventative and other healthcare services the domain of the PCP. Coordinated care between the specialist and the PCP is essential to ensure that all the healthcare needs are met. Regular, effective communication and clear delineation of roles is essential.

Most of the guidelines identified have provided certain recommendations on the nature of follow-up, who should be involved, what type of specialized services ought to be available and what communication tools should be used. Optimal and successful transitions can be facilitated using tools such as a Survivorship Care Plan (SCP). A SCP is a comprehensive and individualized treatment summary and care plan, comprised of information on the patient's diagnosis, cancer treatments and the ongoing follow-up care and monitoring required. Its proposed components are listed in Table 18.3. The goal is to generate a plan that is personalized to a patient's specific disease, treatments and identified needs. Ideally, the SCP should go beyond surveillance recommendations for recurrence, and address side effects, risk reduction and health promotion strategies. While data to support the effectiveness of SCPs is still needed, SCPs have the potential to support appropriate healthcare practices by survivors and healthcare providers, and enhance team communication.

In 2011, the Cancer Journey Survivorship Expert Panel published an evidence-based pan-Canadian guideline outlining 11 recommendations for the organization and care delivery structure for survivorship services in Canada, and a further eight recommendations for psychosocial and supportive care interventions, articulating the current clinical priorities and providing a comprehensive roadmap for the design and delivery of quality cancer survivorship care (Table 18.4). These recommendations can provide a framework to groups looking to establish survivorship care and services in resource-constrained settings. However, they will need to be adapted and redefined within the local context of care.

Table 18.3 Elements of a survivorship care plan recommended by the Institute of Medicine (IOM) of the National Academies (USA)

- Cancer type, treatments received and their potential consequences
- Specific information about the timing and content of recommended follow-up
- Recommendations about preventive practitioners and how to maintain health and well-being
- Information about legal protections regarding employment and access to health insurance
- Availability of psychosocial services in the community

Adapted from Hewitt ME, Stovall E, Greenfield S, National Cancer Policy Board (US) Committee on Cancer Survivorship: Improving Care and Quality of Life (2006). *From Cancer Patient to Cancer Survivor: Lost in Transition*. Washington, D.C: National Academies Press.

Table 18.4 Survivorship services for adult cancer populations: A pan-Canadian guideline

Organization and care delivery structure for survivorship services	Psychosocial and supportive care interventions
Access to survivorship services to meet a broad range of needs	Supporting healthy lifestyle behaviours
Support during the transition to extended survival	Use health behaviour theory-based approaches
Treatment summary and follow-up care plan	Management of psychosocial concerns and distress
Care models and coordination of survivorship services	Monitoring for symptoms and late and long-term effects
Screening for distress and evidence-based practice	Management of concerns about sexual health
Support active engagement of survivors in self-management	Management of post-treatment fatigue
Survivorship education for healthcare providers	Management of vasomotor symptoms
Promoting awareness of survivorship issues	Management of disruption in sleep–wake patterns
Leadership in research	
Evaluation of services	
Inclusive health public policy	

Adapted from Howell D et al (2011). *Curr Oncol* 18(6):e265–e281.

Survivorship care in low and middle income countries

LMICs face the triple burden of injuries and communicable and non-communicable diseases. Notably, they must also deal with 80% of the global cancer burden, yet receive only 5% of global financial resources for the disease. They are particularly challenged to address chronic illness within a resource-constrained and deeply fragmented healthcare system. The chronicity of survivorship is an area that few LMICs have faced or tackled, and knowledge about specific needs and appropriate approaches is scarce. Developing comprehensive cancer care programs in LMICs, of which survivorship is but one component, necessitates resource allocation based on country-specific needs. For this reason, international conversation and shared learning is required.

In 2005, the Breast Health Global Initiative (BHGI), an alliance and network of governmental and non-governmental organizations dedicated to breast cancer prevention, treatment and research, held the Global Summit Consensus Conference on International Breast Healthcare. This summit provided a forum for breast cancer survivors and advocates from 12 countries to describe their experiences with breast cancer and advocacy in their home countries. This allowed for commonalities and differences amongst survivors from different countries to be explored and for strategies to be developed to advance survivorship advocacy globally. As a result of this initiative, three consensus statements on resource-stratified recommendations to address the supportive care needs of curative (during treatment and survivorship) and metastatic breast cancer patients have been published.

An important goal of the survivorship movement is to eliminate the 'fatalism cycle', which has been described in the breast cancer literature from LMICs. This refers to the self-defeating phenomenon in which breast cancer stigma and fatalism lead to late presentation to a healthcare provider, resulting in poorer outcomes with fewer survivors to put a face to the disease and further propagation of stigma and fatalism. Recently, community-based organizations, non-governmental organizations and other grassroots initiatives have begun to emerge from within LMICs, to interrupt this cycle. For example, the Medical Women Association of Tanzania disseminates evidence-based cancer information to increase public awareness of common cancers in Tanzania, dispelling myths, correcting misconceptions and promoting adaptive health-seeking behaviours. As well, organizations from within Europe and North America have begun to support the development of survivorship programs in LMICs. For example, Reach to Recovery International (RRI), a network of breast cancer support groups, offers a 'twinning' programme, whereby new groups may use the support and expertise of an established group in order to build their own programme.

Multiple stakeholder involvement – including governments, industry and the public – and the adoption of a diagonal approach for the optimal use of human and physical resources at the primary and secondary levels, are required for effective, comprehensive cancer care in LMICs.

Box 18.2 Breast cancer survivorship in Mexico: A case study

Mexico is an upper–middle income country that is taking steps to address the challenge of cancer in ways that will increase survival and generate a need for survivorship services. As of 2007, all Mexican women have access to an extensive package of breast cancer treatments under the national health insurance programme Seguro Popular, introduced in 2004 as part of a major health-reform process.

With more women being treated and surviving the disease, there is recognition that cost-effective survivorship care is needed. In response to this challenge, in October 2013, a coalition of hospitals, academic institutions and the private sector hosted an international seminar to inform Mexican institutions on best practices in breast cancer survivorship care.

'Breast Cancer and Survivorship: Challenges and Responses' was led by Tómatelo a Pecho AC and the Mexican Health Foundation, and brought together patients, advocates and international experts from leading institutions, representing experiences from the USA, Canada, England, Costa Rica, Bangladesh and India. The seminar highlighted the importance of survivorship care in the context of the epidemiological profile of breast cancer in Mexico, and the need for both institutional and legal responses.

The National Cancer Institute of Mexico unveiled a pilot programme that will provide young women with breast cancer comprehensive treatment and survivorship care, with the goal of expanding and informing a national approach.

Mexico provides an example of an upper–middle income country that is taking steps to address the challenge of chronic illness in ways that will increase survival and generate a need for survivorship services (Box 18.2).

Survivorship research priorities and challenges

Survivorship research is a relatively new field of study, the first paper being published in 1984. However, over the past two decades, the number of articles on cancer survivorship appearing in the literature has grown substantially, including the development of survivor-specific journals such as the *Journal of Cancer Survivorship: Practice and Research* established in 2007. Funding opportunities for survivorship research are also slowly growing. Despite this, the majority of the evidence regarding late effects of cancer has been learned through the long-term follow-up of participants enrolled in clinical trials of cancer treatments. Evidence regarding the frequency, intensity and type of follow-up required for cancer survivors remains sparse and the development of optimal evidenced-based surveillance practices is a research priority. Most of our knowledge about adult survivors comes from small, single institution, cross-sectional studies. There is little long-term (>10 years) outcome data. The majority of studies have been conducted with breast cancer survivors and there has been very little research on other types of cancers. Outcomes for culturally diverse or disadvantaged populations of survivors have been underrepresented in survivorship research. Survivors over 65 years of age are also poorly represented in the literature despite the fact that they represent two-thirds of cancer survivors.

Moving forward, there is a need to develop research programmes which examine and seek to understand the concerns and issues faced by cancer survivors and to identify effective and sustainable models of care. This will require the development of new and novel epidemiological methods and large investments of time and money. *Descriptive and analytical epidemiologic research* is needed within all cancer sites in order to delineate the natural history of survivorship and document the impact of treatment on long-term outcomes, i.e. the incidence and prevalence of physical and psychological late effects, second cancers and their associated risk factors. The prospective longitudinal study of long-term physical effects is needed to supplement what is currently known from cross-sectional studies and can include such problem areas as CRDC, cardiac and endocrine dysfunction, premature menopause and the effects of co-morbidities and ageing on these adverse outcomes. Psychosocial outcomes include distress, coping, sexuality and body image, and return to work. Large collaborative comprehensive databases will need to be developed, and maintained, where collected data can be stored to support survivorship research. This will likely require multicentre cohorts and coordinated efforts through clinical trials, cooperative groups and population-based registries. With these data, models and tools to assist in risk identification after primary treatment can be developed and will be most beneficial to providers and survivors. *Interventional research*, which includes analytical study designs of cost-effective and therapeutic or lifestyle interventions to ameliorate physical, emotional, social and practical side effects of cancer and its treatment, is also urgently needed. Clinical trials using innovative hybrid designs such as nested case–control, case–cohort, and pragmatic preference trials will likely be required. It will be important for newly developed and tested interventions to be generalizable to a wide range of settings outside of tertiary care centres, take into account preferences of survivors and use a variety of modalities that can be implemented by both healthcare providers and peers. Finally, there is an important need for *health services research* to define optimal care delivery, including the type or components of care delivered, the manner in which that care is delivered and by who, and the efficacy of various models of care. The economic effect of cancer on the survivor and family, and the health and quality of life outcomes resulting from diverse patterns of care and service delivery settings must be examined. Determining the cost of delivery of many of the interventions that are found to improve quality of life and functioning is an important, but often prohibitively expensive, addition to a typical behavioural intervention study.

There are numerous challenges to moving the survivorship research agenda forward. Cancer treatments are constantly changing. New drugs and new combinations of treatment will have unknown effects on new generations of survivors. New tools and techniques to monitor and evaluate cancer's impact on individuals and their families and society over time are needed. Finding a balance between the need to identify emerging chronic and late effects of newer therapies and treating the impact of the older ones is a fundamental challenge for the research community. Another challenge is to develop new ideas and strategies to answer complex research questions, and these are more likely to arise from the multiple perspectives, skills and approaches of interdisciplinary team-based research, an approach actively encouraged by many health research institutes, including the Canadian Institutes of Health Research (CIHR), the Medical Research Council (MRC) and the National Cancer Institute (NCI). Economic constraints will continue to pose barriers to survivorship research investment, so attempts need to be made to leverage existing research mechanisms by redirecting their focus to survivorship issues, forming novel partnerships among philanthropic and government funding agencies, and establishing new focused research consortiums, e.g. the Canadian Cancer Survivorship Research Consortium (CCSRC; www.ccsrc.ca) and the European Collaborative Group on Cancer Survivorship (ECGCS; www.ecgcs.eu).

Survivorship education and capacity-building priorities

Professional education and training

Post-treatment survivorship care is a relatively new concept. Few primary healthcare professionals have had formal education and training in survivorship. Significant efforts must be made by clinicians and healthcare professional educators to raise awareness of the issues facing survivors, and explore healthcare provider knowledge and skill gaps that impact the quality of care delivered. Educational needs assessments can be done in a variety of ways, but must be used in the design and provision of education and training opportunities for practitioners to improve or maintain their practice competencies. The effectiveness of these education programmes should be routinely evaluated and the content shared broadly.

The healthcare needs of cancer survivors are complex and are best met by an interdisciplinary team of healthcare providers including, but not limited to, physicians, nurses, radiation therapists, rehabilitation therapists, psychosocial specialists, dieticians and genetic counsellors. There appears to be a significant demand for such education and the response has been particularly strong in the USA. A growing number of live and on-line courses are being developed by various professional societies and organizations, particularly for US family physicians, medical oncologists and nurses. However, these suffer from the drawback of being unidisciplinary in their focus. Calls for health professional education reform emphasize the need to develop programmes that have members of the practice team learning together. Survivorship care is provided by a number of interdisciplinary teams that form depending on the need. The education and training opportunities for interdisciplinary survivorship education need to be expanded.

Healthcare providers require easily accessible, just-in-time survivorship information, tools and support at the bedside to guide clinical practice decisions. On-line survivorship information aimed at healthcare providers' practice needs should be made widely available.

Lists of topic areas deemed 'essential' have been generated by various authors and groups. Apart from a focus on the issues of general survivorship, including models of care delivery, prevention of second cancers and health promotion, the content of these lists overlaps significantly with what would be considered a comprehensive general oncology curriculum. In general, these lists do not articulate the level of knowledge, skills or attitudinal change expected of the learners, a necessary step in competency-based education planning. In Canada, there is not yet developed or endorsed a comprehensive competency based curriculum that can serve as a guide for program development. This curriculum would be an essential first step before advocating the integration of survivorship education into current health professional undergraduate and graduate curricula. It could then be shared in free on-line peer-reviewed health education repositories such as the Health Education Assets Library (www.healcentral.org). As educators and clinicians identify and build the essential curriculum to support survivorship care, they should adopt strategies that allow the worldwide dissemination of educational programmes, products and services. This will accelerate capacity building in locally underserved areas and will also help to bridge the educational needs in LMICs.

Patient and family education

Self-management refers to the individual's ability to manage the physical and psychological consequences, and lifestyle changes inherent in living with a chronic condition. Successful self-management requires sufficient knowledge of the condition, its causes, treatment options and their subsequent problems, as well as the application of the necessary skills to maintain adequate functioning, reduce health-risk behaviours and enhance coping skills. Providing relevant and practical information, education and support has been shown to mediate meaningful changes in behaviour and lifestyle to promote health and mitigate a number of persistent and late effects such as fatigue, insomnia, CRCD, weight gain, pain and lymphoedema.

Clinicians can provide self-management support through a variety of methods including peer counselling, psychoeducation and professional coaching. In the recently published pan-Canadian Guideline for survivorship services, special note is made of the need to develop healthcare provider education to support survivor self-management, including skills in assessment, motivational interviewing and self-efficacy assessment.

Those developing patient education programmes and materials must respond to a variety of learning styles and preferences, literacy levels, language choices and multicultural needs. Information resources should be used to distribute survivorship information in readily accessible and user friendly formats, and leverage the benefits of on-line strategies. Comprehensive cancer patient education programmes require an organizational commitment and guidelines are available to guide cancer education services. The Ontario Framework describes nine core elements required for a comprehensive patient education service.

The active engagement of survivors in effective self-management is key to improving system capacity to provide quality survivorship care. Approaches require adaptation to the local cultural and healthcare context.

Survivorship advocacy

A diagnosis of cancer thrusts patients and their families into an unfamiliar and complex system of diagnostic investigation, multiple consultations and challenging treatments. The ability to advocate for themselves along the trajectory of care is an important skill set that helps to ensure optimal treatment and support. Maintaining this continuum of survivor advocacy, as described by the National Coalition for Cancer Survivorship (NCCS), is a central purpose of the survivorship movement. Such advocacy has been instrumental in the achievement of many improvements in cancer prevention, treatment and research, and in greater societal understanding and acceptance of the disease and those affected by it.

Survivorship advocacy includes personal advocacy, community advocacy and public interest advocacy. Personal advocacy is focused on self-empowerment, whereby patients become informed healthcare consumers and play an active role in the decision-making around their care. Successful survivor-advocates quickly learn to obtain accurate information about their condition, seek second opinions, access support services and demand clear explanations. Community advocacy involves survivors coming together to support each other as they face their cancer diagnosis and treatment. This may include the formation of support groups, arranging public speaking events, and the establishment of cancer patient organizations and community-based, non-governmental organizations. Public interest advocacy refers to participation by survivors in the public policy process at the local, national or international level. A successful example of this form of advocacy was seen in the lobbying efforts by cancer survivors to eliminate discriminatory insurance rules that disadvantage people with cancer histories.

The framework of survivorship advocacy has been highly effective in the Western context, particularly for breast and cervical cancer. However, cancers with poorer prognoses, such as pancreatic or lung cancers, are numerically much less represented in survivorship advocacy efforts. Similarly, cancer patients in LMICs often make their first presentation to the healthcare system when their disease is already advanced, leaving fewer survivors to lead the survivorship advocacy movement. The application of the NCCS survivorship advocacy model in LMICs has been further challenged by the limited infrastructure and resources, as well as cultural and linguistic differences. In fact, there is no direct translation of the word 'advocacy' in many languages and it has been difficult to provide culturally relevant and sensitive translations of the available survivorship material.

Conclusion

The issues of living well with and beyond cancer begin at diagnosis and continue throughout life. Life after cancer treatment holds diverse and often unexpected challenges, influenced by a significant number of clinical, personal and societal factors. Existing cancer care delivery systems have limited capacity to accommodate the growing numbers of cancer survivors, addressing the range of their physical, psychosocial and practical needs. This chapter has addressed the priorities and challenges of post-treatment adult survivorship clinical care, research, education and advocacy that should be considered both at an individual and organizational level to build capacity for quality survivorship care across variably resourced settings around the world.

Recommended reading

Ahles TA, Root JC, Ryan EL (2012) Cancer and cancer treatment-associated cognitive change: An update on the state of the science. *J Clin Oncol* 30(30):3675.

Barlow J, Wright C, Sheasby J, Turner A, Hainsworth J (2002) Self-management approaches for people with chronic conditions: a review. *Patient Educ Counsel* 48(2):177–187.

Cancer Care Ontario's Patient Education Program Committee & Program In Evidence-Based Care (PEBC) (2006). *Establishing Comprehensive Cancer Patient Education Services: A Framework to Guide Ontario Cancer Education Services*. 20-1. Toronto: Cancer Care Ontario.

Cardoso F, Bese N, Distelhorst SR *et al.* (2013) Supportive care during treatment for breast cancer: resource allocations in low- and middle-income countries. A Breast Health Global Initiative 2013 consensus statement. *Breast* 22(5):593–605.

Cleary J, Ddungu H, Distelhorst SR *et al.* (2013) Supportive and palliative care for metastatic breast cancer: resource allocations in low- and middle-income countries. A Breast Health Global Initiative 2013 consensus statement. *Breast* 22(5):616–627.

Davies NJ, Batehup L, Thomas R (2011) The role of diet and physical activity in breast, colorectal, and prostate cancer survivorship: A review of the literature. *Br J Cancer* 105:S52–S73.

Errico KM, Rowden D (2006) Experiences of breast cancer survivor-advocates and advocates in countries with limited resources: A shared journey in breast cancer advocacy. *Breast J* 12:S111–S116.

Ferlay J, Shin HR, Bray F, Forman D, Mathers C, Parkin DM (2010) *GLOBOCAN 2008 v1.2, Cancer Incidence and Mortality Worldwide: IARC CancerBase No. 10*. Lyon: International Agency for Research on Cancer. Available at http://globocan.iarc.fr. [Accessed November 2013].

Feuerstein M, Ganz PA, eds. (2011) *Quality Health Care for Cancer Survivors: Practice, Policy and Research*. Springer.

Ganz PA, Yip CH, Gralow JR, *et al.* (2013) Supportive care after curative treatment for breast cancer (survivorship care): Resource allocations in low- and middle-income countries. A Breast Health Global Initiative 2013 consensus statement. *Breast* 22(5):606–615.

Glim M, Gorman M (2011) Survivorship advocacy. In: Lester J, Schmitt P, Oncology Nursing Society, eds. *Cancer Rehabilitation and Survivorship: Transdisciplinary Approaches to Personalized Care*. Pittsburgh: Oncology Nursing Society:391.

Grassi L, Riba M (2012) *Clinical Psycho-Oncology: An International Perspective: An International Perspective*. Chichester: Wiley Blackwell.

Hewitt ME, Stovall E, Greenfield S, National Cancer Policy Board (US) Committee on Cancer Survivorship: Improving Care and Quality of Life (2006) *From Cancer Patient to Cancer Survivor: Lost in Transition*. Washington, D.C: National Academies Press.

Howell D, Hack TF, Oliver TK *et al.* (2012) Models of care for post-treatment follow-up of adult cancer survivors: A systematic review and quality appraisal of the evidence. *J Cancer Survivor* 6(4):359–371.

Kangas M, Bovbjerg DH, Montgomery GH (2008) Cancer-related fatigue: A systematic and meta-analytic review of non-pharmacological therapies for cancer patients. *Psychol Bull* 134(5):700–741.

Knaul FM, Gralow JR, Atun R, Bhadelia A (2012) *Closing the Cancer Divide: An Equity Imperative*. Boston, MA: Harvard Global Equity Initiative.

Mullan F (1985) Seasons of survival: reflections of a physician with cancer. *N Engl J Med* 313(4):270–273.

Richards M, Corner J, Maher J (2011) The National Cancer Survivorship Initiative: New and emerging evidence on the ongoing needs of cancer survivors. *Br J Cancer* 105(Suppl 1):S1–S4.

Rowland JH, Bellizzi KM (2008) *Cancer Survivors and Survivorship Research: A Reflection on Today's Successes and Tomorrow's Challenges*. Elsevier Health Science.

19 Rehabilitation

Theresa A. Gillis[1,2] and Kerry Tobias[3]

[1]Oncology Rehabilitation Services, Helen F. Graham Cancer Center, Christiana Care Health System, Wilmington, DE, USA
[2]Department of Rehabilitation Medicine, Jefferson Medical College, Philadelphia, PA, USA
[3]Supportive Care and Survivorship, University of Arizona Cancer Center—Phoenix, Dignity Health, St. Joseph's Hospital and Medical Center Phoenix, AZ, USA

Introduction

Rehabilitation interventions are beneficial for cancer patients throughout the course of their care. Any plan of care which addresses function, mobility, independence and well-being indicates a rehabilitative intent. One typically considers consultation with physical therapy, occupational therapy, speech pathology and psychology specialists as rehabilitation; however, the use of flexibility and stretching exercises, breathing techniques and relaxation strategies also constitute rehabilitative efforts. Physical modalities such as heat, cold, massage, stretch, acupuncture or acupressure, electrical stimulation, biofeedback and movement therapies, such as yoga or tai chi, are also rehabilitative and restorative treatments.

Fluctuating levels of health and independence are typical throughout the course of living with cancer, and sudden downturns, slow recoveries, as well as cumulative injury and debility must be anticipated and addressed throughout the patient's course of care and indeed, lifetime.

Activities of daily living

The basic tasks of eating, bathing, dressing, toileting and transferring are part of everyone's daily life. Independence in activities of daily living (ADLs) is considered to be a component of quality of life and health. Consistent measures of independence are employed when assessing performance status and thus gauging patients' eligibility for, and ability to tolerate, cancer treatment. The Karnofsky Performance Scale and Eastern Cooperative Oncology Group (ECOG) Performance Status Scale are two examples of these measures.

Basic ADLs are rarely reviewed in detail during the oncological physician encounter; patients rarely volunteer this information unless specifically asked. However, patients who require much assistance from others may disrupt the function and roles of those caring for them. Fear of becoming a burden to others is recognized as one of the major anxieties of those with advanced cancer. Loss of independence is viewed as a diminishment in quality of life.

Cancer rehabilitation specifically addresses and attempts to maximize each ADL. Rehabilitationists also use consistent measures of function in order to accurately describe independence; typically each domain of function is graded on the degree of assistance provided by others for that specific activity. These measures help demonstrate improvements of function resulting from rehabilitation interventions, and can also be used to convey the effort or burden required from others. Instrumental ADLs (IADLs) are skills which an individual may utilize to function within a community or to fulfil a role (Tables 19.1 and 19.2). Improved abilities in these activities are important contributors to perceptions of improved quality of life.

Common rehabilitation diagnoses in cancer care

Peripheral neuropathy
Deficits, symptoms and findings
- Symmetrical changes in sensation are more common than complaints of weakness
- Typically, feet are affected earlier than fingers
- Pain: distal limb severe cold, burning, tingling, squeezing or other dysaesthesias
- Balance deficits affecting ambulation
- Impaired fine motor skills alter performance of basic or advanced ADLs
- Skin breakdown due to sensory loss
- Proprioceptive loss
- Autonomic neuropathy: orthostasis, dystrophic skin and nail changes, sweating or loss of sweating

---

UICC Manual of Clinical Oncology, Ninth Edition. Edited by Brian O'Sullivan, James D. Brierley, Anil K. D'Cruz, Martin F. Fey, Raphael Pollock, Jan B. Vermorken and Shao Hui Huang. © 2015 UICC. Published 2015 by John Wiley & Sons, Ltd.

Table 19.1 Activities of daily living (ADLs)

- Bathing/washing
- Dressing
- Eating (chewing and swallowing)
- Feeding (moving food from plate to mouth)
- Mobility: walking, use of wheelchair, transferring from sitting to standing, etc.
- Bowel and bladder management (awareness of need to eliminate)
- Toileting (completing the task of emptying bowel and bladder)
- Communication

Diagnostic considerations

- Typically progressive with repeated exposure to neurotoxic medications
- Concomitant neuropathic insults may be present and additive:
  - Diabetes
  - Excessive alcohol consumption
  - Arteriopathy associated with tobacco use or atherosclerotic disease
  - Vitamin B1, B6 and B12 or other nutritional deficiencies
  - Hereditary neuropathy (e.g. Charcot–Marie–Tooth disease):
- Electromyography/nerve conduction studies (EMG/NCS) are insensitive to small fibre pathology; a normal study does not rule out the presence of neuropathy
- EMG/NCS can help diagnose co-existing radiculopathy or plexopathy if asymmetrical complaints are present or the diagnosis is in doubt.
- Chemotherapeutic agents associated with polyneuropathy (Table 19.3)

Rehabilitation

- Gait and balance training, utilizing various walking surfaces, elevations, stairs, side step, weave and other skills
- Pain control: opioid and non-opioid analgesics, anticonvulsants and antidepressants
- 'Desensitization therapy' using massage, stretch, vibration, temperature, pressure, elastic gloves or socks

Table 19.2 Instrumental activities of daily living (IADLs)

- Ability to use telephone
- Laundry
- Shopping
- Food preparation
- Mode of transportation (public transport or drives self independently)
- Housekeeping
- Responsibility for own medications
- Ability to handle finances

Source: Lawton MP, Brody EM (1969) Assessment of older people: Self-maintaining and instrumental activities of daily living. *Gerontologist* 9:179–186. Reproduced wtih permission of Oxford University Press.

Table 19.3 Chemotherapeutic agents associated with polyneuropathy

Common

- Platinum agents: carboplatin, cisplatin, oxaliplatin
- Thalidomide, lenalidomide
- Vinca alkaloids: vinblastine, vincristine, vinorelbine
- Taxanes: docetaxel, paclitaxel
- Ixabepilone
- Bortezomib

Less common

- Cytarabine
- 5-Fluorouracil
- Etoposide
- Gemcitabine
- Ifosfamide
- Suramin
- Procarbazine

- Counter-stimulation therapy: electrical stimulation distally or at spinal level
- Acupuncture
- Safety/injury precautions
- Fine motor task practice
- Compensatory strategies and technology, e.g. larger handles, elastic shoelaces, voice-recognition software if unable to type

Cancer fatigue
Deficits, symptoms and findings

- Fatigue is not resolved with rest, sleep or inactivity, and persists despite correction of sleep hygiene or restoration of sleep pattern
- Absence of objective muscular weakness or debility
- Cognitive symptoms or physical symptoms may predominate, co-exist with equal severity or alternate
- Onset is insidious rather than sudden
- Often experienced with chemotherapy and radiation therapy
- Mood disorders are not necessarily present at onset, but depression and/or anxiety may develop as fatigue persists
- Lack of motivation
- Declining social interaction
- Decreased mental acuity: concentration, memory, focus
- Increasing difficulty performing ADLs
- Dyspnoea with exertion

Diagnostic considerations

- Assess for presence of encephalopathy
- Assess for anaemia; correction of mild anaemia typically does not resolve complaint
- Consider hypoxaemia and pulmonary embolism as a possible cause or contributor
- Question sleep and breathing patterns for indications of obstructive sleep apnoea

- Explore possible metabolic derangements: hyperbilirubinaemia, hyperglycaemia, vitamin deficiencies, etc.
- Evaluate nutrition and hydration status
- Consider possibility of chronic occult infection
- Assess for decompensation of chronic cardiac or pulmonary disease
- Review medications: excessive benzodiazepines, opioids or other depressants
- Overuse of alcohol alters sleep patterns and reduces restorative sleep

Rehabilitation
- Low-grade aerobic exercise programme, land- or water-based
- Progressive strength and resistance training
- Sleep hygiene: regular schedule for bedtime, dark environment, no television, music or computer screen distractions, low noise or 'white noise'
- Correction of medication or nutritional factors
- Correction of hypoxaemia
- Consideration of therapeutic stimulant medication trials
- Cognitive therapy
- Practice focus and attention; games and skills building memory, overcoming distractions
- 'Mindfulness' activities, such as yoga, tai chi, meditation

Spinal accessory nerve injury

The spinal accessory nerve (cranial nerve XI) innervates the trapezius and sternocleidomastoid muscles. The trapezius is the major muscle of scapular stabilization and the key muscle enabling overhead reach of the arm.

Causes
- Frequently injured during cervical lymph node biopsies and radical and modified radical cervical lymph node dissections
- Tumour infiltration of cervical nodes or the trapezius muscle itself
- Chronic radiation injury: late effect of cervical node or cervical spine radiation

Diagnosis
- Asymmetrical posture: drooping of affected shoulder, affected shoulder protracted
- Inability to symmetrically elevate the ipsilateral scapula
- Lateral displacement of scapula with cephalomedial rotation of the inferior angle and caudal rotation of the acromion and glenoid
- Weakness rather than paralysis suggests partial injury or neuropraxia and more favourable prognosis
- Absence of findings of other brachial plexus or peripheral nerve injury

Rehabilitation
- Stretch ipsilateral pectoralis muscle to restore scapular retraction range of motion
- Active scapular retraction: strengthening of rhomboideus and any remaining functioning trapezius fibres
- Minimize stretch of shoulder capsule: restrict lifting/carrying/pushing with affected arm
- Avoid reach at/above shoulder height to prevent impingement of the rotator cuff between the acromion process and the humeral head
- Support weight of arm with arm rests
- Avoid sling use as these promote pectoral contracture, internal rotation of the humerus and scapular protraction
- Scapular orthotics, compression vests or garments are sometimes helpful but patients may not tolerate the localized chest pressure required to successfully support the scapula

If the nerve is visualized during surgery and known to be transected, ipsilateral trapezius function loss is permanent and rehabilitation goals will focus on compensatory strategies to allow vocational requirements and avocational interests to be completed. More commonly, the nerve is preserved but manipulated, devascularized or under traction, and the extent of the neuropraxic injury, and timing and prognosis for recovery is uncertain. The rehabilitation goal is to reduce the injury to the shoulder capsule and rotator cuff tendons while awaiting neural recovery.

Lymphoedema

Causes
- Radiation of proximal lymphatics
- Node dissection
- Surgical scarring
- Postocclusive; proximal deep venous thrombosis creates venous stasis and secondary lymphatic overload in the affected limb

Diagnostic considerations
- Evaluate for venous thrombosis and thromboembolic risk
- Venous stasis and/or congestive heart failure present
- Dependent positioning and inactivity as contributing factors
- Nutritional abnormality, protein–calorie malnutrition or liver dysfunction causing generalized anasarca
- Presence of neural injury from polyneuropathy, peripheral nerve or plexus dysfunction results not only in reduced muscle activity but also reduced sensation, elevating the risk of injury and subsequent infection

Rehabilitation
- Protection of skin integrity, hydration/moisture, treatment of dermatitis
- Patient education on skin protection, including avoidance of hair removal or shaving affected areas, techniques for safe nail care, and reduced exposure to sunburn, burns, cuts and other insults to skin integrity
- Massage and stretch of restrictive scarring in the affected limb or lymphatic basin
- Mobilization of lymph fluid by skilled lymphatic massage

- Compression of affected area with low-stretch bandaging or use of snug garments to cover affected areas; for the pelvis, bicycling-type compression shorts may be useful; for the chest, a snug camisole or compression shirt
- Fitted compression sleeve or stocking for extremity lymphoedema
- Pneumatic sequential compression pump

Post-thoracotomy syndrome

These impairments are often present after thoracotomies for lung and oesophageal tumours, but may also occur with other thoracic malignancies and surgical procedures.

Deficits, symptoms and findings
- Dysaesthesias of chest wall and/or axilla
- Neuritic pains along course of affected intercostal nerve
- Less commonly, pleuritic pain on the affected side
- Localized weakness of intercostals or serratus with chest deformity: 'bulge', 'swelling', 'mass' causing patient concern
- Exertional dyspnoea and exercise intolerance
- Positional dyspnoea: if diaphragmatic movement is compromised, bending and squatting reduce intrathoracic volume and impede normal breathing
- Altered scapular stability and shoulder function:
  - If long thoracic nerve injury or significant serratus anterior resection, the medial border of the scapula is posteriorly displaced ('posterior winging')
  - If the spinal accessory nerve is injured or the trapezius is resected, the scapula is laterally displaced with the acromion caudally rotated ('lateral winging')

Rehabilitation
- Massage of restrictive or hypersensitive scarring
- Neuropathic pain management: tricyclic secondary amines, selective serotonin norepinephrine reuptake inhibitors (SSNRIs), calcium channel modulators (gabapentin, pregabalin), anticonvulsants
- Compression garment: elastic vest or compression shirt may help relieve pain
- Electrical stimulation (TENS)
- Acupuncture
- Stretch of the pectoralis, serratus or other tight musculature
- Strengthening of spinal extensors, abdominal obliques, trapezius
- Progressive exercise: treadmill, stationary bicycle, aquatic or other means of improving endurance and activity tolerance

Dysphagia

Causes
- Common impairment during treatment of cancers, particularly head & neck cancers
- Tumour infiltration or surgical resection of tumour may disrupt motor functions of the tongue, epiglottis, pharynx and oesophagus
- Fibrotic scarring of the pharynx and surrounding structures following local radiation therapy
- Pain associated with tumours of the oropharynx, nasopharynx or oesophagus
- Mucositis and stomatitis; associated with radiation therapy, infection (candidiasis, herpes simplex virus), chemotherapy (e.g. methotrexate, 5-fluorouracil)
- Neurological: debility/generalized weakness, paraneoplastic syndromes, cerebellar or brainstem tumours, or tumours affecting functions of cranial nerves V, VII, IX, X or XII

Impairments and symptoms
- Pain
- Xerostomia
- Weight loss
- Psychosocial distress: social isolation, costs of non-oral nutrition, anxiety, depression

Rehabilitation
- Treatment and healing of mucositis
- Speech pathology assessment and plan of care
- Daily exercises: jaw and tongue base range of motion exercises, effortful swallow exercises, tongue holding manoeuvre, Mendelsohn manoeuvre, super supraglottic swallow. Patients are encouraged to practice these exercises daily during and after treatment
- Compensatory postures, e.g. chin tuck and rotation towards the damaged side reduces the pharyngeal space on the weaker side and enhances propulsion by the stronger side
- Alternation of liquid or wet foods with dry foods
- Sensory stimulation: cold foods or utensils, utensil pressure on the tongue
- Altered textures and densities: thickened liquids, soft or puréed foods may be required temporarily or long term
- Alternative feeding: nasogastric or percutaneous gastric feedings

Amputation and limb salvage

The treatment decision between amputation and limb salvage is primarily determined by the nature of the tumour itself. What is the extent of surgery required for optimal cancer control? How is this tumour likely to behave with regard to local progression and distant metastasis? However, the rehabilitationist familiar with amputee care and functional mobility can provide a valuable perspective to this discussion. The rehabilitationist also can provide detailed, meaningful insight to the patient on what to expect functionally and psychologically during recovery from these treatments.

Rehabilitation considerations
- Expected residual limb length: very proximal amputations (high trans-femoral, hip disarticulation; high trans-humeral,

shoulder disarticulation) are typically less likely to be successful prosthetic limb users.
- Patients with dysvascular tissue may be unable to tolerate the focal pressure of a prosthetic limb
- Co-morbid diseases (chronic obstructive pulmonary disease, severe peripheral neuropathy, scleroderma) may create additive impairments which impede successful prosthetic use
- Co-existing functional limitations (e.g. poor vision, severe upper extremity impairments) may slow the rehabilitation process
- Quality of life: a lengthy limb salvage process with multiple surgical revisions may be unacceptable to a patient when compared to amputation and rapid recovery of mobility
- Likely prognosis based on primary tumour:
  - A poorly differentiated, aggressive and/or highly likely to metastasize tumour may lead the team to recommend amputation so that function and quality of life are maximized over a possibly shorter lifespan
  - A tumour with more indolent behaviour may be more appropriate for limb salvage surgery

Amputation

Amputation postoperative care
- Postoperative dressing choices are influenced by skin integrity, co-morbid conditions and prognosis for prosthetic fitting as well as available resources and skills (Table 19.4)
- Oedema control speeds healing and allows earlier fitting with prosthesis
- Even in non-prosthetic candidates, oedema control is beneficial to reduce pain
- Frequent visualization of the wound may be desirable in previously irradiated tissues or those with dysvascular tissue

Preparation for prosthesis
- Emotional adjustment: reluctance to look at or touch area
- Social adjustment: fear of being seen by others, fear of rejection
- Return to avocational and vocational activities
- Management of pain including phantom pain
- Prevention of contractures, management of radiation-associated fibrosis and/or lymphoedema
- Prevention of pressure ulcers
- Safe mobility with assistive device or wheelchair
- Safe performance of ADLs

Limb salvage
Typically entails loss of bone, nerve and muscle, and may entail significant soft tissue defects or scarring.

Rehabilitation goals
- Promote healing
- Recover active range of motion and strength when neurological function permits
- Preserve passive range of motion for hygiene
- Use of orthotics for support, alignment and protection to promote function of the limb

Upper limb
- Replacement or reconstruction of shoulder joints typically is not possible
- Tikhoff–Linberg procedure or other humeral reconstruction may allow preservation of an arm if the brachial plexus or most peripheral nerves can be spared
- Orthotics for shoulder mobility or glenohumeral stability are rarely successful functionally or tolerated for long-term use

Table 19.4 Comparison of immediate postoperative amputation dressings

	Soft dressing	Semirigid			Rigid	
Material	Elastic bandages	Paste	Air cast	Silicone sleeve	Plaster cast	Thermoplastic
Cost	+	+	++	+++	++	+++
Wound visibility	Every 4 hours with rewrapping	Weekly	Daily	Daily	Weekly	Daily
Oedema control	+	++	++		+++	
Patient effort	Learn skilled wrapping technique Compliance with frequent wrapping	None	Cast inflation/ deflation Device hygiene		None	Device hygiene
Staff effort	Trained staff, frequent reapplication	Trained staff	Minimal		Highly trained	
Limb protection	+	++	+		+++	
Function impact	Light weight Permits easy mobility of proximal joints				Proprioception from residual limb Weight-bearing on residual limb May be heavy May limit proximal joint movements	

- Distal orthoses can align the wrist and place fingers in the optimal position to maximize function
- Manage lymphoedema
- Protect insensate skin

Lower limb
- Lumbosacral plexus, radicular or peripheral nerve surgical resection or injury may be entailed because of the tumour location
- Control of distal oedema
- Protection of insensate skin
- Management of neuritic pain when present
- *Pelvic reconstruction and internal hemipelvectomy*:
  - Initially may have restrictions on hip range of motion which can affect sitting and supine positioning
  - Weight-bearing and resistance exercise are highly specific to the surgery and reconstructive elements in place. Allograft bone reconstructions typically require lengthy periods of limited weight-bearing and reduced resistance
  - Elevated risks of decubitus and pressure ulcer formation
  - Sensory and motor loss is common either through neurological injury or loss of the muscle compartment
- *Anterior thigh*:
  - Quadriceps (full or partial) resection reduces knee extension strength, knee stability during gait and stair climbing and descent
  - Leg may be stabilized in knee-extended position with a locking knee brace
  - Thigh, knee and medial calf (saphenous nerve) dysaesthesias are common with femoral nerve injury or resection
- *Posterior thigh*:
  - Less functional loss entailed with hamstring resection
  - Increased risk of sciatic nerve injury with loss of ankle dorsi- and plantar flexion
  - Ankle–foot orthosis restores functional positioning for safe and efficient gait
  - Prevention of ankle foot drop contracture
- *Knee and distal resections*:
  - Frequently entail tibial or peroneal nerve injury or loss
  - Bracing with ankle–foot orthoses allows excellent functional mobility, usually without need for an assistive device

Pelvic floor dysfunction: Incontinence and sexuality concerns

Weak muscles in the pelvic floor triangle affect bowel and bladder function independent of nerve involvement. This needs to be distinguished from spinal cord/nerve causes or upper motor neurone causes (brain metastases, pre-existing dementia, pre-existing stress incontinence).

Other causes of sexual dysfunction need to be considered as well: medications; hypogonadism from hormonal treatment for specific cancers or from prolonged opioid use; depression/anxiety; body image concerns; dyspareunia.

Causes
- Prostate surgery
- Pelvic radiation: tissue atrophy and fibrosis
- Gynaecological surgery
- Medications (SSRIs, beta-blockers, etc.)
- Orchiectomy
- Rectal surgery
- Chemotherapy/hormonal therapy causing vaginal atrophy; decreased testosterone levels and libido

Diagnostic considerations
- Urodynamic testing
- Patient history (will also rule out pre-existing incontinence)
- Erectile dysfunction
- Bowel/bladder incontinence
- Change in bowel function/pattern
- Development of chronic cystitis
- Development of proctitis
- Dyspareunia
- Diarrhoea/constipation

Rehabilitation
- Pelvic floor muscle exercises (Kegel exercises): active retraining
- Electrical stimulation with rectal probe: passive retraining
- Vaginal dilators
- Vaginal lubricants
- Biofeedback
- Psychological counselling (body image considerations; erectile dysfunction)
- Erectile dysfunction medications (phosphodiesterase 5 [PDE5] inhibitors)
- Pain medications
- Nutritional counselling and diet modification

Consideration in rehabilitation should also be given in counselling to decrease bladder irritants/stimulants such as caffeine-containing substances which increase urination; and smoking cessation. Patients with bowel incontinence should avoid pro-motility agents or foods. High-fibre diets, adequate fluid intake, physical exercise and laxatives are appropriate in patients with constipation.

Cognitive impairment

Causes
- Primary brain tumours
- Brain metastases
- Radiation
- Chemotherapy ('chemo brain')
- Fatigue
- Pre-existing, undiagnosed mild dementia or Parkinson disease
- Medications
- Non–cancer-related concomitant medical problems (stroke, pre-existing mild traumatic brain injury)
- Hydrocephalus

- Infection/sepsis
- Hypotension
- Anaemia

Diagnostic considerations
- Patient history to obtain baseline of cognitive functioning (may have to enlist family members or caregivers to obtain baseline)
- Incontinence
- Mood changes (irritability, anger)
- Memory loss/lapse
- Neuropsychological testing
- Functional Independence Measure scale
- Anaemia
- Recent or new medication changes
- Inadequate cardiac perfusion (e.g. hypotension)
- Balance/gait impairments
- Depression (may be causing slower thought/cognitive processing)
- Perseveration
- Speech/swallowing difficulties

Rehabilitation
- Enlisting use of memory aids (weekly pill boxes for medication management, encourage use of notebook for recording symptoms and physician recommendations)
- Cognitive skills retraining
- Aerobic physical exercise
- Focus on ADLs
- Gait/balance retraining (will need cueing and repetition within this training)
- Safety assessment (will determine if 24-hour care is needed)
- Speech/swallow assessment (appropriate food consistency modifications if dysphagia present; communication aids such as picture board or pen/paper for writing if dysphasia present)
- Focus on structuring activity scheduling/pacing
- Creation of low sensory stimulation environment to avoid distraction and agitation
- Visual assessment and adaptations

Spinal cord compression

Causes
- Primary spinal, pelvic or sacral tumour
- Bone metastases with epidural extension
- Leptomeningeal carcinomatosis
- Compression fractures
- Paraneoplastic syndromes may mimic the symptoms of spinal cord compression

Diagnostic considerations
The severity of impairment and rapidity of onset may indicate the need for neurosurgical intervention to preserve/prevent further loss of function and deficits.
- Loss of bowel/bladder function
- Limb weakness
- Sensory loss
- Pain
- Limb oedema
- Structural/postural change
- Gait dysfunction
- Falls
- Cauda equina syndrome
- Conus medullaris syndrome
- Presence of decubitus ulcers (may be first indication of weakness in offloading weight from sacrum/buttocks area or sensory loss)

Rehabilitation recommendations depend upon the spinal cord level of injury; this level helps to determine what functional level to expect the patient to achieve or maintain. Cervical cord compression will typically compromise upper extremity strength sufficiently to alter bed mobility and transfers, and dramatically impair mobility, often necessitating use of a wheelchair. If substantial lower limb strength remains despite the cervical injury, balance may still be quite compromised; a walker may enable functional mobility. Determination of the dominant hand will influence choices for adaptive devices for ADLs. Large areas of insensate or poorly sensate skin will require frequent turns in bed and repositioning in a chair to prevent skin breakdown and ulcer development.

Cervical spine involvement with cord or multiple root level injury can also lead to dramatic pulmonary compromise. The diaphragm is innervated by C3–C5 via the phrenic nerves and involvement at those levels can decrease its function, leading to development of atelectasis, pneumonia or dyspnoea.

Truncal involvement at the thoracic level can affect abdominal muscles and respiratory accessory muscles. Consideration then needs to be made regarding posture and truncal stability while sitting. An elastic abdominal binder or rigid thoracic orthosis may enable better sitting balance and improved safety during transfers. Patients with significant thoracic pain may not tolerate the pressure of a spinal orthosis. Transitions from lying to sitting and sitting to standing may be very difficult for patients with thoracic level cord injury; standing will not be feasible without sufficient hip extensor and gluteal strength.

Rehabilitation
- Gait and balance/proprioceptive training
- Use of assistive devices for ambulation and/or ADLs
- Home health assessment for adaptive equipment needed at home or home modifications (e.g. ramp if needed for any steps to enter the home, installation of grab bars in the bathroom)
- Bowel/bladder management (need to determine whether there is upper or lower motor neurone deficit for establishing appropriate regimen)
- Oedema management
- Deep vein thrombosis (DVT) prophylaxis
- Abdominal muscle strengthening
- Postural aid (either soft abdominal binder or more rigid brace) to help with sitting and ambulation

- Lower extremity strengthening
- Upper extremity strengthening for transfers
- Pain control facilitates functional movement
- Steroidal taper when able:
  - To avoid development of steroid-induced myopathy, causing proximal muscle weakness (particularly the hip extensors) and further worsening of the patient's already compromised function
  - Development of steroid myopathy does not depend on length of time of being on steroids or dose
- Wound care if decubitus ulcers present
- Pulmonary care if appropriate: deep breathing exercises to encourage use of accessory muscles, use of incentive spirometry, resisted cough, pursed-lip breathing, etc.

Cord compression can occur in the absence of motor weakness or bowel/bladder dysfunction. Severe pain can prevent a patient's participation in an adequate motor exam or detailed sensory evaluation. Pain is the earliest and most sensitive indicator of impending cord compression, and spinal pain in a cancer patient should always raise concerns for cord compression or impending cord compression.

Late effects of cancer treatment

Long-term injury can occur from cancer treatments and late effects of treatment can be associated with significant declines in function and quality of life. Rehabilitation interventions are often effective in combating the limitations and managing symptoms (Table 19.5).

Patients who experience late sequelae of treatment often experience mood disorders, with frustration that the cancer experience has permanently changed them, anxiety for the risk of developing further impairments as time goes by, anger that the cancer treatment has harmed them and other negative emotions frequently voiced. In addition to physical and pharmacological interventions, psychological care may be very helpful.

Table 19.5 Rehabilitation for late effects of cancer treatment

Impairment	Causative agent examples	Rehabilitative interventions
Osteoporosis	Corticosteroid Radiation Oestrogen and testosterone manipulation	Weight-bearing exercise
Cardiac injury	Adriamycin Radiation of left breast or chest wall	Aerobic exercise
Lung injury Pulmonary fibrosis Radiation fibrosis	Radiation of lung or chest wall Bleomycin	Aerobic exercise Resistance exercise Breathing exercise: pursed-lip, forced cough, diaphragmatic breathing skills
Plexus injury	Radiation Progressive surgical scarring	Upper limb: • Orthoses • Slings Lower limb: • Gait assist devices • Orthoses
Spinal cord injury	Radiation Intrathecal chemotherapy	PT, OT See Chapter 15
Lymphoedema	Radiation Surgery	Complex decongestive physiotherapy
Chemotherapy-induced neuropathy	Platinum agents Vinca alkaloids Taxanes See Table 19.3	Pain control: medications; desensitization therapies Balance and strengthening exercises See Chapter 15
Cognitive and memory deficits	Brain radiation Chemotherapy agents	Neuropsychological testing Cognitive retraining Memory aids
Fatigue	Radiation Nutritional deficits Untreated depression	Nutritional optimization Low-grade aerobic and resistance exercise programme

Recommended reading

Ahles TA, Saykin AJ, Furstenberg CT et al. (2002) Neuropsychologic impact of standard-dose systemic chemotherapy in long-term survivors of breast cancer and lymphoma. *J Clin Oncol* 20(2):485–493.

CuccurulloSJ, ed. (2004) *Physical Medicine and Rehabilitation Board Review*, Demos:628–643.

Delbrück H (2007) *Rehabilitation and Palliation of Cancer Patients*. Springer.

Dietz JH Jr, (1982) *Rehabilitation Oncology*. Chichester: John Wiley & Sons.

Dworkin RH (2012) In: SimpsonDM, McArthurJC, eds. *Neuropathic Pain: Mechanisms, Diagnosis and Treatment*. New York: Oxford University Press.

Lehman JF, DeLisa JA, Warren CG (1978) Cancer rehabilitation: assessment of need, development and evaluation of a model of care. *Arch Phys Med Rehabil* 59:410–419.

McKinley WO, Conti-Wyneken AR, Vokac C, Cifu DX (1996) Rehabilitative functional outcome of patients with neoplastic spinal cord compression. *Arch Phys Med Rehabil* 77(9):892–895.

National Collaborating Centre for Cancer (UK) (2008) Metastatic spinal cord compression: diagnosis and management of patients at risk of or with metastatic spinal cord compression. Cardiff: National Collaborating Centre for Cancer (UK) (NICE Clinical Guidelines, No. 75.):25–28.

Oechsle K, Jensen W, Schmidt T et al. (2011) Physical activity, quality of life, and the interest in physical exercise programs in patients undergoing palliative chemotherapy. *Support Care Cancer* 19(5):613–619.

Olson E, Cristian A (2005) The role of rehabilitation medicine and palliative care in the treatment of patients with end-stage disease. *Phys Med Rehabil Clin North Am* 16(1):285–305.

Rankin J, Robb K, Murtagh N, Cooper J, Lewis S (2008) *Rehabilitation in Cancer Care*, Oxford: Wiley Blackwell.

Schuurs, A, Green HJ (2013) A feasibility study of group cognitive rehabilitation for cancer survivors: enhancing cognitive function and quality of life. *Psycho-Oncology* 22:1043–1049.

Terzoni S, Montanari E, Mora C, Ricci C, Destrebecq A (2013) Reducing urine leakage after radical retropubic prostatectomy: pelvic floor exercises, magnetic innervation or no treatment? A quasi-experimental study. *Rehabil Nurs* 38:153–160

Winningham ML, Barton-Burke M (2000) *Fatigue in Cancer: A Multidimensional Approach*. Jones & Bartlett Learning.

Yanga EJ, Lima J-Y, Rahb UW, Kim YB (2012) Effect of a pelvic floor muscle training program on gynecologic cancer survivors with pelvic floor dysfunction: A randomized controlled trial. *Gynecol Oncol* 125(3):705–711.

PART 2: Site-specific multidisciplinary cancer management

20 Lung

Suresh S. Ramalingam[1], Felix Fernandez[2], Kristin A. Higgins[3], William F. Auffermann[4] and Fadlo R. Khuri[1]

[1]Department of Hematology and Medical Oncology, Emory University, Winship Cancer Institute, Atlanta, GA, USA
[2]Division of Thoracic Surgery, Department of Surgery, Emory University, Winship Cancer Institute, Atlanta, GA, USA
[3]Department of Radiation Oncology, Emory University, Winship Cancer Institute, Atlanta, GA, USA
[4]Department of Radiology, Emory University, Winship Cancer Institute, Atlanta, GA, USA

Summary	Key facts

Introduction	- Accounts for 12.9% of all cancers:
	  - 1.8 million new cases of lung cancer worldwide in 2012
	  - Most common cancer in men
	  - Nearly 600,000 new cases in women each year
	- Accounts for 18% of all cancer-related deaths:
	  - 1.6 million deaths due to lung cancer in 2012
	- Nearly 85% of all lung cancers are related to cigarette smoking
	- Other risk factors include exposure to asbestos, radon, second-hand smoke and industrial carcinogens
	- Nearly 85% of patients have non-small cell lung cancer (NSCLC):
	  - NSCLC includes adenocarcinoma, squamous cell carcinoma and large cell histology
	- Small cell lung cancer (SCLC) accounts for approximately 15% of lung cancers

Presentation	- Lung cancer is diagnosed at an advanced stage in the majority of patients - Presenting symptoms include cough, chest pain, haemoptysis, weight loss, fatigue and dyspnoea: - Diagnosis is often delayed as the presenting symptoms are often attributed to co-morbid conditions - Paraneoplastic syndromes can be the presenting feature in some patients

Scenario	- *Stage I or II NSCLC*: surgery followed by adjuvant chemotherapy for tumours of >4 cm or lymph node involvement
	- *Stage IIIA NSCLC*: preoperative chemotherapy followed by surgery or definitive chemoradiotherapy
	- *Stage IIIB NSCLC*: concurrent chemotherapy with radiation
	- *Stage IV NSCLC*:
	  - Platinum-based chemotherapy for patients without a targetable mutation
	  - Targeted therapy for patients with *EGFR* mutation or *ALK* gene rearrangement
	- *Limited-stage SCLC*:
	  - Platinum-based chemotherapy with concurrent radiation
	  - Prophylactic cranial radiation upon completion of systemic therapy
	- *Extensive-stage SCLC*: platinum + etoposide chemotherapy followed by prophylactic cranial irradiation (PCI) in responding patients

Trials	- Winton *et al.* (2005) *N Engl J Med* 352(25):2589–2597:
	  - Cisplatin-based adjuvant chemotherapy versus observation for Stage IB and II NSCLC
	- Lynch *et al.* (2004) *N Engl J Med* 350(21):2129–2139:
	  - *EGFR* mutation predicts for sensitivity to EGFR tyrosine kinase inhibitors
	- Schiller *et al.* (2002) *N Engl J Med* 346(2):92–98:
	  - Comparison of platinum-based combination chemotherapy in advanced NSCLC
	- Soda *et al.* (2007) *Nature* 448:561–566:
	  - *ALK* gene rearrangements in NSCLC
	- Maemondo *et al.* (2010) *N Engl J Med* 362(25):2380–2388:
	  - Comparison of gefitinib versus chemotherapy in patients with *EGFR*-mutated NSCLC

UICC Manual of Clinical Oncology, Ninth Edition. Edited by Brian O'Sullivan, James D. Brierley, Anil K. D'Cruz, Martin F. Fey, Raphael Pollock, Jan B. Vermorken and Shao Hui Huang. © 2015 UICC. Published 2015 by John Wiley & Sons, Ltd.

Introduction

Historically, the prognosis for lung cancer patients was uniformly poor. Recent advances in lung cancer diagnosis and treatment have led to improved survival and quality of life for a subset of patients with all stages of lung cancer. Optimal management of lung cancer requires multidisciplinary teams of cancer professionals including thoracic surgeons, medical oncologists, radiation oncologists, pathologists and radiologists, along with good nursing care.

Incidence, aetiology and screening

Incidence

Lung cancer is the second most common cause of cancer in both males and females, and the most common cause of cancer-related death in the USA. Lung cancer causes over four times as many cancer-related deaths as the next four most common forms of cancer combined. In 2011, approximately 220,000 people were diagnosed with lung cancer and nearly 160,000 people died of lung cancer in the USA. It is estimated that approximately 1.6 million people die of lung cancer per year worldwide.

Aetiology (Table 20.1)

Tobacco smoke has been demonstrated to contain at least 50 different carcinogens. Heavy use of tobacco is estimated to increase the risk of developing lung cancer by about 20-fold. Cigarette smoking caused about 100 million deaths in the 20th century, and it is estimated that even more will die as a result of tobacco use in the 21st century. In the USA, the incidence of lung cancer has been decreasing since the 1980s, correlating with decreased use of tobacco after the 1964 Surgeon General's report linking cigarette smoking to lung cancer. However, tobacco use in many parts of the world remains high, particularly in Asia. Second-hand tobacco smoke exposure also contributes to the development of lung cancer.

Table 20.1 Risk factors for lung cancer

Risk factor	Comments
Cigarette smoking	85% of all patients with lung cancer. Nearly 50% of lung cancer patients are former smokers
Exposure to radiation	Seen in breast cancer and lymphoma survivors
Occupational/environmental exposures	Asbestos exposure increases risk of lung cancer. Radon exposure is associated with lung cancer
Infections	Risk of lung cancer appears higher in patients with human immunodeficiency virus (HIV) disease

Table 20.2 US National Lung Screening Trial

Screened population	Age 55–74 years; 30-pack year smoking history; Former smokers should have quit within 15 preceding years
Intervention	Low-dose CT scan versus chest radiograph at baseline and annually for 2 years
Results	Higher rate of positive screening with CT over chest radiograph (27% vs 9%) at baseline. Approximately 4% with positive screen had lung cancer. Reduction in lung cancer mortality by 20% with CT scan. Overall reduction in mortality by 6.7% with CT scan

Screening

Results from the US National Lung Screening Trial (NLST) (Table 20.2) indicate that there is an improvement in mortality rate for high-risk patients screened yearly for lung cancer using low-dose computed tomography (CT) screening relative to chest radiography screening. Given these results, several clinical and patient advocacy groups in the USA have recommended routine screening for patients at high risk for lung cancer, based on the criteria and methodology of the NLST. However, given the high false-positive rate, variability in cancer growth rates and cost, the clinical implications of this study are still being evaluated.

Pathology

Lung cancers grow from a microscopic single abnormal cell or small group of abnormal cells to large macroscopic masses that may be many centimetres in diameter. Most lung cancers originate from the bronchial epithelium and are termed carcinomas. Primary non-carcinoma lung cancers are less common and include: carcinoid, pulmonary blastomas (more common in younger patients) and sarcomas. Early lung cancers measuring <3 cm in diameter often manifest as pulmonary nodules. A pulmonary nodule is defined as 'a

Table 20.3 NSCLC and SCLC histology and prevalence

Histology	Prevalence	Comments
Non-small cell lung cancer		
Adenocarcinoma	40–50%	Has surpassed squamous histology as the most common subtype. Positive staining for thyroid transcription factor 1 (TTF-1) or napsin-1 by Immunohistochemistry
Squamous cell carcinoma	20–30%	Positive staining for p63 or p40
Large cell carcinoma	5–10%	Often harbours neuroendocrine features
NSCLC-NOS	5–10%	
Small cell lung cancer		
	10–15%	Decreasing in incidence. Stains positively for neuroendocrine markers

rounded opacity, well or poorly defined, measuring up to 3 cm in diameter'. Abnormal lung tissues range in histological grade from mildly atypical cells to aggressive cancers. Lesions such as atypical adenomatous hyperplasia are considered to be preinvasive lesions, with a continuum of cellular atypia through adenocarcinoma.

Historically, lung cancers were often grouped into two categories: SCLC and NSCLC. This grouping was related to the fact that historically, NSCLCs were all treated similarly, with less regard for the subtype and tumour-specific biomarkers. NSCLC histology includes adenocarcinoma, squamous cell carcinoma and large cell neuroendocrine carcinoma as its subtypes (Table 20.3). With advances in molecular diagnostics and therapies, the type of cancer and presence of specific molecular markers are critical determinants for therapy, and traditional classification systems, while still used, often do not convey sufficient information. However, lung cancer prognosis and treatment is still strongly correlated with the stage at which cancer is diagnosed.

The doubling time for lung cancer typically ranges from approximately 20 days for aggressive lesions to ~400 days for indolent adenocarcinomas. Ground-glass nodules are a notable exception to this rule, and their doubling times have been documented to be as long as 884 days (~2.4 years). This presents difficulties with regards to diagnosis (based on growth rate) and early detection using screening.

Diagnostic work-up

The work-up for suspected lung cancers is dependent on the probability that the lesion in question is malignant and/or the stage of disease at presentation. Early lung cancers often present as small indeterminate pulmonary nodules (Table 20.4). The management of nodules differs depending on whether they are solid (soft tissue attenuation) or sub-solid (less than soft tissue attenuation without obscuration of the underlying lung architecture on CT). Pulmonary nodules often occur due to current or prior infection, although they may be the manifestation of early cancer. Results from the NLST (see Table 20.3) showed that of all nodules detected, ~95% were false positives and were non-cancerous. For larger nodules, CT characteristics of concern for malignancy include: irregular margins, spiculation, invasion of adjacent structures, lymphadenopathy and distant metastases.

Sub-solid pulmonary nodules have a more detailed management algorithm, due to the spectrum of potential aetiologies and variable growth rates of cancers with this appearance. A new algorithm for the management of small sub-solid nodules was published in 2013. Ground-glass nodules of >5 mm should be followed for at least 3–4 years to document stability.

Staging work-up (Table 20.5)

Establishing the diagnosis and determination of histological subtype requires a diagnostic biopsy. The most accessible site of the tumour that is amenable to biopsy is chosen for diagnostic purposes. In most cases the approach involves a transthoracic biopsy with CT guidance or transbronchial biopsy. Though a fine needle aspirate is usually sufficient for biopsy, the contents are not adequate to conduct molecular tests. Therefore, core needle biopsy is recommended whenever possible. In recent years, even after histological diagnosis is established with a biopsy, additional biopsy to procure tissue for molecular testing is gaining ground among patients and physicians. Cytology from pleural or pericardial fluid can also lead to the diagnosis of lung cancer, though this might be inadequate for molecular testing. In patients with pleural effusion, the diagnostic yield from

Table 20.4 Evaluation of pulmonary nodules

Nodule	Follow-up
Nodule <8 mm	CT scan in 3–6 months for follow-up. If stable for 2 years, no further follow-up necessary
Nodule >8 mm	Requires further work-up with PET scan and/or biopsy

Table 20.5 Staging work-up

Test	Comments
CT chest	• Determines size of lesions, lymph node enlargement and presence of effusions • Should include visualization of the liver and adrenal glands
PET–CT scan	• Used for staging • Evaluation of pulmonary nodules with sensitivity and specificity of 97% and 78%, respectively • Evaluation of mediastinal lymph node status • Not helpful for lesions of <10 mm in size • Replaces the need for a separate bone scan to evaluate for skeletal metastasis
MRI brain	• Indicated for patients with central nervous system (CNS) symptoms • Recommended for patients with T3 or nodal involvement before surgical resection • CT brain with contrast is an alternative if MRI brain is not available
MRI chest	• Indicated to characterize anatomy of certain tumours before surgical resection • Helpful to determine invasion of major structures such as aorta and brachial plexus
Bone scan	• Indicated in patients with symptoms of bone metastasis • Not necessary if patient has already undergone PET scan
Pulmonary function tests	• To determine pulmonary reserve capacity in patients for whom surgical resection of early-stage disease is planned

cytology is 50–70%. If the specimen is non-diagnostic after two thoracentesis procedures, thoracoscopy with biopsy is recommended to establish the diagnosis. Ascertainment of pleural fluid cytology might be necessary in certain instances to determine the stage in patients with otherwise localized disease. Biopsy from bone lesions is unsuitable for molecular testing and should be done only for diagnostic purposes.

Staging the mediastinum

Before surgery is performed, staging the mediastinum is an essential aspect of managing early-stage NSCLC.

Invasive thoracic staging

The presence or absence of mediastinal nodal metastases is of major importance in determining prognosis, assessing resectablity and selecting the appropriate treatment strategy for primary lung cancer. Enlarged lymph nodes identified on CT or positron emission tomography (PET) scan require histological confirmation. It is debatable as to whether all patients require invasive mediastinal staging prior to surgical resection, or other local treatment modality such as stereotactic body radiotherapy (SBRT), which involves delivering targeted radiation to the tumour with minimal exposure to surrounding normal tissues. Only 5–15% of cases with peripheral T1 tumours with a negative mediastinum on CT and/or PET have mediastinal nodal metastases.

Transbronchial needle aspiration (TBNA)

TBNA allows staging of the mediastinum during diagnostic bronchoscopy. Sensitivity is dependent on lymph node size, location and needle size. On-site cytopathological analysis is associated with a higher likelihood of obtaining a malignant diagnosis. This technique is best suited for large, clinically positive lymph nodes.

Endobronchial ultrasound (EBUS)

Linear-array ultrasound technology combined with TBNA techniques allows EBUS fine needle aspiration (FNA) of mediastinal and hilar lymph node stations. EBUS-FNA is superior in performance to TBNA. Overall sensitivity of EBUS-FNA approaches 90%.

Oesophageal endoscopic ultrasonography (EUS)

EUS-FNA is complimentary to EBUS-FNA. This modality allows sampling of inferior pulmonary ligament, perioesophageal and subcarinal lymph node stations (9, 8 and 7). Stations 2 and 4 are difficult to sample. The yield for combined EBUS-FNA and EUS-FNA has been shown to exceed 90% in obtaining a tissue diagnosis of lung cancer when present.

Mediastinoscopy

Cervical mediastinoscopy is the standard procedure for invasive mediastinal staging of lung cancer. It is now commonly performed with the assistance of video technology (video mediastinoscopy). Mediastinoscopy allows for sampling or removal of lymph node stations 2, 4, 7 and often 10. The complication rate is 2% with few life-threatening complications. With video mediastinoscopy, sensitivity and specificity exceed 97%.

Anterior mediastinotomy

An anterior mediastinotomy (Chamberlain procedure) provides access to stations 5 and 6 (aortic and aortopulmonary window), generally not accessible with standard cervical mediastinoscopy. This is performed through an incision in the left second or third intercostal space, or through an excision of the second costal cartilage.

Video-assisted thoracic surgery (VATS)

VATS provides an alternative to an anterior mediastinotomy for staging stations 5 and 6. In addition, VATS allows for access to lymph node stations 8 and 9. On the right side, subcarinal and paratracheal lymph nodes can be evaluated. Finally, the pleural cavity and primary tumour may also be assessed with VATS.

Table 20.6 UICC TNM stage grouping and summary: Lung

Stage grouping			
Occult carcinoma	TX	N0	M0
Stage 0	Tis	N0	M0
Stage IA	T1a, b	N0	M0
Stage IB	T2a	N0	M0
Stage IIA	T2b	N0	M0
	T1a, b	N1	M0
	T2a	N1	M0
Stage IIB	T2b	N1	M0
	T3	N0	M0
Stage IIIA	T1a, b, T2a, b	N2	M0
	T3	N1, N2	M0
	T4	N0, N1	M0
Stage IIIB	T4	N2	M0
	Any T	N3	M0
Stage IV	Any T	Any N	M1

For all pN categories higher than pN1MI, at least one lymph node metastasis must exceed 2.0 mm.

TNM categories	
TX	Positive cytology only
T1	≤3 cm
T1a	≤2 cm
T1b	>2–3 cm
T2	Main bronchus <2 cm from carina, invades visceral pleura, partial atelectasis
T2a	>3–5 cm
T2b	>5–7 cm
T3	>7 cm; parietal pleura, chest wall, diaphragm, pericardium, mediastinal pleura, main bronchus
	<2 cm from carina, total atelectasis, separate nodule(s) in same lobe
T4	Mediastinum, heart, great vessels, carina, trachea, oesophagus, vertebral body; separate tumour nodule(s) in a different ipsilateral lobe
N1	Ipsilateral peribronchial, ipsilateral hilar
N2	Ipsilateral mediastinal, subcarinal
N3	Contralateral mediastinal or hilar, scalene or supraclavicular
M1	Distant metastasis
M1a	Separate tumour nodule(s) in a contralateral lobe; pleural nodules or malignant pleural or pericardial effusion
M1b	Distant metastasis

Staging and prognostic grouping

UICC TNM staging
See Table 20.6.

Prognostic factors
See Tables 20.7, 20.8 and 20.9.

Table 20.7 Prognostic factors in surgically resected NSCLC

Prognostic factors	Tumour related	Host related	Environment related
Essential	T category N category Extracapsular nodal extension	Weight loss Performance status	Resection margins Adequacy of mediastinal dissection
Additional	Histological type Grade Vessel invasion Tumour size	Gender	
New and promising	Molecular/ biological markers	Quality of life Marital status	

Table 20.8 Prognostic risk factors in advanced (locally-advanced or metastatic) NSCLC

Prognostic factors	Tumour related	Host related	Environment related
Essential	Stage Superior vena cava obstruction (SVCO) Oligometastatic disease Number of sites	Weight loss Performance status	Chemotherapy Targeted therapy
Additional	Number of metastatic sites Pleural effusion Liver metastasis Haemoglobin Lactate dehydrogenase (LDH) Albumin	Gender Symptom burden	
New and promising	Molecular/biological markers	Quality of life Marital status Anxiety/ depression	

Table 20.9 Prognostic risk factors in SCLC

Prognostic factors	Tumour related	Host related	Environment related
Essential	Stage	Performance status Age Co-morbidity	Chemotherapy Thoracic radiotherapy Prophylactic cranial radiotherapy
Additional	LDH Alkaline phosphatase Cushing syndrome M0 – mediastinal involvement M1 – number of sites Brain or bone involvement White blood cell count (WBC)/platelet count		
New and promising	Molecular/biological markers		

Treatment philosophy

Scenario	Treatment philosophy
Stage I or II NSCLC	• Surgery, followed by adjuvant chemotherapy for tumours of >4 cm or lymph node involvement
Stage IIIA NSCLC	• Preoperative chemotherapy followed by surgery or definitive chemoradiotherapy
Stage IIIB NSCLC	• Concurrent chemotherapy with radiation
Stage IV NSCLC	• Platinum-based chemotherapy for patients without a targetable mutation • Targeted therapy for patients with *EGFR* mutation or *ALK* gene rearrangement
Limited-stage SCLC	• Platinum-based chemotherapy with concurrent radiation • Prophylactic cranial radiation upon completion of systemic therapy
Extensive-stage SCLC	• Platinum + etoposide chemotherapy followed by prophylactic cranial irradiation (PCI) in responding patients

Treatment

Surgery

Non-small cell lung cancer

Surgical management is an important component of multimodality therapy for early-stage lung cancer. For patients with localized NSCLC, surgery is recommended in those who are medically fit and have an adequate pulmonary reserve capacity.

Surgery	Description
Stage IA	• Lobectomy by either VATS or thoracotomy, with sampling of mediastinal nodes: 　▪ VATS lobectomy is safe, has a similar complication rate and shorter length of hospital stay compared to thoracotomy • 5-year survival rate of 73–92% with surgery • No advantage to complete mediastinal dissection over nodal sampling
Stage IA, small peripheral tumours (<2 cm)	• Role of sub-lobar resection is under evaluation and may be offered to patients with limited pulmonary reserve capacity • Anatomical segmentectomy is favoured over a non-anatomical wedge resection when performing a sub-lobar pulmonary resection • Intraoperative brachytherapy with ^{125}I to the surgical margin following a sub-lobar pulmonary resection does not decrease local tumour recurrence
Stage IB (T2aN0)	• Lobectomy is standard therapy • Centrally located tumours or those that cross the fissure into adjacent lobes may require a pneumonectomy or sleeve resection • 5-year survival rate is 55–60%
Stage II	• Lobectomy is standard therapy • Pneumonectomy or sleeve resection is utilized as necessary • Incomplete resection is not beneficial • For T3 tumours, *en bloc* resection of tumour invasion into the chest wall, diaphragm, mediastinal pleural or parietal pericardium is indicated if an R0 resection is attainable • 5-year survival rates are approximately 35–45%
Superior sulcus tumours (Pancoast)	• Chemotherapy and radiation followed by surgery • Standard radiation dose is 45 Gy • Surgery is contraindicated in patients with brachial plexus involvement more extensive than C8 and T1, presence of N2 or N3 disease

Surgery	Description
Stage IIIA	• For T3N1 or T4N0–1 NSCLC, surgery followed by chemotherapy is recommended • Upfront surgery is not recommended for patients with N2 disease • Induction chemotherapy or chemoradiotherapy followed by surgery is recommended for N2 disease • Trimodality therapy is not optimal for patients who require a pneumonectomy • Surgery is not recommended for patients with bulky N2 disease or multistation involvement
Stage IIIB/IV	• Surgery has a limited role • May be beneficial for patients with solitary brain metastasis and a peripheral lung tumour • Surgery can be considered for oligometastatic disease, following systemic therapy for patients with indolent disease biology

Small cell lung cancer

Surgical intervention is not considered standard therapy for SCLC. Operative therapy may be considered in patients with peripheral Stage I (N0) SCLC confirmed by rigorous preoperative staging. Only approximately 5% of SCLC will meet such criteria, as the majority of patients present with locally-advanced or metastatic disease. Adjuvant therapy with a cisplatin-based regimen is recommended following resection, given the high metastatic potential of these tumours. Some physicians have advocated preoperative chemotherapy followed by surgery for certain patients with peripheral SCLC and node negative disease. For pathological Stage I SCLC treated with surgery along with induction or adjuvant chemotherapy, 50% 5-year survival rates may be achieved.

Radiotherapy
Non-small cell lung cancer

Radiation therapy plays a major role in the treatment of patients with lung cancer. Combined chemotherapy and radiation is associated with a cure rate of approximately 20% in patients with Stage III surgically unresectable NSCLC.

Radiotherapy	Description
Stage I (unresectable due to medical co-morbid illness*)	• SBRT is recommended for peripheral lesions • Local control rate of nearly 90% with SBRT in T1–2N0 disease
Stages I and II	• No role for radiation in patients with negative surgical margins • Detrimental hazard ratio was observed with postoperative radiotherapy in Stages I and II NSCLC • For microscopically positive margins after surgery, 60 Gy of EBRT is recommended
Stage IIIA, N2 positive, planned for surgery	• Radiotherapy may be used with chemotherapy for selected patients as induction therapy • Standard preoperative radiation is 1.8 Gy/day to 45 Gy/day
Stage IIIA, N2 positive, surgically resected	• No proven role for radiotherapy • 50–54 Gy of EBRT may be considered after adjuvant chemotherapy for patients with multistation N2 disease • Limit target volumes to inclusion of ipsilateral hilum, bronchial stump and high-risk nodal regions
Stage IIIA/B, surgically unresectable disease	• EBRT of 60–66 Gy with concomitant platinum-based chemotherapy is standard • Sequential chemoradiotherapy is utilized for patients with poor performance status • Higher doses of radiotherapy are not recommended • No role for induction chemotherapy • If node negative: clinical tumour volume (CTV) = gross tumour volume (GTV) + 5 mm (up to 8 mm) • If node positive: CTV = GTV + 5 mm (up to 8 mm) and involved nodes + 3–5 mm
Stage IV	• Palliation of airway obstruction or haemoptysis: ▪ GTV may = CTV but depending on extent of disease, all gross tumour need not be included in the CTV • Pain control by radiation to painful bone metastatic sites • Treatment of brain metastasis • For spinal cord compression related to tumour

*Reasons for inoperability include a baseline FEV_1 of <40%, a predicted postoperative FEV_1 of <30% or a severely limited diffusion capacity.

In recent years, SBRT has been widely adopted for the management of early-stage NSCLC when surgery is not feasible. The SBRT technique involves one to five treatments with high-dose radiation in which the tumour is localized stereotactically (Table 20.10). SBRT is initially delivered utilizing a body frame, which provides a 3D coordinate system in which the tumour can be localized; however, modern techniques typically rely on image-guided radiation therapy (IGRT; i.e. cone-beam CT) to localize the tumour prior to treatment delivery. Recurrence in regional lymph node stations after SBRT is approximately 10–15%, while distant failure develops in approximately 25%.

Of particular importance when choosing a dose fractionation regimen is whether the tumour is centrally located (within 2 cm of the bronchial tree or mediastinal structures). Increased toxicity has been demonstrated with centrally located tumours when 18 Gy × 3 has been used; however, recent data indicate that central tumours can be safely treated with a dose reduction, such as 10 Gy × 5. The ongoing RTOG 0813 trial is evaluating the optimal fractionation for centrally located tumours. SBRT is generally not recommended for tumours of over 5 cm in size. Relative to standard radiation fractionation (1.8–2 Gy/day to 60–66 Gy), local control and disease-free survival are increased with the SBRT technique. Lung SBRT should only be undertaken in a radiation oncology department with a robust radiation physics programme. Important technical factors required for the safe delivery of SBRT include adequate immobilization, control of tumour motion with respiration, and quality assurance of radiation plans prior to treatment delivery.

The role of elective nodal irradiation (ENI) in NSCLC continues to evolve. RTOG 0515, a phase II study utilizing PET–CT in the delineation of radiation treatment volumes, demonstrated that rates of elective nodal failure were 2% when radiation volumes covered PET-positive disease only. Current RTOG protocols have shifted to an ENI approach.

The role of targeted agents in Stage III lung cancer is currently under investigation. For patients with unresectable, non-metastatic lung cancer and a known *EGFR* mutation or *ALK* translocation, the current standard of care is radiation with concurrent chemotherapy; however, the use of targeted agents in this patient population is under investigation.

Table 20.10 Doses for SBRT

Cumulative dose (Gy)	Number of fractions	Tumour characteristics
25–34	1	Peripheral tumours <2 cm
45–60	3	Peripheral tumours
48–50	4	Peripheral tumours <5 cm, <1 cm from chest wall
50–55	5	Central tumours, peripheral tumours <1 cm from chest wall
60–70	8–10	Central tumours

Stage IV NSCLC

Radiation therapy is reserved for palliation of symptomatic metastases in Stage IV lung cancer, including bone, brain and thoracic sites. Radiation therapy is approximately 80% effective in achieving a reduction in pain from bone metastases. A variety of radiation fractionation regimens are appropriate for palliation of bone metastases, including 8 Gy × 1, 4 Gy × 5 and 3 Gy × 10. Radiation is also useful for bulky thoracic tumours that lead to central obstruction of the airway or haemoptysis, and can effectively reduce pain in lesions that extend into the chest wall. For thoracic radiation, dose fractionation of 30–35 Gy in 10–14 fractions is recommended for patients with a good performance status and no or minimal disease outside the lung, who are likely to have a longer life expectancy, as higher dose regimens have been associated with modest improvements in overall survival. In patients with a poor performance status, 17 Gy in two fractions or 20 Gy in five fractions can be used. Concurrent chemotherapy with palliative thoracic radiation is not supported in the literature and not recommended due to increased toxicity. For patients with brain metastases, whole-brain radiation is generally recommended, typically 20–37.5 Gy in 5–15 fractions, with consideration of a stereotactic radiosurgery (SRS) boost in patients with a good performance status and one to three brain metastases. SRS is a technique that delivers high doses of radiation to the tumour with minimal exposure to surrounding normal tissues.

In patients with an isolated metastasis or limited number of metastatic sites, prospective studies have demonstrated prolonged survival with SBRT to sites of distant metastases and definitive treatment of thoracic disease. This approach can be considered in patients with a good performance status and low-volume metastatic disease.

Spinal cord compression and, to a lesser extent, compression of the superior vena cava are considered urgent clinical scenarios in which local therapy should be rapidly initiated. In spinal cord compression, if a patient has a single area of compression and a life expectancy of >3 months, decompressive laminectomy and spine stabilization should be performed followed by spinal radiation. In multilevel spinal cord compression and in patients with a poor performance status, immediate radiation should be pursued.

Small cell lung cancer
Early SCLC (T1–2N0)

Approximately 5% of all patients with SCLC are diagnosed with T1–2N0 tumours; in this clinical scenario, patients should undergo surgical resection after assessment of the mediastinum to ensure occult nodal disease is not present. This should be followed by systemic therapy and consideration of prophylactic cranial irradiation (PCI). If N2 disease is present after surgery, mediastinal radiation should be delivered.

Limited-stage SCLC ($T_{any}N_{any}M0$)

Definitive chemoradiation should be employed to treat patients with limited-stage SCLC. Concurrent chemoradiation is preferred to sequential treatment, and radiation should begin within delivery of the first two cycles of chemotherapy. The optimal radiation fractionation is unknown. Daily radiation to 45 Gy is inferior to 45 Gy delivered twice daily; however, it is unknown if twice-daily radiation to 45 Gy (1.8 Gy/day delivered over 3 weeks) is superior to daily radiation to higher doses (60–70 Gy). This question is being investigated in the CALGB 30610/RTOG 0538, a randomized trial comparing 45 Gy twice daily over 3 weeks to 70 Gy daily over 7 weeks, with concurrent cisplatin and etoposide. The role of ENI continues to evolve; however, recent data indicate that when using PET-based radiation planning, elective nodal failure rates are <5%. Ongoing randomized trials including CALGB 30610/RTOG 0538 have omitted ENI. The most significant grade 3 toxicity of concurrent chemoradiation is oesophagitis, which occurs in approximately 25% of patients receiving 45 Gy twice daily. Overall survival at 5 years for patients receiving definitive chemoradiation is approximately 25%. Patients achieving a complete response to therapy should receive PCI, as it decreases development of brain metastases and leads to an absolute improvement in overall survival of approximately 5%. PCI treatment should be given to 25 Gy in 10 fractions, or 30 Gy in 10–15 fractions. Doses up to 36 Gy have been shown to lead to higher rates of neurotoxicity and death in a randomized trial compared to 25 Gy, and should not be used.

Extensive-stage SCLC ($T_{any}N_{any}M1a/M1b$ or T3/T4 with separate nodules not fitting within a treatable radiation field)

The primary treatment for extensive-stage SCLC is systemic therapy. Thoracic radiation (see Box 20.1) has been shown to decrease thoracic failure and improve overall survival in some studies. Ongoing randomized trials are investigating the use of thoracic radiation after systemic therapy. Patients achieving a partial response to systemic therapy should receive PCI, as it has been shown to improve overall survival. Accepted PCI dose regimens are similar to those utilized in limited-stage SCLC: 25 Gy in ten fractions or 30 Gy in 10–15 fractions.

In patients with brain metastases, whole-brain radiation should be utilized (20–37.5 Gy in 5–15 fractions). If patients were given PCI previously, a second course of whole-brain radiation can be employed at a lower dose, typically 20 Gy in ten fractions. SRS generally should not be used as a first approach to brain metastases in SCLC, as micrometastatic seeding of the brain is very high in SCLC and the risk for further intracranial failure is high. SRS can be considered after recurrence of intracranial disease in patients with a history of PCI or whole-brain radiotherapy. Palliative radiation for painful symptomatic metastatic sites is commonly used, with fractionation regimens similar to those used in NSCLC.

Systemic therapy
Advanced-stage non-small cell lung cancer
Systemic therapy plays an important role in the treatment of nearly all stages of NSCLC. In advanced-stage disease, systemic therapy is the treatment modality of choice (see Boxes 20.2 and 20.3), whereas in earlier stages of the disease, it is given in conjunction with local therapy. Systemic therapy refers to the use of cytotoxic agents and molecularly targeted agents that have recently been incorporated into the treatment paradigm of NSCLC. Chemotherapeutic agents used commonly for lung cancer include platinum compounds, taxanes, gemcitabine, pemetrexed and vinorelbine (Table 20.11). Erlotinib, gefitinib and afatinib are small molecule tyrosine kinase inhibitors (TKIs) that inhibit the epidermal growth factor receptor (EGFR). Crizotinib, a recently approved agent, targets the anaplastic lymphoma kinase (ALK) tyrosine kinase. In addition, a number of

> **Box 20.1** Thoracic radiation planning and delivery
>
> - All patients undergoing definitive treatment should undergo CT-based radiation planning with 3D conformal radiation planning
> - PET–CT, where available, should be used when defining radiation volumes for patients undergoing curative treatment
> - Tumour motion with respiration should be assessed, ideally with 4D CT
> - If tumour motion is significant, attempts to decrease motion should be made with techniques including gated treatment or abdominal compression to dampen motion
> - Treatment planning software should include the use of heterogeneity corrections
> - IGRT is recommended for SBRT treatment and 3D/intensity-modulated radiation therapy (IMRT)-based treatments with steep dose gradients
> - If motion assessment is not available, a planning target volume (PTV) margin of 1 cm circumferentially and 1.5 cm superior/inferior may be appropriate. However, this should not be combined with a large CTV margin

> **Box 20.2** Systemic therapy in advanced-stage disease
>
> - Platinum compounds are the cornerstone of therapy:
>   - Cisplatin and carboplatin have comparable survival effects in advanced NSCLC
>   - Carboplatin-based therapy has a better tolerability profile compared to cisplatin-based regimens
>   - Carboplatin is easier to administer in the outpatient setting
>   - Platinum-based two-drug combinations are recommended
> - Paclitaxel, nab-paclitaxel, docetaxel, gemcitabine, pemetrexed, vinorelbine and irinotecan are all acceptable combination partners for platinum in advanced NSCLC:
>   - Combination of cisplatin + pemetrexed is superior to cisplatin + gemcitabine in adenocarcinoma, but inferior in squamous histology
>   - Combination of three cytotoxic agents is more toxic and does not improve survival

Box 20.3 Systemic therapy in surgically unresectable, locally-advanced NSCLC

- Concurrent chemotherapy with radiation is the recommended approach for patients with a good performance status
- Cisplatin + etoposide and carboplatin + paclitaxel are two of the most commonly used chemotherapy regimens
- Use of induction chemotherapy is not recommended prior to radiotherapy
- For patients with a poor performance status, sequential chemoradiotherapy is better tolerated
- Incidence of oesophagitis is higher with concurrent therapy than with sequential therapy
- With concomitant chemoradiotherapy, the 5-year survival rate is approximately 20% with a median survival of 17–20 months

new agents are presently under development for the treatment of specific molecular subsets of NSCLC.

Multiple randomized clinical trials have established the superiority of platinum-based two-drug combinations over single-agent therapy for advanced NSCLC patients. This benefit appears to be primarily limited to patients with a good performance status (ECOG score 0 or 1), although recent studies show that certain patients with poor performance status (ECOG score 2) might also benefit from combination regimens. Frequently used combination regimens include carboplatin + paclitaxel, carboplatin + docetaxel, cisplatin + pemetrexed, cisplatin + gemcitabine, cisplatin + vinorelbine and carboplatin + nab-paclitaxel. In the Japanese patient population, the combination of cisplatin + irinotecan is widely used for advanced NSCLC.

The comparative efficacy of various combinations has been tested in several randomized studies. In ECOG 1594, patients were randomized to one of four different platinum-based chemotherapy

Table 20.11 Chemotherapy regimens for first-line therapy of advanced NSCLC

Regimen	Dosage	Reference
Cisplatin + vinorelbine	Cisplatin 100 mg/m^2 Day 1 Vinorelbine 25 mg/m^2 Days 1, 8, 15 and 21 every 28 days	Wozniak et al. (1998) J Clin Oncol 16(7):2459–2465
Cisplatin + gemcitabine	Cisplatin 100 mg/m^2 Day 1 Gemcitabine 1250 mg/m^2 Days 1 and 8 every 21 days	Cardenal et al. (1999) J Clin Oncol 17(1):12–18
Cisplatin + gemcitabine	Cisplatin 100 mg/m^2 Day 1 Gemcitabine 1000 mg/m^2 Days 1, 8 and 15 every 28 days	Sandler et al. (2000) J Clin Oncol 18(1):122–130
Cisplatin + paclitaxel	Cisplatin 80 mg/m^2 Day 1 Paclitaxel 175 mg/m^2 Day 1 every 21 days	Smit et al. (2003) J Clin Oncol 21(21):3909–3917
Cisplatin + docetaxel	Cisplatin 75 mg/m^2 Day 1 Docetaxel 75 mg/m^2 Day 1 every 21 days	Fossella et al. (2003) J Clin Oncol 21(16):3016–3024
Cisplatin + pemetrexed	Cisplatin 75 mg/m^2 Day 1 Pemetrexed 500 mg/m^2 Day 1 every 21 days	Scagliotti et al. (2008) J Clin Oncol 26(21):3543–3451
Carboplatin + paclitaxel	Carboplatin AUC 6 Day 1 Paclitaxel 225 mg/m^2 Day 1 every 21 days	Schiller et al. (2002) N Engl J Med 346(2):92–98
Carboplatin + weekly paclitaxel	Carboplatin AUC 6 Day 1 Paclitaxel 100 mg/m^2 Day 1, 8 and 15 every 21 days	Belani et al. (2008) J Clin Oncol 26(3):468–473
Carboplatin + paclitaxel + bevacizumab	Carboplatin AUC 6 Day 1 Paclitaxel 200 mg/m^2 Day 1 Bevacizumab 15 mg/kg Day 1 every 21 days	Sandler et al. (2006) N Engl J Med 355(24):2542–2550
Carboplatin + nab-paclitaxel	Carboplatin AUC 6 Day 1 Nab-paclitaxel 100 mg/m^2 Days 1, 8 and 15 every 21 days	Socinski et al. (2012) J Clin Oncol 30(17):2055–2062
Carboplatin + gemcitabine	Carboplatin AUC 5 Day 1 Gemcitabine 1100 mg/m^2 Days 1 and 8 every 28 days	Iaffaioli et al. (1999) J Clin Oncol 17(3):921–926
Carboplatin + pemetrexed	Carboplatin AUC 6 Day 1 Pemetrexed 500 mg/m^2 Day 1 every 21 days	Scagliotti et al. (2005) Clin Cancer Res 11 (2 Pt 1):690–696

Table 20.12 Maintenance therapy agents

Pemetrexed	• Improves survival when used as either 'switch' or 'continuation' maintenance* • Modest improvement in overall survival • Not recommended for squamous histology
Erlotinib	• Improves survival when used as switch maintenance • Benefit was mainly in patients who achieved stable disease with platinum-based chemotherapy compared to those with a partial or complete response • Robust PFS in patients with *EGFR* mutation with the use of erlotinib
Bevacizumab	• Monoclonal antibody against vascular endothelial growth factor (VEGF) • Approved for first-line therapy of patients with advanced non-squamous NSCLC in combination with platinum-based chemotherapy • After four to six cycles of combination therapy, bevacizumab is continued as monotherapy for maintenance

*Switch maintenance refers to introduction of a new agent that was not part of the first-line combination regimen, whereas continuation refers to using one of the first-line therapy components as maintenance therapy.

regimens. The response rate, progression-free survival (PFS) and overall survival were comparable for all four regimens, with the only differences being related to toxicity issues. More recently, the regimen of cisplatin + pemetrexed was compared to cisplatin + gemcitabine in a phase III study for first-line therapy of advanced NSCLC. The cisplatin + pemetrexed regimen was non-inferior in the overall population, but was superior in patients with non-squamous histology, based on a prespecified analysis. In patients with squamous histology, the cisplatin + gemcitabine regimen was superior to cisplatin + pemetrexed. Therefore, ascertainment of specific histological subtype is important for the use of the cisplatin + pemetrexed combination regimen.

Platinum-based two-drug combinations result in a response rate of approximately 30–40% and a median PFS of approximately 3.5–6 months in advanced-stage NSCLC. The median overall survival is approximately 8–11 months with a 1-year survival rate of 40–50%. Prognostic factors include both clinical and molecular characteristics associated with the cancer. The clinical factors include performance status, female sex, never-smoking status and serum haemoglobin levels. *EGFR* mutation status has recently emerged as a molecular factor that is associated with a favourable survival in advanced NSCLC.

Maintenance therapy

Maintenance therapy refers to the use of single-agent therapy following four to six cycles of combination chemotherapy. It is used until disease progression or patient intolerance. The optimal maintenance agent should have minimal toxicity, be easy to administer in the outpatient setting and improve survival. Erlotinib and pemetrexed are approved maintenance therapy agents (Table 20.12). For patients who receive bevacizumab in combination with chemotherapy, continuation of bevacizumab as maintenance monotherapy is recommended. Use of maintenance therapy should be based on patient choice, symptom burden, tolerance of prior therapy and performance status.

In first-line therapy for advanced NSCLC, four to six cycles of combination chemotherapy are considered optimal. Randomized studies that compared administration of three or four cycles of chemotherapy to continuation of therapy until progression demonstrated comparable efficacy outcomes, but unfavourable toxicity results for the latter approach. More recently, clinical trials have evaluated the use of single-agent therapy for maintaining response to first-line combination chemotherapy among patients who achieve either an objective response or stable disease. Since maintenance therapy is often given for an extended number of cycles, an agent with proven efficacy, low cumulative toxicity and favourable tolerability would be considered ideal.

The use of maintenance therapy must be individualized to patients based on performance status, patient preference and toxicities associated with prior chemotherapy. For some patients, a treatment 'holiday' following combination chemotherapy with close surveillance would be appropriate. This is supported by observations that the benefit from maintenance therapy can be achieved with salvage therapy as long as patients receive active therapy upon disease progression. The lack of data supporting improvement in patient quality of life with maintenance therapy is another factor that calls for careful selection of patients for maintenance therapy.

Salvage therapy

Salvage therapy is appropriate for patients who develop disease progression following first-line therapy (Table 20.13). Docetaxel

Table 20.13 Chemotherapy regimens for second-line therapy of advanced NSCLC

Regimen	Dosage	Reference
Docetaxel	75 mg/m² Day 1 every 21 days	Fossella *et al.* (2000) *J Clin Oncol* 18(12):2354–2362
Pemetrexed	500 mg/m² Day 1 every 21 days	Hanna *et al.* (2004) *J Clin Oncol* 22(9):1589–1597
Erlotinib	150 mg daily	Shepherd *et al.* (2005) *N Engl J Med* 353(2):123–132
Gefitinib	250 mg daily	Kim *et al.* (2008) *Lancet* 372:1809–1818

was the first agent to be approved for salvage therapy. When given at a dose of 75 mg/m² every 3 weeks, docetaxel improves response rate and survival over best supportive care. It also confers improvements in symptoms related to lung cancer when used as salvage therapy. Pemetrexed has also demonstrated efficacy for salvage therapy of non-squamous NSCLC. A randomized study compared pemetrexed to docetaxel for salvage therapy of advanced NSCLC. The efficacy parameters were non-inferior and the safety profile was more favourable with pemetrexed. The incidences of hospitalization, myelosuppression and alopecia were lower with pemetrexed. Based on a *post hoc* analysis by histology, the efficacy of pemetrexed was found to be restricted to patients with non-squamous histology. Hence, it is only indicated for the treatment of non-squamous NSCLC.

Erlotinib has also been approved by the FDA for salvage therapy of advanced NSCLC. It was compared to placebo in patients with advanced NSCLC who had disease progression following one or two prior chemotherapy regimens. There was an improvement in overall survival (6.7 months vs 4.7 months) and response rate (9% vs <1%) with erlotinib. Diarrhoea and skin rash were the most common toxicities associated with erlotinib. Initial studies of erlotinib were conducted in patients regardless of their molecular status. Following the discovery of sensitizing mutations in *EGFR*, recent studies have evaluated the efficacy of erlotinib based on the presence or absence of mutations. While it is clear that patients with certain mutations in *EGFR* derive robust benefits from erlotinib, its efficacy in patients with wild-type *EGFR* is relatively modest. Therefore, the optimal salvage therapy for patients with wild-type *EGFR* is still evolving.

A number of new agents are presently being tested for salvage therapy of advanced NSCLC. The use of combination regimens for salvage therapy has failed to demonstrate survival benefit and is therefore not considered standard.

Targeted therapy

Antiangiogenic therapy. Angiogenesis is critical for cancer progression and metastasis. A number of factors that mediate the balance between promotion and inhibition of angiogenesis have been described in the setting of cancer. Activation of the vascular endothelial growth factor (VEGF) signalling pathway promotes angiogenesis as a major contributor to tumour growth and metastasis. Strategies to inhibit angiogenesis by blocking VEGF or its receptors have been extensively studied in NSCLC.

Bevacizumab is a monoclonal antibody against VEGF. A randomized clinical trial demonstrated improved survival in patients with advanced non-squamous histology when it was given in combination with carboplatin + paclitaxel compared to chemotherapy alone. A second randomized study in a similar patient population that added bevacizumab to cisplatin + gemcitabine met its primary endpoint of a statistically significant improvement in PFS, but did not result in improved survival. These trials led to the approval of bevacizumab by the US FDA and the EMA for first-line therapy of advanced non-squamous NSCLC.

Box 20.4 *EGFR* mutations

- Observed in nearly 15% of Caucasian and 40% of Asian patients
- More common in never-smokers and women
- Observed in adenocarcinoma patients but not in other histological subtypes
- Most mutations are localized to exon 19 or 21 of the *EGFR* gene
- Prognostic for improved survival and predictive of benefit from both chemotherapy and EGFR tyrosine kinase inhibitors
- Screening for *EGFR* mutation is considered standard in patients with newly diagnosed advanced-stage lung adenocarcinoma
- Use of immunohistochemistry and FISH for *EGFR* mutation are not recommended to make treatment decisions
- Preferred first-line therapy for patients with activating *EGFR* mutations is EGFR inhibitors

---

Safety data are now available to advocate the use of bevacizumab following appropriate local therapy to the brain such as whole-brain radiotherapy or SRS. The combination of bevacizumab with thoracic radiation is not recommended since a few cases of tracheoesophageal fistula have been reported in this setting. The higher incidence of adverse events with bevacizumab-based combinations in elderly patients (>70 years) calls for careful selection of patients based on clinical factors such as performance status and co-morbid conditions. Efforts to identify predictive biomarkers to select patients for bevacizumab have been unsuccessful to date.

A number of small VEGF receptor TKIs have been studied as monotherapy and in combination with standard therapies in advanced NSCLC. Sorafenib, sunitinib, vandetanib, axitinib and motesanib have all failed to demonstrate improvement in survival upon administration with standard chemotherapy, despite modest single-agent activity in NSCLC. The use of agents that disrupt existing vasculature, referred to as vascular disrupting agents, has also yielded disappointing results in advanced NSCLC.

In the present days, molecular testing for *EGFR* mutations (see Box 20.4) is recommended for all patients with lung adenocarcinoma. For advanced NSCLC patients with an activating mutation, EGFR TKIs are recommended for first-line therapy (Table 20.14). If *EGFR* mutation is not observed, the patient is best served with first-line chemotherapy. In most settings it would take approximately 1–2 weeks to obtain the results of *EGFR* mutation testing. If the clinical course of the patient does not allow this wait, then initiation of chemotherapy followed by utilization of EGFR TKIs in either the maintenance or salvage therapy setting is appropriate.

The efficacy of EGFR inhibitors appears to be comparable regardless of whether they are used in the first-line therapy, maintenance therapy or salvage therapy settings. Response

Table 20.14 EGFR inhibitors in clinical use

Gefitinib (250 mg/day)	• Reversible EGFR inhibitor • Superior PFS and response rate compared to platinum-based chemotherapy in advanced NSCLC patients with *EGFR* mutation • Diarrhoea and skin rash are the common adverse events • Only indicated in patients with activating EGFR mutations
Erlotinib (150 mg/day)	• Reversible EGFR inhibitor • Improvement in PFS and response rate (RR) over platinum-based chemotherapy • Has not been directly compared to other EGFR inhibitors • Also approved for patients regardless of mutation status in salvage therapy setting
Afatinib (40 mg/day)	• Irreversible EGFR inhibitor • Also inhibits ErbB2 and ErbB4 • Improved PFS and RR over and pemetrexed in advanced NSCLC patients with *EGFR* mutation • Higher incidence of mucositis, diarrhoea and skin rash than the reversible EGFR inhibitors

Box 20.5 Crizotinib in advanced NSCLC

- Indicated for patients with ALK positivity by FISH assay
- Administered at a dose of 250 mg twice a day
- Results in response rate of approximately 60% and a median PFS of 10 months
- Preferred for use in first-line, maintenance or second-line therapy
- In a randomized trial, crizotinib was superior to salvage chemotherapy in ALK-positive patients: improved response rate and PFS

rates of approximately 50–70% and a median PFS of 8–12 months have been observed with EGFR inhibitors in randomized clinical trials of patients with sensitizing mutations in exon 19 or 21. Acquired resistance to EGFR inhibitors develops from secondary mutations in exon 20 (*T790*) in approximately 60% of patients, or by activation of alternative pathways. Activation of the MET pathway contributes to resistance in approximately 10% of patients. There have also been reports of the development of SCLC in response to EGFR inhibitor therapy. In <5% of patients, *de novo T790* mutations are present in addition to sensitizing mutations in exon 19 or 21. The clinical efficacy of EGFR inhibitors in patients with *de novo T790* mutations is not well known. For patients who develop resistance from *T790* mutations, specific inhibitors are presently under development. Combination approaches to delay resistance such as by using inhibitors of MET with EGFR inhibition are also under evaluation.

ALK inhibition. Gene rearrangement involving the *ALK* gene was reported recently in patients with NSCLC. A number of fusion partners that associate with ALK lead to dominant signalling by this pathway, thus rendering this a molecular driver for a subset of approximately 5% of patients with lung adenocarcinoma. Crizotinib, an inhibitor of ALK, MET and ROS1 tyrosine kinases, has demonstrated robust anticancer activity in patients with *ALK*-positive NSCLC (see Box 20.5).

Despite the robust efficacy, resistance to crizotinib develops from a variety of mechanisms, most prominent of which are the development of new 'gatekeeper' mutations and the activation of alternate non–ALK-dominant pathways. A number of second-generation ALK inhibitors are presently under development to overcome resistance to crizotinib. LDK 378 belongs to this class of agents and has demonstrated a response rate of nearly 70% in patients with ALK-positive disease following emergence of resistance to crizotinib. Heat shock protein 90 inhibitors have also demonstrated activity in ALK-positive NSCLC and could be used as another strategy to overcome resistance. Ongoing studies are evaluating the role of ALK inhibitors in earlier stages of NSCLC.

In all the trials conducted to date, ALK status was evaluated by fluorescent *in situ* hybridization (FISH) test and positivity defined as the presence of a fusion gene in at least 15% of the cells. More recent studies have demonstrated the utility of ALK protein detection by immunohistochemistry as a screening test before the FISH assay.

Other molecular abnormalities in NSCLC. The discovery of *EGFR* mutations and *ALK* gene rearrangement has paved the way for further development of individualized therapies in NSCLC. Recent studies have documented *ROS1* gene rearrangements in approximately 1% of lung adenocarcinoma patients. This subset of patients also responds to crizotinib therapy with a robust response rate of nearly 70%. *RET* gene fusion abnormalities have also been detected in nearly 1% of lung adenocarcinoma patients. Other uncommon mutations in lung adenocarcinoma include *HER2*, *B-RAF* and phosphoinositide 3-kinase (*PI3K*). Studies are presently ongoing to evaluate targeted therapies for these individual molecular subsets of patients. Nearly two-thirds of patients with lung adenocarcinoma have a dominant mutation or gene rearrangement that can be used to guide therapy. Similar efforts to identify mutations in squamous cell histology are underway. Molecular abnormalities reported in squamous cell carcinoma include *PI3K*, fibroblast growth factor receptor (*FGFR*) amplification and discoid domain receptor (*DDR2*) mutation. As a result of these molecular classification efforts, the treatment landscape for NSCLC has undergone major changes. Testing the diagnostic tumour tissue for molecular abnormalities to guide therapy is highly recommended for patients with lung adenocarcinoma.

Early-stage NSCLC

The treatment of early-stage NSCLC has gradually evolved from single modality therapy to multimodality therapy over the past two decades (see Box 20.6). This has largely been due to studies that have documented improved cure rates with the integration

> **Box 20.6** Role of adjuvant chemotherapy in early-stage NSCLC
>
> - Cisplatin-based two-drug combinations are recommended
> - Indicated for patients with lymph node involvement and/or tumour size >4 cm
> - Four cycles of therapy recommended
> - Chemotherapy should begin within 6–8 weeks from the time of surgery
> - Chemotherapy may be detrimental in patients with Stage IA disease
> - Use of carboplatin is unproven in this setting

of systemic therapy for nearly every stage of NSCLC. Cisplatin-based combination chemotherapy is now considered standard therapy for surgically resected Stage II and IIIA NSCLC. In several randomized clinical trials, administration of four cycles of adjuvant chemotherapy following surgery resulted in an absolute improvement in the 5-year survival rate of 5–15%. The benefit from adjuvant chemotherapy appears to be proportional to the risk of recurrence following surgery based on tumour size and nodal involvement. The majority of clinical trials have evaluated the regimen of cisplatin + vinorelbine for adjuvant therapy and hence this has emerged as a regimen of choice for adjuvant chemotherapy. The benefit from third-generation chemotherapy agents such as taxanes, gemcitabine and pemetrexed has not been established in the adjuvant therapy setting, although these agents are tolerated well and have shown comparable activity to vinorelbine in patients with advanced-stage NSCLC.

Stage IIIA NSCLC with mediastinal nodal disease includes a very heterogeneous group of patients based on number of involved nodes, number of stations and size of the nodes. Therefore, treatment options should be individualized with input from all involved specialties. Randomized studies have documented an improvement in survival for neoadjuvant chemotherapy followed by surgery versus surgery alone. Chemoradiotherapy followed by surgery has also yielded favourable results compared to surgery alone. The added utility of radiotherapy in the preoperative setting has not been fully established, although it can be beneficial for certain patient subsets. A recent study that randomized patients to chemoradiotherapy followed by surgery versus the former alone failed to demonstrate a survival advantage for the surgical group, but disease-free survival was improved in the tri-modality therapy group. Patients who underwent a pneumonectomy following chemoradiotherapy had a poor outcome due to a high 30-day mortality following surgery. Therefore, the tri-modality approach is not considered optimal for patients who require a pneumonectomy. Patients who achieve clearance of the mediastinal lymph nodes with induction therapy are most likely to benefit from subsequent surgery. The use of EBUS-guided biopsy allows for restaging the mediastinum after neoadjuvant therapy to assess the role of surgery in these patients. For patients with multistation N2 disease and/or bulky nodal disease, chemoradiotherapy alone is considered adequate therapy.

Small cell lung cancer

SCLC is characterized by a rapid disease course with initial responsiveness to chemotherapy. It is diagnosed at an advanced stage in the majority of patients. Systemic chemotherapy is the recommended treatment for patients with SCLC (see Box 20.7 and Table 20.15). Platinum-based combination regimens are used to treat both limited and extensive stages of SCLC. The combination of cisplatin + etoposide is the most commonly used treatment regimen for first-line therapy of SCLC. This regimen results in a response rate of approximately 50–70% and a median survival of nearly 10 months.

Despite the initial sensitivity to chemotherapy, patients with extensive-stage SCLC develop disease progression in

> **Box 20.7** Chemotherapy in SCLC
>
> - Cisplatin + etoposide is the preferred regimen for limited-stage SCLC
> - Carboplatin can be substituted for cisplatin in extensive-stage SCLC
> - In the Japanese patient population, use of cisplatin + irinotecan is efficacious and superior to cisplatin + etoposide; in the Western patient population, it was not superior
> - No role for high-dose chemotherapy or dose-dense therapy
> - Four cycles of chemotherapy are considered optimal
> - Median PFS is approximately 4–6 months with an overall survival of 8–11 months
> - In limited-stage SCLC, earlier initiation of radiotherapy along with chemotherapy is preferred over delayed radiotherapy
> - Topotecan is approved for salvage chemotherapy
> - Effectiveness of topotecan is restricted to patients with 'sensitive' relapse

Table 20.15 Commonly used chemotherapy regimens for SCLC

Cisplatin + etoposide	Cisplatin 75 mg/m^2 Day 1 Etoposide 100 mg/m^2 Days 1, 2 and 3 Every 21 days	Sundstrom et al. (2002) J Clin Oncol 0(24):4665–4672
Cisplatin + irinotecan	Cisplatin 60 mg/m^2 Day 1 Irinotecan 60 mg/m^2 Days 1, 8 and 15 Every 28 days	Noda et al. (2002) N Engl J Med 346(2):85–91
Carboplatin + etoposide	Carboplatin AUC 6 Day 1 Etoposide 100 mg/m^2 Days 1, 2 and 3 Every 21 days	Quoix et al. (2001) Ann Oncol 12(7):957–966

approximately 4–6 months. Topotecan is the only agent approved for salvage therapy for SCLC, based on a randomized study that demonstrated improved symptom control for this drug, although there was no improvement in overall survival. The efficacy of topotecan is limited to patients with sensitive disease, defined as responsiveness to a platinum-based combination regimen with at least a 60-days interval from the time of last chemotherapy until disease progression. In patients with refractory disease to first-line chemotherapy, there are no proven approaches and therefore enrolment in a clinical trial or supportive care is considered optimal. Amrubicin, an anthracycline derivative, has demonstrated activity in refractory SCLC, but a phase III study failed to demonstrate any advantage over topotecan.

There have been no major improvements to systemic therapy of SCLC in the past two decades. Several targeted agents including inhibitors of angiogenesis, *Bcl-2* and *c-Kit*, have been studied without much success. Recently, with genomic sequencing approaches, a variety of novel targets have been identified in SCLC. These observations provide new therapeutic opportunities to improve the outcome for patients with SCLC.

Post-treatment assessments

Many patients treated for lung cancer will experience either local or distant recurrence. Recurrence often occurs at multiple sites and is rarely curable. The main goal of follow-up is early identification of recurrent disease (or second primary cancer) while still small and treatable.

Post-treatment follow-up	Description
Early-stage disease	• No evidence-based guidelines are available • Imaging study every 6 months is reasonable for the first 2 years, followed by annual evaluations • History and physical exam every 3–6 months
Locally-advanced Stage III disease	• Imaging study every 3–6 months for 2 years, followed by less frequent follow-up • Annual imaging after 5 years
Advanced-stage disease	• *On systemic therapy:* ▪ CT scans every two to three cycles of therapy ▪ No role for PET scan in surveillance • *On treatment 'holiday':* CT scan every 3 months

It is to be noted that practice patterns vary widely regarding the imaging modality and frequency due to the lack of evidence-based guidelines. The role of PET–CT scan in patients with treated lung cancer has not been studied adequately for it to be used in routine practice.

Controversies

The growing understanding of the biology of lung cancer and the development of new treatment approaches has improved the outcomes for patients with all stages of lung cancer. However, several controversies still remain that are being addressed by ongoing and planned clinical trials.
- *Early-stage disease:*
  - Lobectomy versus sub-lobar resection for small primary tumours
  - Role of SBRT versus surgery
  - Chemotherapy versus chemoradiotherapy as induction treatment in N2-positive disease
  - Role of postoperative radiotherapy in resected N2-positive disease
  - Use of targeted therapy for oncogene addicted tumours
- *Advanced-stage disease:*
  - Role of maintenance therapy in advanced NSCLC
  - Multiplex versus targeted mutation testing
  - Use of chemotherapy with concurrent EGFR inhibitors in patients with activating *EGFR* mutation
  - Role of EGFR inhibitors in patients with wild-type tumours

An important clinical issue relates to optimal follow-up of patients with surgically resected early-stage NSCLC and for patients with Stage III disease following definitive therapy. Varying strategies are presently being used including CT scans and PET scans at varying intervals ranging from every 3 months to annual surveillance. There are presently no evidence-based guidelines for surveillance. The Eastern Cooperative Oncology Group (ECOG) is planning a randomized clinical trial to address this issue.

Phase III clinical trials

See Table 20.16.

Table 20.16 Phase III clinical trials

Trial	Issue addressed
ECOG 1505 (NCT 00324805)	• Role of bevacizumab in combination with adjuvant chemotherapy for early-stage NSCLC
ALCHEMIST (EGFR and ALK) (NCT 02194738)	• Role of targeted therapy in early-stage disease
ECOG 5508 (NCT 01107626)	• Optimal maintenance therapy in advanced-stage non-squamous NSCLC
LUNG ART Trial (NCT 00410683)	• Use of postoperative radiotherapy in patients with resected Stage IIIA N2-positive disease
LUX Lung 7 Study (NCT 01466660)	• Comparison of afatinib to gefitinib in advanced NSCLC patients with an activating *EGFR* mutation

Recommended reading

Albain KS, Swann RS, Rusch VW et al. (2009) Radiotherapy plus chemotherapy with or without surgical resection for stage III non-small-cell lung cancer: a phase III randomised controlled trial. *Lancet* 374:379–386.

Brandman S, Ko JP (2011) Pulmonary nodule detection, characterization, and management with multidetector computed tomography. *J Thorac Imaging* 26:90–105.

Curran WJ, Jr., Paulus R, Langer CJ et al. (2011) Sequential vs. concurrent chemoradiation for stage III non-small cell lung cancer: randomized phase III trial RTOG 9410. *J Natl Cancer Inst* 103:1452–1460.

Darling GE, Allen MS, Decker PA et al. (2011) Randomized trial of mediastinal lymph node sampling versus complete lymphadenectomy during pulmonary resection in the patient with N0 or N1 (less than hilar) non-small cell carcinoma: results of the American College of Surgery Oncology Group Z0030 Trial. *J Thorac Cardiovasc Surg* 141:662–670.

Douillard JY, Rosell R, De Lena M et al. (2008) Impact of postoperative radiation therapy on survival in patients with complete resection and stage I, II, or IIIA non-small-cell lung cancer treated with adjuvant chemotherapy: the adjuvant Navelbine International Trialist Association (ANITA) Randomized Trial. *Int J Radiat Oncol Biol Phys* 72:695–701.

Hanna N, Shepherd FA, Fossella FV et al. (2004) Randomized phase III trial of pemetrexed versus docetaxel in patients with non-small-cell lung cancer previously treated with chemotherapy. *J Clin Oncol* 22:1589–1597.

Hotta K, Matsuo K, Ueoka H et al. Meta-analysis of randomized clinical trials comparing Cisplatin to Carboplatin in patients with advanced non-small-cell lung cancer. *J Clin Oncol* 22:3852–3859.

Kwak EL, Bang YJ, Camidge DR et al. (2010) Anaplastic lymphoma kinase inhibition in non-small-cell lung cancer. *N Engl J Med* 363:1693–1703.

Lynch TJ, Bell DW, Sordella R et al. (2004) Activating mutations in the epidermal growth factor receptor underlying responsiveness of non-small-cell lung cancer to gefitinib. *N Engl J Med* 350:2129–2139.

MacMahon H, Austin JH, Gamsu G et al. (2005) Guidelines for management of small pulmonary nodules detected on CT scans: a statement from the Fleischner Society. *Radiology* 237:395–400.

Mok TS, Wu YL, Thongprasert S et al. (2009) Gefitinib or carboplatin-paclitaxel in pulmonary adenocarcinoma. *N Engl J Med* 361:947–957.

National Lung Screening Trial Research T, Aberle DR, Adams AM et al. (2011) Reduced lung-cancer mortality with low-dose computed tomographic screening. *N Engl J Med* 365:395–409.

Pignon JP, Tribodet H, Scagliotti GV et al. (2008) Lung adjuvant cisplatin evaluation: a pooled analysis by the LACE Collaborative Group. *J Clin Oncol* 26:3552–3559.

Ramalingam SS, Owonikoko TK, Khuri FR (2011) Lung cancer: New biological insights and recent therapeutic advances. *CA Cancer J Clin* 61:91–112.

Ravenel JG, Mohammed TL, Movsas B et al. ACR Appropriateness Criteria(R) noninvasive clinical staging of bronchogenic carcinoma. *J Thorac Imaging* 25:W107–111.

Sandler A, Gray R, Perry MC et al. (2006) Paclitaxel-carboplatin alone or with bevacizumab for non-small-cell lung cancer. *N Engl J Med* 355:2542–2550.

Scagliotti GV, Parikh P, von Pawel J et al. (2008) Phase III study comparing cisplatin plus gemcitabine with cisplatin plus pemetrexed in chemotherapy-naive patients with advanced-stage non-small-cell lung cancer. *J Clin Oncol* 26:3543–3551.

Schiller JH, Harrington D, Belani CP et al. (2002) Comparison of four chemotherapy regimens for advanced non-small-cell lung cancer. *N Engl J Med* 346:92–98.

Shepherd FA, Dancey J, Ramlau R et al. Prospective randomized trial of docetaxel versus best supportive care in patients with non-small-cell lung cancer previously treated with platinum-based chemotherapy. *J Clin Oncol* 18:2095–2103.

Timmerman R, Paulus R, Galvin J et al. (2010) Stereotactic body radiation therapy for inoperable early stage lung cancer. *JAMA* 303:1070–1076.

21 Breast

Ivo A. Olivotto[1], Caroline Lohrisch[2] and Christopher Baliski[3]

[1]Division of Radiation Oncology, University of Calgary and Tom Baker Cancer Centre, Calgary, AB, Canada
[2]Division of Medical Oncology, University of British Columbia and BC Cancer Agency, Vancouver, BC, Canada
[3]Division of Surgical Oncology, University of British Columbia and BC Cancer Agency, Kelowna, BC, Canada

Summary	Key facts
Introduction	- >1 million women globally are diagnosed with breast cancer each year - Large geographical variation in incidence: developed countries have a two to three times higher incidence than the least developed countries
Presentation	- Palpable localized breast masses are most common - Asymptomatic, small invasive cancers and ductal carcinoma *in situ* (DCIS) are common in mammographically-screened populations - Locally-advanced disease accounts for 5–10% of cases in developed countries and >50% of cases in the least developed countries - Even in developed countries, about 5% of women present with metastatic disease

Scenario	- *Early-stage disease:*
	  - Treatment is with curative intent
	  - Surgery is the single most important intervention
	  - Breast conserving surgery (BCS) followed by radiation therapy (RT) is equivalent to mastectomy
	  - Adjuvant locoregional RT improves local control and survival for node-positive women after mastectomy or BCS
	  - Most patients benefit from adjuvant systemic therapy
	  - Choice of adjuvant systemic therapy is based on extent of disease, patient age, oestrogen receptor (ER) and human epidermal growth factor receptor 2 (HER2) status, and a limited number of other prognostic factors
	- *Locally-advanced disease:*
	  - Treatment is with curative intent
	  - Usually start with systemic therapy (chemotherapy and/or hormone therapy depending on ER, HER2, age and co-morbidities):
	    - >75% of patients have stable disease or respond to systemic therapy but <40% achieve a pathological complete response
	  - Both mastectomy and locoregional RT should follow systemic therapy
	- *Metastatic disease at first presentation or at relapse:*
	  - Treatment is with palliative intent
	  - Initial treatment frequently achieves symptom improvement and sometimes there is prolongation of survival but cure is not currently achievable
	  - If ER positive, treatment is sequential use of hormone therapy, chemotherapy and intermittent, symptom-directed RT or surgery
	  - If ER negative, or there is symptomatic visceral disease, or if the disease was initially ER positive but becomes hormone resistant, chemotherapy should be tried
	  - HER2-positive cancers benefit from the addition of anti-HER2 therapy to chemotherapy
	  - Surgery and RT are useful in selected patients with symptoms from local masses or infiltrative lesions which are amenable to resection or stabilization (chest wall, brain, bone, etc.)

Trials	- Multiple large trials and meta-analyses of the randomized trials are available to inform decision-making

Introduction

Breast cancer is the most frequent female cancer, especially in 'developed' countries. Breast cancer has a long natural history and many patients (>50%) with localized disease at diagnosis may be cured by definitive surgery. There is a wealth of data from prospective randomized trials dating from the 1950s to inform decisions about appropriate surgery, radiation, hormone therapies and chemotherapies. This chapter focuses on the management of patients (99% of whom will be women) with a diagnosis of *in situ* or invasive breast cancer, including those with recurrent or metastatic disease. Other sources should be consulted for detailed recommendations about prevention and screening for breast cancer.

Incidence, aetiology and screening

Incidence, aetiology and screening	Description
Incidence	• Lifetime (to age 90 years) risk of breast cancer among average-risk women in developed countries is about 9% • Risk is one-half to one-third as high in less developed countries

Aetiology	• Oestrogen exposure and advancing age are the primary inciting factors
	 • Greatest risk factors for breast cancer are female gender and increasing age
	 • Prolonged unopposed oestrogen exposure (due to early menarche, late menopause, nulliparity, or >5 years of postmenopausal hormone replacement therapy) increases risk
	 • Other risk factors:
	   ▪ Mutation in the *BRCA1* or *2* genes
	   ▪ Family history of breast cancer in first-degree relatives
	   ▪ Postmenopausal obesity
	   ▪ Previous exposure of the breasts to RT, e.g. during curative treatment of Hodgkin disease or paediatric cancer

Screening	• Early detection of smaller breast cancers enables more effective treatment and results in a lower rate of death from breast cancer

Incidence and aetiology

- Incidence of breast cancer varies geographically:
  - Breast cancer is over three times more common in North America and Western Europe (85–100 cases per 100,000 women) than in the least developed countries (20–30 cases per 100,000 women in Eastern Africa and South-Central Asia)
- Breast cancer is a disease of women (100:1 female-to-male ratio)
- Incidence increases with advancing age, higher socio-economic status, increasing median body mass index of the population and duration of uninterrupted oestrogen exposure
- Breast cancer is increased in women:
  - Whose first pregnancy was after age 30 years
  - Who have not had any deliveries
  - Who use postmenopausal hormones for >5 years
  - Who have had an early menarche or late menopause
- Dietary factors associated with postmenopausal obesity increase the risk of a breast cancer diagnosis, possibly mediated by increased inflammatory state, insulin-like growth factor-induced proliferation or the conversion of glucocorticoids into oestrogen in adipose tissues:
  - Studies have failed to demonstrate that fat-restricted diets can prevent breast cancer
- Tamoxifen, other antioestrogens and aromatase inhibitors decrease the risk of developing ER-positive breast cancer by about 40–60% over 5–10 years
- Most reliable breast cancer prevention strategy is bilateral mastectomy, which many women and families find unacceptable:
  - Not recommended for breast cancer prevention for women at average risk for breast cancer

Screening

- Simple and potentially readily accessible interventions such as healthcare provider physical examination or teaching women to perform breast self-examination have not resulted in earlier-stage disease at diagnosis
- Mammographic screening of asymptomatic women at increased risk of breast cancer on the basis of family history (if younger than age 50 years) or age (50–75 years) with a mammogram every 2 years results in earlier diagnosis and a 15–25% reduction in breast cancer deaths a decade or so later
- Breast screening with mammography is recommended in jurisdictions where breast cancer is common and resources are available for this priority
- Mammographic screening programmes require:
  - Substantial attention to quality control (to avoid excess radiation or poor quality images)
  - Staff training to ensure appropriate patient positioning during the mammogram
  - Diagnostic care pathways to efficiently and appropriately investigate abnormal mammographic findings
  - Availability of effective but not excessive treatment of early-stage breast cancer

Pathology

The vast majority of breast tumours arise from the ductal–lobular system (around 90% of invasive breast cancers). Rarely, patients present with primary lymphomas, sarcomas or phylloides tumours of the breast. Key prognostic factors include the extent of nodal involvement, tumour size, histological grade, presence of lymphatic or vascular invasion, degree of expression of hormone receptors and over-expression of HER2 (see Table 21.2).

Pathology	Description

Ductal carcinoma (75%)	• Show ductal features not otherwise specified (NOS):
	  ▪ Cells are cuboidal to irregular and tend to be cohesive
	  ▪ Histological grade is assigned based on variation in degree of tubule formation, mitotic count (number of mitoses per high power field) and nuclear pleomorphism, with a 1–3-point scale for each
	• Tubular, mucinous and colloid cancers (1% each) are variants of ductal carcinoma that express predominantly a tubular, mucin-producing or solid growth pattern, respectively
	• Papillary variants generally have a better prognosis, while micropapillary variants have an inferior prognosis compared to usual ductal histology
	• Medullary cancer is characterized by small cells with intense nuclear pleomorphism and usually a surrounding inflammatory cell infiltrate
	• Inflammatory cancers (3–5%) may be of ductal or lobular origin:
	  ▪ Characterized by diffuse spread within lymphatic channels of the breast and skin producing hot, red and often thickened or oedematous skin
	  ▪ Bulky nodal spread is often present at diagnosis

Lobular carcinoma (15%)	• Characterized by small, rounded, non-cohesive cells that spread through tissue planes as single cells or columns of cells • Usually ER positive
Metaplastic cancers (<1%)	• Show elements of both epithelial and mesenchymal malignant differentiation, including osteogenic or other sarcomatous elements, within a background of ductal carcinoma • Rarely ER or HER2 positive
Squamous cancers (<1%)	• May arise from ductal structures and should be distinguished from squamous carcinoma arising from the skin • Rarely ER or HER2 positive
Paget disease of the nipple (<1%)	• Intraepithelial spread of adenocarcinoma cells that presents as a reddish or eczematous rash or weeping on the nipple or areola • Frequently associated with an underlying invasive or *in situ* cancer • Natural history of the underlying lesion will dominate the clinical course and should dictate management
Phylloides tumours (<1%)	• Mixed epithelial and stromal cellular proliferation that presents as a breast mass, often located in the posterior half of the breast • Degree of malignancy is based on the cellularity of the stromal component, appearance of infiltration at the edge of the tumour and mitotic activity • Should be managed as for a sarcoma with wide excision

Presentation

Breast cancer may present due to:
- A mammographic abnormality in asymptomatic women:
  - DCIS accounts for 20–30% of mammographically-detected breast cancers
- A mass or symptom in the breast or regional nodes
- Symptoms from metastatic disease such as bone pain, anorexia, weight loss or chest symptoms.

Presentation	Description
Non-palpable mammographic abnormality	• Common presentation in jurisdictions where screening with mammograms is performed • Detection rate varies from 1 to 15 cases per 1000 women screened, depending on the woman's age, her family history, the length of time since her previous mammogram and the quality or performance characteristics of the screening service • Approximately 20–30% of mammogram detected breast cancers will be DCIS • Median tumour size of mammogram-detected invasive cancers is ≤1.5 cm and the majority of patients (>80%) have no involvement of axillary lymph nodes • Patients with node-negative, ER-positive, mammogram-detected breast cancer have a 10-year life expectancy that exceeds 85% with definitive local therapy alone

Symptomatic breast cancer	• Most patients, even those in developed countries with ready access to mammograms, present with a symptom they notice themselves
	• Most common presentation is a unilateral new lump in the breast:
	  ▪ Usually described as a painless, hard, mobile mass without overlying skin changes
	• Breast cancer may be tender or painful; a vague mass (especially if lobular histology); fixed to the chest wall; or involving the skin by direct extension or diffuse lymphatic invasion
	• A palpable breast cancer mass usually does not demonstrate noticeable growth over an interval of a few weeks to 3 months, but frequently shows signs of growth over an interval of 6 months to a year
	• Absence of growth or change over even a few months or the presence of pain are *not* reassurances that a breast mass is not cancer
	• Other presentations that should lead to a suspicion of breast cancer include:
	  ▪ Any unilateral breast change such as swelling or shrinkage, skin oedema or erythema
	  ▪ A mass in the axilla without any breast changes, including negative breast imaging
	  ▪ Unilateral nipple discharge (rare), especially if the discharge is bloody, comes from a single milk duct or is associated with an underlying mass:
	    ○ More commonly, nipple discharge is physiological or associated with a benign papilloma of a proximal milk duct
	  ▪ Scaling or an eczematous-like change on the nipple

Symptoms from metastatic disease	• Even in countries with well-developed breast screening programmes and breast cancer awareness among the population, approximately 3–5% of breast cancers will have metastatic disease at diagnosis:
	  ▪ Rate is higher in jurisdictions where there is less focus on early detection
	  ▪ Metastases most commonly involve the bones, mediastinal lymph nodes, lungs, liver or brain
	  ▪ Symptoms will depend on the location and extent of the metastases

Natural history

Natural history		Description

Presentation	Local	• Clinically detected/apparent:
		  ▪ Mass in breast: usually painless
		  ▪ Nipple discharge: infrequent
		  ▪ Change in breast shape or size: infrequent
		  ▪ Skin erythema or ulceration: infrequent; sign of locally-advanced disease
		  ▪ Palpable nodes: infrequent; sign of locally-advanced disease
		  ▪ Bilateral: lobular histology most frequently
		• Screening or mammogram detected:
		  ▪ Architectural distortion
		  ▪ Malignant calcifications
		  ▪ With or without palpable mass and nodes

	Metastatic	• Bone: pain • Liver: abdominal pain, weight loss, malaise, anorexia • Lung: shortness of breath, cough • Brain: headache, nausea, seizure • Peritoneal/ovary: bloating, bowel obstruction

Natural history		Description
Routes of spread	Local	• Single focus in the breast: most common • Multifocal: several foci in same breast quadrant • Multicentric: several foci in different breast quadrants • Skin: erythema, oedema, tethering, ulceration, bleeding • Chest wall: skin tethering or ulceration, infiltration of chest wall musculature
	Regional	• Sentinel node in the axilla • Non-sentinel axillary nodes • Internal mammary chain nodes, especially if the primary tumour is located in the medial or central part of the breast and the axillary nodes are involved • Infraclavicular or supraclavicular nodes

	Metastatic	• Bone
		• Liver
		• Lung:
		  ▪ Parenchyma
		  ▪ Pleura, effusions
		• Brain
		  ▪ HER2+ and triple negative histology predominantly
		• Ovaries, peritoneum:
		  ▪ Lobular histology predominantly
		• Other

Diagnostic work-up

All patients with suspected breast cancer should have tissue obtained for diagnosis and to evaluate ER and HER2 overexpression status. Higher-stage disease and systemic symptoms are the most reliable predictors of distant metastases. Staging investigations are generally unrewarding and are not recommended in patients with low clinical stage disease and who have no systemic symptoms. Figure 21.1 provides a synopsis of the approach to initial diagnosis, staging and treatment.

Assuming the patient presents with localized or asymptomatic breast cancer, the following are indicated:

Breast imaging

Each patient should have a complete history, physical examination and bilateral mammograms. The goal is to assess the extent of abnormality in the breast relative to the breast volume. This assessment will influence the indications, technique and location for biopsy and the suitability for breast conservation.
- Frequently, an ultrasound of the breast is useful to characterize a mass as solid or cystic and to guide a core-needle biopsy for tissue diagnosis
- Breast MRI is not routinely recommended or necessary to establish the diagnosis or plan optimal surgery:
  - It may be considered selectively if there is:
    - Multifocal disease and breast conserving surgery (BCS) is still planned
    - Concern about chest wall invasion, or
    - Discrepancy between the physical examination and breast imaging based on mammograms and ultrasound
- Contralateral breast should be evaluated because 1–2% of patients present with synchronous contralateral disease
- Bilateral mammograms should also be done for men presenting with breast cancer

Tissue diagnosis

All patients should have a tissue diagnosis, even if they present with metastatic disease. Obtaining a tissue diagnosis prior to definitive surgery enables the patient and her physician(s) to make more informed decisions about treatment options and enables more efficient use of operating room time and effort.
- Optimal approach is to perform an ultrasound-guided, core needle biopsy prior to definitive surgery
- Patients with non-palpable mammographic abnormalities (not identified on ultrasound) should undergo a vacuum-assisted, stereotactic core biopsy if available, or alternatively have a fine-wire localization-directed biopsy
- If the primary lesion is palpable, a core biopsy may be performed without ultrasound guidance
- A core biopsy is superior to a fine needle aspiration (FNA) because more definitive histology can be obtained and the ER and HER2 status of the tumour can be assessed:
  - Patients presenting with T4 disease (involving skin or the chest wall) should either have a core needle biopsy or an incisional biopsy

Axillary lymph node staging

Most patients with invasive breast cancer should have a pathological assessment of the axillary lymph nodes. Exceptions

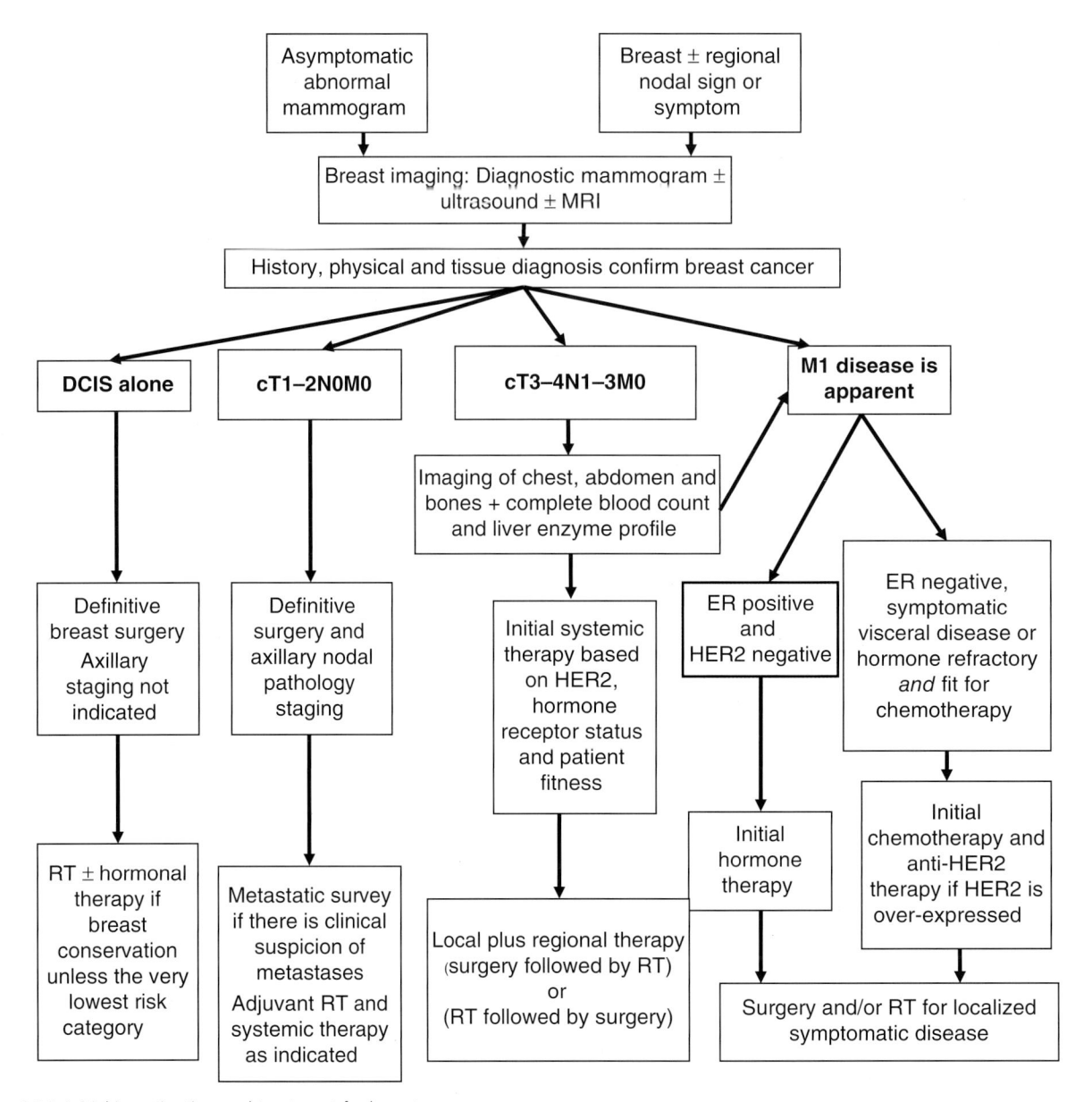

Figure 21.1 Initial investigation and treatment for breast cancer.

include patients presenting with metastatic or supraclavicular disease or such extensive breast disease that management will not be influenced by the axillary pathology.
- Patients with bulky, matted or fixed nodes should have a core biopsy or FNA of the nodal mass at the same time as core biopsy of the primary lesion:
  - May be useful to confirm that the primary and nodal disease have congruent ER and HER2 statuses
- Patients with suspicious palpable but mobile nodes (N1) should have a level I–II axillary dissection for both pathological staging and to improve local control
- Patients with T1–3 primary tumours and no palpable lymph nodes should be managed with sentinel node biopsy or an axillary lymph node dissection (if there is no or limited capacity or experience in the centre to perform a sentinel lymph node biopsy)
- Consideration may be given to preoperative, ultrasound assessment of regional lymph nodes if there is a T2–4 primary tumour and no palpable axillary disease:
  - Ultrasound-guided core biopsy or FNA should then be performed if enlarged or abnormal nodes are identified
- To reduce the risk of false-negative findings, sentinel lymph node biopsy should be performed by an experienced team including nuclear medicine, surgery and pathology specialists:
  - Team should have demonstrated a <10% false-negative rate within a consecutive series of at least 30 sentinel node biopsies followed by formal axillary dissection

Investigations to exclude metastases and determine fitness for definitive treatment

The primary investigations are a complete history and physical examination with particular attention to the breast, axilla and supraclavicular regions.

- If the history and physical examination do not suggest distant spread, and the primary tumour by physical examination and imaging is T1N0, then no further investigations or at most a chest X-ray are required prior to definitive treatment
- If chemotherapy is being considered, a complete blood count, liver enzyme profile and serum creatinine should be done
- If the primary is T3 or T4 or the patient has clinical or pathological nodal spread, a bone scan, liver imaging, chest X-ray and blood work as above should be done
- If there are evident distant metastases including to the supraclavicular nodes, by history or physical examination, then bone, liver and lung imaging is indicated along with blood work to screen for adequate organ function:
  - A tumour marker (CA15.3) may be elevated and helpful in monitoring response to therapy in the metastatic setting
- Imaging of the brain is indicated if the patient has neurological symptoms:
  - Breast cancers that are HER2 positive or are 'triple negative' (negative for ER, PR and HER2) have a higher propensity to spread to the brain
  - There should be a high index of suspicion for brain metastases if the patient with an HER2-positive or triple negative cancer describes even subtle neurological symptoms, but a 'routine' or screening CT of the brain is not indicated

Staging and prognostic risk grouping

UICC TNM staging

See Table 21.1.

Table 21.1 UICC TNM categories and stage grouping: Breast

TNM categories			
Tis	*In situ*		
T1	≤2 cm		
T1mi	≤0.1 cm		
T1a	>0.1–0.5 cm		
T1b	>0.5–1.0 cm		
T1c	>1.0–2.0 cm		
T2	>2–5 cm		
T3	>5 cm		
T4	Chest wall/skin ulceration, skin nodules, inflammatory		
T4a	Chest wall fixation		
T4b	Skin ulceration, satellite skin nodules, skin oedema		
T4c	Both T4a and T4b		
T4d	Inflammatory carcinoma		
N0	No regional lymph node metastasis		
N1	Mobile axillary	pN1mi	Micrometastasis >0.2 mm to 2 mm
		pN1a	1–3 axillary nodes
		pN1b	Internal mammary nodes with microscopic/macroscopic metastasis by sentinel node biopsy but not clinically detected
		pN1c	1–3 axillary nodes and internal mammary nodes with microscopic/macroscopic metastasis by sentinel node biopsy but not clinically detected
N2a	Fixed axillary	pN2a	4–9 axillary nodes
N2b	Internal mammary clinically apparent	pN2b	Internal mammary nodes, clinically detected, without axillary nodes
N3a	Infra-clavicular	pN3a	≥10 axillary nodes or infraclavicular
N3b	Internal mammary and axillary	pN3b	Internal mammary nodes, clinically detected, >3 axillary nodes and internal axillary mammary nodes with microscopic metastasis by sentinel node biopsy but not clinically detected
N3c	Supraclavicular	pN3c	Supraclavicular nodes
M1	Distant Metastasis		

Stage grouping			
Stage 0	Tis	N0	M0
Stage IA	T1*	N0	M0
Stage IB	T0, T1*	N1mi	M0
Stage IIA	T0, T1*	N1	M0
	T2	N0	M0
Stage IIB	T2	N1	M0
	T3	N0	M0
Stage IIIA	T0, T1*	T2 N2	M0
	T3	N1, N2	M0
Stage IIIB	T4	N0, N1, N2	M0
Stage IIIC	Any T	N3	M0
Stage IV	Any T	Any N	M1

*T1 includes T1mi.

Prognostic factors

Both prognostic and predictive factors are relevant to treatment decision-making in early-stage breast cancer. A number of validated prognostic markers exist but they are not sufficiently discriminatory to accurately identify cancers that are cured with local therapy alone. As a result, many patients with early-stage breast cancer receive unnecessary systemic therapy. However, the alternative, under-treatment of potentially curable disease, is associated with greater harm from a population perspective.

Table 21.2 lists the prognostic factors that influence survival, locoregional control, and/or treatment tolerance, and should be considered during treatment planning of patients without documented metastatic disease.

Patients with evident metastatic disease should be evaluated for:
- Hormone receptor and HER2 status which are both prognostic and predictive of response to targeted therapy
- Age, co-morbidities, performance status, disease-free interval (time from initial breast cancer diagnosis to metastatic recurrence) and disease burden at the time of relapse, which influence treatment options and the duration of survival after a diagnosis of metastases.

A number of validated tools provide both prognostic and predictive information to guide local and systemic therapy decisions in early-stage disease.
- Most widely available and important prognostic tool is an adequate pathology report from the primary surgery of the breast and axilla:
  - Report should contain the essential tumour-related factors listed above
  - Quality control for ER and HER2 testing ensures reproducibility and accuracy of results, on which systemic therapy recommendations are made:
    - ER is most frequently tested by immunohistochemistry (IHC) and is most commonly reported using the 8-point Allred score (based on an assessment of the percentage of cells which stain for the ER receptor and the intensity of the stain)
    - HER2 testing may be by IHC (a 0–3-point intensity score) or by gene amplification studies using fluorescent *in situ* hybridization (FISH) or chromogenic *in situ* hybridization (CISH) or both:
      IHC score 0 or 1+: considered negative for HER2
      IHC 3+: considered positive
      IHC 2+: considered indeterminate and should be subjected to FISH or CISH to determine whether the *HER2* gene is amplified
- Adjuvant! Online (adjuvantonline.com) uses patient characteristics (age, co-morbidity score) and information from the pathology of the excised cancer (size, number of involved axillary nodes, ER status, histological grade) to provide estimates of recurrence risk and benefits from various systemic therapies
- Oncotype Dx Recurrence Score Assay®, Mammaprint, PAM50 and IHC4 are tissue-based assays that provide prognostic and some predictive information
- Several nomograms, including the Memorial Sloan Kettering breast nomogram (http://www.mskcc.org/cancer-care/adult/breast/prediction-tools) can provide estimates of further axillary nodal involvement based on the presence of disease in sentinel nodes coupled with histopathological features of the primary cancer
- The Van Nuys Prognostic Index estimates the risk of in-breast recurrence following BCS for DCIS based on four factors: patient age, tumour size, margin width and pathological classification

Table 21.2 Prognostic factors for breast cancer

Prognostic factors	Tumour related	Host related	Environment related
Essential	ER HER2 receptor Histological grade Number and percentage of involved nodes Tumour size Presence of lymphatic or vascular invasion (LVI+) Surgical resection margin status	Age Menopausal status	Prior radiation involving the chest or mediastinum (e.g. for Hodgkin disease)
Additional	Progesterone receptor Tumour profiling UPA, PAI-1	*BRCA1* or *2* mutation Obesity	Use of postmenopausal hormone replacement therapy
New and promising	Ki-67	Level of activity or exercise Single nucleotide polymorphisms (SNPs) associated with drug metabolism or action	

- Other tools, such as IBTR! (http://160.109.101.132/ibtr) are being designed to estimate local recurrence risk after BCS for invasive breast cancer and to estimate the absolute benefit of adding whole-breast radiation therapy (WBRT)

Treatment philosophy

- Curative-intent therapy includes multidisciplinary assessment involving surgical, medical and radiation oncology opinions to tailor treatment to the patient's extent of disease and personal preferences
- Most patients require combinations of locoregional and systemic interventions with the goal of eliminating the primary tumour and reducing the risk of recurrence from regional or systemic metastases, while avoiding over-treatment
- Palliative-intent therapy focuses on symptom management and may achieve some survival prolongation

Treatment guidelines

There are a number of well-established and regularly revised treatment guidelines for breast cancer.
- NCCN: The National Comprehensive Cancer Network has general breast cancer management guidelines which also address a number of special topics: http://www.nccn.org/professionals/physician_gls/f_guidelines.asp#breast
- ASCO: The American Society of Clinical Oncology periodically publishes guidelines on particular aspects of cancer care. Among them are:
  - Breast Cancer Follow-Up and Management After Primary Treatment: American Society of Clinical Oncology Clinical Practice Guideline Update
  - ASCO Endorsement of the CCO Practice Guideline on Adjuvant Ovarian Ablation in the Treatment of Premenopausal Women with Early-Stage Invasive Breast Cancer
  - ASCO Clinical Practice Guideline Update on the Role of Bone-Modifying Agents in Metastatic Breast Cancer
  - ASCO Clinical Practice Guideline: Update on Adjuvant Endocrine Therapy for Women with Hormone Receptor-Positive Breast Cancer
  - ASCO-CAP Guideline Recommendations for Immunohistochemical Testing of Estrogen and Progesterone Receptors in Breast Cancer
  - American Society of Clinical Oncology 2007 Update of Recommendations for the Use of Tumor Markers in Breast Cancer
  - ASCO-CAP Guideline Recommendations for Human Epidermal Growth Factor Receptor 2 Testing in Breast Cancer
  - ASCO Guideline Recommendations for Sentinel Lymph Node Biopsy in Early-Stage Breast Cancer
  - Postmastectomy Radiotherapy: Clinical Practice Guidelines of the American Society of Clinical Oncology
- A number of other institutions and professional bodies produce guidelines for physicians treating breast cancer; frequently available publicly and can be located by searching the Internet using terms such as 'breast cancer, guidelines, therapy, management'

Treatment

Local therapy

Local therapy by type and extent of disease	Description
Lobular carcinoma *in situ* (LCIS)	- May be an incidental finding with other breast pathology or found at the time of breast reduction surgery - Should be treated by excisional biopsy if it is the sole pathology - Is a marker for an increased risk of new disease (DCIS or invasive cancer) in either breast with a risk of approximately 1% per year - If LCIS is extensive and the woman has a high likelihood of living another 20+ years, and especially if there is also a first-degree family history of breast cancer, then she may elect for bilateral mastectomy for breast cancer prevention - If there is a family history of breast cancer, the patient has a good life expectancy and is motivated for treatment but declines mastectomy, tamoxifen 20 mg daily (pre- or post-menopausal women) or exemestane 25 mg (postmenopausal women) daily for 5 years are options to reduce risk - No established role for RT or chemotherapy

(continued)

Local therapy by type and extent of disease	Description
Ductal carcinoma *in situ* (DCIS) without invasive cancer (Tis)	<ul><li>Typically identified on a screening mammogram alone or admixed with invasive carcinoma:<ul><li>May also present as a palpable mass</li></ul></li><li>Pathological extent of disease is often greater than the distribution of calcifications seen on a mammogram</li><li>DCIS should be excised with clear margins</li><li>Excision specimen should be marked with ink and serially sectioned at 3-mm intervals</li><li>Mastectomy is an option for any patient with DCIS</li><li>Axillary dissection is not necessary</li><li>Sentinel node biopsy is reasonable especially for larger or high-grade disease, but is not mandatory:<ul><li>Patients undergoing mastectomy should be considered for sentinel node biopsy in case incidental invasive disease is found on pathology</li></ul></li><li>Excision alone and regular mammographic follow-up may be sufficient if all of the following are present:<ul><li>Disease is unifocal, small (<1.5 cm or fewer than five contiguous 3-mm serial sections of an excision specimen)</li><li>Widely excised (>5 mm between disease and the closest inked margin or with an entirely clear re-excision)</li><li>No grade 3 histological features or comedo-necrosis</li><li>Patient is postmenopausal</li></ul></li><li>If the disease is very extensive (>7 cm; close or positive margins on a second attempt at wide excision) or segmental mastectomy is expected to result in a poor cosmetic outcome, then mastectomy is recommended</li><li>If the disease is >1.5 cm but <7 cm, or has grade 3 histology even if <1.5 cm, then WBRT should follow a local excision with clear margins</li><li>Tamoxifen 20 mg/day for 5 years may be added for motivated patients with moderate-risk disease after BCS:<ul><li>Impact on long-term survival is minimal so if the patient experiences toxicity that adversely affects quality of life, there should be a low threshold to discontinue hormone therapy</li></ul></li><li>Aromatase inhibitors likely have similar efficacy to tamoxifen but have not been evaluated in randomized trials</li><li>No role for chemotherapy</li></ul>
Invasive breast cancer	
pT1–2pN0 disease *without* high-risk features (see Box 21.1)	<ul><li>Surgical removal is the primary treatment</li><li>No advantage to preoperative as compared with postoperative systemic therapy</li><li>No role for RT if treated with mastectomy unless the final surgical margin is involved with invasive cancer</li><li>BCS followed by WBRT is equivalent to mastectomy in terms of local control and survival, and is superior to mastectomy in terms of body image:<ul><li>Standard of care is to include the patient and family in decision-making, and to respect the patient's preference for BCS + WBRT or mastectomy</li></ul></li><li>BCS alone results in a higher rate of local recurrence, metastases and death from breast cancer compared with BCS + WBRT:<ul><li>WBRT reduces the risk of local recurrence by approximately 70%</li><li>Approximately one in four 'unnecessary' local recurrences translates into a breast cancer death</li><li>To optimize survival, WBRT should be offered to most women with invasive cancer following BCS</li></ul></li><li>Absolute benefit of WBRT varies with the baseline risk of local recurrence:<ul><li>Factors that increase the risk of local recurrence include younger age, presence of high-grade or ER-negative disease, lymphovascular invasion, multifocal or larger tumour size, involved margins, lobular histology or extensive *in situ* disease if not widely excised</li><li>Adjuvant hormone therapy decreases the risk of local recurrence in patients with hormone receptor-positive cancers</li></ul></li><li>WBRT following BCS delivered with 40–42.5 Gy in 15–16 fractions is equivalent to 50 Gy in 25 fractions in terms of local control, survival, normal tissue effects and cosmesis; is more convenient for the patient; and less resource intensive for the healthcare system:<ul><li>Short fractionation should be the standard for most women</li><li>If the breast is very large or there are postoperative complications that predict for greater fibrosis, such as infections, significant oedema or dependent erythema, then a dose biologically lower than 50 Gy in 25 fractions should be used for the whole breast, such as 45 Gy in 25 fractions</li><li>If 45 Gy in 25 fractions is used for WBRT, all patients should receive a boost to the primary tumour site delivering 10–16 Gy in five to eight fractions</li></ul></li></ul>

Local therapy by type and extent of disease	Description

	• Even with 'standard' WBRT doses of 40–42.5 Gy in 15–16 fractions or 50 Gy in 25 fractions, a supplemental 'boost' dose of radiation should be added to the primary site following WBRT if the patient is younger than 50 years or the distance from invasive or *in situ* disease to the nearest inked surgical margin is <2 mm:
	  ▪ Boost dose may be 10 Gy in four to five fractions or 16–20 Gy in eight to ten fractions
	  ▪ Higher boost doses increase the risk of skin telangiectasia and cosmetic deterioration
	• Studies are ongoing, but women with *all* of the characteristics in Box 21.2 might reasonably be considered to have a <5% 5-year risk of local recurrence with BCS alone:
	  ▪ Adding WBRT will further reduce the risk of local recurrence but the impact on 10-year survival will likely be ≤1%
	  ▪ Some women may elect to avoid WBRT for such a small survival gain
	• Before considering not using WBRT, *all* the factors in Box 21.2 should be present
	• Accelerated partial breast irradiation (APBI) is still (in 2015) experimental:
	  ▪ 3D conformal RT at a dose of 38.5 Gy in ten fractions delivered twice per day caused increased grade 1–2 toxicity and a significantly worse cosmetic outcome compared with WBRT
	  ▪ 3D conformal, external beam APBI with the dose and techniques used in major North American clinical trials is not recommended
	• Brachytherapy APBI techniques are more conformal:
	  ▪ There are small studies that support equivalence of brachytherapy to WBRT in terms of local control and survival; however, most women treated in such trials had a low risk of breast recurrence even without RT
	  ▪ Safe brachytherapy requires considerable expertise and specialized equipment that is not available in many centres, and should not be done unless the care provider has demonstrated low rates of toxicity and maintains expertise
	  ▪ Provider should be expected to perform 20 or more brachytherapy procedures annually to maintain sufficient clinical expertise
	• Intraoperative APBI requires specialized equipment:
	  ▪ Since the pathological status is not known at the time of treatment, approximately 25% of patients still require WBRT after surgery
	  ▪ 5-year outcomes demonstrate that patients who received intraoperative RT alone following BCS had high local recurrence rates compared to patients treated with WBRT
	  ▪ Long-term outcomes from such techniques are awaited

pT1–2pN0 disease *with* high risk features (see Box 21.1) and T1–2pN1 disease	• Surgical management of the primary includes tumour excision with negative margins and sentinel lymph node biopsy if the surgical team has demonstrated sufficient experience and proficiency
	• If the axillary nodes are clinically abnormal, are shown to contain disease on preoperative biopsy or there are more than two pathologically positive sentinel nodes, an axillary dissection is recommended
	• BCS is appropriate and should always be followed with adjuvant WBRT unless the patient is participating in a clinical trial that includes written informed consent quantifying the local and distant recurrence risks of avoiding WBRT
	• WBRT following BCS delivered with 40–42.5 Gy in 15–16 fractions is equivalent to 50 Gy in 25 fractions in terms of local control, survival, normal tissue effects and cosmesis, and is more convenient for the patient and less resource intensive for the health system:
	  ▪ Short fractionation should be the standard for most women
	  ▪ If the breast is very large or has postoperative complications that predict for greater fibrosis, such as infections, significant oedema or dependent erythema, then a dose biologically lower than 50 Gy in 25 fractions should be used for the whole breast such as 45 Gy in 25 fractions
	  ▪ If 45 Gy in 25 fractions is used, all patients should receive a boost of 10–16 Gy in five to eight fractions
	• Even with 'standard' WBRT doses of 42.5 Gy in 16 fractions or 50 Gy in 25 fractions, a supplemental 'boost' dose of radiation should be added to the primary site following WBRT if the patient is younger than age 50 years or the distance from invasive or *in situ* disease to the nearest margin is <2 mm:
	  ▪ Boost dose may be 10 Gy in four to five fractions or 16–20 Gy in eight to ten fractions
	  ▪ Higher boost doses increase the risk of skin telangiectasia and cosmetic deterioration
	• Regional nodal RT added to WBRT, and chest wall plus regional nodal RT following mastectomy, should be used to improve locoregional control, reduce the risk of distant metastases and improve survival for women with a moderate risk of locoregional recurrence who are also receiving adjuvant systemic therapy
	• Following BCS, regional nodal RT should be added to WBRT if the patient has involved nodes, including if pN1mic
	• Following BCS with negative axillary lymph nodes, it is reasonable to add regional nodal RT to WBRT if there are three or more 'high-risk' features, especially if no axillary dissection
	• Following mastectomy, chest wall plus nodal RT should be used if the patient has involved nodes or if the disease is pN0 but there are three or more 'high-risk' features

(continued)

Local therapy by type and extent of disease	Description

Clinical or pathological T3–4 or N2–3 breast cancer	• Combination of surgical excision plus RT significantly improves locoregional control compared with using either modality alone
	• Even with effective systemic therapy, the risk of locoregional recurrence exceeds 30% if the patient is treated with mastectomy or RT, and is significantly reduced if both modalities are used
	• There is little evidence that adjuvant RT improves survival for patients with this stage of disease even though locoregional recurrence risk is significantly reduced
	• Patients with T1–2N2–3 disease may be treated with BCS + WBRT + regional nodal RT:
	  ▪ Nodal RT should include the full axilla, supraclavicular and internal mammary regions
	• Patients with T3–4 or clinical N2 disease should generally be treated with preoperative systemic therapy followed by mastectomy and full locoregional RT:
	  ▪ Sequence of mastectomy and RT will not influence rates of locoregional control or survival, but may affect morbidity
	  ▪ This sequence should be influenced by whether the patient will have immediate reconstruction:
	    ○ If there will not be immediate reconstruction, the recommended sequence is mastectomy followed by RT
	    ○ If immediate reconstruction is planned, it is recommended that RT precedes the mastectomy
	    ○ Reconstruction should preferentially include a tissue transfer procedure to avoid the frequent occurrence of capsular contracture that follows implant reconstruction in combination with RT

Metastatic disease (M1) at presentation	• In general, the patient should be treated with supportive care and systemic therapy:
	  ▪ Surgery or RT to the primary or nodal areas should be reserved for the relief of symptomatic or progressive disease
	  ▪ Some retrospective studies have suggested that excision of the primary tumour in combination with systemic therapy may improve survival if the extent of distant metastases is very limited, but such an approach should be considered experimental until confirmed by prospective trials
	• Palliative or 'toilet' mastectomy may be considered if there is extensive or ulcerated local disease without clinically apparent nodal or supraclavicular disease:
	  ▪ Mastectomy is rarely useful if there is also extensive nodal disease, in which case RT and systemic therapy should be used
	• Palliative RT should be used if the primary tumour is ulcerated, bleeding, threatening skin, painful or if there are palpable or symptomatic lymph nodes that do not respond to systemic therapy:
	  ▪ 35 Gy in ten fractions is convenient, often effective and reasonably tolerated
	• Surgery may also be useful at the sites of selected distant metastases:
	  ▪ Examples include treatment or prevention of pathological fractures, isolated brain metastases, drainage of effusions, etc.

Box 21.1 High-risk features for T1–2pN0 breast cancer

- Age <40 years
- Grade 3 histology
- Lack of ER expression
- HER2 over-expression
- Lymphatic or vascular invasion

All predict for an increased risk of future distant metastases and death from breast cancer. Combinations of two or more of these factors are associated with a 15% or higher risk of locoregional recurrence after mastectomy or with BCS unless RT is used.

Box 21.2 Factors should *all* be present before ruling out the use of WBRT

- Age: 60 years and older
- Axillary nodes: pathologically assessed and free of metastases
- Primary tumour: unifocal, ER positive, grade 1–2, ductal carcinoma
- Surgical pathology:
  - Tumour size ≤1.5 cm
  - Excision with 5-mm or wider margins
  - Surrounding *in situ* disease is not extensive
- Patient:
  - Fit for and willing to take adjuvant hormone therapy for 5 years
  - Well-informed and consent is documented

Systemic therapy

There are three main types of systemic therapy: hormone therapy, chemotherapy and biological therapy.

- *Adjuvant hormone therapy* should be considered for all patients with hormone receptor-positive breast cancer:
  - Absolute benefit is greatest in patients with higher stage cancers and cancers with stronger ER expression
- *Adjuvant chemotherapy* should be considered for fit patients with T1–2N0 cancers with high-risk features (Box 21.1) and is recommended for higher stage cancers:
  - Optimal adjuvant chemotherapy is multiagent, with four to eight cycles given over 3–6 months
  - Active regimens include those containing anthracyclines, taxanes, or both, and classical cyclophosphamide + methotrexate + 5-fluorouracil (CMF)
  - Antiemetics are essential for anthracycline and cyclophosphamide-containing regimens
  - Granulocyte-colony stimulating factor (G-CSF) is required for some regimens and is recommended for others
- Patients with HER2 over-expressing cancers should be treated with adjuvant chemotherapy plus anti-HER2 therapy:
  - Adjuvant anti-HER2 therapy may be given concurrently with the non-anthracycline portion of chemotherapy (preferred) and/or following completion of chemotherapy
  - Combining anti-HER2 therapy with anthracyclines increases the risk of cardiac toxicity
- Treatment for metastatic disease is dependent on the hormone receptor and HER2 status of the cancer, burden of disease and degree of symptoms:
  - Hormone therapy for metastatic, hormone receptor-positive disease should be continuous until disease progression
  - Chemotherapy for metastatic disease may be single agent or multiagent; choice depends on prior drug exposure, disease-related symptoms, burden of disease, patient co-morbidity, age and preference
- Palliative chemotherapy may be continuous; however, cumulative toxicity often limits the duration of chemotherapy and there is no convincing evidence that continuous therapy enhances survival compared to symptom-directed intermittent chemotherapy
- In patients with bone metastases, bone targeted therapy has a modest effect on delaying skeletal-related events (pain, fracture, cord compression) with no effect on overall survival
- Anti-HER2 therapy added to chemotherapy is indicated for HER2+ breast cancer with regional or metastatic disease
- Targeting the mTOR pathway and ER pathway simultaneously may control disease for longer than hormone therapy alone in patients with hormone receptor-positive cancer that has been previously exposed to hormone therapy:
  - Other pathways and receptors are being investigated as targets for specific therapies

Systemic therapy	Description

Early disease	- Intent of therapy is curative
	- DCIS: intermediate, high grade, ER-positive DCIS treated with BCS:
	  - 5 years of tamoxifen is an option to reduce recurrence risk and contralateral disease risk
	- Invasive disease: high-risk features include any of age <40 years, grade 3, hormone receptor negative, HER2+, lymphatic and/or venous invasion, node positive
	- *T1–2, with no high-risk features*:
	  - Hormone therapy (5 years):
	    - *Premenopausal*: tamoxifen and/or ovarian suppression/oophorectomy
	    - *Menopausal*: aromatase inhibitor during some part (or all) of 5-year therapy, with tamoxifen for the remainder
	  - Chemotherapy: benefit is generally considered to be minimal and it is not indicated
	- *T1–2, with any high-risk features*:
	  - Hormone therapy (5–10 years): for hormone receptor-positive cancers; starts after chemotherapy:
	    - *Premenopausal*: tamoxifen and/or ovarian suppression/oophorectomy
	    - *Menopausal*: aromatase inhibitor during some part (or all) of 5 years of therapy, with tamoxifen for the remainder; the benefit of continuing aromatase inhibitor therapy is still under investigation in 2015
	  - Multiagent chemotherapy (3–6 months):
	    - Anthracycline + taxane preferred if node positive, HER2+ or hormone receptor negative
	    - Anthracycline-free regimen if prior anthracyclines or significant cardiac risk factors
	  - Anthracycline without taxane or taxane without anthracycline and CMF are preferred for older patients and/or patients with low or no nodal disease burden
	  - Anti-HER2 therapy:
	    - 1 year, for HER2+ cancers; optimally started during the non-anthracycline portion of chemotherapy
	    - Cardiac toxicity risk increases if anti-HER2 therapy is given with anthracyclines
	    - Safe to give concurrently with adjuvant RT and hormone therapy
	    - Periodic cardiac function surveillance during therapy is recommended
	    - If left ventricular dysfunction develops, especially if symptomatic, interruption until resolution, or permanent discontinuation of anti-HER2 therapy is recommended

(continued)

Systemic therapy	Description
Advanced, non-metastatic disease	- Intent of therapy is curative
- Preoperative systemic therapy can facilitate curative surgery by shrinking the cancer in the breast and axilla
- *T3–4 or N2–3*:
- Hormone therapy for 5–10 years for hormone receptor-positive cancers:
- Starts after chemotherapy
- May be substituted for preoperative chemotherapy in frail/elderly patients with hormone receptor-positive cancer for a period of 4–6 months, with close follow-up
- Preoperative shrinkage of the primary is generally less with hormone therapy than with chemotherapy
- Choice of hormone therapy is based on menopausal status as outlined for the adjuvant setting above
- Preoperative multiagent chemotherapy for about 6 months:
- An anthracycline + taxane is recommended, unless prior anthracycline or significant cardiac risk factors exist, in which case an anthracycline-free regimen should be used
- Anti-HER2 therapy:
- As described above for early disease
- May be started preoperatively and continued postoperatively
Metastatic disease	- Intent of therapy is palliative
- Focus should be symptom control to enhance quality of life:
- Some survival prolongation may occur
- Control of pain, counselling for psychological distress and community healthcare support as patients decline in function and independence are important
- *Hormone receptor-positive, HER2-negative cancers*:
- Treatment should include hormone therapy:
- Can cause volume reduction of metastases; however, stable disease is also an important clinical benefit
- Cancers eventually become insensitive to hormone therapy
- Continuous, sequential hormone therapy should be given until disease becomes hormone insensitive, or is bulky and symptomatic or demonstrates rapid progression
- Sequential non–cross-resistant chemotherapy should be offered for hormone-insensitive cancers; bulky symptomatic disease; and/or rapidly progressive disease:
- Treatment to progression, prohibitive toxicity or plateau in tumour response is recommended
- *Hormone receptor and HER2 negative cancers*:
- Sequential non–cross-resistant chemotherapy should be used for patients with bulky symptomatic or rapidly progressive disease:
- Treat to progression, prohibitive toxicity or plateau in tumour response is recommended
- *HER2-positive cancers*:
- Benefit from anti-HER2 therapy
- Chemotherapy combined with anti-HER2 therapy is the standard
- Anti-HER2 therapy should be continued beyond chemotherapy until disease progression, at which time new chemotherapy should be added and the same or different anti-HER2 therapy continued
- Cardiac function surveillance is optional but anti-HER2 therapy should be discontinued if symptomatic left ventricular dysfunction develops
- Hormone therapy is generally less effective in HER2-positive than in HER2-negative cancers which are ER positive:
- May be considered instead of chemotherapy plus anti-HER2 combination in patients wishing to postpone chemotherapy and who have disease which is hormone receptor-positive and of low burden
- Patients electing observation or endocrine therapy alone should be followed closely
- May be added to maintenance anti-HER2 therapy once chemotherapy is stopped in women with ER-positive cancers
- Specific management of particular sites of disease:
- *Bone metastases*: bone-modifying agents (bisphosphonate or RANK-ligand inhibitor) reduce cancer-related skeletal complications such as pain, need for radiation, pathological fracture, hypercalcaemia and cord compression:
- These agents have no impact on overall survival
- RT provides effective pain relief for bony pain and is recommended for treatment of cord compression from bony metastases
- For uncomplicated bone metastases (no fracture or threat of cord compression), RT with a single fraction is recommended

Systemic therapy	Description

	- *Symptomatic fluid collections*:
	  ○ Ascites: periodic paracentesis
	  ○ Pleural effusions: periodic thoracentesis, pleurodesis or Pleurex catheter if symptomatic
	  ○ Pericardial effusions: periodic pericardiocentesis or pericardial window
	- *Bowel obstruction*: peritoneal and omental metastases may lead to bowel obstruction:
	  ○ Infrequently resolved with systemic therapy or surgery as it is often multilevel
	  ○ A decision to support patients with total parental nutrition during a trial of systemic therapy should be undertaken with clear expectations outlined about when futility will be declared with a transition to terminal care
	- *Central nervous system disease*:
	  ○ Patients presenting with symptomatic brain or leptomeningeal metastases should be given corticosteroids promptly to reduce the oedema which is largely responsible for symptoms; steroids can be tapered to discontinuation after definitive treatment
	  ○ Up to four brain metastases: consider surgical resection or stereotactic radiosurgery:
	  Use of whole-brain radiation varies by jurisdiction
	  Whole-brain radiation will delay the development of subsequent brain metastases but may not alter survival compared with repeated stereotactic therapy
	  ○ Multiple, unresectable brain metastases: whole brain radiation is recommended
	  ○ Leptomeningeal spread: radiation, intrathecal chemotherapy and high-dose systemic methotrexate can provide temporary relief of symptoms; this form of disease is frequently poorly or transiently responsive to treatment
	- *Uveal metastases and periorbital tissue infiltration*: radiation is often useful to palliate symptoms

Post-treatment assessment

There are four main goals of follow-up after treatment for early-stage breast cancer.
- *Surveillance for recurrence:*
  - Periodic history and physical examination are recommended, with the frequency decreasing as the interval from diagnosis increases
  - Routine imaging (other than annual mammograms) and blood work (including tumour markers) are *not* recommended in the absence of concerning signs or symptoms
  - Detection of asymptomatic metastases does not improve survival or benefit patients
- *Surveillance for a new breast cancer:*
  - In patients who have not undergone bilateral mastectomy, annual mammography is recommended
  - Screening the chest wall or reconstructed breast with mammograms after mastectomy is not recommended
- *Compliance with endocrine therapy:*
  - Studies suggest that rates of compliance with hormone therapy drop over time
  - Benefits of endocrine therapy to reduce breast cancer recurrence cannot accrue to patients not taking it
  - Reminders by physicians have been associated with increased compliance
- *Assessment and support of patients with ongoing or late toxicities from therapy which are amenable to intervention:*
  - Cardiac dysfunction:
    ○ May develop following exposure to anthracyclines and to anti-HER2 therapy:
    ○ Medical management to maximize left ventricular function should be considered
    ○ Endocrine therapy may also have an adverse effect on coronary artery health and cholesterol and triglyceride levels
    ○ If adjuvant RT included the anterior heart, there may be an increased risk of coronary artery disease ≥15 years later
  - Secondary malignancies may develop following exposure to chemotherapy (leukaemia and myelodysplastic syndrome), to radiation (lung, skin) and to tamoxifen (endometrium):
    ○ Should be treated using the same principles as cancers in those organs which arise without precipitating causes
    ○ Angiosarcoma presenting as small red to bluish 'blood blisters' on the irradiated skin occurs in approximately 1 in 1000 women treated with BCS and WBRT
  - Permanent and/or premature menopause may result from chemotherapy which in turn can affect libido, mood, weight, bone health, heart health and quality of life:
    ○ Addressing such effects requires a variety of counselling and medical interventions and benefits from multidisciplinary input

- Bone density:
  - Premature menopause (from oophorectomy or chemotherapy) and aromatase inhibitors can accelerate normal bone mineral density losses that occur as women age
  - Osteoporosis and fragility fractures are slightly increased as a result
  - Women should be counselled to take therapeutic doses of vitamin D and calcium
  - Exercise may also mitigate bone mineral loss
- Peripheral sensory neuropathy can last a number of months after taxane chemotherapy, and can be permanent:
  - Occasionally, pain medication is required
- Lymphoedema may develop after axillary dissection and/or axillary radiation:
  - Prompt intervention with compression garments and/or massage will limit worsening

Controversies

Over treatment

To maximize the cure rate for early-stage breast cancer, adjuvant therapies have been developed based on benefits demonstrated in populations of patients. However, the ability to select which patients in the population actually need the therapy is limited by the lack of specificity of prognostic markers. As a result, many patients receive treatment that may not be required.

Prognostic tools do not provide adequate discrimination of who does not need radiation, chemotherapy and/or hormone therapy. Predictive oncology is a critical partner to prognostic information, to identify who will and will not benefit from certain types of adjuvant therapy. Predictive tools, such as the OncotypeDx Recurrence Score Assay®, are under study to determine whether they will more accurately predict lack of benefit from chemotherapy than histopathological and patient characteristics. Investigations are also ongoing to validate the ability to identify women with a very low likelihood of local failure if radiation is omitted after BCS.

Duration of adjuvant therapy
Endocrine therapy

Several studies support a small survival benefit with 10 years of hormone therapy when tamoxifen is given for the first 5 years to women with hormone receptor-positive breast cancer. However, the majority of women are cured by 5 years from diagnosis. Tools to predict those most likely to benefit from extended hormone therapy are lacking.

Studies of 10 years of therapy included only a small number of premenopausal women, so it is difficult to determine the benefit in younger women.

Menopausal women frequently receive an aromatase inhibitor during some or all of the first 5 years of hormone therapy: studies exploring the value of continuing hormone therapy for another 5 years in this setting have not reported results as of 2015.

Anti-HER2 therapy

One year of anti-HER2 adjuvant therapy is the standard of care. This is based on four large, randomized trials of chemotherapy with or without trastuzumab. Two years of anti-HER2 therapy did not improve relapse-free survival compared to 1 year. One large study of 6 months of anti-HER2 therapy did not provide sufficient evidence to change the standard of care. Several ongoing studies are exploring shorter courses of therapy.

Use of two anti-HER2 therapies with chemotherapy as compared to one is under study in the adjuvant setting.

Biomarker testing

Fundamental to prognosis and breast cancer treatment decisions are the ER and HER2 status of invasive breast cancers. The most frequent method to determine ER and HER2 is IHC. IHC testing is subject to variable interpretation and reproducibility. Pathology labs should have quality assurance standards and measures to ensure high internal and external consistency of IHC testing. Labs with high volumes of ER and HER2 testing and with quality assurance programmes in place are more likely to produce consistently accurate results. Regionalization of pathology laboratory testing should be promoted.

Adjuvant bisphosphonates

Several studies have examined the role of adjuvant bisphosphonate therapy to prevent bone recurrence after early-stage breast cancer:
- Trials of clodronate have shown conflicting results
- Trials of zoledronic acid have shown a small effect among women who are menopausal either naturally or as part of their breast cancer treatment.

Universal use of adjuvant bisphosphonates in menopausal women has not been adopted pending confirmatory evidence of benefit.

Special circumstances

Male breast cancer
- Breast cancer in men occurs infrequently (male-to-female incidence ratio is 1:100)
- Treatment principles are similar to those outlined for women of similar age and co-morbidity
- Men with a *BRCA1* or *2* mutation have an increased lifetime risk of breast cancer and prostate cancer

- An hereditary cause and genetic evaluation should be considered in families with both male and female breast cancer, or male breast cancer and a family history of ovarian cancer (see below)

Breast cancer arising in pregnancy
- Breast cancer arising in pregnancy is uncommon
- Management depends on the stage of pregnancy and extent of the cancer
- Management should be multidisciplinary and include obstetrics and neonatology input
- If the cancer is operable, the preferred first step is surgery
- Breast conservation is appropriate if technically feasible
- Axillary dissection is preferred to sentinel node biopsy if surgery is performed in the first trimester as no dye or radioactive tracer is needed, which may have unknown consequences for the fetus:
    - Sentinel lymph node biopsy is considered safe after the first trimester
- Radiation should be delayed until after delivery
- Hormone therapy should be delayed until after delivery
- Anti-HER2 therapy should be delayed until after delivery
- Need for chemotherapy should be assessed from histopathological characteristics, in the usual way
- Among patients in whom chemotherapy is indicated, this should be delayed until at least the second trimester because fetal malformations may occur if chemotherapy is given during organogenesis in the first trimester
- Doxorubicin + cyclophosphamide combinations are the most well-documented chemotherapy drugs administered in pregnancy
- Limited data on the safety of paclitaxel
- Mild intrauterine growth restriction appears to be the only consistent detriment to the baby when doxorubicin + cyclophosphamide (AC) combination chemotherapy is used in the second or third trimester.
- For cancers diagnosed early in the third trimester of pregnancy, the safest course of action for mother and baby may be early (34+ weeks) delivery of the pregnancy before starting chemotherapy
- If the diagnosis is late in the third trimester, it may be safest to delay all therapy for breast cancer (including surgery) until after a planned, early (34+ weeks) delivery
- Patients presenting with locally-advanced disease may undergo chemotherapy from the second trimester, with surgery prior to or after delivery

Hereditary breast cancer
- 5–10% of all breast cancers have a defined hereditary cause
- Most hereditary breast cancers arise in individuals with a BRCA1 or 2 mutation:
    - Prevalence of BRCA1 and 2 mutations in a geographical area depends on the ethnic diversity of the population:
        - High prevalence among Ashkenazi Jews and certain other 'founder' or isolated populations such as in Iceland and Quebec, Canada
    - BRCA1 and 2 mutations result in increased breast and ovarian cancer risk in an autosomal dominant manner with variable penetrance
    - Women with a BRCA1 mutation have a 50–65% lifetime risk of developing breast cancer and a 35–45% risk of developing ovarian cancer
    - Women with a BRCA2 mutation have a 40–60% chance of developing breast cancer and a 15–25% risk of ovarian cancer
    - Men with a BRCA1 or 2 mutation carry an increased risk of breast (6%) and prostate cancer (25–35%)
    - Second, contralateral breast cancers occur among 35% of BRCA1 and 25% of BRCA2 mutation carriers within 25 years of a first breast cancer
    - BRCA1 mutation breast cancers are frequently, although not exclusively, ER, PR, and HER2 negative (triple negative)
- Other germline genetic mutations, such as Li-Fraumeni (TP53 mutation) and Cowden (PTEN mutation) syndromes are also associated with an increased lifetime risk of breast cancer, but are less prevalent in the population
- There are likely other germline mutations responsible for hereditary breast cancers that are not yet discovered
- Hereditary breast cancer should be suspected if there are multiple cases of breast and/or ovarian cancer in a bloodline, particularly if any of the diagnoses were in individuals younger than age 50 years
- Where testing is available, it is most rewarding to screen individuals whose personal and family cancer histories suggest an elevated likelihood of a BRCA mutation:
    - BRCA mutation testing can result in a positive test (known deleterious mutation identified), negative test (no mutation) or indeterminate test (unclassified variant mutation identified with unclear clinical implications)
- Prophylactic bilateral mastectomy and bilateral salpingo-oophorectomy is recommended as the most effective method of prevention among women with a confirmed BRCA1 or 2 mutation
- Increased frequency of breast screening and patient breast self-examination are recommended for confirmed mutation carriers who elect not to undergo mastectomy
- There are insufficient data to know the impact of chemoprevention (tamoxifen, exemestane) on breast cancer risk reduction among confirmed BRCA mutation carriers

Management of isolated locoregional recurrence
- An isolated local recurrence following BCS and RT may be curable with local therapy and should be treated by mastectomy
- Staging investigations to rule out distant metastases should be performed

- Isolated local recurrence following BCS that was not followed initially with RT should be excised and the breast should receive RT if the woman remains interested in breast conservation
- Isolated chest wall recurrence following mastectomy without RT should be excised if feasible without removing muscle or bone, and the chest wall plus nodal areas should be treated with RT:
  - If the chest wall appears involved on imaging, then surgical excision should involve an *en bloc* resection, or consideration can also be given to neoadjuvant chemotherapy which may allow a less aggressive surgical approach
- If a local recurrence occurs on the chest wall after mastectomy + RT, excision and systemic therapy should be used:
  - Repeat RT may be feasible for palliative purposes, especially if there is a long interval between the original RT and diagnosis of recurrence
- If a patient presents with isolated axillary recurrence without a prior axillary dissection, it should be treated surgically and usually followed with RT
- If a patient presents with local plus nodal disease, it is usually a marker that systemic spread is imminent:
  - Systemic therapy based on age, co-morbidities and prior systemic treatment should be considered
  - If the patient has not had the sites of recurrence already treated with RT, then excision of mobile disease followed by RT to the breast/chest wall plus nodal areas is recommended in addition to systemic therapy
- It is unclear whether (and how much) 'secondary adjuvant' systemic therapy is beneficial after a local or regional recurrence that has been completely removed or treated with RT:
  - Hormone therapy should be used if the recurrence or original cancer was ER positive
  - Chemotherapy may be reasonable if the woman is young, fit, motivated and, especially, if she did not receive chemotherapy at the time of her initial treatment

Breast reconstruction after mastectomy
- Breast reconstruction following or concurrent with mastectomy is an option for women where available:
  - Goal is to restore self-image and improve quality of life
  - Not all women are interested in breast reconstruction
- Prior to embarking on reconstruction the woman and plastic surgeon should have a realistic discussion of likely outcomes, the woman should be emotionally and physically healthy, and she should understand the risks and potential complications
- It is often possible to create a breast mound that looks similar to the opposite side while the woman is clothed:
  - In patients with large breasts, a contralateral breast reduction may be used to achieve symmetry
- Timing of the reconstruction should be discussed by a multidisciplinary team so that it does not interfere with optimal therapy for the breast cancer
- Most often the reconstructive process involves two or more surgical procedures
- Implant reconstruction often involves insertion of a subpectoral tissue expander, gradual inflation of the tissue expander over several months and then removal of the expander and insertion of a silicone- or saline-filled prosthesis:
  - Increasingly, single-step implant reconstruction is being used with dermal allografts or combination implant plus tissue transfer techniques
- Tissue-transfer reconstruction involves harvesting skin, fat, muscle and its blood supply from one part of the body and transferring it to the chest wall:
  - Typical donor sites are the abdomen (transverse rectus-abdominus muscle flap [TRAM]) or posterior chest wall (latissimus dorsi flap)
  - Successful outcomes require expertise in microsurgical techniques
  - Very slim women may not be suitable for tissue transfer reconstruction because their donor sites may have insufficient tissue
  - Previous lower abdominal incisions may restrict the option of TRAM flaps
- Obese women and smokers are at higher risk of wound and operative complications and may not be suitable for reconstruction
- Patients with implant reconstruction are at risk of capsular contracture:
  - Risk is higher if the patient has had RT before or after the implant reconstruction
  - For that reason, if RT has already been used or is planned, a tissue-transfer type of reconstruction is preferred
- Follow-up or surveillance mammography of a reconstructed breast is not recommended since there is no remaining breast tissue:
  - However, abnormalities arising in a reconstructed breast may be investigated by mammogram, ultrasound and/or MRI for diagnostic purposes

Exercise and weight reduction
- Obesity is associated with an increased incidence of breast cancer and worse survival following breast cancer
- Modest weight reduction for overweight women, and exercise for all women may offer some protection against recurrence following treatment for breast cancer

Phase III clinical trials

See Table 21.3.

Table 21.3 Phase III clinical trials

Trial name	Results
Local therapy	
Early Breast Cancer Trialists' Cooperative Group meta-analysis of breast conservation trials Darby et al. (2011) Lancet 378:1707–1716	• Over 10,000 patients randomized in 17 trials of BCS with or without RT • RT decreased the risk of local recurrence and distant metastases, and improved survival compared to BCS alone • Absolute benefit from RT varied with the *a priori* risk of local recurrence • Approximately one extra breast cancer death results from every four to five 'preventable' local recurrences • Young age was associated with a higher risk of local recurrence overall but the chance of survival and of local recurrence were equivalent with mastectomy or BCS + RT • Tables available as appendices to the on-line version of the manuscript identify that only the oldest patients with small tumours and receiving hormone therapy would be expected to have a breast recurrence risk of <5% at 10 years without RT
Early Breast Cancer Trialists' Collaborative Group meta-analysis of post-mastectomy trials Clarke et al. (2005) Lancet 366:2087–2106; EBCTCG, McGale et al. (2014) Lancet 383;2127–2135	• Adjuvant locoregional RT reduced the risk of local and regional recurrence and also decreased the risk of death from breast cancer among women with involved axillary lymph nodes • Among women with pN0 disease who received RT (a treatment that is not generally recommended today) and survived >10 years, there was an increased risk of cardiovascular mortality • Most trials that showed a survival advantage from adjuvant RT included the internal mammary nodes in the treatment volume
European Organization for Research and Treatment of Cancer (EORTC) 22881-10882 Boost Trial Bartelink et al. (2007) J Clin Oncol 25:3259–3265	• 5316 patients were randomized to receive a boost of 16 Gy in eight fractions or not following BCS with negative margins and WBRT • With a median follow-up of 10.8 years, the risk of local recurrence was reduced in all subgroups, but the absolute gain was larger in younger women • Boost RT should be added following BCS and WBRT in women aged 50 years and younger
Canadian Hypofractionation Trial Whelan et al. (2010) N Engl J Med 362:513–520; subsequent commentary Haviland et al. (2010) N Engl J Med 362:1843–1844	• 42.5 Gy in 16 fractions was compared to 50 Gy in 25 fractions following BCS • 10-year follow-up demonstrated equivalent outcomes in terms of local control, survival, acute and late normal tissue toxicity and cosmesis • An unplanned subset analysis questioned whether hypofractionation was less effective among patients with grade 3 disease, but this was subsequently refuted by an analysis from the UK hypofractionation trials
UK START Trials Haviland et al. (2013) Lancet Oncol. 14:1086–1094	• 40 Gy in 15 fractions had fewer side effects than 50 Gy in 25 fractions and comparable local control and survival. • 40–42.5 Gy in 15–16 daily fractions is more convenient for women, is less costly for the healthcare system and should be considered the 'standard' following BCS
American College of Surgeons Oncology Group (ACOSOG) Z0011 trial Giuliano et al (2011) JAMA 305:569–575 International Breast Cancer Study Group (IBCSG) trial Galimberti et al. (2013) Lancet Oncol 14:297–305	• 813 patients (half of the intended target) were randomized to axillary dissection or no further surgery following BCS and a sentinel lymph node biopsy that recovered one or two pathologically positive nodes • No significant difference in locoregional recurrence, distant metastases or overall survival with a median follow-up of 6 years • Similar findings were reported by the IBCSG investigating the value of axillary dissection after a sentinel node biopsy with micrometastases
Systemic therapy	
Early Breast Cancer Trialists' Collaborative Group meta-analysis for chemotherapy and hormone therapy (2005) Lancet 365:1687–1717	• Comprehensive meta-analysis of randomized controlled trials of chemotherapy showed that 6 months of anthracycline-based chemotherapy reduced mortality by 38% in women aged <50 years and by 20% in women aged 50–69 years, irrespective of ER status, nodal status and other tumour characteristics • Similarly, 5 years of tamoxifen reduced mortality by 31% after ER-positive breast cancer irrespective of age, chemotherapy and tumour characteristics • Oophorectomy or ovarian suppression, when given as the only adjuvant systemic therapy, reduced mortality by about 13% • Impact of oophorectomy was attenuated when chemotherapy was also given

(continued)

Table 21.3 (Continued)

Trial name	Results
Role of adjuvant taxanes according to biomarker profile and nodal status Hayes et al. (2007) N Engl J Med 357:1496–1506; De Laurentiis et al. (2008) J Clin Oncol 26:444–453	• Combined analyses of several trials of anthracycline versus anthracycline plus taxane chemotherapy showed a significant survival advantage for adding a taxane to the treatment of HER2-positive and ER-negative early-stage breast cancers • A meta-analysis of taxane-containing adjuvant regimens showed a 15% survival advantage for the addition of taxanes, either sequentially or concurrently, to anthracyclines in the treatment of node-positive disease
Impact of adjuvant aromatase inhibitors in hormone receptor positive breast cancer Dowsett et al. (2009) J Clin Oncol 28:509–518	• A meta-analysis of trials of adjuvant hormone therapy in menopausal women showed a 23% risk reduction in recurrence by replacing 5 years of tamoxifen with 5 years of an aromatase inhibitor as adjuvant therapy for ER-positive breast cancer, but no overall survival benefit with a median follow-up of 6 years • Combining 2–3 years of tamoxifen with 2–3 years of an aromatase inhibitor reduced recurrence by 40% and mortality by 21% • However, the absolute benefit was just a 3% improvement in recurrence-free survival in either strategy
Impact of adding trastuzumab to adjuvant chemotherapy for HER2 positive breast cancer Viani et al. (2007) BMC Cancer 7:153	• This pooled analysis of five randomized trials reported a 48% reduction in mortality with the addition of trastuzumab to chemotherapy for HER2-positive early-stage breast cancer • Cardiac toxicity was 2.5 times greater in patients who received trastuzumab, but overall rates were low (4.5% in the trastuzumab groups)

Areas of research

- Optimal approach to targeted therapy in HER2-positive early and metastatic breast cancer
- Optimal duration of hormone therapy in ER-positive early breast cancer
- Predictive tools to reliably identify cancers likely not to benefit from chemotherapy
- Optimal management of the axilla when the sentinel node is positive
- Role of stem cells in breast cancer genesis, progression and spread
- Factors that drive or predict progression from atypical ductal hyperplasia or ductal carcinoma in situ into invasive cancer
- Identification of new targeted drugs to compliment hormone and chemotherapy efficacy
- Identification of women who can avoid RT after BCS
- Pharmacogenomics to identify individuals at risk for specific treatment-related toxicities

Recommended reading

Bartelink H, Horiot JC, Poortmans PM et al. (2007) Impact of a higher radiation dose on local control and survival in breast-conserving therapy of early breast cancer: 10-year results of the randomized boost versus no boost EORTC 22881–10882 trial. J Clin Oncol 25:3259–3265.

Clarke M, Collins R, Darby S et al. (2005) Effects of radiotherapy and of differences in the extent of surgery for early breast cancer on local recurrence and 15-year survival: an overview of the randomised trials. Lancet 366:2087–2106.

De Laurentiis M, Cancello G, D'Agostino D et al. (2008) Taxane-based combinations as adjuvant chemotherapy of early breast cancer: a meta-analysis of randomized trials. J Clin Oncol 26:444–453.

Dowsett M, Cuzick J, Ingle J et al. (2009) Meta-analysis of breast cancer outcomes of adjuvant trials of aromatase inhibitors versus tamoxifen. J Clin Oncol 28:509–518.

Early Breast Cancer Trialists' Collaborative Group (2005) Effects of chemotherapy and hormone therapy for early breast cancer on recurrence and 15-year survival: an overview of the randomised trials. Lancet 365:1687–1717.

Early Breast Cancer Trialists' Collaborative Group, Darby S, McGale P et al. (2011) Effect of radiotherapy after breast-conserving surgery on 10-year recurrence and 15-year breast cancer death: meta-analysis of individual patient data for 10,801 women in 17 randomised trials. Lancet 378:1707–1716.

Early Breast Cancer Trialists' Collaborative Group, McGale P, Taylor C et al. (2014) Effect of radiotherapy after mastectomy and axillary surgery on 10-year reccurence and 20-year breast cancer mortality: meta-analysis of individual patient data for 8135 women in 22 randomised trials. Lancet 383:2127–2135.

Giuliano AE, Hunt KK, Ballman KV et al. (2011) Axillary dissection vs. no axillary dissection in women with invasive breast cancer and sentinel node metastases: a randomized clinical trial. JAMA 305:569–575.

Galimberti V, Cole BF, Zurrida S et al. (2013) Axillary dissection versus no axillary dissection in patients with sentinel-node micrometastases (IBCSG 23-01): a phase 3 randomised controlled trial. Lancet Oncol 14:297–305.

Haviland JS, Owen JR, Dewar JA, et al. (2013) The UK standardisation of breast radiotherapy (START) trials of radiotherapy hypofractionation for treatment of early breast cancer: 10-year follow-up results of two randomised controlled trials. Lancet Oncol. 14:1086–1094.

Hayes DF, Thor AD, Dressler LG et al. (2007) HER2 and response to paclitaxel in node positive breast cancer. N Engl J Med 357:1496–1506.

Viani GA, Afonso SL, Stefano EJ, De Fendi LI, Soares FV (2007) Adjuvant trastuzumab in the treatment of HER2 positive early breast cancer: a meta-analysis of published randomized trials. BMC Cancer 7:153.

Whelan TJ, Pignol JP, Levine MN et al. (2010) Long-term results of hypofractionated radiation therapy for breast cancer. N Engl J Med 362:513–520.

22 Liver

Eddie K. Abdalla[1], Emile Brihi[2] and Hady Ghanem[3]

[1]Department of Surgery, The Lebanese American University, Beirut, Lebanon
[2]Divsion of Radiation Oncology, The Lebanese American University, Beirut, Lebanon
[3]Division of Medical Oncology, The Lebanese American University, Beirut, Lebanon

Summary	Key facts

Introduction	- *Incidence*:
	  - Worldwide liver cancer is the fifth and seventh most common cancer in men and women, respectively
	  - Worldwide it is the third most common cause of cancer death (estimated 694,000 deaths from liver cancer in 2008 with mortality-to-incidence ratio of 0.93)
	- *Epidemiology*:
	  - 85% of cases in the developing world (especially East/Southeast Asia, Middle/Western Africa)
	  - Low rates in developed regions and Latin America, with the exception of Southern Europe
	  - Related in most, but importantly not all, cases to cirrhosis of any cause, including hepatitis B infection and alcohol abuse (falling incidences), hepatitis C infection and non-alcoholic steatohepatitis (NASH; rising incidences), and less common causes
	- *Pathology*:
	  - 'Liver cancer' specifically refers to hepatocellular carcinoma; a second type of primary liver cancer (cholangiocarcinoma) is considered separately in Chapter 23.1
	  - Microscopically well-to-poorly differentiated with four types: fibrolamellar, adenoid, giant cell and clear cell
	  - Macroscopically (more clinically relevant) may be nodular or infiltrative
	  - *Note*: pathology does not dictate treatment except for the fibrolamellar subtype

Presentation	- Co-existing presence of cirrhosis impacts clinical presentation:
	  - In patients with underlying liver disease, signs and symptoms related to functional hepatic reserve predominate (portal hypertension, jaundice, ascites, encephalopathy)
	  - In patients with preserved liver function, presentation may relate to tumour bulk, malaise, weight loss, fever, anorexia or constitutional symptoms
	  - Spontaneous rupture occurs in up to 10% in some areas (sub-Saharan Africa and Southeast Asia); paraneoplastic syndromes and symptoms related to metastases (e.g. bone pain) may occur

Scenario	- Limited or multifocal tumours in patients with normal liver, as well as small lesions in patients with well-compensated cirrhosis treated by liver resection - Early liver cancer in more advanced cirrhosis treated by liver transplantation - Small lesions in cirrhotic livers may be treated with ablative techniques - Single or multiple lesions may be treated with arterial embolization when surgery/transplantation is not feasible - Systemic therapy is limited to sorafenib (phase III trial data)
Trials	- Two randomized controlled trials (RCTs) showed transarterial chemoembolization (TACE) and transarterial bland embolization (TAE) to prolong survival in unresectable liver cancer - PRECISION V (RCT) showed drug-eluting beads with doxorubicin (DEB-TACE) are as efficacious as conventional TACE, but with fewer side effects overall and better efficacy in patients with more advanced disease - SHARP trial showed sorafenib prolongs survival by nearly 3 months compared to placebo for advanced liver cancer - RCT demonstrated surgical 'anterior approach' to right hepatectomy for large (>5 cm) liver cancers results in improved perioperative outcomes and longer survival than conventional right hepatectomy - Data synthesized from Bismuth by Mazzaferro has led to the adoption of the 'Milan' criteria for transplantation in cirrhotic patients with liver cancer: one tumour of up to 5 cm in diameter, or up to three tumours of up to 3 cm in diameter

UICC Manual of Clinical Oncology, Ninth Edition. Edited by Brian O'Sullivan, James D. Brierley, Anil K. D'Cruz, Martin F. Fey, Raphael Pollock, Jan B. Vermorken and Shao Hui Huang. © 2015 UICC. Published 2015 by John Wiley & Sons, Ltd.

Introduction

Liver cancer (hepatocellular carcinoma) is not a homogenous disease. In the majority of patients, it develops in fibrotic/cirrhotic livers (approximately 80%), and cirrhosis, regardless of aetiology, represents the strongest predisposing factor for liver cancer. The behaviour of liver cancer is as variable as the known causes of the disease. Similarly, mechanisms of carcinogenesis likely differ between causes of liver cancer, even differing between common causes such as hepatitis B virus (HBV)- and hepatitis C virus (HCV)-related cirrhosis. Doubling time for liver cancer can vary from a few weeks to several months, and the natural history of untreated disease varies further, depending on the stage at presentation and the degree of underlying liver disease. The prognosis is poor for untreated liver cancer, even for early-stage disease in some cases, particularly when the liver disease is advanced – which is commonly the case worldwide.

Unlike for other tumour types, treatment is primarily dictated by liver functional reserve and patient performance status, and only secondarily by tumour extent. Most liver cancer patients have competing causes of death – liver cancer and underlying liver disease. These variations in biology and combinations of problems (cancer and liver disease) make treating this disease highly complex.

Removal of the tumour is the treatment most likely to result in long-term survival, with reported 5-year survival rates of 50% and higher after liver resection and up to 70% after orthotopic liver transplantation when indicated. The mortality-to-incidence ratio is 0.93, although many patients die of complications of liver disease and not of liver cancer.

Incidence, aetiology and screening

Incidence, aetiology and screening	Description

Incidence (Table 22.1)	- Fall in known causes of liver cancer (hepatitis B and alcohol abuse), however:
	  - Two-fold rise in overall incidence between 1980 and 1998 and a 37% increase in mortality between 1997 and 2001 in the USA
	  - Similar increase in incidence in the UK and France
	  - Apparent link to rising incidence of hepatitis C and of non-alcoholic steatohepatitis (NASH)

Aetiology	- *Infections*:
	  - Hepatitis B
	  - Hepatitis C

Incidence, aetiology and screening	Description

	- *Cirrhosis*:
	  - Alcohol
	  - Autoimmune hepatitis
	  - Primary biliary cirrhosis
	  - Cryptogenic cirrhosis
	  - NASH-related cirrhosis
	- *Exposures*:
	  - Androgenic steroids
	  - Aflatoxins
	  - N-nitrosylated compounds, pyrrolizidine alkaloids, thorotrast
	- *Metabolic diseases*:
	  - Haemochromatosis
	  - Alpha-1-antitrypsin (A1AT) deficiency
	  - Wilson disease
	  - Porphyria cutanea tarda
	  - Glycogen storage diseases types 1 and 3
	  - Galactosaemia
	  - Citrullinaemia
	  - Hereditary tyrosinaemia
	  - Familial cholestatic jaundice
	  - NASH without cirrhosis

Screening (Fig. 22.1)	- Whether screening reduces mortality from liver cancer is controversial, even in high risk populations; however, most agree screening is of value
	- The American Association of Liver Diseases (AASLD) guidelines suggest surveillance in:
	  - Asian men >40 years old
	  - Asian women >50 years old
	  - Patients with HBV and cirrhosis
	  - Africans and North American Blacks
	  - Patients with a family history of liver cancer
	  - All patients with cirrhosis
	- Screening methods:
	  - Liver ultrasonography every 6 months (AASLD recommendation)
	  - Alpha-fetoprotein (AFP) serum testing is *not* recommended by AASLD because of the absence of data and variability of AFP testing
	  - However, recommended by National Comprehensive Cancer Network (NCCN) and others
	  - AFP + ultrasound increases detection but also false positives and therefore is *not* recommended
	  - Computed tomography (CT) is *not* recommended because of elevated false-positive rates, potential risk associated with radiation exposure over time and lack of cost-effectiveness

Table 22.1 Estimated numbers of cases of and deaths from liver cancer worldwide (Globocan data through November 2012)

Numbers ('000)	Cases	Deaths
World – both sexes	749	695
World – men only	523	478
World – women only	226	217
More developed regions	122	114
Less developed regions	625	579
WHO Africa region (AFRO)	44	42
WHO Americas region (PAHO)	51	49
WHO East Mediterranean region (EMRO)	13	12
WHO Europe region (EURO)	65	66
WHO Southeast Asia region (SEARO)	67	62
WHO Western Pacific region (WPRO)	504	460
USA	21	17
China	401	371
India	19	17
European Union (EU-27)	47	46

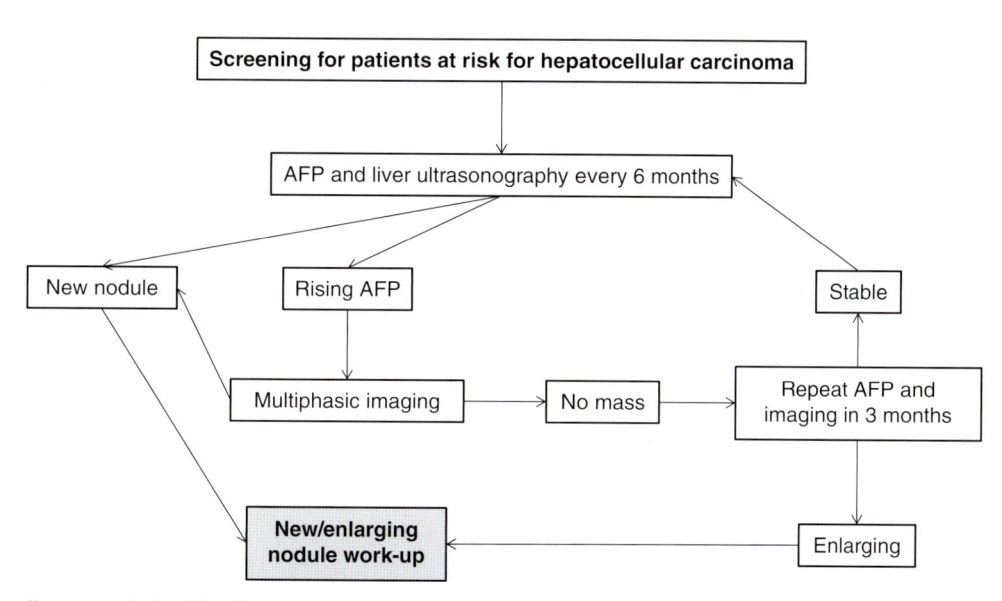

Figure 22.1 Generally accepted algorithm for screening patients at risk for hepatocellular carcinoma using alpha-fetoprotein (AFP) and imaging

Pathology

Histological variations in liver cancer (which can range from well-differentiated to undifferentiated, anaplastic lesions) are of minimal importance with regard to the treatment of liver cancer, with the exception of the fibrolamellar subtype. Tumour grade may contribute to prognostic stratification; it is interesting that although the macroscopic morphological types (nodular, massive, diffuse) contribute to prognostic stratification, they are not currently part of any formal staging system.

Pathology	Description

Overview	• Typical liver cancer (well and moderately differentiated) comprises tumour cells recognizable as hepatocytic in origin (architectural types are described below):
	  ■ May contain cytoplasmic inclusions
	  ■ Hepatitis B surface antigen-positive staining if hepatitis B is active
	  ■ A1AT immunohistochemistry (IHC) stain positive in about 75% of cases
	  ■ AFP IHC stain positive in 60–80% of patients
	  ■ Reliably have bile pigment within tumour cells (or formation of bile canaliculi on electron microscopy)
	• Poorly differentiated tumours may contain:
	  ■ Small, completely undifferentiated cells
	  ■ Spindle cells with sarcoma-like appearance; stroma can be highly vascularized and appear angiosarcoma-like
	  ■ Giant pleomorphic cells, totally disorganized with bizarre cells, abundant cytoplasm, often multiple nuclei or atypical mitoses
	• Vascular invasion is common in all types of liver cancer

Liver cancer architectural growth patterns (well- and moderately-differentiated liver cancer)	• Microtrabecular, macrotrabecular, compact, acinar, clear cell, mixed • Architectural growth pattern not associated with outcome or treatment (except for fibrolamellar) • *Microtrabecular pattern*: seen most often in non-cirrhotic livers: ■ Trebuclae are made up of several layers of tumour cells separated by vascular channels that may resemble sinusoids surrounded by a sheath of connective tissue • *Acinar (or pseudoglandular) pattern*: the cells surround 'lumina' and often contain bile plugs • *'Clear cell' liver cancers*: rare but have cytoplasmic glycogen excess and appear micrographically very similar to clear cell renal cancer • *Macrotrabecular pattern*: seen most often in cirrhotic livers

Liver cancer histological grading, microscopic growth interface	• Grade, particularly Edmondson's classification (low, intermediate, high), correlates to survival and probability of intrahepatic metastasis:
	  ■ May correlate to surrounding liver parenchyma (higher grade most often in cirrhotic livers, although this point is debated)
	• Microscopic growth interface (between tumour and liver parenchyma) may be sinusoidal, replacing, pseudocapsular or capsular:
	  ■ Capsule associated with lower grade and better survival but overall, growth interface not clearly independently prognostic

Vascular invasion	• One of the most important macro- and micro-scopic features of liver cancer which forms the backbone of prognosis and thus staging:
	  ■ Macroscopic vascular invasion usually associated with death <2 years from resection
	  ■ Microscopic VI (vascular invasion) is predictive of outcome from resection and transplantation
	• Associated with increasing tumour size, higher histological grade and higher mitotic rate (>4–10 mitoses/10 HPF)

Macroscopic growth patterns	• Much more important than microscopic architectural type with regard to outcome
	• *Nodular type*:
	  ■ Type most often resectable
	  ■ Three subtypes with increasing frequency of microvascular invasion:
	    ○ Single nodular type, well defined (often cirrhotic); 14% microvascular invasion
	    ○ Single nodular type with extranodular growth (25% microvascular)
	    ○ Contiguous multinodular type (70% microvascular)
	• *Massive type*: poorly demarcated, usually >10 cm in size, often younger, non-cirrhotic patients with portal vein tumour thrombi
	• *Diffuse type*: multiple small nodules of up to 1 cm throughout hepatic parenchyma; uniquely in cirrhotic patients, associated with portal thrombosis (70%) and nodal metastasis (50%) with grim prognosis

Fibrolamellar liver cancer	• Macroscopically, 80–90% are large, well circumscribed and heterogeneous with a central scar (up to 75%) • Microscopically, well-differentiated, polygonal very large malignant-appearing hepatocytes with deeply eosinophilic cytoplasm and macronucleoli: ■ Cord-like trabeculae of tumour cells are usually surrounded by thick fibrous bands in parallel (lamellar) formation without cirrhosis • Typically occurs in younger patients without cirrhosis • AFP typically normal

Presentation

Presentation	Description

Patients with cirrhosis	• Presence of and severity of cirrhosis impacts clinical presentation of liver cancer
	• In moderate/severe cirrhosis: symptoms of liver failure and portal hypertension predominate:
	  ▪ Progressive jaundice, ascites; jaundice may be:
	    ○ Hepatocellular (90%), related to hepatic insufficiency; most patients with this feature die within 10 weeks of presentation
	    ○ Related to hepatitis activation
	    ○ Related to neoplastic obstruction of bile ducts
	  ▪ Encephalopathy or tremors, confusion, mild disturbance of consciousness
	  ▪ Peripheral stigmata of liver insufficiency, e.g. oedema, palmar erythema, caput medusa
	  ▪ Variceal bleeding
	• May be due to:
	  ▪ Intrinsic liver disease (cirrhosis)
	  ▪ Portal invasion by tumour
	  ▪ Budd Chiari – hepatic venous obstruction:
	    ○ Usually presents with sudden, severe oedema, tense ascites and tender hepatomegaly
	    ○ Extension of thrombus to the right atrium can lead to dyspnoea and sudden death

Patients without cirrhosis	• Hepatomegaly from tumour mass
	• Pleural effusion
	• Arterial bruit on abdominal auscultation (related to bruit)
	• Constitutional symptoms (can be related to cirrhosis or advanced disease at presentation): weight loss, fever, anorexia, malaise, dysphagia, mild abdominal distension
	• Right upper quadrant pain with right shoulder pain (common manifestation when tumour stretches liver capsule)
	• Acute, severe pain and hypotension due to rupture:
	  ▪ Can occur spontaneously or after abdominal trauma
	  ▪ Most common cause of spontaneous haemoperitoneum in sub-Saharan Africa and Southeast Asia (10%)
	• Paraneoplastic syndromes: hypoglycaemia (metabolic or due to production of insulin growth factor 2 [IGF-2]), hypercalcaemia (parathyroid hormone-related protein), erythrocytosis (erythropoietin), thrombocytosis (thrombopoetin), gynaecomastia (independent of cirrhosis), hypercholesterolaemia, cryofibrinogenaemia, dysfibrinogenaemia, carcinoid syndrome
	• Cutaneous manifestations (non-specific but have been described), including porphyria cutanea tarda, dermatomyositis and others
	• Metastases: bone (causing pain or fracture), lungs, meninges or brain, adrenal glands, lymph nodes (abdominal or thoracic)

Natural history

Most patients with liver cancer have two competing causes of death – cirrhosis and cancer. Further, the behaviour of liver cancer is as variable as the known causes of the disease. Doubling time can vary from a few weeks to several months, and the natural history of untreated disease varies further, depending on the stage at presentation and the degree of underlying liver disease. The prognosis is poor for untreated liver cancer, even for early-stage disease, particularly when liver disease is advanced. The mortality-to-incidence ratio is 0.93, although many patients die of complications of liver disease and not of liver cancer.

Natural history		Description
Presentation	Local	• In contrast to other diseases, localized versus metastatic does not define the natural history or presentation of liver cancer

(continued)

Natural history		Description

		• Localized liver cancer in patient with preserved liver function – *tumour dominates presentation*:
		  ■ Often incidental or found on imaging for non-specific mild abdominal discomfort
		  ■ Common triad of symptoms: right upper quadrant pain radiating to the shoulder, abdominal mass and weight loss.
		    □ Abdominal mass with or without arterial bruit on auscultation (from arteriovenous fistula)
		  ■ Hepatomegaly or mild respiratory symptoms because of hemidiaphragm elevation
		  ■ Symptoms related to tumour growth/features of advanced malignancy such as weight loss, dysphagia, fever, anorexia, malaise (constitutional syndrome) usually with abdominal distension
		  ■ Rarely presents with acute abdomen due to tumour rupture
		  ■ Budd–Chiari syndrome with oedema, ascites and tender hepatomegaly if thrombus occludes vena cava
		• Localized liver cancer in patient with poor liver function – *liver dominates presentation* (tumour found on exam for liver):
		  ■ Signs and symptoms of liver failure and portal hypertension: progressive jaundice, ascites, tremors, confusion and disturbances of consciousness or frank encephalopathy
		  ■ Peripheral stigmata of liver insufficiency such as ankle oedema, palmar erythema or caput medusa
		  ■ Variceal bleeding, gastropathy

	Metastatic	• Presentation related to metastases directly (rarely does this overshadow liver-related symptoms) • Bone pain or pathological fracture (osteolytic bone metastases) • Neurological presentation due to brain or meningeal metastases • Lung metastases rarely symptomatic but can produce cough, dyspnoea or haemoptysis • Paraneoplastic syndromes (may be a metastatic or local tumour, uncommon without knowledge of primary tumour) including: hypoglycaemia (metabolic or due to production of IGF-2), hypercalcaemia (parathyroid hormone-related protein), erythrocytosis (erythropoietin), thrombocytosis (thrombopoetin), gynaenocomastia (independent of cirrhosis), hypercholesterolaemia, cryofibrinogenaemia, dysfibrinogenaemia and carcinoid syndrome • Cutaneous manifestations (non-specific but have been described) including porphyria cutanea tarda, dermatomyosistis and others

Routes of spread	Local	• Portal spread is most common:
		  ■ Portoportal spread causes intrahepatic metastases
		  ■ Portal extension (tumour thrombus) occludes portal branches, and can extend to contralateral liver and extrahepatically, causing acute changes in portal pressure
		• Hepatic venous extension (tumour thrombus) also frequent:
		  ■ If reaching vena cava, symptoms as described above
		• Direct extension:
		  ■ To gall bladder, diaphragm, stomach, colon

	Regional	• To lymph nodes in order of frequency (common for fibrolamellar subtype; less common for classical liver cancer):
		  ■ Coeliac
		  ■ Porta hepatis
		  ■ Para-aortic
		  ■ Portocaval
		  ■ Mediastinal
		  ■ Cardiophrenic

	Metastatic	• Haematogenous, in order of frequency:
		  ■ Lung
		  ■ Bone (vertebral body, ribs, skull most common)
		  ■ Adrenal glands
		  ■ Other: brain, meninges, peritoneum, skin, muscle

Diagnostic work-up

- Work-up of large versus small liver nodules differs, but both focus on patient characteristics, liver characteristics, imaging studies, serum studies and, when indicated, biopsy
- Liver nodules in cirrhotic patients discovered on screening ultrasound that are not definitively benign cysts or haemangioma and mandate work-up as indicated below
- Newly diagnosed liver lesions with venous invasion, hypervascular in the arterial phase of CT or magnetic resonance imaging (MRI), associated with elevated AFP (especially >200 ng/mL) are liver cancer until proven otherwise
- Hypervascular lesions in non-cirrhotic livers evoke consideration for liver cancer especially in patients with other risk factors such as HBV infection
- Newly diagnosed nodules on screening ultrasound prompt multiphasic imaging (see Fig. 22.2):
  - If no mass, repeat AFP and imaging in 3 months
  - If enlarging, work-up
  - If stable, resume standard follow-up
  - If nodule confirmed, work-up

Diagnostic work-up	Description

Liver nodules >1 cm	• Multiphase, multidetector CT or dynamic multiphase contrast-enhanced MRI of the liver is the first step:
	  ▪ If early arterial filling with venous or delayed washout of contrast present, diagnosis is liver cancer
	  ▪ If classic washin/washout not present, perform second multiphasic study (if CT done first, then MRI; if MRI done first, then CT):
	    ○ If second study shows classical arterial hypervascularity and venous/delayed washout, then diagnosis is liver cancer
	• If both MRI and CT fail to show classical imaging, then biopsy is indicated where clinically required to guide therapy:
	  ▪ Biopsy, properly performed, has an extremely low risk of negative effects on patients; needle track seeding is exceedingly rare (far <2%) and bleeding is rare
	  ▪ If biopsy is non-diagnostic, repeat imaging and continue follow-up algorithm or rebiopsy

Liver nodules <1 cm	• If suspicion is high, then follow algorithm in Fig. 22.2 as for masses >1 cm
	• If AFP is elevated, particularly >200 ng/mL, then follow algorithm in Fig. 22.2 as for masses >1 cm
	• If suspicion is low and/or AFP is low, repeat liver ultrasound is indicated:
	  ▪ If stable, continue surveillance
	  ▪ If increasing in size or imaging character changes, then pursue multiphasic imaging and/or biopsy

Liver nodules 1–2 cm	• Varying recommendations (AASLD vs European Association for the Study of the Liver [EASL] vs others), but most recommend utilization of two modalities (CT and MRI) for characterization:
	  ▪ If both reveal classical arterial enhancement and late washout, liver cancer is the diagnosis
	  ▪ Biopsy can be considered as appropriate
	• Some liver cancers are mixed hepatocellular/cholangiocellular tumours:
	  ▪ Varying imaging characteristics and varying patterns of elaboration of tumour markers (e.g. AFP and carbohydrate antigen 19-9 [CA19-9])
	  ▪ When indicated, biopsy may be required to guide therapy

Patient evaluation after liver cancer diagnosis confirmed	• Evaluation of liver function (cirrhotic patients):
	  ▪ Classification according to Child–Pugh (CP) class (see Table 22.3) and/or Model of End-stage Liver Disease (MELD)/Pediatric End-stage Liver Disease [PELD], or MELD adjusted for children
	  ▪ Child–Pugh (CP) classification considers total bilirubin and albumin, presence and degree of ascites, encephalopathy and prothrombin time/international normalized ratio (INR) (see Table 22.3)
	    ○ Operative mortality rates (abdominal operations) for CP classes A, B and C are approximately 10%, 30% and 92%, respectively.
	    ○ CP class A patients without portal hypertension can be considered for a variety of hepatic resection options
	    ○ CP class B patients may tolerate minor resections
	    ○ CP class C patients are generally not considered candidates for hepatic resection
	    ○ Risk for other treatments (radiofrequency ablation [RFA], embolization) also correlate to CP class in terms of risk for both complications and mortality
	    ○ CP may be combined with indocyanine green retention

(continued)

Diagnostic work-up	Description
	<ul><li>MELD estimates mortality at 3 months awaiting liver transplantation:<ul><li>Combines bilirubin, creatinine and INR in a mathematical formula</li><li>Liver cancer patients receive additional points to reduce wait time for transplantation</li><li>Effective for allocation for liver transplant but no more effective than CP in predicting outcome of liver resection</li></ul></li><li>Portal hypertension:<ul><li>May be significant even in CP class A and MELD low patients</li><li>Increases risk for hepatic insufficiency and failure after hepatectomy</li><li>May be assessed by hepatic venous pressure gradient but most assess clinical/radiological signs, including splenomegaly, abdominal collaterals, thrombocytopenia (platelet count <100,000/mm^3), presence of oesophagogastric varices as predictors of occult portal hypertension</li></ul></li><li>Other tests:<ul><li>Urea-nitrogen synthesis rate, galactose elimination capacity, bromsulphalein and aminopyrine breath tests, and indocyanine green (ICG) clearance assess global liver function; none in routine use and all lack specific indications</li><li>For major resection, liver volumetry is used to assess liver remnant volume and to predict function</li><li>When therapy is being considered, some or all of the following may be considered:</li></ul></li><li>Blood type and antibody screen, panel reactive antibody (PRA)</li><li>Full hepatitis profile, to include serum HCV-RNA titres, HCV genotype, HBV-DNA, hepatitis B 'e' antigen and antibody</li><li>Full autoimmune markers to include iron and copper studies, immune protein electrophoresis</li><li>Cancer markers, i.e. AFP, carcinoembryonic antigen (CEA), prostate-specific antigen (PSA), CA19-9</li><li>Complete blood count (CBC), complete metabolic panel to include magnesium and phosphate</li><li>Coagulation studies, i.e. INR, fibrinogen levels</li><li>Cytomegalovirus (CMV) status, varicella titres, cryptococcal antibodies</li><li>Arteriography and lipiodol CT are rarely used in the era of high-quality CT and MRI multiphasic imaging</li><li>Diagnostic laparoscopy, although invasive, may be used in some patients with large or ruptured tumours, and those in whom assessment of the liver is needed in preparation for surgery</li></ul>
Evaluation for surgery	<ul><li>CT chest to rule out lung metastases, adrenal and peritoneal metastases</li><li>Role for positron emission tomography (PET) evolving with existing and new radionuclides; not standard for work-up of liver cancer</li><li>CT or MRI abdomen is part of work-up to rule out adrenal metastases; CT better to rule out peritoneal carcinomatosis</li><li>Resection considered in all patients with sufficient hepatic reserve when all disease can be resected (even multiple tumours, bilateral tumours) but leave an adequate liver remnant</li><li>Resection considered in very highly selected cases with solitary bone metastases, with portal or hepatic venous thrombosis</li><li>Preoperative assessment with liver volumetry, and in some regions indocyanine green retention stratifies safe resection extent and allows consideration of preoperative strategies to improve perioperative and long-term outcomes of resection (e.g. use of TACE and/or portal vein embolization)</li><li>Oesophago-gastroduodenoscopy (EGD) is occasionally used to assess for varices, but CT evaluates anatomical causes of severe portal hypertension that would impact selection for surgery</li></ul>
Evaluation for liver transplantation	<ul><li>CT chest, abdomen and pelvis to rule out metastases</li><li>EGD typically required because most who undergo transplantation have portal hypertension and varices which may require treatment before transplant</li><li>Colonoscopy generally required in patients >35 years of age to rule out polyps or cancer</li><li>Ultrasound of liver with Doppler studies to measure pressure in the portal system</li><li>If female, mammography and Pap smear</li><li>Cardiac echo and usually cardiac stress test</li><li>Chest radiography and examinations of sinuses and teeth to rule out potential infectious sources</li></ul>
Evaluation for locoregional therapies	<ul><li>E.g. percutaneous ablation, arterial chemoembolization, external beam radiotherapy (EBRT)</li><li>Metastatic work-up</li><li>Assessment of liver function</li></ul>

Diagnostic work-up	Description

Staging work-up	• Candidates for resection/transplantation and patients who have very advanced liver disease may not be staged using a single system or algorithm
	• Accurate staging provides prognostic data but also may aid in selecting patients for specific treatments
	• The 2010 Americas Hepato-Pancreato-Biliary Association consensus was to use the Barcelona Clinic Liver Cancer (BCLC) for unresectable and TNM (specifically UICC/American Joint Committee on Cancer [AJCC]) for resectable/transplantable liver cancer
	• AASLD recommends only BCLC (in contrast to above)
	• Cancer of the Liver Italian Program (CLIP) classification:
	  ■ Uses CP classification of liver function, tumour morphology (both size and number of nodules), AFP level and presence or absence of portal vein thrombosis (see Table 22.4)
	  ■ Patients with CLIP scores of 0, 1, 2, 3 and 4 have median survival times of 36, 22, 9, 7 and 3 months, respectively
	  ■ Not as applicable to patients who present with early-stage disease who are eligible for surgical resection
	• BCLC classification system:
	  ■ Developed as a 'staging system' for liver cancer, but it has been criticised as being a treatment algorithm because it allocates treatments based on performance status and disease extent
	  ■ Conversely, as a system which incorporates both liver function and tumour extent, the BCLC is valuable for classifying patients who are not candidates for surgical therapies
	• UICC TNM staging (see Table 22.2):
	  ■ Only staging system validated in patients treated with liver resection and liver transplantation

Tumour markers	• AFP is the most commonly used serum marker:
	  ■ Normal in 20–40% of patients with small liver cancer
	  ■ Can be elevated (even to 500 ng/mL) in cirrhotic patients without liver cancer, particularly when INR and aspartate aminotransferase level is elevated and necroinflammatory activity is high
	  ■ Usually normal in patients with fibrolamellar liver cancer
	  ■ AFP > normal (in most labs 20 ng/mL): sensitivity for diagnosis of liver cancer of 41–65% and specificity of 80–94%
	  ■ AFP >200 ng/mL with characteristic imaging: sensitivity for diagnosis of liver cancer nearly 100%
	  ■ Trend for its use to aid in diagnosis and follow-up of patients with liver cancer
	• Des-gamma-carboxy prothrombin (DCP) (also called protein induced by vitamin K absence/antagonist-II [PIVKA-II]):
	  ■ Used primarily in Japan
	  ■ Present in up to 90% of patients with liver cancer
	  ■ PIVKA-II for diagnosis of liver cancer: sensitivity approximately 65% and specificity approximately 75%
	  ■ Sensitivity of PIVKA-II at 250 mAU/mL is 95% for liver cancer
	  ■ May be useful in detection of recurrence after treatment
	  ■ May be used in combination with AFP to increase sensitivity

Staging and prognostic grouping

The complexity of liver cancer patients leads to the need for several systems to classify and prognosticate patients. The gold standard is the UICC (unified) TNM staging system, although this largely pathological system applies mainly to patients who are candidates for surgical therapies (hepatic resection and liver transplantation). Consensus suggests using UICC TNM staging for surgical patients, and BCLC for non-surgical patients. However worldwide, and in the literature, several systems are discussed and these systems are integrated into recommendations and thus are briefly described here (although others exist).

Post-resection/post-transplantation pathological factors dominate staging and prognostic risk stratification for classical liver cancer when interventions are considered (resection/transplantation). Vascular invasion and degree of invasion (macrovascular invasion vs microvascular invasion), tumour number, tumour size and the presence of cirrhosis/fibrosis in the associated underlying liver are independent predictors of survival following surgery for liver cancer. These formulate the basis for the UICC TNM staging system for liver cancer. It is of note that the UICC TNM staging system is the only staging system validated in cohorts of patients both in the West and in the East, who have undergone liver resection and liver transplantation.

In contrast, prognosis in patients with severe underlying liver disease and who are not candidates for resection/transplantation is dominated primarily by clinical factors (CP classification,

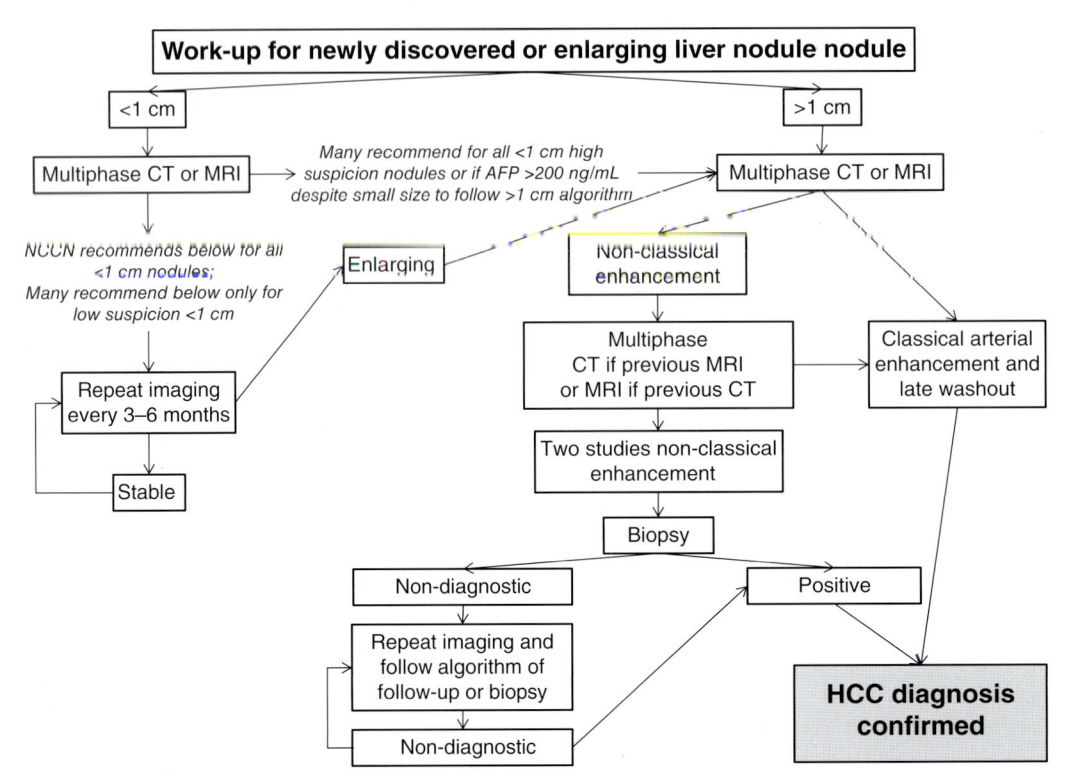

Figure 22.2 Detailed algorithm for work-up of a new or enlarging liver nodule in cirrhotic liver.
HCC, hepatocellular carcinoma; NCCN, National Comprehensive Cancer Network.

Table 22.2 UICC TNM categories and stage grouping: Hepatocellular carcinoma TNM categories

TX	Primary tumour cannot be assessed
T0	No evidence of primary tumour
T1	Solitary tumour without vascular invasion
T2	Solitary tumour with vascular invasion or multiple tumours (none >5 cm)
T3a	Multiple tumours >5 cm
T3b	Single tumour or multiple tumours of any size that invades a major branch of portal or hepatic vein
T4	Direct invasion of adjacent organs other than the gall bladder or with perforation of visceral peritoneum
NX	Regional lymph nodes cannot be assessed
N0	No regional lymph node metastasis
N1	Regional lymph node metastasis
M0	No distant metastasis
M1	Distant metastasis
F0*	Ishak Grade 0–4 fibrosis (none to moderate)
F1*	Ishak Grade 5–6 fibrosis (severe fibrosis/cirrhosis)

*F score is not formally included in assessment of stage, but the staging manual recommends notation of F score because the F score stratifies prognosis for each stage grouping.

Stage grouping			
Stage I	T1	N0	M0
Stage II	T2	N0	M0
Stage IIIA	T3a	N0	M0
Stage IIIB	T3b	N0	M0
Stage IIIC	T4	N0	M0
Stage IVA	Any T	N1	M0
Stage IVB	Any T	Any N	M1

AFP, portal thrombosis assessed on imaging, global tumour extent within the liver) reflected in the clinical staging systems (CLIP, Okuda, BCLC).

UICC TNM staging

TNM staging is based on data that reveal that prognosis is distinctly different in patients who have undergone liver resection or transplantation based on tumour size, presence and degree of vascular invasion, extrahepatic invasion and extrahepatic metastasis (Table 22.2). The key points are:
- Tumour size does not impact prognosis if vascular invasion is absent

- Tumour multiplicity does impact prognosis based on tumour size
- Vascular invasion (microvascular or major vascular) prominently impacts prognosis
- Extrahepatic metastasis portends poor prognosis, whether in a lymph node, peritoneum or another solid organ
- Although the prognosis for patients with major vascular invasion and invasion of extrahepatic organs is similar, these remain separate stages (IIIB and IV, respectively).

Child–Pugh classification

The Child-Pugh (CP) classification (Table 22.3) permeates the literature on cirrhosis and liver cancer management and is central to its therapeutic decision-making.

Table 22.3 Child–Pugh classification of hepatic functional reserve

Clinical or laboratory measurement	1 point	2 points	3 points
Encephalopathy (grade)	0 (absent)	1–2	3–4
Ascites	Absent	Slight	Poorly controlled
Bilirubin (mg/dL)	<2.0	2.0–3.0	>3.0
Albumin (g/dL)	>3.5	2.8–3.5	<2.8
International normalized ratio (INR)	<1.7	1.7–2.2	>2.3

Each feature is assigned 1, 2, or 3 points: class A: 5–6 points; class B: 7–9 points; class C: 10–15 points.
Adapted from Pugh et al (1973). The British Journal of Surgery 60(8): 646–9.

Cancer of the Liver Italian Program (CLIP)

CLIP (Table 22.4) is widely used independently, as is discussed by NCCN, and integrated with serum factors (e.g. with IGF-1) with interesting results for unresectable patients.

Table 22.4 Cancer of the Liver Italian Program (CLIP) Staging System

Category	Score		
	0	1	2
Child–Pugh classification	A	B	C
Tumour morphology	Uninodular; extension ≤50%	Multinodular; extension ≤50%	Massive or extension >50%
Alpha-fetoprotein (ng/mL)	<400	≥400	
Portal vein thrombosis	Absent	Present	

Each patient is assigned a score (from 0 to 6) by adding the points from the four categories listed.
Adapted from The Cancer of the Liver Italian Program (CLIP) Investigators. A new prognostic system for hepatocellular carcinoma: a retrospective study of 435 patients. Hepatology 28, 751–755 (1998).

Okuda staging system

Okuda staging (Table 22.5) is somewhat similar to CP but incorporates tumour extent.

Table 22.5 Okuda staging system

		Points
Tumour extent (% liver involvement)	>50%	1
	<50%	0
Ascites	Yes	1
	No	0
Serum albumin	<3 g/dL	1
	>3 g/dL	0
Serum bilirubin	>3 mg/dL	1
	<3 mg/dL	0
Okuda stage	I	0
	II	1 or 2
	III	3 or 4

Adapted from Okuda et al. (1985) Cancer 56:918–928.

Barcelona Clinic Liver Cancer (BCLC) staging

The BCLC staging system is best described as an algorithm which allocates patients to treatments based on two levels of evaluation: (1) performance status and CP classification and (2) number/size/portal invasion of liver cancer.
- Patients with normal performance status and preserved liver function, normal portal pressure, normal bilirubin and very small single liver cancer are allocated to resection
- Patients with normal performance status and liver function but increased portal pressure or three nodules of up to 3 cm are allocated to transplantation or RFA (designated as 'curative therapies')

This allocation of patients is (appropriately) criticised because many more patients are candidates for surgery and experience long survival than those allocated to surgical therapies by BCLC. Patients with mildly altered performance status or CP class are allocated to TACE or systemic therapy (sorafenib) as 'palliative therapies', again eliciting criticism because many patients in the intermediate categories can be treated with 'curative therapies' and experience long-term survival. Advanced-stage patients (with regard to performance status, CP class and tumour classification) are allocated to symptomatic treatment.

Prognostic factors

See Table 22.6.

Table 22.6 Prognostic factors for liver cancer

Prognostic factors	Tumour related	Host related	Environment related
Essential	Major vascular invasion* Microvascular invasion* Size >5 cm Multiple (vs single) Tumour differentiation	Fibrosis of underlying liver* Tumour growth rate Patient performance status at diagnosis Liver function Degree of portal hypertension	*Treatment factors*: Post-resection residual disease (R0,1,2) Post-ablation residual disease Post-embolization residual disease
Additional	AFP level DCP/PIVKA-II level	Hepatitis activity	
New and promising	5-gene score (genetic profile) Cancer stem cell markers Circulating microRNA, DNA, circulating cancer cells	IGF-1 combined with CLIP Regulatory T cells C-reactive protein (CRP), interleukin 10 (IL-10), vascular endothelial growth factor (VEGF), neutrophil-to-lymphocyte ratio, MnSOD (magnesium superoxide dismutase)	

*Dominant prognostic factors in resected/transplanted patients.

Treatment philosophy

Unlike for other cancers, local versus regional versus distant does not solely direct therapy; instead the underlying liver function and resulting performance status of the patient dictate therapy (Fig. 22.3).

```
HCC treatment once diagnosis is confirmed
                    ↓
         Multidisciplinary work-up
This algorithm groups patients into three areas. Specific recommendations must be carefully tailored to the
patient, tumour and liver (reserve) and thus are not amenable to 'algorithmic' summary with excessive detail
```

No metastatic disease present*

- Resectable / Adequate liver reserve / No specific limits on tumour number/size → **Hepatic resection**
  A proportion of patients who will undergo hepatic resection may be advised to undergo preparation with arterial or portal embolization
  *Resection is *rarely* considered if limited metastatic disease present

- Solitary tumour ≤5 cm or up to 3 tumours ≤3 cm and no macrovascular invasion and no extrahepatic disease → **Liver transplantation**
  Bridge therapy as indicated by anticipated wait time to transplantation

- Unresectable/untransplantable → **Locoregional therapy**
  Locoregional therapy may include
  - In situ ablation
  - Transarterial chemoembolization
  - Radiotherapy
  - Combination

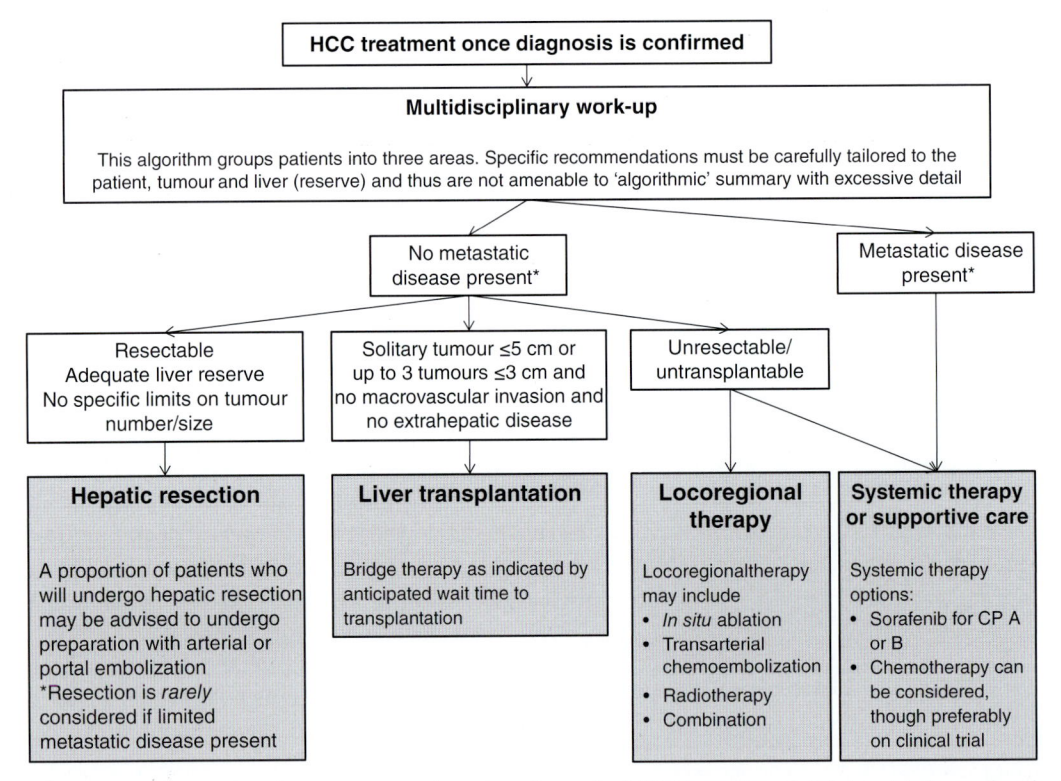

Metastatic disease present* → **Systemic therapy or supportive care**
Systemic therapy options:
- Sorafenib for CP A or B
- Chemotherapy can be considered, though preferably on clinical trial

Figure 22.3 Hepatocellular carcinoma (HCC) treatment overview when diagnosis of HCC is confirmed. This is not to be confused with a treatment algorithm but rather shows the types of patients treated by each modality: surgery, transplantation, other locoregional therapies and systemic/supportive care.

CP, Child–Pugh class.

Many patients are harmed by delivery of any therapy for the cancer (e.g. those with advanced cirrhosis with very atrophic livers, ascites and portal hypertension); in these patients supportive care is superior to any antitumoural therapy. Others with more extensive tumour but preserved liver function are candidates for aggressive resection strategies. Transplantation is a highly effective therapy for patients with advanced liver disease and early cancer, but fails as a therapeutic modality in those with advanced liver cancer (vascular invasion, extensive intrahepatic disease, any extrahepatic disease). Locoregional therapies (percutaneous ablation and TACE) can be used to control, and occasionally (but rarely) cure liver cancer in patients who are not candidates for resection or transplantation; these therapies can also be used as adjuncts to or preparation for resection or transplantation.

Scenario	Treatment philosophy	
	Preserved performance status	*Compromised performance status*
Local, preserved liver function	• Solitary or multiple, single or bilateral, complete resection leaving adequate functional liver remnant possible: 　▪ Partial hepatectomy • Solitary or multiple, single or bilateral, complete resection leaving adequate functional liver remnant *not possible*: 　▪ Consider locoregional therapy vs combined therapies (e.g. resection plus ablation) vs sorafenib (systemic therapy)	• Locoregional therapy vs sorafenib vs investigational therapy vs symptomatic treatment
Local, compromised liver function	• Solitary liver cancer up to 5 cm in diameter or up to three liver cancers of up to 3 cm in diameter, and suitable candidate (based on age and availability of donor liver): 　▪ Liver transplantation • Beyond above criteria: 　▪ Arterial embolization vs sorafenib	• Supportive care
Regional	• Nodal metastases from liver cancer are considered 'metastatic' *except* fibrolamellar subtype • If typical liver cancer, then treat as metastatic: 　▪ *Note*: nodes are frequently enlarged in cirrhosis; thus, enlarged nodes alone do not diagnose metastatic nodes 　　○ Imaging characteristics and or biopsy may be necessary to establish diagnosis of nodal metastases • If fibrolamellar subtype, then resection of liver and nodes	
Metastatic	• Preserved liver function (CP A or B), sorafenib • Compromised liver function: supportive care • Clinical trials as available • For fibrolamellar subtype: resection is indicated for primary and metastases, including lung; lymph nodes when complete resection is feasible	
Recurrent	• Consider local therapy including resection and locoregional therapy as liver function and performance status permit • If locoregional therapies are not possible, then sorafenib or supportive care • For fibrolamellar subtype, recurrent liver, lung and nodes are iteratively resected	
Follow-up	• Varies depending on therapy delivered 　▪ After surgery/transplantation or locoregional therapy: cross-sectional imaging and serum studies three times per year for 2 years, then twice per year thereafter 　▪ During sorafenib therapy: re-image every 2–3 months	

Treatment

Surgery

Surgery	Description
Early disease	**First choice when possible: complete resection** • Partial hepatectomy (does not treat liver disease): 　▪ *Pros*: can be considered in large, multinodular and bilateral liver cancer, occasionally if portal/hepatic vein thrombosis 　▪ *Cons*: limited by liver function 　▪ *Risks*: hepatic dysfunction, recurrence in remnant liver

(continued)

Surgery	Description

	• Liver transplantation:
	  ▪ *Pros*: treats liver disease, useful in advanced cirrhosis, may improve disease-free survival
	  ▪ *Cons*: limited to early liver cancer (Milan criteria; see below) without vascular invasion and limited by donor organ availability
	  ▪ *Risks*: recurrence in transplant liver, immunosuppression-related risks (and mortality; lifelong)
	Second choice when resection/transplantation is not possible
	• Arterial embolization:
	  ▪ *Pros*: can be considered in large, multinodular and bilateral liver cancer, minimally invasive
	  ▪ *Cons*: limited by liver function, rarely curative, usually has to be repeated
	  ▪ *Risks*: liver dysfunction, frequently must be repeated
	• Ablation therapies:
	  ▪ *Pros*: can be administered via laparotomy, laparoscopy or percutaneously
	  ▪ *Cons*: limited to oligonodular liver cancer, and lesions usually <5 cm, best ≤3 cm
	  ▪ Somewhat limited by liver function, but apply to marginal liver function patients
	  ▪ *Risks*: local recurrence, recurrence in remnant liver, abscess
	• EBRT:
	  ▪ Usually for one to three tumours, usually with CP A
	  ▪ *Risks*: radiation hepatitis, liver insufficiency, local recurrence
	• Embolization and ablation can be used as adjunct to resection or bridge to transplantation

Advanced non-metastatic	• Resect if possible based on liver functional reserve using advanced techniques and combined therapies (e.g. arterial + portal embolization) • Consider appropriate locoregional therapy (embolization or EBRT) • Sorafenib for CP A or B if locoregional therapy not possible • Clinical trial or supportive care otherwise
Metastatic	• Highly selected cases, resection of liver and metastasis (e.g. solitary bone metastasis) • Sorafenib (CP A or B) • Supportive care or clinical trial otherwise

Hepatic resection

- Must be fit for major surgery
- Indicated for:
  - CP A, no portal hypertension
  - Solitary mass, no vascular invasion on imaging (NCCN and AASLD indication)
  - Adequate liver remnant can be preserved
- Controversial (but can be considered):
  - CP B, controlled portal hypertension
  - Multifocal lesions but resectable with adequate remnant
  - Major vascular invasion
  - Other highly selected cases (e.g. solitary bone metastases)
- If major resection is considered and underlying liver disease is present, portal vein embolization (or TACE followed by portal embolization) should be considered
- Under study: adjuvant sorafenib after resection

Advances in anaesthetic and surgical techniques, in addition to improved patient selection and preparation for surgery, have contributed to improvements in the outcome and safety of liver resection for liver cancer. Recognition that specific aspects of surgical technique impact outcome has led to the development and study of approaches that enhance the probability not only of a good surgical outcome, but also a better oncological outcome. Established techniques include the use of low central venous pressure anaesthesia, intraoperative ultrasonography (IOUS) and hepatic vascular occlusion. Increasingly accepted approaches include portal-oriented anatomical resection, the anterior approach with hanging manoeuver for major resection, and parenchymal transaction techniques that permit complete resection of tumours with less blood loss.

Many patients require advanced preparation for surgery, including assessments of the functional reserve of the liver specifically in the setting of the planned resection. When major resection is considered (defined as resection of more than two or better defined as resection of more than three anatomical segments of the liver), three-dimensional volumetry of the liver that will remain after resection (the future remnant liver [FLR]) is considered standard. When the liver function is preserved and portal pressure absent, preoperative portal vein embolization (deliberate occlusion of the portal branches supplying the liver to be resected) is performed; the resulting portal flow diversion to the FLR induces a shift in liver volume and function to the FLR. Subsequent resection has been shown to be safer after portal vein embolization when applied appropriately based on volumetric criteria. Many centres perform iterative TACE followed by portal vein embolization, particularly for large right liver cancer, as this leads to excellent perioperative outcomes and evidence suggests better oncological outcomes than resection without TACE + portal vein embolization (emerging data).

Finally, surgical technique matters with liver cancer. Right lesions should be resected with an anterior approach (the liver is divided *in situ* without mobilization; then after complete separation of the liver and vessels, the tumourous liver is liberated from the hypochondrium) as prospective data reveal improved outcomes with this technique. Outcome from smaller resections is improved by portal-oriented resection versus simple wedge resection when liver function permits, as data from several series and meta-analyses demonstrate.

These examples reiterate that treatment of liver cancer does not easily conform to an algorithm – even defining 'resectable' has become more difficult, because it relates less to the size and number of tumours, and more to the condition of the patient and liver. Application of multidisciplinary assessment and management requires significant experience with liver cancer, in particular with resection of liver cancer.

Liver transplantation

Advanced cirrhosis often eliminates liver resection as an option for treatment of liver cancer. In such cases, liver transplantation can be considered, although only a very small fraction of all patients with liver cancer worldwide undergo liver transplantation. Indications for liver transplantation are guided by the seminal proposal of Bismuth, which was subsequently formalized by Mazzaferro *et al.*, to include patients with a solitary liver cancer of <5 cm or a maximum of three tumours, each <3 cm, without macroscopic vascular involvement or distant disease (see Box 22.1). These selection criteria, known as the *Milan criteria*, have resulted in 5-year survival rates of 71–75% in some centres and of about 60% in registry data from Europe and the USA.

The major advantages of liver transplantation include both treatment of underlying liver disease and complete removal of the 'field at risk' for development of *de novo* cancer. These advantages are counterbalanced by the 13% 1-year mortality rate in adults, the severe shortage of organ donors, and the cost and morbidity of life-long immunosuppression. Progression of liver cancer while waiting for a suitable donor organ can lead to 'drop-out' or loss of opportunity for transplantation; in fact, the rate of tumour progression is reported to be 15–33% in patients waiting for liver transplantation. Progression and drop-out while waiting worsen the outcomes of liver transplantation: the 2-year intention-to-treat survival rate is 84% for patients with 62 days of waiting time, but only 54% for patients with 162 days of waiting time. Recent intention-to-treat analyses of a large cohort of patients found 5-year survival rates of 47–62%, far below the 70% survival rates which are frequently quoted.

Expansion of the limits of the morphological selection criteria for liver transplantation has been considered, while some have suggested incorporating biological factors such as grading and genotyping. A detailed discussion of the pros and cons of these controversial approaches is beyond the scope of this chapter, but the encouraging results of early studies are balanced by the difficulties in identifying good prognosis tumours among patients with liver cancer beyond the Milan criteria.

Outcomes following liver transplantation for early liver cancer are excellent, yet have changed little since the standardized application of the Milan criteria for liver transplantation (see above). Mortality for liver transplantation remains an issue of concern, with some series initially reporting up to 22% 90-day mortality rates primarily related to immunosuppression-related complications, which have fallen closer to 2% in more modern series.

> **Box 22.1** Indications for liver transplantation
>
> - Cirrhotic patients with poor liver function who meet Milan criteria (single lesion ≤5 cm or two or three lesions of ≤3 cm)
> - Controversial:
>   - Patients beyond Milan criteria who fall into Milan after 'bridge therapy' such as TACE
>   - Patients with preserved liver function within Milan criteria (some recommend transplantation, others resection with reconsideration for transplantation after resection)
> - Under study:
>   - Extended indications (see text)
>   - Adjuvant sorafenib after transplantation

Locoregional therapies

Consideration for locoregional therapy is made in the setting of a multidisciplinary team which considers resection and transplantation as first options. When resection and transplantation are considered inappropriate, locoregional therapies may apply. Further, some locoregional therapies (specifically *in situ* ablation and TACE) may be used as part of a strategy to control tumours (bridge) to transplantation, to down-stage to transplantable status (still controversial) or in the case of TACE, as a step toward resection in some cases.

Locoregional therapies	Description

***In situ* ablation**	• *Indications*:
	  ▪ CP A, CP B
	  ▪ All lesions must be accessible (preferably, although not necessarily, percutaneously or laparoscopically) to ablation with a margin of normal tissue (except percutaneous alcohol ablation for very small lesions)
	  ▪ All lesions must be sufficiently far from major vascular, biliary and extrahepatic structures to permit complete ablation
	  ▪ Ideally tumours should be ≤3 cm
	  ▪ If 3–5 cm, consider TACE + ablation

(continued)

Locoregional therapies	Description

	• *Controversial*:
	  ■ CP C can be considered but ablation volumes should be small
	• Under study:
	  ■ Adjuvant sorafenib after RFA

Transarterial chemoembolization	• *Indications*:
	  ■ CP A and B
	  ■ All lesions accessible to arterially directed therapy without non-target embolization
	• *Contraindications*:
	  ■ Liver dysfunction/failure/death risk increases progressively from CP A to C. Thus, CP C rarely considered and if so, highly selective, small volume embolization
	  ■ Generally contraindicated with main portal vein thrombosis (although useful in patients with segmental thrombosis)
	  ■ Generally contraindicated when bilirubin >3 mg/dL (except very small, super-select TACE)
	  ■ ^{90}Y-microsphere radioembolization (discussed below) is generally contraindicated when bilirubin >2 mg/dL (increased risk for liver failure)
	• Under study:
	  ■ Current evidence reveals no benefit from adjuvant sorafenib after TACE, although new studies (concurrent sorafenib) are being considered

Ablative therapies

Advantages of ablative therapies are generally low morbidity and potential for percutaneous treatment. The major disadvantages of all ablation techniques are the difficulties with evaluating treatment margins and the need to obtain negative treatment margins in three dimensions and almost universal local recurrence. Ultimately, most agree that despite limitations of ablative strategies to completely destroy liver cancer, the effect in cirrhotic patients is to adequately control small tumours. These patients have a competing risk for death (liver failure), and ablation can safely control tumours without high risk for the development of liver failure. Certainly, when resection can be offered, it is a better oncological treatment than ablation, but if resection comes at the cost of liver failure, this better 'oncological' treatment comes at an unacceptable risk. Thus again, the treatments must respect the two problems in cirrhotic patients with liver cancer – liver disease and cancer.

Ablative therapies	Description
Percutaneous ethanol injection (PEI)	• Oldest, best-known and best-studied ablative therapy for liver cancer (and least expensive) • Injection of absolute ethanol via a fine needle under imaging guidance leads to cellular dehydration, necrosis and vascular thrombosis, causing tumour cell death • Essentially used exclusively for very small (<2 cm) liver cancer or those abutting vascular structures in locations contraindicating heat ablation (see below)

Radiofrequency ablation (RFA)	• Most utilized alternative mode of ablative therapy
	• Uses heat to destroy tumours: a needle electrode inserted into the tumour delivers a high-frequency alternating current, which generates rapid vibration of ions, frictional heat and, ultimately, coagulative necrosis
	• Similar efficacy for <2-cm liver cancer, but much better for tumours of 2–5 cm than PEI
	• Radiological complete ablation correlates with 70% local persistence in explant studies, yet clinical control rates are excellent as is overall survival
	• *Drawbacks*:
	  ■ Cost, higher rate of complications compared to PEI (0–12%), which can include pneumothorax, pleural effusion, haemorrhage, subcapsular haematoma, haemobilia, biliary stricture and liver abscess
	  ■ Treatment-related mortality rate of up to 1%

Microwave ablation	• Newer technology, similar limitations to RFA but slightly faster and with slightly more consistent ablation volumes • Future study will differentiate role for microwave versus RFA

Transarterial therapies

For liver cancer not amenable to RFA, liver resection or transplantation, especially when multifocal, transarterial therapies can be considered. This approach is attractive for liver cancer because of the preferential arterial blood supply to liver cancer, which enables delivery of anatomically targeted treatments while (theoretically) sparing hepatic parenchyma and thus allowing treatment with fewer hepatic and systemic side effects. TACE is also used as a modality to control (or perhaps to down-size) liver cancer for patients awaiting liver transplantation.

Three categories of intra-arterial therapies for liver cancer have been used. All involve delivery of intra-arterially targeted embolic and/or (chemo)therapeutic agents into the liver or selectively into hypervascular liver tumours: (1) bland embolic particles; (2) chemotherapy (as an infusion or more commonly with an embolic component); and, more recently, (3) radioactive particles.

Transarterial therapies	Description
Bland embolization	• Largely supplanted by TACE and DEB-TACE since Barcelona RCT (see below)
Transarterial chemoembolization (TACE)	• Traditionally chemotherapy mixed with the fatty carrier/embolic particle lipiodol which concentrates in tumoursEvidence does not point to a clear drug (cisplatin vs doxorubicin vs combination) as the ideal and this remains the choice of the treating physician • Select (tumour only) embolization is preferred over lobar or whole liver embolization • Angiographic endpoint remains the choice of the treating physician (drug is delivered and the artery terminally embolized with permanent material versus delivery of drug-bearing solution leaving continued arterial inflow or followed by placement of a temporary plug)
Transarterial chemoembolization with drug-eluting beads (DEB-TACE)	• Delivery of beads without occlusion of inflow vessels • High levels of drug delivered to tumours • Recently shown to be equal to traditional TACE but with fewer side effects and perhaps has advantage in poor liver disease patients
Radioembolization (^{90}Y-microspheres)	• Safe, low toxicity • High cost • Associated with special anatomical constraints (shunting to lung must be limited to avoid radiation toxicity to lungs) • May be option for patients with portal vein thrombosis • Specific indications await study but often the whole liver can be treated in a single setting with good tumour control • Can be performed in the outpatient setting (no post-embolization syndrome of fever, nausea and pain)

Radiotherapy

EBRT has emerging utility in the treatment of liver cancer, especially for liver cancer with portal tumour thrombus, and is established for the treatment of bone metastases. Whole-liver radiation is not effective for any liver disease and may be associated with radiation hepatitis. Newer methods using conformal, '4D' planning techniques and proton therapy are promising for tumour control, and radiation therapy can provide palliative, symptomatic relief in highly selected patients with liver cancer. Interest is increasing in selective internal radiation therapy or radioembolization (discussed above in the Transarterial therapies section).

Radiotherapy (EBRT)*	Description
Early	• Most lesions can be considered for EBRT using 3D conformal or stereotactic body radiotherapy techniques • EBRT is indicated when ablation or embolization are contraindicated or have failed • Generally, CP A but some CP B patients can be safely treated
Advanced non-metastatic	• EBRT for patients with portal vein thrombosis is increasingly used
Metastatic	• EBRT for symptomatic bone metastases

*Specific guidelines for treatment have not been established for radiotherapy for liver cancer. As little as 30 Gy and as much as ~90 Gy have been delivered depending on tumour location with acceptable toxicity and tumour control rates.

Box 22.2 Sorafenib

Sorafanib, an oral multikinase inhibitor, blocks tumour cell proliferation through an antiangiogenic effect derived from blockade of VEGF receptors 2 and 3, and blockade of platelet-derived growth factor-β.

Sorafenib is the first drug to be approved for treatment of advanced liver cancer, and despite its modest effect (extending survival by only a few weeks, typically without even a radiographic response; see SHARP trial in the Phase III clinical trials section), this advance has opened the door to a new treatment approach to liver cancer using molecularly targeted agents and other treatment combinations.

From a surgical perspective, there is interest in sorafenib as a post-treatment adjuvant therapy following TACE, RFA or resection; each is being assessed in an ongoing clinical trial.

There is some interest in an antiviral effect of sorafenib on HCV, but this remains to be confirmed.

Sorafenib leads to higher rates of progressive liver dysfunction in CP B cirrhotic patients than CP A patients, and generally should not be used when bilirubin is more than three times the upper limit of normal.

Systemic therapy

Systemic therapies remain difficult to deliver in patients with advanced liver disease, but advances in targeted therapies continue to open doors to new treatment approaches that could enable down-sizing pretreatment or adjuvant post-treatment systemic approaches to reduce risk for recurrence after definitive therapy (see Box 22.2). Many molecularly targeted agents are under study for liver cancer, although advances in systemic treatment for this disease continue to move slowly.

Systemic therapy	Description
Early	• No role

Advanced non-metastatic	• Sorafenib 400 mg by mouth twice daily until progression
	• Not part of established guidelines but often considered in high-volume centres:
	  ■ Highly selected cases of liver cancer with normal liver function may respond to systemic chemotherapy with doxorubicin alone or PIAF (platinum + interferon-α 2b + adriamycin [doxorubicin] + fluorouracil [FU]) immunochemotherapy, although treatment is toxic and response rates vary; a small proportion of cases will downsize to resectable (26% response rate, 8% complete pathological response)
	  ■ Fibrolamellar liver cancer may respond to 5-FU + interferon combination immunochemotherapy

Metastatic	• Sorafenib 400 mg by mouth twice daily until progression
	• Bone metastases can be palliated with EBRT when symptomatic
	• Not part of established guidelines but often considered in high-volume centres:
	  ■ Highly selected patients with preserved liver function: consider doxorubicin or PIAF as above
	  ■ Selected patients with fibrolamellar liver cancer: consider 5-FU and interferon

Treatment of fibrolamellar liver cancer

- Surgery is the mainstay of treatment: resection and transplantation
- Lymphadenectomy is mandatory (in stark contrast to conventional liver cancer)
- Surgery for nodal and lung metastases at diagnosis and at recurrence is of value
- May respond to 5-FU + interferon-α systemic chemotherapy (controversial)
- Survival following resection is up to 65%
- Survival following orthotopic liver transplantation is 50%

Controversies

Diagnosis and staging questions

Controversy remains regarding the role of biopsy in liver cancer. Advocates quote a very low needle tract seeding rate when the proper technique is used (<2%), low false-positive rate and potential to perform molecular studies on biopsy material. Critics site needle tract seeding and inhomogeneity of large tumours, i.e. tumours may contain regions of lower and higher grade which may be difficult to target separately and may lead to under- or over-assessment of the aggressiveness of the tumour. This has been a particular point of discussion with regard to incorporating grade into the transplant eligibility assessment.

The importance of the 2-cm size cut-off for staging has been raised by the Liver Cancer Study Group of Japan. Emerging data suggest that the T1 classification (solitary tumour of any size without vascular invasion) should also include solitary liver cancer ≤2 cm with or without vascular invasion because both have a favourable survival rate following resection. This may be addressed in future updates of the TNM staging system.

Locoregional therapy

Many controversies and questions surround locoregional therapy. Some are less critical, e.g. which chemotherapeutic agents or combinations should be used in TACE. Results are fairly similar around the world, although the utilization of DEBs has created significant interest because of evidence of similar efficacy but lower toxicity than with traditional TACE.

Also, among the embolic therapies is the emergence of radioembolization. This is similar to traditional TACE but utilizes particles embedded with yttrium-90. Selection for radioembolization continues to require evaluation by a multidisciplinary team of hepatologists, oncologists, surgeons and interventional radiologists. Of interest is the relatively low toxicity, potential to treat patient with significant tumour burden (often in a single setting rather than multiple sessions as for classic or DEB-TACE), and relatively limited side effects. The extremely high cost and certain anatomical constraints (pass-through of the radioactive material to the lung in some patients with shunting) limit the utility of the treatment. A specific role for radioembolization has not yet been defined, although yttrium-90 microsphere radioembolization is safe; its role is emerging as a suitable alternative to TACE, specifically for down-staging/bridging to transplantation or resection, for patients with portal vein thrombosis and those with advanced disease but preserved liver function. Absence of level I data for ^{90}Y-microsphere radioembolization compared to other regional therapies limits specific recommendations, although organizations such as the NCCN include it as an option in guidelines.

In situ ablation (RFA and microwave primarily) is debated as an alternative to resection in limited but resectable liver cancer. A few studies suggest superiority of ablation over resection with regard to outcome, primarily due to lesser negative impact on liver function. Recent meta-analysis of published data, however, revealed that resection is superior to ablation (specifically RFA) for treatment of liver cancer in comparable patients in terms of overall and disease-free survival, perhaps with similar overall survival for the subgroup with very small tumours (≤2 cm). Further study will clarify the role for resection versus RFA in patients who are candidates for both therapies. No controversy exists regarding ablation in patients unsuitable for laparotomy or liver resection because of co-morbidity or liver dysfunction. Finally, emerging data suggest that some patients may benefit from combined TACE + ablation versus ablation alone; the specific subgroup of patients who will benefit is not yet defined, although it is usually considered for larger tumours (3–5 cm).

Liver resection

Debate rages over resection versus transplantation of Milan criteria patients; however, this debate is largely theoretical because of the limited availability of donor organs for all patients in this category. Advocates of resection cite similar oncological outcomes in patients with preserved liver function who undergo resection and transplantation, as well as the discrepancy between organ supply and demand, problems associated with liver transplantation such as graft rejection, recurrent viral hepatitis, immunosuppression-related opportunistic infections, long-term medical complications, and the potential value of liver resection followed by 'salvage' transplantation for tumour recurrence or deterioration of the hepatic function or recurrence of liver cancer. Transplant advocates insist that disease-free survival is better with transplantation, focus on the beneficial effect of transplantation on cirrhosis and portal hypertension, as well as cancer and risk for degradation of liver function after resection.

Following from this debate is that concerning resection as a 'bridge' to transplantation. Currently, patients on transplant list can expect to wait >6 months to undergo 'bridge' therapy designed to prevent progression of liver cancer while awaiting transplantation. Following a report of resection as a bridge, controversy raged in the literature and at scientific meetings on this issue. Advocates of the resection bridge tout the advantage of avoiding immunosuppression, good disease control, uncommon recurrence outside transplant criteria and reasonable morbidity with subsequent good transplant outcomes. Critics suggest no benefit to resection before transplantation and increased morbidity of the transplant operation. Concern that recurrence after resection would be outside transplantable criteria is also expressed.

Open versus laparoscopic resection is an area of ongoing discussion. Laparoscopic liver resection is clearly safe, and some suggest that it may become a standard of care for liver cancer. Data are simply not sufficient to make a recommendation in this regard; thus open and laparoscopic approaches to resection can be considered valid alternatives for those with sufficient experience.

Liver transplantation

Currently, liver transplantation is the standard therapy for liver cancer within Milan criteria in patients with compromised liver function (CP B and C). Several groups have sought to expand the Milan criteria to include patients with larger or more numerous tumours, citing similar outcomes for selected patients within wider criteria groups (e.g. UCSF: single tumour of ≤6.5 cm, up to three tumours of ≤4.5 cm and cumulative tumour size of ≤8 cm; Pittsburgh: based on lymph node status, metastasis, vascular invasion, tumour size and bilaterality). Insufficient data exist to clarify which patients will benefit from transplantation beyond Milan criteria; thus, no international organization has adopted clear criteria outside Milan criteria except for in selected United Network for Organ Sharing (UNOS) regions as part of an effort to study the outcomes.

A second area of controversy is the criteria that should be used to select patients with liver cancer for living donor transplantation. Many groups advocate (and are) transplanting patients far beyond Milan criteria when a living donor is willing to provide an organ. This is criticized primarily because of the dual risk – for donor and recipient – and because of the risk without clearly defined benefit for patients often well beyond the Milan criteria. Post living-donor transplant management is also criticized. How should a living donor recipient be managed in the event of transplant-related complications such as primary organ dysfunction or acute rejection? Does this patient, not initially a transplant candidate, move to the top of the list and take a cadaveric organ ahead of another person legitimately on the list? This is a raging controversy.

Finally, regarding extended criteria, some patients downstage with bridge therapy (RFA, TACE, resection). Controversy exists with regard to placement of these patients on the waiting list for transplantation with some revised priority based on treated liver cancer.

In practice, liver resection and liver transplantation are complementary, not competing, treatments. Patients with preserved hepatic function are generally considered for liver resection as first-line treatment. Conversely, those with poor liver function and early liver cancers are eligible for liver transplantation. The problem of more advanced liver cancers arising in the setting of advanced cirrhosis remains unsolved by either liver resection or liver transplantation.

Phase III clinical trials

See Table 22.7.

Table 22.7 Phase III clinical trials

Trial name	Results
Local therapy	
TACE vs best supportive care (BSC) (Hong Kong) Lo et al. (2002) *Hepatology* 35(5):1164–1171	• TACE (cisplatin, lipiodol and gelatine sponge for unresectable liver cancer) repeated every 2–3 months until contraindication or progression • TACE improves survival for unresectable liver cancer despite risk for degradation in liver function (3-year overall survival for TACE 26% vs 3% for BSC) • TACE relative risk of death 0.49 (95% CI 0.29–0.81) vs BSC; $P = 0.006$ • More advanced disease than in following RCT of TACE vs. TAE from Barcelona
TACE vs TAE vs BSC (Barcelona Liver Cancer Group) Llovet et al. (2002) *Lancet* 359:1734–1739	• TACE (doxorubicin, lipiodol and gelatine sponge for unresectable liver cancer), repeated at Month 2, Month 6 and then every 6 months until contraindication or progression • TACE improves survival over best supportive care (BCS) (3-year OS TACE 29% vs 11% BSC) • TACE relative risk of death 0.45; 95% CI 0.25–0.81 vs BSC; $P = 0.02$
PRECISION V Lammer et al. (2010) *Cardiovasc Intervent Radiol* 33(1):41–52	• 212 patients with CP A/B cirrhosis and large/multinodular unresectable, non-metastatic liver cancer randomized to TACE (doxorubicin) or drug-eluting beads (DEB; doxorubicin) • Primary endpoint: EASL tumour response at 6 months • Overall, DEB was not superior ($P = 0.11$) to TACE in terms of complete response rate (27% vs 22%), objective response rate (52% vs 44%) or disease control rate (63% vs 52%) • In CP B, ECOG 1, bilobar disease and recurrent disease, DEB associated with superior objective response rate vs TACE ($P = 0.038$) • DEB was associated with significantly less liver toxicity ($P < 0.0001$) and a lower rate of doxorubicin-related toxicity ($P = 0.0001$)
Adjuvant systemic therapy	
TACE sorafenib Kudo et al. (2011) *Eur J Cancer* 47(14):2117–2127	• Adjuvant sorafenib initiated >9 weeks after TACE did not prolong time to progression (TTP) in patients who responded to TACE (median TTP with sorafenib 5.4 months vs placebo 3.7 months [HR 0.87; 95% CI 0.70–1.09; $P = 0.252$]) • HR (sorafenib/placebo) for overall survival was 1.06
Interferon-α 2b adjuvant post resection Chen et al. (2012) *Ann Surg* 255(1):8–17	• 53 weeks of adjuvant interferon-α 2b did not impact recurrence-free survival (RFS) post curative resection of viral hepatitis-related liver cancer (median RFS for interferon-α 2b was 42.2 months [95% CI 28.1–87.1] vs control 48.6 months [95% CI 25.5 to infinity]; $P = 0.828$, log-rank test)
Advanced disease and metastatic disease	
SHARP trial Llovet et al. (2008) *N Engl J Med* 359:378–390	• Sorafenib vs BCS for advanced liver cancer (70% macroscopic vascular invasion or extrahepatic disease or both) but >95% CP A and >90% ECOG performance status 0 or 1 • Median overall survival for sorafenib 10.7 months vs 7.9 months BSC (HR = 0.69; 95% CI 0.55–0.87; $P < .001$) • Time to progression was prolonged (5.5 months vs 2.8 months, respectively) • Side effects, including significant diarrhoea, hand-and-foot syndrome and fatigue, were not insignificant • Subset analysis suggested some greater benefit in hepatitis C patients compared to patients with other aetiologies of liver cancer

Trial name	Results
Asia-Pacific Sorafenib Study Cheng et al. (2009) Lancet Oncol 10(1):25–34	• Similar to SHARP except only Asian patients, of a younger median age and predominantly HBV-related liver cancer with symptoms and more advanced disease • Median overall survival for sorafenib 6.5 months vs 4.2 months for BSC (HR = 0.68; 95% CI 0.50–0.93; $P = 0.014$) • Notable compared to SHARP was lower survival in both arms but similar magnitude of benefit for sorafenib (2.8 months in SHARP, 2.3 months in Asia-Pacific)
Doxorubicin vs PIAF Yeo et al. (2005) J Natl Cancer Inst 97(20):1532–1538	• Patients with unresectable liver cancer • PIAF associated with double the RR (20.9% vs 10.5%), but no impact on survival (median survival for doxorubicin 6.83 months [95% CI 4.80–9.56] vs PIAF 8.67 months [95% CI 6.36–12.00]; $P = 0.83$) • 28% of PIAF patients down-staged to resectable cancer vs 12% with doxorubicin

Areas of research

- *Prevention*:
  - Hepatitis C vaccine
  - Improved therapies for chronic viral hepatitis
  - Develop therapies for non-viral hepatitis, especially NASH
  - Develop improved early screening tests
- *Treatment*:
  - Expanding surgical resection options with newer techniques (multistage resection, preoperative portal vein embolization, combined arterial and portal embolization pre-resection)
  - Expanding transplantation options with combined therapies and better disease assessment to allow transplantation for liver cancer beyond current criteria
  - Expanding intra-arterial therapies with new methods of chemotherapy delivery (DEBs) and delivery of intra-arterial radiotherapy (yttrium-90)
  - Refining radiotherapy and developing/discovering radio-sensitizers
  - Development of post-resection, post-embolization, post-transplantation adjuvant therapies (trials with sorafenib adjuvant therapy are ongoing)
  - Exploration of new systemic therapies, particularly targeted therapies with drugs like bevacizumab (anti-VEGF antibody) and erlotinib (epidermal growth factor receptor [EGFR]-targeted reversible tyrosine kinase inhibitor)
- *Staging, prognosis and other treatments*:
  - Tumour genetic profiling
  - Cancer stem cell markers
  - Circulating microRNA, DNA, cancer cells
  - Regulatory T-cell modulation and therapy

Recommended reading

Bruix J, Sherman M; American Association for the Study of Liver Diseases (2011) Management of hepatocellular carcinoma: An update. *Hepatology* 53(3):1020–1022.

Burak KW, Kneteman NM (2010) An evidence-based multidisciplinary approach to the management of hepatocellular carcinoma (liver cancer): the Alberta liver cancer algorithm. *Can J Gastroenterol* 24(11):643–650.

El-Serag HB (2011) Hepatocellular carcinoma. *N Engl J Med* 365:1118–1127.

Gordon-Weeks AN, Snaith A, Petrinic T, Friend PJ, Burls A, Silva MA (2011) Systematic review of outcome of downstaging hepatocellular cancer before liver transplantation in patients outside the Milan criteria. *Br J Surg* 98(9):1201–1208.

Han KH, Kudo M, Ye SL et al. (2011) Asian consensus workshop report: expert consensus guideline for the management of intermediate and advanced hepatocellular carcinoma in Asia. *Oncology* 81(Suppl 1):158–164.

HRSA/OPTN (United States Department of Health and Human Services, Health Resources and Services Administration/Organ Procurement and Transplantation Network) Policies. Available at http://optn.transplant.hrsa.gov/policiesAndBylaws/policies.asp

Huang J, Yan L, Cheng Z et al. (2010) A randomized trial comparing radiofrequency ablation and surgical resection for HCC conforming to the Milan Criteria. *Ann Surg* 252:903–912.

Jarnagin W, Chapman WC, Curley S et al. (2010) Surgical treatment of hepatocellular carcinoma: expert consensus statement. *HPB (Oxford)* 12(5):302–310.

Liu CL, Fan ST, Cheung ST et al. (2006) Anterior approach versus conventional approach right hepatic resection for large hepatocellular carcinoma. *Ann Surg* 244:194–203.

Mazzaferro V, Regalia E, Doci R et al. (1996) Liver transplantation for the treatment of small hepatocellular carcinomas in patients with cirrhosis. *N Engl J Med* 334(11):693–699.

Mazzaferro V, Bhoori S, Sposito C et al. (2011) Milan criteria in liver transplantation for hepatocellular carcinoma: an evidence-based analysis of 15 years of experience. *Liver Transpl* 17(Suppl 2):S44–57.

Minagawa M, Ikai I, Matsuyama Y, Yamaoka Y, Makuuchi M (2007) Staging of hepatocellular carcinoma assessment of the Japanese TNM and UICC/AJCC TNM Systems in a cohort of 13,772 patients in Japan. *Ann Surg* 245:909–922.

NCCN Clinical Practice Guidelines in Oncology, Hepatobiliary Cancers Version 1.2013. Available at http://www.nccn.org/professionals/physician_gls/pdf/hepatobiliary.pdf

Okuda K, Ohtsuki T, Obata H et al. (1985) Natural history of hepatocellular carcinoma and prognosis in relation to treatment. *Cancer* 56:918–928.

Pugh RNH, Murray-Lyon IM, Dawson JL, Pietroni MC, Williams R (1973) Transection of the oesophagus for bleeding oesophageal varices. *Br J Surg* 60(8):646–649.

Ribero D, Abdalla EK, Thomas MB, Vauthey JN (2006) Liver resection in the treatment of hepatocellular carcinoma. *Expert Rev Anticancer Ther* 6(4):567–579.

Schwarz RE, Abou-Alfa GK, Geschwind JF, Krishnan S, Salem R, Venook AP (2010) Nonoperative therapies for combined modality treatment of hepatocellular cancer: expert consensus statement. *HPB* 12:313–320.

The Cancer of the Liver Italian Program (CLIP) Investigators (1998) A new prognostic system for hepatocellular carcinoma: a retrospective study of 435 patients. *Hepatology* 28:751–755.

Vauthey JN, Lauwers GY, Esnaola NF *et al.* (2002) Simplified staging for hepatocellular carcinoma. *J Clin Oncol* 20(6):1527–1536.

Vauthey JN, Ribero D, Abdalla EK *et al.* (2007) Outcomes of liver transplantation in 490 patients with hepatocellular carcinoma: validation of a uniform staging after surgical treatment. *J Am Coll Surg* 204(5):1016–1027; discussion 1027–1028.

Vauthey JN, Dixon E, Abdalla EK *et al.* (2010) Pretreatment assessment of hepatocellular carcinoma: expert consensus statement. *HPB* 12:289–299.

Zhou Y, Xu D, Wu L, Li B. (2011) Meta analysis of anatomic resection versus nonanatomic resection for hepatocellular carcinoma. *Langenbecks Arch Surg* 396(7):1109–1117.

23.1 Biliary tract

Rory L. Smoot[1], Christopher L. Hallemeier[2], Robert R. McWilliams[3] and Mark J. Truty[1]

[1]Hepatobiliary and Pancreatic Surgery, Mayo Clinic, Rochester, MN, USA
[2]Radiation Oncology, Mayo Clinic, Rochester, MN, USA
[3]Medical Oncology, Mayo Clinic, Rochester, MN, USA

Summary	Key facts

Introduction	• *Incidence*:
	   ▪ Highly variable based on region
	   ▪ Highest incidence in Asian countries
	• *Epidemiology*:
	   ▪ Identified risk factors: inflammatory, infectious, exposure and precursor lesions

Presentation	• Obstructive jaundice and/or elevated liver enzymes most common:
	   ▪ Work-up includes CT scan of chest, abdomen, pelvis as well as biliary imaging with either MRCP or ERCP
	• Most cases are metastatic or locally advanced at the time of diagnosis:
	   ▪ Limited treatment options in advanced cases

Scenario	• Local treatment is surgical resection: ▪ Preoperative biliary drainage and/or preoperative portal vein embolization may be necessary • Locally-advanced perihilar tumours may be amenable to neoadjuvant chemoradiation and liver transplantation in highly selected individuals at specialized centres • Locally advanced distal tumours and metastatic distal and hilar tumours are treated with systemic chemotherapy if the patient's performance status allows

Trials	• ABC-02 trial; Valle *et al.* (2010) *N Engl J Med* 362(14):1273–1281:
	   ▪ Cisplatin and gemcitabine combination was superior to gemcitabine therapy alone in advanced biliary tract cancer
	• SWOG S0809; Ben-Josef *et al.* (2014) *J Clin Oncol* 32(5 Suppl):Abstract 4030:
	   ▪ Preliminary results of phase II single-arm trial demonstrated favourable outcomes with adjuvant capecitabine + gemcitabine followed by chemoradiation

Introduction

Cholangiocarcinoma can arise from the biliary epithelium anywhere within the biliary tract (Fig. 23.1.1). Extrahepatic cholangiocarcinoma refers to cancers arising near or from the main bifurcation (hilar cholangiocarcinoma) or within the common bile duct (distal cholangiocarcinoma) (Fig. 23.1.2). Klatskin tumour is a name that has in the past been used for hilar cholangiocarcinomas. Jaundice is the most common presenting sign, and most tumours are inoperable at the time of diagnosis; however, surgical resection offers the only chance for cure. Recent experience with neoadjuvant chemoradiation and liver transplantation for hilar cholangiocarcinoma has demonstrated encouraging results in highly selected individuals.

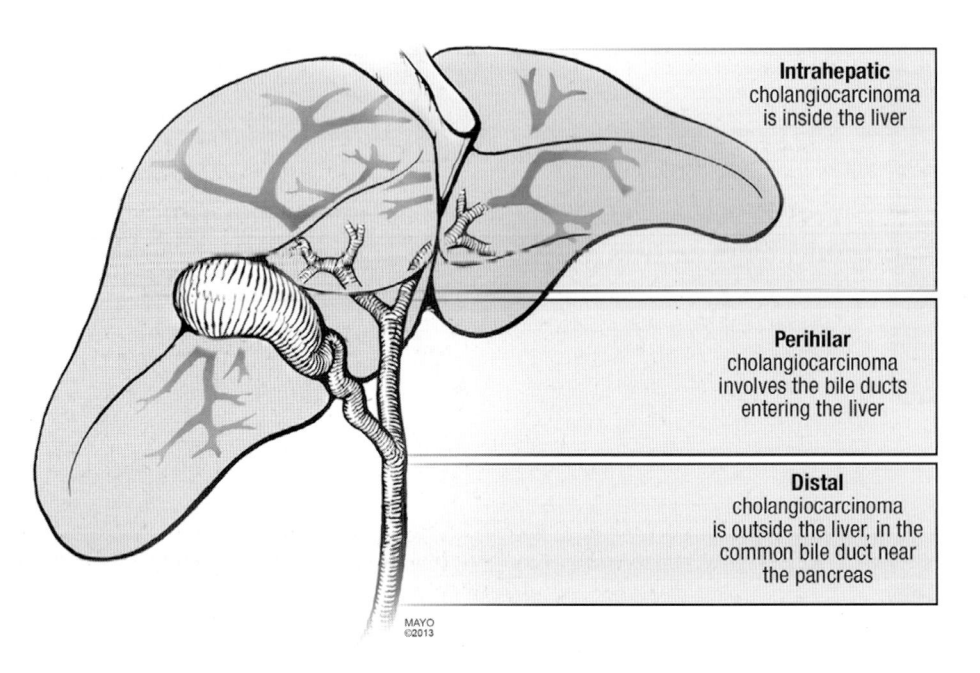

Figure 23.1.1 Locations of different types of cholangiocarcinoma.

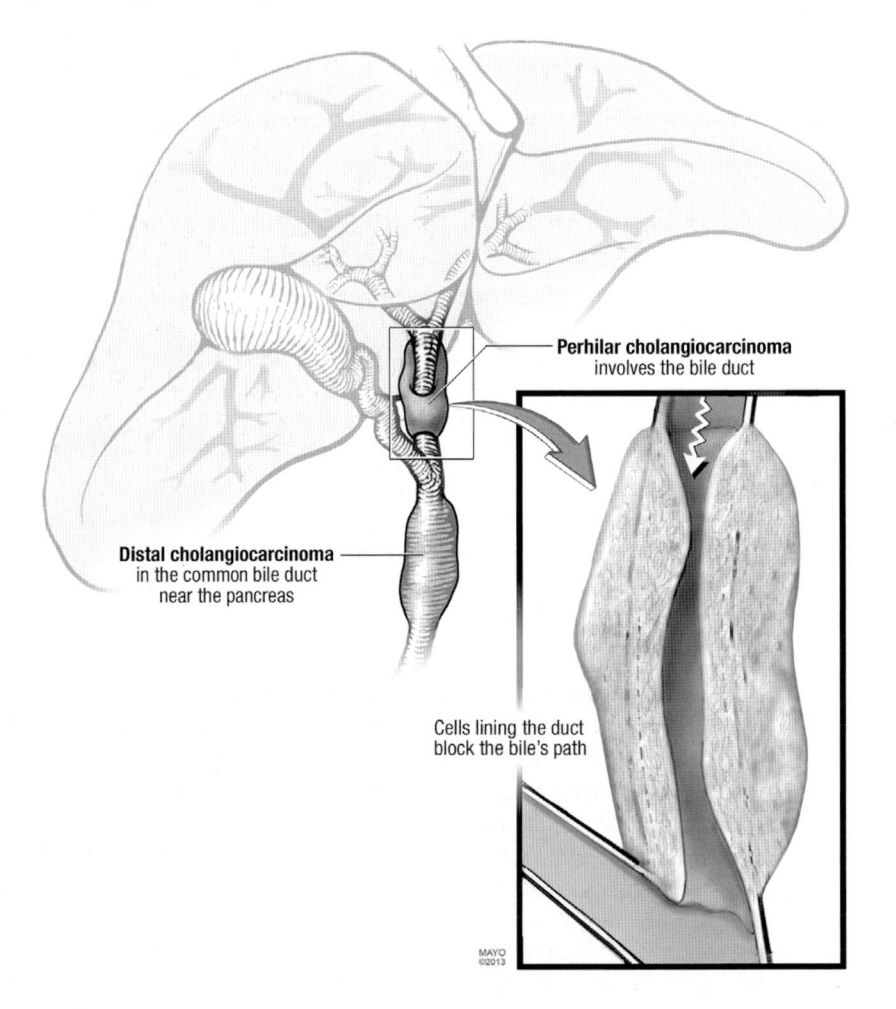

Figure 23.2.2 Hilar and distal cholangiocarcinoma.

Incidence, aetiology and screening

Incidence, aetiology and screening	Description
Incidence	- Significant regional variation - From 0.1 cases per 100,000 to >3 cases per 100,000

Aetiology	- *Inflammatory*:
	  - Primary sclerosing cholangitis (PSC)
	- *Infectious*:
	  - Recurrent pyogenic cholangitis (RPC)
	  - Chronic liver fluke infection
	- *Exposure*:
	  - Thorotrast contrast agent (no longer in use)
	- *Predisposing factors*:
	  - Choledochal cyst
	  - Biliary adenoma

Screening	- In the setting of known infections/inflammatory conditions (RPC, PSC):
	  - Consider US or MRI/MRCP every 6–12 months
	  - Consider CA19-9 every 6–12 months

Pathology

Cholangiocarcinomas are adenocarcinomas and have three main subtypes: sclerosing, nodular and papillary. Perineural and lymphovascular involvement and spread are common.

Pathology	Description
Sclerosing type	- Most common subtype: - More commonly hilar than distal - Infiltration and fibrosis are hallmarks - Overlap with nodular subtype
Nodular type	- Intraductal projection of tumour common (Fig. 23.1.3.) - Nodular growth pattern - Overlap with sclerosing subtype
Papillary type	- Least common subtype: - More commonly distal than hilar - Intraductal growth pattern - Better prognosis

Presentation

- Jaundice most common:
  - Acholic stools
  - Pruritus
- General malaise/weight loss
- Distal cholangiocarcinoma can present with pancreatitis
- Advanced cases can present with pain and/or gastric outlet obstruction

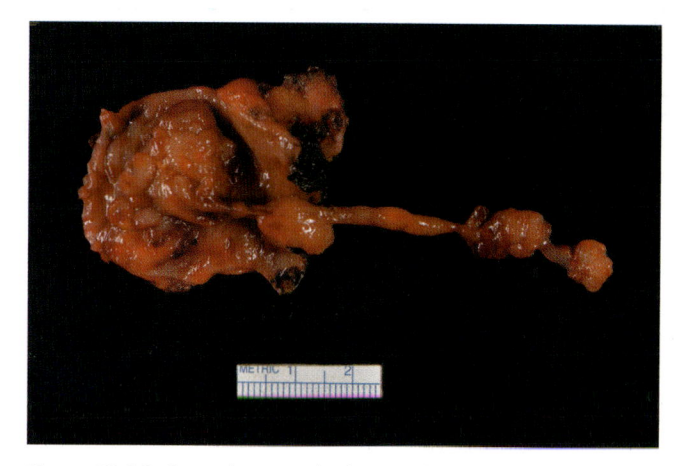

Figure 23.1.3 Gross photograph of resected mid-duct 'nodular' subtype with intraductal tumour extension.

Natural history

Less than half of patients with cholangiocarcinoma are resectable at the time of diagnosis secondary to metastases or vascular involvement at the liver hilum precluding resection.

Natural history		Description
Presentation	Local	- Hilar tumours typically present with jaundice and/or pruritus - Distal tumours may present with jaundice or pancreatitis - May be discovered secondary to work-up for elevated liver function tests or incidentally discovered mass on imaging
	Metastatic	- Metastatic tumours may present with pain and weight loss in addition to local symptoms
Routes of spread	Local	- Hilar tumours invade directly into the liver - Lymphovascular and perineural invasion/spread is common - Lymph node involvement and encasement of local vascular structures is common: - Encasement of vascular structures in hilar tumours can lead to occlusion and secondary hepatic atrophy
	Regional	- Lymph node involvement in the hepatoduodenal ligament (hilar tumours) and posterior pancreatic lymph nodes (distal) is common - Intrahepatic metastases from distal and hilar tumours
	Metastatic	- Liver - Lung - Peritoneum

Diagnostic work-up

Diagnostic work-up	Description
Work-up	Work-up likely initiated for elevated liver function tests or mass on imaging • MRI with MRCP (hilar tumours) to assess extent of biliary involvement • Percutaneous transhepatic cholangiography (PTC) with tube placement and brushings (hilar tumours): 　▪ Demonstrates upper extent of biliary tract involvement 　▪ Drain side of liver expected to be remain after resection 　▪ Takes the place of endoscopic retrograde cholangio-pancreatography (ERCP) for hilar tumours: 　　– ERCP often preferentially used in distal tumours • ERCP (distal tumours): 　▪ ERCP facilitates stenting and brushing for cytology in distal tumours and can be used for hilar tumours if MRCP and PTC unavailable • CT chest/abdomen/pelvis: 　▪ Assesses resectability/staging • Cytology often non-diagnostic from brushings • Percutaneous biopsy *not* recommended unless tissue diagnosis needed for chemotherapy in metastatic/palliative cases • Consider IgG subtypes to rule out IgG4 cholangiopathy
Tumour markers	CA19-9 (sialylated Lewis (a) antigen) 　▪ False negatives (10% non-secretors) 　▪ False positives (elevated with biliary obstruction/inflammation) 　▪ Not particularly useful for screening 　▪ Can assist in diagnosis but does have prognostic indications and elevation is associated with metastatic disease and early recurrence post resection 　▪ Useful in some cases for monitoring response and recurrence

Staging and prognostic grouping

UICC TNM staging

See Tables 23.1.1 and 23.1.2.

Table 23.1.1 Stage grouping and summary: Perihilar bile ducts and intrahepatic bile ducts

Stage grouping: Perihilar bile ducts			
Stage 0	Tis	N0	M0
Stage I	T1	N0	M0
Stage II	T2a, T2b	N0	M0
Stage IIIA	T3	N0	M0
Stage IIIB	T1, T2, T3	N1	M0
Stage IVA	T4	N0, N1	M0
Stage IVB	Any T	Any N	M1

Summary: Perihilar bile ducts	
T1	Ductal wall
T2a	Beyond ductal wall
T2b	Adjacent hepatic parenchyma
T3	Unilateral branches of portal vein or hepatic artery
T4	Main portal vein; bilateral branches; common hepatic artery; second-order biliary radicals bilaterally; unilateral second-order biliary radicals with contralateral portal vein or hepatic artery involvement
N1	Nodes along cystic duct, common bile duct, common hepatic artery, portal vein
M1	Distant metastasis

Stage grouping: Intrahepatic bile ducts			
Stage I	T1	N0	M0
Stage II	T2	N0	M0
Stage III	T3	N0	M0
Stage IVA	T4	N0	M0
Stage IVB	Any T	N1	M0
	Any T	Any N	M1

Summary: Intrahepatic bile ducts	
T1	Solitary without vascular invasion
T2a	Solitary with vascular invasion
T2b	Multiple
T3	Perforates visceral peritoneum or invades adjacent extrahepatic structures
T4	Periductal invasion
N1	Regional
M1	Distant metastasis

Table 23.1.2 UICC TNM categories and stage grouping: Gall bladder and cystic duct

TNM categories	
T1	Lamina propria or muscular layer
T1a	Lamina propria
T1b	Muscular layer
T2	Perimuscular connective tissue
T3	Serosa, one organ, and/or liver
T4	Portal vein, hepatic artery, or two or more extrahepatic organs
N1	Along cystic duct, common bile duct, common hepatic artery, portal vein

Stage grouping			
Stage 0	Tis	N0	M0
Stage I	T1	N0	M0
Stage II	T2	N0	M0
Stage IIIA	T3	N0	M0
Stage IIIB	T1, T2, T3	N1	M0
Stage IVA	T4	Any N	M0
Stage IVB	Any T	Any N	M1

TNM staging for hilar cholangiocarcinoma incorporates depth of invasion but also the extent of involvement of hilar structures (hepatic artery, portal vein and bile duct). The main determinant of prognosis is resectability (see Table 23.1.3) and preoperative staging systems have been suggested that have demonstrated the ability to predict resectability and thus correlate with median survival. Lymph node involvement portends a poor prognosis and patients with nodal metastases at the time of resection are Stage IIIb or higher (hilar) and Stage IIb or higher (distal).

Prognostic factors

See Table 23.1.3.

Table 23.1.3 Prognostic risk factors in biliary tract carcinoma

Prognostic factors	Tumour related	Host related	Environment related
Essential	Resectable	ECOG status	Residual disease (R0, R1, R2)
Additional	Lymph node metastases		
New and promising	*FGFR2* mutations		

Treatment philosophy

Scenario	Treatment philosophy

Local disease	• For resectable hilar tumours this entails extended hepatic resection with biliary reconstruction, and lymphadenectomy:
	  ▪ Preoperative drainage (PTC) is common, draining lobes of liver to remain
	  ▪ Preoperative portal vein embolization (PVE) is often necessary to facilitate hypertrophy of the liver remnant and thereby avoid postoperative liver insufficiency
	• For distal tumours this entails a pancreatico-duodenectomy (Whipple):
	  ▪ May require portal venous resection and reconstruction
	• Adjuvant therapy (chemotherapy and/or chemoradiation) can be considered for patients with R1 resection and/or node-positive disease

Regional disease	• For locally-advanced (unresectable) hilar tumours liver transplantation may be possible:
	  ▪ Specialized centres offer neoadjuvant chemoradiation followed by restaging and transplantation
	  ▪ Strict criteria for tumour size and work-up (*no* percutaneous biopsy)
	• For unresectable and untransplantable tumours the goal of care is symptom control:
	  ▪ Stenting biliary obstruction versus palliative surgical bypass (distal tumours)
	  ▪ Chemotherapy ± chemoradiation if ECOG status allows

Metastatic disease	• Goals of care are symptom control:
	  ▪ For hilar tumours: stenting versus PTC
	  ▪ For distal tumours: stenting versus palliative surgical bypass
	  ▪ Palliative chemotherapy if ECOG status allows
	  ▪ Palliative radiotherapy to sites of local or metastatic disease
	• Clinical trials as available

(continued)

Scenario	Treatment philosophy
Recurrent disease	• Recurrent disease is treated with chemotherapy and symptom control as possible
Follow-up	• Following surgical resection CT chest/abdomen/pelvis at regular intervals: ▪ Every 6 months for first 2 years

Treatment

Surgery

Surgery	Description

Early disease	• Hilar cholangiocarcinoma:
	    ▪ Extended hepatectomy with biliary reconstruction and lymphadenectomy:
	      – Preoperative biliary drainage is common with PTC draining lobe remaining following resection
	    ▪ Preoperative PVE is often necessary to facilitate hypertrophy of liver remnant to avoid postoperative liver insufficiency
	• Distal cholangiocarcinoma:
	    ▪ Whipple pancreatico-duodenectomy
	    ▪ ± Preoperative biliary stenting (ERCP)

Advanced non-metastatic disease	• Liver transplantation following neoadjuvant chemoradiation (hilar tumours) • For advanced distal tumours: palliative surgical bypass (hepatico- and gastro-jejunostomy) may be indicated
Metastatic disease	• No surgical options in hilar tumours • For advanced distal tumours: palliative surgical bypass (hepatico- and gastro-jejunostomy) may be indicated

Radiotherapy

Radiotherapy	Description
Early disease	• Adjuvant chemoradiation may be considered, particularly for patients with R1 margins or lymph node-positive disease: ▪ 50.4–54 Gy, with concurrent 5-fluorouracil (5-FU)–capecitabine/gemcitabine

Advanced non-metastatic disease	• Neoadjuvant chemoradiation as part of the liver transplantation protocol (Mayo Clinic regimen):
	    ▪ 45 Gy external beam
	    ▪ Brachytherapy boost
	• Chemoradiation may be considered

Metastatic disease	• Palliative radiotherapy to sites of local or metastatic disease

Systemic therapy

Systemic therapy	Description
Early disease	• Adjuvant chemotherapy alone or chemoradiotherapy may be considered, particularly for patients with R1 margins or lymph node-positive disease • No standard adjuvant chemotherapy regimen

Advanced non-metastatic disease	Gemcitabine + cisplatin regimen:
	    ▪ Based on ABC-02 trial data:
	      – Cisplatin 25 mg/m^2 and gemcitabine 1000 mg/m^2 on Days 1 and 8, every 3 weeks

Metastatic disease	Gemcitabine + cisplatin regimen:
	    ▪ Based on ABC-02 trial data:
	      – Cisplatin 25 mg/m^2 and gemcitabine 1000 mg/m^2 on Days 1 and 8, every 3 weeks

Controversies

The controversies in the treatment for cholangiocarcinoma concern preoperative biliary drainage. Studies have demonstrated increased episodes of sepsis and postoperative complications with preoperative biliary drainage; however, other studies have found no increase in these complications. Symptomatic patients (cholangitis, pruritus, malabsorption) are likely to benefit from preoperative biliary drainage; however, this decision should be individualized for each patient.

For local disease treated with surgical resection, the role of adjuvant therapy (chemotherapy and/or chemoradiation) and optimal regimens remain undefined. Additionally, the use of liver transplantation for locally-advanced hilar cholangiocarcinoma has met with controversy. Initial attempts at liver transplantation for hilar cholangiocarcinoma were met with unacceptably high recurrence rates. Contemporary protocols for neoadjuvant chemoradiation in highly selected patients have demonstrated good results and locally-advanced cholangiocarcinoma is considered an indication for liver transplantation at centres with these protocols in place. The lack of randomized data for resectable patients has also precluded consensus on neoadjuvant or adjuvant therapy. Some practitioners are extrapolating data from pancreas adenocarcinoma therapy, while others utilize gemcitabine and cisplatin in this role. Until randomized data are generated to determine a standard of care, there will continue to be inconsistency in the management of these patients at high risk for recurrence.

Phase III clinical trials

See Table 23.1.4.

Table 23.1.4 Phase III clinical trials

Trial name	Results
Local disease	
	• No reported phase III trials in resectable disease
Advanced disease and metastatic disease	
ABC-02 Valle et al. (2010) N Engl J Med 362(14):1273–1281	• Cisplatin + gemcitabine regimen associated with increased overall and progression-free survival as compared to gemcitabine alone
Lee et al. (2012) Lancet Oncol 13(2):181–188	• Addition of erlotinib to the gemcitabine + oxaliplatin regimen did not increase overall survival: ▪ Subgroup analysis of patients with cholangiocarcinoma demonstrated increased progression-free survival with addition of erlotinib

Areas of research

Areas of research in cholangiocarcinoma focus on chemotherapy options. Molecular studies examining the role of inflammation and cell death mechanisms in this tumour type are attempting to elucidate new targets for therapy. For instance, the recent identification of fusions in *FGFR2* in cholangiocarcinoma may be promising for the identification of a molecular subgroup of patients for therapy with FGF inhibitors.

Recommended reading

Ben-Josef E, Guthrie K, El-Khoueiry A, Corless C, Zalupski M (2014) SWOG S0809: A phase II trial of adjuvant capecitabine (cap)/gemcitabine (gem) followed by concurrent capecitabine and radiotherapy in extrahepatic cholangiocarcinoma (EHCC) and gallbladder carcinoma (GBCA). *J Clin Oncol* 32(5 Suppl):Abstract 4030.

Bragazzi MC, Cardinale V, Carpino G et al. (2012) Cholangiocarcinoma: epidemiology and risk factors. *Transl Gastrointest Cancer* 1:21–32.

Darwish Murad S, Kim WR, Harnois DM et al. (2012) Efficacy of neoadjuvant chemoradiation followed by liver transplantation for perihilar cholangiocarcinoma at 12 US centers. *Gastroenterology* 143(1):88–98.

Hochwald SN, Burke EC, Jarnagin WR, Fong Y, Blumgart LH (1999) Association of preoperative biliary stenting with increased postoperative infectious complications in proximal cholangiocarcinoma. *Arch Surg* 134(3):261–266.

Jarnagin, WR, Fong Y, DeMatteo RP, Gonen M et al. (2001) Staging, resectability, and outcome in 225 patients with hilar cholangiocarcinoma. *Ann Surg* 234(4):507–517.

Khan SA, Davidson BR, Goldin RD et al. (2012) Guidelines for the diagnosis and treatment of cholangiocarcinoma: an update. *Gut* 61:1657–1669.

Lee J, Park SH, Chang HM et al. (2012) Gemcitabine and oxaliplatin with or without erlotinib in advanced biliary tract cancer: a multicentre, open-label, randomized, phase 3 study. *Lancet Oncol* 13(2):181–188.

Nuzzo G, Guiliante F, Ardito F et al. (2012) Improvement in perioperative and longterm outcome after surgical treatment of hilar cholangiocarcinoma. *Arch Surg* 147(1):26–34.

Rea DJ, Munoz-Juarez M, Farnell MB et al. (2004) Major hepatic resection for hilar cholangiocarcinoma: analysis of 46 patients. *Arch Surg* 139(5):514–523.

Valle J, Wasan H, Palmer DH et al. (2010) Cisplatin plus gemcitabine versus gemcitabine for biliary tract cancer. *N Engl J Med* 362(14):1273–1281.

Wang Q, Gurusamy KS, Lin H, Xie X, Wang C (2008) Preoperative biliary drainage for obstructive jaundice. *Cochrane Database Syst Rev* (3):CD005444.

23.2 Pancreas

Rory L. Smoot[1], Christopher L. Hallemeier[2], Robert R. McWilliams[3] and Mark J. Truty[1]

[1]Hepatobiliary and Pancreatic Surgery, Mayo Clinic, Rochester, MN, USA
[2]Radiation Oncology, Mayo Clinic, Rochester, MN, USA
[3]Medical Oncology, Mayo Clinic, Rochester, MN, USA

Summary	Key facts

Introduction	- *Incidence*:
	  - Variable based on region
	  - Highest incidence in developed countries
	- Mortality rates are essentially similar regardless of region as survival rates for pancreatic carcinoma are very low
	- *Epidemiology*:
	  - Identified risk factors: smoking, hereditary pancreatitis, genetic predisposition

Presentation	- Obstructive jaundice and weight loss most common, hyperglycaemia - Most cases are metastatic or locally advanced/unresectable at the time of diagnosis: - Work-up includes cross-sectional imaging to assess for metastatic disease (chest/abdomen/pelvis) ± biliary drainage and/or biopsy confirmation
Scenario	- Local disease treatment is surgical resection in fit patients - Following surgical resection, adjuvant chemotherapy prolongs survival - Unresectable tumours (borderline/locally advanced) may be amenable to resection following neoadjuvant chemotherapy ± chemoradiation in selected individuals - Metastatic cancers are treated with systemic chemotherapy if the patient's performance status allows

Trials	- PRODIGE 4/ACCORD 11; Conroy *et al.* (2011) *N Engl J Med* 13(2):181–188:
	  - Combination chemotherapy (FOLFIRINOX) as compared with gemcitabine as first-line therapy in patients with metastatic pancreatic cancer resulted in significantly improved overall survival, progression-free survival and response rates
	- MPACT; Von Hoff *et al.* (2013) *N Engl J Med* 369(18):1691–1703:
	  - In patients with metastatic pancreatic adenocarcinoma, nab-paclitaxel + gemcitabine significantly improved overall survival, progression-free survival and response rates compared to gemcitabine alone
	- ECOG 4201 (under-accrued); Loehrer *et al.* (2008) *J Clin Oncol* 26:214s:
	  - In patients with localized but unresectable pancreatic adenocarcinoma, gemcitabine + radiotherapy compared to gemcitabine alone resulted in improved survival but increased toxicity
	- CONKO-001; Oettle *et al.* (2013) *JAMA* 310(14):1473–1481:
	  - Use of adjuvant post-resection gemcitabine for 6 months compared with observation alone resulted in increased overall and disease-free survival
	- ESPAC-1; Neoptolemos *et al.* (2004) *N Engl J Med* 350(12):1200–1210:
	  - Adjuvant fluorouracil had a significant survival benefit in patients with resected pancreatic cancer

UICC Manual of Clinical Oncology, Ninth Edition. Edited by Brian O'Sullivan, James D. Brierley, Anil K. D'Cruz, Martin F. Fey, Raphael Pollock, Jan B. Vermorken and Shao Hui Huang. © 2015 UICC. Published 2015 by John Wiley & Sons, Ltd.

Introduction

Pancreatic tumours are classified according to their cell type of origin, structure and behaviour. The exocrine pancreas is comprised of ductular and acinar cells that secrete enzymatic fluids needed for digestion. The majority of exocrine pancreatic cancers are adenocarcinomas and account for >90% of all pancreatic malignancies. Pancreatic ductal adenocarcinoma (PDAC) is an invasive epithelial gland-forming malignancy with at least focal ductal differentiation with a characteristic intense desmoplastic stromal reaction (Fig. 23.2.1). Although most commonly arising in the pancreatic head (two-thirds of cases), these adenocarcinomas also arise in the neck, body and tail of the pancreas, and also diffusely involve the entire gland. Jaundice and weight loss are the most common presenting signs, and most tumours are metastatic at the time of diagnosis. In those with clinically apparent localized disease, surgical resection offers the only chance for long-term survival. However, distant recurrence is common post resection; thus, most patients are likely systemically micrometastatic upon presentation and this correlates with tumour size, biomarker level (CA19-9) and cancer-associated symptoms (i.e. pain, cachexia, etc.) (Fig. 23.2.2). Newer systemic regimens have shown significantly improved response rates but with higher toxicity profiles. Recent experience with preoperative therapy (neoadjuvant) has shown encouraging results in those with initial clinically non-metastatic disease.

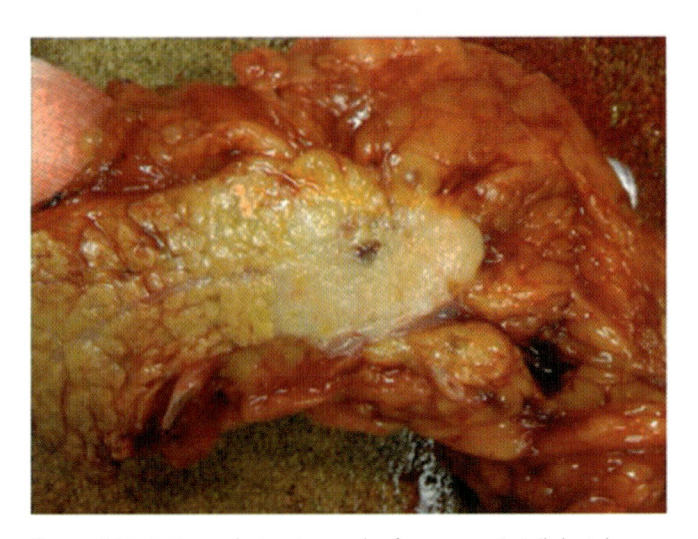

Figure 23.2.1 Gross photomicograph of a pancreatic tail ductal adenocarcinoma.

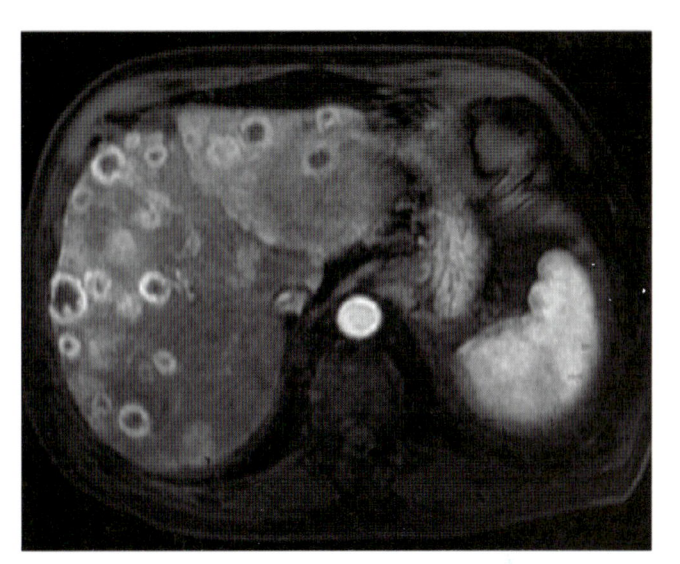

Figure 23.2.2 Computed tomography of a patient 3 months a seemingly curative resection for diffuse liver metastases.

Incidence, aetiology and screening

Incidence, aetiology and screening	Description
Incidence	• Rates for new PDAC cases have not changed significantly between 2002 and 2011: 　▪ Incidence: 　　○ Age-standardized ratio (ASR) per 100,000 for women 10.9 　　○ ASR per 100,000 for men 14.0 　▪ 1.5% lifetime risk in absence of other risk factors • Death rate: 　▪ ASR per 100,000 for women 9.6 　▪ ASR per 100,000 for men 12.5 　▪ Rising on average by 0.4% each year • Geographical variation: 　▪ PDAC is a disease of developed countries with highest incidence in the Americas and Europe, and lowest in North Africa and South Asia 　▪ In the USA, PDAC has the 12th highest incidence of all cancers, but is the third leading cause of cancer death 　▪ Despite variable incidence, survival is uniformly low

Incidence, aetiology and screening	Description

Aetiology	- *Host factors*:
	  - Age: PDAC is most frequently diagnosed among people aged 60–80 years (80%); rare before 40 years
	  - Gender: male-to-female incidence ratio 1.3
	- *Genetic factors*:
	  - Germline mutations: BRCA 2, BRCA 1, CDKN2A, mismatch repair genes,
	  - Polymorphisms: ABO gene – non-O blood type
	  - Cancer syndromes: familial melanoma, hereditary pancreatitis, familial adenomatous polyposis, Lynch syndrome (hereditary non-polyposis colorectal cancer [HNPCC]), Peutz–Jeghers, ataxia telangiectasia
	  - Family history: two or more affected first-degree relatives (unrelated to cancer syndromes)
	  - Hereditary pancreatitis: 50-fold increased risk
	- Exposures: tobacco, organochlorine, cadmium
	- Predisposing conditions: diabetes, chronic pancreatitis
	- Excessive alcohol intake
	- Nutritional factors (possible): high red meat/saturated fat intake, low fruit/vegetable intake, cooking methods, dietary carcinogens
	- Obesity and lack of physical activity
	- Precursor lesions:
	  - Intraductal papillary mucinous tumours (IPMN)
	  - Pancreatic intraepithelial neoplasia (PanIN)
	  - Mucinous cystic neoplasm (MCN)

Screening	- No effective role for screening in asymptomatic patients without significant risk factors
	- Consider screening in high-risk individuals:
	  - Individuals affected by hereditary pancreatitis
	  - Verified germline mutation carrier or those with high-risk syndromes
	  - Significant family history (two or more affected first-degree relatives)
	  - Presence of precursor lesions (PanIN, IPMN, MCN) with high-risk features
	  - Consider endoscopic ultrasound (EUS)/computed tomography (CT)/magnetic resonance imaging (MRI)

Pathology

PDAC arises from and is phenotypically similar to pancreatic duct epithelia, with mucin production and expression of a characteristic cytokeratin pattern. Adenosquamous, undifferentiated (anaplastic) carcinoma, mucinous non-cystic, signet ring cell carcinoma and mixed ductal/endocrine carcinoma are considered histological variants (subtypes) of ductal adenocarcinoma because most of these carcinomas contain some foci showing neoplastic glands with ductal differentiation.

Pathology	Description
Adenocarcinoma	- Ductal adenocarcinoma is the most common subtype - Well-to-moderately differentiated and characterized by well-developed glandular structures that recapitulate normal pancreatic ductal elements embedded in highly desmoplastic stroma, accounting for their firm consistency
Adenosquamous carcinoma	- Rare subtype characterized by the presence of mucin-producing glandular elements and squamous components (at least 30%), and anaplastic and spindle cell foci - More aggressive than adenocarcinoma with associated worse survival even in localized resectable cases
Undifferentiated (anaplastic) carcinoma	- Also referred to as giant cell carcinoma, pleomorphic large cell carcinoma and sarcomatoid carcinoma - Composed of large eosinophilic pleomorphic and/or spindle cells in poorly cohesive formations with scanty fibrous stroma with small foci of atypical glandular elements - High mitotic activity as well as perineural, lymphatic and blood vessel invasion is found in almost all cases and the prognosis of undifferentiated carcinoma is worse than that of poorly differentiated ductal adenocarcinoma of the pancreas - Presence of osteoclast-like giant cells might have a more favourable prognosis

Pathology	Description
Mucinous non-cystic carcinoma	• Also referred to as colloid or gelatinous carcinoma • Very uncommon carcinoma marked by large pools of mucin account for >50% of these tumours • Not to be confused with mucinous cystic carcinomas that have a significantly improved prognosis
Signet ring cell carcinoma	• Extremely rare adenocarcinoma composed almost exclusively of mucin-filled cells with extremely poor prognosis regardless of therapy • Gastric cancer should be excluded before making this diagnosis
Mixed ductal-endocrine carcinoma	• Characterized by a mixture of ductal and endocrine cells (at least one-third) • Exceptionally rare but these mixed carcinomas behave like typical ductal adenocarcinomas

Presentation

- Dependent on tumour location and stage
- Painless jaundice, acholic stools, pruritis, weight loss, abdominal/back pain, malaise
- Advanced cases can present with gastric outlet obstruction or ascites
- 70% of cases have a diabetes history of <2 years
- Acute pancreatitis, migratory thrombophlebitis, hypoglycaemia and hypercalcaemia are other less typical presentations

Natural history

Approximately 50% of all patients with pancreatic adenocarcinoma present with distant metastasis at diagnosis. Only 15–20% have tumours localized to the pancreas radiographically and considered anatomically potentially resectable.

Natural history		Description
Presentation	Local	• Head tumours typically with painless jaundice • Localized body/tail tumours are often incidentally identified on imaging for other indications as these are typically silent while still localized • Abdominal pain/bloating or back pain are common symptoms
	Metastatic	• May present with pain, unexplained weight loss in addition to local symptoms
Routes of spread	Local	• Carcinomas of the head of the pancreas usually invade the bile duct and/or pancreatic duct, resulting in stenosis and proximal dilatation of both duct systems • Extrapancreatic tumour invasion is common with involvement and/or encasement of local vascular structures, perineural sheaths, retroperitoneal tissues and gastroduodenal invasion

	Regional	• Lymphatic spread of pancreatic carcinomas depends on tumour location with head tumours typically involving the superior/inferior and anterior/posterior pancreatico-duodenal nodal basins:
		  ▪ Hepatoduodenal, common hepatic, coeliac trunk, mesenteric and para-aortic nodes involved with more distant nodal metastases
		• Carcinomas of the body and tail typically are found in the superior/inferior pancreatic body/tail and splenic hilus lymph node basins:
		  ▪ Some proximal tumours found in coeliac, mesenteric root and para-aortic basins
		• Cancer cells may also spread via lymphatic channels to the pleura and lung

	Metastatic	• Liver • Lung • Peritoneum • Bone • Brain

Diagnostic work-up

Diagnostic work-up	Description

Work-up	• Initiated for jaundice, mass on imaging or clinical suspicion:
	  ▪ Thorough history and physical examination
	  ▪ Assessment of performance and nutritional status
	  ▪ Review of anatomical, biological and conditional resectability criteria to determine treatment sequencing (Fig. 23.2.3)
	• Contrast-enhanced multiphasic CT and/or MRI:
	  ▪ Identification of distant metastases, peritoneal carcinomatosis/ascites and locoregional tumour/vascular involvement
	• EUS ± fine needle aspiration (FNA) cytology of mass
	• Endoscopic retrograde cholangiography for biliary stenting and cytological brushings
	• Consider IgG subtypes to rule out IgG4 autoimmune pancreatitis

Tumour markers	• CA19-9 (sialylated Lewis (a) antigen):
	  ▪ False negatives (10% non-secretors)
	  ▪ False positives (elevated with biliary obstruction/inflammation)
	  ▪ Not particularly useful for screening:
	    ○ Can assist in diagnosis
	  ▪ Has prognostic indications: elevation associated with metastatic disease and early recurrence post resection
	  ▪ Useful in some cases for monitoring response and recurrence
	• Carcinoembryonic antigen (CEA), CA125:
	  ▪ Addition of these biomarkers to CA19-9 may improve diagnostic accuracy; however, typically only elevated in advanced cases

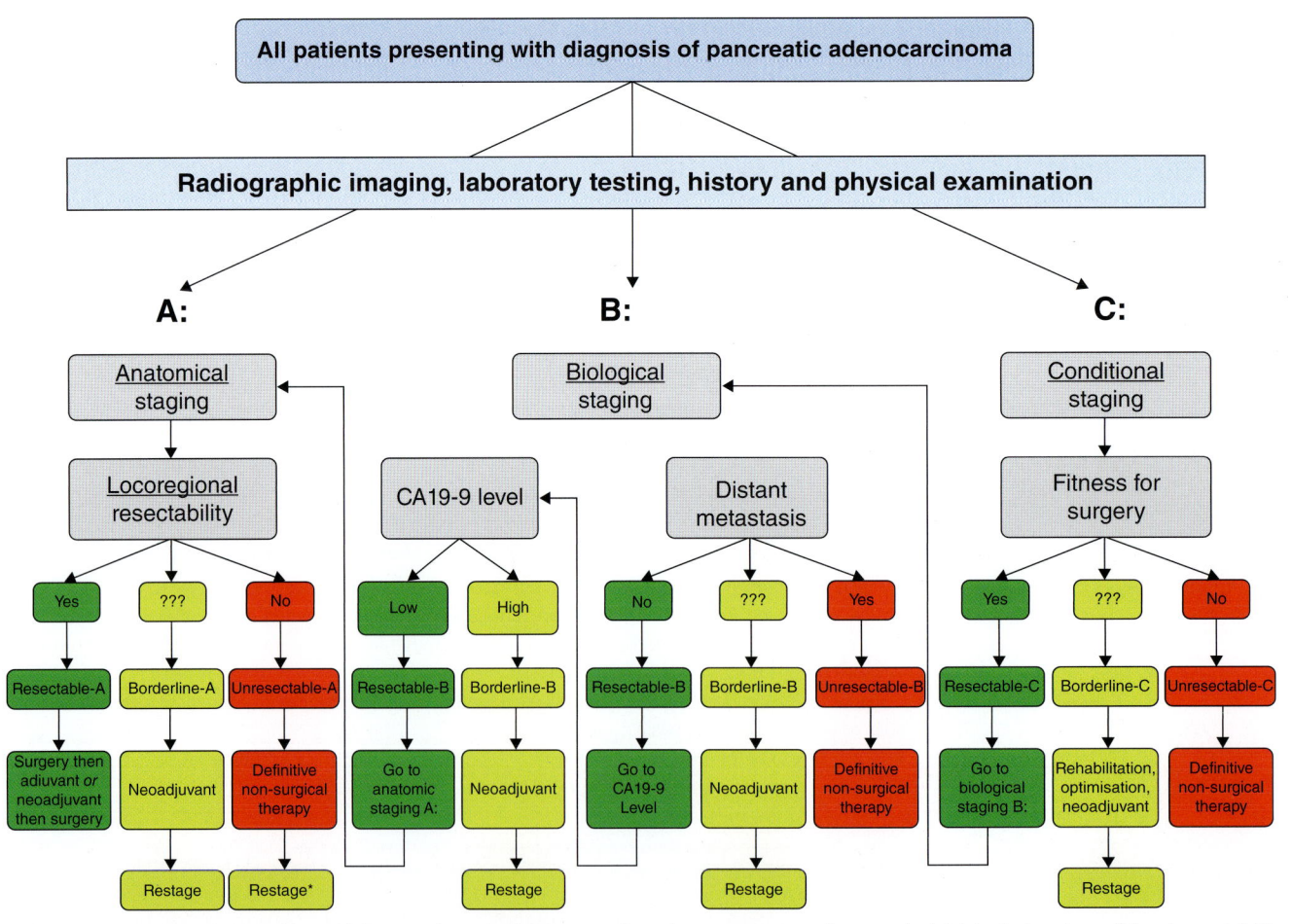

Figure 23.2.3 Proposed treatment guidelines and sequencing strategy based on assessment of anatomical, biological and conditional resectability criteria.*

*Some patients with locally advanced unresectable tumors on anatomical staging may be downstaged to potentially resectable with modern neoadjuvant therapies.

Staging and prognostic factors

UICC TNM staging
TNM staging for PDAC incorporates tumour size, regional lymph node metastases and distant metastases (Table 23.2.1).

Table 23.2.1 UICC TNM categories and stage grouping: Pancreas

TNM categories	
T1	Limited to pancreas ≤2 cm
T2	Limited to pancreas >2 cm
T3	Beyond pancreas
T4	Coeliac axis or superior mesenteric artery
N1	Regional

Stage grouping			
Stage 0	Tis	N0	M0
Stage IA	T1	N0	M0
Stage IB	T2	N0	M0
Stage IIA	T3	N0	M0
Stage IIB	T1, T2, T3	N1	M0
Stage III	T4	Any N	M0
Stage IV	Any T	Any N	M1

Prognostic factors
The main determinant of prognosis is absence of distant disease and anatomical resectability (Table 23.2.2).

Table 23.2.2 Prognostic risk factors for pancreatic cancer

Prognostic factors	Tumour related	Host related	Environment related
Essential	Distant metastases	ECOG status	Post-resection residual disease or margin status (R0, R1, R2)
Additional	Lymph node metastases CA19-9 level	Postoperative morbidity	Adjuvant therapy
New and promising	hENT1 expression	Modified Glasgow prognostic score (C-reactive protein [CRP] and albumin) Neutrophil-to-lymphocyte ratio (NLR)	Pathological response to neoadjuvant therapy

Treatment philosophy

Scenario	Treatment philosophy
Localized disease	• For localized head/uncinate tumours: pancreatico-duodenectomy is recommended in fit patients: 　▪ Preoperative biliary drainage via an endoscopic stent if resection is delayed 　▪ May require portal/superior mesenteric vein (SMV) venous resection and reconstruction 　▪ Patients must have adequate performance status • For localized body/tail tumours: distal pancreatectomy is recommended • Postoperative adjuvant systemic therapy ± external beam radiation • Neoadjuvant therapy for otherwise localized resectable tumours is institutionally dependent • Clinical trials as available
Borderline/locally advanced disease	• For anatomically borderline/locally-advanced tumours, resection may be possible: 　▪ Specialized centres offer neoadjuvant therapy followed by restaging and subsequent resection 　▪ High likelihood of vascular resection/reconstruction • For locally unresectable tumours: 　▪ Goal is treatment of occult systemic disease and subsequent locoregional tumour/symptom control 　▪ Durable endoscopic or surgical palliation of biliary and/or gastric outlet obstruction 　▪ Systemic chemotherapy and locoregional chemoradiation • Clinical trials as available
Metastatic disease	• Goals of care are palliative: 　▪ Adequate biliary/gastrointestinal stenting versus surgical bypass 　▪ Palliative chemotherapy if ECOG status allows • Clinical trials as available

(continued)

Scenario	Treatment philosophy
Recurrent disease	- Treated with chemotherapy and symptom control as possible - Locoregional therapy possible for select patients with isolated recurrences: - In general, re-resection of recurrences does not improve survival - Clinical trials as available
Follow-up	- Following surgical resection, cross-sectional imaging (CT and/or MRI) of chest/abdomen/pelvis at regular intervals: - Every 6 months - CA19-9 (in secretors)

Treatment

Surgery

Surgery	Description

Early disease	- Head tumours:
	  - ± Preoperative biliary drainage
	  - Pancreatico-duodenectomy (Whipple)
	  - ± Venous resection
	  - Regional lymphadenectomy
	- Body/tail tumours:
	  - Distal pancreatectomy/splenectomy
	  - Regional lymphadenectomy
	- Total pancreatectomy when necessary for adequate margins
	- Diagnostic laparoscopy prior to formal exploration for identification of radiographically occult metastasis
	- Postoperative adjuvant systemic therapy
	- Neoadjuvant therapy for otherwise localized resectable tumours is institutionally dependent
	- Clinical trials as available

Advanced non-metastatic disease	- Neoadjuvant strategy for possible surgical down-staging in select patients - Induction systemic chemotherapy ± chemoradiation - Highly selective utilization of various forms of radical pancreatic resection ± complex vascular resection for negative margins - Clinical trials as available
Metastatic disease	- No oncological benefit from palliative resection for metastatic cases

Radiotherapy

Radiotherapy	Description

Early disease	Adjuvant chemoradiation:
	- Controversial, but considered with R1 margins or positive lymph nodes following resection (Hopkins Hospital–Mayo Clinic collaborative study)
	- Total dose and fractionation varies by institution:
	  - Clinical target volume (CTV) is typically the tumour bed, any possible microscopic residual disease and high-risk peripancreatic nodes (coeliac, superior mesenteric, porta hepatis and para-aortic nodes may also be included)
	  - Typical doses are 45–54 Gy in 1.8-Gy fractions
	- Various radiosensitizers (gemcitabine, fluorouracil, capecitabine, etc.)
	- Typically combined with systemic therapy
	Neoadjuvant chemoradiation protocol varies by institution, however:
	- CTV is typically the gross tumour and involved nodes with a 0.5–1-cm margin:
	  - Limited volume elective nodal irradiation may be employed
	- Typical doses are 45–50.4 Gy in 1.8-Gy fractions:
	  – Some centres employ hypofractionated schedules
	- Various radiosensitizers (gemcitabine, fluorouracil, capecitabine, etc.)

Radiotherapy	Description

Advanced non-metastatic disease	- Locoregional chemoradiation is more effective than radiation alone (Gastrointestinal Tumor Study Group (GITSG)-9273, ECOG 4201):
	  - Total dose and fractionation varies by institution
	    - CTV is typically the gross tumour and involved nodes with a 0.5–1-cm margin:
	      - Limited volume elective nodal irradiation may be employed
	    - Typical doses are 45–54 Gy in 1.8-Gy fractions
	      - Some centres employ hypofractionated schedules
	  - Various radiosensitizers (gemcitabine, fluorouracil, capecitabine, etc.)
	  - Typically combined with initial induction systemic therapy
	  - Emerging data suggest stereotactic body radiation (SBRT) may be an option in select cases at experienced institutions, although further data are needed before this can be routinely recommended
	- Neoadjuvant chemoradiation protocol varies by institution
	- Radiation therapy can control locoregional complications in select patients

Metastatic disease	- No standard role for radiation therapy in the metastatic setting - Palliation of symptoms from locoregional spread or metastases

Systemic therapy

Systemic therapy	Description
Early disease	- Surgical resection is the mainstay for localized disease - Adjuvant post-resection gemcitabine given at an IV dose of 1000 mg/m^2 over 30 minutes on Days 1, 8 and 15, every 4 weeks for 6 months
Advanced non-metastatic disease	- Various systemic regimens (see below) in neoadjuvant or definitive treatment strategy - Various chemoradiation (see above) in neoadjuvant or consolidated definitive strategy: - Strong tendency in Europe to replace chemoradiation by chemotherapy alone in this setting

Metastatic disease	- FOLFIRINOX regimen:
	  - Irinotecan 180 mg/m^2 + oxaliplatin 85 mg/m^2 + leucovorin 400 mg/m^2 + 5-fluorouracil (5-FU) bolus 400 mg/m^2 IV, then 2400 mg/m^2 over 46 hours of each 2-week cycle
	- Gemcitabine + nab-paclitaxol:
	  - Gemcitabine 1000 mg/m^2 + nab-paclitaxel 125 mg/m^2 weekly for three of 4 weeks
	- Single-agent gemcitabine:
	  - Gemcitabine 1000 mg/m^2 weekly for three of 4 weeks

Controversies

Although most would agree that neoadjuvant therapy is appropriate for non-metastatic locally unresectable (borderline/locally advanced) pancreatic adenocarcinoma, the utilization of such strategies in otherwise localized resectable cancers is controversial but gaining interest. Benefits of upfront therapy prior to resection include lower positive margin rates (positive margin resections are highly associated with lower survival), early treatment of micrometastatic disease and selection of patients who would not benefit from resection (a significant proportion of surgically resected patients develop early systemic recurrence), and the ability of patients to receive all recommended therapy prior to potentially morbid resectional procedures (up to 40% of patients do not receive complete recommended adjuvant therapy due to surgical complications or poor performance status). Non-randomized single institutional studies have shown equivalent or potentially improved results with upfront therapy and such a strategy may allow a higher proportion of patients to receive full cancer treatment therapy versus a surgery-first approach. There are several trials underway specifically addressing this topic in both localized and borderline/locally-advanced cancer utilizing a variety of neoadjuvant strategies with systemic chemotherapy and/or locoregional radiation therapies.

Additional controversy exists over the type of resection as minimally invasive procedures are becoming more common for pancreatectomy; also, how these procedures compare to traditional open resections in terms of short (margin status, adequacy of lymphadenectomy) and long-term (recurrence and overall survival) oncological metrics.

Table 23.2.3 Phase III clinical trials

Trial name	Results
Local disease	
Doi et al. (2008) Surg Today 38(11):1021–1028	• Resection is superior to chemoradiation for resectable locally invasive pancreatic cancer
Adjuvant systemic therapy	
CONKO-001 Oettle et al. (2013) JAMA 310(14):1473–1481	• Among patients with macroscopic complete removal of pancreatic cancer, the use of adjuvant gemcitabine for 6 months compared with observation alone resulted in increased overall and disease-free survival • Long-term follow-up (>10 years) showed strong support for the use of gemcitabine in this setting
ESPAC-1 Neoptolemos et al. (2004) N Engl J Med 350(12):1200–1210	• Adjuvant fluorouracil gave a significant survival benefit in patients with resected pancreatic cancer • Adjuvant chemoradiotherapy had a deleterious effect on survival, although there are major criticisms of the radiotherapy schedule/technique and study methodological design
ESPAC-3 Neoptolemos et al. (2010) JAMA 304(10):1073–1081	• Compared with the use of fluorouracil + leucovorin, gemcitabine did not result in improved overall survival in patients with completely resected pancreatic cancer
Advanced disease and metastatic disease	
PRODIGE 4/ACCORD 11 Conroy et al. (2011) N Engl J Med 13(2):181–188	• Combination chemotherapy regimen consisting of oxaliplatin + irinotecan + fluorouracil + leucovorin (FOLFIRINOX) as compared with gemcitabine as first-line therapy in patients with metastatic pancreatic cancer resulted in significantly improved overall and progression-free survival, and marked response rates • Although currently considered 'standard of care', this regimen is associated with significant toxicities and is not suitable for all patients with metastatic disease
MPACT Von Hoff et al. (2013) N Engl J Med 369(18):1691–1703	• In patients with metastatic pancreatic adenocarcinoma, nab-paclitaxel + gemcitabine significantly improved overall survival, progression-free survival and response rates compared to gemcitabine alone
ECOG 4201 Loehrer et al. (2008) J Clin Oncol 26:214s	In patients with localized but unresectable pancreatic adenocarcinoma, gemcitabine plus radiotherapy compared to gemcitabine alone resulted in improved survival but increased toxicity • Study was under-accrued and stopped early

Phase III clinical trials

See Table 23.2.3.

Areas of research

As there are no effective screening methods for pancreatic cancer and the majority of patients present with distant metastasis, the identification of early-stage disease biomarkers will most likely result in the greatest improvement in survival for patients.

Other areas of research in pancreatic cancer focus on chemotherapeutics, predicting therapeutic responses prior to treatment, cancer vaccines and targeted therapies for an individualized treatment approach.

Recommended reading

Conroy T, Desseigne F, Ychou M et al. (2011) FOLFIRINOX versus gemcitabine for metastatic pancreatic cancer. N Engl J Med 364(19):1817–1825.

Doi R, Imamura M, Hosotani R et al. (2008) Surgery versus radiochemotherapy for resectable locally invasive pancreatic cancer: final results of a randomized multi-institutional trial. Surg Today 38(11):1021–1028.

Hsu CC, Herman JM, Corsini MM et al. (2010) Adjuvant chemoradiation for pancreatic adenocarcinoma: the Johns Hopkins Hospital-Mayo Clinic collaborative study. Ann Surg Oncol 2010;17(4):981–990.

Katz MH, Marsh R, Herman JM et al. (2013) Borderline resectable pancreatic cancer: need for standardization and methods for optimal clinical trial design. Ann Surg Oncol 20(8):2787–2795.

Loehrer P, Powell M, Cardenes H (2008) A randomized phase III study of gemcitabine in combination with radiation therapy versus gemcitabine alone in patients with localized, unresectable pancreatic cancer: E4201. J Clin Oncol 26:214s.

Moore MJ, Goldstein D, Hamm J et al. (2007) Erlotinib plus gemcitabine compared with gemcitabine alone in patients with advanced pancreatic cancer: a phase III trial of the National Cancer Institute of Canada Clinical Trials Group. J Clin Oncol 25(15):1960–1966.

Neoptolemos JP, Stocken DD, Friess H et al. (2004) A randomized trial of chemoradiotherapy and chemotherapy after resection of pancreatic cancer. N Engl J Med 350(12):1200–1210.

Neoptolemos JP, Stocken DD, Bassi C et al. (2010) Adjuvant chemotherapy with fluorouracil plus folinic acid vs gemcitabine following pancreatic cancer resection: a randomized controlled trial. *JAMA* 304(10):1073–1081.

Oettle H, Neuhaus P, Hochhaus A *et al.* (2013) Adjuvant chemotherapy with gemcitabine and long-term outcomes among patients with resected pancreatic cancer: the CONKO-001 randomized trial. *JAMA* 310(14):1473–1481.

The Gastrointestinal Tumor Study Group (1979) A multi-institutional comparative trial of radiation therapy alone and in combination with 5-fluorouracil for locally unresectable pancreatic carcinoma. The Gastrointestinal Tumor Study Group. *Ann Surg* 189(2):205–208.

Thomas RM, Truty MJ, Nogueras-Gonzalez GM *et al.* (2012) Selective reoperation for locally recurrent or metastatic pancreatic ductal adenocarcinoma following primary pancreatic resection. *J Gastrointest Surg* 16(9):1696–1704.

Truty MJ, Thomas RM, Katz MH *et al.* (2012) Multimodality therapy offers a chance for cure in patients with pancreatic adenocarcinoma deemed unresectable at first operative exploration. *J Am Coll Surg* 215(1):41–51; discussion 42.

Von Hoff DD, Ervin T, Arena FP *et al.* (2013) Increased survival in pancreatic cancer with nab-paclitaxel plus gemcitabine. *N Engl J Med* 369(18):1691–1703.

24 Oesophagus

Wentao Fang[1], Zhigang Li[2], Teng Mao[1], Jun Liu[3] and Xufeng Guo[1]

[1] Department of Thoracic Surgery, Shanghai Chest Hospital, Jiaotong University Medical School, Shanghai, China
[2] Department of Cardiothoracic Surgery, Changhai Hospital, Second University of Military Medicine, Shanghai, China
[3] Department of Radiation Oncology, Shanghai Chest Hospital, Jiaotong University Medical School, Shanghai, China

Summary	Key facts
Introduction	• Squamous cell carcinoma (SCC) from squamous epithelium of the cervical and thoracic oesophagus: still the predominant histology in the Eastern world • Adenocarcinoma (AC) mainly from Barrett's oesophagus at the lower thoracic oesophagus or oesophagogastric junction: incidence rising rapidly in Western populations
Presentation	• Dysphagia is the most common presenting symptom • May be detected during endoscopic follow-up for Barrett's oesophagus or in endemic populations showing a high incidence of the disease • Oligophagia, body weight loss and hoarseness are signs of advanced disease
Scenario	• Endoscopic therapy is warranted for accurate staging and management of early disease • Surgery gives the only chance of cure for localized thoracic SCC • For AC and locally-advanced SCC, induction chemoradiation or chemotherapy improves survival • Definitive chemoradiation is preferred to surgery in cervical lesions
Trials	• Paucity of phase III trials in oesophageal SCC

Incidence, aetiology and screening

Oesophageal cancer is the eighth most common cancer worldwide and the sixth most common cause of death from cancer. Oesophageal cancers mainly include squamous cell carcinomas (SCC) arising from the squamous epithelium lining the cervical and thoracic oesophagus, and adenocarcinomas (AC) arising from the adenoepithelium at the oesophagogastric junction or from the metaplastic epithelium at the lower thoracic oesophagus. Other histology subtypes such as small cell carcinomas or basaloid carcinomas are very rare. Other malignancies include melanoma, sarcoma, carcinosarcoma, etc. Gastrointestinal stromal tumours (GIST) are rarely seen in the oesophagus.

The 5-year survival rate for all patients with oesophageal cancer is only 17%, with better survival for local (33.7%) or regional (16.9%) compared to distant (2.9%) disease at presentation. Recent advances in diagnosis and staging, improvement in surgical techniques and introduction of multimodal therapies have led to small but significant improvement in survival.

Incidence, aetiology and screening	Description

Incidence	- Huge variation in the epidemiological pattern between different regions of the world:
	  - SCC used to be the dominant histological type of oesophageal cancer worldwide, but while it remains the most common type in East Asia, its incidence has slowly decreased over the past three decades in Western populations
	  - AC has shown a clear increasing trend (attributed to gastroesophageal reflux disease [GERD])
	- Global incidence:
	  - Eighth most common cancer worldwide
	  - Two to four times more common in men than in women:
	    - Age standardized ratio (ASR) for women: 4.2 per 100,000
	    - ASR for men: 10.1 per 100,000
	- Mortality: the sixth most common cause of death from cancer:
	  - ASR for women: 3.4 per 100,000
	  - ASR for men: 8.5 per 100,000
	  - Highest mortality rates are found in both sexes in Eastern and Southern Africa, and in Eastern Asia

Aetiology	- Alcohol and tobacco consumption, poor dietary hygiene, human papillomavirus (HPV) infection and low socioeconomic status may be responsible for SCC - Cause of the dramatic increase of AC in Western populations is unknown, but is suspected to be associated with the increased prevalence of GERD, obesity and Barrett's oesophagus
Screening	- Endoscopic screening for SCC may be useful only in regions where the disease is endemic - Endoscopic follow-up may detect high-grade dysplasia (HGD; carcinoma *in situ*) in GERD

Presentation

- No or slight non-specific symptoms (such as hiccups) in early stage
- Typical dysphagia in local disease (retrosternal or epigastric discomfort [non-specific])
- Pain (invasion into surrounding structures), hoarseness (recurrent laryngeal nerve involvement by metastatic lymph nodes), loss of body weight (poor dietary intake)
- Enlarged cervical lymph nodes
- Rarely presents as upper gastrointestinal (GI) bleeding, rupture into airway or chest cavity

Pathology and natural history

Pathology and natural history	Description

Squamous cell carcinoma	- Malignant epithelial tumour with squamous cell differentiation, microscopically characterized by keratinocyte-like cells with intercellular bridges and/or keratinization
	- Most common histology subtype in East Asia (>90%), decreasing in Western nations
	- 3:1 male-to-female ratio
	- Median age at presentation 60–70 years
	- 60–70% locally advanced (>T3) at presentation with symptoms
	- Early and frequent lymphatic involvement:
	  - >30% when invading submucosa
	  - 50–70% in locoregional diseases
	  - Most frequently at cervicothoracic junction nodes (recurrent laryngeal nerve nodes) for tumours in the upper and middle thoracic oesophagus, or at paracardial and left gastric nodes for tumours in the lower thoracic oesophagus
	- Distant spread presents late, most commonly seen in the liver, lung and bone

(continued)

Pathology and natural history	Description

	- Survival:
	  - Overall 5-year survival: <20%
	  - 30–40% after complete surgical resection
	  - T category:
	    - Confined to submucosa: 80%
	    - Muscularis propria: 50%
	    - Invasion beyond adventitia: 30%
	  - N category:
	    - No lymph node involvement: 50%
	    - Regional nodal involvement: 30%
	    - Multiple station or field involvement: <10%

Adenocarcinoma	- Typically papillary and/or tubular
	- A few tumours are of the diffuse type and show rare glandular formations and sometimes signet ring cells
	- Most common histological type in Western countries; rare in Asia and Africa
	- 7:1 male-to-female ratio
	- Average age at diagnosis around 65 years
	- Occurs predominantly in Caucasian males of industrialized countries, with a marked trend of increasing incidence
	- Most important aetiological factor is chronic GERD, leading to Barrett-type mucosal metaplasia, the most common precursor lesion of AC
	- Oesophageal carcinomas with glandular differentiation are typically located in the distal oesophagus
	- Dysphagia is often the first symptom:
	  - May be associated with retrosternal or epigastric pain
	- Tumour spread:
	  - First locally and then infiltrate the oesophageal wall
	  - Distal spread to the stomach may occur
	  - Most commonly metastasizes to para-oesophageal and paracardial lymph nodes, lesser curvature of the stomach and coeliac nodes
	  - Distant metastases occur late, most commonly seen in lung, liver and bone
	- Survival:
	  - Overall 5-year survival: 20–25%
	  - Stage I tumours in 60–70%, stage III in 5–10%

Small cell carcinoma	- Arise from multipotential cells of the basal layer:
	  - Cells may be small with dark nuclei of a round or oval shape and scanty cytoplasm, or be larger with more cytoplasm (intermediate cells) forming solid sheets and nests
	- Represents 0.15–2.4% of all oesophageal tumours:
	  - Most tumours located in the middle-to-distal oesophagus
	- Male-to-female ratio 1.5:1
	- Mean age at presentation around 60 years
	- Role of surgery remains undefined; chemotherapy increases survival
	- Prognosis remains poor, with median survival 4.2–18.5 months

Sarcoma	- Mesenchymal tumour of the oesophagus:
	  - Accounts for 0.2% of malignant oesophageal tumours
	  - Mostly located in the distal oesophagus (45%)
	- Carcinosarcomas of mixed histology, most often with SCC, is not uncommon
	- Typically multinodular or polypoid lesions, arising from the submucosa:
	  - Less commonly plaque-like masses
	- Presenting symptoms are non-specific to other oesophageal malignancies, and include dysphagia (75%), weight loss (50%) and chest pain (45%)
	- 5-year survival >70% after R0 resection:
	- Dismal long-term survival if not resected completely

Pathology and natural history	Description
Melanoma	- Arise from a zone of atypical junctional proliferation of melanocytes and often present adjacent to the invasive tumour, although it may not be observed in advanced disease
- Much more commonly metastatic than primary, representing 0.1–0.5% of all malignant oesophageal tumours:
- Mostly seen in the middle-to-distal oesophagus
- Usually single, pigmented, polypoid lesions:
- Growth is typically expansile rather than infiltrative
- Extremely poor prognosis:
- Median survival 14.4 months, with 5-year survival <5%
- Long-term survival can only be expected for Stage Ia

Diagnostic work-up

Diagnostic work-up	Description
Work-up	- Initial work-up for diagnosis: upper GI barium swallow, endoscopy and biopsy for histological confirmation
- Clinical evaluation:
- Chest and abdomen computed tomography (CT) scan with oral and intravenous (IV) contrast
- Endoscopic ultrasonography (EUS) for depth of invasion and lymph node involvement
- Endoscopic mucosal resection (EMR) or endoscopic submucosal dissection (ESD) may improve the accuracy of staging for early superficial lesions
- Positron emission tomography (PET)/CT recommended for lymphatic involvement and potential distant metastasis
- Fine needle biopsy under ultrasonography guidance or EUS for better nodal staging
- Bone scan, brain magnetic resonance imaging (MRI) when metastasis suspected
- Nutritional assessment
Tumour markers	- Usually elevated in locally advanced or late stage
- May be helpful during follow-up, e.g. carcinoembryonic antigen (CEA)
- No role in diagnosis
- Value only for prognosis and follow-up
- Genetic abnormalities are potential biomarkers for tumour growth, invasion and metastasis; these include *p53*, *HER2*, *cyclin D1* and *EGFR*

Staging and prognostic grouping

It is of critical importance to make a careful and thorough evaluation before treatment so that therapeutic strategies can be tailored to the disease as well as the patient.

UICC TNM staging and prognostic grouping

Prognoses of oesophageal cancers are related to their histological types as well. The 7th edition requires that tumours invading the oesophagogastric junction (Siewert types I and II) be classified as oesophageal cancers. The stage grouping of SCC and ACs are now separated (Table 24.1). Also, both tumour grade and location are now incorporated into prognostic grouping, especially in early diseases.

Table 24.1 UICC TNM categories (oesophagus, including oesophagogastric junction), stage grouping (oesophagus and oesophagogastric junction) and prognostic grouping (squamous cell carcinoma and adenocarcinoma)

TNM categories: Oesophagus (includes oesophagogastric junction)	
T1	Lamina propria (T1a), submucosa (T1b)
T2	Muscularis propria
T3	Adventitia
T4a	Pleura, pericardium, diaphragm
T4b	Aorta, vertebral body, trachea
N1	1–2 regional
N2	3–6 regional
N3	≥7 regional
M1	Distant metastasis

(continued)

Table 24.1 (Continued)

Stage grouping: Carcinomas of the oesophagus and oesophagogastric junction			
Stage 0	Tis	N0	M0
Stage IA	T1	N0	M0
Stage IB	T2	N0	M0
Stage IIA	T3	N0	M0
Stage IIB	T1, T2	N1	M0
Stage IIIA	T4a	N0	M0
	T3	N1	M0
	T1, T2	N2	M0
Stage IIIB	T3	N2	M0
Stage IIIC	T4a	N1, N2	M0

Prognostic grouping: Squamous cell carcinoma					
	T	N	M	Grade	Location*
Group 0	Tis	0	0	1	Any
Group IA	1	0	0	1, X	Any
Group IB	1	0	0	2, 3	Any
	2, 3	0	0	1, X	Lower, X
Group IIA	2, 3	0	0	1, X	Upper, middle
	2, 3	0	0	2, 3	Lower, X
Group IIB	2, 3	0	0	2, 3	Upper, middle
	1, 2	1	0	Any	Any
Group IIIA	1, 2	2	0	Any	Any
	3	1	0	Any	Any
	4a	0	0	Any	Any
Group IIIB	3	2	0	Any	Any
Group IIIC	4a	1, 2	0	Any	Any
	4b	Any	0	Any	Any
	Any	3	0	Any	Any
Group IV	Any	Any	1	Any	Any

Prognostic grouping: Adenocarcinoma				
	T	N	M	Grade
Group 0	Tis	0	0	1
Group IA	1	0	0	1, 2, X
Group IB	1	0	0	3
	2	0	0	1, 2, X
Group IIA	2	0	0	3
Group IIB	3	0	0	Any

	1, 2	1	0	Any
Group IIIA	1, 2	2	0	Any
	3	1	0	Any
	4a	0	0	Any
Group IIIB	3	2	0	Any
Group IIIC	4a	1, 2	0	Any
	4b	Any	0	Any
	Any	3	0	Any
Group IV	Any	Any	1	Any

Note: *Lower, middle and upper correspond to the intrathoracic thirds of the oesophagus.

Prognostic factors

The major prognostic factors for oesophageal cancer are still anatomical: depth of tumour invasion and extent of lymphatic or haematological spread of the disease (Table 24.2).

Table 24.2 Prognostic factors for survival in oesophageal cancer

Prognostic factors	Tumour related	Host related	Treatment related
Essential	Depth of invasion Lymph node involvement Presence of lymphovascular invasion (LVI)	Performance status Age Nutritional status	Quality of surgery Multimodality approach
Additional	Tumour grading Tumour location	Economic status	Nutritional support
New and promising	CEA VEGF-C HER2		

Prognosis of SCC of the oesophagus has been reported to be worse than that of AC. Long-term survival is mainly achieved in patients with early disease and who are physically fit for treatment. A multimodality approach with a curative intent improves the chance of cure.

Given the difference in aetiology, epidemiology, biological characteristics, presentation and prognosis, treatment strategies for SCC and AC of the oesophagus will be discussed separately.

SQUAMOUS CELL CARCINOMA

Treatment philosophy

As most SCC of the thoracic oesophagus are already at a locally-advanced stage upon presentation, the goal of management should be decided by prognostic factors based on the efficacy of currently available treatment modalities. Complete surgical resection of the primary lesion as well as involved locoregional lymph nodes provides the best chance of cure. Effective induction therapies, including chemotherapy or concurrent chemoradiation, help down-stage the disease and improve the rate of radical resection and the probability of prolonged survival. When long-term survival is not expected, treatment should be directed at improving quality of life through better local control and restoration of oral intake. Concurrent chemoradiation or radiation alone is helpful in achieving this goal. Endoscopic procedures like stenting carry minimal risk and are highly effective in relieving dysphagia associated with oesophageal carcinomas of the thoracic oesophagus.

Scenario: SCC	Treatment philosophy

High-grade dysplasia/T1a	• Endoscopic therapy (either endoscopic mucosal resection [EMR] or endoscopic submucosal dissection [ESD]) is strongly recommended as first-line therapy
	• Purposes of endoscopic therapy include diagnosis, staging and treatment:
	  ▪ Often difficult to differentiate between low-grade dysplasia and HGD, or between HGD and invasive SCC on biopsy specimens
	  ▪ In addition to the resection margin after EMR, histological examination of depth of invasion is mandatory, as lymphatic involvement is rare in HGD or T1a but may occur in 20–30% of T1b lesions

T1b–3/N0–1	• For cervical oesophageal cancer (<5 cm from the cricopharyngeus):
	  ▪ Definitive chemoradiation is preferred as first-line treatment
	  ▪ Surgery is reserved for the salvage setting
	• Surgery gives the best chance of cure for thoracic oesophageal tumours:
	  ▪ Long-term survival is only feasible where complete surgical resection can be achieved
	  ▪ Subtotal oesophagectomy together with systemic lymph node clearance offers accurate staging, radical resection and optimal chance of local control
	• Even in radically resected tumours without lymph node involvement (pN0), locoregional recurrence is still the major pattern of treatment failure:
	  ▪ Therefore, adjuvant therapies may be beneficial in high-risk patients, including those with upper thoracic or T3–4 disease, LVI or submucosal metastasis
	• Induction may be considered, but evidence for this is not as strong as it is for AC
	• For T1b lesions, definitive chemoradiation is a reasonable alternative in patients who are unfit for surgery

T4/N2–3	• Surgery should *not* be recommended as the first-line therapy, as survival rate is very low (around 10%) even with adjuvant therapies:
	  ▪ Prognosis is extremely poor in T4b or N3 disease
	  ▪ Effective induction therapy may be the only hope of improving survival
	• Concurrent chemoradiation has the highest response rate (RR) (>80%; and 30% complete response [CR]):
	  ▪ Induction chemotherapy is less effective (60–70% RR and 10% CR), but is better tolerated than chemoradiation
	• In patients with multistation lymphatic involvement, induction chemotherapy may be preferred as it is difficult to give radiation to the entire mediastinum and the superior abdomen
	• Given the high relapse rate in Stage III disease, postoperative chemotherapy or chemoradiation should be recommended to patients without induction therapy

M1	• Distant lymph node involvement (supraclavicular or retroperitoneal) may respond to concurrent chemoradiation (3-year survival 20%)
	• When presenting with distant organ metastasis, the chance of long-term survival is extremely low:
	  ▪ RR to systemic chemotherapy is often very low
	  ▪ Treatment is mainly aimed at alleviating symptoms and improving quality of life:
	    ○ Radiation is most effective in this setting
	• Endoscopic stenting is safe and effective in relieving dysphagia and restoring oral intake

(continued)

Scenario: SCC	Treatment philosophy

Recurrent diseases	• Locoregional recurrence after surgery:
	  ▪ Reoperation is often technically impossible for local recurrence
	  ▪ Chemoradiation or radiation alone is often the only choice for relapse in the anastomosis, original tumour bed or regional lymph node
	• Locoregional disease after chemoradiation:
	  ▪ Salvage surgery may be considered for medically fit patients, but is technically demanding and carries a high risk of morbidity and mortality
	• Metastatic disease on follow-up:
	  ▪ Chemotherapy may be tried but the RR is unsatisfactory:
	    ○ For liver metastasis, interventional therapies are more effective and better tolerated
	    ○ Supportive care is often the best choice
	  ▪ Radiation may be considered for bone metastasis to relieve pain and prevent secondary complications
	  ▪ Surgery or radiation can be considered for a solitary metastasis

Follow-up	• After surgery with or without induction therapy:
	  ▪ Cervical ultrasound (US) scan, chest and abdominal CT scan, barium swallow and serum tumour marker (CEA) measurement
	  ▪ Endoscopy is recommended to rule out potential failure at the anastomosis, extent and consequences of reflux
	• After chemoradiation:
	  ▪ Periodic endoscopy is mandatory to look for potential local recurrence
	  ▪ CT scan is not sensitive in detecting local recurrence but is helpful for lymph node relapse or distant organ dissemination
	  ▪ ^{18}F-FDG-PET scan is recommended when recurrence is suspected
	  ▪ Persistent elevated tumour marker level is often indicative of recurrence

Treatment

Surgery

Surgery and endoscopic intervention: SCC	Description

High-grade dysplasia	• Endoscopic therapy: EMR or ESD
	  ▪ Endoscopic resection for lesions of <75% circumferential involvement to avoid stricture formation:
	    ○ Multifocal lesions should be carefully ruled out by narrow band imaging (NBI) or chromoendoscopy
	  ▪ Ablation for circumferential lesions:
	    ○ Radiofrequency ablation is preferred because of its lower incidence of stricture

T1a	• Endoscopic resection:
	  ▪ EMR or ESD preferred to surgery, especially for T1a without lymphatic involvement
	  ▪ When invasion through the muscularis mucosae or into superficial submucosa is suspected, the indication for endoscopic therapy is relative because of the potential for nodal metastases (8%) in high-risk patients (LVI positive or poor differentiation histology)
	  ▪ Repeated endoscopic resection attempts are acceptable for local recurrent T1a and a positive resection margin
	• Oesophagectomy:
	  ▪ Indicated for patients with circumferential lesions, high-risk patients (LVI or poor differentiation histology) or evidence of node metastasis

Surgery and endoscopic intervention: SCC	Description

T1bN0	• Oesophagectomy with systemic lymph nodes dissection:
	  ▪ At least two-field (thoracoabdominal) lymph node dissection is recommended to ensure accurate staging and radical removal of disease
	  ▪ Minimally invasive oesophagectomy (MIE, including robotic): as long as standard oncological and dissection principles are not compromised, similar survival results can be expected with improved early postoperative recovery
	• Endoscopic resection:
	  ▪ EMR or ESD may be considered, with or without radiation, for those who cannot tolerate surgery or chemoradiation

T1b–3/N0–1	• Oesophagectomy with systemic lymph node dissection (either after induction or followed by adjuvant chemotherapy, radiotherapy or chemoradiation)
	  ▪ Approaches: transthoracic oesophagectomy (TTE) is the most widely adopted approach:
	    ○ Right thoracotomy (Ivor–Lewis) is preferred to enable *en bloc* oesophagectomy and complete two-field lymph node dissection
	    ○ McKeown approach with cervical anastomosis provides a safer resection margin for upper thoracic tumours and enables cervical (three-field) lymph node dissection
	    ○ Left thoracotomy (Sweet) approach is indicated only in lower thoracic and abdominal oesophageal lesions
	    ○ MIE: thoracoscopic and/or laparoscopic Ivor–Lewis or McKeown; feasible in experienced hands
	    ○ Transhiatal oesophagectomy (THE) is more feasible in lesions close to the thoracic inlet or oesophagogastric junction
	  ▪ Conduits:
	    ○ Stomach is the most commonly used conduit for reconstruction
	    ○ Colon and jejunum can be candidates in case of an unusable stomach or recurrence
	  ▪ Routes of reconstruction:
	    ○ When cervical anastomosis is required, no significant difference in swallowing function is found between orthotopic and retrosternal routes, except that leak rate is higher in the latter
	  ▪ Lymph nodes dissection:
	    ○ Extended two-field lymph node dissection is recommended for all SCC of the thoracic oesophagus
	    ○ For patients with upper thoracic lesions or increased risk of cervical involvement, three-field dissection may improve staging accuracy, local control and long-term survival
	    ○ At least 12–15 nodes from the mediastinum and superior abdomen should be harvested to achieve adequate nodal staging in patients without induction therapy

T4/N2–3	• Not recommended as first-line therapy as survival is dismal even with adjuvant therapies, especially in T4b or N3 • May be considered after effective induction therapy or in salvage settings
M1	• Generally contraindicated

Radiotherapy
See Box 24.1.

Box 24.1 Radiotherapy techniques

- CT scans, barium swallow, EUS, PET or PET/CT if available should be reviewed before treatment
- Recommend contrast-enhanced CT and 3D treatment planning. 4D CT is encouraged to create an ITV (internal target volume) from the clinical target volume (CTV)
- Clinical data are now emerging to support the role of intensity-modulated radiation therapy (IMRT) in oesophageal cancer
- Radiation techniques:
  - Gross target volume (GTV): primary tumour and involved regional lymph nodes
  - CTV: expansion of tumour GTV, nodal GTV and elective nodal regions:
    - Tumour CTV is defined as the primary tumour + 3–4 cm craniocaudal margin and a 1-cm radical expansion
    - Nodal CTV is defined as a 1-cm expansion from the nodal GTV and should also include elective nodal regions

- Elective nodal regions depend on the location of the primary tumour in the oesophagus:
  Cervical oesophagus: include bilateral supraclavicular nodes, para-oesophageal nodes and higher cervical nodes if disease involvement is suspected
  Upper thoracic oesophagus: include bilateral supraclavicular nodes and para-oesophageal nodes
  Middle thoracic oesophagus: include para-oesophageal lymph nodes
  Lower thoracic oesophagus and oesophagogastric junction: include para-oesophageal nodes, lesser curvature nodes and coeliac nodes
- Planning target volume (PTV): expansion should be 0.5–1 cm from the CTV
- PTV dosage:
  - For squamous cell carcinoma:
    - Neoadjuvant therapy: 4000–5000 cGy (180–200 cGy/day)
    - Definitive therapy: 5000–6000 cGy (180–200 cGy/day)
    - PORT: 4500–5000 cGy (180–200 cGy/day)
  - For adenocarcinoma:
    - Neoadjuvant therapy: 4140–5040 cGy (180–200 cGy/day)
    - Definitive therapy: 5000–5040 cGy (180–200 cGy/day)
    - PORT: 4500–5040 cGy (180–200 cGy/day)

Radiotherapy: SCC	Treatment

Cervical oesophagus	- Cervical oesophageal cancer (<5 cm from the cricopharyngeus)
	  - Definitive chemoradiation is recommended as first-line treatment
	  - Radiation alone only in patients unable to tolerate chemoradiation for palliative purpose

Early disease (HGD and T1a)	- No role

Local disease (T1b–3/N0–1)	- Concurrent chemoradiation is the most effective induction modality in down-staging and may prolong survival in responders:
	  - Radiation alone for induction has been shown to be ineffective either in increasing respectability or improving survival
	- Definitive chemoradiotherapy (concurrent or sequential) is an acceptable alternative for those who are medically unfit for or who decline surgery, with a curative intent
	- Chemotherapy delivered concurrently with radiation has been shown to improve local control and survival:
	  - Radiation alone should only be considered in patients who are medically unfit for or refuse surgery, and who are unable to tolerate chemotherapy or chemoradiation, as palliative treatment
	- For patients revealed as node positive after complete resection without preoperative treatment, chemoradiation is preferred to chemotherapy alone when tolerable
	- Postoperative radiation therapy (PORT) is mainly indicated for positive resection margins (R1) or residual tumour (R2):
	  - Randomized trials of adjuvant radiation alone without chemotherapy failed to show any survival benefit despite improvement in locoregional control
	  - PORT may be considered in high-risk radically resected pN0 patients, including those with upper thoracic lesions and deeper depth of invasion (above T3), poorly differentiated histology and/or LVI:
	    - PORT tailored to insufficient lymphatic clearance has shown benefit in improving local control

Locally-advanced disease (T4/N2–3)	- Induction chemoradiation may down-stage T4 or N2–3 diseases and increase the chance of cure by surgery - For patients with extensive nodal involvement (multistation or multifield), definitive chemoradiation is a reasonable alternative
Metastatic disease (M1)	- Concurrent chemoradiation has a role where there is distant nodal involvement (supraclavicular or retroperitoneal) - Radiation is the best available measure for relieving pain from bone metastasis - Local therapy such as stereotactic body radiation therapy (SBRT) may be considered for a solitary metastasis
Recurrent disease	- Concurrent chemoradiation is most effective in treating locoregional relapse after surgery, especially nodal recurrence

Systemic therapy

See Table 24.3.

Systemic therapy: SCC	Description
Early disease (HGD and T1a)	• No role

Local disease (T1b–3/N0–1)	• In conjunction with radiation (concurrent chemoradiation) preferred
	• Induction chemotherapy also may prolong survival in responders:
	  ■ RR is lower than concurrent chemoradiation (pathological complete response [PCR] 5–10%), but toxicity is also much lower:
	  ■ For patients with multistation nodal involvement, chemotherapy alone may be more applicable
	• Adjuvant chemotherapy improves disease-free survival in patients with lymph node metastasis after radical resection:
	  ■ May also be considered in high-risk, radically-resected pN0 patients, including those with upper thoracic lesions, poor cell differentiation histology and deeper depth of invasion (above T3)

Locally-advanced disease (T4/N2–3)	• In conjunction with radiation (concurrent chemoradiation) • Induction chemotherapy may down-stage and give the chance of surgical cure for T4 or N2–3 diseases: ■ For patients with extensive nodal involvement (multistation or multifield), chemotherapy alone may be more applicable than concurrent chemoradiation
Metastatic disease (M1)	• Chemotherapy may be tried but has low efficacy; as yet no survival benefit has been shown • Systemic chemotherapy is ineffective in dealing with liver metastasis, which is the most common site of involvement in SCC • Biological and targeted therapies are under study in Stage IV diseases
Recurrent disease	• Concurrent chemoradiation is most effective in treating locoregional relapse, especially nodal recurrence • Oral maintenance chemotherapy can be tried to control disease progression

Table 24.3 Systemic therapy regimens

Regimens for induction chemoradiation	• Paclitaxel + carboplatin:
	  ■ Paclitaxel: 50 mg/m^2 IV on Day 1
	  ■ Carboplatin: AUC 2 IV on Day 1
	  ■ Weekly for 5 weeks
	• Cisplatin + fluorouracil:
	  ■ Cisplatin: 75–100 mg/m^2 IV on Days 1 and 29
	  ■ Fluorouracil: 750–1000 mg/m^2 IV continuous infusion over 24 hours on Days 1–4 and 29–32
	  ■ 35-day cycle
	• For SCC, consider novibine + cisplatin:
	  ■ Novibine: 25 mg/m^2 IV on Days 1, 8, 22 and 29
	  ■ Cisplatin: 75 mg/m^2 IV on Days 1 and 22
	  ■ Cycled every 21 days for two cycles
	• For AC, consider oxaliplatin + fluorouracil:
	  ■ Oxaliplatin: 85 mg/m^2 IV on Day 1
	  ■ Leucovorin: 400 mg/m^2 IV on Day 1
	  ■ Fluorouracil: 400 mg/m^2 IVP on Day 1
	  ■ Fluorouracil: 800 mg/m^2 IV continuous infusion over 24 hours on Days 1 and 2
	  ■ Cycled every 14 days for three cycles with radiation and three cycles after radiation

Regimens for definitive chemoradiation:	• Cisplatin + fluorouracil:
	  ■ Cisplatin: 75–100 mg/m^2 IV on Day 1
	  ■ Fluorouracil: 750–1000 mg/m^2 IV continuous infusion over 24 hours on Days 1–4
	  ■ Cycled every 28 days for two to four cycles: two cycles with radiation followed by two cycles of consolidation without radiation

(continued)

Table 24.3 (Continued)

	• Paclitaxel + carboplatin:
	   ■ Paclitaxel: 50 mg/m² IV on Day 1
	   ■ Carboplatin: AUC 2 IV on Day 1
	   ■ Weekly for 5 weeks
	• For AC, consider:
	   ■ Oxaliplatin + fluorouracil:
	      ○ Oxaliplatin: 85 mg/m² IV on Days 1, 15 and 29 for three doses
	      ○ Fluorouracil: 180 mg/m² IV on Days 1–33
	      or
	   ■ Oxaliplatin 85 mg/m² IV on Day 1
	      ○ Leucovorin 400 mg/m² IV on Day 1
	      ○ Fluorouracil 400 mg/m² IVP on Day 1
	      ○ Fluorouracil 800 mg/m² IV continuous infusion over 24 hours on Days 1 and 2
	   ■ Cycled every 14 days for three cycles with radiation and three cycles after radiation

Regimens for induction or adjuvant chemotherapy	• ECF (epirubicin + cisplatin + fluorouracil):
	   ■ Epirubicin: 50 mg/m² IV on Day 1
	   ■ Cisplatin: 60 mg/m² IV on Day 1
	   ■ Fluorouracil: 200 mg/m² IV continuous infusion over 24 hours on Days 1–21
	   ■ Cycled every 21 days for three cycles preoperatively and three cycles postoperatively
	• Fluorouracil + cisplatin:
	   ■ Fluorouracil: 800 mg/m² IV continuous infusion over 24 hours on Days 1–5
	   ■ Cisplatin: 100 mg/m² IV on Day 1
	   ■ Cycled every 28 days for two to three cycles preoperatively and three to four cycles postoperatively for a total of six cycles
	• Paclitaxel + carboplatin:
	   ■ Paclitaxel: 175 mg/m² IV on Day 1
	   ■ Carboplatin: AUC 5 IV on Day 1
	   ■ Cycled every 21 days for two cycles preoperatively and two cycles postoperatively

Controversies

Lymph node dissection

Although there have been no strictly designed phase III trials, retrospective data from large samples with long-term follow-up have demonstrated that systemic lymph node dissection increases the accuracy of staging, and improves local control and survival of oesophageal SCC. One major change in the 7th edition of the UICC TNM staging system is that nodal status is stratified according to the number of nodes involved, instead of just as with or without nodal involvement as in the 6th edition. This requires that at least 12–15 lymph nodes are harvested for accurate staging. The extent of dissection should be tailored to the pattern of lymph node involvement according to the location and depth of invasion of the primary lesion, as well as patient's performance status. For SCC of the thoracic oesophagus invading beyond the submucosa (T1b or above), dissection of nodes along the bilateral recurrent nerves and those around the oesophagogastric junction and left gastric artery is mandatory. These nodes are often the first site of metastasis and carry a high rate of involvement. Neck (three-field) dissection may be beneficial for upper thoracic lesions and those with nodal involvement at the superior mediastinum. However, its oncological benefit must be weighed against the potential risks such as increased recurrent nerve palsy.

Minimal invasive oesophagectomy versus open oesophagectomy

There has been no consensus as to whether MIE is oncologically equivalent to open oesophagectomy. The published literature to date has shown that MIE may be superior to open thoracotomy in terms of perioperative morbidity, especially cardiopulmonary complications, and length of postoperative hospitalization. MIE is safe and applicable in early-stage lesions, and may be beneficial for patients with decreased cardiopulmonary reserve. The number of lymph nodes procured is comparable to that with open approaches. Generally speaking, MIE is a feasible option for surgically resectable patients, as long as the standard oncological and dissection principles of oesophagectomy are not compromised.

Neoadjuvant chemoradiation versus neoadjuvant chemotherapy

Neoadjuvant chemoradiation and chemotherapy have been used for locally-advanced oesophageal cancers. In a meta-analysis, both were shown to be beneficial in prolonging survival. The complete response rates are 20–30% after concurrent chemoradiation, but only 5–10% after chemotherapy alone. However, treatment-related morbidity and mortality are also much lower after chemotherapy. Another important factor is the extent of lymphatic spread. Lymph node metastasis in SCC of the thoracic oesophagus occurs early and may longitudinally involve the cervical, mediastinal and superior abdominal regions. This makes it difficult to encompass the entire range of lymphatic drainage in radiation field planning. For patients with multiple nodal metastases, especially those at multiple stations or in multiple fields, chemotherapy as a systemic treatment modality may be more appropriate.

Modalities utilized in endoscopic therapy for superficial SCC: EMR, ESD or ablation

There are three major reasons why EMR or ESD is favoured over ablation in SCC:

1. It is often difficult to differentiate between low-grade dysplasia and HGD, or between HGD and invasive SCC on biopsy specimen
2. In addition to the resection margin, histological confirmation of depth of invasion is mandatory for SCC, as lymphatic involvement is rare in HGD or T1a lesions but may occur in as high as 20–30% of cases of T1b
3. Superficial lesions of squamous cell histology are usually localized rather than diffuse, as in AC arising from Barrett's oesophagus.

Phase III clinical trials
See Table 24.4.

OESOPHAGEAL OR OESOPHAGOGASTRIC JUNCTION ADENOCARCINOMA

Treatment philosophy

The 7th UICC staging system designated that AC invading into the oesophagogastric junction should be staged and treated as oesophageal cancer. Most AC are located either in the lower thoracic oesophagus near or at the oesophagogastric junction. Treatment should be determined by location and staging of the tumour, as well as the general condition of the patient.

Table 24.4 Phase III clinical trials: Squamous cell carcinoma

Trial reference	Results
Kato et al. (1991) Ann Thorac Surg 51:931–935	• Three-field lymph node dissection increased survival for thoracic oesophageal carcinoma
Ando et al. (2003) J Clin Oncol 21:4592–4596	• Postoperative adjuvant chemotherapy with cisplatin and 5-fluorouracil (5-FU) is better than surgery alone in preventing relapse in oesophageal SCC
Bosset et al. (1997) N Engl J Med 337:161–167	• Preoperative chemoradiotherapy did not improve overall survival in squamous cell oesophageal cancer, but did prolong disease-free survival
Lee et al. (2004) Ann Oncol 5:947–954	• Although preoperative chemoradiotherapy induced high clinical and pathological responses, there was no statistically significant benefit in overall and disease-free survival
Ando et al. (2012) Ann Surg Oncol 19:68–74	• Preoperative chemotherapy with 5-FU/cisplatin improved 5-year survival as compared to postoperative adjuvant chemotherapy in SCC

Complete resection gives the best chance of cure for local diseases. Given that most AC located at the oesophagogastric junction originate from Barrett's oesophagus, endoscopic therapy is often the first-line treatment for superficial lesions. For locally-advanced diseases, effective induction with chemotherapy or concurrent chemoradiation helps down-stage the disease and improves the rate of radical resection and the probability of prolonged survival. Definitive chemoradiation is a reasonable alternative to surgery, especially in patients who are medically unfit for surgery. When treatment with curative intent is not feasible, either because of advanced disease or poor general condition of the patient, management should focus on restoring oral intake and improving quality of life. Palliative radiation and endoscopic procedures are often useful and effective in this setting.

Scenario: AC	Treatment philosophy
High-grade dysplasia	• Endoscopic therapy is recommended, including either EMR or ablation

T1a	• Endoscopic resection of all visible lesions, followed by ablation of residual Barrett's oesophagus
	• Oesophagectomy is reserved for:
	  ▪ Long-segment Barrett's oesophagus or a circumferential lesion when a high possibility of endoscopic therapeutic complications such as stricture formation is foreseen
	  ▪ High-risk patients (poorly differentiated tumour, LVI or suspicion of lymph node involvement)

(continued)

Scenario: AC	Treatment philosophy

T1bN0	- Oesophagectomy:
	  - Siewert tumour type should be assessed in all surgical candidates to determine the approach, extent of resection and lymph node dissection:
	    - Siewert type III lesions are considered gastric cancers (see also Chapter 25)
	  - Transthoracic approaches are preferred as they give more accurate staging
	- For those who are medically unfit for surgery, EMR followed by ablation should be considered:
	  - Concurrent chemoradiation may be considered for tumours with poor prognostic features (LVI, poorly differentiated histology, positive EMR margin and lesion size >2 cm)

T1bN+ T2–4aN0–N+	- Neoadjuvant treatment (chemotherapy or preferably concurrent chemoradiation) followed by surgery provides the best chance of cure - Definitive chemoradiation for patients who decline or who are unfit for surgery - Oesophagectomy could be the first choice in low-risk patients with lesions of <2 cm and well-differentiated histology, and without obvious nodal involvement. - Adjuvant chemoradiation, if not given preoperatively, is recommended after R1–R2 resection or if N+ disease is revealed after surgery: - Preoperative adjuvant chemotherapy is recommended - For patients who are medically unfit for surgery and unable to tolerate chemoradiation or chemotherapy, palliative radiation or best supportive care (BCS) should be considered
T4b	- Definitive chemoradiation, sequential or preferably concurrent - Palliative radiation or BCS for patients who are unable to tolerate chemotherapy
Metastatic disease	- Chemotherapy if Karnofsky performance score is ≥60 or ECOG performance score is ≤2 - BCS if Karnofsky performance score is <60 or ECOG performance score is ≥3
Recurrent disease	- For locoregional-only recurrence after surgery in patients not given preoperative chemotherapy or chemoradiation, concurrent chemoradiation or chemotherapy is recommended if the patient is medically fit: - Re-resection may be considered but is often difficult - Chemotherapy and/or BCS for distant metastasis

Follow-up	- If asymptomatic:
	  - Every 3–6 months for 1–2 years
	  - Every 6–12 months for 3–5 years
	  - Annually for >5 years
	- Imaging (including US, CT scan or barium swallow), upper GI endoscopy and blood chemistry profile, as clinically indicated
	- Tumour marker may be helpful

Treatment

Surgery and endoscopic intervention

Surgery and endoscopic intervention: AC	Description

High-grade dysplasia Barrett's oesophagus	- Endoscopic therapy:
	  - Barrett's oesophagus with HGD or histologically unidentifiable superficial lesions:
	    - Histologically-confirmed HGD and all visible lesions (focal nodules) should be resected, rather than ablated under endoscopy
	    - Complete removal of all Barrett's metaplastic epithelium by EMR or ablation is highly recommended (radiofrequency ablation [RFA], cryoablation, photodynamic therapy [PDT]). RFA is favoured because of its low risk of stenosis and high efficacy for complete eradication
	- Oesophagectomy:
	  - Reserved for patients who are unfit for endoscopic therapy or failure after endoscopic therapy
	  - Risk and benefit need to be carefully weighted, as oesophagectomy is associated with a much higher morbidity and mortality than endoscopic therapy (2% mortality, 40% in-hospital complications) and significant impact on quality of life

Surgery and endoscopic intervention: AC	Description

T1a	- Endoscopic therapy is recommended as the first-line therapy for low-risk patients (no evidence of LVI, lymph node metastasis or poorly differentiated histology):
	  - Endoscopic resection of all visible lesions, with total eradication of flat Barrett's epithelium with ablation or EMR
	  - Endoscopic US prior to EMR is recommended for accurate staging
	- Oesophagectomy:
	  - Reserved for high-risk patients: long-segment Barrett's oesophagus, visible lesions with characteristics of polypoid mass, or excavated or ulcerative lesions, LVI positive, suspected lymph node involvement, poorly differentiated histology
	  - Treatment failure or inappropriate indication of endoscopic therapy (high possibility of endoscopic therapeutic complications such as stricture)

T1bN0	- Oesophagectomy:
	  - Acceptable surgical approaches:
	    - Ivor–Lewis oesophagectomy (laparotomy + right thoracotomy) for middle/lower thoracic and Siewert type I tumour
	    - McKeown oesophagectomy (right thoracotomy + laparotomy + cervical anastomosis) for upper/middle thoracic tumour
	    - Sweet–Churchill oesophagectomy (left thoracic transdiaphragmatic approach) is a reasonable option for lower thoracic and Siewert type I tumour
	    - Laparotomy with total gastrectomy and distal oesophagectomy for Siewert type II tumour
	    - Transhiatal oesophagectomy (laparotomy + cervical anastomosis, with or without mediastinoscopy assistance): Similar survival results compared to transthoracic approaches have been reported, but staging may be less accurate
	    - Minimally invasive Ivor–Lewis or McKeown oesophagectomy (including hybrid procedures or robot assisted) is preferred as cardiopulmonary morbidity is lower
	  - Extent of lymph node dissection:
	    - Extensive lymph node dissection can ensure more accurate staging, but survival benefit is controversial
	- Endoscopic therapy is a reasonable alternative in patients who are unfit for surgery:
	  - Concurrent chemoradiation following endoscopic therapy should be considered in high-risk patients (LVI, poorly differentiated histology)

T1bN+
T2–4aN0–N+
	- *En bloc* resection with extensive lymph node dissection after induction therapies (chemotherapy or concurrent chemoradiation)
	- Oesophagectomy:
	  - Surgical approach:
	    - Compared with transhiatal oesophagectomy, the transthoracic approach can improve the accuracy of staging and locoregional disease control, but the survival benefit is less definite
	    - Transhiatal oesophagectomy is a reasonable choice for lower thoracic or Siewert I tumours after effective induction
	    - Laparoscopic total gastrectomy is recommended in Siewert type II tumours for better clearance of abdominal lymph nodes
	  - Lymph node dissection:
	    - Systemic lymph node dissection can ensure more accurate staging and better assessment of treatment response to induction therapies
	    - At least 12–15 lymph nodes should be removed to achieve adequate nodal staging in patients not given induction therapy

T4 M1	- Surgical resection is generally contraindicated - Palliative resection with residual tumour will lead to quick relapse and, possibly, poorer survival

Local recurrence	- Salvage oesophagectomy:
	  - Repeated endoscopic procedures are feasible for limited local recurrence after initial endoscopic therapy or metachronous superficial lesions (HGD/T1a)
	  - Local recurrence after oesophagectomy: re-resection of locally recurrent oesophageal carcinoma is technically demanding and associated with considerable morbidity:
	    - Long-term survival is possible in patients after complete re-resection
	  - Local recurrence after definitive chemoradiation: the morbidity and mortality of salvage oesophagectomy are higher than with oesophagectomy in the neoadjuvant setting:
	    - Long-term disease-free interval (>2 years) and good performance status predict a better prognosis

Radiotherapy

See Box 24.1.

Radiotherapy: AC	Description
Early disease (HGD and T1a)	• No role
T1bN0	• Concurrent chemoradiation only in patients who are unfit for surgery, or with poor prognostic factors after endoscopic therapy (LVI, poorly differentiated histology, positive EMR margin and/or maximum tumour diameter >2 cm)
T1bN+ T2–4aNx	• Radiation alone may be considered for those who are medically unfit for surgery, refuse surgery or unable to tolerate chemotherapy or chemoradiation, as palliative treatment • Concurrent chemoradiation is the most effective induction modality in down-staging, and significantly prolongs survival in responders • Definitive chemoradiation (concurrent or sequential) is an acceptable alternative for those who are medically unfit for or who decline surgery, with a curative intent
T4b	• Definitive chemoradiation is the standard treatment if the patient can tolerate it • Radiation alone may be used with palliative intent in patients who are unable to tolerate chemotherapy or chemoradiation
Postoperative radiation therapy	• Adjuvant chemoradiation is the standard of care for patients with a positive node revealed at surgery, or after R1 or R2 resection, if not given preoperatively • Radiation alone is only considered in patients who are unable to tolerate chemotherapy or chemoradiation
Metastatic disease	• Radiotherapy may be considered with palliative intent to relieve symptoms such as dysphagia or bone pain • Concurrent chemoradiation may be useful in selected cases of distant nodal involvement (supraclavicular or retroperitoneal)
Recurrent disease	• Concurrent chemoradiation is the most effective treatment for locoregional relapse after surgery, especially nodal recurrence, in patients without prior chemoradiation

Systemic therapy

See Table 24.3.

Systemic therapy: AC	Description
High-grade dysplasia Stage Ia	• No role
T1bN0	• Chemotherapy in conjunction with radiation may be considered for patients who are unfit for surgery or with poor prognostic features (LVI, poorly differentiated histology, positive EMR margin and lesion size >2 cm)
T1bN+ T2–4aNx	• Chemotherapy in conjunction with radiation (concurrent chemoradiation) is preferred to chemotherapy alone for induction • For patients who decline or who are unfit for surgery, concurrent chemoradiation is preferred for definitive treatment • Induction chemotherapy may prolong survival in responders: ▪ RR is lower than for concurrent chemoradiation (PCR 5–10%) but toxicity is also much lower • Preoperative adjuvant chemotherapy after radical resection is recommended
T4b	• In conjunction with radiation (concurrent chemoradiation)
Metastatic disease	• Chemotherapy if Karnofsky performance score of ≥60 or ECOG performance score of ≤2
Recurrent disease	• Chemotherapy alone or in conjunction with radiation is recommended for locoregional-only recurrence after surgery in patients who have not received prior chemotherapy or chemoradiation

Controversies

Endoscopic therapy: EMR, ESD or ablation
Unlike superficial lesions of squamous cell histology, early-stage AC of the distal oesophagus and oesophagogastric junction mostly arises from Barrett's epithelium and is caused by GERD. Therefore, as well as complete removal of the cancerous lesion, all Barrett's epithelium around these lesions should be treated effectively to remove occult synchronous lesions and sites with neoplastic potential. Close follow-up after endoscopic therapy is mandatory for evaluation of treatment results and detection of metachronous or recurrent tumour.

Extent of lymph node dissection
Pattern of lymphatic involvement in AC located at the distal oesophagus and oesophagogastric junction is different from that in SCC of the thoracic oesophagus. Metastasis in the neck and upper mediastinum is comparatively rare. On the other hand, involvement of abdominal nodes is a common phenomenon, making dissection of perigastric nodes important and mandatory for accurate staging and radical resection. For Siewert type II tumours, a D2 dissection including removal of coeliac nodes may be more desirable. Mediastinal involvement is reported to be as high as 20% in Siewert type I tumours, and dissection of para-oesophageal and subcarinal nodes in the mid and lower mediastinum through a transthoracic approach is recommended. Similarly, at least 12–15 nodes should be harvested to ensure the accuracy of staging.

Transhiatal oesophagectomy *or* transthoracic oesophagectomy
A variety of approaches have been used for distal oesophageal and oesophagogastric junction AC and there is no one-fit-for-all procedure. Selection of approach should be based on the following considerations:
1 To ensure a clear proximal and distal resection margin
2 To facilitate radical lymphadenectomy of potentially involved areas
3 To make an easy and safe reconstruction of the upper digestive tract.

Thus, Ivor–Lewis or THE is the most widely applied procedure for oesophagothoracic and Siewert type I tumours, whereas the TEE approach or laparotomy with distal oesophageal resection through the hiatus is preferred for most Siewert type II tumours.

Minimally invasive or open procedures
For oesophageal or Siewert type I AC, large single-centre experience and one multicentre phase II trial have shown that MIE is safe and feasible, with lower perioperative morbidity and mortality but similar oncological outcomes as compared to open oesophagectomy. For Siewert type II tumours, there are currently only sporadic small case reports for laparoscopic total gastrectomy with transhiatal distal oesophagectomy.

Phase III clinical trials
See Table 24.5.

Table 24.5 Phase III clinical trials: Adenocarcinoma

Trial reference	Results
Van Hagen et al. (2012) N Engl J Med 366:2074–2084	• Preoperative chemoradiotherapy improved survival among patients with potentially curable oesophageal or oesophagogastric junction cancer
Tepper et al. (2008) J Clin Oncol 26:1086–1092	• Long-term survival advantage with chemoradiotherapy followed by surgery
Ychou et al. (2011) J Clin Oncol 29:1715–1721	• In patients with resectable AC of the lower oesophagus and oesophagogastric junction, perioperative 5-FU/cisplatin chemotherapy significantly increased the curative resection rate, overall and disease-free survival
Burmeister et al. (2005) Lancet Oncol 6:659–668.	• Compared with surgery alone, preoperative 5-FU/cisplatin chemoradiotherapy does not improve overall or progression-free survival for patients with resectable oesophageal cancer
Stahl et al. (2009) J Clin Oncol 27:851–856	• Although the study was closed early, results pointed to a survival advantage for preoperative chemoradiotherapy compared with preoperative chemotherapy in AC of the oesophagogastric junction

Recommended reading

Allum WH, Stenning SP, Bancewicz J et al. (2009) Long-term results of a randomized trial of surgery with or without preoperative chemotherapy in esophageal cancer. *J Clin Oncol* 27:5062–5067.

Ando N, Iizuka T, Ide H et al. (2003) Surgery plus chemotherapy compared with surgery alone for localized squamous cell carcinoma of the thoracic esophagus: a Japan clinical oncology group study. *J Clin Oncol* 21:4592–4596.

Ando N, Kato H, Igaki H et al. (2012) A randomized trial comparing postoperative adjuvant chemotherapy with cisplatin and 5-fluorouracil versus preoperative chemotherapy for localized advanced squamous cell carcinoma of the thoracic esophagus. *Ann Surg Oncol* 19:68–74.

Bosset JF, Gignoux M, Triboulet JP et al. (1997) Chemoradiotherapy followed by surgery compared with surgery alone in squamous-cell cancer of the esophagus. *N Engl J Med* 337:161–167.

LBiere SS, van Berge Henegouwen MI, Maas KW et al. (2012) Minimally invasive versus open oesophagectomy for patients with oesophageal cancer: a multicentre, open-label, randomised controlled trial. Lancet 379:1887–1892.

Lee JL, Park SI, Kim SB et al. (2004) A single institutional phase III trial of preoperative chemotherapy with hyperfractionation radiotherapy plus surgery versus surgery alone for resectable esophageal squamous cell carcinoma. Ann Oncol 15:947–954.

Luketich JD, Pennathur A, Awais O et al. (2012) Outcomes after minimally invasive esophagectomy: review of over 1000 patients. Ann Surg 256:95–103.

Malthaner RA, Wong RK, Rumble RB et al. (2004) Neoadjuvant or adjuvant therapy for resectable esophageal cancer: a systematic review and meta-analysis. BMC Med 2:35.

Nguyen NT, Follette DM, Wolfe BM, Schneider PD, Roberts P, Goodnight JE Jr. (2000) Comparison of minimally invasive esophagectomy with transthoracic and transhiatal esophagectomy. Arch Surg 135:920–925.

Orringer MB, Marshall B, Chang AC. (2007) Two-thousand transhiatal esophagectomies. Ann Surg 246:363–374.

Pennathur A, Farkas A, Krasinskas AM et al. (2009) Esophagectomy for T1 esophageal cancer: outcomes in 100 patients and implications for endoscopic therapy. Ann Thorac Surg 87:1048–1055.

Pouliquen X, Levard H, Hay JM et al. (1996) 5-Fluorouracil and cisplatin therapy after palliative surgical resection of squamous cell carcinoma of the esophagus: a multicenter randomized trial. French Associations for Surgical Research. Ann Surg 223:127–133.

Siewert JR, Stein HJ. (1996) Adenocarcinoma of the gastroesophageal junction: classification, pathology and extent of resection. Dis Esophagus 9:173–182.

Siewert JR, Feith M, Werner M, Stein HJ (2006) Adenocarcinoma of the esophagogastric junction. Results of surgical therapy based on anatomical/topographic classification in 1,002 consecutive patients. Ann Surg 232:353–361.

Sjoquist KM, Burmeister BH, Smithers BM et al. (2011) Survival after neo-adjuvant chemotherapy or chemoradiotherapy for resectable oesophageal carcinoma: an updated meta-analysis. Lancet Oncol 12:681–692.

Tepper J, Krasna MJ, Niedzwiecki D et al. (2008) Phase III trial of trimodality therapy with cisplatin, fluorouracil, radiotherapy, and surgery compared with surgery alone for esophageal cancer. J Clin Oncol 26:1086–1092.

van Hagen P, Hulshof MC, van Lanschot JJ et al. (2012) Preoperative chemoradio-therapy for esophageal or junctional cancer. N Engl J Med 366:2074–2084.

Watanabe H, Kato H, Tachimori Y (2000) Significance of extended systemic lymph node dissection for thoracic esophageal carcinoma in Japan. Recent Res Cancer Res 155:123–133.

Xiao ZF, Yang ZY, Liang J et al. (2003) Value of radiotherapy after radical surgery for esophageal carcinoma: a report of 495 patients. Ann Thorac Surg 75:331–336.

Yamamoto H (2007) Technology insight: endoscopic submucosal dissection of gastrointestinal neoplasms. Nat Clin Pract Gastroenterol Hepatol 4:511–520.

25 Stomach

Takeshi Sano[1], Savtaj S. Brar[2], James Brierley[3] and Jan B. Vermorken[4]

[1]Cancer Institute Hospital, Tokyo, Japan
[2]Department of Surgery, Mount Sinai Hospital, Toronto, ON, Canada
[3]Department of Radiation Oncology, The Princess Margaret Cancer Centre, University of Toronto, Toronto, ON, Canada
[4]Department of Medical Oncology, Antwerp University Hospital, Edegem, Belgium

Summary	Key facts

Introduction	- *Incidence*:
	  - Fourth most common cancer worldwide
	  - Age-standardized incidence per 100,000: men 19.8 and women 9.1
	    - Age standardized death rates per 100,000: men 14.3 and women 6.9
	- *Epidemiology*:
	  - Large regional difference in incidence, decreasing worldwide:
	    - Highest in Eastern Asia, lowest in North America
	  - Persistent *Helicobacter pylori* infection is a known causative factor

Presentation	- *Local disease*:
	  - Peptic ulcer-like pain, anaemia, nausea, weight loss, dysphagia
	- *Metastatic disease*:
	  - Ascites, liver mass, Virchow's supraclavicular nodes, back pain

Scenario	- *Local disease*:
	  - Endoscopic resection for appropriately selected T1 tumours
	  - Gastrectomy with limited lymphadenectomy (D1 or D1+)
	- *Regional disease*:
	  - Gastrectomy with limited or extended lymphadenectomy (D1+ or D2)
	  - Pre- and/or post-operative chemotherapy or chemoradiotherapy
	- *Metastatic disease*:
	  - Systemic chemotherapy
	  - Palliative surgery for bleeding or obstructing tumours
	  - Stenting for stenosis at cardia or pylorus
	- *Follow-up*:
	  - No evidence of prognostic improvement by postoperative surveillance

Trials	- Dutch D1/D2 trial (n = 711; D1 vs D2 lymphadenectomy); Bonenkamp et al. (1999) *N Engl J Med* 340(12):908–14; Songun et al. (2010) *Lancet Oncol* 11(5):439–449
	  - No difference in overall survival but lower gastric cancer-related death rate in D2 group
	- INT0116 trial (n = 556; surgery vs adjuvant chemoradiotherapy); Macdonald et al. (2001) *N Engl J Med* 345(10):725–730; Smalley et al. (2012) *J Clin Oncol* 30(19):2327-2333:
	  - Adjuvant chemoradiotherapy significantly improved survival
	- MAGIC trial (n = 503; surgery vs perioperative chemotherapy); Cunningham et al. (2006) *N Engl J Med* 355(1):11–20:
	  - Perioperative chemotherapy significantly improved survival
	- ACTS-GC trial (n = 1059; surgery vs adjuvant chemotherapy); Sakuramoto et al. (2007) *N Engl J Med* 357(18):1810-1820; Sasako et al. (2001) *J Clin Oncol* 29(33):4387-4393:
	  - Postoperative chemotherapy significantly improved survival
	- ToGA trial (n = 594; chemotherapy with or without trastuzumab); Bang et al. (2010) *Lancet* 376:687–697:
	  - Trastuzumab significantly prolonged survival in patients with a metastatic HER2-positive tumour

UICC Manual of Clinical Oncology, Ninth Edition. Edited by Brian O'Sullivan, James D. Brierley, Anil K. D'Cruz, Martin F. Fey, Raphael Pollock, Jan B. Vermorken and Shao Hui Huang. © 2015 UICC. Published 2015 by John Wiley & Sons, Ltd.

Introduction

Cancer of the stomach arises from gastric mucosa and is mostly adenocarcinoma. Gastric cancer was once the most common cancer worldwide, but incidence is decreasing especially in developed countries. This trend seems to be closely related to the rapid decrease of *Helicobacter pylori* infection. In most countries, patients with gastric cancer frequently present with advanced disease and prognosis is generally poor. On the other hand, in Japan and Korea where the disease incidence is high and screening programmes with access to endoscopy are well established, gastric cancer is often diagnosed in early stages and the majority of new patients are cured by surgical or endoscopic treatment alone.

Incidence, aetiology and screening

Incidence, aetiology and screening	Description

Incidence	- Common cancer worldwide:
	  - Fourth most common cancer following lung, breast and colorectal cancer, with 0.9 million new patients per year (2008)
	  - Second most common cause of cancer death following lung cancer, with 0.7 million deaths per year (2008)
	  - Global incidence and death rate:
	    - Age standardized ratio (ASR) per 100,000 for men 19.8 and 14.3
	    - ASR per 100,000 for women 9.1 and 6.9
	- Large regional difference in incidence (ASR for men):
	  - High in Eastern Asia (42.4) and Central-Eastern Europe (22.2)
	  - Low in South-Central Asia (6.7), Western Europe (9) and USA (5.9)
	  - Approximately 60% arises in Eastern Asia (China, Japan, Korea, Mongolia)
	- Decreasing across the world:
	  - In proportion to the decrease of *H. pylori* infection rates

Aetiology	- Aetiology is multifactorial: pathogenic, environmental and host genetic factors are known:
	  - Hereditary gastric cancers seen in Lynch syndrome or hereditary diffuse gastric carcinoma (HDGC) syndrome account for only 1–3% of all gastric cancers
	- Chronic atrophic gastritis caused by persistent infection of *H. pylori* (Cag-A type) is the most important background for gastric carcinogenesis in the non-cardiac, distal stomach
	- Risk factors:
	  - Definite: *H. pylori* infection, smoking
	  - Probable: salt-preserved/high-salt foods
	  - Possible: processed meat, smoked and grilled meat, chili pepper

Screening	- Available only in high-incidence countries (Japan and South Korea):
	  - Double contrast barium study and/or endoscopy
	  - Selective endoscopy in people with seropositivity of *H. pylori* and positive pepsinogen test for atrophic gastritis
	- Mutations in the *CDH1* tumour suppressor gene (E-cadherin gene) are found in families of HDGC:
	  - Close endoscopic surveillance or prophylactic total gastrectomy is considered

Pathology

Gastric cancer is mostly adenocarcinoma originating from the glandular epithelium of the gastric mucosa. Non-epithelial tumours include gastrointestinal stromal tumour (GIST), smooth muscle tumour or neurogenic tumour. Compared with colorectal cancer, gastric carcinoma shows marked morphological diversity both macroscopically and histologically. Even within a single tumour, histological heterogeneity is quite common.

Pathology	Description

Intestinal type (Lauren)	• Histological features:
	  ▪ Characterized by a predominance of glandular epithelium with cells similar to intestinal columnar cells
	  ▪ Usually sharply demarcated by a pushing margin ('expanding type' as per Ming's classification)
	• Common clinical features:
	  ▪ Arises in older patients, located in the distal stomach, forms Borrmann type I or II, and metastasizes to the liver
	• Mostly corresponds to papillary and tubular adenocarcinoma in the Japanese classification

Diffuse type (Lauren)	• Histological features:
	  ▪ Composed of scattered, poorly cohesive cells or small clusters of cells with wide and diffuse infiltration:
	    ○ Cells may contain mucus and can show typical signet ring cell appearance
	  ▪ Usually diffusely spreading with an ill-demarcated margin ('infiltrating type' as per Ming's classification)
	• Common clinical features:
	  ▪ Arises in younger patients, located in the proximal gastric body, forms Borrmann type III or IV, and metastasizes to the peritoneum
	• Mostly corresponds to poorly differentiated adenocarcinoma, signet ring cell carcinoma and mucinous adenocarcinoma in the Japanese classification

Mixed type	• Lauren's intestinal-type and diffuse-type structures often co-exist in a tumour:
	  ▪ For clinical purposes, these tumours are usually classified as diffuse type
	  ▪ For epidemiological and histogenetic studies, they may be classified according to the predominant structures

Other classifications	• Histological grading (TNM classification):
	  ▪ G1: well differentiated
	  ▪ G2: moderately differentiated
	  ▪ G3: poorly differentiated
	  ▪ G4: undifferentiated
	  ▪ G1 and G2 can be grouped as low grade, G3 and G4 as high grade
	  ▪ In mixed type tumours, the highest grade determines the category

Natural history

Gastric carcinoma arises in the mucosa and seldom metastasizes until it penetrates the muscularis mucosae. Risk of lymph node metastasis, the most common type of metastasis in gastric cancer, begins when the tumour invades the submucosa, and becomes more frequent and extensive as the tumour invades deeper. Extensive lymphatic spread often results in systemic disease such as bone or lung metastasis. Once the tumour penetrates the serosa, peritoneal dissemination becomes common, especially in diffuse-type tumours. Liver metastasis occurs predominantly in intestinal-type tumours. When a tumour directly infiltrates the retroperitoneum, it may spread within this space and obstruct the urinary tract and/or rectum causing 'frozen pelvis'.

Natural history		Description

Presentation	Local	• *Early disease*:
		  ▪ Usually asymptomatic and incidentally detected during endoscopy for dyspeptic/reflux disease
		  ▪ Peptic ulcer symptoms (hunger pain relieved by meals) or bleeding due to peptic ulceration in superficial gastric cancer
		• *Advanced disease*:
		  ▪ Anaemia due to chronic or active tumour bleeding
		  ▪ Early satiety, nausea, vomiting, appetite loss, weight loss, due to obstructive tumour or gastric motility disturbance
		  ▪ Palpable mass in the upper abdomen

	Metastatic	• Ascites • Back pain due to retroperitoneal tumour invasion (sometimes causing hydronephrosis) or para-aortic lymph node involvement • Palpable liver mass or lymph nodes in the left supraclavicular fossa (Virchow's nodes) • Jaundice due to direct or lymphatic invasion of the hepatoduodenal ligament

(continued)

Natural history		Description

Routes of spread	Local	• Direct tumour invasion:
		   ▪ Contiguous extension: oesophagus, duodenum, lesser/greater omenta
		   ▪ Trans-serosal invasion to adjacent organs: liver, pancreas, colon, diaphragm, hepatoduodenal ligament
		   ▪ Retroperitoneal infiltration: left adrenal gland, ureters

	Regional	• Lymph node metastasis: ▪ Perigastric nodes → those around the coeliac axis and its branches → para-aortic nodes → thoracic duct → venous circulation

	Metastatic	• Liver metastasis:
		   ▪ Via portal vein
		• Peritoneal metastasis:
		   ▪ Trans-serosal tumour dissemination
		• Extra-abdominal metastasis (lung, bone, skin):
		   ▪ Haematogenous route via either the portal vein or the lymphatic thoracic duct
		   ▪ Lymphatic or direct infiltration to the lung and/or pleura

Diagnostic work-up

Diagnostic work-up	Description

Work-up	• For primary tumour assessment:
	   ▪ Endoscopy with biopsy is the first and definitive diagnostic modality
	   ▪ Double contrast barium swallow is complementary: can be useful for the diagnosis of linitis plastica
	   ▪ Endoscopic ultrasonography (EUS) is useful for T staging and diagnosis of perigastric lymphadenopathy
	• For assessment of metastasis:
	   ▪ Computed tomography (CT)
	   ▪ Abdominal ultrasonography
	   ▪ Magnetic resonance imaging (MRI) is complementary: can be useful to detect liver and bone lesions
	   ▪ Staging laparoscopy with peritoneal cytology
	   ▪ Value of fluorodeoxyglucose-positron emission tomography (FDG-PET) is relatively limited due to low sensitivity in histologically diffuse tumours
	• Patient assessment before surgery:
	   ▪ American Society of Anesthesiologists (ASA) classification score
	   ▪ Electrocardiography (ECG) and stress testing
	   ▪ Chest X-ray and pulmonary function testing
	• Patient assessment before chemotherapy:
	   ▪ ECOG performance status
	   ▪ Neutrophil counts and creatinine clearance in addition to routine blood chemistry

Tumour markers	• CEA, CA19-9, CA72-4:
	   ▪ Serum levels are associated with tumour stage and patient survival
	   ▪ No role in screening, but useful for detecting recurrence and distant metastasis
	• CA125, sialyl Tn antigens (STN):
	   ▪ Often elevated in peritoneal metastasis

Staging and prognostic grouping

UICC TNM staging

T category is defined according to the depth of tumour invasion (Table 25.1). Distinction between T1a (tumour invades lamina propria) and T1b (tumour invades submucosa) is essential for considering the indication of endoscopic tumour resection. N category is defined according to the number of regional lymph node metastasis. Metastasis in non-regional lymph nodes such as the retropancreatic or para-aortic is M1 disease. It is recommended that at least 16 lymph nodes are examined for N staging. When peritoneal cytology reveals cancer cells, it is categorized as M1, and in this setting surgery is R1.

Prognostic risk factors

See Table 25.2.

Table 25.1 UICC TNM categories and stage grouping: Stomach

TNM categories

T1	Lamina propria (T1a), submucosa (T1b)
T2	Muscularis propria
T3	Subserosa
T4a	Perforates serosa
T4b	Adjacent structures
N1	1–2 nodes N2
	3–6 nodes N3a
	7–15 nodes N3b
	16 or more
M1	Distant metastasis

Stage grouping

Stage 0	Tis	N0	M0
Stage IA	T1	N0	M0
Stage IB	T2	N0	M0
	T1	N1	M0
Stage IIA	T3	N0	M0
	T2	N1	M0
	T1	N2	M0
Stage IIB	T4a	N0	M0
	T3	N1	M0
	T2	N2	M0
	T1	N3	M0
Stage IIIA	T4a	N1	M0
	T3	N2	M0
	T2	N3	M0
Stage IIIB	T4b	N0, N1	M0
	T4a	N2	M0
	T3	N3	M0
Stage IIIC	T4a	N3	M0
	T4b	N2, N3	M0
Stage IV	Any T	Any N	M1

Table 25.2 Prognostic factors for survival in gastric adenocarcinoma

Prognostic factors	Tumour related	Host related	Environment related
Essential	T category N category M category HER2 status		Residual disease: R0, R1 or R2
Additional	Tumour site: cardia or distal stomach Histological type Vessel infiltration	Age	Extent of resection
New and promising	Molecular profile	Race: Asian or non-Asian	

Adapted from NCCN Clinical Practice Guidelines in Oncology: Esophageal and Esophago-gastric Junction Cancers. Version 1.2013 NCCN.org.

R0 resection is essential for cure. Adjuvant and/or neoadjuvant chemotherapy improves survival after R0 resection of T2–4 gastric cancer. Several studies focusing on ethnicity show the survival of Asian gastric cancer patients is better than it is for non-Asian patients treated in the same institution or region.

Treatment philosophy

Surgery plays the central role in the treatment of potentially curable gastric cancer. Surgical treatment should consist of gastrectomy with adequate resection margins and appropriate lymphadenectomy. Pre- and/or post-operative chemotherapy or chemoradiotherapy should be considered according to tumour stage. Careful tumour assessment and multidisciplinary team evaluation are essential for the determination of the treatment strategy.

For advanced disease with unresectable local extension or distant metastasis, chemotherapy should be considered first. Palliative surgery should be limited to obstructive or bleeding tumours. Non-curative, reduction surgery has no evidence of survival benefit and may simply reduce patient quality of life and chemotherapy compliance.

Scenario	Treatment philosophy
Local disease only	• Endoscopic resection (endoscopic submucosal dissection [ESD]): 　▪ T1 gastric cancers satisfying specific criteria (see Treatment section) 　▪ Histological confirmation of the resected specimen is mandatory • Gastrectomy with limited lymphadenectomy (D1/D1+): 　▪ Sufficient resection margin of the stomach 　▪ Histological examination of at least 16 nodes for proper staging

Scenario	Treatment philosophy

Regional	• Gastrectomy with lymphadenectomy (D1/D1+):
	  ▪ R0 resection
	  ▪ Postoperative adjuvant chemotherapy or chemoradiotherapy to be considered
	• Gastrectomy with extended lymphadenectomy (D2):
	  ▪ By experienced surgeons at high-volume centres
	  ▪ Postoperative adjuvant chemotherapy to be considered
	• Neoadjuvant chemotherapy:
	  ▪ Followed by gastrectomy with lymphadenectomy (D1/D1+/D2) and postoperative chemotherapy
	  ▪ Pretreatment staging laparoscopy to be considered to rule out peritoneal metastasis

Metastatic	• Systemic chemotherapy
	• Palliative surgery:
	  ▪ Gastrectomy for bleeding and/or obstructing tumours
	  ▪ Gastro-jejunostomy for obstructing tumours
	• Radical surgery in exceptional situations:
	  ▪ E.g. solitary liver metastasis
	• Stenting for stenosis:
	  ▪ Cardia or pyloric stenosis

Recurrent	• Systemic chemotherapy • Palliative surgery: ▪ Bypass or ileostomy/colostomy for obstruction • Radical surgery in exceptional situations, e.g. solitary liver metastasis

Follow-up	• After curative endoscopic resection for T1a tumours:
	  ▪ Annual endoscopy for local recurrence or new lesions
	  ▪ Abdominal US or CT for regional recurrence
	• After R0 surgery for Stage I disease:
	  ▪ Annual abdominal US or CT and tumour markers
	  ▪ Biennial endoscopy of the remnant stomach
	• After R0 surgery for Stage II/III disease:
	  ▪ Biannual abdominal US or CT and tumour markers
	  ▪ Biennial endoscopy of the remnant stomach

Treatment

Surgery

Surgery and endoscopic resection	Description

Early disease	• Note that T1 disease is often underestimated by endoscopy or EUS and that absence of lymph node metastasis cannot be determined during surgery
	• Gastrectomy with D1 or D1+ lymphadenectomy:
	  ▪ Distal gastrectomy for tumours in the distal two-thirds
	  ▪ Total gastrectomy for tumours involving the proximal one-third
	  ▪ Proximal gastrectomy for tumours limited to the proximal one-third
	  ▪ Option: pylorus-preserving gastrectomy for tumours limited to the middle one-third
	  ▪ Dissection of the perigastric nodes and those along the left gastric artery
	
	Endoscopic resection
	• Endoscopic mucosal resection (EMR) or ESD:
	  ▪ Tumours that satisfy all the following criteria have a very low possibility of lymph node metastasis ('absolute indications' for endoscopic resection):
	    ○ Differentiated adenocarcinoma without ulcerative findings
	    ○ Depth of invasion is mucosa (this should be confirmed histologically on the resected specimen)
	    ○ 2 cm or smaller in diameter

Surgery and endoscopic resection	Description
	■ Experienced endoscopists may apply ESD to the following tumours ('expanded indications'): 　○ T1a, differentiated type, no ulcerative findings, >2 cm in diameter 　○ T1a, differentiated type, with ulcerative findings, ≤3 cm in diameter 　○ T1a, undifferentiated type, no ulcerative findings, ≤2 cm in diameter
Advanced non-metastatic disease	• Gastrectomy with D2 lymphadenectomy: 　■ Technically demanding procedure and consideration should be given to it being performed by an experienced surgeon at a specialized institution 　■ Distal or total gastrectomy with sufficient resection margins (grossly 5 cm) 　■ Total gastrectomy with lower oesophagectomy for Siewert type III tumour with limited oesophageal invasion 　■ In addition to the perigastric and left gastric artery lymph nodes, those along the hepatic and splenic artery should be dissected 　■ Splenectomy or pancreato-splenectomy is associated with high operative morbidity and mortality 　　○ Procedure should be limited to the tumours directly infiltrating these organs in which combined resection is necessary for R0 resection 　■ For tumours invading the pancreatic head, pancreato-duodenectomy may be considered only when R0 resection can be achieved, but this scenario is rare • Gastrectomy with D0/D1 lymphadenectomy followed by chemoradiotherapy: 　■ In the situation where D2 gastrectomy cannot be safely performed
Metastatic	• Palliative surgery is associated with high operative morbidity and mortality 　■ Should be considered only for fit patients with urgent symptoms such as bleeding or obstruction • Palliative gastrectomy: 　■ Distal gastrectomy for obstructing and/or bleeding distal tumours • Bypass surgery for obstructing tumours: 　■ Gastro-jejunostomy for distal tumours 　■ Ileostomy or colostomy for bowel obstruction

Radiotherapy

Radiotherapy	Description
Advanced non-metastatic disease	• Adjuvant chemoradiotherapy after curative gastrectomy with limited lymphadenectomy (D0/D1): 　■ 4500 cGy in 25 fractions, 5 days per week 　■ Fluorouracil 425 mg/m^2 + leucovorin 20 mg/m^2 for 5 days, before and after chemoradiotherapy • Trials of preoperative chemoradiation are underway but are considered experimental
Metastatic disease	• Palliative irradiation: 　■ Chronic continuous bleeding from unresectable gastric cancer may be stopped by irradiation 　■ Pain: local or from metastases, especially bone

Systemic therapy

Systemic therapy	Description
Advanced non-metastatic	• Perioperative chemotherapy (three cycles preoperatively and three cycles postoperatively): 　■ ECF (epirubicin + cisplatin + fluorouracil): 　　○ Epirubicin: 50 mg/m^2 IV on Day 1 　　○ Cisplatin: 60 mg/m^2 IV on Day 1 　　○ Fluorouracil: 200 mg/m^2 IV continuous infusion over 24 hours on Days 1–21

(continued)

Systemic therapy	Description

	- ECF modifications:
	  - EOF: oxaliplatin 130 mg/m² IV on Day 1 instead of cisplatin
	  - ECX: capecitabine 625 mg/m² PO b.i.d. on Days 1–21 instead of fluorouracil
	  - EOX: oxaliplatin + capecitabine instead of cisplatin + fluorouracil
	- Postoperative chemotherapy after D2 gastrectomy:
	  - Capecitabine + oxaliplatin (cycled every 21 days for eight cycles):
	    - Capecitabine: 1000 mg/m² PO b.i.d. on Days 1–14
	    - Oxaliplatin: 130 mg/m² IV on Day 1
	  - S-1 (cycled every 42 days for eight cycles):
	    - S-1 given 80–120 mg/m² PO b.i.d. on Days 1–28 in Asian population
	    - Dose may need to be carefully adjusted because of possible difference in pharmacokinetics

Metastatic disease	- Two-drug regimens are preferred
	- Three-drug regimens are reserved for medically fit patients with good performance status
	- Trastuzumab can be added for HER2-positive adenocarcinoma:
	  - Trastuzumab with chemotherapy (capecitabine + cisplatin [XP] or 5-fluorouracil + cisplatin [FP])
	    - Trastuzumab: 8 mg/kg IV on Day 1 of cycle 1, then 6 mg/kg IV every 21 days
	- First-line therapy:
	  - DCF (docetaxel + cisplatin + fluorouracil, cycled every 21 days):
	    - Docetaxel: 75 mg/m² IV on Day 1
	    - Cisplatin: 75 mg/m² IV on Day 1
	    - Fluorouracil: 750 mg/m² IV continuous infusion over 24 hours on Days 1–5
	  - DCF modifications in dose or drugs
	  - ECF and ECF modifications (see Perigastric chemotherapy above)
	  - FP (cycled every 28 days):
	    - Cisplatin: 100 mg/m² IV on Day 1
	    - Fluorouracil: 1000 mg/m² IV continuous infusion over 24 hours daily on Days 1–5
	  - XP (cycled every 21 days):
	    - Cisplatin: 80 mg/m² IV on Day 1
	    - Capecitabine: 1000 mg/m² PO b.i.d. on Days 1–14
	- Second-line therapy: selection depends on prior therapy and performance status:
	  - Docetaxel: 75–100 mg/m² IV on Day 1, cycled every 21 days
	  - Paclitaxel: 80 mg/m² IV on Days 1, 8 and 15 every 4 weeks
	  - Irinotecan: 150 mg/m² IV on Days 1 and 15 every 4 weeks

Controversies

D1, D2 or more lymphadenectomy for potentially curable gastric cancer

D2 lymphadenectomy was proposed by Japanese surgeons in 1960s, but its efficacy was not properly evaluated until the Dutch D1/D2 and the British MRC D1/D2 trials started in the late 1980s. Both trials failed to show survival benefit for D2, but highlighted significant operative morbidity and mortality mostly related to pancreato-splenectomy which was a necessary part of D2 for total gastrectomy in these trials. Modified D2 without splenectomy was carefully introduced by specialist surgeons in the West achieving low operative mortality, and the 15-year follow-up of the Dutch trial showed significantly reduced gastric cancer deaths in the D2 group. Currently, the ESMO guidelines and the NCCN guidelines recommend D2 lymphadenectomy for potentially curable gastric cancer by specialist surgeons in high-volume centres. More extended lymphadenectomy, D2 + para-aortic dissection, was studied in a Japanese randomized trial and its superiority over D2 alone was rejected.

Transhiatal or transthoracic approach for oesophagogastric junctional tumours

The surgical approach to oesophagogastric tumours is controversial. A Japanese randomized trial for Siewert types II and III showed that the left thoracoabdominal approach had higher operative morbidity but lower survival than the transhiatal approach, especially in Siewert type III tumours. In contrast, a Dutch randomized trial comparing right thoracotomy and the transhiatal approach to the lower oesophageal adenocarcinoma (Siewert types I and II) suggested survival benefits from thoracotomy, especially in Siewert type I tumours with a limited number of lymph node metastasis. In both trials, survival with Siewert type II tumours was similar between the transhiatal and the transthoracic approaches. Middle-to-lower mediastinal lymphadenectomy seems necessary for type I oesophageal carcinoma, but is too invasive and adds little benefit for type III gastric cancer.

Pre- or post-operative chemotherapy or chemoradiotherapy for potentially curable gastric cancer

Following the three pivotal randomized trials listed below, various regimens of chemotherapy or chemoradiotherapy are being evaluated in either peri- or post-operative settings. Preoperative chemotherapy is becoming increasingly favoured and almost all ongoing phase III trials have been designed with at least an arm of preoperative therapy. Three-drug regimens are used in many trials in an attempt to achieve down-grading and down-sizing of the tumour. Exclusion of patients with peritoneal disease by staging laparoscopy is essential for radiotherapy. The best multimodal approach should be sought by carefully designed randomized trials with clear targets.

Phase III clinical trials

See Table 25.3.

Table 25.3 Phase III clinical trials

Trial name	Results
Local disease	
Dutch D1/D2 trial Bonenkamp et al. (1999) N Engl J Med 340(12):908–14; Songun et al. (2010) Lancet Oncol 11(5):439–449	• 996 patients were randomized before surgery and 711 underwent curative resection (380 D1, 331 D2) at 80 hospitals. No adjuvant therapy was given: 　▪ A Japanese specialist surgeon participated in D2 training 　▪ Operative morbidity/mortality were significantly higher in the D2 group (43% vs 10%) than in the D1 group (25% vs 4%) 　▪ Morbidity/mortality in the D2 group was mostly attributed to splenectomy • No significant difference in overall survival (OS) between the groups • 15-year follow-up showed significantly lower locoregional recurrence and gastric cancer-related death rates in D2 than in D1
Taipei D1/D3 trial Wu et al. (2006) Lancet Oncol 7(4):309–315	• 221 patients were randomized after surgical exploration (110 D1, 111 D3) at a single institution. No adjuvant therapy was given: 　▪ 'D3' in this trial is almost identical to D2 in the current Japanese classification 　▪ Three experienced surgeons performed the surgery 　▪ There were no operative deaths in the trial • 5-year OS was significantly better in D3 than in D1
JCOG9501 trial Sasako et al. (2008) N Engl J Med 359(5):453–462	• 523 patients were randomized after surgical exploration (263 D2, 260 D2 + para-aortic nodal dissection [PAND]) at 24 Japanese institutions. No adjuvant therapy was given: 　▪ Operative morbidity was slightly higher in D2 + PAND group (28% vs 21%) but mortality was 0.8% in both groups • No difference in overall or recurrence-free survival between the groups
Adjuvant systemic treatment	
INT0116 Macdonald et al. (2001) N Engl J Med 345(10):725–730; Smalley et al. (2012) J Clin Oncol 30(19):2327–2333	• 556 patients (pathological Stage IB to IV/M0, after R0 resection) were randomized to surgery only or to surgery + chemoradiotherapy (45 Gy): 　▪ Majority of patients underwent limited lymphadenectomy (54% D0, 36% D1, 10% D2) 　▪ 85% had histological lymph node metastasis • 3-year median survival time and survival of adjuvant chemoradiotherapy group (36 months, 50%) were significantly better than in the surgery-only group (27 months, 41%): 　▪ First site of recurrence was more locoregional in the surgery-only group 　▪ Significant survival advantage was confirmed after 10-year follow-up
MAGIC trial Cunningham et al. (2006) N Engl J Med 355(1):11–20	• 503 patients (clinical Stages II–IV/M0) were randomized to either surgery only or to perioperative chemotherapy (ECF × 3 + surgery + ECF × 3): 　▪ Lower oesophageal adenocarcinoma was included in the last part of the trial • 5-year overall and progression-free survival rates were significantly better in the chemotherapy group (OS 36.3%) than in surgery-only group (OS 23.0%). 　▪ 28% of the surgery-only group turned out to be non-curative at laparotomy 　▪ Operative mortality was similar between the groups 　▪ Postoperative chemotherapy was completed in 41.6% of the group

(continued)

Table 25.3 (Continued)

Trial name	Results
ACTS-GC Sakuramoto et al. (2007) N Engl J Med 357(18):1810–1020, Sasako et al. (2011) J Clin Oncol 29(33):4387–4393	• 1059 patients (pathological Stages II and III, after D2 gastrectomy) were randomized to surgery only or to adjuvant S-1 chemotherapy: ▪ For enrolment peritoneal lavage cytology had to be negative for cancer ▪ 89% had histological lymph node metastasis • 3-year OS rate was significantly better in the chemotherapy group (80.1%) than in surgery only group (70.1%): ▪ Significant survival advantage was confirmed after 5-year follow-up (5-year OS 71.7% vs 61.1%)
Advanced and metastatic disease	
ToGA trial Bang et al. (2010) Lancet 376:687–697	• 594 patients with metastatic disease and HER2 positive were randomized to trastuzumab + chemotherapy or chemotherapy alone: ▪ 22% of all patients screened were HER2 positive ▪ 73.7% of randomized patients had intestinal-type cancer • OS was significantly better with trastuzamab + chemotherapy than chemotherapy alone (median 13.8 vs 11.1 months) ▪ Trastuzamab + chemotherapy was associated with improved progression-free survival ▪ High expression of HER2 protein was associated with better survival in patients treated with trastuzamab + chemotherapy compared to low expression
REAL-2 Cunningham et al. (2008) N Engl J Med 358(1):36–46	• 1002 patients (unresectable or metastatic) were randomized in a two-by-two trial design to three-drug chemotherapy (ECF or ECX vs EOF or EOX): ▪ Included patients with oesophageal and oesophagogastric junction cancer but most patients had adenocarcinoma ▪ 77.3% of patients had metastatic disease • OS was improved with EOX (11.2 months) compared to ECF (9.9 months) in secondary analysis: ▪ Non-inferiority of capecitabine and oxaliplatin compared with FP in primary analysis ▪ 1-year survival with ECF, ECX, EOF and EOX was 37.7%, 40.8%, 40.4% and 46.8%, respectively
Second-line RCT Kang et al. (2012) J Clin Oncol 30(13):1513–1518	• 202 patients with metastatic disease were randomized (2:1) to receive second-line chemotherapy (SLC; docetaxel or irinotecan) or best supportive care (BSC) ▪ All failed prior treatment with one- or two-drug chemotherapy regimens ▪ 59% had responded to prior chemotherapy with subsequent failure • OS (median) was better with SLC (5.3 months) than with BSC (3.8 months): ▪ No significant difference in OS between irinotecan and docetaxel ▪ Subsequent therapy beyond doxetacel/irinotecan was given to 40% of patients in the SLC arm and 22% in the BSC arm: ○ Increased OS (median 8.0 vs 3.7 months)

Areas of research

Molecular targeted therapy

As of 2013, trastuzumab for HER2-positive tumours is the only molecular targeted agent with established evidence of survival benefit in patients with gastric cancer. Numerous randomized trials using various agents have failed to show survival benefit, partly because of the heterogeneous nature of gastric tumours. Combination or sequential therapies will be further tested.

Recommended reading

Bang YJ, Cutsem EV, Feyereislova A et al. (2010) Trastuzumab in combination with chemotherapy versus chemotherapy alone for treatment of HER2-positive advanced gastric or gastro-oesophageal junction cancer (ToGA): a phase 3, open-label, randomized controlled trial. Lancet 376:687–697.

Cunningham D, Allum WH, Stenning SP et al. (2006) Perioperative chemotherapy versus surgery alone for resectable gastroesophageal cancer. N Engl J Med 355(1):11–20.

Cunningham D, Starling N, Rao S et al. (2008) Capecitabine and oxaliplatin of advanced esophagogastric cancer. N Engl J Med 358(1):36–46.

Degiuli M, Sasako M, Ponti A et al. (2014) Randomized clinical trial comparing survival after D1 or D2 gastrectomy for gastric cancer. Br J Surg 101(2):23–23.

Gotoda T, Yanagisawa A, Sasako M et al. (2000) Incidence of lymph node metastasis from early gastric cancer: estimation with a large number of cases at two large centers. Gastric Cancer 3(4):219–225.

Hiki N, Nunobe S, Kubota T et al. (2013) Function-preserving gastrectomy for early gastric cancer. Ann Surg Oncol 20(8):2683–2692.

Isomoto H, Shikuwa S, Yamaguchi N et al. (2009) Endoscopic submucosal dissection for early gastric cancer: a large-scale feasibility study. Gut 58(3):331–336.

Japanese Gastric Cancer Association (2011) Japanese gastric cancer treatment guidelines version 3. *Gastric Cancer* 14(2):113–123.

Jeurnink SM, Steyerberg EW, van Hooft JE *et al.* (2010) Surgical gastrojejunostomy or endoscopic stent placement for the palliation of malignant gastric outlet obstruction (SUSTENT study): a multicenter randomized trial. *Gastrointest Endosc* 71(3):490–499.

Kang JH, Lee SI, Lim DH *et al.* (2012) Salvage chemotherapy for pretreated gastric cancer: a randomized phase III trial comparing chemotherapy plus best supportive care with best supportive care alone. *J Clin Oncol* 30(13):1513–1518.

Leake PA, Cardoso R, Seevaratnam R *et al.* (2012) A systematic review of the accuracy and utility of peritoneal cytology in patients with gastric cancer. *Gastric Cancer* 15(Suppl 1):S27–37.

Lee J, Lim DH, Kim S *et al.* (2012) Phase III trial comparing capecitabine plus cisplatin versus capecitabine plus cisplatin with concurrent capecitabine radiotherapy in completely resected gastric cancer with D2 lymph node dissection: the ARTIST trial. *J Clin Oncol* 30(3):268–273.

Macdonald JS, Smalley SR, Benedetti J *et al.* (2001) Chemoradiotherapy after surgery compared with surgery alone for adenocarcinoma of the stomach or gastroesophageal junction. *N Engl J Med* 345(10):725–730.

NCCN Treatment Guidelines in Oncology: Gastric Cancer Version 2.2013. Available at NCCN.org

Omloo JM, Lagarde SM, Hulscher JB *et al.* (2007) Extended transthoracic resection compared with limited transhiatal resection for adenocarcinoma of the mid/distal esophagus: five-year survival of a randomized clinical trial. *Ann Surg* 246(6):992–1000.

Sakuramoto S, Sasako M, Yamaguchi T *et al.* (2007) Adjuvant chemotherapy for gastric cancer with S-1, an oral fluoropyrimidine. *N Engl J Med* 357(18):1810–1820.

Sasako M, Sano T, Yamamoto S *et al.* (2006) Left thoracoabdominal approach versus abdominal-transhiatal approach for gastric cancer of the cardia or subcardia: a randomised controlled trial. *Lancet Oncol* 7(8):644–651.

Sasako M, Sano T, Yamamoto S *et al.* (2006) D2 lymphadenectomy alone or with para-aortic nodal dissection for gastric cancer. *N Engl J Med* 359(5):453–462.

Songun H, Putter EMK, Kranenbarg M *et al.* (2010) Surgical treatment of gastric cancer: 15-year follow-up results of the randomised nationwide Dutch D1D2 trial. *Lancet Oncol* 11(5):439–449.

Wu CW, Hsiung CA, Lo S *et al.* (2006) Nodal dissection for patients with gastric cancer: a randomised controlled trial. *Lancet Oncol* 7(4):309–315.

26.1 Colon and rectum

Rob Glynne-Jones[1], Gina Brown[2], Ian Chau[2] and Brendan J. Moran[3]

[1]Radiotherapy Department, Mount Vernon Centre for Cancer Treatment, Mount Vernon Hospital, Northwood, UK
[2]Department of Radiology, Royal Marsden Hospital, London & Surrey, UK
[3]Department of Surgery, Hampshire Hospitals Foundation Trust, Basingstoke, Hampshire, UK

Summary	Key facts
Introduction	- Colorectal cancer (CRC) is the third commonest cancer worldwide after lung and breast cancer - CRC is the second commonest cause of death after lung cancer and was responsible for >200,000 deaths in Europe in 2008 - Median age at diagnosis is >70 years
Presentation	- Up to 20% of CRC still presents as an emergency, usually as obstruction **Colon cancer** - Early stages of CRC may be asymptomatic or be associated with vague abdominal discomfort and flatulence, minor changes in bowel habit, with or without rectal bleeding - Left-sided colonic cancer may cause constipation alternating with diarrhoea, nausea and vomiting, abdominal pain, loss of weight, rectal bleeding and obstructive symptoms - Right-sided colon cancer tends more commonly to cause vague discomfort and an abdominal mass, anaemia as a result of chronic blood loss, fatigue and weight loss **Rectal cancer** - Rectal bleeding, change in bowel habit, frequency of defaecation, pain and anaemia are common: - These symptoms are not specific and occur frequently in benign conditions
Scenario	**Colon cancer** - *Localized*: surgery - *Regional*: chemotherapy prolongs survival if nodal involvement - *Metastatic*: role for surgery if oligometastatic. Otherwise systemic therapy **Rectal cancer** - *Localized*: surgery - *Regional*: preoperative adjuvant therapy - *Metastatic*: role for surgery if oligometastatic; otherwise systemic therapy

Trials	**Colon cancer**
	- André *et al*. (2009) *J Clin Oncol* 27:3109–3116:
	  - Adding oxaliplatin to 5FU significantly improved 5-year disease-free survival and 6-year overall survival in the adjuvant treatment of Stage II or III colon cancer
	- Alberts *et al*. (2012) *JAMA* 307:1383–1393:
	  - For patients with Stage III resected colon cancer, cetuximab with adjuvant mFOLFOX6 compared with mFOLFOX6 alone did not result in an improved disease-free survival
	Rectal cancer
	- Kapiteijn *et al*. (2001). *N Engl J Med* 345:690–692:
	  - Demonstrated superior local control from the addition of SCPRT to mesorectal excision in rectal cancer
	- Sauer *et al*. (2004). *N Engl J Med* 351:1731–1740:
	  - Demonstrated superiority of preoperative compared to postoperative therapy in rectal cancer
	- Bujko *et al*. (2004) *Radiother Oncol* 72:15–24:
	  - Demonstrated similar results for long-course CRT and SCPRT in rectal cancer

UICC Manual of Clinical Oncology, Ninth Edition. Edited by Brian O'Sullivan, James D. Brierley, Anil K. D'Cruz, Martin F. Fey, Raphael Pollock, Jan B. Vermorken and Shao Hui Huang. © 2015 UICC. Published 2015 by John Wiley & Sons, Ltd.

Colon and rectum

Incidence, aetiology and screening

Incidence, aetiology and screening	Description
Incidence	• Colorectal cancer (CRC) is the third commonest cancer worldwide after lung and breast cancer: 　▪ Commonest is moderately differentiated adenocarcinoma of the rectum derived from epithelial cells 　▪ Malignant melanoma, neuroendocrine tumours, gastrointestinal stromal cell tumours (GIST) and squamous cell cancers are rare cancers in the colon, rectum or anus • CRC is the second commonest cause of death after lung cancer and was responsible for >200,000 deaths in Europe in 2008 • 142,820 men and women (73,680 men and 69,140 women) were projected to be diagnosed with and 50,830 men and women to die from cancer of the colon and rectum in 2013 in the USA • Incidence of CRC increases with age, with 92% occurring in people aged 50 years and over and 80% occurring in people aged 60 and over: 　▪ Median age at diagnosis is >70 years
Aetiology	• See Table 26.1.1 and text
Screening	• Inherited cancers are much rarer in the rectum than in the right side of the colon • Randomized controlled clinical trials have shown that both annual screening and biennial screening for occult blood significantly reduce the rate of death from CRC • The National Screening Programme in the UK using occult blood has resulted in an increased incidence detection rate with more early detection

Table 26.1.1 Risk factors for CRC

Increase risk	Protective
Excess of red/processed meat	Diet (high fibre)
Tobacco smoking	Exercise
Alcohol excess	Regular use of aspirin/non-steroidal anti-inflammatory drugs (NSAIDs)
Sedentary lifestyle/lack of exercise	Metformin
Inflammatory bowel disease (ulcerative colitis and Crohn's disease)	Acetylcholine esterase (ACE) inhibitors
Diabetes (type 2) with a possible role of hyperinsulinaemia and insulin-like growth factors (IGF)	Turmeric
Lack of vitamin D	Calcium-rich foods
Prior radiotherapy for prostate cancer (rectal cancer only)	Postmenopausal hormone replacement therapy in women

Incidence and epidemiology

Worldwide CRC is the third most common cancer after lung and breast cancer with 1.23 million cases representing approximately 10% of the total cancer burden. The incidence of CRC is higher in developed areas of the world (the USA, Canada, Western Europe, Scandinavia, New Zealand, Australia) and lower in Asia, Africa and South America (with the exception of Argentina and Uruguay). For reasons which are poorly understood, men have a slightly higher risk of developing CRC than women. About 20% of patients with rectal cancer present with metastatic disease at the time of diagnosis, and a further 25% will subsequently develop metastases. The crude incidence of rectal cancer (as defined by a tumour with its lower edge within 15 cm of the anal verge on rigid sigmoidoscopy) in the European Union is approximately 35% of the total CRC incidence (15–25 per 100,000 per year). The mortality is 4–10 per 100,000 per year with the lower figures valid for females, the higher for males. The risk increases with age. Median age at diagnosis is about 70 years or slightly above in most European countries.

Emigration from a low-risk to a high-risk area confers the risk of CRC in the adopted country, suggesting the importance of environmental factors in CRC.

Risk factors with increasingly strong evidence but still inconsistent for CRC are given in Table 26.1.1.

Hereditary component (colorectal)

CRC is a genetically heterogeneous disease with two distinct recognized pathways leading to the development of cancer: chromosomal instability and the microsatellite instability (MSI) pathway.

The lifetime risk of developing CRC for any individual is approximately 5%. About 5% of CRC may be recognized to be of hereditary origin, but up to a further 30% might have a hereditary factor.

The descriptive clustering used to define families with an increased lifetime risk/hereditary predisposition (Amsterdam criteria) has been modified over time.

Patients diagnosed with CRC should be questioned as to family history regarding colonic polyps, CRC and any type of cancer (in first- and second-degree relatives). If an individual has first-degree relatives who developed CRC at an age younger than 50 years, the risk of CRC is increased two-fold,

> **Box 26.1.1** Genetic conditions associated with an increased risk of CRC
>
> **Familial adenomatous polyposis**
> - Inherited as an autosomal dominant trait with variable penetrance
> - Familial adenomatous polyposis coli (*APC*) gene has been localized to chromosome 5q21
> - Clinical diagnosis of classical FAP relies on the identification of >100 colorectal adenomas
> - Correlated with 100% lifetime risk of developing CRC, usually before 25 years of age
>
> **Lynch syndrome**
> - Reflects mutations in several different genes and is inherited in an autosomal dominant pattern
> - Approximately 3–5% of CRC are due to Lynch syndrome
> - Clinical criteria (Amsterdam, Bethesda) in the context of a suggestive personal or family history prompt screening for microsatellite instability (MSI) and/or immunohistochemistry (IHC) for mismatch repair proteins (MMRs):
>   - Variations in the MMR genes *MLH1*, *MSH2*, *MSH6*, *PMS2* or *EPCAM* increase the risk of developing Lynch syndrome
>   - MSI is observed in approximately 15% of sporadic tumours and in almost all Lynch syndrome cases
>   - Most cases identified by IHC are sporadic and caused by methylation of *MLH1* as opposed to germline mutations
>   - MSI is found in >90% of cases of CRC with Lynch syndrome compared with approximately 15% of sporadic cases
> - Some patients with Lynch syndrome do not demonstrate a significant family history and are older than 50 years of age
> - Although mutations in the genes predispose individuals to CRC, not all who carry these mutations will develop CRC
> - Also associated with an increased risk of cancers of the stomach, small bowel, liver and bile duct, and brain
> - Genetic spectrum includes Muir–Torre syndrome and Turcot syndrome
>
> **Attenuated FAP (AFAP)**
> - Suspected when a person has a history of >20, but <100, adenomatous colon polyps:
>   - Total number of colon polyps is usually <100, with 30 being average
> - Follows an autosomal dominant inheritance pattern
> - A blood test can detect a mutation in the *APC* gene
> - Clinical diagnosis is based on the following criteria:
>   - At least two relatives with 10–99 adenomas at age >30 years, or
>   - One case with 10–99 adenomas at age <30 years
>   - A first-degree relative with CRC and a few adenomas, but no family members with >100 adenomas before the age of 30 years
> - Polyps and cancer of the stomach and small intestine are also seen in families with AFAP, but there is a lower chance of developing desmoid tumours
> - Risks of those with AFAP developing CRC are considered to be similar to those associated with classical FAP, but the overall cancer risks may be lower
>
> **Peutz-Jeghers syndrome**
> - Associated with multiple polyps in the digestive tract, increased pigmentation around the mouth and on the hands, and an increased risk of other cancers
>
> **Gardner syndrome**
> - Associated with osteomas (bony tumours) of the jaw and soft tissue tumours including fibromas
>
> **MYH-associated polyposis**
> - Associated with a risk of developing multiple colonic polyps which may increase the risk of CRC

and the risk is further increased if cancer developed at a young age (<45 years). There is a three- to four-fold increased risk of CRC with two affected first-degree relatives. The risk increases further if other close relatives have developed CRC.

Some genetic conditions are associated with an increased risk of CRC (see Box 26.1.1):
- Familial adenomatous polyposis (FAP)
- Lynch syndrome (formerly hereditary non-polyposis CRC [HNPCC])
- Other genetic family syndromes (Peutz–Jeghers syndrome [PJS], Gardner syndrome and MYH-associated polyposis (MAP).

The molecular characterization of human colon and rectal cancer continues to advance (Cancer Genome Atlas Network 2012).

Individuals with a higher than average risk of CRC may benefit from referral to specialist cancer genetics services and early detection strategies, i.e. screening.

Prevention

Prophylactic total colectomy is the standard of care in patients with classical FAP, and can even be discussed with some patients with an attenuated form.

Specific dietary or pharmacological interventions are not yet recommended in individuals with Lynch syndrome to prevent the development of CRC, although data are accumulating to support the regular use of aspirin.

Prophylactic total colectomy in otherwise healthy individuals with mutations is not recommended, although some advocate prophylactic gynaecological surgery in female carriers after childbearing is completed. If subtotal colectomy is undertaken, regular endoscopic surveillance every 6–12 months is recommended to detect rectal adenoma recurrence.

Screening

Malignant transformation from adenoma to carcinoma is believed to require years rather than months and is thought to account for the development of the majority of CRC. The purpose of screening is to eradicate potential cancers while they are still in the benign stage of the adenoma–carcinoma sequence. Screening also increases the likelihood of diagnosing existing cancers while they are still in an early, easily treatable stage.

- CRC is potentially amenable to secondary prevention by one-off or regular screening, because detection and removal of an adenomatous polyp can prevent subsequent development of a CRC
- If CRC is diagnosed while still at a localized stage (i.e. confined to the wall of the bowel), 5-year survival is likely to be extremely favourable (in the region of 90%), but falls to 66% for Stage III (i.e. disease with lymph node involvement)

- The principle of the benefits of colonoscopic and flexible sigmoidoscopic screening is widely accepted, yet the large numbers of colonoscopies required demands considerable resources, and existing guidelines tend not to provide estimates of resource implications.

Patients with average risk for CRC who should be considered for colonoscopy include those with:

- No symptoms and age 50–75 years
- No symptoms requesting screening
- Persistent change in bowel habit for >6 weeks
- Rectal and anal bleeding
- Unexplained abdominal pain
- Unexplained iron deficiency anaemia.

Methods of screening include (see Box 26.1.2):
- Faecal occult blood (FOB), etc.
- Rigid proctosigmoidoscopy
- Flexible sigmoidoscopy
- Colonoscopy.

Screening of high-risk patients

People at increased risk for CRC include those with affected first-degree relatives, those with a family history of FAP or Lynch syndrome, and those with a personal history of adenomatous polyps, CRC or inflammatory bowel disease (IBD) (see Box 26.1.3).

Box 26.1.2 Methods of screening

Faecal occult blood
- Three prospective, randomized controlled clinical trials showed that screening with a guaiac-based faecal occult blood test (FOBT) significantly decreased mortality:
  - In the UK screening programme is performed from age 60 years, every other year by testing two samples from each of three consecutive stools:
    - If any of the three sample findings are positive, the patient is recommended to have the entire colon studied via colonoscopy or flexible sigmoidoscopy and CT Colonography
  - Significant false positives and false-negatives
- Stool DNA screening (SDNA): uses polymerase chain reaction of sloughed mucosal cells in the stool and evaluates genetic alterations
- Faecal immunochemical test (FIT): uses a monoclonal antibody assay to identify human haemoglobin:
  - More specific for lower gastrointestinal tract lesions because the globin molecule is broken down during passage through the upper gastrointestinal tract

Rigid proctosigmoidoscopy
- Can generally be performed without an anaesthetic
- Allows direct visualization of the lower bowel and any potential lesion
- Provides an estimate of the size of the lesion and degree of obstruction
- Biopsies can be obtained
- Can determine the degree of fixation
- Gives an accurate measurement of the distance of the lesion from the anal verge (which assists in deciding the most appropriate operation)

Flexible sigmoidoscopy
- Evidence based on several randomized controlled trials:
  - In the UK a prospective randomized study of >100,000 patients showed that a single flexible sigmoidoscopy in individuals aged 55–64 years reduced CRC incidence by 33% and mortality by 43%
- Should be performed every 5 years
- Any lesions identified should be biopsied
- Some lesions beyond the reach of the sigmoidoscope may be missed

CT colonography (CTC)
- After bowel preparation, the thin-cut axial colonic images are collated from prone and supine positions with a high-speed helical CT scanner
- Images are reconstituted into a 3D replica of the entire colon and rectum
- Provides a good visualization of the entire colon (including views of the flexures and haustral folds)
- Patients with positive findings should undergo colonoscopic evaluation

Colonoscopy
- Allows full visualization of the colon if complete to the caecum, and excision and biopsy of any lesions
- Optimal follow-up strategy for evaluating patients with a positive FOBT
- Some polyps and small lesions can be missed because of blind corners and mucosal folds
- Visualization of the caecum cannot always be achieved
- Fibre-optic flexible colonoscopy is recommended every 5–10 years

Box 26.1.3 Screening of high-risk patients

First-degree relative affected
- Screening at age 40 rather than 50 years
- Colonoscopy often recommended as initial screening test, particularly if the relative was diagnosed with cancer at a young age

Family history of FAP
- Genetic counselling/testing is recommended to determine whether the individual is a gene carrier
- Current tests are approximately 80% accurate (in 20% the mutation cannot be identified)
- Genetic testing is useful only if the test result is a true positive or true negative (i.e. mutation present in other family members not identified in the individual being tested)
- Flexible sigmoidoscopy should be offered to known gene carriers and is often performed every 2 years from the age of 12–14 years
- When adenomas are found, annual colonoscopy is appropriate
- In those with an indeterminate carrier status, yearly screening to look for polyps from the age of 18–20 years and continued lifelong
- When polyposis develops, consider colectomy

Screening for extracolonic manifestations
- There is an association with upper gastrointestinal adenomas, thyroid cancers and desmoid tumours
- If colorectal polyposis is diagnosed from age 25 to 30 years, upper gastrointestinal endoscopy should be performed every 5 years until adenomas are detected:
  - *Note*: gastrointestinal adenomas may also develop more distally in the jejunum and ileum
- Screening for thyroid cancer should be performed by ultrasonography of the neck
- Regular physical examination and if masses palpated, abdominal CT should be considered to pick up desmoids tumours

Family history of Lynch syndrome
- Genetic counselling/testing recommended for individuals whose family histories meet the updated Amsterdam criteria
- Individuals with documented Lynch syndrome should undergo colonoscopy every 1–2 years when aged 20–40 years of age, and every year after 40 years of age
- Flexible sigmoidoscopy is not recommended since cancers tend to be located on the right side of the colon

Personal history of adenomatous polyps
- Patients who have adenomatous polyps removed during colonoscopy should have a repeat examination at 1–3 years
- If examination reveals no abnormalities, i.e. no polyps present, follow-up at 5 years

Personal history of CRC
- Patients who have CRC and undergo resection for cure should have a colonoscopy within 1 year
- If examination reveals no abnormalities, i.e. no polyps present, follow up at 5 yearly until aged 80-85 (depending on fitness)

Personal history of IBD
- Surveillance colonoscopy with testing for dysplastic changes as a marker for future development of CRC in patients with long-standing IBD
- Colonoscopy every 1–2 years after 8–10 years of diffuse disease or after 10–15 years of localized disease
- Random biopsies are performed at specific intervals throughout the colon and rectum
  - Total colectomy is recommended when high-grade dysplasia is present

Pathology and molecular biology

Pathology	Description
Adenocarcinomas	• 90–95% of large-bowel cancers • Characterized by cuboidal or columnar epithelia with variable differentiation and variable amounts of mucin
Mucinous adenocarcinoma	• Defined by the presence of >50% extracellular mucin • Tendency to intracoelomic spread • More commonly seen in younger patients • Associated with a worse prognosis
Signet ring cell carcinoma	• Uncommon variant of mucinous carcinoma, accounting for 1% of colorectal adenocarcinomas

Other tumour types	• Include:
	  ▪ Carcinoid tumours
	  ▪ Poorly differentiated neuroendocrine carcinomas
	  ▪ Squamous cell carcinomas
	  ▪ Undifferentiated carcinomas
	• Non-epithelial tumours, such as GIST, sarcomas and lymphomas, are very rare

- CRC arise from dysplastic adenomatous polyps in the majority of cases in a multistep process involving the inactivation of a variety of tumour suppressor and DNA repair genes, along with simultaneous activation of oncogenes:
  - These changes drive transformation from normal colonic epithelium to adenomatous polyp to invasive CRC
- Germline mutations occur in the well-characterized inherited colon cancer syndromes:
  - A single germline mutation in the *APC* tumour suppressor gene is responsible for the dominantly inherited syndrome
- Sporadic cancers arise from a stepwise accumulation of somatic genetic mutations
- Clinical expression of the disease is seen when the inherited mutation of one *APC* allele is followed by a second hit mutation or deletion of the second allele
- Ulcerative colitis and Crohn's colitis are associated with an increased risk of CRC with an interim step of dysplastic epithelium
- Spread of rectal cancer is to local lymph nodes and via the vasculature to the liver and lungs and, uncommonly, to bone and the brain

Diagnostic work-up

Diagnostic work-up	Description

Work-up	• Digital rectal examination: helps to assess low rectal lesions and estimate sphincter function
	• Rigid/flexible sigmoidoscopy/colonoscopy and biopsy is required for histopathological examination:
	  ▪ Tumours with distal extension to ≤15 cm (as measured by rigid sigmoidoscopy) from the anal margin are classified as rectal, more proximal tumours as colonic
	  ▪ Examination under anaesthetic (EUA) is necessary on occasion for low rectal or anal cancer to inspect and to obtain biopsy
	• Whole-body computed tomography (CT) to determine whether there is metastatic disease
	• Pelvic magnetic resonance imaging (MRI) is mandatory for initial staging of rectal cancer and anal cancer and/or transrectal endoscopic ultrasound (TRUS)
	• Other options include positron emission tomography (PET) scan and carcinoembryonic antigen (CEA)

Tumour markers	• CEA

Initial local invasion is facilitated by circumferential growth with subsequent lymphatic, perineural and extramural vascular, and eventually haematogenous and transcoelomic spread.

Locoregional recurrence from colon cancer can occur at the site of anastomosis, in the resection bed, paracolic gutter or in retroperitoneal (para-aortic, paracaval) lymph nodes.

The most common site of distant metastasis is the liver, followed by the lungs (especially in low rectal cancer). Other sites include bone, adrenal glands, spleen and brain, although metastases can spread to any organ.

Preoperative staging of colon cancer
- Colonoscopy and biopsy should be performed prior to surgery if possible
- For staging of colon tumours, CT is recommended as the best modality:
  - CT-determined T stage (ctT) can be used to stratify patients into good and poor prognosis, and patients with depth as spread >5 mm have a greater likelihood of having node-positive disease
  - CT is poor in identifying nodal disease and significantly weaker than ctT using substaging by CT to identify high-risk node-positive patients
- CT thorax, abdomen and pelvis is recommended as the main modality of choice for assessment of metastatic disease
- For patients with suspicious lesions on CT, further imaging by MRI and/or PET-CT may be helpful in characterizing and diagnosing metastatic disease, particularly in the liver

Preoperative staging of rectal cancer
Magnetic resonance imaging
- Preoperative multidisciplinary team discussion of MRI rectal cancer findings leads to improved outcomes – through better selection of high-risk patients for preoperative therapy and improved surgical planning
- Current guidelines for preoperative imaging of rectal cancer recommend MRI for local staging and CT chest, abdomen and pelvis for detection of distant metastases (as above)
- High-resolution MRI (pixel size 0.6 × 0.6 mm and voxel size ≤1 mm³ on T2-weighted images) enables optimal results for rectal tumour staging
- An MRI reporting proforma that includes all the known prognostic MRI staging features should be performed:
  - Measured depth of extramural tumour spread beyond the rectal muscularis propria which correlates very precisely with corresponding histopathology measurements:
    - Increasing depth of spread beyond 5 mm is associated with worsening disease-free survival
  - Distance of ≤1 mm to the mesorectal fascia (MRF) is associated with a high risk of circumferential surgical margin involvement and an increased risk of local recurrence
  - MRI depiction of tumour signal extending into the extramural vessels (mrEMVI) – seen in 30–40% of staged rectal cancers:
    - EMVI is associated with an increased risk of local recurrence and/or metastatic disease
  - Low rectal tumours – accurately defining the relationship of the tumour to the sphincter complex and demonstrating threatened resection margins:
    - Staging enables distinction of the two potential planes for surgery: (1) the total mesorectal excision (TME) plane, which enables intersphincteric dissection of low tumours and in some cases avoidance of a permanent stoma, and (2) the extralevator plane, which ensures a more radical removal of the sphincter complex
    - Latter should be considered if tumour encroaches on the plane between the rectal wall and the distal levator/puborectalis sling and external sphincter to avoid a positive surgical margin
  - Nodal staging is possible with MRI in rectal cancer, but lacks sensitivity and a tendency to overstage nodes when using size criteria
    - Mixed signal intensity and irregular borders are the features on MRI predicting nodal involvement with the greatest accuracy

FDG-PET-CT
- Not used routinely for initial staging, but can be helpful for equivocal evidence of metastatic disease
- May be useful if MRI staging detects gross extramural vascular invasion or pathologically enlarged common iliac or lateral pelvic nodes outside the MRF
- More sensitive than CT in helping to rule out extrahepatic metastases, particularly in para-aortic nodes or patients with synchronous liver metastases on CT, who are being assessed for curative liver surgery

Measurement of response after preoperative chemoradiation
- None of the currently available imaging modalities (ERUS, MRI, CT) reliably predicts complete pathological response
- High-resolution MRI assessment of tumour regression (TRG), which evaluates the proportion of fibrosis versus residual tumour signal, is a reliable method of assessing response:
  - Patients with mrTRG 1 and 2 show virtual eradication of tumour
  - Survival outcomes for mrTRG 1 and 2 are equivalent to complete pathological response
- MRI assessment of shrinkage of tumour away from the MRF can be assessed and is an independent preoperative predictor for the risk of local recurrence:
  - MRI agreement for pathological prognosis using mrT and TRG assessment is good, with good interobserver reproducibility
  - Volume and RECIST shows poorer agreement with pathology response and poorer interobserver agreement
- mrTRG is useful for assessing the potential circumferential resection margin (CRM) and distinguishing between good and poor response to treatment
  - Current treatment strategies, however, do not take into account findings of mrTRG
- MRI should be performed after 4–6 weeks following completion of chemoradiation (CRT), although studies investigating the optimum timing of imaging and surgery are underway
- Diffusion-weighted MRI is unproven compared with high-resolution MRI in assessing response and predicting outcomes
- Role of FDG-PET-CT in the assessment of response is still under investigation

Pathology reporting of a surgical specimen

A pathology proforma should be employed to ensure a comprehensive report, and on this the pathologist should describe:
- TNM staging (documenting TNM version used)
- Extent of penetration beyond the muscularis propria in millimetres
- Degree of differentiation
- Presence of mucin if >50%
- All distal and circumferential margins, the mesenteric and antimesenteric borders, and the completeness of resection
- Any evidence of perforation
- Total number of lymph nodes found and number of involved lymph nodes
- Extramural vascular invasion
- Lymphovascular invasion
- Perineural invasion.

The Guidelines of the Royal College of Pathologists in the UK are widely used for reporting rectal cancer (Box 26.1.4).

Box 26.1.4 Guidelines for reporting rectal carcinoma (adapted from Royal College of Pathologists guidelines)

Preparation and assessment of specimen

Macroscopic
- Macroscopic examination of the quality of the TME specimen is critical and of prognostic significance as an indicator of the quality/adequacy of radical surgical resection
- Specimen, particularly the anterior and posterior surfaces, should be photographed to allow categorization into three grades (within the mesorectal plane, the intramesorectal plane and the muscularis propria plane)
- Any perforation, defects in the specimen and the plane of surgical dissection should be described
- Abdominoperineal resection specimen

Microscopic
- Surgically created margin surfaces are inked
- Specimen is not opened and the area of the tumour left intact to allow assessment of CRM involvement, without distortion introduced by opening the bowel
- Specimen should be fixed in formalin for at least 72 hours
- Tumour (for a distance of 2 cm above and below) should be thinly sliced (3–5 mm) and slices photographed to document the plane of surgical dissection as regards CRM
- Distance of direct tumour spread outside the muscularis propria should be recorded and the area in which the tumour spreads closest to the CRM should be identified macroscopically
- Blocks should be taken from the area closest to the tumour/CRM and other areas where tumour extends to within <3 mm of the margin:
  - Other blocks should be taken to include at least five blocks of tumour to confirm the presence or absence of extramural venous invasion
- At least 12 lymph nodes should be assessed:
  - Number of lymph nodes needed to accurately stage preoperatively-treated cases is unknown
- *Circumferential resection margin*:
  - Most important resection margin for rectal cancer is the CRM, which is in effect the MRF if the surgeon performs a TME along the MRF unless the tumour involves or grows within 1 mm of the fascia when TME alone is insufficient
  - Important to report the exact measurement of tumour to the CRM in millimetres
    - Extent of the CRM is an important predictor of local failure and distant metastases in patients – and should preferably be >2 mm
    - Increased risk for local recurrence, distant metastases and poorer survival if the CRM is involved or <1 mm
    - If a positive lymph node or a tumour deposit is closer to the margin, a second CRM measurement should be made and reported
- *Distal margin*:
  - Minimal acceptable extent of the distal surgical margin remains a matter of debate, although some suggest 5–10 mm is acceptable if CRT has been delivered

Classification of rectal primary tumour after preoperative therapy
- *Tumour regression grading (TRG)*:
  - Observer dependent and poorly reproducible
  - Has not yet demonstrated independent prognostic value in large randomized trials and is not routinely recommended to be reported
- *Pathological complete response (PCR)*:
  - Uncertain prognostic value regarding disease-free or overall survival
  - Should be documented in a standardized fashion:
    - At least five tissue blocks should be taken from the area of macroscopic tumour
    - If there is no tumour in these blocks, the whole area should be further blocked and if there is still no tumour in these blocks, three levels should be cut to exclude the presence of viable tumour

Staging and prognostic grouping

UICC TNM staging
See Table 26.1.2.

Table 26.1.2 UICC TNM categories and stage grouping: Colon and rectum

TNM categories	
Submucosa	
T2	Muscularis propria
T3	Subserosa, pericolorectal tissues
T4a	Visceral peritoneum
T4b	Other organs or structures
N1a	1 regional
N1b	2–3 regional
N1c	Satellite(s) without regional nodes
N2a	4–6 regional
N2b	7 or more regional
M1a	1 organ
M1b	>1 organ, peritoneum

Stage grouping			
Stage 0	Tis	N0	M0
Stage I	T1, T2	N0	M0
Stage II	T3, T4	N0	M0
Stage IIA	T3	N0	M0
Stage IIB	T4a	N0	M0
Stage IIC	T4b	N0	M0
Stage III	Any T	N1, N2	M0
Stage IIIA	T1, T2	N1	M0
	T1	N2a	M0
Stage IIIB	T3, T4a	N1	M0
	T2, T3	N2a	M0
	T1, T2	N2b	M0
Stage IIIC	T4a	N2a	M0
	T3, T4a	N2b	M0
	T4b	N1, N2	M0
Stage IVA	Any T	Any N	M1a
Stage IVB	Any T	Any N	M1b

Overall 5-year survival rates for rectal cancer are:
- Stage I: 90%
- Stage II: 60–85%
- Stage III: 27–60%
- Stage IV: 5–10% (improving year by year).

Fifty per cent of patients develop recurrence, which may be local, distant or both.

Prognostic and predictive biomarkers and other risk factors
See Box 26.1.5 and Table 26.1.3.
- Knowledge is accumulating on the prognostic and predictive biomarkers (blood, tumour tissue) to guide selection of drugs and individual treatment strategies, but in practice *KRAS* is the only validated biomarker for CRC

Box 26.1.5 Biomarkers for early, advanced and metastatic disease, efficacy of chemotherapy and toxicity

Early colorectal cancer
- No evidence for any predictive marker for the efficacy of adjuvant chemotherapy
- Some pooled analyses have suggested a detrimental effect for adjuvant treatment with 5-fluorouracil (5-FU) in patients with Stage II MSI-H/dMMR tumours, but this finding has not been confirmed in randomized trials (PETACC 3, QUASAR)
- Insufficient data with respect to the impact of germline versus sporadic MMR defects

Advanced/metastatic colorectal cancer
- Associated with poor prognosis and less favourable outcome with chemotherapy:
  - Elevated alkaline phosphatase (ALP) and lactate dehydrogenase (LDH), high white cell count, low serum albumin
  - More than one site of disease
  - Poor performance status
- *Epithelial growth factor receptor (EGFR) inhibitors*:
  - *KRAS* mutation precludes efficacy of treatment with anti-EGFR antibodies and *KRAS* status determination is therefore mandatory before treatment
  - *BRAF*, *NRAS*, *PI3K*, *PTEN* and *EGFR* mutations, and EGFR ligands (epiregulin, amphiregulin) expression are not yet robust markers
- *Vascular endothelial growth factor (VEGF) inhibitors*:
  - No predictive marker for antiangiogenic agents such as bevacizumab or aflibercept
- *Epithelial growth factor receptor inhibitors*:
  - *KRAS* mutation precludes efficacy of treatment with anti-EGFR antibodies and *KRAS* status determination is therefore mandatory before treatment

Efficacy of chemotherapy
- Topoisomerase-1 (Topo-1) overexpression is believed to be predictive for the efficacy of treatment with irinotecan, but randomized trials have conflicting results
- *ERCC1* (excision repair cross-complementing gene 1) polymorphisms, thymidine phosphorylase (TP) and thymidylate synthase (TS) expression are thought to be associated with efficacy of oxaliplatin and 5-FU chemotherapy, respectively, but are not routinely used to select treatment

Toxicity
- *Dihydropyrimidine dehydrogenase (DPD)*:
  - DPD deficiency (0.3–1.5% of patients) results in reduced drug clearance and prolonged exposure to fluoropyrimidines:
    - Homozygosity for DPD deficiency is rare (0.1% of patients)
    - In cases of DPD deficiency there is a risk of rapid and lethal toxicity with fluoropyrimidines from diarrhoea, myelosuppression, mucositis and stomatitis.
      - Oral prodrugs of 5-FU such as capecitabine, S1 and UFT oral produce similar effects, but routine testing for DPD deficiency prior to starting fluoropyrimidines is not generally performed
      - If severe toxicity from 5-FU is observed, testing for DPD deficiency is recommended, before administering further 5-FU
      - In proven homozygous DPD deficiency, further administration of 5-FU is contraindicated, and can be replaced by raltitrexed in the advanced setting
      - Heterozygous enzyme deficiency dose reduction for 5-FU/oral fluoropyridimines may be appropriate, but an exact dose reduction guideline is not available
- *Cytadine deaminase* (CDA):
  - Activates the oral prodrug capecitabine
  - Variants in the *CDA* promoter region increase cytidine deaminase expression, and may be associated with an increased risk of diarrhoea with capecitabine chemotherapy
- UGT1A1 *polymorphism*:
  - Homozygosity for a *UGT1A1*28* allele leads to lower UGT1A1 expression, reduced SN38 glucuronidation and higher risk of irinotecan-induced toxicity
  - If severe toxicity potentially related to treatment with irinotecan occurs, testing for *UGT1A1* polymorphisms should be considered:
    - This is particularly important when irinotecan is used at high doses (300–350 mg/m^2)

Table 26.1.3 Prognostic factors for survival in differentiated colorectal cancer

Prognostic factors	Tumour related	Host related	Environment related
Essential	T category N category M category Circumferential margin (rectal cancer)	Age	Screening programme
Additional	Vascular/lymphatic invasion Perineural invasion Grade Tumour budding Perforation KRAS MSI BRAF	Race	Socioeconomic status Centre volume and experience
New and promising	Molecular profile		

- Status of high-frequency microsatellite instability (MSI-H) or mismatch repair deficiency (dMMR) and *KRAS*-codon 12 or G13D or *BRAF* mutation is gaining strengthening relevance, but each requires further validation as a prognostic marker for early and advanced CRC
- However, apart from MSI in the adjuvant setting and *KRAS* in advanced disease, no biomarkers can be used to make therapeutic decisions
- Patients expressing MSI-H/dMMR have a recognized better prognosis in Stage II and III than low-frequency MSI (MSI-L) or microsatellite stable (MSS) patients
- Genomic signatures have a potentially high prognostic value, but are currently not robust enough to guide decision-making on adjuvant treatment

Treatment philosophy

CRC is one of the commonest solid tumours, and is responsible for considerable clinical morbidity and mortality.

The definitive management of both colon and rectal cancer relies on resection of the bowel with the adjacent draining lymph nodes. Patterns and sites of recurrence following a notionally 'curative' resection are different for colon and rectal carcinoma. Rectal cancer has a higher risk of locoregional failure; colon cancer tends to recur within the abdominal cavity in the peritoneum, but also in other distant sites such as the lung, liver and bone.

In about 75% of patients with CRC, all macroscopic disease can be surgically resected. Despite this high resectability rate, a further 30–40% who have undergone surgery with apparently complete excision will subsequently succumb to locally recurrent or metastatic disease. Hence adjuvant radiation or systemic therapies are appropriate at this time in high-risk patients to reduce the risk of recurrence. Surgical resection of local recurrence or metastases may be appropriate in selected patients; otherwise systemic chemotherapy can control the disease, provide substantial symptom palliation and to some extent prolong survival. Selection of chemotherapy for patients diagnosed with metastatic CRC should be individualized according to the use, form and timing of previous chemotherapy, integrating the goal of treatment, potential toxicity, performance status and co-morbidity. Between 20% and 30% of patients will be found to have metastatic disease at the time of diagnosis, but a limited number may still be potentially curable with treatment.

Total mesorectal excision (TME) is now a universally accepted standard surgical technique for 'resectable' rectal cancer and is the single-most important advance in reducing rates of local recurrence in the last 25 years. Early rectal cancer may be adequately treated by local excision, avoiding major surgery. Radiotherapy and chemoradiotherapy have a recognized role for locally-advanced and unresectable rectal cancers, but currently there is debate regarding intermediate-risk rectal tumours; some guidelines recommend preoperative therapy for all Stage II and III rectal cancers, but this may result in undue morbidity for patients with a low risk of recurrence, while other guidelines such as ESMO guidelines (see below) are more selective based on a preoperative MRI scan. Proactive combined modality treatment (chemotherapy, radiotherapy, resection of metastases) has increased survival in selected cases. In easily resectable cancers, short course preoperative radiotherapy (5 × 5 Gy) and neoadjuvant chemoradiotherapy (NCRT) are equivalent in terms of reducing local recurrence, but with little influence on overall survival. In the low rectum, where defects in the specimen and perforation were common, careful preoperative assessment of the safety of the intersphincteric plane and the selective use of NCRT where the plane is unsafe results in better histopathological outcomes (CRM involvement rates and ypTN stage). There is a controversial role for postoperative adjuvant chemotherapy. Metastatic disease is amenable to treatment with palliative cytotoxic chemotherapy using fluoropyrimidines, oxaliplatin or irinotecan ± biological agents.

Scenario			Treatment philosophy
Colon	Surgical candidate	Stages I – III	• Surgical resection of primary tumour and mesentery • Postoperative chemotherapy offered to patients with Stage III
		Stage IV	• Surgical resection of primary tumour and mesentery ± metastases • Preoperative chemotherapy • Chemotherapy ± the targeted drugs (bevacizumab ± cetuximab/panitumumab)
	Non-surgical candidate	Stages I–IV	• Stenting • Chemotherapy ± a targeted drug (bevacizumab/cetuximab/panitumumab) • Radiotherapy
Rectum	Surgical candidate	Stage I, low risk: • <3 cm • <30% circumference of the bowel • Moderately or well differentiated	• Local excision may be curative, especially by more accurate technique of transanal endoscopic microsurgery (TEM) • Excised specimen should be seen as a 'Big biopsy' and risk of nodal involvement further assessed
		Stage I, high risk	• Surgical resection using TME principles: ▪ Preoperative radiation therapy (especially short-course preoperative radiotherapy [SCPRT] optional)

		Stages II–III	• Surgical resection with the following options:
			  ▪ Preoperative CRT
			  ▪ Postoperative chemotherapy
			  ▪ Postoperative CRT

Scenario		Treatment philosophy

	Stage IV	• Surgical resection with following additional options:
		  ▪ Preoperative CRT
		  ▪ Postoperative chemotherapy, bevacizumab, cetuximab
		  ▪ Preoperative chemotherapy,
		  ▪ Postoperative CRT

Non-surgical candidate	Stages I–IV	• Chemotherapy • Monoclonal antibodies • Stenting • Radiotherapy

Recommendations for preoperative radiotherapy in rectal cancer are given in Table 26.1.4.

Table 26.1.4 Recommendations for preoperative radiotherapy in rectal cancer

Position	Stage	Recommendation
Upper third >10 cm from anal verge	T4b Peritoneal or adjacent structures	Consider CRT
Mid-third 5–10 cm from anal verge	T3b*, MRF**negative	CRT or SCPRT
	MRF positive or lateral lymph nodes	CRT
Lower third <5 cm from anal verge	T2 MRF positive	Consider CRT
	T3b, MRF negative	CRT or SCPRT
	MRF positive or lateral lymph nodes	CRT

*T3b = ≥5 mm invasion into the mesorectal fat.
**MRF positive or negative, potential for mesorectal fascia involvement or positive circumferential margin.
Adapted from Schmoll H et al. (2012).

Treatment

Surgery

Surgery	Description

Colon cancer	• Multiple large randomized trials have convincingly established laparoscopic colonic resection as a safe and acceptable method of treating cancer of the colon
	• Surgery is increasingly performed by laparoscopic techniques
	• Most cases can have colonic reconstruction and thus avoid a stoma
	• Complete pan-proctocolectomy is feasible if needed (e.g. multiple CRC or severe dysplasia in colitis) and a neorectum created using a 'J pouch' constructed from the small bowel
	• Mortality (<3–5%) and morbidity are low for elective surgery
	• Approximately 20% of cases still present as an emergency (usually from obstruction) where colonic intraluminal stenting may be used as palliation or a 'bridge to surgery' or facilitate the administration of systemic therapy:
	  ▪ Stents should be used with caution
	    ○ Can migrate with response to chemotherapy or radiation, leading to potential for obstruction, perforation or pain
	• Enhanced recovery after surgery (ERAS) has been developed, trialled and popularized in open and laparoscopic colonic resection:
	  ▪ Main elements are patient and carer education, no mechanical bowel preparation, minimal trauma, restricted intraoperative fluids, no drains or nasogastric tubes, early removal of urinary catheter, early feeding (1–2 days) and targeted mobilization focusing on early discharge

(continued)

Surgery	Description
Rectal cancer	- More complex than for colon cancer
- Rectum is conventionally divided into three parts, defined from the anal verge as:
- Lower rectum: <5 cm
- Middle rectum: 5–10 cm
- Upper rectum: >10 cm
- Mechanical bowel preparation recommended but other enhanced recovery methods are applicable
- Principles of TME have optimized outcomes
- Accurate 'local extension' staging is crucial with selective neoadjuvant radiotherapy or chemoradiotherapy in patients with predicted involved or threatened MRF margins in the upper rectum or sphincter complex in the low rectum
- Stents should not be used for obstructing mid or low rectal cancers because they can give rise to sensations of tenesmus and they migrate easily (see above)
- Low rectal cancer (defined as a tumour with its lower edge at, or below, the origins of the levator origins on the pelvic sidewall as visualized on MRI or CT) particularly problematic as reduced or no protective mesorectum at this level:
- Many low rectal cancers require complete rectal excision by abdominoperineal excision (APE):
- APE for an advanced low rectal cancer should follow the principles of an Extra Levator (ELAPE)
- ELAPE is a concept of wide excision through the extralevator plane and does not require the prone jack-knife position
- Anal and rectal function are impaired after rectal resection and reconstruction and the effects are worse when surgery is preceded by neoadjuvant therapy:
- A short colon 'J pouch' of 5–7 cm or a side-to-end technique improves function
- A temporary diverting stoma is recommended for most patients who have a low rectal or coloanal reconstruction after rectal cancer surgery:
- Temporary stoma is reversed at 2–3 months following confirmation of a healed anastomosis by a water-soluble contrast study
- Laparoscopic rectal surgery is feasible but less effective than for colon cancer due to difficulties in pelvic dissection, problems with stapling guns needed for reconstruction and often the need for a defunctioning stoma which negates some of the benefits of a minimally access approach
Metastatic and recurrent disease	- *Liver or lung metastases*:
- PET scan may be useful to exclude other less obvious sites of unresectable disease
- Resection should be considered providing the primary has or can be completely resected and there are no unresectable extrahepatic or extrapulmonary metastases:
- Metastases are resectable based on extent of disease, hepatic or pulmonary anatomical constraints, sufficient residual hepatic or pulmonary function
- Ablative techniques including stereotactic radiation may be considered if metastases are technically not surgically resectable
- In highly selected patients with unresectable disease, preoperative chemotherapy may be considered
- Survival after metastatectomy is in the region of 20–40%
- *Pelvic recurrence*:
- Local recurrence is more common in rectal cancer than in colon cancer:
- Disease recurs in 5–30% of patients, usually in the first year after surgery
- Factors that influence the development of recurrence include surgeon variability, grade and stage of the primary tumour, location of the primary tumour and ability to obtain negative margins
- Surgical therapy may be attempted for recurrence and includes pelvic exenteration or APE in patients who have had a previous sphincter-sparing procedure:
- Pelvic exenteration which may include partial sacrectomy may be appropriate in well-motivated patients with no evidence of metastatic or recurrent disease elsewhere with an overall survival of >40% at 4 years in carefully selected patients
- Preoperative chemotherapy and radiation if not previously given:
- If preoperative radiation previously given, further preoperative chemotherapy and radiation with hyperfractionated radiotherapy is usually tolerable and may be appropriate to achieve a curative resection
- Patients with isolated anastomotic recurrence fair better than those with other isolated pelvic recurrences

Unresectable cancer

Clinical features which may indicate surgery may not be curative and the patient has an unresectable cancer are:
- Persistent buttock/sciatic nerve pain
- Bilateral ureteral obstruction
- Extensive fixation to lateral pelvic side wall (according to CT/MRI or at surgery on trial dissection)
- Sacral involvement above S2 (resection produces spinal instability or postoperative complications)

- Bilateral lymphoedema or bilateral venous thrombosis (indicating encasement of major vascular structures)
- Multiple peritoneal metastasis or metastasis fixed to or invading vital structures.

Management is discussed under palliative care; it may include palliative radiotherapy, palliative chemotherapy, stent and best supportive care. Aim of palliative therapy is the prolongation of survival and the improvement of quality of life.

Systemic therapy

Although some metastases can be resected, the efficacy of systemic chemotherapy is pivotal to determining outcome of patients with metastatic CRC. Metastases typically present within 3 years of the initial diagnosis. The 5-year survival rate for metastatic colorectal disease without resection is <10%. Systemic chemotherapy can control the disease, provide substantial symptom palliation and to some extent prolong survival. However, the median survival in randomized studies (with fit patients) until recently has almost invariably been <24 months. Hence, there is an urgent need for predictive biomarkers to optimize efficacy of chemotherapy and minimize toxicity (see above).

The current integration of molecularly targeted drugs into the treatment of CRC, the development of sophisticated technologies for characterizing individual tumours, and the potential for individual patient molecular profiling underlines the potential for personalized medicine. Introduction of the mutational status of the *KRAS* oncogene as the first predictive marker into clinical care is an important step towards the personalization of treatment in CRC.

Some sites of metastatic disease (i.e. bone and ovary) appear to respond less favourably to systemic chemotherapy. With the introduction of numerous new agents, overall survival in metastatic CRC patients has nearly doubled during the past 10 years. Yet, why some patients respond to chemotherapy and others do not, remains poorly understood.

Cytotoxic agents
- Evidence from the 1980s suggested that palliative chemotherapy should be used early and not be delayed until symptoms arise if the aim is to maintain quality of life
- The intravenous fluoropyrimidine 5-fluorouracil (5-FU) represents the mainstay of treatment for patients with advanced and metastatic CRC:
  - Toxicity depends on the method of administration (bolus or prolonged venous infusion):
    - Bolus administration causes more myelotoxic effects, diarrhoea and mucositis
    - Dose-limiting toxic effects of prolonged infusion of 5-FU include hand–foot syndrome
- Meta-analyses initially confirmed a higher response rate with the addition of leucovorin to 5-FU and a small overall survival advantage
- More recently, combinations of cytotoxic chemotherapy using oxaliplatin or irinotecan have been integrated and are commonly used
- A French randomized phase III trial compared the sequence of FOLFOX (oxaliplatin + 5-FU + leucovorin) followed by FOLFIRI (irinotecan + leucovorin) or the reverse order in metastatic CRC, and showed no significant difference in median survival for either strategy
- Other alternatives to 5-FU include the oral fluorinated pyrimidine capecitabine, UFT and S-1, which have simplified the administration of fluoropyrimidine chemotherapy in CRC
- Many different strategies are possible with these available cytotoxic agents:
  - Sequential use of cytotoxic chemotherapy starting with a single agent
  - Using two- or three-drug combinations upfront.
    - Current multiple combinations of chemotherapy are more complex, and hence associated with greater toxicity, but are observed to be modifying the patterns of disease
  - Treating to progression with or without a maintenance component, or employing a stop-and-go strategy
  - Integrating the biological agents either upfront or as maintenance:
    - There are four monoclonal antibodies which can be integrated into systemic chemotherapy

Chemotherapy regimens are numerous; details are beyond the scope of this chapter but are available in treatment guidelines such as the NCCN guidelines (http://www.nccn.org/professionals/physician_gls/f_guidelines.asp).

Chemotherapy regimens concurrent with radiation are:
- 5-FU infusion: 200–250 mg/m^2/day throughout radiation
- Capecitabine: 825–900 mg/m^2 b.i.d., 5 days per week.

Systemic therapy	Description

Intensive neoadjuvant chemotherapy prior to preoperative SCPRT or CRT	- Prior to SCPRT or CRT:
	  - In locally-advanced tumours with a high risk of metastatic disease:
	    - Neoadjuvant chemotherapy ± the targeted drugs (bevacizumab and/or cetuximab), followed by CRT and subsequent radical surgery have been explored in phase II studies
	    - Neoadjuvant chemotherapy followed by preoperative CRT remains an investigational approach and is not recommended outside clinical trials

(continued)

Systemic therapy	Description

	- Instead of local radiation:
	  - Small studies have explored the use of neoadjuvant combination chemotherapy with FOLFOX + bevacizumab and without CRT in cancers which are considered easily resectable
	  - Further studies in this setting are ongoing, but the use of neoadjuvant chemotherapy alone is not recommended outside clinical trials

Postoperative adjuvant treatment for colon cancer	- Improves survival for Stage III disease
	- May improve survival in some patients with Stage II colon cancer
	- Postoperative radiation/CRT should only be considered for selected T4 cancers with residual disease following surgery
	- High-risk features such as T4, poor differentiation, bowel perforation and extramural venous invasion have been used to guide the use of adjuvant chemotherapy in Stage II disease:
	  - Patients with MMR gene-deficient Stage II tumour have a low risk of disease relapse and therefore may not require adjuvant chemotherapy
	- FOLFOX, oxaliplatin + capecitabine, and capecitabine are all recognized standard adjuvant treatment options
	- Benefit of oxaliplatin-based doublet adjuvant chemotherapy may be less in patients aged >70 years or with Stage II disease:
	  - Single-agent fluoropyrimidines could be used in these groups of patients
	- Elderly patients (>70 years) derive the same magnitude of benefit from adjuvant chemotherapy for Stage III colon cancer and therefore it should be offered to those who are medically fit

Postoperative CRT + adjuvant chemotherapy for rectal cancer	- Preoperative CRT is more effective and has less acute and long-term toxicity than postoperative CRT
	- Patients with rectal cancer who have not received preoperative CRT should be considered for postoperative CRT and chemotherapy for the following indications:
	  - Involved circumferential margin (CRM+)
	  - Poor quality TME specimen suggesting that residual microscopic tumour may still reside within the patient
	  - Defects or a perforation in the tumour area or extranodal deposits
	- Postoperative CRT is delivered for a total of 6 months with either oral capecitabine or intravenous 5-FU (bolus or continuous infusion) and concomitantly with radiotherapy (e.g. 50 Gy, 1.8–2.0 Gy/fraction) either initially or during third and fourth cycle
	- Postoperative CRT allows better selection of high-risk patients based on pathological staging, but is associated with increased toxicity probably because the small bowel may be tethered within the pelvis
	- In a small randomized trial in patients who underwent abdomino-perineal excision, the disease-free survival rate at 10 years was significantly higher in the early radiotherapy arm than in the late radiotherapy arm (63% vs 40%; $P = 0.043$), suggesting that CRT should be administered as early as possible in the postoperative setting
	- Patients who refuse or are too frail or with excess co-morbidity to be considered for radical surgery after local excision of a rectal cancer can be offered postoperative CRT, although data supporting this approach is limited:
	  - These patients are often those for whom local excision of a pT1 tumour shows adverse histopathological factors (involved margins, poor differentiation, sm3 and lymphovascular invasion) or pathology shows to be pT2
	  - Their risk for local recurrence is considered to be high even if a full-thickness negative margin has been achieved

Postoperative (adjuvant) chemotherapy for rectal cancer	- In contrast to colon cancer, data from randomized trials in rectal cancer investigating the efficacy of adjuvant chemotherapy after preoperative CRT and surgery have been hampered by small numbers of patients and conflicting results - In the USA, standard adjuvant treatment for locally-advanced rectal cancer is usually 5-FU + leucovorin, or capecitabine or FOLFOX, although there is little firm evidence for this approach - Adjuvant chemotherapy should ideally commence as early as possible after recovery from surgery up to a maximum of 8–12 weeks following surgery - Stage II patients, i.e. those with upper rectal pT3N0 tumours after TME with 12 lymph nodes examined and an adequate CRM, are considered low risk and are not usually offered postoperative adjuvant treatment

Systemic therapy	Description

Palliative chemotherapy	• Palliative treatment involves a combination of specialist treatments (such as palliative surgery, chemotherapy and radiation), symptom control and psychosocial support
	• Chemotherapy has improved in the past decade:
	  ▪ Seven drugs are approved by the FDA for the treatment of metastatic CRC, many of which are used in combination
	  ▪ National Comprehensive Cancer Network (NCCN) guidelines offer 12 different possible drug combinations as options for first-line treatment in patients with metastatic CRC
	  ▪ Newer cytotoxic drugs such as oxaliplatin and irinotecan have improved the overall survival of metastatic CRC patients
	  ▪ Modern drug combinations produce a median survival consistently in the region of 18–24 months:
	    ○ Median overall survival for patients with unresectable metastatic CRC who receive best supportive care alone is approximately 5–6 months
	• Primary resection of metastases or resection after combination therapy and down-sizing of lesions offers a chance for cure for some patients:
	  ▪ Long-term survival is infrequent once metastatic disease has been diagnosed and is limited mainly to patients who are suitable for resection of metastases
	• *Combination treatment*:
	  ▪ Optimal sequence of therapy (FOLFOX followed by FOLFIRI or the reverse sequence) for metastatic CRC has been addressed in randomized trials, but no particular sequence has demonstrated an advantage in terms of response rates or overall survival
	  ▪ Optimal sequence of using biological agents (Box 26.1.6) is also unclear, but patients exposed to all cytotoxic and biological drugs may now have a median survival of >30 months

---

Box 26.1.6 Biological agents in palliative chemotherapy

VEGF (bevacizumab and aflibercept)
- *Bevacizumab*:
  - Can be combined with both FOLFIRI and FOLFOX and this has shown survival benefit over cytotoxic drugs alone
  - Can be used in first- or second-line treatment or continuing from first- to second-line treatment with different cytotoxic drug platforms
  - Needs to be given with cytotoxic drugs
  - During an intensive chemotherapy-free period, can only be used as maintenance therapy when combined with 5-FU or capecitabine
- *Aflibercept*:
  - Combined with FOLFIRI has improved survival in second-line setting after failure of oxaliplatin-based chemotherapy

Anti-human epidermal growth factor receptor (EGFR) (cetuximab and panitumumab)
- EGFR is overexpressed in about 70% of patients with metastatic CRC and has been considered a poor prognostic factor
- Cetuximab and panitumumab are monoclonal antibodies (chimeric human–mouse and fully human, respectively) that block the ligand-binding site of the EGFR
- Cetuximab and panitumumab bind to the extracellular domain of the EGFR on normal and tumour cells, and competitively inhibit the binding of EGF and other ligands, thus inhibiting cell growth and induction of apoptosis
- Mutations in *KRAS* are present in 40–50% of patients and predict resistance to cetuximab or panitumumab, although a wild-type *KRAS* does not ensure response to these treatments
- Cetuximab and panitumumab can be combined with oxaliplatin- or irinotecan-based chemotherapy
- For cetuximab, oxaliplatin is increasingly recognized as a suboptimal partner and irinotecan-based chemotherapy is preferred
- Unlike bevacizumab, both cetuximab and panitumumab demonstrate single-agent activity and can be used without cytotoxic drugs

Radiotherapy

Detailed and dogmatic definitions of radiotherapy treatment fields are beyond the scope of this chapter. There are significant differences in approach within Europe and the USA, but in general the clinical target volume should include:

- Primary tumour
- Entire mesorectum
- Any sites of likely nodal involvement (mesorectal nodes, presacral nodes and potentially obturator and internal iliac nodes)

- External iliac nodes need only be included if an anterior organ such as the urinary bladder, prostate or female sexual organs are macroscopically involved to such an extent that there is a risk of involvement of these lymph node stations.

Intraoperative radiotherapy (IORT) is a form of localized radiation, which remains an investigational treatment for very locally-advanced and locoregionally recurrent rectal cancers. The techniques of high dose rate endoluminal brachytherapy (HDBRT) or IORT as a local boost also remain experimental.

There are two common schedules for delivering preoperative radiotherapy:
- SCPRT with 25 Gy in five fractions, 5 Gy per fraction followed by immediate surgery
- Long-course CRT with 45–50.4 Gy in 25–28 fractions, 1.8 Gy per fraction, with surgery after a 4–12-week interval:
  - CRT can convert borderline resectable and fixed unresectable lesions into resectable lesions
  - CRT uses protracted infusions of 5-FU which are delivered via a portable infusion pump during pelvic radiation therapy or its oral equivalents such as capecitabine or UFT
  - A boost dose to the primary tumour can be administered to enhance shrinkage, enabling a total dose of 55.4 Gy to be administered (if required).

SCPRT versus CRT
- SCPRT and CRT are considered equivalent in terms of efficacy and late toxicity for resectable cancers where down-sizing is not necessary and there is no threat that the tumour extends up to or beyond the MRF
- In this setting, SCPRT is quicker, easier and more cost-effective
- For more locally-advanced tumours, where tumour extends up to or beyond the MRF, CRT is considered necessary

Preoperative versus postoperative CRT
- Randomized studies have demonstrated that preoperative CRT compared to postoperative adjuvant CRT significantly reduces local recurrence rates, with less acute and long-term toxicity
- Some surgeons believe that preoperative CRT is preferable because it facilitates down-sizing and also enables a higher rate of sphincter-saving surgery

Optimal timing of surgery after radiotherapy
- After SCPRT (5 × 5 Gy), the standard interval to surgery is 3–7 days following radiation:
  - Longer intervals of 10–14 days are associated with more morbidity and even a higher risk of mortality and are not recommended
- Optimal interval between completion of preoperative CRT and surgery has never been proven, but most consider this should be 4–12 weeks
- SCPRT with delayed surgery in fit patients (6–8 weeks) appears safe, but long-term results are not available and hence this strategy remains experimental
- However, for elderly (>80 years) or frail patients who are unsuitable for chemotherapy and intended for SCPRT as an alternative, surgery can safely be delayed to 8 weeks

External beam radiation for palliation
- Patients who present with locally advanced rectal cancer or recurrent disease often experience pelvic pain secondary to involvement of nerve structures within the pelvis, or from involvement of the sacrum
- Bleeding is also common
- Radiotherapy with 20–60 Gy as palliation can relieve pain and bleeding in 75% of patients for a short median duration of 6–9 months
- Radiotherapy either alone or combined with chemotherapy currently plays an integral role in the multimodal treatment of rectal cancer, particularly in potentially resectable disease

Normal tissue complications
Individual factors, such as genetic predisposition, co-morbidities such as systemic lupus, diabetes and hypothyroidism, medications (statins and ACE inhibitors) and lifestyle choices (e.g. diet and smoking habits), can all affect normal tissue complication risk from radiation.

Identification of the relevant factors for each endpoint, and incorporation of these factors into the dose–volume-based models, will undoubtedly improve the prediction of sequelae.

Quality of life
- Data on long-term quality of life is sparse after surgery, but appears satisfactory to patients despite objective impairment of sphincter function and a risk of faecal incontinence
- Sexual and urinary function may also be compromised
- Efforts should be made to better document quality of life and late effects
- Adverse late effects appear to relate mostly to total radiation dose received and timing of radiation (postoperative CRT is more morbid)

Follow-up and surveillance
- Optimal form, investigations, duration and intensity of follow-up after curative surgery for CRC remain a matter of debate
- ASCO and ESMO European guidelines are proactive
- Many recommend 6-monthly assessment for the first 3 years, followed by annual visits for a further 2 years:
  - Surveillance includes the assessment of long-term toxicities (e.g. neuropathy after oxaliplatin), clinical examination, CT scan of the chest and abdomen, and regular CEA testing for early detection of potentially resectable locoregional, hepatic or pulmonary recurrences on a 6-monthly basis
- Colonoscopy should be performed at initial diagnosis, or within 6 months if the patient presents with obstruction, then subsequently every 5 years, providing there are no abnormal findings

Survivorship
- Patients should be encouraged to improve their lifestyle by maintaining a healthy weight, performing regular physical activity, quitting smoking, acceptance of moderate alcohol use and the adoption of a healthy diet, which have been shown to lower the risks of recurrence
- There is increasing support for the development of nurse-led, late effects/survivorship clinics for patients who have received pelvic radiotherapy
- Effectiveness of pelvic floor exercises and/or biofeedback training in patients who experience faecal urgency and incontinence has been reported

Palliative care
- Palliation of the dying patient with CRC can be difficult
- Symptoms of large bowel obstruction are often difficult to control
- Pain due to recurrent pelvic tumour can be severe and debilitating:
  - Expertise in combinations of opiate and non-opiate pain relief, sedatives and anxiolytics is required
  - Nerve blocks and re-irradiation may be feasible
- Fistulae are not uncommon and surgical diversion procedures may be appropriate in patients with reasonable life-expectancy

Controversies
- What is the optimal timing of chemotherapy for patients with metastatic CRC who are asymptomatic, i.e. what is the value of early chemotherapy versus delaying the treatment until there are symptoms?
- Sequential versus combination therapy
- For symptomatic metastatic disease, what is the optimal duration of chemotherapy?
- Optimal time for surgery (4–12 weeks) in terms of minimizing surgical morbidity and maximizing response after neoadjuvant treatment remains unclear:
  - Some groups have investigated extending the interval between CRT and surgery or filling this interval with further chemotherapy to enhance response
- Accuracy of standard imaging (ERUS, CT, MRI and PET-CT) and novel imaging methods, such as diffusion-weighted MRI and PET-CT, in determining that the complete pathological response reported for 15% of patients has been achieved, is under investigation; this is currently insufficiently robust:
  - Identifying a complete response to neoadjuvant therapy remains a challenge
- Optimal treatment of small early tumours (cT1) (contact therapy/local excision/radical surgery) remains a matter of debate
- In the event of a primary rectal cancer presenting with synchronous metastases:
  - Does the primary tumour need to be resected?
  - What is the optimal sequence, type and length of the optimal treatment?

Phase III clinical trials

See Table 26.1.5.

Table 26.1.5 Phase III clinical trials

Trial reference	Results
Systemic therapy in colon cancer	
Alberts *et al.* (2012) *JAMA* 307:1383–1393	• For patients with Stage III resected colon cancer, cetuximab with adjuvant mFOLFOX6 compared with mFOLFOX6 alone did not result in an improved disease-free survival
André *et al.* (2009) *J Clin Oncol* 27:3109–3116	• Adding oxaliplatin to IV5FU2 significantly improved 5-year disease-free survival and 6-year overall survival in the adjuvant treatment of Stage II or III colon cancer
Haller *et al.* (2011) *J Clin Oncol* 29:1465–1471	• Addition of oxaliplatin to capecitabine improves disease-free survival in patients with Stage III colon cancer
Preoperative therapy in rectal cancer	• No published phase III trials where all elements are optimized, namely good quality imaging (including MRI), TME within the mesorectal plane, precision radiotherapy and modern pathology techniques (whole-mount) in rectal cancer
Kapiteijn *et al.* (2001) *N Engl J Med* 345:690–692	• Demonstrated superior local control from the addition of SCPRT to mesorectal excision in rectal cancer
Sauer *et al.* (2004) *N Engl J Med* 351:1731–1740	• Demonstrated superiority of preoperative compared to postoperative therapy in rectal cancer
Bujko *et al.* (2004) *Radiother Oncol* 72:15–24	• Demonstrated similar results for long-course CRT and SCPRT in rectal cancer
Braendengen *et al.* (2008) *J Clin Oncol* 26:3687–3694	• CRT improved local control, time to treatment failure and cancer-specific survival compared with radiotherapy alone in patients with non-resectable rectal cancer

Areas of research

- Future approaches include:
  - Incorporation of novel cytotoxic and biological agents into CRT schedules and adjuvant chemotherapy regimens
  - More sophisticated radiation techniques, such as the use of brachytherapy, IORT and intensity-modulated radiotherapy with an accelerated concomitant radiation boost
  - Gene and protein expression profiling

Recommended reading

Atkin WS, Valori R, Kuipers EJ et al. (2012) European guidelines for quality assurance in colorectal cancer screening and diagnosis. First Edition – Colonoscopic surveillance following adenoma removal. Endoscopy 44(Suppl 3):SE151–163.

Bernstein TE, Endreseth BH, Romundstad P et al. (2009) Circumferential resection margin as a prognostic factor in rectal cancer. Br J Surg 96:1348–1357.

Brenner H, Chang-Claude J, Rickert A, Seiler CM, Hoffmeister M (2012) Risk of colorectal cancer after detection and removal of adenomas at colonoscopy: population-based case-control study. J Clin Oncol 30(24):2969–2976.

Cecil TD, Sexton R, Moran BJ, Heald RJ (2004) Total mesorectal excision results in low local recurrence rates in lymph node-positive rectal cancer. Dis Colon Rectum 47:1145–1149.

de Jong AE, Vasen HF (2006) The frequency of a positive family history for colorectal cancer: a population-based study in the Netherlands. Neth J Med 64(10):367–370.

Fazio VW, Zutshi M, Remzi FH et al. (2007) A randomized multicenter trial to compare long-term functional outcome, quality of life, and complications of surgical procedures for low rectal cancers. Ann Surg 246:481–488.

Fleshman J, Sargent DJ, Green E et al. (2007) Laparoscopic colectomy for cancer is not inferior to open surgery based on 5-year data from the COST Study Group trial. Ann Surg 246:655–662.

Greenberg JA, Shibata D, Herndon JE 2nd et al. (2008) Local excision of distal rectal cancer: An update of cancer and leukemia group B 8984. Dis Colon Rectum 51:1185–1191.

Holm T, Ljung A, Häggmark T, Jurell G, Lagergren J (2007) Extended abdominoperineal resection with gluteus maximus flap reconstruction of the pelvic floor for rectal cancer. Br J Surg 94(2):232–238.

Jimeno A, Messersmith WA, Hirsch FR et al. (2009) KRAS mutations and sensitivity to epidermal growth factor receptor inhibitors in colorectal cancer: Practical application of patient selection. J Clin Oncol 27:1130–1136.

Levin B, Lieberman DA, McFarland B et al. (2008) Screening and surveillance for the early detection of colorectal cancer and adenomatous polyps, 2008: A joint guideline from the American Cancer Society, the US Multi Society Task Force on Colorectal Cancer, and the American College of Radiology. CA Cancer J Clin 58:130–160.

Lynch HT, de la Chapelle A (2003) Hereditary colorectal cancer. N Engl J Med 348:919.

MERCURY Study Group (2007) Extramural depth of tumour invasion at thin section MR in patients with rectal cancer. Results of the MERCURY Study. Radiology 243:132–139.

Marijnen CA, van Gijn W, Nagtegaal ID et al. (2010) The TME trial after a median follow-up of 11 years. Presented at: 52nd Annual ASTRO Meeting; November 1, 2010; San Diego, CA. Abstract 1.

Quirke P, Dixon MF, Durdey P, Williams NS (1986) Local recurrence of rectal cancer due to inadequate surgical resection. Lancet 2:996.

Quirke P, Steele R, Monson J et al.; MRC CR07/NCIC-CTG CO16 Trial Investigators; NCRI Colorectal Cancer Study Group (2009) Effect of the plane of surgery achieved on local recurrence in patients with operable rectal cancer: a prospective study using data from the MRC CR07 and NCIC-CTG CO16 randomised clinical trial. Lancet 373:821–828.

Sauer R, Liersch T, Merkel S et al. (2012) Preoperative versus postoperative chemoradiotherapy for locally advanced rectal cancer: Results of the German CAO/ARO/AIO-94 randomized phase III trial after a median follow-up of 11 years. J Clin Oncol 30:1926–1933.

Schmoll H et al. (2012) ESMO Consensus Guidelines for management of patients with colon and rectal cancer. A personalized approach to clinical decision making. Ann Oncol 23(10):2479–2516.

Siena S, Sartore-Bianchi A, Di Nicolantonio F et al. (2009) Biomarkers predicting clinical outcome of epidermal growth factor receptor-targeted therapy in metastatic colorectal cancer. J Natl Cancer Inst 101:1308–1324.

Sinicrope FA, Sargent DJ (2009) Clinical implications of microsatellite instability in sporadic colon cancers. Curr Opin Oncol 21:369–373.

Tol J, Koopman M, Cats A et al. (2009) Chemotherapy, bevacizumab, and cetuximab in metastatic colorectal cancer. N Engl J Med 360:563–572.

Wong R, Tandan V, De Silva S, Figueredo A (2007) Preoperative radiotherapy and curative surgery for the management of localized rectal cancer. Cochrane Database Syst Rev (2):CD002102.

26.2 Anus

Rob Glynne-Jones[1], Gina Brown[2], Ian Chau[2] and Brendan J. Moran[3]

[1]Radiotherapy Department, Mount Vernon Centre for Cancer Treatment, Mount Vernon Hospital, Northwood, UK
[2]Department of Radiology, Royal Marsden Hospital, London & Surrey, UK
[3]Department of Surgery, Hampshire Hospitals Foundation Trust, Basingstoke, Hampshire, UK

Summary	Key facts
Introduction	<ul><li>Incidence is increasing throughout the world, particularly in females</li><li>Overall 5-year survival is 65% in the USA for males and 70% for females, but has changed little over the past two decades:<ul><li>Prognosis is worse for men <50 years old; may reflect HIV infection in young men</li><li>Localized disease is associated with an 80% 5-year survival rate, regional nodes with a 57% survival rate and distant disease with only a 17% survival rate</li></ul></li><li>Usually spreads in a locoregional manner within, and outside, the anal canal</li><li>Systemic spread at diagnosis is observed in <10% of cases</li></ul>
Presentation	<ul><li>Diagnosis is often delayed because seemingly trivial symptoms (bleeding, itching, mucous discharge and discomfort) are non-specific and can be attributed to benign conditions, such as haemorrhoids or anal fissures</li><li>Findings of a palpable mass, a non-healing ulcer or anal pain are common</li><li>Patients may also present with faecal incontinence</li><li>Occasionally, patients present with awareness of enlarged inguinal lymph nodes</li><li>Small, early cancers are sometimes diagnosed serendipitously following the removal of anal skin tags</li></ul>
Scenario	<ul><li>Primary aim of treatment is to achieve locoregional control and preserve anal function, with the best possible quality of life</li><li>*Early Stage I cancers at the anal margin*:<ul><li>Local excision (with careful examination of margins)</li></ul></li><li>*Stage I–III*:<ul><li>Definitive CRT</li></ul></li><li>*Stage IV*:<ul><li>No curative treatment</li><li>Options:<ul><li>Palliative radiation</li><li>Palliative chemotherapy</li><li>Combinations of chemotherapy and radiotherapy</li><li>Stoma</li></ul></li></ul></li></ul>
Trials	<ul><li>Combinations of 5-FU–based chemoradiotherapy (CRT) and other cytotoxic agents (usually mitomycin C [MMC]) have been established as the standard of care:<ul><li>Complete tumour regression in 80–90% of patients, with locoregional failures approximately 15%</li></ul></li></ul>

UICC Manual of Clinical Oncology, Ninth Edition. Edited by Brian O'Sullivan, James D. Brierley, Anil K. D'Cruz, Martin F. Fey, Raphael Pollock, Jan B. Vermorken and Shao Hui Huang. © 2015 UICC. Published 2015 by John Wiley & Sons, Ltd.

Incidence, aetiology and screening

Incidence, aetiology and surveillance	Description

Incidence	- Squamous cell cancers of the anus (SCCA) are rare:
	  - Incidence of 1 in 100,000
	  - Accounts for 1–2% of digestive tract tumours and 2–4% of colon, rectal and anal tumours
	- Median age at presentation is 50–64 years; rare below 20 years of age:
	  - Incidence increases with age in women
	- It was projected that 7060 men and women (2630 men and 4430 women) in the USA will be diagnosed with, and 880 men and women will die from, cancer of the anus, anal canal and anorectum in 2013

Aetiology	- SCCA is common in the human immunodeficiency virus-positive (HIV+) population - SCCA is also strongly associated with human papillomavirus (HPV types 16–18) infection - Immune suppression in transplant recipients - Use of immunosuppressants such as long-term corticosteroids - Tobacco smoking - Autoimmune disorders - Social deprivation - Inflammatory bowel disease (Crohn's disease) - No recognized hereditary component

Screening and prevention	- *Screening*:
	  - Programmes using anal cytology and high-resolution anoscopy have been proposed for high-risk populations (men who have sex with men [MSM] and HIV-positive women)
	  - No randomized control study has yet demonstrated the advantage of screening in high-risk populations
	- *Prevention*:
	  - A recent meta-analysis indicated that 80% of anal cancers might also be prevented with prophylactic quadrivalent HPV vaccine (against HPV types 6, 11, 16 and 18)
	  - Vaccination has no role when invasive SCC is present

Pathology and molecular biology

Anal intraepithelial neoplasia

- Anal cancer may arise from a precursor dysplastic lesion – anal intraepithelial neoplasia (AIN), also known as anal squamous intraepithelial lesions (SIL):
  - Prevalence of AIN in the general population is low, but high in MSM
- Progression from AIN 1 and 2 to AIN 3 is uncommon, as is progression from AIN 3 to invasive malignancy in immunocompetent patients, but appears more likely in immunosuppressed patients and is influenced by HIV seropositivity, low CD4 count and serotype of HPV infection
- Both synchronous and metachronous HPV-related vaginal and cervical intraepithelial and malignant squamous lesions are frequent and should be screened for in younger women

Histology

The anal canal extends from the anorectal junction to the anal margin. It has a complex anatomical structure, with the main components being the internal and external sphincter muscles. The anal margin is the pigmented skin immediately surrounding the anal orifice, extending laterally to a radius of approximately 5 cm.

- Histological confirmation is mandatory as other histologies, i.e. adenocarcinoma, melanoma, gastrointestinal stromal tumours, poorly differentiated neuroendocrine tumours and lymphoma occur at this site
- Histological grading is important:
  - Cancers arising in the anal canal are often poorly differentiated SCC
  - Tumours arising at the anal margin are more likely to be well differentiated.
  - Subject to interobserver variability
  - Considerable heterogeneity is seen in larger tumours
- Histological subclassifications of basaloid, transitional, spheroidal and cloacogenic cell cancers no longer have any additional confirmed bearing on management
- In very poorly differentiated cancers, cases of rectal adenocarcinoma can be distinguished by positivity for CK 18, 20 and CDX2, in contrast to CK 14, which favours SCCA

Diagnostic work-up

- Assessment and treatment should be carried out in specialized centres
- Symptoms, other relevant medical conditions, current medications and predisposing factors should be documented
- Examination should include:
  - Digital rectal examination (DRE)
  - In women, particularly those with low anteriorly placed tumours, a vaginal exam
  - Palpation of the inguinal nodes is important, particularly the superficial inguinal nodes
  - Examination under anaesthetic (EUA) is necessary on occasion for inspection and to obtain a biopsy
- Suspicious lesions should always be biopsied
- Standard work-up includes proctoscopy
- Imaging:
  - Whole-body computed tomography (CT) to determine whether there is metastatic disease

- Pelvic magnetic resonance imaging (MRI) is mandatory for locoregional staging
- Other options include positron emission tomography (PET) and squamous cell carcinoma antigen (SCCAg) testing
- If histology is unknown, a colonoscopy can be performed to assess pathology in the proximal bowel, although unlike for colorectal adenocarcinoma, synchronous lesions are not reported for SCCA

Staging work-up
- SCCA has a low rate of distant metastases at presentation
- *Imaging* should include:
  - MRI pelvis:
    - If not available, endoanal ultrasound (EUS)
  - CT thorax, abdomen and pelvis
  - PET-CT with ^{18}F-fluorodeoxyglucose (FDG-PET-CT) can identify involved lymph nodes, particularly in immunocompetent patients, and is recommended in the current National Comprehensive Cancer Network (NCCN) treatment guidelines
- *Further investigations*:
  - Biopsy, either by needle or excisional biopsy, can clarify clinically involved inguinal nodes or those enlarged to >10 mm on CT or MRI
  - Sentinel lymph node biopsy (SLNB) can reveal micrometastatic spread of disease:
    - May be more accurate than diagnostic imaging, but has not been systematically evaluated
  - HIV testing is recommended for patients with anal cancer

Staging and prognostic grouping

UICC TNM staging
See Table 26.2.1.
- Nodal involvement of anal canal lesions differs from that of anal margin tumours
- Involvement of the internal or external sphincter muscles alone is not classified as T4

Table 26.2.1 UICC TNM categories and stage grouping: Anal canal

TNM categories	
T1	≤2 cm
T2	>2–5 cm
T3	>5 cm
T4	Adjacent organ(s)
N1	Perirectal
N2	Unilateral internal iliac/inguinal
N3	Perirectal and inguinal, bilateral internal iliac/inguinal
M1	Distant metastasis

Prognostic factors
See Table 26.2.2.

Table 26.2.2 Prognostic factors for outcome in anal cancer

Prognostic factors	Tumour related	Host related	Environment related
Essential	T, N and M category	Age Male gender	Cigarette smoking Social deprivation
Additional	Skin ulceration Sphincter involvement Primary tumour size >5 cm	Immune suppression Long-term corticosteroids HIV	
New and promising	Squamous cell carcinoma antigen (SCCAg)	Concomitant herpes simplex virus (HSV) Haemoglobin level	

Treatment philosophy

The primary aim of treatment is to achieve locoregional control and preserve anal function, with the best possible quality of life.

Scenario	Treatment philosophy
Early Stage I cancers at the anal margin	• Local excision (with careful examination of margins)
Stage I–III	• Definitive CRT

Stage IV	• No curative treatment
	• Options:
	  ▪ Palliative radiation
	  ▪ Palliative chemotherapy
	  ▪ Combinations of chemotherapy and radiotherapy
	  ▪ Stoma

Stage grouping			
Stage 0	Tis	N0	M0
Stage I	T1	N0	M0
Stage II	T2, T3	N0	M0
Stage IIIA	T1, T2, T3	N1	M0
	T4	N0	M0
Stage IIIB	T4	N1	M0
	Any T	N2, N3	M0
Stage IV	Any T	Any N	M1

Treatment

Surgery

- Early cancers at the anal margin may be adequately treated by local excision
- Until the introduction of definitive CRT, abdominoperineal excision (APE) was recommended for anal cancers (except those small enough for local excision):
  - Primary APE was associated with local failure in up to half of cases and 5-year survival rates in the region of 50–70% were reported
  - Today, primary APE may be offered to patients previously irradiated in the pelvic region or, more uncommonly, on patient preference
- There is an accepted role for surgical salvage for refractory or recurrent disease

Chemoradiotherapy

Evidence supporting the effectiveness of CRT as a radical treatment has been provided by multiple phase II and case series studies. Subsequent randomized trials have established the optimal regimen, although no individual randomized study has directly compared surgery versus CRT. Recommendations are based on the results of phase II and now six randomized phase III trials (EORTC 22861, UKCCCR ACT I, RTOG 87-04, RTOG 98-11, ACCORD-03, CRUK ACT II) (see Table 26.2.3).

- Synchronous CRT (SCRT), as the primary modality, is superior to radiotherapy alone:
  - 5-Fluorouracil (5-FU) and MMC (see Box 26.2.1) combined with radiotherapy are recommended rather than 5-FU + cisplatin, MMC + cisplatin, any single drug or three drugs
  - Cisplatin in combination with infused 5-FU and radiation does not improve complete response rates or local control compared to MMC, and does not reduce overall toxicity (but does result in less myelotoxicity)
  - Phase II studies and data extrapolated from randomized trials in rectal cancer suggest that capecitabine is a potential alternative to infused 5-FU
- Addition of neoadjuvant chemotherapy (NACT) prolongs the overall treatment time and has led to inferior local control, disease-free survival (DFS) and colostomy-free survival:
  - Should not be given outside clinical trials
- Additional maintenance/consolidation chemotherapy following CRT has not impacted on local control, DFS or overall survival (OS):
  - Should not be given outside clinical trials
- Toxicity from CRT is substantial, with high rates of acute skin toxicity and gastrointestinal toxicity (often requiring treatment breaks):
  - Treatment breaks may decrease the efficacy of radiation
  - Patients should be encouraged to stop smoking before therapy, because smoking enhances acute and late toxicity
- Optimal radiation dose and fractionation remains uncertain because randomized trials have not described the patterns/sites of local failure (within, marginal to or outside of the field of radiotherapy):
  - Examples of volumes and doses used in published phase III studies are given in Box 26.2.2
  - These studies were conducted before the era of intensity-modulated radiotherapy (IMRT) and the optimal schedules, optimal radiation dose, technique, duration of gap and chemotherapy choice remain uncertain
- IMRT offers the ability to conform the radiation dose to the shape of the target and thereby reduce the dose to normal tissues, such as the bowel, bladder, skin, genitalia and femurs, whilst allowing delivery of varying doses to different parts of the target
- For small tumours (T1), some investigators have used external beam radiotherapy alone, followed by a small volume

---

Box 26.2.1 Example chemotherapy regimens

- Based on ACT II:
  - MMC 12 mg/m^2 (max. 20 mg) on Day 1
  - 5-FU 1000 mg/m^2 on Days 1–4 and 29–32 concurrently with radiation
- Based on RTOG 98-11:
  - MMC 10 mg/m^2 on Days 1 and 29 (not to exceed 20 mg per course)
  - 5-FU 1000 mg/m^2/day by continuous infusion on Days 1–4 and 29–32

Box 26.2.2 Example radiation volumes and doses

- Based on ACT II study:
  - Phase I: all pelvic nodes below common – dose of 30.6 Gy in 1.8-Gy fractions
  - Phase II: primary tumour and involved regional lymph nodes – 50.4 Gy in 1.8-Gy fractions over 5½ weeks
- Based on RTOG 98-11:
  - Phase I: pelvis, anus, perineum and inguinal nodes, with the superior field border at L5–S1 and the inferior border to include the anus with a minimum margin of 2.5 cm around the anus and tumour –30.6 Gy in 17 fractions
  - Phase II: superior field extent reduced to the bottom of the sacroiliac joints and 14.4 Gy given in eight fractions (total dose of 45 Gy in 25 fractions/5 weeks), with additional field reduction for node-negative inguinal nodes after 36 Gy
  - Phase III: for T3, T4, node-positive disease or patients with T2 residual disease – after 45 Gy, an additional boost of 10–14 Gy in 2-Gy fractions (total dose of 55–59 Gy in 30–32 fractions over 5.5–6.5 weeks) (intended)

boost either with photons, electrons or interstitial implantation
- Brachytherapy has been advocated to increase dose to the primary tumour, but requires considerable expertise to avoid radionecrosis due to an unsatisfactory dose distribution

Considerations for immunocompromised patients

- Immunocompromised patients are at higher risk for developing anal carcinoma
- Patients with a positive HIV status may experience increased toxicity with combined chemotherapy and radiation
- A CD4+ cell count of <200/μL in HIV-positive patients is associated with higher rates of toxicity
- Use of IMRT may benefit this patient subset

Palliative chemotherapy

- Precise choice of chemotherapy is often influenced by the prior CRT regimen
- Systemic chemotherapy with a combination of 5-FU + cisplatin remains the most commonly used palliative regimen
- Responses can be sustained, but do not represent a cure
- Other agents such as a taxane are sometimes effective and single-centre series show response rates of 20–60% in first line

- Over-expression of epidermal growth factor receptor (EGFR) is common in SCCA, but *KRAS* and *BRAF* mutations appear rare, so there may be a therapeutic role for EGFR inhibition:
  - Data on the efficacy of biological agents combined with CRT are awaited

Survivorship

Women should be warned regarding the risk of vaginal stenosis, and be counselled as to the use of vaginal dilators.

Palliative care

- Pain due to recurrent pelvic tumour can be extreme, and requires expertise in combinations of opiate and non-opiate pain relief, sedatives and anxiolytics
- Nerve blocks and re-irradiation may be feasible
- Fistulae from the bladder or rectum may require surgical diversion procedures in patients with reasonable life-expectancy

Phase III clinical trials

See Table 26.2.3.

Table 26.2.3 Phase III clinical trials

Trial reference	Results
UKCCCR (1996) *Lancet* 348:1049–1054	- 585 patients - At median follow-up of 42 months, a 46% reduction (95% CI 0.42–0.69; $\chi = 24.6$; $P < 0.0001$) in the risk of local treatment-failure (locoregional failure and need for colostomy) using combined modality treatment (CMT) with 5-FU/MMC and radiotherapy, compared to that achieved by radiotherapy alone (61% vs 39% at 3 years)
Bartelink et al. (1997) *J Clin Oncol* 15(5):2040–2049	- Similar design - Restricted to T3/4 and T1–4N+ tumours - Local control also improved with CRT (68% vs 55% at 3 years)
RTOG-8704 Flam et al. (1996) *J Clin Oncol* 14(9):2527–2539	- Demonstrated the advantage of adding two courses of MMC at a dose of 10 mg/m^2 when combined with radiotherapy in terms of complete tumour regression and improved colostomy-free survival (CFS) over irradiation and 5-FU alone - At 4 years, the CFS rate was 71% vs 59% for the MMC arm compared to the 5-FU-alone arm, respectively, and DFS was 73% vs 51%, respectively
RTOG 98-11 Gunderson et al. (2012) *J Clin Oncol* 30(35):4344–4351; Ajani et al. (2008) *JAMA* 299(16):1914–1921	- Assigned 682 patients to either neoadjuvant 5-FU + cisplatin for two cycles prior to concurrent CRT with 5-FU + cisplatin (n = 341), or the standard arm of concurrent CRT with 5-FU and MMC (n = 341) - DFS, locoregional control and distant relapse or OS were not improved in the neoadjuvant cisplatin-based chemotherapy arm - More mature follow-up suggests the outcome for cisplatin was significantly inferior
ACCORD 03 Peiffert et al. (2012) *J Clin Oncol* 30(16):1941–1948	- Tested two cycles of NACT with 5-FU + cisplatin, and also radiation dose escalation in a factorial 2 × 2 trial design in 307 patients with SCC >40 mm in size and/or with pelvic or inguinal involved nodes - No benefit in CFS at doses >59 Gy or for the use of NACT

(continued)

Table 26.2.3 (Continued)

Trial reference	Results
ACT II James et al. (2013) Lancet Oncol 14(6):516–524.	• Recruited 940 patients • Patients received 5-FU (1000 mg/m²/day on Days 1–4 and 29–32) and radiotherapy (50.4 Gy in 28 daily fractions), and were randomized to receive MMC (12 mg/m² on Day 1; n = 471) or CDDP (60 mg/m² on Days 1 and 29; n = 469) • A second randomization directed two courses of consolidation therapy (n = 448) at 5 and 8 weeks after CRT (5-FU/CDDP, i.e. Weeks 11 and 14), or no consolidation (n = 446) • Neither strategy, i.e. CRT with CDDP vs CRT with MMC, nor chemotherapy consolidation with CDDP was more effective for achieving cCR, reducing tumour relapse or cancer-specific deaths compared with the standard of MMC/CRT

Phase III clinical trials have established 5-FU–based CRT combined with other cytotoxic agents (MMC) as the standard of care.

Recommended reading

Anal Carcinoma. Version 3.2014. NCCN.com. Available at http://www.nccn.org/professionals/physician_gls/pdf/anal.pdf

Bentzen AG, Guren MG, Vonen B et al. (2013) Faecal incontinence after chemoradiotherapy in anal cancer survivors: Long-term results of a national cohort. *Radiother Oncol* 108(1):55–60.

Glynne-Jones R et al. (2010) Anal cancer: ESMO Clinical Practice Guidelines for diagnosis, treatment and follow-up. On behalf of the ESMO Guidelines Working Group. *Ann Oncol* 21(Suppl 5): v87–v92.

Jemal A, Simard EP, Dorell C et al. (2013) Annual Report to the Nation on the Status of Cancer, 1975–2009, featuring the burden and trends in human papillomavirus(HPV)-associated cancers and HPV vaccination coverage levels. *J Natl Cancer Inst* 105(3):175–201.

Kachnic LA, Winter K, Myerson RJ et al. (2013) RTOG 0529: A phase 2 evaluation of dose-painted intensity modulated radiation therapy in combination with 5-fluorouracil and mitomycin-C for the reduction of acute morbidity in carcinoma of the anal canal. *Int J Radiat Oncol Biol Phys* 86(1):27–33.

Lampejo T, Kavanagh D, Clark J et al. (2010) Prognostic biomarkers in squamous cell carcinoma of the anus: a systematic review. *Br J Cancer* 103(12): 1858–1869.

Matzinger O, Roelofsen F, Mineur L et al. (2009) Mitomycin C with continuous fluorouracil or with cisplatin in combination with radiotherapy for locally advanced anal cancer (European Organisation for Research and Treatment of Cancer phase II study 22011-40014). *Eur J Cancer* 45(16):2782–2791.

Mullen JT, Rodriguez-Bigas MA, Chang GJ et al. (2007) Results of surgical salvage after failed chemoradiation therapy for epidermoid carcinoma of the anal canal. *Ann Surg Oncol* 14:478–483.

Myerson RJ, Garofalo MC, El Naqa I et al. (2009) Elective clinical target volumes for conformal therapy in anorectal cancer: a radiation therapy oncology group consensus panel contouring atlas. *Int J Radiat Oncol Biol Phys* 74(3):824–830.

Ng M, Leong T, Chander S, Chu J et al. (2012) Australasian Gastrointestinal Trials Group (AGITG) Contouring Atlas and Planning Guidelines for Intensity-Modulated Radiotherapy in Anal Cancer. *Int J Radiat Oncol Biol Phys* 83(5):1455–1462.

Scholefield JH, Castle MT, Watson NF (2005) Malignant transformation of high-grade anal intraepithelial neoplasia. *Br J Surg* 92(9):1133–1136.

Sebag-Montefiore D, James R, Meadows H (2012) The pattern and timing of disease recurrence in squamous cancer of the anus: Mature results from the NCRI ACT II trial. *J Clin Oncol* 30(Suppl):abstract 4029.

27 Prostate

Malcolm Mason[1], Howard Kynaston[1] and Robert Jones[2]

[1]Institute of Cancer and Genetics, School of Medicine, Cardiff University, Cardiff, UK
[2]Institute of Cancer Sciences, University of Glasgow, Glasgow, UK

Summary	Key facts
Introduction	• Most prostate cancers are adenocarcinomas • A few are small cell carcinomas derived from neuroendocrine cells • Most common in men over 60 years of age
Presentation	• Localized disease is frequently asymptomatic • Diagnosed after a prostate-specific antigen (PSA) measurement: ◦ May be diagnosed after investigation for lower urinary tract symptoms • Metastatic disease may present with bone pain or with spinal cord compression • Usual work-up includes transrectal ultrasound scan (TRUS) and biopsy • Imaging includes magnetic resonance imaging (MRI) of prostate plus bone scan if metastatic disease is suspected • Spinal cord compression requires imaging of the spine (MRI, computed tomography [CT] or myelogram) to accurately diagnose the level of compression

Scenario	• Localized disease may be treated by surgery (radical prostatectomy) or by radiotherapy (external beam or brachytherapy):
	  ◦ External beam radiotherapy is often combined with androgen deprivation therapy (ADT)
	  ◦ In low-risk cases, patients may opt for surveillance and then have treatment if there are signs of progression
	• First-line treatment for metastatic disease is with ADT (luteinizing hormone-releasing hormone [LHRH] agonist or orchiectomy most commonly)
	• Spinal cord compression requires immediate treatment with surgery or radiotherapy
	• Second-line treatments for metastatic disease include docetaxel and additional hormone-based therapies

Trials	• Two randomized trials of population screening by serial PSA assessment do not support its widespread introduction • Two randomized trials of surgery versus watchful waiting suggest that some men benefit from immediate intervention, but do not inform about the benefits versus active surveillance • Randomized trials of radiotherapy indicate that higher doses (>70 Gy) are better than lower doses, and that the combination of radiotherapy + ADT is optimum, particularly for patients with intermediate or high-risk disease • Randomized trials have indicated that docetaxel, abiraterone, enzalutamide, radium-223 and cabazitaxel all improve survival for men with metastatic castration-resistant disease: ◦ Sipuleucel-T is another therapy with similar efficacy, but it is not widely available

Introduction

The majority of prostate cancers are adenocarcinomas, with a few being small cell carcinomas of neuroendocrine origin. The disease is most commonly diagnosed in men over 60 years of age. In the pre-PSA era, around 50% of new presentations were with metastatic disease, but this is now less common in populations with access to PSA testing. There is a disparity between changes in the incidence of and the mortality from prostate cancer over time, indicating that there is over-diagnosis and over-treatment using current criteria. Conversely, metastatic prostate cancer is still incurable, and accounts for the vast majority of deaths from this disease.

UICC Manual of Clinical Oncology, Ninth Edition. Edited by Brian O'Sullivan, James D. Brierley, Anil K. D'Cruz, Martin F. Fey, Raphael Pollock, Jan B. Vermorken and Shao Hui Huang. © 2015 UICC. Published 2015 by John Wiley & Sons, Ltd.

Incidence, aetiology and screening

Incidence, aetiology and screening	Description

Incidence	- Second most common incident cancer in men worldwide:
	  - In 2008, estimated 899,000 cases
	- Sixth most common cause of cancer mortality in men worldwide:
	  - In 2008, estimated 258,000 deaths
	- Wide variation in international incidence and death rates:
	  - High mortality rates are observed in the Caribbean, parts of South America and sub-Saharan Africa
	  - Geographical differences in incidence are mainly due to differences in PSA testing, which is common in high-income countries, particularly the USA

Aetiology	- Only well-established risk factors are older age, Black race/ethnicity and family history of the disease - Westernized diet, sedentary lifestyle and obesity may also play a role
Screening	- Routine screening for prostate cancer by PSA testing is not currently recommended worldwide: - Two large studies of prostate cancer screening, one in Europe and one in the USA, demonstrated either a small or no overall benefit to patients - Many countries have a high prevalence of PSA testing which results in high levels of case finding - Shared decision-making between patient and health professional is recommended when considering PSA testing in asymptomatic men - May be of greater benefit in high-risk groups, such as men with a very strong family history of prostate cancer in multiple generations and/or early onset below 55 years, or African–American race

Pathology and natural history

Pathology and natural history	Description

Adenocarcinoma	- Pathology is usually described by the Gleason grading system:
	  - Assigns a score of 1–5 to each of the two most prevalent patterns in the tumour (1 = best, 5 = worst)
	  - Two scores are usually combined to give a 'sum score', e.g. Gleason 3 + 3 = 6
	  - Gleason sum scores of ≤6 are considered low risk, 7 intermediate and 8–10 high risk
	- Adenocarcinomas typically metastasize to pelvic lymph nodes and to bone, especially the axial skeleton, pelvis and long bones

Neuroendocrine carcinoma	- Tendency to metastasize early and to widespread sites, including lymph nodes and viscera - Tend to have a poorer prognosis than adenocarcinomas and respond less well to ADT

Presentation

- Elevated PSA in:
  - Asymptomatic men
  - Men with urinary symptoms and/or urinary retention
- Abnormal prostate gland on rectal examination
- Bone pain if metastatic spread to bones
- Renal failure if ureteric obstruction
- Spinal cord compression presents as leg weakness, sensory or sphincter disturbance, often combined with back pain

Diagnostic work-up

Diagnostic work-up	Description
Work-up	- Serum PSA - DRE for clinical stage - Prostate biopsy using TRUS scanning: - Provides histopathological diagnosis and Gleason score - Localized disease is often categorized into low, intermediate and high risk, e.g. D'Amico classification (Table 27.1) - Local staging by MRI scan improves accuracy, especially when multiparametric MRI is used - Bone scan in high-risk cases to look for bony metastases

Tumour markers	- PSA:
	  - Serine protease produced by the prostate gland
	  - All men have detectable levels and normal serum ranges are age-dependent
	  - Benign and malignant conditions can cause elevated levels
	  - The higher the level, the greater the risk that prostate cancer is present and the more likely it is to be of a higher stage

Table 27.1 d'Amico risk classification for non-metastatic prostate cancer

	T category	Gleason sum score	PSA (ng/mL)
Low risk	T1–2a	<6	<10
Intermediate risk	T2b	7	10–20
High risk	>T2b	≥8	>20

Data source: D'Amico (1998)

Staging and prognostic grouping

UICC TNM staging
See Table 27.2.

Table 27.2 UICC TNM categproes, stage grouping and prognostic grouping: Prostate

TNM categories	
T1	Not palpable or visible
T1a	≤5%
T1b	>5%
T1c	Needle biopsy
T2	Confined within prostate
T2a	Less than one-half of one lobe
T2b	More than one-half of one lobe
T2c	Both lobes
T3	Through prostatic capsule
T3a	Extracapsular
T3b	Seminal vesicle(s)
T4	Fixed or invades adjacent structures: external sphincter, rectum, levator muscles, pelvic wall
N1	Regional lymph node(s)
M1a	Non-regional lymph node(s)
M1b	Bone(s)
M1c	Other site(s)

Stage grouping

Stage I	T1, T2a	N0	M0		
Stage II	T2b, T2c	N0	M0		
Stage III	T3	N0	M0		
Stage IV	T4	N0	M0		
	Any T	N1	M0		
	Any T	Any N	M1		

Prognostic grouping

Group I	T1a–c	N0	M0	PSA <10	Gleason ≤6
	T2a	N0	M0	PSA <10	Gleason ≤6
Group IIA	T1a–c	N0	M0	PSA <20	Gleason 7
	T1a–c	N0	M0	PSA ≥10 <20	Gleason ≤6
	T2a	N0	M0	PSA ≥10 <20	Gleason ≤6
	T2a	N0	M0	PSA <20	Gleason 7
	T2b	N0	M0	PSA <20	Gleason ≤7
Group IIB	T2c	N0	M0	Any PSA	Any Gleason
	T1–2	N0	M0	PSA ≥20	Any Gleason
	T1–2	N0	M0	Any PSA	Gleason ≥8
Group III	T3a, b	N0	M0	Any PSA	Any Gleason
Group IV	T4	N0	M0	Any PSA	Any Gleason
	Any T	N1	M0	Any PSA	Any Gleason
	Any T	Any N	M1	Any PSA	Any Gleason

Note: When either PSA or Gleason score is not available, grouping should be determined by T category and whichever of either PSA or Gleason score is available. When neither is available, prognostic grouping is not possible and stage grouping should be used.

Prognostic factors
See Table 27.3.

Table 27.3 Prognostic factors for prostate cancer

Prognostic factor	Tumour related	Host related	Environment related
Essential	Gleason sum score TNM stage PSA level	Co-morbidity Age Performance status	
Additional	Alkaline phosphatase (if bone metastases) % involvement of cores on biopsy and number of positive cores		

Treatment philosophy

Scenario	Treatment philosophy

Localized disease only	• Main aim of treatment is to prevent future morbidity and mortality from prostate cancer whilst minimizing the acute and chronic toxicity of therapy
	• As many men with localized prostate cancer will die of other causes without having suffered significant symptoms from prostate cancer, immediate treatment of the local tumour is not always necessary
	• Management options include:
	  ▪ Radical prostatectomy
	  ▪ External beam radiotherapy (EBRT) ± prior, concomitant and subsequent ADT
	  ▪ Brachytherapy
	  ▪ Active surveillance (close monitoring followed by any of the above if the disease progresses)
	• Focal therapies (ablative therapy to the involved part of the prostate only) using cryotherapy or high-intensity frequency ultrasound are experimental
	• Treatment for low-risk disease (e.g. PSA ≤10 ng/mL, Gleason ≤6, T1–2aN0M0) is likely to result in long-term disease-free survival (DFS) for the majority (>90%) of men
	  ▪ DFS percentage is lower for intermediate- or high-risk disease

Locally-advanced disease	• Main aim of treatment is to prevent or delay morbidity and mortality from prostate cancer
	• As these men are at high risk, they generally require immediate treatment where this is appropriate
	• Management options include:
	  ▪ EBRT with prior (neoadjuvant) and post (adjuvant) ADT:
	    ○ Around 90% will remain disease free 7 years after treatment
	  ▪ Radical prostatectomy ± adjuvant ADT and ± adjuvant radiotherapy should only be performed in carefully selected patients, and by highly experienced surgeons
	  ▪ ADT alone
	• In cases of significant co-morbidity, particularly where the patient's life expectancy from that co-morbidity is short, it may be appropriate to defer ADT until such a time that there are significant symptoms (watchful waiting):
	  ▪ In a patient fit enough to receive radiotherapy, the use of ADT alone is insufficient

Pelvic nodal metastases present	• Main aim of treatment is to delay morbidity from prostate cancer • Unclear whether radiotherapy to pelvic lymph nodes offers any prolongation of life • Patients may be treated with ADT if pelvic lymph node metastases are present • No level I evidence that radiotherapy to pelvic nodes is beneficial, but very fit patients with small volume lymph node disease can be treated with ADT + radiotherapy to the whole pelvis and the prostate • See above for further information about radiotherapy

Metastatic disease at presentation	• Aims of treatment are to improve current symptoms (if any), delay further symptoms and prolong survival
	• As all treatments are associated with side effects and as cure is not possible, maintaining overall quality of life is an important consideration
	• Most patients should begin treatment immediately with ADT by surgical or medical castration (± an androgen receptor antagonist, e.g. bicalutamide, which is generally continued lifelong):
	  ▪ Although most men are sensitive to castration therapy, the disease nearly always develops resistance (castration-resistant prostate cancer [CRPC])
	  ▪ At this point, additional therapies may be added (see below)
	  ▪ Maximal androgen deprivation (MAB), in which an oral antiandrogen is added to an LHRH agonist, has been extensively studied:
	    ○ Offers a statistically significant, but extremely small, additional benefit at the expense of greater toxicity and higher cost
	    ○ Not routinely used in many parts of the world

Recurrent disease after radical local treatment	• Aims of treatment are to delay or prevent morbidity and mortality from prostate cancer whilst minimizing the side effects of treatment
	• Treatment depends on the extent and characteristics of the disease, and the nature of the prior treatment
	• Treatment options include:
	  ▪ Salvage prostatectomy
	  ▪ Radiotherapy to the prostate bed
	  ▪ ADT
	• Other locally ablative therapies (e.g. cryotherapy or high-intensity frequency ultrasound) are experimental

Scenario	Treatment philosophy

Progressive metastatic disease after castration therapy	• Aims of treatment of metastatic CRPC are to improve current symptoms (if any), to delay future symptoms and to prolong survival
	• Overall quality of life remains an important consideration
	• Treatment options include:
	  ▪ Best supportive care:
	    ○ EBRT to symptomatic bone metastases, analgesia, zoledronic acid, denosumab, corticosteroids
	  ▪ Additional ADT:
	    ○ Androgen receptor antagonists, e.g. bicalutamide, enzalutamide
	    ○ Androgen biosynthesis inhibitors, e.g. abiraterone
	  ▪ Cytotoxic chemotherapy (docetaxel, cabazitaxel, mitoxantrone)
	  ▪ Systemic radionucleotides, e.g. radium-223, strontium-89

Follow-up	• Follow-up patterns vary according to the stage of the disease, co-morbidities and nature of prior treatment • PSA testing is often used as an indicator of recurrent or progressive disease, but clinical observations, radiological findings and (in the case of active surveillance) repeat prostate biopsy may be more important features of follow-up • Some patients with a rising PSA have very slowly progressing disease, and observation may be preferable to immediate treatment if the patient is clinically well

Treatment guidelines

There are three well-respected guidelines available and freely accessible over the internet:

- UK NICE guidelines (2014). Available at http://www.nice.org.uk/cg58
- US NCCN guidelines. Available at http://www.nccn.org/professionals/physician_gls/PDF/prostate.pdf
- European Association of Urology guidelines. Available at http://www.uroweb.org/guidelines/online-guidelines

In all instances, guidelines do not replace clinical judgement, and many patients with prostate cancer are frail, elderly or have significant co-morbidities. In all cases the benefits and the risks must be weighed:

- Special care should be exercised with the use of hormone therapy in a patient with severe cardiovascular disease or diabetes
- For patients with metastatic disease, the risks posed by their prostate cancer will often outweigh the risks posed by the potential side effects of ADT

Treatment

Surgery

Surgery	Description
Localized disease T1–3a	• Radical prostatectomy for low-, intermediate- and high-risk disease • In intermediate- and high-risk disease, staging lymphadenectomy of the pelvic lymph nodes is undertaken • Patients with high-risk disease may benefit from adjuvant radiotherapy (± additional ADT): ▪ Ongoing trials are underway • Salvage radiotherapy ± ADT is used for PSA recurrent disease in the absence of metastases

Radiotherapy

Radiotherapy	Description
Localized disease only	• Target volume includes the prostate and seminal vesicles ± the pelvic lymph nodes • Acceptable dose schedules include 74 Gy in 37 fractions over 7½ weeks to 78 Gy in 40 fractions over 8 weeks, or 55 Gy in 20 fractions over 4 weeks, provided that conformal radiotherapy is used
Locally-advanced disease	• Target volume includes the prostate, seminal vesicles and pelvic lymph nodes • Dose schedules: as above • Radiotherapy should be combined with ADT, commencing 4–6 months before radiotherapy, and continued during and after radiotherapy for a further 3 years (see below)
Pelvic lymph node metastases	• Small volume lymph node metastases can be treated with a combination of ADT and EBRT (as above for locally-advanced disease): ▪ Duration of ADT should be lifelong

(continued)

Radiotherapy	Description
Recurrent disease after radical prostatectomy	• Target volume is the prostate bed only • Dose of 66 Gy in 33 fractions over 6 weeks is appropriate

Metastatic disease	• Radiotherapy for metastatic disease is palliative and given to relieve symptoms:
	  ▪ Bone pain can be treated with a single 8-Gy fraction of radiotherapy to the affected area
	  ▪ Local symptoms in patients with metastases due to disease in the prostate can be treated with EBRT to the prostate
	    ○ A palliative dose can be used, such as 36 Gy in six fractions over 6 weeks, treating with one fraction per week

Systemic therapy

Systemic therapy	Description

Localized disease	• Systemic therapy, including ADT, has no role as monotherapy
	• Adjuvant ADT has a limited role following radical prostatectomy:
	  ▪ Except in selected patients, such as those with lymph node positive disease
	  ▪ No proven role as neoadjuvant before prostatectomy
	• ADT has a role prior to EBRT in patients with intermediate- and high-risk localized disease:
	  ▪ Started 4–6 months prior to radiotherapy
	  ▪ May consist of monoagent bicalutamide or an LHRH agonist
	  ▪ In patients with high-risk localized disease, should be continued after completion of radiotherapy for a total of 3 years
	• Chemotherapy should not be used in this indication

Locally-advanced disease	• Androgen deprivation (either bicalutamide alone [150 mg daily], LHRH agonist alone or a combination of these, in which case the dose of bicalutamide should be 50 mg once daily) should be used prior to, during and after EBRT:
	  ▪ Started 4–6 months prior to radiotherapy
	  ▪ Continued for a total of 3 years in the absence of disease progression
	• In patients for whom radical treatment is not appropriate, androgen deprivation may be given alone:
	  ▪ Options include bicalutamide alone or LHRH agonist ± an antiandrogen
	• Chemotherapy should not be used in this indication

PSA failure after radical local therapy	• May be managed by local salvage radiotherapy, provided there is no evidence of lymph node or other metastatic disease:
	  ▪ Treatment volume is the prostate bed
	  ▪ Dose is lower than for primary radical radiotherapy (e.g. 64 Gy in 32 fractions over 6.5 weeks, or equivalent)
	  ▪ Approach has been shown to result in biochemical (PSA) control, but as yet no definite proof of improved survival
	  ▪ Unknown whether additional ADT is beneficial in the context of salvage radiotherapy
	• In the absence of metastases, ADT may be used where the PSA is rising in the absence of ongoing castration therapy:
	  ▪ Continuous androgen deprivation or intermittent use of LHRH agonists may be used in this setting
	  ▪ Where intermittent androgen deprivation is used, the LHRH agonist should be given for at least 8 months until the PSA falls to normal levels, whereupon it may be withdrawn and the patient's PSA monitored at 3-monthly intervals
	    ○ When the PSA rises above 10 ng/mL, the LHRH agonist should be re-introduced for a further 8 months
	    ○ This cycle is repeated until emergence of castration resistance or other signs of disease progression, whereupon the LHRH agonist should be continued indefinitely

Failure of initial ADT in the absence of metastatic disease	• For patients with a rising PSA despite ongoing castration therapy, consider adding an antiandrogen (e.g. bicalutamide 50 mg once daily) • For patients progressing despite ongoing monoagent antiandrogen therapy, consider castration therapy with an LHRH agonist followed by withdrawal of the antiandrogen (withdraw 2 weeks later to protect against possible tumour flare) • Where dual androgen blockade (LHRH agonist in combination with antiandrogen) has failed, the androgen receptor antagonist should be withdrawn as this change may bring about a fall in the PSA • Other treatments, such as chemotherapy, abiraterone and corticosteroids, are of no proven value in the absence of metastatic disease, so patients failing castration and dual androgen blockade should be closely monitored for signs of metastatic disease before considering further systemic therapy (see below)

Systemic therapy	Description

Metastatic disease: initial treatment	- First-line treatment should include continuous, lifelong castration therapy:
	  - Surgical (bilateral orchidectomy), or
	  - Medical:
	    - LHRH agonist, e.g. goserelin, leuprorelin, histrelin, triptorelin (dose and schedule as per individual product) alone
	    - LHRH agonist in combination with an antiandrogen, e.g. bicalutamide 50 mg once daily, or
	    - LHRH antagonist alone (degarelix, loading dose 240 mg SC, followed by 80 mg SC every 4 weeks)
	    - Antiandrogen monotherapy is not satisfactory treatment for metastatic disease; however, where LHRH agonists are to be used to treat metastatic disease, it is recommended to administer an antiandrogen (e.g. bicalutamide 50 mg once daily) for 1 week before and 2 weeks after first dose to protect against tumour flare. This is not necessary with an LHRH antagonist

Metastatic disease: after failure of ADT	- Patients whose disease is progressing despite ongoing castration therapy (as manifested by rising PSA or the appearance of new or enlarging metastases clinically or at imaging) are considered to have CRPC
	- In cases where the patient is receiving an antiandrogen (e.g. bicalutamide) in addition to castration therapy, this should be withdrawn for at least 6 weeks before concluding castration resistance:
	  - In some cases, bicalutamide can become agonistic, and the PSA may fall after withdrawal ('withdrawal response')
	  - Castration therapy (e.g. an LHRH agonist) should continue lifelong
	- Where a patient has not previously failed a non-steroidal antiandrogen, then addition of such a drug (e.g. bicalutamide 50 mg once daily) is an option, although the benefits are modest:
	- Abiraterone acetate (1000 mg once daily) in combination with prednisone (5 mg b.i.d.) or Enzalutamide 160 mg once daily are options for patients with metastatic CRPC irrespective of prior docetaxel exposure
	- Docetaxel (75 mg/m^2 by infusion every 21 days) in combination with prednisone (5 mg b.i.d. continuously) for up to ten cycles has been shown to improve survival in men with metastatic CRPC when compared to mitoxantrone and prednisone:
	  - Unclear whether it is better to give this treatment early and so delay or prevent significant symptoms, or whether it is safe to delay this treatment and await symptomatic progression
	  - Data suggest that both asymptomatic and symptomatic patients may benefit from docetaxel, and so the decision to proceed with chemotherapy should be made after an informed discussion with the patient, taking into consideration the pace of disease progression, the patient's expectations of treatment regarding the trade-off between outcome and toxicity, and alternative treatment options which may be available
	  - As the dose-limiting toxicity of docetaxel is neutropenia, patients should be made aware of the risk of neutropenic sepsis and inpatient facilities to manage this event should be available if required:
	    - Other toxicities may be cumulative (such as fatigue and neuropathy) and so careful clinical review should be made prior to commencing each cycle of treatment
	- Mitoxantrone (12 mg/m^2 every 21 days by IV injection) with prednisone (5mg twice daily) for up to ten cycles is an alternative to docetaxel for some symptomatic men for whom docetaxel is not appropriate:
	  - Although generally well tolerated, it causes cumulative cardiotoxicity, limiting its use in men with prior cardiac damage:
	    - Cardiac ejection fraction should be carefully monitored in patients receiving this treatment
	- For patients progressing following prior docetaxel there are a number of options:
	  - Abiraterone acetate (1000 mg once daily) in combination with prednisone (5 mg b.i.d.) is licensed and is an option for those patients who have not previously failed this treatment
	  - Enzalutamide (160 mg once daily until progression) is also proven to be effective in this situation and has the advantages of not requiring concomitant use of corticosteroids (although these are permissible and safe) and being safe to take with food
	  - There are few data examining the benefits of enzalutamide in patients who have previously failed abiraterone and *vice versa*, although, by their mechanisms of action, a degree of cross-resistance is expected
	  - Cabazitaxel (25 mg/m^2 every 21 days by IV infusion) + prednisone (5 mg twice daily) for up to ten cycles has been shown to improve survival when compared to mitoxantrone + prednisone in patients who have previously received docetaxel:
	    - Like docetaxel, the main dose-limiting toxicity is neutropenia, and consideration should be given to using primary prophylactic granulocyte-colony stimulating factor (G-CSF, e.g. pegfilgrastim 6 mg on Day 2 of each cycle by SC injection) in patients at high risk

(continued)

Systemic therapy	Description

	• Immunotherapy using a process of extracorporeal immune stimulation called sipuleucel-T has been shown to prolong survival in men with metastatic castration-resistant prostate cancer:
	    ▪ Due primarily to technical limitations, this is currently only licensed in the USA
	    ▪ Although the optimal timing of this treatment relative to other therapies (such as chemotherapy) is unclear, it is likely that the greatest benefits from this approach will accrue to those patients receiving it relatively early in the course of metastatic CRPC
	• Bone-seeking radioisotopes such as strontium-89 (1.5–2.2 MBq/kg) or more recently radium-223 (50 kBq/kg every 4 weeks for six cycles) can also be used for men with symptoms of bone metastases:
	    ▪ Radium is preferred if it is available
	    ▪ These treatments can only be delivered in centres where there are appropriate resources in place for the management and handling of radioisotopes
	• A group of supportive care drugs whose role is primarily in delaying bone-related complications ('skeletal-related events'): need for palliative radiotherapy, increased need for analgesia, pathological fracture and spinal cord compression:
	    ▪ Bisphosphonates (primarily zoledronate 4 mg every 28 days by IV infusion)
	    ▪ More recently, denosumab (120 mg by SC injection every 28 days):
	        ○ Denosumab was more effective than zoledronate in a head-to-head comparison
	• Other acceptable treatments with low-level evidence of efficacy:
	    ▪ Low-dose corticosteroids, especially dexamethasone (0.5 mg once daily)
	    ▪ Ketoconazole in combination with corticosteroids may be used but is toxic
	    ▪ Synthetic oestrogens (e.g. diethylstilbestrol 1 mg once daily) can sometimes be beneficial, but carry a significant risk of thrombosis and are usually given with some form of anticoagulation (e.g. aspirin 75 mg once daily) and should be used with care in patients at risk of vascular events such as stroke or cardiovascular disease

Post-treatment assessment

For patients with *localized disease*:
- PSA levels should be monitored after surgery:
  - Should remain <0.1 ng/mL
  - Measurable and/or rising PSA levels after surgery indicate biochemical recurrence
  - Salvage therapy, including prostate bed radiotherapy ± ADT should be considered
- PSA should be monitored after radiotherapy:
  - If the patient is on concomitant or adjuvant hormone therapy, the PSA may rise following discontinuation and this does not necessarily indicate treatment failure
  - PSA failure after radiotherapy is defined according to the ASTRO 'Phoenix' definition, i.e. a rise by ≥2 ng/mL above the nadir (defined as the lowest PSA achieved) after radiotherapy ± short-term hormonal therapy
- Repeat biopsy of the prostate following radiotherapy may be difficult to interpret.

For patients with *metastatic disease*:
- Castration therapy should, in general, be continued indefinitely
- Systemic therapy for advanced disease should not, in general, be switched on the basis of changes in PSA alone:
  - Increases in PSA within the first 12 weeks of initiation of a new line of treatment are often not indicative of true disease progression
- Changes in symptoms and imaging of distant metastases should be used to guide changes in systemic treatment of metastatic CRPC
- Tumour 'flare' (the appearance of new lesions on bone scan in the absence of true progression) may arise during the first 12 weeks or more:
  - Where there is doubt, treatment should be continued and further, subsequent evidence of disease progression should be sought (e.g. the appearance of further new lesions on a subsequent bone scan at least 6 weeks later).

Continuing care

In addition to the specific treatments described elsewhere, attention should be paid to the following:
- Adequate pain control for bone pain due to bone metastases:
  - May include the adequate use of opiate analgesia
  - Palliative radiotherapy is usually extremely effective and may be given to a wide field as an 8-Gy single fraction
- Use of a nephrostomy or a suprapubic catheter may be required in some instances of urinary tract obstruction due to malignant disease, but suitable patients require careful selection
- Spinal cord compression is an ever-present risk for men with spinal bone metastases, and a high level of awareness by patient and doctor is strongly recommended.

Controversies

- Role of population-based screening for prostate cancer
- Optimal management of patients with clinically localized prostate cancer

- Optimal sequencing of systemic therapies in metastatic CRPC, particularly the optimal timing of chemotherapy initiation

Phase III clinical trials

See Table 27.4.

Areas of research

- Identification of biomarkers to distinguish indolent from aggressive disease in patients with apparently organ-confined prostate cancer
- Optimization of surgery, radiotherapy and focal therapies for localized disease
- Randomized comparison of surgery, radiotherapy and active monitoring in localized disease
- Benefits of additional systemic therapy for patients with high-risk localized or metastatic disease from starting first-line ADT
- Identification of molecular predictive markers to prioritize choice of systemic treatments for metastatic disease at the individual patient level
- Novel therapies for CRPC

Table 27.4 Phase III clinical trials

Trial name	Results
MRC RT01 Dearnaley et al. (2007). Lancet Oncol 8(6):475–487	• For patients with low-, intermediate- and high-risk localized disease, dose-escalated radiotherapy (74 Gy) results in better progression-free survival compared with lower dose (64 Gy)
EORTC 22863 Bolla et al. (2010) Lancet Oncol 11(11):1066–1073	• For patients with high-risk localized and locally-advanced disease, radiotherapy + hormone therapy improves overall survival compared with radiotherapy alone for locally-advanced disease
SPCG-7 Widmark et al. (2009). Lancet 373:1174–1174	• For patients with high-risk localized and locally-advanced prostate cancer, the addition of radiotherapy to ADT improved disease-specific and overall survival
PR3/PR07 Warde et al. (2011). Lancet 378:2104–2111	• For patients with high-risk localized and locally-advanced prostate cancer, the addition of radiotherapy to ADT improved disease-specific and overall survival
S9346(INT-0162) Hussain et al. (2013). N Engl J Med 368(14):1314–1325	• For patients with castrate-refractory, metastatic disease, intermittent androgen deprivation failed to demonstrate non-inferiority compared to continuous ADT in men who had had an initially good response to ADT
TAX327 Tannock et al. (2004). N Engl J Med 351:1502–1512	• For patients with castrate-refractory, metastatic disease, 3-weekly docetaxel + prednisone improved survival compared with mitoxantrone + prednisone in metastatic CRPC • Weekly docetaxel alone did not
TROPIC de Bono M et al. (2010). Lancet 376:1147–1154	• For patients with castrate-refractory, metastatic disease, 3-weekly cabazitaxel + prednisone prolonged survival compared to mitoxantrone + prednisone in patients who had previously received docetaxel
COU-AA-301 de Bono et al. (2011). N Engl J Med 364:1995–2005	• For patients with castrate-refractory, metastatic disease, abiraterone acetate + prednisone improved survival compared to placebo + prednisone in patients who had previously received docetaxel
COU-AA-302 Ryan et al. (2013). N Engl J Med 368(2):138–148	• For patients with castrate-refractory, metastatic disease, abiraterone acetate + prednisone improved radiographic progression-free survival compared to placebo + prednisone in asymptomatic or minimally symptomatic patients who had not previously received docetaxel
AFFIRM Scher et al. (2012). N Engl J Med 367(13):1187–1197	• For patients with castrate-refractory, metastatic disease, enzalutamide improved survival compared to placebo in patients who had previously received docetaxel
ALSYMPCA Parker et al. (2013). N Engl J Med 369(3):213–223	• For patients with castrate-refractory, metastatic disease, radium-223 improved survival compared to placebo in men with symptomatic bone metastases and CRPC who had previously received docetaxel or for whom docetaxel was not appropriate

Recommended reading

Andriole GL, Crawford ED, Grubb RL et al. (2009) Mortality results from a randomized prostate cancer screening trial. N Engl J Med 360:1310.

Bolla M, Tienhoven VT, Warde P et al. (2010) External irradiation with or without long-term androgen suppression for prostate cancer with high metastatic risk: 10-year results of an EORTC randomised study. Lancet Oncol 11(11):1066–1073.

Bolla M, van Poppel H, Tombal B et al. (2012) Postoperative radiotherapy after radical prostatectomy for high-risk prostate cancer: long-term results of a randomised controlled trial (EORTC trial 22911). Lancet 380:2018–2027.

Berthold DR, Pond GR, Roessner M et al. (2008) Treatment of hormone-refractory prostate cancer with docetaxel or mitoxantrone: relationships between prostate-specific antigen, pain, quality of life response and survival in the TAX 327 study. Clin Cancer Res 14:2763–2767.

D'Amico AV, Whittington R, Malkowicz SB et al. (1999) A pre-treatment nomogram for prostate specific antigen recurrence following radical prostatectomy or external beam radiation therapy for clinically localized prostate cancer. J Clin Oncol 17:168–172.

Dearnaley DP, Sydes MR, Graham JD et al. (2007) Escalated-dose versus standard-dose conformal radiotherapy in prostate cancer: first results from the MRC RT01 randomised controlled trial. Lancet Oncol 8(6):475–487.

de Bono JS, Logothetis CJ, Molina A et al. (2011) Abiraterone and increased survival in metastatic prostate cancer. N Engl J Med 364:1995–2005.

de Bono JS, Oudard S, Ozguroglu M et al. (2010) Prednisone plus cabazitaxel or mitoxantrone for metastatic castration-resistant prostate cancer progressing after docetaxel treatment: a randomised open-label trial. Lancet 376:1147–1154.

Ferlay J et al. (2010) GLOBOCAN 2008, cancer incidence and mortality worldwide: IARC CancerBase No 10. Lyon: International Agency for Research on Cancer.

Fizazi K, Carducci M, Smith M et al. (2011) Denosumab versus zoledronic acid for treatment of bone metastases in men with castration-resistant prostate cancer: a randomised, double-blind study. Lancet 377:813–822.

Hussain M, Tangen CM, Berry DL et al. (2013) Intermittent versus continuous androgen deprivation in prostate cancer. N Engl J Med 368(14):1314–1325.

Parker C, Nilsson S, Heinrich D et al. (2013) Alpha emitter radium-223 and survival in metastatic prostate cancer. N Engl J Med 369(3):213–223.

Ryan CJ, Smith MR, de Bono JS et al. (2013) Abiraterone in metastatic prostate cancer without previous chemotherapy. N Engl J Med 368(2):138–148.

Saad F, Gleason DM, Murray R et al. (2002) A randomized, placebo-controlled trial of zoledronic acid in patients with hormone-refractory metastatic prostate carcinoma. J Natl Cancer Inst 94(19):1458–1468.

Scher HI, Fizazi K, Saad F et al. (2012). Increased survival with enzalutamide in prostate cancer after chemotherapy. N Engl J Med 367(13):1187–1197.

Schroder FH, Hugosson J, Roobol MJ et al. (2009) Screening and prostate cancer mortality in a randomized European study. N Engl J Med 360:1320.

Tannock IF, Osoba D, Stockler MR et al. (1996) Chemotherapy with mitoxantrone plus prednisone or prednisone alone for symptomatic hormone-resistant prostate cancer: A Canadian randomized trial with palliative end points. J Clin Oncol 14:1756–1764.

Tannock IF, de Wit R, Berry WR et al. (2004) Docetaxel plus prednisone or mitoxantrone plus prednisone for advanced prostate cancer. N Engl J Med 351:1502–1512.

Widmark A, Klepp O, Solberg A et al. (2009) Endocrine treatment, with or without radiotherapy, in locally advanced prostate cancer (SPCG-7/SFUO-3): an open randomised phase III trial. Lancet 373:1174–1174.

Warde P, Mason M, Ding K et al. (2011) Combined androgen deprivation therapy and radiation therapy for locally advanced prostate cancer: a randomised, phase 3 trial. Lancet 378:2104–2111

28 Bladder and other urothelium

Gillian M. Duchesne[1], Shomik Sengupta[2] and Ian D. Davis[3]

[1]Sir Peter MacCallum Department of Oncology, University of Melbourne, Melbourne, Victoria, Australia
[2]Urology Department, Austin Health and Austin Department of Surgery, University of Melbourne, Heidelberg, Victoria, Australia
[3]Monash University and Eastern Health, Victoria, Australia

Summary	Key facts
Introduction	- Can arise anywhere along the urinary tract from the kidneys down to the urethra: - Commonest site of occurrence is the bladder, where they comprise the majority of histological types - Highest incidence in developed nations - Strong correlation with smoking
Presentation	- Urological symptoms, e.g. dysuria, haematuria, frequency, pain - Systemic symptoms, e.g. weight loss with disseminated disease

Scenario	- *Non-muscle invasive disease*:
	  - Local resection
	  - Intravesical chemotherapy or Bacillus Calmette-Guerin (BCG)
	  - Ongoing cystoscopic surveillance
	- *Muscle-invasive disease*:
	  - Radical cystectomy with urinary diversion ± neoadjuvant systemic chemotherapy, and possible adjuvant chemotherapy
	  - Bladder-preserving chemoradiation with cisplatin-based radiosensitization in selected cases

Trials	- Phase III trials have established the role of intravesical chemotherapy for non-invasive disease and systemic chemotherapy in the management of muscle-invasive disease - No recent phase III trials of primary treatment modality

Introduction

Urothelial cancers, previously known as transitional cell carcinomas (TCC), can arise anywhere in the urothelium from the renal pelvis down to the proximal urethra and prostatic ducts. Squamous carcinomas are associated with squamous metaplasia of the transitional epithelium caused by chronic irritation, and adenocarcinomas occur rarely, most often in the urachal remnant. The urinary bladder is the predominant site of urothelial malignancy.

Incidence, aetiology and screening

Incidence, aetiology and screening	Description
Incidence	- Urothelial carcinoma represents about 3% of malignancies worldwide and 2% of cancer deaths - Statistics clouded due to inclusion of some upper tract urothelial cancers in 'kidney and renal pelvis' and variable collection of non–muscle-invasive bladder cancer data

(continued)

UICC Manual of Clinical Oncology, Ninth Edition. Edited by Brian O'Sullivan, James D. Brierley, Anil K. D'Cruz, Martin F. Fey, Raphael Pollock, Jan B. Vermorken and Shao Hui Huang. © 2015 UICC. Published 2015 by John Wiley & Sons, Ltd.

Incidence, aetiology and screening	Description
	• 14-fold variation in incidence internationally: 　▪ Higher in more developed nations; highest in Europe, North America, Northern Africa 　　○ High versus low incidence areas: 　　　– Age standardized ratio (ASR) per 100,000 for men: 16.6 versus 5.4 　　　– ASR per 100,000 for women: 3.6 versus 1.4 • Global mortality: 　▪ ASR per 100,000 for men 4.6 versus 2.6 　▪ ASR per 100,000 for women 1.0 versus 0.7 　▪ Mortality rates between 1997 and 2006 in the USA were stable in males and fell in females
Aetiology	• Smoking: risk proportionate to duration and intensity of exposure • Occupational chemical exposure: aromatic amines • Drug exposure: cyclophosphamide, phenacetin • Chronic irritation, e.g. infection, schistosomiasis, bladder stone or long-term catheter: generally associated with risk of squamous cell carcinoma • Urachal remnant may develop adenocarcinoma
Screening	Limited value

Pathology

- Majority (>90%) are pure urothelial carcinoma (previously known as TCC):
  - May have papillary or sessile morphology
- Variant histology may be found, including squamous, glandular (adenocarcinoma), sarcomatoid or micropapillary differentiation
- Other pathology: small cell carcinoma, sarcoma, carcinosarcoma, lymphoma, metastases, e.g. melanoma
- Depth of invasion is a key histological prognostic factor
- Use of molecular markers to assist with diagnosis and prognostic determination is currently limited:
  - Apparent divergence of molecular and genetic profiles between early papillary and sessile cancers, with convergence as the cancer progresses to become more invasive and/or metastatic

Presentation and natural history

Presentation and natural history	Description
Presentation	• Local symptoms: 　▪ Haematuria (macroscopic or microscopic), urinary frequency, urgency, strangury, infection 　▪ Pain or detectable mass if locally advanced • Symptoms of metastatic disease, e.g. pain, weight loss
Natural history	• Most lesions are non-muscle invasive and have limited lethal potential • Muscle invasive cancers have a significant metastatic potential and a poor prognosis • High probability of recurrence after transurethral resection: 　▪ Can be modified by additional therapy and smoking cessation • Critical differences in behaviour between non–muscle-invasive and invasive cancers, and between low-grade/high-grade pathology 　▪ Low-grade/non-invasive cancers tend to recur locally (50–70% risk over 10 years) but not progress 　▪ High-grade/muscle-invasive cancers invade locally and metastasize

Diagnostic work-up

Diagnostic work-up	Description
Initial evaluation of apparently localized disease	• Urinary cytology • Examination under anaesthetic • Bladder imaging: ultrasound, contrast computed tomography (CT) scan or magnetic resonance imaging (MRI) of the pelvis: limited value • Cystoscopy and tissue biopsy: 　▪ Preferably maximal transurethral resection for bladder lesions • Upper tract imaging: 　▪ Ultrasound, intravenous urography (IVU) or CT – intravenous pyelogram protocol, retrograde pyelogram • Upper tract endoscopy: 　▪ Usually by retrograde ureteropyeloscopy 　▪ Only if abnormalities suspected on imaging • Assessment of renal function

Bladder and other urothelium

Diagnostic work-up	Description
After initial diagnostic work-up: for high-grade or locally-advanced disease, to determine stage and appropriate management	• As above, plus • Assessment of renal function, haemoglobin, liver function and alkaline phosphatase (ALP) • CT abdomen and pelvis • Chest radiography ± CT scan • Whole-body bone scan (if clinical suspicion of metastasis or raised ALP) • Other imaging as clinically indicated • Assessment for suitability for ileal conduit or neobladder or bladder-preserving treatment • Multidisciplinary review

Staging and prognostic grouping

UICC TNM staging
Each individual tumour site of urothelial carcinoma has a specific staging system (Table 28.1).

Prognostic factors
Prognostic factors are given for urothelial carcinoma of the bladder (Tables 28.2 and 28.3). Evidence of application to other tumour types and sites is very limited, although it may be reasonable to extrapolate the behaviour of carcinomas elsewhere in the urothelium from the bladder cancer literature. Disease at other sites, e.g. the ureter, often presents at a more advanced stage, worsening the prognosis.

With established metastatic disease, visceral metastasis is associated with a poorer prognosis.

Table 28.1 UICC TNM categories and stage grouping: Urinary bladder; renal pelvis, ureter; and urethra

TNM categories: Urinary bladder	
Ta	Non-invasive papillary
Tis	*In situ*: 'flat tumour'
T1	Subepithelial connective tissue
T2	Muscularis
T2a	Inner half
T2b	Outer half
T3	Beyond muscularis
T3a	Microscopically
T3b	Extravesical mass
T4	Prostate, uterus, vagina, pelvic wall, abdominal wall
T4a	Prostate, uterus, vagina
T4b	Pelvic wall, abdominal wall
N1	Single
N2	Multiple
N3	Common iliac
M1	Distant metastasis

Stage grouping: Urinary bladder			
Stage 0a	Ta	N0	M0
Stage 0is	Tis	N0	M0
Stage I	T1	N0	M0
Stage II	T2a, b	N0	M0
Stage III	T3a, b	N0	M0
	T4a	N0	M0
Stage IV	T4b	N0	M0
	Any T	N1, N2, N3	M0
	Any T	Any N	M1

TNM categories: Renal pelvis, ureter	
Ta	Non-invasive papillary
Tis	*In situ*
T1	Subepithelial connective tissue
T2	Muscularis
T3	Beyond muscularis
T4	Adjacent organs, perinephric fat
N1	Single ≤2 cm
N2	Single >2–5 cm, multiple ≤5 cm
N3	>5 cm
M1	Distant metastasis

Stage grouping: Renal pelvis, ureter			
Stage 0a	Ta	N0	M0
Stage 0is	Tis	N0	M0
Stage I	T1	N0	M0
Stage II	T2	N0	M0
Stage III	T3	N0	M0
Stage IV	T4	N0	M0
	Any T	N1, N2, N3	M0
	Any T	Any N	M1

TNM categories: Urethra	
Ta	Non-invasive papillary, polypoid or verrucous
Tis	*In situ*
T1	Subepithelial connective tissue
T2	Corpus spongiosum, prostate, periurethral muscle
T3	Corpus cavernosum, beyond prostatic capsule, anterior vagina, bladder neck
T4	Other adjacent organs
Urothelial (transitional cell) carcinoma of prostate (prostatic urethra)	
Tis pu	*In situ*, prostatic urethra
Tis pd	*In situ*, prostatic ducts
T1	Subepithelial connective tissue
T2	Prostatic stroma, corpus spongiosum, periurethral muscle
T3	Corpus cavernosum, beyond prostatic capsule, bladder neck (extraprostatic extension)
T4	Other adjacent organs (bladder)
N1	Single ≤2 cm
N2	>2 cm or multiple

Stage grouping: Urethra			
Stage 0a	Ta	N0	M0
Stage 0is	Tis	N0	M0
	Tis pu	N0	M0
	Tis pd	N0	M0
Stage I	T1	N0	M0
Stage II	T2	N0	M0
Stage III	T1, T2	N1	M0
	T3	N0, N1	M0
Stage IV	T4	N0, N1	M0
	Any T	N2	M0
	Any T	Any N	M1

Table 28.2 Prognostic factors for progression to invasive disease in superficial bladder cancer (Ta, T1, Tis)

Prognostic factor	Tumour related	Host related	Environment related
Essential	Grade T stage Carcinoma *in situ* (Cis) Number of lesions Previous recurrences	Age Performance status Other co-morbidities	Extent of transurethral resection (Intravesical chemotherapy reduces recurrence but limited evidence for reducing progression)
Additional	Tumour size Recurrence at 3-month check	Gender Continued tobacco use	
Novel/promising	p53 NMP22 FGFR3 mutation status COX-2 (especially upper tract) Claudin protein family members DNA methylation status Lymphovascular invasion Extent of invasion (T1*microinvasive* or T1*extensive invasive*)		

Table 28.3 Prognostic factors for metastatic risk and survival in invasive, locally-advanced and/or node positive bladder cancer (T2–4N0–1)

Prognostic factors	Tumor related	Host related	Environment related
Essential	T stage N stage	Age Performance status ALP Other co-morbidities	Surgical margin status
Additional	Grade Histological type Lymphovascular invasion Concomitant Cis Tumour size Hydronephrosis	Haemoglobin Response of primary to chemotherapy	Extent of lymph node resection Proportion (density) of involved lymph nodes
Novel/promising	p53, p63, p21 (for long-term bladder preservation) Rb protein Ki67 EGF receptor HER2 expression E-cadherin Microvessel density Treatment resistance mechanisms (ERCC1, BRCA1 or MMR mutations)	Certain germline single-nucleotide polymorphisms (SNPs)	

With established metastatic disease, visceral metastasis is associated with a poorer prognosis.

Treatment philosophy

The goals of treatment depend on the site, grade and stage, and type of the cancer, and the age/performance status and life expectancy of the patient. For example, some elderly patients or those with significant co-morbidities with apparently localized but muscle-invasive disease may not be considered suitable for curative treatment because of the potential risks and morbidity of treatment. The scenarios below specifically apply to urothelial carcinoma of the bladder, with the concepts reasonably extrapolated to the other tumour sites/types, except where indicated.

Scenario	Treatment philosophy

Non-muscle invasive low-grade urothelial carcinoma (Ta)	• Local (intravesical) manoeuvres:
	  ▪ Transurethral resection
	  ▪ Intravesical cytotoxic chemotherapy:
	    ○ Immediate post-surgical use (6–24 hours) reduces recurrence risk
	  ▪ Intravesical BCG:
	    ○ Used in limited cases, e.g. for frequent or numerous recurrences
	• Aims:
	  ▪ Chemotherapy to prevent or reduce risk of recurrence (frequent)
	  ▪ BCG to reduce risk of recurrence or progression of stage or grade (rare)
	  ▪ Maintain organ function

Non-muscle invasive high-grade urothelial carcinoma (Ta or T1 or Cis)	• Local (intravesical) manoeuvres:
	  ▪ Transurethral resection (may be repeated to ensure full clearance and exclude understaging)
	  ▪ Intravesical BCG
	  ▪ Intravesical chemotherapy
	• Failure of intravesical treatment may require more radical treatment as for muscle-invasive disease (see below)
	• Aims:
	  ▪ To prevent or reduce risk of recurrence, progression of stage or grade
	  ▪ To maintain organ function

(continued)

Scenario	Treatment philosophy
Muscle-invasive localized (and some locally-advanced) carcinomas	• Consideration of both local and potential systemic treatment is required: 　▪ Curative cystectomy with diversion (continent or otherwise) + lymphadenectomy 　▪ Preoperative neoadjuvant chemotherapy 　▪ Bladder-preserving chemoradiation 　　○ Not for squamous carcinoma or adenocarcinoma, or if significant carcinoma in situ component 　▪ Adjuvant chemotherapy 　▪ Possible postoperative radiation therapy (residual pelvic disease) • Aims: to eliminate primary and occult systemic disease, whilst optimizing functional outcomes and organ preservation where possible
Metastatic disease	• Treatment of systemic disease, as well as symptomatic local disease if present: 　▪ Local measures for the primary tumour as required for symptom control 　▪ Systemic chemotherapy 　▪ Localized palliative radiation therapy, e.g. for pain or bleeding 　▪ Adequate analgesia • Aims: 　▪ To control local and systemic symptoms in incurable disease 　▪ To maintain quality of life and possible prolongation of life
Locally-recurrent or -advanced disease	• Salvage cystectomy for recurrence following primary chemoradiation • Palliative diversion: if cystectomy not technically feasible or deemed risky • Palliative transurethral resection of bladder tumour (TURBT) if elderly or unfit (i.e. not a candidate for radical treatment) • Urethral catheter placement for bladder drainage • Ureteric stent or nephrostomy tube placement for relief of renal obstruction • Palliative or curative radiation therapy or chemoradiation • Aims: 　▪ To control local symptoms 　▪ As a second attempt at cure for those having salvage cystectomy after bladder-preserving therapy
Follow-up	• Cystoscopic surveillance after management of primary tumour • For those at risk of metastasis or as clinically indicated: clinical examination, chest radiography, CT scan abdomen and pelvis, bone scan • Aims: to detect and treat local recurrence and early small volume metastasis

Routine multidisciplinary discussion of all patients with disease beyond non-muscle-invasive is optimal practice.

Treatment

Surgery	Description
Ta, T1, Tis	• TURBT: for initial diagnosis and definitive therapy • Followed by intravesical BCG or chemotherapy for high-grade or T1 disease • Radical cystectomy indicated for salvage of failed intravesical treatment
T2–4N0–1	• TURBT for initial diagnosis • Radical cystectomy with pelvic lymphadenectomy for cure or occasionally palliation • Urinary diversion may be by means of an ileal conduit or continent reservoir • Chemotherapy should be considered for use as a neoadjuvant or adjuvant to surgery
Metastatic	• TURBT for initial diagnosis: 　▪ May be repeated for palliation • Palliative urinary diversion may be considered • Radical cystectomy usually not undertaken since risks and morbidity outweigh potential benefits

Radiation therapy

Radiation therapy	Description
Ta, T1, Tis	• Limited role

T–T4N0 curative	• Radiation therapy may be considered as an alternative to cystectomy where surgery is contraindicated or refused by the patient:
	  ▪ Should be used in combination with radiosensitizing chemotherapy if the patient is fit enough
	• Planned cystoscopy after two-thirds of a curative radiation dose may identify poor responders and permit early cystectomy
	• External beam irradiation with organ-sparing techniques, such as image-guided, 3D conformal or intensity modulated therapy, enhance treatment accuracy and reduce morbidity
	  ▪ Used together with radiosensitizing cytotoxic drugs if patient is fit enough:
	    ○ Cisplatin (or carboplatin if renal function poor), or
	    ○ 5-fluorouracil + mitomycin C
	• Clinical target volume (CTV):
	  ▪ Urinary bladder either full or empty with 1.5-cm expansion to planning target volume (PTV) preferably imaged with CT scan
	  ▪ Pelvic nodes are not specifically targeted, but perivesical nodes will be included in the CTV
	  ▪ Adaptive radiotherapy based on 'on-treatment' volumetric imaging can allow individualization of target margins and field size, and potentially reduce toxicity
	  ▪ Minimum of four fields is recommended
	• Radiation dose: 64 Gy in 32 fractions, 5 days per week:
	  ▪ Accelerated fractionation schedules are under investigation
	• Patients failing this bladder-preserving technique should be considered for salvage cystectomy for isolated local recurrence or residual disease

Locally-advanced, palliative therapy	• Simple two field or 3D conformal three or four field • 35 Gy in ten fractions over 2 weeks *or* 21 Gy in three fractions over 1 week • Aim: to relieve or prevent local symptoms
Metastatic disease	• For symptomatic metastasis

Systemic therapy

Systemic therapy	Description
Ta, T1, Tis	• Systemic therapy has no benefit • Cytotoxic intravesical BCG and/or cytotoxic chemotherapy should be considered

T2–4N0–2/NxM0	• *Neoadjuvant chemotherapy*:
	  ▪ Recommended but still used relatively infrequently in routine practice
	  ▪ Cochrane review (2008):
	    ○ Provides approximately 5% absolute survival benefit (45–50% 5-year median survival; HR 0.86; 95% CI 0.77–0.95; $P = 0.003$)
	    ○ More recent data including 3047 patients in 12 randomized controlled trials (RCTs): HR 0.89; 95% CI 0.81–0.98; $P = 0.02$.
	    ○ Most trials in Cochrane review (2008) include clinical Stage T2; probably higher relative benefit in more advanced disease
	    ○ Most trials reviewed were N0 or Nx; one trial included up to N2
	    ○ Pathological clinical response is observed in 7–38% of cases
	  ▪ Advantages:
	    ○ Patient more likely to complete planned treatment
	    ○ Patient might not be fit for adjuvant therapy if surgical complications develop

(continued)

Systemic therapy	Description
	- *Adjuvant chemotherapy*: 　- Cochrane review (2008): 　　○ Provides approximately 9% absolute survival benefit (approximately 50–60% 3-year median survival; HR 0.75; 95% CI 0.60–0.96; $P = 0.019$) 　　○ 34% of patients were N1–2 　　○ More recent data including 939 patients in nine RCTs: HR 0.75; 95% CI 0.63–0.90; $P = 0.002$ 　- Advantages: 　　○ Treatment is based on pathological stage 　　○ Surgery is not delayed due to chemotherapy toxicity or lack of response - Key points regarding chemotherapy: 　- Strongest data are from older and more toxic chemotherapy regimens (e.g. MVAC, CMV, dose-dense CMV) that are now not often used in the metastatic setting. 　- Many groups use gemcitabine + cisplatin based on non-inferiority in the metastatic setting and much better tolerability: 　　○ Level 1 evidence is lacking for use of this combination either in the neoadjuvant or adjuvant situation 　- Cisplatin is superior to carboplatin but many patients are unsuitable for cisplatin due to renal impairment or other co-morbidities: 　　○ Use of carboplatin-based regimens or carboplatin as a single agent is not supported by evidence and any benefit is likely to be smaller than with cisplatin-based regimens - Management of upper tract urothelial cancers is based on extrapolation from work in bladder cancer, but there is little evidence to support this - Management of non-urothelial bladder cancers remains controversial and is based on extrapolation from other histologically-similar cancers or those of similar embryological derivation
Metastatic disease	- Cisplatin-based chemotherapy combinations are active and improve progression-free and overall survival: 　- Complete responses can be observed - Gemcitabine + cisplatin is the regimen of choice: 　- Similar efficacy to MVAC (methotrexate + vinblastine + doxorubicin + cisplatin) and is better tolerated - Carboplatin is probably inferior to cisplatin in this setting - Management in the second-line setting and beyond is largely experimental: 　- Vinflunine has some activity but the phase III trial comparing it to supportive care did not achieve the primary objective of a gain of 2 months in median survival - Other drugs with reported activity include ifosfamide, paclitaxel, gemcitabine monotherapy and pemetrexed: 　- Nab-paclitaxel appears promising but requires further investigation 　- Non-platinum combinations such as gemcitabine + paclitaxel have been used with some activity observed but also toxicity - Antiangiogenic and epidermal growth factor receptor (EGFR)-based therapies have not yet demonstrated benefit - Immunotherapeutic approaches such as inhibition of CTLA-4 or the PD1 axis are under investigation - All patients require holistic management and will often benefit from early involvement of palliative care services to support quality of life during and after treatment

Post-treatment assessment

Post-treatment assessment	Description
Ta, T1, Tis	- Cystoscopy: usually at 3 months post diagnosis - Upper tract imaging repeated after 2 years for high-grade tumours: 　- Not required for low-grade disease given very low risk of upper tract involvement
T2–4N0–1	- Assessment to focus on surveillance for cancer recurrence as well as ongoing functional outcomes (issues include infection, calculi, obstruction, haematuria, incontinence, sexual function): usually 3 months post treatment - Clinical review - Laboratory assessment: full blood examination (FBC or FBE), urea electrolyte and creatinine (UEC), liver function tests (LFTs), vitamin B12 (reduced absorption), urine microbiology as indicated, urine cytology - Imaging: chest X-ray or CT, abdominopelvic ultrasound or CT - Cystoscopy (if treated with chemoradiation)
Metastatic disease	- Clinical review - Laboratory assessment: FBE, UEC, LFTs, calcium, phosphate - Imaging: chest X-ray or CT, abdominopelvic CT

Continuing care

Continuing care	Description

Ta, T1, Tis	• Maintenance schedule for intravesical BCG:
	  ▪ Improves efficacy of treatment
	  ▪ Optimal regimen has not been established; various protocols exist (e.g. single-dose BCG monthly for 12 months)
	  ▪ With time, morbidity of treatment increases
	• Cystoscopy: usually 3–6 monthly for 1–2 years, with frequency reduced to annually if free of recurrences:
	  ▪ Continued until disease free for 10 years
	• Upper tract imaging repeated every 2 years for high-grade tumours

T2–4N0–1	• Assessment to focus on surveillance for cancer recurrence as well as ongoing functional outcomes from urinary diversion (issues include infection, calculi, obstruction, haematuria, incontinence, sexual function): initially 3–6 monthly, with reduced frequency to annually over time if no concerns • Clinical review • Laboratory assessment: FBE, UEC, LFTs, vitamin B12, urine microbiology, urine cytology • Imaging: chest X-ray or CT, abdominopelvic ultrasound or CT • Cystoscopy for patients treated with chemoradiation
Metastatic disease	• Clinical review • Symptom management • Detection and treatment of progressive disease

Controversies

- *Surgery*:
  - Use and schedule for maintenance intravesical BCG
  - Role and timing of radical surgery for high-grade non–muscle-invasive disease
  - Uptake and extent of lymphadenectomy during cystectomy
  - Use of minimally invasive approaches for radical cystectomy (e.g. robotic surgery); reproducibility outside expert centres
- *Radiation oncology*:
  - Ongoing refinement of patient selection for bladder-preserving techniques rather than cystectomy
  - Defining the place of pre- or post-operative radiation therapy after contemporary surgical techniques (e.g. neobladder) for high-risk disease
  - Optimizing the combined chemoradiation schedules in terms of choice of radiosensitizing drug to use and the drug sequencing with radiation
- *Medical oncology*:
  - How to improve uptake and routine use of perioperative (neoadjuvant and/or adjuvant) chemotherapy in the setting of surgery
  - Optimal chemotherapy regimen in neoadjuvant and adjuvant settings
  - Timing of adjuvant therapy and longest acceptable delay between surgery and commencement of treatment
  - Management of patients unsuitable for cisplatin
  - Management of metastatic disease in the second-line setting and thereafter
  - Optimal management of metastatic upper tract disease
  - Management of non-urothelial cancers

Phase III clinical trials

See Table 28.4.

Table 28.4 Phase III clinical trials

Trial reference	Results
Surgery	
Bochner et al (2014) *Eur Urol* [Epub ahead of print]	• Memorial Sloan Kettering Cancer Center single-institution trial of robotic vs open cystectomy • No significant differences in terms of pathological stage, length of stay, 90-day complication rates or quality of life at 3 or 6 months

(continued)

Table 28.4 (Continued)

Trial reference	Results
Oddens et al. (2013) Eur Urol 63(3):462–472	• EORTC trial of standard vs one-third dose BCG in patients with intermediate-to-high risk Ta and T1 urothelial carcinoma • Higher recurrence risk for lower dose, but not a lower toxicity • Three years of maintenance BCG reduced recurrence compared to 1 year of maintenance among high-risk but not intermediate-risk patients
de Reijke et al. (2005) J Urol 173(2):405–409	• Intravesical BCG vs epirubicin for CIS of the bladder • No difference in the complete response (CR) rate • Longer time to recurrence after CR and lower CIS recurrence rate with BCG • Numerous other trials have compared intravesical BCG and chemotherapy, generally finding that BCG is somewhat superior to chemotherapy in reducing recurrence, but also causes more adverse effects
Lamm et al. (2000) J Urol 163(4):1124–1129	• Landmark SWOG study of maintenance BCG • Improved recurrence-free and progression-free survival when added to standard induction therapy for CIS and papillary urothelial carcinoma • Other trials have since replicated this result, leading to maintenance therapy becoming standard of care
Oosterlinck et al. (1996) J Urol 149:749–52	• Instillation of a single dose of intravesical chemotherapy immediately after TURBT reduces the recurrence risk • This finding has been replicated in numerous other trials, leading to this becoming standard of care
Radiation oncology	
Coppin et al. (1996) J Clin Oncol 14 (11):2901–2907	• Canadian trial of 99 patients randomized to radiation or preoperative radiation ± cisplatin radiosensitization • Radiosensitization improved local control in the pelvis • It did not improve overall survival, because of its failure to influence the distant metastatic rate
Duchesne et al. (2000) Int J Radiat Oncol Biol Phys 47(2) 379–388	• MRC UK trial of palliative radiation therapy for incurable cancer, 3 × 7 Gy vs 10 × 3.5 Gy • No clinically significant differences in symptom control • This trial set the benchmark for rates of symptom control
Horwich et al. (2005) Radiother Oncol 75(1): 34–43	• Royal Marsden Hospital trial of accelerated radiation therapy in invasive bladder cancer compared to conventional scheduling • No improvement in local control • Increased toxicity
Medical oncology	
Loehrer et al. (1992) J Clin Oncol 10(7):1066–1073	• Cooperative Group study of MVAC vs single agent cisplatin for metastatic bladder urothelial carcinoma • MVAC was superior for response rate, duration of remission and overall survival
Harker et al. (1985) J Clin Oncol 3(11):1463–1470	• NCOG study of CMV for metastatic bladder urothelial carcinoma • 28% CR and 28% partial response (PR) rates • Median duration of CR was 9 months • Median overall survival was 8 months
von der Maase et al. (2000) J Clin Oncol 18(17):3068–3077	• Multigroup study of MVAC vs gemcitabine + cisplatin (GC) in locally-advanced or metastatic bladder urothelial carcinoma • GC was not superior to MVAC for overall survival, but toxicity was significantly less with GC
Von der Maase et al. (2005) J Clin Oncol 23(21):4602–4608	• Long-term follow-up • Overall survival and progression-free survival were similar for GC vs MVAC
Sternberg et al. (2006) Eur J Cancer 42(1):50–54	• EORTC protocol 30924 • Locally advanced or metastatic UC • High-dose MVAC with granulocyte-colony stimulating factor (G-CSF) support vs standard MVAC • Well tolerated • Borderline significant reduction in the risk of progression or death

Areas of research

- *Surgery*:
  - Optimization of intravesical treatment for high-risk non–muscle-invasive disease
  - Optimal surveillance schedule and improving acceptability of surveillance for non–muscle-invasive disease
  - Optimal integration of radical surgery with systemic neoadjuvant or adjuvant therapy
  - Role and extent of lymphadenectomy, as in the following two trials:
    - NCT01215071: Prospective randomized study to compare extensive with limited lymphadenectomy in the surgical treatment of bladder cancer (AUO, Germany)
    - RAZOR (randomized open vs robotic cystectomy) trial
  - Optimal training and service delivery strategies
- *Radiation oncology*:
  - Personalizing radiation fractionation schedules according to tumour profile
  - How best to combine radiation therapy with other agents, e.g. novel biological therapies
  - Evaluating the efficacy of adaptive radiation therapy techniques
- *Medical oncology*:
  - Biological differences between upper and lower tract cancers
  - Development of clinically useful biomarkers predictive of response
  - Development of active 'targeted' therapies
  - Immunology and immunotherapy
  - Supportive care and quality of life

Recommended reading

Advanced Bladder Cancer Meta-analysis Collaboration (2004) Neoadjuvant chemotherapy for invasive bladder cancer. *Cochrane Database Syst Rev* (1):CD005246.

Babjuk M, Burger M, Zigeuner R, et al (2013) EAU guidelines on non-muscle-invasive urothelial carcinoma of the bladder: update 2013. *Eur Urol.* 64(4):639-53.

Bambury RM, Rosenberg JE (2013) Advanced urothelial carcinoma: overcoming treatment resistance through novel treatment approaches. *Front Pharmacol* 4:3

Biagioli MC, Fernandez DC, Spiess PE, Wilder RB (2013) Primary bladder preservation treatment for urothelial bladder cancer. *Cancer Control* 20(3):188–199.

Clark PE, Agarwal N, Biagioli MC *et al.* (2013) NCCN Clinical Practice Guidelines in Oncology: Bladder cancer. Version 1, 2013. *J Natl Compr Cancer Network* 11(4):446–475.

Elbe JN, Sauter G, Epstein JI, Sesterhenn IA (2004) Tumours of the urinary system. In: *WHO Classification of Tumours: Pathology and Genetics of Tumours of the Urinary System and Male Genital Organs.* Lyon: IARC Press:59–168.

Jemal A, Bray F, Center MM *et al.* (2011) Global cancer statistics. *CA-Cancer J Clin* 61:69–90.

Mitin T, Shipley WU, Efstathiou JA *et al.* (2013) Trimodality therapy for bladder conservation in treatment of invasive bladder cancer. *Curr Urol Rep* 14(2):109–115.

Pezaro C, Liew MS, Davis ID (2012) Urothelial cancers: using biology to improve outcomes. *Expert Rev Anticancer Ther* 12:87–98.

Resnick MJ, Bassett JC, Clark PE (2013) Management of superficial and muscle-invasive urothelial cancers of the bladder. *Curr Opin Oncol* 25(3):281–288.

Roupret M, Babjuk M, Comperat E (2013) European guidelines on upper tract urothelial carcinomas: 2013 update. *Eur Urol* 63(6):1059–1071.

Sengupta S, Blute ML (2006) The management of superficial bladder cancer. *Urology* 67(s1):48–54.

Shelley MD, Barber J, Wilt T, Mason MD (2008) Surgery versus radiotherapy for muscle invasive bladder cancer. *Cochrane Database Syst Rev* (1):CD002079.

Smith ND, Castle EP, Gonzalgo ML *et al.* (2015) The RAZOR (randomized open vs robotic cystectomy) trial: study design and trial update. *Br J Urol Int* 115(2):198–205.

Tilki D, Brausi M, Colombo R *et al.* (2013) Lymphadenectomy for bladder cancer at the time of radical cystectomy. *Eur Urol* 64(2):266–276.

Tjokrowidjaja A, Lee C, Stockler MR (2013) Does chemotherapy improve survival in muscle-invasive bladder cancer (MIBC)? A systematic review and meta-analysis (MA) of randomized controlled trials (RCT). *J Clin Oncol* 31(Suppl):abstract 4544.

Vale CL: Advanced Bladder Cancer Meta-analysis Collaboration (2006) Adjuvant chemotherapy for invasive bladder cancer (individual patient data). *Cochrane Database Syst Rev* (2):CD006018.

29 Kidney

J. E. Ferguson III[1], W. Kimryn Rathmell[2] and Eric M. Wallen[1]

[1]Department of Urology, University of North Carolina School of Medicine, Chapel Hill, NC, USA
[2]Department of Medicine, Division of Hematology-Oncology, University of North Carolina School of Medicine, Chapel Hill, NC, USA

Summary	Key facts
Introduction	• Incidence is increasing due in part to incidental discovery secondary to increased utilization of cross-sectional imaging for common symptoms • Survival rates for kidney cancer have been increasing for both localized and advanced disease
Presentation	• Asymptomatic: ▪ Often incidentally discovered on cross-sectional imaging for other complaints • Advanced disease presentation includes a classical triad of haematuria, flank pain and flank mass • Other presenting symptoms related to metastatic disease or systemic cytokine release in advanced setting: fatigue, weight loss, fever, night sweats, cough, haemoptysis, skeletal pain or fracture, jaundice, neurological symptoms

Scenario	• *Localized*: surgical removal or ablation associated with high rates of cure
	• *Metastatic*:
	  ▪ Variable depending on histological subtype
	  ▪ For clear cell histology: immunotherapy or targeted therapy ± cytoreductive nephrectomy or resection of solitary metastases
	• Resistant to traditional chemotherapy (except rare non-renal cell variant kidney tumours such as collecting duct carcinoma, renal medullary carcinoma, urothelial tumours, Xp11 translocation carcinomas)
	• Radiotherapy primarily plays a role in palliation or management of central nervous system (CNS) metastatic disease

Trials	• Phase III trials have confirmed efficacy of systemic targeted therapy, cytoreductive nephrectomy in metastatic disease for selected patient groups, and equivalence of partial versus radical nephrectomy for small renal masses (SRM) • Current trials are evaluating new systemic agents for metastatic disease, the benefit of cytoreductive nephrectomy in the targeted agent era, the benefit of adjuvant or neoadjuvant approaches, and the benefit of stereotactic radiotherapy

Introduction

Cancers of the kidney can arise from any of the cell lineages found in the kidney. Transitional or urothelial cell carcinoma and Wilms tumour of childhood are covered in Chapters 28 and 57, respectively. This chapter focuses on renal cell carcinoma (RCC), which, depending on the histological subtype, can arise from cells in the proximal or distal tubules. Several very rare tumours also arise in the kidney from the collecting duct and renal medulla. These cancers (collecting duct carcinoma and renal medullary carcinoma) represent disease entities that are highly distinct from RCC, and should be considered unrelated to RCC. Additionally, other cancers can arise in the kidney, such as lymphoma (primary lymphoma of the kidney) and sarcomas (liposarcoma, RMS). In addition, other cancers, including colon, lung and breast cancers, can metastasize to the kidney.

When renal cancer is suspected upon imaging, biopsy is usually not performed prior to surgical excision, but alternate entities such as those listed above should always be considered in the differential, particularly when the radiographic appearance is not typical for a renal cortical origin. Cross-sectional imaging (preferably computed tomography [CT] scan) plays an important role in differentiating solid from cystic masses, and their

UICC Manual of Clinical Oncology, Ninth Edition. Edited by Brian O'Sullivan, James D. Brierley, Anil K. D'Cruz, Martin F. Fey, Raphael Pollock, Jan B. Vermorken and Shao Hui Huang. © 2015 UICC. Published 2015 by John Wiley & Sons, Ltd.

malignant potential. Solid masses are more likely to be malignant than cystic masses, and the larger the mass, the more likely its malignant potential. Components of soft tissue within cysts or complex cystic lesions increase the risk of malignancy.

Pre- and post-intravenous (IV) contrast CT scans are used to identify enhancing lesions (defined by a change of >15 HU), which also raises suspicion of malignancy. Of enhancing masses of >3 cm, 80% are malignant.

Incidence, aetiology and screening

Incidence, aetiology and screening	Description

Incidence	- 15th most common cancer worldwide:
	  - Sixth most common cancer in American men
	  - 65,000 new cases in the USA annually
	- Incidence is increasing in Western countries along with increasing rates of cross-sectional imaging, although disease-specific survival is improving

Aetiology	- Average age at presentation: sixth to seventh decade
	- Black race: 10–20% higher incidence
	- Gender: male-to-female ratio 3:2
	- Smoking, obesity, hypertension, acquired cystic renal disease from end-stage renal disease (ESRD)
	- Hereditary forms (<3% of cases):
	  - Familial oncocytoma (non-malignant)
	  - Von Hippel–Lindau disease (VHL) (clear cell, *VHL* gene)
	  - Birt–Hogg–Dubé syndrome (BHD) (clear cell, chromophobe, oncocytoma, *FLCN* gene)
	  - Hereditary clear cell (*BAP1* gene)
	  - Tuberous sclerosis (RCC and angiomyolipoma [AML]; *TSC1* or *TSC2* gene)
	  - Hereditary papillary RCC (*MET* gene)
	  - Hereditary leiomyomatosis and RCC (papillary type 2, *FH* gene)

Screening	- None for average risk
	- ESRD with acquired cystic renal disease:
	  - 1–2% lifetime incidence of RCC
	  - Periodic ultrasound or CT/magnetic resonance imaging (MRI) after third year on dialysis if long life expectancy
	- VHL patients:
	  - Biannual ultrasound or CT/MRI beginning at age 20 years
	  - Refer for risk management of other disease sequelae such as CNS haemangioblastomas

Pathology and natural history

Histology is determined after surgical resection or biopsy, and represents only a minor component of overall prognosis. However, as the clear cell subtype is uniquely responsive to systemic therapies, histological subtype is particularly important in the metastatic setting. There are rare histological subtypes that confer a decidedly poor prognosis.

Pathology and natural history	Description

Clear cell (70% of RCC)	- Common chromosomal sporadic mutation of VHL tumour suppressor, leading to increased levels of hypoxia-inducible factors (HIFs) which promote transcription of angiogenic proteins such as vascular endothelial growth factor (VEGF), its receptor (VEGFR) and others
	- Hypervascular:
	  - Nests or sheets of clear cells with delicate vascular network
	  - Vascular invasion is common.
	- Bleeding from CNS metastases is common with anticoagulation:
	  - Always perform an MRI before initiating anticoagulants
	- Aggressive behaviour more common than for papillary or chromophobe subtypes
	- Tumour shrinkage is common with targeted molecular therapy (antiangiogenic agents that target VEGF or VEGFR)
	- 10–20% response rate to immunotherapy
	- Common in VHL disease (inherited), with patients developing hundreds or thousands of tumours

(continued)

Pathology and natural history	Description
Papillary (15–20%)	• Hypovascular: ▪ Papillary structures with single layer of cells around a fibrovascular core • Type 1 (basophilic cells with low-grade nuclei): good prognosis • Type 2 (eosinophilic cells with high-grade nuclei): worse prognosis • Commonly multicentric (40% of cases) • Associated with ESRD and acquired cystic kidney disease
Chromophobe (5%)	• 'Plant cell' with pale cytoplasm, perinuclear clearing or 'halo', nuclear 'raisins' and prominent cell borders • Generally good prognosis unless sarcomatoid features or metastatic • Closely associated with and commonly misdiagnosed as oncocytoma • More common in BHD syndrome
Unclassified (2%)	• Varied primary histology, but usually highly undifferentiated • Generally poor prognosis
Xp11 translocation carcinoma (very rare)	• Occurs in children, teens and young adults • Aggressive and rapidly progressive • Histology can mimic sarcomatoid clear cell RCC • May respond to cytotoxic chemotherapy
Collecting duct carcinoma (<1%)	• Complex, highly infiltrative cords within inflamed, desmoplastic stroma • Poor prognosis. >50% metastatic at presentation • May respond to cytotoxic chemotherapy
Renal medullary carcinoma (<1%)	• Seen exclusively in patients with sickle cell trait or sickle cell disease • Poorly differentiated cells with lace-like appearance: ▪ Inflammatory infiltrate • Dismal prognosis: mean survival is 15 weeks • Responsive to palliative combination cisplatin-based chemotherapy

Benign masses (oncocytoma, angiomyolipoma)	• 10–20% of suspicious SRM after surgical removal
	• *Oncocytoma*:
	  ▪ Nests of polygonal cells with a granular eosinophilic cytoplasm
	    ○ Can be difficult to differentiate from chromophobe RCC
	    ○ No imaging features differentiate oncocytoma from RCC:
	      – Oncocytoma can co-exist with RCC
	      – Thus, even biopsy-proven oncocytomas should raise suspicion for malignancy
	• *Angiomyolipoma*:
	  ▪ Mix of blood vessels (angio), smooth muscle (myo) and fat cells (lipo)
	  ▪ Fat on CT scan or ultrasound is suggestive of diagnosis, although fat-poor AML do exist
	  ▪ Associated with tuberous sclerosis
	  ▪ Rate of spontaneous haemorrhage increases with size, especially >4 cm
	• Both have an excellent prognosis, but can cause local symptoms due to growth, necessitating surgical treatment
	• Complex renal cysts:
	  ▪ Cysts with internal septations, wall thickening and calcification have a risk of malignancy

The most important prognostic factor for localized RCC is size/T stage, with small tumours confined to the kidney having a low probability of metastatic disease and an excellent prognosis after surgical resection. Localized tumours of <4 cm have a 5-year survival of 90–100%, whereas metastatic disease has a 5-year survival of only 0–10%. Unfortunately, despite the increasing detection of surgically curable tumours, 25% of cases still present after metastasis has already occurred. For patients with metastatic clear cell RCC, integrated staging systems have been validated that synthesize stage, functional status, Fuhrman grade and laboratory derangements in an attempt to identify patients with good prognosis who would benefit from aggressive therapy. Histological subtyping is important to identify patients with the clear cell subtype, as this subtype is more responsive to available systemic therapies. Further, in a handful of cases, the rare histological subtypes of collecting duct and medullary RCC portend a uniformly poor prognoses.

Increased use of cross-sectional imaging in developed countries has resulted in an increase in the detection of small, early-stage renal masses. In fact, localized tumours now represent 70% of new diagnoses. With the understanding that roughly 20% of SRM are benign, 60% are indolent RCC and 20% are potentially aggressive RCC, there is significant interest in determining which SRM can be surveyed safely, and which require removal or ablation. Traditionally, all SRM were removed without biopsy due to the historically unreliable biopsy results. However, the utility of improved biopsy techniques is currently being reconsidered, and active surveillance cohorts (with or without biopsy) have emerged that have given some further insight into growth rates and the natural history of SRM.

RCC metastasizes through haematological and lymphatic routes at equal rates. RCC is relatively unique in its ability to invade the venous system, and tumour thrombus can spread as distally as the right atrium. Importantly, surgical cure is still possible in this scenario, but surgical extirpation in these high-risk situations is associated with increased morbidity and mortality, and requires the involvement of a multispecialty surgical team.

The natural history of metastatic disease can vary significantly from indolent to aggressive. Prognostic scores have been developed to try to differentiate those patients with a favourable prognosis who might benefit from surgical resection of solitary metastases or immunotherapy, such as high-dose interleukin 2 (IL-2) with a chance for durable remission and long-term disease control.

Presentation

- Classically flank pain/mass and haematuria
- Now predominantly asymptomatic:
  - Found incidentally on cross-sectional imaging for other indications
- Microhaematuria, gross haematuria

Diagnostic work-up

Discovery of a renal mass requires a complete work-up (Fig. 29.1).

Once a renal malignancy is suspected, a complete staging algorithm should be followed (Fig. 29.2). Postoperative grade/stage provides prognostic information.

Diagnostic work-up and evaluation	Description

Work-up	- CT or MRI abdomen, without and with IV contrast
	  - Enhancing renal mass defined as an increase of >15 HU between pre- and post-contrast scans
	  - It is difficult on preoperative imaging to predict whether exophytic masses have invaded through the capsule into perinephric fat.
	- Chest X-ray (CXR):
	  - Chest CT, if abnormal CXR or T3 or node positive
	- Blood urea nitrogen (BUN)/creatinine, alkaline phosphatase (ALP), lactate dehydrogenase (LDH), liver function tests (LFTs), calcium, complete blood count (CBC) with differential, urinalysis
	- Document ECOG or Karnofsky performance status
	- If chronic kidney disease (CKD): renal scan to determine differential function and aid in surgical planning
	- If bone pain, elevated Ca or ALP: bone scan (although lytic lesions can lead to false-negative results)
	- If neurological symptoms or metastases on other scans: brain MRI
	- Positron emission tomography (PET) scan is often non-avid for clear cell tumours and should only be ordered and interpreted with caution
	- Biopsy is often not performed if resection is planned:
	  - Core needle biopsy is performed if:
	    - Metastatic disease is suspected
	    - Diagnosis is in question (concern for primary lymphoma, AML or metastasis)
	    - Burden of metastatic disease is high and warrants upfront systemic therapy
	    - Percutaneous ablative local control is planned
	- Up to 20% of RCC patients have a paraneoplastic syndrome (erythrocytosis, hypercalcaemia, non-metastatic elevation in LFTs [Stauffer syndrome], amyloidosis, hypertension, fever):
	  - Importantly, these syndromes resolve with surgical resection and persistence can signify residual disease
	  - For this reason, RCC is referred to as 'the internist's tumour'

Evaluation	**Local disease**
	- Surgical resectability:
	  - Before considering nephron-sparing surgery (discussed below), ipsilateral and contralateral kidney function should be assessed
	  - If function of either is in doubt, renography should be obtained
	Surgical candidacy:
	  - Medical co-morbidities (congestive heart failure, cirrhosis, coronary artery disease, chronic obstructive pulmonary disease)
	  - Past abdominal or renal surgeries (may affect surgical approach)

(continued)

Diagnostic work-up and evaluation	Description
	Metastatic disease • Surgical resectability of primary lesion and any solitary metastases • Fitness for systemic therapy (MSKCC criteria, see Box 29.2)
Tumour markers	None

```
Suspected renal mass on physical exam or radiographic study
                            ↓
         Complete history and physical exam
                            ↓
Complete radiographic characterization of mass. Options include:    Urothelial
  1. Abdominal CT scan without and with IV contrast (preferred)  →  tumour
  2. MRI without and with IV gadolinium                             suspected
  3. Renal ultrasound (can completely characterize simple           (see
     cysts and identify some AMLs)                                  Chapter 28)
                            ↓
                      Renal mass
              ↙                     ↘
           Cystic                   Solid
        ↙        ↘            ↙      ↓      ↘
  Bozniak I–II  Bozniak III/IV  Enhancing  Non-       Fat: AML
  No further                    (malignancy enhancing excise if
  work-up                       suspected)  pseudo-   symptomatic
  (Bozniak IIF,                             tumour    or large
  follow-up                                 confirm
  scans)                                    with
                                            DMSA scan
                       ↓
        Complete diagnostic work-up (Fig. 29.2)
```

Figure 29.1 Work-up algorithm of renal mass.

```
Suspected renal malignancy on dedicated contrast-
            enhanced cross-sectional imaging

Complete staging work-up               Evaluate for para=neoplastic
• Chest imaging (CXR or CT)            syndromes (present in 10–20% of
• Brain MRI if neurological symptoms or cases, confer poorer prognosis,
  Stage IV                             often reversible with successful
• Bone scan/PET often not helpful      treatment):
• If venous invasion suspected, MRI    • Anaemia (CBC)
  abdomen                              • Hypertension
                                       • Hypercalcaemia (complete
 Localized    Metastatic   Suspected     metabolic panel)
                           metastasis* • Stauffer syndrome (non-
 Evaluate for Evaluate for to kidney or  metastatic elevation in LFTs)
 surgical     surgical     lymphoma
 candidacy    candidacy
              and overall    Biopsy
              fitness for
              systemic
              therapy
              Biopsy if
              surgery not
              pursued
```

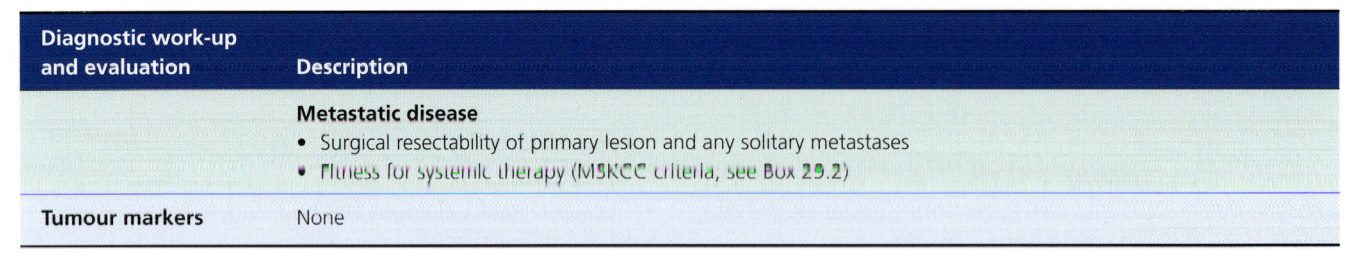

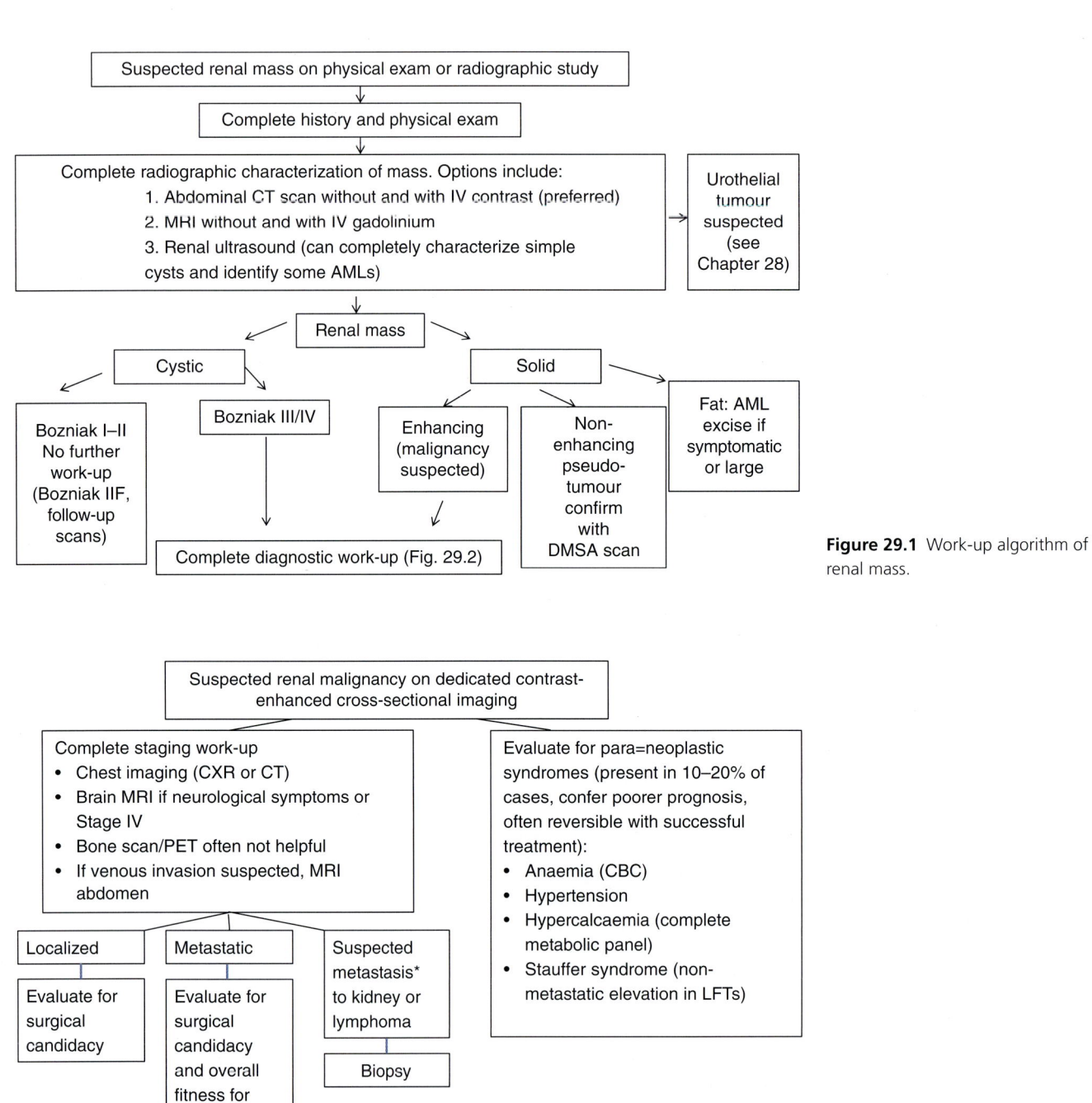

Figure 29.2 Work-up algorithm for suspected renal malignancy.
Primary sites of metastasis to kidney: lung, melanoma, breast, gastrointestinal, pancreas, ovary, testis.

Staging and prognostic grouping

UICC TNM staging
See Table 29.1.

- Stage I – T1N0M0: 90% 5-year survival
- Stage II – T2N0M0: 75–90% 5-year survival
- Stage III – T1–3N1M0 or T3N0–1M0: 60–70% 5-year survival
- Stage IV – T4N0–1 or M1 any N: 10% 5-year survival

Table 29.1 UICC TNM categories and stage grouping: Kidney

TNM categories	
T1	≤7 cm; limited to the kidney
T1a	≤4 cm
T1b	>4 cm
T2	>7 cm; limited to the kidney
T2a	>7–10 cm
T2b	>10 cm
T3	Major veins, perinephric fat
T3a	Renal vein, perinephric fat
T3b	Vena cava below diaphragm
T3c	Vena cava above diaphragm
T4	Beyond Gerota's fascia, ipsilateral adrenal
N1	Single
M1	Distant metastasis

Stage grouping			
Stage I	T1	N0	M0
Stage II	T2	N0	M0
Stage III	T3	Any N	M0
	T1–3	N1	M0
Stage IV	T4	Any N	M0
	Any T	Any N	M1

Prognostic factors

See Table 29.2.

Table 29.2 Prognostic factors for cancers of the kidney

Prognostic factors	Tumour related	Host related	Environment related
Essential	Stage	Surgical candidacy	
Additional	Histological subtype Fuhrman grade (clear cell RCC only) Histological features of necrosis, sarcomatoid histology Symptom score	Performance status Hereditary diseases	Lymph node dissection Adrenalectomy Metastatectomy Immunotherapy/targeted therapy
Investigational	DNA ploidy Genetic alterations Molecular markers		

Treatment philosophy

With the recent stage migration of kidney cancer, patients and physicians now have high expectations for cure, with minimal morbidity and preservation of kidney function. Even in patients with metastatic disease, durable response has been achieved in a minority of highly fit patients with a combination of cytoreductive nephrectomy, immunotherapy and metastatectomy. Surgical resection is a mainstay of treatment in both localized and metastatic cases as RCC is relatively resistant to radiotherapy and chemotherapy. However, recent immunotherapy and targeted therapy regimens have resulted in still moderate, but improved, response rates and extended survival in the setting of metastatic disease.

Scenario	Treatment philosophy
Local disease only	• Surgical excision without biopsy in surgical candidates: ▪ High chance of cure • Ablative therapies for amenable T1a SRM (requires biopsy), including cryotherapy and radiofrequency ablation (RFA) • Active surveillance for SRM (<4 cm) in frail patients (with or without biopsy) or patients with VHL or BHD syndromes
Regional nodal metastases present	• Nephrectomy with lymph node dissection (LND): ▪ LND provides prognostic, but not therapeutic, benefit • Adjuvant therapy trials are ongoing, but there is no evidence to support adjuvant treatment

Metastatic disease (Box 29.1)	• *Solitary*:
	  ▪ Cytoreductive nephrectomy ± metastatectomy + systemic therapy
	• *Multiple*:
	  ▪ Systemic therapy ± cytoreductive nephrectomy in patients with favourable prognosis

Recurrent disease (local vs distant)	• *Local*: re-resection. • *Distant*: surgery/ablation vs systemic therapy ▪ Depends on surgical resectability, symptoms, number of metastases
Follow-up	• Depends on stage and likelihood of recurrence (see below)

Box 29.1 Key points for management of patients with metastatic RCC

- *Never* start anticoagulation without obtaining a brain MRI first in a patient with metastatic or high likelihood of metastatic RCC:
  ▪ Clear cell RCC in particular is highly prone to spontaneous bleeding when treatment with anticoagulation is utilized
- Bone fractures should receive radiation before surgery to prevent bleeding
- Patients with bone metastases should be prescribed calcium, vitamin D and bisphosphonates such as zoledronic acid, or RANK ligand inhibitors (denosumab) to prevent skeletal-related events

Surgery

Surgical resection remains a mainstay of treatment for RCC, even in the setting of metastatic disease.

Surgery	Description

T1a kidney mass	• *Partial nephrectomy* if mass location is amenable:
	  ▪ Open or laparoscopic or robotic
	  ▪ Major complications: urine leak, haemorrhage, infection.
	  ▪ Risk of recurrence at 4 years is 9%, including 3% local recurrence, and 6% distant metastases:
	    ○ Most recurrences occur between 6 and 48 months
	    ○ Recurrence risk increases with stage
	• *Radical nephrectomy* if mass is not amenable to partial nephrectomy:
	  ▪ Complications: infection, haemorrhage
	  ▪ Risk of recurrence: 7%

≥T1b renal mass	• *Radical nephrectomy* (with node dissection if >N0 suspected):
	  ▪ Laparoscopic or open
	  ▪ Adrenalectomy for tumour thrombus to level of adrenal vein, or suspicion of involvement (radiographic or visual)
	• *Partial nephrectomy* if technically feasible

Surgery	Description

Renal vein or inferior vena cava (IVC) thrombus	• Open radical nephrectomy with IVC thrombectomy:
	  ▪ 5-year survival: 45–69%
	  ▪ Complications: high mortality rate (5–10% in high-risk cases)

Locally-advanced disease (T4)	• Despite aggressive surgery (63% negative surgical margins), outcomes are poor (90% mortality rate at 1 year) • Incomplete excision/cytoreductive nephrectomy is not beneficial in these cases: ▪ Thus, if complete excision is not possible, surgical debulking should not be attempted
Metastatic disease	• Cytoreductive nephrectomy in patients with favourable prognosis • Palliative nephrectomy or embolization for haematuria or severe pain ▪ Metastectomy If solitary/oligometastatic, amenable lesions have shown some stability (no evidence of rapid progression) or for symptomatic lesions (especially lung, but also bone and brain)
Solitary recurrence (local)	• If after partial nephrectomy, options include repeat partial nephrectomy, completion radical nephrectomy, cryoablation or RFA • If after radical nephrectomy, should prompt metastatic re-evaluation if resection is considered: ▪ Long-term control in 30–40% of patients
Solitary recurrence (distal)	• Metastectomy can be considered in patients with favourable prognosis and a prolonged disease-free interval • Sites include lung, bone, adrenal and brain • Recurrence in most patients, but long-term progression-free survival has been reported

Surgery/ablative therapies for T1a masses

Traditionally, radical nephrectomy was performed for a kidney mass of any size. Partial nephrectomy was only performed in patients in whom radical nephrectomy would render the patient anephric or high risk for eventual dialysis: patients with solitary kidneys, with bilateral masses, with CKD requiring maximization of residual kidney function or at high risk for recurrence (i.e. patients with VHL syndrome). However, radical nephrectomy has been postulated to increase the risk for CKD and cardiovascular risk, and partial nephrectomy even in the absence of the above indications is now recommended for T1 renal masses to maximize long-term kidney function. Both radical and partial nephrectomy can be performed through open or laparoscopic approaches, although pure laparoscopic partial nephrectomy is technically challenging. Robotic-assisted laparoscopic partial nephrectomy, which facilitates renorrhaphy through a minimally invasive approach, has gained significant popularity and is thought to be oncologically equivalent to open and laparoscopic surgeries. Unfortunately, the robotic surgery system has a high capital cost, limiting its use to specialized surgical centres.

Whether an SRM is amenable to partial nephrectomy is dependent on surgeon discretion. A variety of scoring systems are currently under evaluation that attempt to quantify the surgical difficulty of a partial nephrectomy on the basis of various tumour factors including tumour size and location. Generally, the more difficult tumours to resect are >7 cm, endophytic and abutting the renal hilum and vessels. Because attempted partial nephrectomy of masses with these characteristics has a high rate of complications (Table 29.3), radical nephrectomy

Table 29.3 Major complication rates in procedures for T1 renal masses

Procedure	Complication rate (95% CI)	Recurrence-free survival rate (RFS) (95% CI)	Median tumour size (cm)	Median follow-up (months)
Radiofrequency ablation	6.0 (4.4–8.2)	87 (83–90)	2.7	19
Cryoablation	4.9 (3.3–7.4)	91 (84–95)	2.6	18
Laparoscopic partial nephrectomy	9.0 (7.7–10.6)	98 (97–99)	2.6	15
Open partial nephrectomy	6.3 (4.5–8.7)	98 (97–99)	3.1	47
Laparoscopic radical nephrectomy	3.4 (2.0–5.5)	99 (98–100)	4.6	18
Open radical nephrectomy	1.3 (0.6–2.8)	98 (97–99)	4.8	58

is recommended. Patients should be counselled that if partial nephrectomy is found to be too risky at the time of surgery, radical nephrectomy will be performed.

In partial nephrectomy series, disease recurrence is low and is dependent upon stage. T1 tumours have a 3% local recurrence and 6% distant recurrence, and T3 tumours 0% and 12%, respectively. Recurrences occur between 6 and 48 months postoperatively. Positive surgical margins are identified in 1–5%. However, these patients experience the same progression-free survival as patients with negative surgical margins. Whether this is due to false-positive pathological results, indolent disease or other factors is unclear. Adjuvant therapy has not been proven to be beneficial in this setting. These results are controversial, and negative surgical margins remain a strict goal for this oncological surgery.

Despite the benefits of partial nephrectomy based on multiple retrospective studies, a recent prospective randomized trial comparing partial nephrectomy and radical nephrectomy in patients with a solitary SRM and a normal contralateral kidney found no difference in overall survival at a median of 9.3 years of follow-up. These data may be helpful in counselling patients in resource-poor settings where, due to surgeon training/discretion, radical nephrectomy may be the best surgical option.

For patients with multiple medical co-morbidities that significantly increase their surgical risk, percutaneous ablation of SRM can be considered. RFA and cryoablation have both been utilized. These approaches are indicated for masses of <4 cm, in anatomically favourable positions (posterior and away from the hilum), patients with local recurrence after previous nephron-sparing surgery, and patients with hereditary renal cancer who present with multifocal lesions for which multiple partial nephrectomies might be impossible. Local recurrence rates in cryoablation series with 48 months of follow-up have been 5–10%, representing a slightly higher rate than for surgical excision. Five- and 10-year disease-free survival rates are 78% and 51%, respectively, which is also inferior to those for surgical excision.

In frail patients with competing co-morbidities, active surveillance may be appropriate. The concept of active surveillance is based on the assumption that in some elderly or frail patients with SRM, other competing mortality risks will outweigh that of the SRM. The concerns with such an approach include:
- Inability to accurately predict expected lifespan due to medical co-morbidities
- Inability to accurately predict the natural history of a given tumour based on biopsy results and other prognostic factors
- Potential loss of chance for cure or nephron-sparing approach over time
- Patient reliability in follow-up
- Patient anxiety.

However, in patients with significant co-morbidities or patients who wish to avoid intervention, delaying intervention until masses are >3–4 cm still allows chance for cure at an overall low (~1%) risk for metastasis. The exact protocol for active surveillance has not been determined, but most series recommend serial imaging at 6- or 12-month intervals.

In addition, for patients with VHL disease, active surveillance can also be integrated into the lifelong disease management. Although the histology of these tumours will be clear cell, the growth rate of solid masses in the kidney of these patients can be quite slow. Large, long-term cohort studies have established a '3-cm rule', implying that each lesion in the kidneys of these patients may be safely monitored (biannual imaging) until this threshold is approached. This strategy considers carefully the need to preserve kidney function in these individuals, weighed against the minimal risk for development of metastatic disease for the very small renal tumours, and delays or minimizes the numbers of such interventions these individuals will undergo in their lifetime.

Surgery for T1b masses

For localized renal masses not amenable to partial nephrectomy, radical nephrectomy is the standard treatment. Classically, radical nephrectomy consisted of early ligation of the renal artery and vein, excision of the kidney *en bloc* with the perirenal fat and Gerota's fascia, regional lymphadenectomy and ipsilateral adrenalectomy. Currently, lymphadenectomy is only performed in the setting of enlarged nodes (based on preoperative imaging or intraoperatively) and provides prognostic but not therapeutic benefit. Adrenalectomy is only performed if adrenal involvement is suspected (based on imaging or intraoperative findings) or in high-risk situations such as upper pole tumours of >7 cm or renal vein thrombus involving the adrenal vein. Radical nephrectomy can be performed in an open or laparoscopic fashion, with equivalent oncological outcomes. However, if vena caval thrombus is suspected, the open approach is usually required.

Overall, metastatic recurrence after radical nephrectomy is dependent on tumour stage. For localized tumours, recurrence rates are 7% for T1N0M0, 26% for T2N0M0 and 39% for T3N0M0, with the majority of recurrences occurring in the lung. Recurrence risk is highest over the first 3 postoperative years. The risk of recurrence is markedly increased in node-positive patients.

Tumour thrombus

Due to its hypervascularity, RCC can invade the venous system to form a tumour thrombus. This can occur in 4–10% of cases. These thrombi can extend anywhere from the renal veins to the inferior vena cava and right atrium. Level of extension is best characterized using MRI. Extension above the hepatic veins may require veno-venous or cardiopulmonary bypass (with or without circulatory arrest), open thoracotomy or sternotomy, and specialized surgical teams including vascular, oncological, thoracic and/or cardiac surgeons. Notably, while nephrectomy with IVC tumour thrombectomy carries a significant morbidity compared with nephrectomy alone, 45–70% of patients can be cured with this surgical approach.

Adjuvant therapy

Adjuvant radiotherapy or systemic therapy for completely resected tumours has not been extensively studied and available data with interferon and IFNα have not shown benefit, even in the setting of high risk of recurrence (node positive, high stage or grade). Furthermore, adjuvant radiotherapy in the setting of positive surgical margins has not shown benefit. However, current trials are investigating the newer targeted systemic agents in the adjuvant setting. Until further data are available demonstrating benefit, adjuvant therapy should not be administered outside of the setting of a clinical trial.

Local recurrence

Local recurrence of RCC after radical nephrectomy is rare, occurring in 2–4% of cases. Of these, 60% have concomitant distant metastases, so a thorough metastatic evaluation is required prior to consideration of surgical resection of localized recurrence. However, if isolated, surgical resection can result in long-term cancer-free status in 30–40% of patients.

Local recurrence after partial nephrectomy is also rare, occurring in 1–10% of cases. A significant portion may represent originally multifocal tumours. Treatment options include repeat partial nephrectomy, completion radical nephrectomy, cryo- or radio-ablation, or active surveillance, depending on the tumour characteristics, patient co-morbidities and surgical risk.

Cytoreductive nephrectomy

In the setting of metastatic disease with surgically resectable primary tumour and metastases, cytoreductive nephrectomy before IFNα systemic therapy has a proven survival benefit over IFNα systemic therapy alone (13.6 vs 7.8 months). However, patient selection is critical. Patients who are most likely to benefit are those with lung-only metastases, good prognostic features (discussed below) and good performance status. Trials are currently underway to confirm that cytoreductive therapy prior to systemic antiangiogenic therapy (discussed below) shows the same benefit. Furthermore, benefit in patients with non-clear cell histologies is unclear. Decisions to undertake cytoreductive nephrectomy should be made with the involvement of a multidisciplinary team including medical oncologists with RCC expertise.

Metastatectomy

Most patients with metastatic RCC will not achieve a long-term disease remission with systemic agents. However, retrospective series have shown long disease-free intervals and overall survival in patients undergoing complete resection of solitary or oligometastatic disease. In some series, median 5-year survival rates have approached 35–50%. Predictors of favourable outcome include complete resection, solitary metastasis, age <60 years, metachronous metastasis with a disease-free interval of >1 year after nephrectomy and pulmonary metastases.

Resection of bone and brain metastases is often undertaken with palliative rather than curative intent. Surgical resection is combined with radiation and/or systemic therapy to prevent long bone fractures, spinal cord compression from vertebral metastases, and neurological devastation from solitary brain metastases.

Radiotherapy

External beam radiotherapy (EBRT) for the treatment of primary RCC is controversial, and not commonly utilized. Early studies in the 1960s and 70s evaluating the overall survival benefit of neoadjuvant radiotherapy prior to surgical resection demonstrated conflicting results. Furthermore, studies evaluating the use of adjuvant radiotherapy to the primary site in the setting of high-risk features such as positive surgical margins or positive lymph nodes failed to show a benefit in survival, although local control was improved. However, this resistance to radiotherapy has recently been postulated to be due to the conventional fractionation of traditional EBRT, and more promising results have been demonstrated using stereotactic radioablative approaches with 40 Gy delivered over five fractions with crude local control at 12 months of between 84% and 100%.

Along these same lines, RCC brain metastases are considered unresponsive to fractionated whole-brain radiotherapy with a survival of only 3–4 months. However, stereotactic radiosurgery with Gamma Knife technology provides local control rates of between 83% and 96% and a median survival of 9–13 months. Thus, for patients with symptomatic brain metastases, radiotherapy can provide benefit.

Finally, in patients with RCC metastases to bone, palliative EBRT has been shown to improve bone pain, and when combined with zoledronic acid, to decrease skeletal-related events. In patients with good prognosis (time from nephrectomy to metastasis of >2 years, solitary metastasis and good performance status), surgical excision preceded by EBRT to control intraoperative bleeding is both palliative and can provide long-term disease-free status.

Systemic therapy

Metastatic RCC ranges in behaviour from indolent to highly aggressive. It is important to recognize this difference early to avoid over-treatment in some patients and under-treatment in others. It is also important to recognize that most studies have focused on clear cell RCC and results should not be extrapolated to papillary, chromophobe or other histological subtypes. In order to gauge the pace of an individual patient's disease, a variety of algorithms have been developed that place patients into low-, intermediate- or high-risk groups to estimate the prognosis and tailor the treatment plan to each patient. The most widely used set of risk factors, widely referred to as the MSKCC criteria, is given in Box 29.2.

These prognostic risk groups are important for the evaluation of outcomes in clinical trials, as well as identifying individual favourable-risk patients in clinical practice who are likely to benefit most from aggressive therapies aiming to achieve a disease-free status.

> **Box 29.2** MSKCC risk factors for overall prognosis in the setting of metastatic clear cell RCC
>
> - Karnofsky performance status <80
> - Interval from diagnosis to metastatic disease <1 year
> - LDH > 1.5 × upper limit of normal
> - Elevated corrected calcium
> - Low haemoglobin
>
> | Risk group | Number of risk factors | Prognosis |
> |---|---|---|
> | Favourable | 0 | 2–4-year survival |
> | Intermediate | 1–2 | 1–2-year survival |
> | Poor | 3–5 | 6–12-month survival |

Systemic therapy

The field of treatment for metastatic RCC has undergone a revolution in recent years with the advent of numerous targeted therapies. Several drugs are now on the market and the sequencing of these drugs and use in settings other than progressive metastatic disease is still emerging, along with cohorts of new drugs every year. Cytotoxic chemotherapy is not routinely used for RCC management. It is important to regularly check UpToDate or the NCCN guidelines for updates to the standard of care for management of this complex disease.

Immunotherapy (Box 29.3)

Until 2005, the only approved therapy for the treatment of advanced or metastatic RCC was high-dose IL-2. This treatment is administered in specialty centres and often requires intensive care unit (ICU)-level care during treatment due to treatment-related complications related to capillary leak syndrome (respiratory failure, cardiac failure, hypotension, shock, renal failure, hepatic failure, CNS depression). However, with qualified oversight, the mortality rate associated with this therapy is quite low (<1%). The benefit from IL-2 therapy is that patients who do respond to treatment experience more frequent durable responses that can last for many years. This observation of durable response to IL-2, a non-specific stimulant of T-cell activation, has led many to speculate that RCC is uniquely situated to respond to immune-mediated therapy.

Interferon-α was widely used for clear cell RCC in the era prior to the advancement of targeted therapy. However, this treatment was never approved by the FDA as outcome-based benefits have been difficult to prove in clinical trials. This therapy is no longer widely used alone for RCC, but remains available for selected cases.

Emerging therapies are attempting to harness this immune-mediated activity with more target specificity and fewer side effects. In particular, therapeutics targeting T-cell co-stimulation, a strategy of the immune system to induce tolerance, are emerging in numerous clinical trials. Several targets are undergoing evaluation, including PD-1 and its ligand PD-L1, as well as CTLA4. These targets are considered investigational at this time.

Targeted therapy against VEGF and mTOR signalling pathways (Box 29.4)

Based on the findings related to VHL loss in clear cell tumours and the resultant stabilization of HIF1α and HIF2α, the expression of several key genes is induced and these genes present unique opportunities for targeted therapy. In particular, VEGF is a target of HIF regulation, and the high level expression of VEGF is responsible for the highly vascular nature of clear cell RCC. Numerous agents targeting VEGF or its receptor VEGFR (expressed on endothelial cells) have been developed and tested in phase III clinical trials. Currently approved agents include: sorafenib, sunitinib, pazopanib and axitinib, which are all VEGFR inhibitors with various kinase domain potency, and bevacizumab, a neutralizing VEGF antibody which is approved in conjunction with interferon (Tables 29.4 and 29.5).

> **Box 29.3** Key points for immune therapy for RCC
>
> - High-dose IL-2 is effective but toxic:
>   - Response rates are around 15% with 5% durable response
>   - Should be considered for front-line therapy for young healthy patients with clear cell histology who have a relatively limited extent of metastatic disease and whose primary tumour has been resected
> - Only for use in clear cell subtype
> - Only administered at specialty centres with ICU-level care

> **Box 29.4** Key points for targeted therapy for RCC
>
> - Lead with most potent agent available
> - Sequential use of targeted agents
> - Always consider available clinical trials
> - Therapy selection largely guided by side effect profile

Table 29.4 First- and second-line agents for targeted therapy

Category	First line	Second line
Clear cell, favourable or intermediate risk	Sunitinib Pazopanib Bevacizumab + IFN-α Sorafenib IL-2	Everolimus Axitinib Temsirolimus First-line agents if not already used
Clear cell, poor risk	Temsirolimus	
Non-clear cell	Unknown (clinical trial) Temsirolimus for poor risk	

Table 29.5 Details for agents for targeted therapy for RCC

Agent	Administration	Mechanism of action	Response	Side effects
Sunitinib	50 mg/day PO for 28 days of a 42-day cycle Dose reduction: 37.5 mg/day PO, same schedule	Tyrosine kinase inhibitor (TKI), anti-angiogenesis	30% response rate Median PFS of 11 months vs 5 months for IFN-α	Neutropenia Thrombocytopenia Diarrhoea Hand–foot syndrome Hypertension Fatigue
Pazopanib	800 mg/day PO Dose reduction: 600 mg/day PO to 400 mg/day PO	VEGFR TKI	30% response rate PFS 9.2 months vs 4.2 months for placebo PFS equivalent to sunitinib	Diarrhoea Hepatotoxicity Hypertension Change in skin and hair colour Fatigue
Bevacizumab	10 mg/kg IV every 2 weeks	VEGF neutralizing antibody	30% response rate PFS 10 months vs 5 months for IFN-α	Fatigue Proteinuria Hypertension
Temsirolimus	25 mg IV every week	mTOR inhibitor	OS 11 months vs 7 months for IFN-α	Rash Hyperglycaemia Pneumonitis High cholesterols
Sorafenib	400 mg PO b.i.d. Dose reduction: 400 mg/day PO to 400 mg PO every other day	VEGFR TKI	10% response rate Equivalent PFS to IFN-α	Hand–foot syndrome Diarrhoea Hypertension Hypothyroidism
Axitinib	5 mg PO b.i.d. Dose escalation: 7.5 mg PO b.i.d. to 10 mg PO b.i.d. Dose to hypertension	VEGFR TKI	PFS 7 months vs 5 months for sorafenib	Hypertension Fatigue Hypothyroidism
Everolimus	10 mg/day PO	mTOR inhibitor	PFS 5 months vs 2 months for placebo Second-line after TKI	Stomatitis Rash Fatigue Pneumonitis
IL-2	IV bolus	T-cell activation, and other diverse immune-modulatory effects	5–27%	Significant Mortality ~1% due to capillary leak syndrome Acute kidney injury Hypotension Pulmonary oedema

The other category of currently approved agents is those targeting the mammalian target of rapamycin (mTOR). This central regulator of cell growth is connected to the altered hypoxia response signalling resulting from HIF deregulation. Drugs approved in this class include temsirolimus and everolimus (Table 29.4). The selection of targeted agent relies on evidence-based medicine, and thorough understanding of the clinical settings of each trial is important. For example, patients with brain metastases were excluded from many of these studies.

Post-treatment assessment

There is no level I evidence to guide follow-up protocols. The exact type and timing of surveillance imaging is controversial. The main goal is to detect recurrent disease early when re-resection could offer cure, without subjecting low-risk patients to excessive radiation (Table 29.6). Thus, surveillance in high-risk patients is more intense.

Table 29.6 Recommendations for post-treatment assessment

Stage	Treatment	Office visit, blood work	CXR/CT chest	CT abdomen
pT1	PN/RN	Yearly	CXR yearly for 3 years	At 3–12 months. If negative, yearly imaging for 3 years can be considered (for RN, no further imaging necessary)
pT2	RN/PN	Yearly	CXR yearly for 3 years	At 3–6 months, then every year to Year 5
pT3–4 or N+	RN	At 3–6 months, then every 3–6 months until Year 5	Chest CT at 3–6 months, with CXR or CT every 6 months until Year 3, then yearly until Year 5	At 3–6 months then every 6 months until Year 3, then every 12 months until Year 5

PN, partial nephrectomy; RN, radical nephrectomy.
Adapted from Donat et al. (2013)

Continuing care

- Monitor for hyperfiltration renal injury (24-hour urine protein)
- To protect renal function:
  - Initiate ACEi
  - Weight loss in the obese
  - Low protein/sodium diet
  - Control diabetes mellitus, hypertension, hyperlipidaemia
  - Avoid non-steroidal anti-inflammatory drugs (NSAIDs)
- Early nephrology referral when necessary

Controversies

- Whether partial nephrectomy is beneficial in patients at low risk for eventual end-stage renal disease, especially in resource-poor settings
- Whether positive surgical margins after partial nephrectomy truly confer no added risk
- Whether cytoreductive nephrectomy in the antiangiogenic era is beneficial
- What is the most beneficial systemic therapy for metastatic *non-clear cell* RCC?

Phase III clinical trials

See Table 29.7.

Areas of research

- To investigate the efficacy of adjuvant therapy with targeted agents to prevent recurrence
- To evaluate if there is still benefit to cytoreductive nephrectomy in the targeted therapy era (CARMENA trial)
- To investigate if the utilization of novel biomarkers on renal biopsy can differentiate indolent from aggressive disease
- To develop novel systemic therapies

Table 29.7 Phase III clinical trials

Trial reference	Results
Van Poppel et al. (2010) Eur Urol 59:543–552	• For patients with T1a masses and a normal contralateral kidney, no difference in overall survival between radical and partial nephrectomy
Flanigan et al. (2001) N Engl J Med 345:1655–1669	• For patients with metastatic disease with favourable risk scores, improved overall survival with cytoreductive nephrectomy + IFN-α compared to IFN-α alone
Blom et al. (2009) Eur Urol 55:28–34	• No difference in overall or progression-free survival between radical nephrectomy alone vs nephrectomy + regional lymph node dissection
Hudes et al. (2007) N Engl J Med 356:2271–2281	• In patients with metastatic disease and poor prognosis, improved overall survival for temsirolimus compared with IFN-α
Motzer et al. (2007) N Engl J Med 356:115–124	• Improved progression-free survival for patients with metastatic disease (all risks) treated with sunitinib vs IFN-α

Recommended reading

Cancer Genome Atlas Research Network (2013) Comprehensive molecular characterization of clear cell renal cell carcinoma. *Nature* 499:43–49.

Cancer Genome Atlas Research Network (2013) National Comprehensive Cancer Network (NCCN) clinical practice guidelines in oncology: kidney cancer. V.1.2013 ed.

Blom JH, Van Poppel H, Marechal JM *et al.* (2009) Radical nephrectomy with and without lymph-node dissection: final results of European Organization for Research and Treatment of Cancer (EORTC) randomized phase 3 trial 30881. *Eur Urol* 55:28–34.

Campbell SC, Novick AC, Belldegrun A *et al.* (2009) Guideline for management of the clinical T1 renal mass. *J Urol* 182:1271–1279.

Chawla SN, Crispen PL, Hanlon AL, Greenberg RE, Chen DY, Uzzo RG (2006) The natural history of observed enhancing renal masses: meta-analysis and review of the world literature. *J Urol* 175:425–431.

Donat SM, Diaz M, Bishoff JT *et al.* (2013) Follow-up for Clinically Localized Renal Neoplasms: AUA Guideline. *J Urol* 190:407–416.

Flanigan RC, Salmon SE, Blumenstein BA *et al.* (2001) Nephrectomy followed by interferon alfa-2b compared with interferon alfa-2b alone for metastatic renal-cell cancer. *N Engl J Med* 345:1655–1669.

Heng DY, Chi KN, Murray N *et al.* (2009) A population-based study evaluating the impact of sunitinib on overall survival in the treatment of patients with metastatic renal cell cancer. *Cancer* 115:776–783.

Huang WC, Elkin EB, Levey AS, Jang TL, Russo P (2009) Partial nephrectomy versus radical nephrectomy in patients with small renal tumors–is there a difference in mortality and cardiovascular outcomes? *J Urol* 181:55–61; discussion 61–62.

Hudes G, Carducci M, Tomczak P *et al.* (2007) Temsirolimus, interferon alfa, or both for advanced renal-cell carcinoma. *N Engl J Med* 356:2271–2281.

Jonasch E, Futreal PA, Davis IJ *et al.* (2012) State of the science: an update on renal cell carcinoma. *Mol Cancer Res* 10:859–880.

Motzer RJ, Escudier B, Oudard S *et al.* (2008) Efficacy of everolimus in advanced renal cell carcinoma: a double-blind, randomised, placebo-controlled phase III trial. *Lancet* 372:449–456.

Motzer RJ, Hutson TE, Tomczak P *et al.* (2007) Sunitinib versus interferon alfa in metastatic renal-cell carcinoma. *N Engl J Med* 356:115–124.

Phe V, Yates DR, Renard-Penna R, Cussenot O, Roupret M (2011) Is there a contemporary role for percutaneous needle biopsy in the era of small renal masses? *BJU Int* 109:867–872.

Sutherland SE, Resnick MI, Maclennan GT, Goldman HB (2002) Does the size of the surgical margin in partial nephrectomy for renal cell cancer really matter? *J Urol* 167:61–64.

Van Poppel H, Da Pozzo L, Albrecht W *et al.* (2010) A prospective, randomised EORTC intergroup phase 3 study comparing the oncologic outcome of elective nephron-sparing surgery and radical nephrectomy for low-stage renal cell carcinoma. *Eur Urol* 59:543–552.

Wallen EM, Joyce GF, Wise M (2007) Kidney cancer. In: LitwinMS, SaigalCS, eds. *Urologic Diseases in America*. Los Angeles, CA: National Institute of Diabetes and Digestive and Kidney Diseases (U.S.), National Institutes of Health (U.S.), United States. Department of Health and Human Services, RAND Health.

30 Testicular germ cell tumours

Christian Winter[1], Anja Lorch[3], Carsten Bokemeyer[3], Heinz Schmidberger[4] and Peter Albers[2]

[1]Department of Urology, Malteser-Hospital St. Josef Hospital, Krefeld-Uerdingen, Germany
[2]Department of Urology, University Hospital Dusseldorf, Dusseldorf, Germany
[3]Department of Oncology, Hematology, BMT with Section Pneumology, University Hospital Hamburg-Eppendorf, Hamburg, Germany
[4]Department of Radiation Oncology, University Medical Center Mainz, Mainz, Germany

Summary	Key facts
Introduction	• Most common solid malignancy of young men aged 15–40 years • Divided into two major groups: pure seminoma and non-seminoma (NGGCT) • Pathogenesis still remains largely unknown
Presentation	• Primary tumour in the testis: painless unilateral mass in the scrotum or the casual finding of an intrascrotal mass: ▪ In a minority, the primary tumour manifestation is located extragonadally (retroperitoneum, mediastinum) • Back and flank pain are present in about 11% of cases
Scenario	• Early-stage germ cell tumour (GCT) is treated by individualized risk stratification within a multidisciplinary approach • Individual management (surveillance, chemotherapy, radiotherapy, surgery) has to be balanced according to clinical features and the risk of short- and long-term toxic effects • Metastatic tumours are treated with cisplatin-based combination chemotherapy based on risk stratification according to IGCCCG: ▪ Residual tumour lesions are resected • Relapsed patients are treated with high-dose chemotherapy and salvage resection

Trials	• *Local disease*:
	  ▪ AUO trial AH 01/94, German Testicular Cancer Study Group; Albers *et al.* (2008) *J Clin Oncol* 26(18):2966–2972:
	    ○ 1 × BEP demonstrated superiority over retroperitoneal lymph node resection (RPLND) in non-seminoma GCT (NSGCT) clinical Stage I patients
	  ▪ MRC TE19/EORTC 30982 study; Oliver *et al.* (2005) *Lancet* 366:293–300
	    ○ Phase III trial of carboplatin versus radiotherapy for Stage I seminoma
	    ○ Showed the non-inferiority of carboplatin to radiotherapy in the treatment of Stage I seminoma
	• *Advanced disease*:
	  ▪ Lorch *et al.* (2011) *J Clin Oncol* 29:2178–2184:
	    ○ Conventional-dose versus high-dose chemotherapy as first salvage treatment in GCT patients
	    ○ Five prognostic categories of relapsed patients benefitted from high-dose chemotherapy given as intensification of first salvage treatment

Incidence, aetiology and screening

Malignant tumours of the testis (germ cell tumours [GCT]) are rare, but are the most common cancer among men aged 15–40 years and the leading cause of cancer-related mortality and morbidity in this age group. The majority of patients with testicular cancer present with a primary tumour in the testis, whereas in <5% the primary tumour manifestation is located extragonadally in the retroperitoneum or the mediastinum.

Testicular germ cell tumours

Incidence, aetiology and screening	Description

Incidence	• Worldwide incidence of testicular GCT has doubled in the past 30 years and is still increasing
	• GCT incidence shows marked variation between countries and populations of different ethnic backgrounds:
	  ▪ Age-standardized incidence rate (ASIR) in Scandinavian countries is up to 15.2 new cases per 100,000 males per year
	  ▪ In Japan ASR is only 0.8 new cases per 100,000 males per year
	  ▪ ASIRs from 2002–2006 in the USA were:
	    ○ 5.4 per 100,000 men per year in all men
	    ○ 1.3 per 100,000 men per year in the African–American population
	• GCT age-standardized mortality rate (ASMR) varies widely:
	  ▪ Highest rates for Central America (0.7%), Central and Eastern Europe (0.6%) and Western Asia (0.6%)
	  ▪ Lowest rates for Australia (0.1%) and Eastern Asia (0.1%)

Aetiology	• Pathogenesis of testicular cancer remains largely unknown
	• Established GCT risk factors:
	  ▪ Cryptorchidism/undescended testis (up to 4.8-fold increased risk)
	  ▪ Klinefelter syndrome
	  ▪ Testicular cancer in first-degree relatives
	  ▪ Contralateral tumour
	• Discussed GCT risk factors:
	  ▪ *Perinatal factors*:
	    ○ Maternal older age at pregnancy
	    ○ Maternal *in utero* elevated oestrogen levels
	    ○ Maternal smoking
	    ○ Early life exposure to organic pesticides
	  ▪ *Postnatal factors*:
	    ○ Cannabis exposure
	    ○ High fat intake and dairy products, largely in childhood
	• Inherited susceptibility for testicular cancer:
	  ▪ Eight-fold higher risk in brothers and four-fold higher risk in sons of affected men
	• Genetic mutations:
	  ▪ Evidence for a testicular cancer susceptibility gene, *TGCT1*, located on chromosome Xq27
	  ▪ GCT are also characterized by gain of the short arm of chromosome 12 in almost all cases
	  ▪ Genome-wide association studies in cohorts of GCT patients identified a specific single nucleotide polymorphism (SNP) related to genes including *DMRT1* and *KITLG*

Screening	• Limited use: ▪ If significant family history, testis ultrasound and tumour marker controls may be performed, but there is no consensus

Pathology

Histopathologically, GCT can be divided into two major groups: seminomas and non-seminomas. Major groups and subtypes of testicular GCT are histologically classified according to the World Health Organization (WHO) system (Table 30.1). This classification recognizes three histological subtypes of teratoma: mature, immature and teratomas with malignant transformation. In addition, the finding of any of these histological GCT types within a seminoma defines the tumour as a non-seminoma GCT (NSGCT), primarily because the natural history of these tumours is less favourable than that of a pure seminoma.

Pathology	Description
Seminoma	• Not pluripotent • Appear as sheets of undifferentiated cells that resemble primitive germ cells

Non-seminoma	• Display a variety of histological forms including mixed tumours with seminoma
	• Differentiate along an embryonic lineage (embryonal carcinoma, teratoma, teratocarcinoma) or extra-embryonic tissue components (yolk sac tumour, choriocarcinoma)
	• *Teratomas*:
	  ▪ Special subgroup of NSGCT
	  ▪ Show tremendous histological diversity:
	    ○ Contain a variety of tissue elements derived from all three embryonic germ cell layers
	    ○ Three histological subtypes: mature, immature and teratomas with malignant transformation

Table 30.1 WHO histopathological classification

Germ cell tumours	Histopathological classification: subtypes
Precursor lesions	Intratubular germ cell neoplasia (TIN) Unclassified type (carcinoma in situ)
Seminoma	Seminoma Seminoma with syncytiotrophoblastic cells Spermatocytic seminoma
Non-seminoma (NSGCT)	Embryonal carcinoma Yolk sac tumour Trophoblastic tumours: • Choriocarcinoma, monophasic choriocarcinoma • Placental site trophoblastic tumour • Cystic trophoblastic tumour Teratoma: • Dermoid cyst • Epidermoid cyst • Monodermal teratoma (carcinoid, primitive neuroectodermal tumour [PNET], nephroblastoma-like tumour, others) • Teratoma with somatic-type malignancy Tumours of more than one histological type (mixed forms): • Embryonal carcinoma and teratoma • Teratoma and seminoma • Choriocarcinoma, teratoma and embryonal carcinoma • Others

Adapted from Sobin 2002. Reproduced with permission of Wiley & Sons.

Presentation

- Most GCT patients present with a primary tumour in the testis:
  - Usually appears as a painless unilateral mass in the scrotum or the casual finding of an intrascrotal mass
- In a minority of patients, the primary tumour manifestation is located extragonadally, i.e. in the retroperitoneum or the mediastinum
- Gynaecomastia is present in 7% of men (often in NSGCT)
- Back and flank pain are present in about 11% of cases

Natural history

The natural history is dependent on the subtype of GCT, with non-seminomas usually more aggressive than seminomas. GCT typically remain localized or spread to lymph nodes. The most commonly involved nodes are in the retroperitoneum, and further spread may occur to the mediastinum and supraclavicular fossa. They may occasionally become more aggressive and spread haematogenously to the lungs. Less commonly involved organs include the brain, liver and bone.

Natural history	Description

Testicular intraepithelial neoplasia (TIN)	• Defined as a carcinoma in situ, a malignant preinvasive testicular germ cell lesion:
	  ▪ Without treatment 70% of TIN advance to become definitive GCT within 7 years
	  ▪ Approximately 2.5% of patients with GCT have a TIN in the contralateral testis
	• Malignant transformation of TIN is characterized by growth beyond the basement membrane, eventually replacing most of the testicular parenchyma

Seminoma	• Usually has a much slower doubling time that NSGCT • May recur 2–10 years after initial treatment because of indolent course • Based on the natural history of the disease, curability after multimodality treatment regimens is often declared after 5 years
Non-seminoma	• Doubling time ranges from 10 to 30 days: ▪ Reflected by alterations in serum tumour markers • Most treatment failures followed by mortality occur within the first 2–3 years of diagnosis
Routes of spread	• Tunica albuginea is a natural barrier to local metastasis so it should not be compromised by direct diagnostic scrotal needle biopsy or scrotal violation during primary surgical exploration • Lymphatic spread is the most common cause of metastasis and commonly occurs through the spermatic cord lymphatics to the retroperitoneal lymph node chain: ▪ An exception is pure choriocarcinoma, which may disseminate more frequently through vascular invasion • In rare cases, a direct communication exists between the testicular lymphatics and the thoracic duct, causing a thoracic metastasis without retroperitoneal involvement • Scrotal invasion may present with inguinal metastasis (rare situation)

Diagnostic work-up

In patients in whom a testicular tumour is suspected, the following diagnostic examinations are mandatory:
- Testis inspection and palpation
- Ultrasound of the testes (7.5-MHz transducer)
- Determination of serum tumour markers (see below)
- Surgical exploration:
  - Organ-sparing surgery for small lesions (<30% of testis parenchyma)
  - In lesions encompassing most of the testis: parenchyma orchiectomy
- Contralateral biopsy in patients with high-risk features for testis cancer (testis volume <12 mL, history of cryptorchidism)
- Staging examinations

Diagnostic work-up	Description
Surgical exploration/ orchiectomy	• Orchiectomy is obligatory for suspected tumours: ■ *Exception*: in life-threatening metastatic disease or massive elevation of tumour markers, an orchiectomy should not delay chemotherapy and may be deferred until clinical stabilization (usually at the end of chemotherapy) • Exploration should be performed through an inguinal incision and the spermatic cord divided at the internal inguinal ring if a tumour is found (radical orchiectomy, ablatio testis) • If the diagnosis of testicular cancer is unclear, a biopsy is taken for frozen section histological examination • In small lesions (<30% of parenchyma), organ-sparing surgery should be performed even in patients with a normal contralateral testis to rule out benign or stromal (Leydig cell, Sertoli cell) tumours before orchiectomy is indicated • Organ-sparing surgery should be attempted in special cases like bilateral testicular tumours, metachronous contralateral tumours and tumour in a solitary testis with normal preoperative testosterone levels • Option of organ-sparing surgery must be carefully discussed with the patient and surgery performed in a centre with experience
Contralateral biopsy	• Should be discussed with patients at high risk of contralateral TIN: ■ Risk factors are testicular volume <12 mL, age <40 years, history of maldescensus testis or poor spermatogenesis • New trials have shown no evidence to recommend contralateral biopsy in patients who are not at high risk
Imaging	• Chest X-ray (seminoma clinical Stage I [CS I]) • Computed tomography (CT) scan of the abdomen and pelvis • CT chest (not mandatory for seminoma CS I) • Magnetic resonance imaging (MRI) of the chest and abdomen (only if CT is contraindicated) • CT central nervous system (CNS) (in advanced disease or in the presence of symptoms) • Ultrasound of the liver (only in the presence of symptoms) • Bone scan (only in the presence of symptoms) • Fluorodeoxyglucose-positron emission tomography (FDG-PET) scan in primary staging is not justified

Tumour markers	*Alpha-fetoprotein (AFP)*:
	   ■ Homologue of albumin that acts as a carrier protein in the fetus
	   ■ Half-life of 5 days
	   ■ Normal level <10–15 µg/L
	   ■ Sensitive marker for non-seminomas especially in yolk sac tumours and embryonal carcinoma, and increases in 50–70% of NSGCT patients
	   ■ Rising serum levels indicate persistent GCT, even in the absence of radiographic evidence of disease
	   ■ Elevated AFP occurs in most hepatocellular carcinomas and 10–30% of other gastrointestinal cancers
	   ■ Benign liver disease, in particular hepatitis, and liver damage induced by chemotherapy are often associated with moderately elevated serum levels (may result in misinterpretation)
	• *Human chorionic gonadotropin (hCG)*:
	   ■ Member of the glycoprotein hormone family, which includes luteinizing hormone (LH), follicle-stimulating hormone (FSH) and thyroid-stimulating hormone (TSH)
	   ■ Normal level <2.1 U/L
	   ■ β-subunit of hCG (ß-hCG) is secreted by GCT, especially choriocarcinoma and at low levels by seminoma (<200 IU/L)
	   ■ Increased ß-hCG in 40–60% of NSGCT patients and up to 30% of seminoma patients
	   ■ Important to note that chemotherapy often causes gonadal suppression that increases the ß-hCG levels:
	     ○ Levels increasing from <2 up to 5–8 U/L during chemotherapy are not unusual
	• *Lactate dehydrogenase (LDH)*:
	   ■ Exists as a tetramer that may contain various combinations of two subunits (LDH-A, LDH-B)
	   ■ Subunits can combine in five different isoenzymes (LDH1–5)
	   ■ Expressed in many tissues and elevated levels caused by a wide variety of diseases like haemolysis, meningitis, encephalitis, acute pancreatitis and HIV
	   ■ Useful marker in GCT:
	     ○ Elevated in 80% of patients with advanced GCT and is proportional to tumour volume
	• Other tumour markers *not* routinely recommended:
	   ■ *Placental alkaline phosphatase (PLAP)*:
	     ○ Elevated most frequently in patients with seminoma (60–70%), and less frequently in other GCT forms
	     ○ Concentrations are increased up to 10-fold in smokers, which limits its clinical application
	   ■ *Neurone-specific enolase (NSE)*:
	     ○ Elevated in about 30–50% of patients with seminomas and less often in NSGCT patients

Staging and prognostic grouping

UICC TNM staging

After completion of the diagnostic procedures, the clinical stage (Table 30.2) based on the UICC TNM classification (Table 30.3) and serum tumour markers should be defined.

The International Germ Cell Cancer Collaborative Group (IGCCCG) staging system has been incorporated into the TNM classification and uses histology, location of the primary tumour, location of metastases and pretreatment tumour marker levels in serum as prognostic factors to categorize patients into 'good', 'intermediate' or 'poor' prognosis (Table 30.4). The optimal individual treatment strategy is predicated from the clinical stage and the IGCCCG classification.

Table 30.2 Clinical stages of testicular cancer

Clinical stage	Definition	CS	TNM category (see also Table 30.3)
Stage I (CS I)	Negative lymph nodes (N0) No metastasis (M0)	IA	pT1N0M0S0
		IB	pT2N0M0S0
			pT3 N0 M0 S0
			pT4N0M0S0
		IS	pT1–4N0M0S1–3
Stage II (CS II)	Positive lymph nodes (N+) No metastasis (M0)	IIA	pT1–4N1M0S0
			pT1–4N1M0S1
		IIB	pT1–4N2M0S0
			pT1–4 N2 M0 S1
		IIC	pT1–4N3M0S0
			pT1–4 N3 M0 S1
Stage III (CS III)	Metastasis (M+)	IIIA	pT1–4N1–3M1AS0
			pT1–4N1–3M1AS1
		IIIB	pT1–4N1–3M0S2
			pT1–4N1–3M1AS2
		IIIC	pT1–4N1–3M0S3
			pT1–4N1–3M1AS3
			pT1–4N1–3M1BS0–1

Table 30.3 UICC TNM categories and stage grouping: Testis

TNM categories				
pTis	Intratubular			
pT1	Testis and epididymis, no vascular/lymphatic invasion			
pT2	Testis and epididymis with vascular/lymphatic invasion or tunica vaginalis			
pT3	Spermatic cord			
pT4	Scrotum			
N1	2 cm	pN1	≤2 cm and ≤5 nodes	
N2	>2–5 cm	pN2	>2–5 cm or >5 nodes or extranodal extension	
N3	>5 cm	pN3	>5 cm	
M1a	Non regional lymph nodes or lung			
M1b	Other sites			

Stage grouping				
Stage 0	pTis	N0	M0	S0, SX
Stage I	pT1–4	N0	M0	SX
Stage IA	pT1	N0	M0	S0
Stage IB	pT2–4	N0	M0	S0
Stage IS	Any pT/TX	N0	M0	S1–3
Stage II	Any pT/TX	N1–3	M0	SX
Stage IIA	Any pT/TX	N1	M0	S0
	Any pT/TX	N1	M0	S1
Stage IIB	Any pT/TX	N2	M0	S0
	Any pT/TX	N2	M0	S1
Stage IIC	Any pT/TX	N3	M0	S0
	Any pT/TX	N3	M0	S1
Stage III	Any pT/TX	Any N	M1a	SX
Stage IIIA	Any pT/TX	Any N	M1a	S0
	Any pT/TX	Any N	M1a	S1
Stage IIIB	Any pT/TX	N1–3	M0	S2
	Any pT/TX	Any N	M1a	S2
Stage IIIC	Any pT/TX	N1–3	M0	S3
	Any pT/TX	Any N	M1a	S3
	Any pT/TX	Any N	M1b	Any S

Including S serum tumour markers.

Table 30.4 Prognostic classification of the International Germ Cell Cancer Collaborative Group (IGCCCG)

	NSGCT	Seminoma
Good prognosis	56% of cases 5-year PFS 89% 5-year survival 92% *Criteria:* Testis or primary extragonadal retroperitoneal tumour No non-pulmonary visceral metastases AFP <1000 ng/mL ß-hCG <1000 ng/mL (<5000 IU/L) LDH <1.5 × normal level	90% of cases 5-year PFS 82% 5-year survival 86% *Criteria:* Any primary localization No non-pulmonary visceral metastases Any marker level

	NSGCT	Seminoma
Intermediate prognosis	28% of cases 5-year PFS 75% 5-year survival 80% *Criteria*: Testis or primary extragonadal retroperitoneal tumour No presence of non-pulmonary visceral metastases AFP 1000–10,000 ng/mL and/or ß-hCG 1000–10,000 ng/mL (5000–50,000 IU/L) and/or LDH 1.5–10 × normal levels	10% of cases 5-year PFS 67% 5-year survival 72% *Criteria*: Any primary localization Presence of non-pulmonary visceral metastases (liver, CNS, bone, intestinum) Any tumour marker level
Poor prognosis	16% of cases 5-year PFS 41% 5-year survival 48% *Criteria*: Primary mediastinal GCT with or without testis or primary retroperitoneal tumour Presence of non-pulmonary visceral metastases (liver, CNS, bone, intestinum) and/or AFP >10,000 ng/mL and/or ß-hCG >10,000 ng/mL (50,000 IU/l) and/or LDH >10 × normal level	Does not exist

Prognostic factors

See Table 30.5.

Table 30.5 Prognostic factors for testicular cancer

Prognostic factors	Tumour related	Host related	Environment related
Essential	Histological type T category N category M category Tumour markers (AFP, hCG, LDH) Site of metastases		
Additional	Rate of marker decline	Delay in diagnosis	Physician expertise
New and promising	Copy number of i(12p) p53 Ki-67 Apoptotic index		

Treatment philosophy

Scenario	Treatment philosophy

Testicular intraepithelial neoplasia (TIN) (Fig. 30.1)	• Without treatment, 70% of TIN become definitive GCT within 7 years
	• Once diagnosed in a solitary testis, three treatment options:
	  ▪ Local radiotherapy (20 Gy in single 2-Gy fractions)
	  ▪ Radical orchiectomy
	  ▪ Surveillance

(continued)

Scenario	Treatment philosophy

Seminoma CS I (Fig. 30.1)	• Outcome is usually very favourable even without adjuvant treatment
	• However, approximately 20% of patients with seminoma CS I can relapse if no adjuvant treatment is given, despite normal diagnostic imaging:
	  ■ Risk factors:
	    ○ Size of primary tumour >4 cm and rete testis invasion are risk factors for occult retroperitoneal metastasis (but are not prospectively validated)
	    ○ Patients with both of these risk factors are defined as having *high-risk seminoma* with a relapse rate of up to 32%; the two risk factors can be used to advise patients about their individual treatment options
	    ○ In patients with *low-risk seminoma* stage I (no risk factors), the risk of recurrence is as low as 6–8%
	• Cure rate in patients with CS I seminoma is close to 100% and can be achieved with two accepted strategies:
	  ■ Surveillance (currently the preferred option)
	  ■ Single-agent carboplatin (AUC 7) chemotherapy
	• Adjuvant radiotherapy, because of the risk of late toxicity (e.g. development of secondary malignant neoplasms), is currently not recommended as standard adjuvant treatment

Non-seminoma CS I (Fig. 30.1)	• Up to 50% of patients can relapse if no adjuvant treatment is given
	• *Risk factors*:
	  ■ Vascular or lymphatic tumour invasion (high risk) in the histopathological examination of the primary tumour:
	    ○ High risk: 48% risk of developing metastasis without adjuvant treatment
	    ○ Low risk (absence of tumour invasion): only 14–22% will relapse
	• Treatment recommendation should be risk-adapted depending on the presence or absence of vascular tumour invasion:
	  ■ Cisplatin-based chemotherapy (high-risk patients)
	  ■ Surveillance (low-risk patients, and alternative to cisplatin-based chemotherapy for high-risk patients)
	  ■ Nerve-sparing retroperitoneal lymph node dissection (NS-RPLND) (necessity for this has been questioned by the high effectiveness of cisplatin-based chemotherapy, and preference for active surveillance)

Seminoma CS IIA/B (Fig. 30.2)	• Recommended standard therapy is radiotherapy for CS IIA/B • In CS IIB, cisplatin-based chemotherapy is an alternative to radiotherapy with comparable oncological outcome but higher acute and long-term toxic effects

Non-seminoma CS IIA/B (Fig. 30.2)	• Elevated tumour marker levels: treat according to IGCCCG risk group recommendations with BEP:
	  ■ Where a residual retroperitoneal tumour of ≥1 cm has been detected, a residual tumour resection is mandatory
	• Without elevated tumour markers: treat with primary RPLND, using a nerve-sparing technique if possible, or surveillance strategy:
	  ■ Possible further treatment depends on histological outcome

Seminoma or non-seminoma IIC or III (Fig. 30.3)	• Chemotherapy according to IGCCCG risk classification remains standard treatment
Residual tumour (Fig. 30.3)	• After completing chemotherapy or radiotherapy, an evaluation of tumour markers and imaging investigations are mandatory • *Seminoma patients*: ■ Residual mass of seminoma should not be resected, irrespective of its size, but should be monitored regularly with tumour markers and imaging investigations

	• *Non-seminoma patients*:
	  ■ Residual viable GCT and mature teratoma (chemotherapy-resistant tumour) will progress if untreated
	  ■ Residual tumour resection is necessary when residual radiographic abnormalities after chemotherapy are present, and should be performed within 4 weeks after chemotherapy:
	    ○ If necrosis or mature teratoma is detected, no further treatment
	    ○ If incomplete resection, immature teratoma detected or >10% undifferentiated tumour in the resected specimen: consolidation chemotherapy may be justified

Brain metastasis	• Optimal therapeutic management and its sequence (chemotherapy, radiotherapy, surgery) has not yet been completely defined • Four cycles of chemotherapy followed by cranial radiotherapy appears to be the best evidence-based approach
Relapse/refractory disease	• Standard treatment after first-line chemotherapy is salvage chemotherapy according to Lorch–Beyer prognostic score • High-dose chemotherapy still represents a curative option for patients with subsequent relapse (second relapse) and is considered standard if it has not been used before
Late relapse	• Late relapsing tumours are usually less chemotherapy sensitive • Immediate surgical treatment is the first choice, irrespective of tumour marker levels

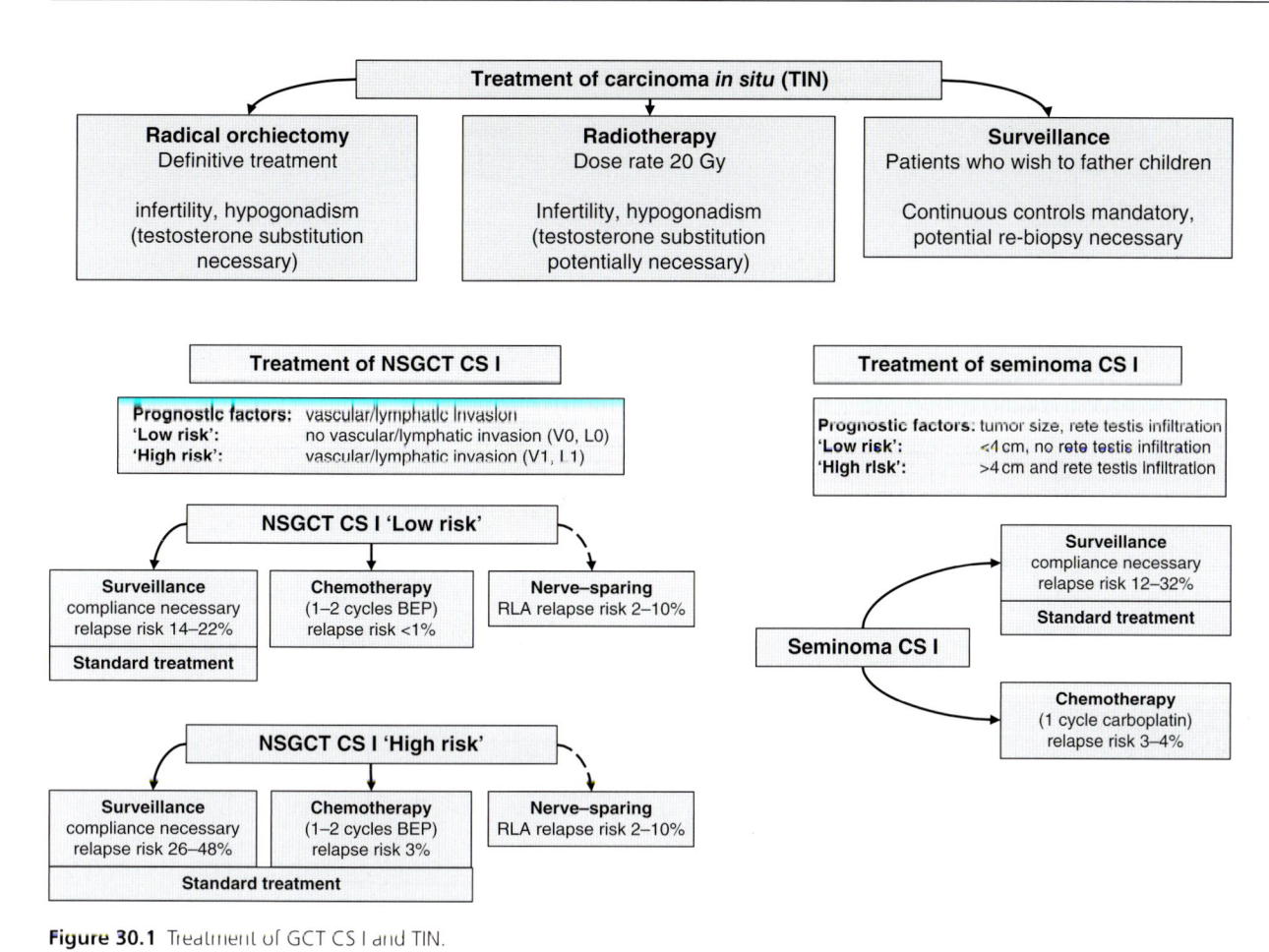

Testicular germ cell tumours

```
                    Treatment of carcinoma in situ (TIN)

    Radical orchiectomy              Radiotherapy                    Surveillance
    Definitive treatment             Dose rate 20 Gy         Patients who wish to father children

    infertility, hypogonadism    Infertility, hypogonadism       Continuous controls mandatory,
    (testosterone substitution   (testosterone substitution      potential re-biopsy necessary
          necessary)              potentially necessary)
```

```
        Treatment of NSGCT CS I                                Treatment of seminoma CS I

Prognostic factors: vascular/lymphatic invasion       Prognostic factors: tumor size, rete testis infiltration
'Low risk':  no vascular/lymphatic invasion (V0, L0)  'Low risk':  <4 cm, no rete testis infiltration
'High risk': vascular/lymphatic invasion (V1, L1)     'High risk': >4 cm and rete testis infiltration

          NSGCT CS I 'Low risk'                                                    Surveillance
                                                                               compliance necessary
                                                                                relapse risk 12–32%
  Surveillance      Chemotherapy       Nerve–sparing
compliance necessary (1–2 cycles BEP)   RLA relapse risk 2–10%                  Standard treatment
 relapse risk 14–22%  relapse risk <1%
                                                             Seminoma CS I
  Standard treatment
                                                                                 Chemotherapy
          NSGCT CS I 'High risk'                                             (1 cycle carboplatin)
                                                                               relapse risk 3–4%
  Surveillance      Chemotherapy       Nerve–sparing
compliance necessary (1–2 cycles BEP)   RLA relapse risk 2–10%
 relapse risk 26–48%  relapse risk 3%

  Standard treatment
```

Figure 30.1 Treatment of GCT CS I and TIN.
RPA, retroperitoneal lymphadenectomy.

Treatment

Testicular intraepithelial neoplasia and testicular cancer CS I (see Fig. 30.1)

Treatment: TIN and CS 1	Description
Testicular intraepithelial neoplasia (TIN)	• Three treatment options: *local radiotherapy* (20 Gy in single 2-Gy fractions), *radical orchiectomy* or *surveillance*: ▪ Radiotherapy and orchiectomy are definitive options, but they cause infertility and may lead to androgen deficiency ▪ Surveillance is justified for fertile patients who wish to father children: ○ Regular evaluation of the TIN-bearing testis by ultrasonography is mandatory ▪ All options should be individually discussed with the patient, including each of their benefits and risks

Seminoma CS I	• Two accepted strategies:
	 ▪ *Single-agent carboplatin (AUC 7) chemotherapy*:
	   ○ Relapse rates of up to 5% (comparable to those for adjuvant radiotherapy in a randomized trail)
	   ○ Reduced long-term toxic effects
	   ○ Acceptance limited by lack of long-term data

(continued)

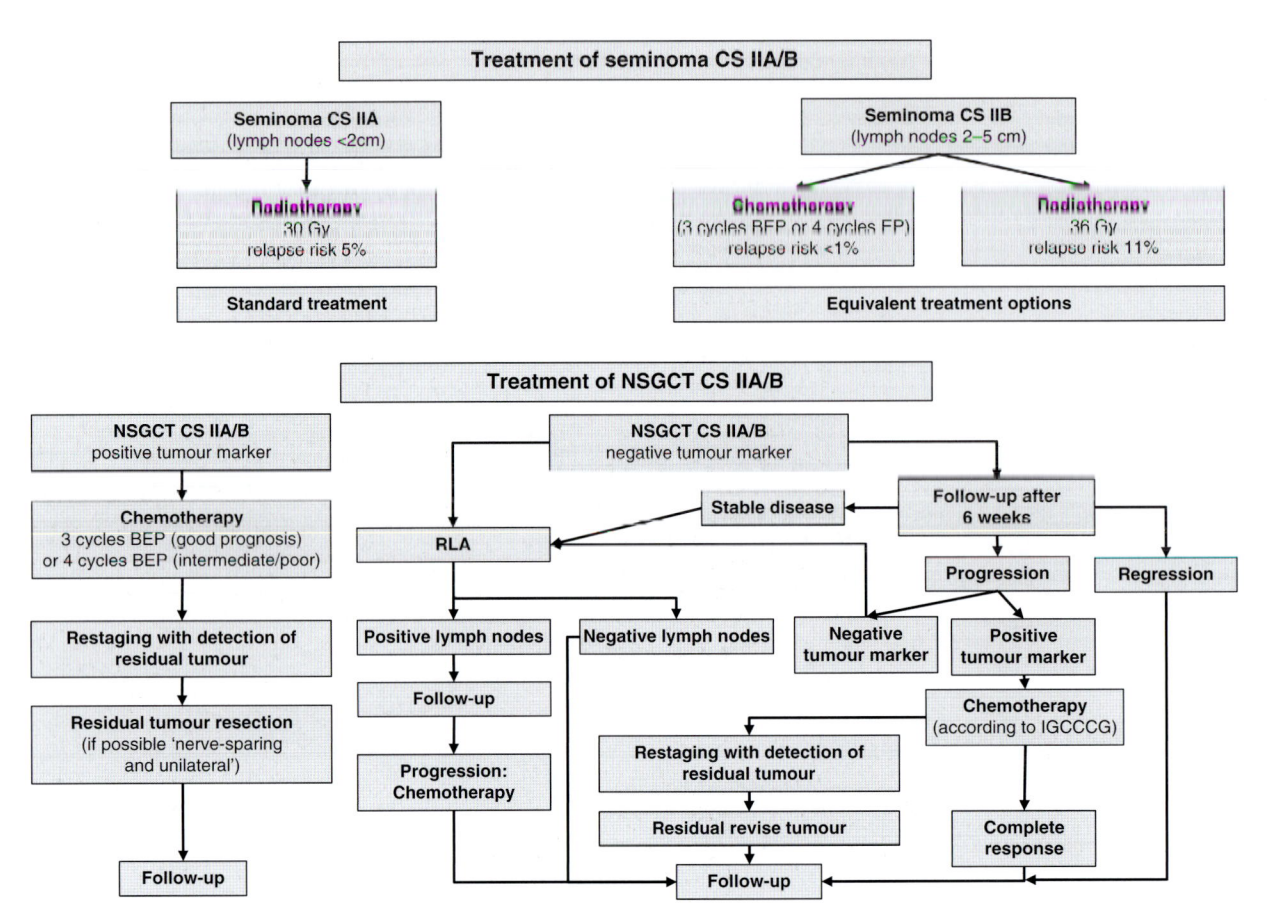

Figure 30.2 Treatment of GCT CS IIA/B.
RPA, retroperitoneal lymphadenectomy.

Treatment: TIN and CS 1	Description

	- *Surveillance* (preferred):
	  ○ Avoids treatment-related morbidity and over-treatment without compromising curability from the use of salvage chemotherapy regimens for relapses, and is a successful strategy in most cases
	  ○ Close and active follow-up for at least 5 years is recommended
	  ○ Small but clinically significant risk of relapse exists >5 years after orchiectomy (late relapse), which suggests a need for long-term surveillance
	  ○ Recommended for patients with low-risk seminoma (risk of recurrence is only 6–8%)
	  ○ Large prospective trials have shown that, independent of risk factors, surveillance is a safe treatment option if patient compliance and regular follow-up examinations are guaranteed
	- *Adjuvant radiotherapy*:
	  ▪ To the retroperitoneum and ipsilateral pelvis has for decades been the treatment and is associated with excellent long-term survival (relapse rate 3.5–5.0%)
	  ▪ However, there is a risk of late toxic effects, particularly the development of secondary malignant neoplasms that result from radiation exposure
	  ▪ Therefore, radiotherapy is currently not recommended as standard adjuvant treatment for patients younger than 40 years old
	  ▪ Since radiation-induced secondary malignancies are less common in patients over the age of 40 years, adjuvant radiotherapy can be an option for this age group

```
Treatment of advanced germ cell tumours
         │
Seminoma/NSGCT CS IIC/CS III
```

'Good prognosis' IGCCCG classification → Chemotherapy 3 cycles BEP or 4 cycles EP → Restaging → Residual tumour (≥1 cm)

'Intermediate/poor prognosis' IGCCCG classification → Chemotherapy 4 cycles BEP or 4 cycles PEI → Inadequate decline of tumour marker after 1–2 cycles chemotherapy → High-dose chemotherapy with stem cell support (2–3 cycle)

Tumour marker normalization

Elevated tumour marker (plateau) ↔ Restaging ↔ Increasing tumour marker

Elevated tumour marker (plateau) → Residual tumour resection → Incomplete resection

Salvage chemotherapy depending on risk factors: 4 cycles PEI/VIP, 4 cycles TIP, or high-dose chemotherapy with stem cell support (preferred)

Detection of necrosis or mature teratoma / Detection of <10% of viable tumour, complete resection / Detection of >10% viable tumour, complete resection

Salvage resection / 'desperation surgery' (after salvage chemotherapy, relapse after salvage chemotherapy, late relapse)

Follow-up ← Consolidation chemotherapy (2 cycles of cisplatin-based chemotherapy)

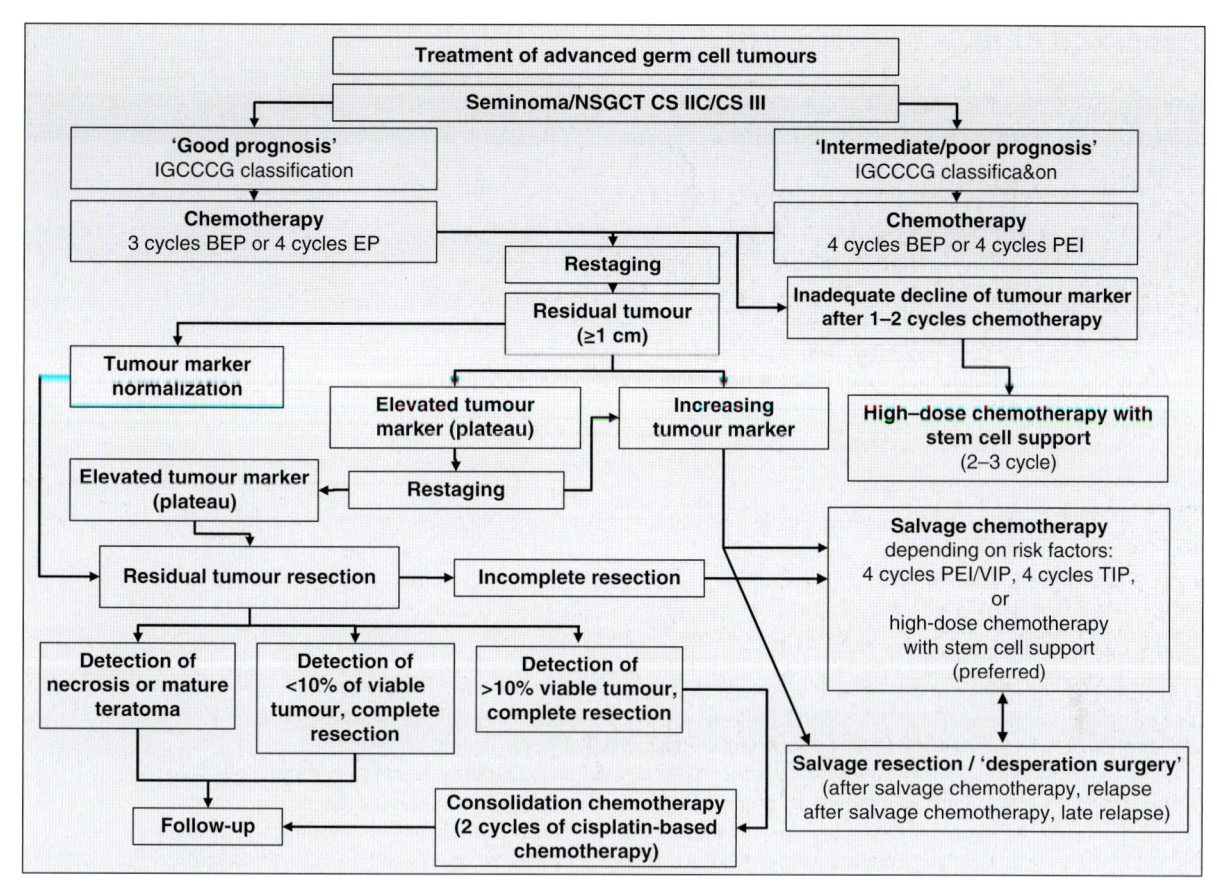

Figure 30.3 Treatment of GCT CS IIC and CS III.

Treatment: TIN and CS 1	Description

Non-seminoma CS I	• Three accepted strategies:
	  ▪ Surveillance
	  ▪ Chemotherapy with one (or two) courses of bleomycin + etoposide + cisplatin (BEP)
	  ▪ Nerve-sparing retroperitoneal lymph node dissection (NS-RPLND)
	• *Low-risk patients (V0/L0)*:
	  ▪ Patients who do not present with vascular or lymphatic tumour invasion (low risk) have a risk of metastasis of only 15%
	  ▪ A surveillance strategy lasting for at least 5 years is recommended if the patient is willing and able to comply
	  ▪ Adjuvant chemotherapy with BEP or NS-RPLND remains the treatment option for patients who are unwilling to undergo surveillance
	• *High-risk patients (V1 and/or L1)*:
	  ▪ Patients who shows a vascular or lymphatic tumour invasion (high risk) have a 48% risk of developing metastasis
	  ▪ Adjuvant chemotherapy with one (or two) cycles of BEP or a surveillance strategy is recommended
	• *Active surveillance*:
	  ▪ Excellent option in all patients (low and high risk)
	  ▪ Overall survival is comparable with the best results reported for primary RPLND or adjuvant chemotherapy
	• *Adjuvant chemotherapy with BEP*:
	  ▪ Two cycles has been reported as a primary treatment with a relapse rate of 3%
	  ▪ Generally, cisplatin-based chemotherapy increases the long-term risks of secondary malignant neoplasms and cardiovascular disease, at least for patients who receive three or more cycles of BEP
	  ▪ One cycle of BEP may be a valid option as initial treatment for all patients with non-seminoma CS I; offers an optimized risk-adapted adjuvant chemotherapy with high cure rate (relapse rates up to 1.3–3.2%; SWENOTECA and GTCSG study data), even in those classified as high risk, and reduced long-term toxic effects
	• *NS-RPLND*:
	  ▪ In Europe, remains a treatment options for those unwilling or unable to undergo surveillance or adjuvant chemotherapy
	  ▪ In these rare cases, surgery should be performed in dedicated referral centres in order to avoid excess morbidity

Testicular cancer CS IIA/B (see Fig. 30.2)

Treatment: CS IIA/B	Description

Seminoma CS IIA/B	• *Seminoma CS IIA*:
	  ▪ Infradiaphragmatic metastasis of <2 cm
	  ▪ Standard therapy is radiotherapy with total doses of 30 Gy
	  ▪ Standard radiation field should be extended from the para-aortic region to the ipsilateral iliac field (hockey-stick field)
	  ▪ Relapse rates are moderate (5%)
	  ▪ Overall survival is almost 100%
	• *Seminoma CS IIB*:
	  ▪ Infradiaphragmatic metastasis 2–5 cm
	  ▪ Standard therapy is radiotherapy with total doses of 36 Gy
	  ▪ Standard radiation field should be extended from the para-aortic region to the ipsilateral iliac field (hockey-stick field)
	  ▪ Lateral field margin should be modified to the size of the lymph nodes with a safety distance of 1.0–1.5 cm
	  ▪ Relapse rates are moderate (11%)
	  ▪ Overall survival is almost 100%
	  ▪ Alternative treatment option is chemotherapy with three cycles of BEP or four cycles of EP

Non-seminoma CS IIA/B	• *Non-seminoma CS IIA/B + positive tumour markers*:
	  ▪ Treatment according to IGCCCG risk group recommendations:
	    ○ 'Good prognosis': three cycles of BEP
	    ○ 'Intermediate' or 'poor prognosis': four cycles of BEP
	  ▪ If residual retroperitoneal tumour of ≥1 cm, a residual tumour resection is mandatory:
	    ○ Surgical margins should not be compromised in an attempt to preserve ejaculation
	    ○ Nerve-sparing techniques and the reduction of the surgical field to a left- or right-sided template are possible to preserve antegrade ejaculation and fertility in patients with marker normalization after chemotherapy and no viable tumour as assessed by frozen-section histology
	• *Non-seminoma CS IIA/B + negative tumour markers*:
	  ▪ Two options: primary *NS-RPLND* or *surveillance strategy* with a 6-week follow-up examination
	  ▪ RPLND serves also as a diagnostic approach to confirm the disease stage
	  ▪ Possible further treatment depends on histological outcome:
	    ○ If undifferentiated embryonal carcinoma is detected, adjuvant chemotherapy with two cycles of BEP is indicated, depending on the extent of the metastatic disease and lymph node density
	    ○ If teratoma is detected, postoperative surveillance is recommended after a complete resection
	  ▪ Surveillance strategy is indicated to evaluate if the retroperitoneal lesion grows, is stable or shrinks:
	    ○ *Rapidly growing lesions and rising tumour markers*: tumour should not be resected but treated with primary BEP chemotherapy according to IGCCCG recommendations (see above)
	    ○ *Progressive or stable disease with negative tumour markers* (teratoma or a growing, undifferentiated malignant tumour is suspected): RPLND or – if feasible – a CT-guided biopsy is indicated
	    ○ *Shrinking lesion* (probably of non-malignant origin): monitor in further follow-up examinations

Testicular cancer CS IIC and III (see Fig. 30.3), residual tumour and brain metastasis

Residual tumour after chemotherapy

Overall, following chemotherapy for residual tumours in patients with non-seminomatous testicular GCT, only 10% of residual masses contain viable cancer, 50% contain mature teratoma and 40% contain necrotic tissue. However, after initial chemotherapy, residual viable GCT and mature teratoma (chemotherapy-resistant tumour) will progress if untreated. Completeness of residual tumour resection is, therefore, an independent and consistent predictive variable of clinical outcome. The size and location of residual masses make residual tumour resection a technically demanding procedure that should be performed by experienced surgeons in dedicated referral centres.

Brain metastasis

Approximately 1–2% of all patients with GCT present with brain metastases. The overall survival of patients with brain metastases at initial diagnosis is poor (30–40%), but it is even worse if brain metastasis occurs as recurrent disease (2–5%). The optimal therapeutic management and its sequence (chemotherapy, radiotherapy, surgery) has not yet been completely defined for patients with brain metastasis. However, chemotherapy is necessary in all of these patients.

Treatment: CS IIC and CS III, residual disease and brain metastasis	Description

Seminoma and non-seminoma CS IIC/III	• Treatment according to IGCCCG risk classification
	• Chemotherapy with BEP, EP or PEI (cisplatin + etoposide + ifosfamide) remains standard treatment
	• *'Good prognosis'*:
	  ▪ Three cycles of BEP or (in cases of bleomycin contraindications) four cycles of EP are recommended
	• *'Intermediate' or 'poor prognosis'*:
	  ▪ Four cycles of BEP or four cycles of PEI should be given
	  ▪ Use of recombinant granulocyte-colony stimulating factor (G-CSF) as primary prophylaxis for complications of neutropenia is generally not recommended for BEP, but can be considered for PEI
	  ▪ Restaging examination has to be performed by imaging after two cycles of chemotherapy
	  ▪ Tumour markers need to be evaluated prior to each next cycle of chemotherapy:
	    ○ In cases of adequate tumour marker decline and stable or regressive tumour manifestation, the initiated chemotherapy should be completed
	    ○ If tumour markers decline but metastases grow (a growing teratoma syndrome is possible), resection of the tumour is obligatory at least directly after completion of chemotherapy
	    ○ In 'poor prognosis' patients in whom tumour markers rise or show inadequately slow decline after the first cycle of BEP chemotherapy, intensification of treatment with a dose-dense regimen or high-dose chemotherapy with autologous stem cell transplantation should be considered

Residual tumour after initial chemotherapy	• After completing chemotherapy, evaluation of tumour markers and imaging investigations are mandatory to detect possible residual tumours
	• *Residual tumour in seminoma*:
	  ▪ Should not be resected, irrespective of its size, but should be monitored regularly by imaging investigations and tumour markers:
	    ○ FDG-PET has a high positive and negative predictive value with regard to the question of remaining vital disease in patients with residual masses after treatment of seminoma
	    ○ If FDG-PET findings are positive, a biopsy is mandatory for histological verification
	    ○ If tumour markers (β-hCG, LDH) are positive in cases of residual lesions, salvage chemotherapy is indicated
	  ▪ Further treatment (surveillance, residual tumour resection, radiotherapy or chemotherapy) should be discussed with the patient on the basis of histopathological results
	• *Residual tumour in non-seminoma*:
	  ▪ Residual radiographic abnormalities are lesions of >1 cm
	  ▪ Resection of residual masses of >1 cm is necessary and should be performed within 4 weeks after chemotherapy:
	    ○ Patients with a complete serological remission and in whom no or minimal residual radiographic abnormalities (<1 cm) are present after chemotherapy can be safely observed without residual tumour resection
	    ○ Residual tumour resection is a technically demanding procedure that should be performed by experienced surgeons in dedicated referral centres
	  ▪ After residual tumour resection with detection of necrosis or mature teratoma with complete resection, no further treatment is required
	  ▪ In cases of incomplete resection of vital carcinoma or immature teratoma, or detection of >10% viable, undifferentiated tumour in the resected specimen, consolidation chemotherapy (e.g. two cycles of conventionally dosed PEI) may be justified

Brain metastasis	• Chemotherapy is necessary in all patients (four cycles)
	• Cranial radiotherapy following systemic chemotherapy improves the overall prognosis compared with chemotherapy alone:
	  ▪ If a complete remission is obtained with chemotherapy, radiotherapy can be omitted
	  ▪ A parallel, whole-brain radiotherapy and chemotherapy strategy should be avoided as it can cause late CNS toxic effects (progressive multifocal leukoencephalopathy/cerebral atrophy)
	  ▪ In case of a residual mass after chemotherapy, local radiotherapy to the residual tumour seems to be sufficient and will avoid late effects to the CNS
	  ▪ To date, the requirement for secondary neurosurgical resection of a solitary residual mass after initial chemotherapy and radiotherapy remains unclear

Relapsed, refractory or late relapse tumours

In patients who relapse or suffer from refractory disease, the standard treatment after first-line chemotherapy is salvage chemotherapy, according to their classification by the Lorch–Beyer prognostic score. This score comprises seven important factors (seminoma vs non-seminoma histology; primary tumour site; response to initial chemotherapy; duration of progression-free interval; AFP marker level at salvage; hCG marker level at salvage; and presence of liver, bone or brain metastases at salvage). Using these factors, five risk groups (very low risk = −1; low risk = 0; intermediate risk = 1–2; high risk = 3–4; and very high risk >5) were identified with significant differences in progression-free and overall survival (Table 30.6).

Late relapse is defined as disease recurrence >2 years after completion of first-line therapy. Patients with late relapse after chemotherapy are particularly difficult to treat and should be managed differently from all other patients with testicular GCT. Late relapsing tumours are usually less chemotherapy sensitive (predominantly yolk sac tumours) and surgical treatment should be the first choice.

Treatment: relapse/refractory disease and late relapse	Description

Relapse/refractory disease	• Standard treatment of relapse or refractory disease after first-line chemotherapy is salvage chemotherapy, either conventional or high dose
	• Patients should be classified according to prognostic score (Lorch–Beyer score; see Table 30.6):
	  ▪ *Good prognostic features*: conventional dose first salvage treatment:
	    ○ Four cycles of PEI/VIP (cisplatin + etoposide + ifosfamide), or
	    ○ Four of TIP (paclitaxel + ifosfamide + cisplatin)
	    ○ Role of high-dose chemotherapy remains controversial as first-salvage treatment
	  ▪ *Intermediate- or high-risk prognostic features*: early intensification of first-line therapy using dose-dense or high-dose chemotherapy with autologous stem cell transplant is recommended:
	    ○ Typically using two or three sequential cycles based on a carboplatin + etoposide backbone (Table 30.7)
	    ○ Recent studies have shown an improvement in survival in patients with poor prognosis from early intensification of first-line chemotherapy with this approach
	    ○ Patients in whom unsatisfactory markers decline after the first course of BEP chemotherapy in particular benefit from dose-intensified chemotherapy (GETUG regimen) or high-dose chemotherapy
	• *Second or subsequent relapse*:
	  ▪ High-dose chemotherapy still represents a curative option
	  ▪ Cisplatin-refractory patients and those failing salvage high-dose therapy should be included in trials
	  ▪ Outside of trials, a combined regimen of gemcitabine + oxaliplatin + paclitaxel has shown considerable activity
	• *Residual tumour after salvage chemotherapy*:
	  ▪ Salvage residual tumour resection should be performed 4–6 weeks after completing salvage chemotherapy and after marker normalization or when a marker plateau is reached
	• *Marker and/or tumour progression after salvage chemotherapy and a lack of other chemotherapeutic options*:
	  ▪ Resection of residual tumours as 'desperation surgery' should be considered

Late relapse	• Surgical treatment should be the first choice if disease is clearly localized and fully resectable (irrespective of tumour marker levels) • If complete resection of the tumour is not feasible, biopsies should be performed for histological assessment • If viable tumour is detected, salvage chemotherapy should be initiated

Table 30.6 Lorch-Beyer score for use in salvage therapy

	Points				
Variables	−1	0	1	2	3
Histology	Seminoma	Non-seminoma			
Primary site		Gonadal	Retroperitoneum		Mediastinum
Response		CR/PRm−	PRm+/SD	PD	
Platinum-free interval (PFI)		>3 months	3 months		
AFP salvage		Normal	<1000	1000	
hCG salvage		<1000	1000		
Liver, bone, brain metastases (LBB)		No	Yes		

CR, complete response; PRm+, partial response with positive markers; PRm−, partial response with negative markers; SD, stable disease; PD, progressive disease.

Table 30.7 Options of conventional salvage chemotherapy

Conventional salvage chemotherapy	Agents	Dosage	Duration of cycles
PEI/VIP	Cisplatin	20 mg/m^2	Days 1–5
	Etoposide	75–100 mg/m^2	Days 1–5
	Ifosfamide	1.2 g/m^2	Days 1–5
TIP	Paclitaxel	250 mg/m^2	24-hour continuous infusion on Day 1
	Ifosfamide	1.5 g/m^2	Days 2–5
	Cisplatin	25 mg/m^2	Days 2–5

Follow-up

The aims of follow-up of patients with germ cell cancer are detection of relapse; diagnosis of as well as prevention of secondary malignancy; early diagnosis; and treatment of physical and psychological morbidity related to germ cell cancer or its therapy.

Follow-up consists of regular clinical examinations, monitoring of serum tumour markers and imaging investigations. The frequency and type of examinations depend on the estimated risk of relapse, the chosen treatment strategy and the time that has elapsed since completion of therapy (Table 30.8). For simplification of the follow-up schedules, GCT patients can be categorized into three groups depending on their risk and pattern of recurrence:
- Seminoma CS I under active surveillance
- Non-seminoma CS I (low-risk group) under active surveillance
- All patients who have received adjuvant or curative treatments and achieved a complete remission.

For treated patients of any stage, the risk of recurrence after 2 years is <2% and hence imaging and visit frequency can be reduced after this interval. Follow-up after 5 years for patients with seminoma or non-seminoma under active surveillance is not supported by high-level evidence.

Clinicians and patients should be aware of the risk of a contralateral second testicular primary tumour. Each follow-up visit should include palpation of the contralateral testis and self-examination should be encouraged. Regular ultrasound should be performed in patients with high-risk factors (testicular maldescensus, atrophy of the remaining testicle, infertility) who have not had a testicular biopsy for exclusion of TIN/CIS.

Follow-up visits should include screening and early diagnosis of late side effects of testis cancer and its treatment: metabolic syndrome, cardiovascular disease, renal function impairment, persistent neurotoxicity, secondary malignancies and hypogonadism.

Table 30.8 Active surveillance for seminoma CS I

Procedure and frequency per year	Year 1	Year 2	Year 3	Year 4	Year 5	Years 6–10
Seminoma CS I						
Clinical examination	4×	4×	2×	2×	2×	Annually
Tumour markers	4×	4×	2×	2×	2×	Annually
Chest X-ray	2×	2×	–	–	–	–
CT abdomen/pelvis	2×	2×	Annually	Annually	Annually	–
Non-seminoma CS I (low risk)						
Clinical examination	6×	6×	4×	2×	2×	Annually
Tumour markers	6×	6×	4×	2×	2×	Annually
Chest X-ray	6×	6×	2×	Annually	Annually	–
CT abdomen/pelvis	Months 4 +12	–	–	–	–	–
Metastatic disease in complete remission						
Clinical examination	4×	4×	2×	2×	2×	Annually
Tumour markers	4×	4×	2×	2×	2×	Annually
Chest X-ray	2×	2×	Annually	annually	annually	–
CT abdomen/pelvis	2×	1×	–	–	–	–

Phase III clinical trials

See Table 30.9.

Table 30.9 Phase III clinical trials

Trial name	Results
Local disease	
AUO trial AH 01/94 Albers et al. (2008) J Clin Oncol 26(18):2966–2972	• Aim was to prove the advantage of one cycle of BEP chemotherapy compared with RPLND in terms of recurrence in NSGCT CS I patients • Between 1996 and 2005 382 patients were randomly assigned to receive either RPLND (n = 191) or one course of BEP (n = 191) • Median follow-up of 4.7 years • Two recurrences in the BEP arm and 15 relapses in the RPLND arm ($P = 0.0011$) • 2-year recurrence-free survival rate between chemotherapy (99.5%) and surgery (91.9%) was 7.59% • Superiority shown of one course of BEP over RPLND performed according to community standards to prevent recurrence
MRC TE19/EORTC 30982 study (ISRCTN27163214) Oliver et al. (2005) Lancet 366:293–300	• Aim was to compare the approaches of radiotherapy with carboplatin chemotherapy in seminoma treatment • 1477 patients from 70 hospitals in 14 countries were randomly assigned to receive radiotherapy (para-aortic strip or dog-leg field; n = 904) or one injection of carboplatin (n = 573); 885 and 560 patients actually received radiotherapy and carboplatin, respectively • Median follow-up of 4 years (interquartile range 3.0–4.9) • Relapse-free survival rates for radiotherapy and carboplatin were similar (96.7% vs 97.7% at 2 years; 95.9% vs 94.8% at 3 years) • Showed the non-inferiority of carboplatin to radiotherapy in the treatment of CS I seminoma
AH-10/04 (unpublished)	• Multicentre trial randomizing patients with high-risk CS I NSGCT based on vascular invasion to adjuvant chemotherapy with either one or two courses of BEP • Patients will be followed for at least 2 years for relapse and at least 5 years for long-term data on toxicity • Number of patients needed per arm is 267 with a follow-up of 2 years regarding the primary endpoint • Primary study endpoint is the 2-year relapse rate; secondary endpoints are disease-specific survival, toxicity and health economic data concerning follow-up • Study closed in 2012 due to insufficient recruitment • Analysis is in process
Advanced disease	

GETUG 13.
Fizazi et al. (2013) J Clin Oncol 31(Suppl):abstract LBA4500
	• Analysis in GCT with poor prognosis and unsatisfactory tumour marker decline under chemotherapy
	• GCT patients with IGCCCG poor prognosis were treated with a first cycle of BEP; AFP and hCG were assessed on Days 18–21:
	  ▪ Patients with a favourable decline continued BEP for a total of four courses (Fav-BEP)
	  ▪ Patients with an unfavourable decline were randomized to receive either BEP (Unfav-BEP) or a dose-dense regimen (Unfav-dose-dense), consisting of paclitaxel/BEP + Day 10 oxaliplatin x two cycles, followed by two cycles of cisplatin + ifosfamide + continuous infusion bleomycin (depending on lung function) + G-CSF.
	• 263 patients were enrolled and 254 were evaluable: 51 (20%) had favourable tumour marker decline (Fav-BEP) and 203 had unfavourable decline (randomized: 105 Unfav-dose-dense arm, 98 Unfav-BEP arm)
	• Prognostic value of early tumour marker decline (Fav-BEP vs Unfav-BEP) was confirmed: 70% vs 48% for 3-year progression-free survival (PFS) ($P = 0.01$), and 84% vs 65% for overall survival (OS) ($P = 0.02$)
	• 3-year PFS was 59% in the Unfav-dose-dense arm vs 48% in the Unfav-BEP arm ($P = 0.05$); 3-year OS were 73% and 65%, respectively
	• Analysis showed a survival advantage for patients with poor-prognosis germ cell cancer and unsatisfactory marker decline after the first cycle of BEP chemotherapy

Lorch et al. (2011) J Clin Oncol 29:2178–2184	• Data on 1984 patients with GCT who experienced progression after at least three cisplatin-based cycles and were treated with either cisplatin-based conventional dose chemotherapy (CDCT) or carboplatin-based high-dose chemotherapy (HDCT) were collected from 38 centres or groups worldwide (retrospective analysis) • 1435 patients (90%) could reliably be classified into one of the following five prognostic categories based on prior prognostic classification: very low (n = 76), low (n = 257), intermediate (n = 646), high (n = 351) and very high risk (n = 105) • Within each of the five categories, PFS and OS after CDCT and HDCT were compared; 773 patients received CDCT and 821 received HDCT

Trial name	Results
	• Hazard ratio for PFS was 0.44 (95% CI 0.39–0.51) stratified on prognostic category, and for OS was 0.65 (95% CI 0.56–0.75), favouring HDCT • Results were consistent within each prognostic category except among low-risk patients, for whom similar OS was observed between the two treatment groups • Analysis suggests a benefit from HDCT given as intensification of first salvage treatment
Oechsle et al. (2013) J Clin Oncol 31(Suppl):abstract 4559	• Aim was to evaluate first salvage treatment and the prognostic categories at first relapse • 144 patients (78% non-seminoma) with relapsed or refractory GCC undergoing first salvage treatment with either conventional (CD-CX) or high-dose chemotherapy with autologous stem cell support (HD-CX) were retrospectively analysed • Subgroups (IPFSG prognostic categories) were: very low risk, low risk, intermediate risk, high risk and very high risk • First salvage treatment consisted of HD-CX in 96 (67%) and CD-CX in 48 patients (33%) • Treatment response was complete response CR/PR– in 60%, PR+/SD in 33% and PD in 7% • After a median follow-up of 21 months (range 0–193 months), 53% of all patients had relapsed and 30% had died, resulting in a median PFS of 7 months (95% CI 0–16) and OS of 47 months (95% CI 21–73) • IPFSG prognostic categories significantly correlated with PFS ($P = 0.001$) and OS ($P = 0.004$) after first salvage treatment in this cohort of patients refractory or relapsed GCC • First salvage treatment with CD– or HD-CX resulted in overall 5-year OS rates of about 50% across all prognostic categories

Recommended reading

Albers P, Siener R, Krege S et al. (2008) Randomized phase III trial comparing retroperitoneal lymph node dissection with one course of bleomycin and etoposide plus cisplatin chemotherapy in the adjuvant treatment of clinical stage I Nonseminomatous testicular germ cell tumors: AUO trial AH 01/94 by the German Testicular Cancer Study Group. J Clin Oncol 26:2966–2972.

Beyer J, Albers P, Altena R et al. (2013) Maintaining success, reducing treatment burden, focusing on survivorship: highlights from the third European consensus conference on diagnosis and treatment of germ-cell cancer. Ann Oncol 24(4):878–888.

Bosl GJ, Motzer RJ (199) Testicular germ-cell cancer. N Engl J Med 337:242–253.

Fosså SD et al. (2007) Noncancer causes of death in survivors of testicular cancer. J Natl Cancer Inst 99:533–544.

Kollmannsberger C, Daneshmand S, So A et al. (2010) Management of disseminated nonseminomatous germ cell tumors with risk-based chemotherapy followed by response-guided postchemotherapy surgery. J Clin Oncol 28:537–542.

Krege S, Beyer J, Souchon R et al. (2008) European consensus conference on diagnosis and treatment of germ cell cancer: a report of the second meeting of the European Germ Cell Cancer Consensus group (EGCCCG): part I. Eur Urol 53:478–496.

Krege S, Beyer J, Souchon R et al. (2008) European consensus conference on diagnosis and treatment of germ cell cancer: a report of the second meeting of the European Germ Cell Cancer Consensus Group (EGCCCG): part II. Eur Urol 53:497–513.

Lorch A, Bascoul-Mollevi C, Kramar A et al. (2011) Conventional-dose versus high-dose chemotherapy as first salvage treatment in male patients with metastatic germ cell tumors: evidence from a large international database. J Clin Oncol 29(16):2178–2184.

Lorch A, Neubauer A, Hackenthal M et al. (2010) High-dose chemotherapy (HDCT) as second-salvage treatment in patients with multiple relapsed or refractory germ-cell tumors. Ann Oncol 21:820–825.

Lorch A, Kollmannsberger C, Hartmann JT et al. (2007) Single versus sequential high-dose chemotherapy in patients with relapsed or refractory germ cell tumors: a prospective randomized multicenter trial of the German Testicular Cancer Study Group. J Clin Oncol 25:2778–2784.

Motzer RJ, Mazumdar M, Bajorin DF, Bosl GJ, Lyn P, Vlamis V (1997) High-dose carboplatin, etoposide, and cyclophosphamide with autologous bone marrow transplantation in first-line therapy for patients with poor-risk germ cell tumors. J Clin Oncol 15:2546–2552.

Oldenburg J, Fosså SD (2009) Late relapse of nonseminomatous germ cell tumours. BJU Int 104:1413–1417.

Oliver RT, Mason MD, Mead GM et al. (2005) Radiotherapy versus single-dose carboplatin in adjuvant treatment of stage I seminoma: a randomised trial. Lancet 366:293–300.

Tandstad T, Dahl O, Cohn-Cedermark G et al. (2009) Risk-adapted treatment in clinical stage I nonseminomatous germ cell testicular cancer: the SWENOTECA management program. J Clin Oncol 27:2122–2128.

Winter C, Albers P (2011) Testicular germ cell tumors: pathogenesis, diagnosis and treatment. Nat Rev Endocrinol 7(1):43–53.

Winter C, Raman JD, Sheinfeld J, Albers P (2009) Retroperitoneal lymph node dissection after chemotherapy. BJU Int 104:1404–1412.

31 Penis

Juanita Crook[1], Lance Pagliaro[2] and Curtis Pettaway[3]

[1]British Columbia Cancer Agency, Department of Radiation Oncology and Developmental Radiotherapeutics, Cancer Center for the Southern Interior, Kelowna, BC, Canada
[2]Department of Genitourinary Medical Oncology, University of Texas M. D. Anderson Cancer Center, Houston, TX, USA
[3]Department of Urology, University of Texas M. D. Anderson Cancer Center, Houston, TX, USA

Summary	Key facts
Introduction	• Squamous cell carcinoma is the most common penile cancer • Risk factors include presence of high-risk human papillomavirus (HPV) types, tobacco products, phimosis, increasing age and premalignant lesions
Presentation	• Usually occurs on glans and foreskin • Majority of patients are uncircumcised • Presents with asymptomatic mass under phimotic foreskin, discharge or lesion on glans or foreskin • Tumour biopsy or circumcision for tissue diagnosis and to expose entire glans • Physical exam to determine primary tumour and inguinal node assessment • Staging with physical examination, imaging and biopsy as appropriate
Scenario	• Disease limited to foreskin is managed with circumcision alone • Penile conserving options are preferable • WD Tis-T1/T2: penile conserving surgery or radiation • MD/PD or T3: primary tumour surgery or radiation as appropriate along with surgical staging of inguinal nodes with superficial inguinal lymph node dissection (SILND) or dynamic sentinel node biopsy (DSNB) • Locally advanced: preoperative chemotherapy or chemoradiation therapy
Trials	• Paucity of phase III clinical trials • Most evidence is level III, published experience from single centres spanning several decades

Aetiology, incidence and screening

Cancer of the penis is most commonly of squamous cell origin and involves the glans and/or prepuce and coronal sulcus. Human papillomavirus (HPV) high-risk types 16 and 18 can be isolated in about 50% of cases. Premalignant lesions include HPV-related erythroplasia of Queyrat, Bowen disease, bowenoid papulosis, Bushke–Lowenstein tumour and non–HPV-related lichen sclerosis, cutaneous horn, leukoplakia and pseudoepitheliomatous, keratotic and micaceous balanitis. Non-squamous penile malignancies are rare and include basal cell carcinoma, melanoma, extramammary Paget disease and adenosquamous carcinoma. The penis is rarely the site of metastatic lesions; when they occur these usually involve the shaft, from primary tumour sites such as the prostate, bladder, kidney or testis. Lymphoma and leukaemia have also been reported to involve the penile shaft. Such metastatic lesions may present as priapism.

UICC Manual of Clinical Oncology, Ninth Edition. Edited by Brian O'Sullivan, James D. Brierley, Anil K. D'Cruz, Martin F. Fey, Raphael Pollock, Jan B. Vermorken and Shao Hui Huang. © 2015 UICC. Published 2015 by John Wiley & Sons, Ltd.

Penis

Incidence, aetiology and surveillance	Description
Incidence	• Occurs in about 1 in 100,000 men in the developed world but incidence >10-fold higher in parts of Asia, Africa and South America • Neonatal circumcision to prevent phimosis is protective in regions where poor hygiene is a problem • Increasing incidence with increasing age: most common in sixth to seventh decade
Aetiology	• High-risk HPV types 16 and 18 most common • Increasing age • Tobacco products (i.e. smoking, chewing) • Phimosis • History of penile warts, rash, trauma • Premalignant lesions (see Pathology)
Screening	• Public awareness and self-examination are important

Pathology and natural history	Description

Squamous cell carcinoma	• 95% of penile carcinomas:
	  ▪ 48% glans
	  ▪ 25% prepuce
	  ▪ 9% glans and prepuce
	  ▪ 6% coronal sulcus
	  ▪ 2% shaft only

Lichen sclerosis: balanitis xerotica	• Glans or foreskin, meatal stenosis, phimosis, up to 6% develop cancer over time
Verrucous Buschke–Lowenstein	• Low grade; decreased metastatic potential • Large destructive exophytic masses • Carcinoma may co-exist in up to 50% of cases
Bowenoid papulosis	• Papules on shaft • Intraepithelial neoplasia • Rarely progresses to invasion
Bowen disease	• Crusted lesion on shaft • Intraepithelial neoplasia • Progresses to invasion in about 5% of cases
Erythroplasia of Queyrat	• Red lesion on glans • Intraepithelial neoplasia • Progression to invasion in up to 30%
Melanoma	• Pigmented lesion on glans, shaft • Aggressive behaviour
Metastatic lesion	• Mass in penile corpora in patient with advanced disease from other site

Presentation

- Mass under unretractable foreskin
- Discharge, bleeding from phimotic foreskin
- Non-healing sore, rash
- Palpable inguinal nodes

Diagnostic work-up

Diagnostic work-up	Description

Work-up	• Biopsy for diagnosis
	• Dorsal slit or circumcision often reveals the previously undetected mass
	• Evaluation of inguinal nodes by:
	    ▪ Clinical exam
	    ▪ Computed tomography (CT) scan
	    ▪ Superficial inguinal lymph node dissection (SILND)
	    ▪ Dynamic sentinel node biopsy (DSNB)
	• Screen for metastatic disease with abdominal CT and chest X-ray
	• Penile magnetic resonance imaging (MRI) or ultrasound may assist in evaluation of corporal invasion
	• Fluorodeoxyglucose-positron emission tomography (FDG-PET) in patients with proven metastasis may be valuable

Staging and prognostic grouping

UICC TNM stage

With respect to the primary tumour, because grade and the presence of vascular invasion are established prognostic markers in predicting the risk of subsequent inguinal metastasis, TNM now stratifies pT1 stage by presence (pT1b) or absence (pT1a) of high-grade tumours or vascular invasion. In addition, prostatic invasion (a rare finding) is now included in the pT4 designation (Table 31.1).

Of considerable importance is that clinical and pathological nodal staging descriptors are now available to better predict prognosis before definitive therapy. The prognosis worsens for patients with greater degrees of palpable adenopathy (i.e. unilateral vs bilateral vs fixed mass) or positive nodes on imaging versus those with clinically negative inguinal lymph nodes. Cases with a single positive node are now stratified from those with multiple or bilateral nodes. The new TNM system further recognizes the ominous prognosis associated with extranodal extension of cancer or a fixed inguinal mass.

In the European Association of Urology (EAU) guidelines, risk prognostic stratification groups among cN0 patients are:
- Gp 1 (low risk): pTis, pTaG1–2, pT1G1
- Gp 2 (intermediate risk): pT1G2
- Gp 3 (high risk): pT2 or greater or G3

Table 31.1 UICC TNM categories and stage grouping: Penis

TNM categories		
Tis	Carcinoma *in situ*	
Ta	Non-invasive verrucous carcinoma	
T1	Subepithelial connective tissue	
T1a	Without lymphovascular invasion, not G3–4	
T1b	With lymphovascular invasion, or G3–4	
T2	Corpus spongiosum, cavernosum	
T3	Urethra	
T4	Other adjacent structures	
N1	Single palpable mobile unilateral inguinal	pN1 Single inguinal
N2	Palpable mobile multiple or bilateral inguinal	pN2 Multiple/bilateral inguinal
N3	Fixed inguinal or pelvic	pN3 Pelvic or extranodal
M1	Distant metastasis	

Stage grouping			
Stage 0	Tis	N0	M0
	Ta	N0	M0
Stage I	T1a	N0	M0
Stage II	T1b	N0	M0
	T2	N0	M0
	T3	N0	M0
Stage IIIA	T1, T2, T3	N1	M0
Stage IIIB	T1, T2, T3	N2	M0
Stage IV	T4	Any N	M0
	Any T	N3	M0
	Any T	Any N	M1

Table 31.2 Prognostic factors for survival for squamous cell carcinoma

Prognostic factor	Tumour related	Host related	Environment related
Essential	Differentiation Lymphovascular space invasion Invasion of the corpora	History of genital condylomas Lichen sclerosis PUVA	Poor hygiene
Additional	HPV/p16 (presence may confer better prognosis)	Smoking HIV/immune suppression	
New and promising	p53 (predicts for lymph node metastases) FGFR		

Prognostic factors

The essential prognostic factors for squamous cell carcinoma are tumour related and often difficult to obtain from biopsy material alone. Tumour differentiation, invasion of the corpora and the presence of lymphovascular invasion are all predictive of regional nodal metastases which is itself the strongest predictor of survival (Table 31.2).

Treatment philosophy

Early-stage, well-differentiated cancers of the penis can be effectively managed with local therapy, and attention should be paid to preservation of penile function and morphology when feasible. Penile conservation is recommended for Tis, Ta–T1 and G1–2 lesions, and can be considered for G3 T1 or T2 lesions (tumour is <4 cm) and for selected T3 tumours. Laser surgery for Tis and T1 tumours yields satisfactory local control and cosmesis. Locally-advanced penile cancer is a highly lethal malignancy that requires a multimodality approach, often combining total or partial penectomy and lymph node dissection, systemic chemotherapy and pelvic and inguinal irradiation.

Sexuality and expectations should be discussed with the patient and his partner when deciding on primary management.

Scenario	Treatment philosophy
Local disease only	• Topical therapy for carcinoma *in situ* • Laser ablation • Moh's surgery • Wide local excision • Circumcision • Radiotherapy (brachytherapy or external beam) • Amputation
Regional nodal metastasis: at risk or present	• SILND or DSNB for patients at risk of occult nodal metastasis • Lymphadenectomy with curative intent, inguinal (ILND) ± pelvic lymph node dissection (PLND) • With neoadjuvant chemotherapy for more advanced disease (N2, N3) • Chemoradiotherapy for selected cases
Distant metastatic disease present	• Chemotherapy/radiotherapy for palliation • Supportive care
Recurrent disease	• No standard second-line chemotherapy

Follow-up after definitive therapy	• *Primary tumour:*
	  ▪ Physical exam every 3 months for 2 years for penile conservation, then every 6 months until Year 5, annual Years 5–10
	  ▪ Physical exam every 6 months for 2 years for amputation, then yearly up to Year 5
	• *Inguinal nodes:*
	  ▪ pN+: CT abdomen/pelvis every 3 months for patients treated for lymph node metastasis for 2 years, then every 6 months up to Year 5
	  ▪ pN0: physical exam or CT scan every 6 months for 2 years, then yearly up to Year 5
	  ▪ pNx (observation): physical exam or CT scan every 3 months for 2 years, then every 6 months up to Year 5

Treatment

Surgery

Surgical resection to achieve negative surgical margins remains an important therapeutic strategy in penile cancer. Recently, organ preserving strategies (Fig. 31.1) have played an increasing role in the therapy of patients with low-stage, low-grade, distal lesions. Amputation remains the gold standard for local control among advanced primary tumours. Inguinal lymphadenectomy is curative among patients with minimal unilateral metastases in the absence of extranodal extension of cancer or pelvic metastasis. Among patients with advanced regional metastasis, response to neoadjuvant chemotherapy along with surgical resection can provide durable survival.

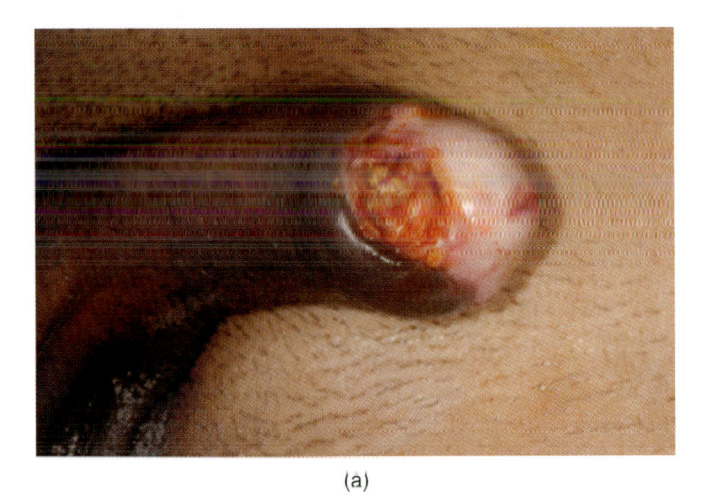

Surgery	Description

Early	• Primary tumour:
	  ▪ Penile glans:
	    ○ Tis–T1: laser therapy, glans resurfacing, glansectomy
	    ○ T2: minimal, glansectomy
	  ▪ Penile foreskin:
	    ○ Tis–T1: surgical excision, laser therapy
	• Inguinal nodes (cN0):
	  ▪ Low risk (Tis–T1 grade 1): observation in reliable patients
	  ▪ Intermediate risk (T1 grade 2, no lymphovascular invasion): SILND, DSNB or observation
	  ▪ High risk (T1b, T2–4): SILND or DSNB

Advanced disease	• Primary tumour:
	  ▪ T2–3: partial or total penectomy
	  ▪ T4: consider neoadjuvant chemotherapy prior to surgical resection
	• Inguinal nodes:
	  ▪ cN1: unilateral <4 cm: ipsilateral ILND or ilioinguinal dissection, contralateral SILND or DSNB
	  ▪ cN2: consider neoadjuvant chemotherapy, then post-chemotherapy bilateral ilioinguinal dissection with initial bilateral presentation, or as for cN1 if multiple unilateral nodes
	  ▪ cN3: as above with wide resection of surrounding skin as needed with myocutaneous flap reconstruction on the affected side

Metastatic disease	• Usually no role among patients with distant metastasis • Palliative groin/pelvic dissection can be considered in selected cases to prevent vascular complications

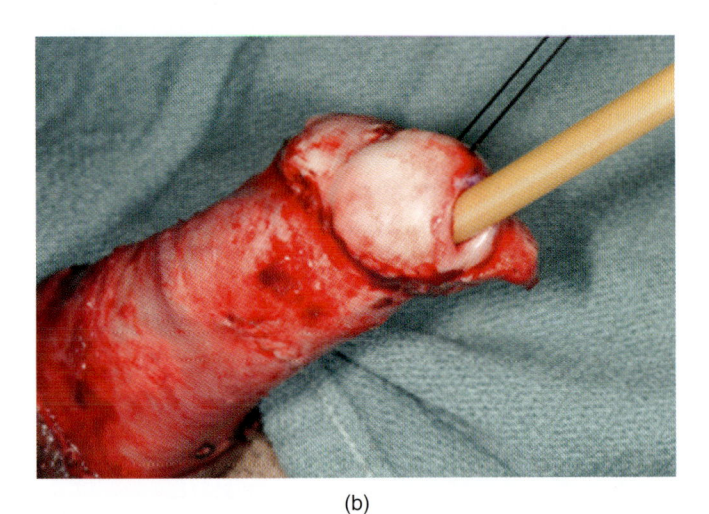

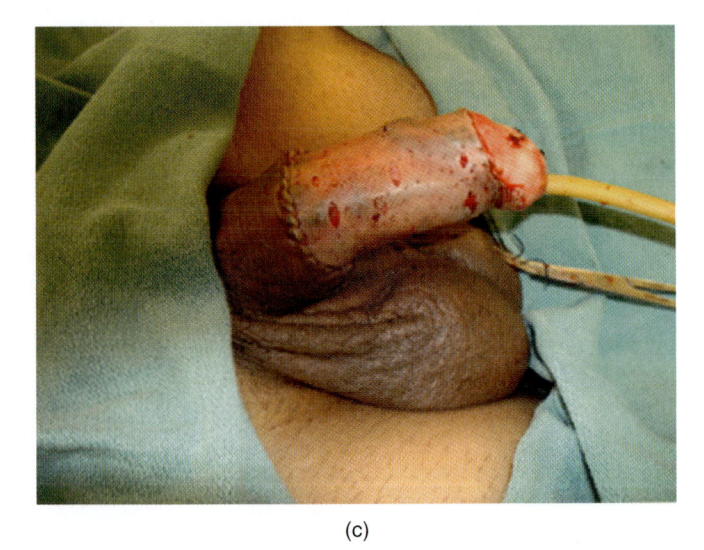

Figure 31.1 (a–c) Penile preserving surgery: 46-year-old male post glans-sparing partial penectomy with a skin graft for skin coverage.

Radiotherapy

As is the case for squamous carcinomas in other body sites, squamous carcinoma of the penis is a radiosensitive and radiocurable tumour. The philosophy is similar to that for the surgical approach, with treatment directed locally with appropriate margins for an early-stage primary tumour. Low-dose rate interstitial brachytherapy (Fig. 31.2) appears to be more effective than external beam radiotherapy, with penile preservation rates at 5 years of 85%, although an external beam approach is more versatile for more extensive lesions. Patients with high-risk pathological features should be considered for surgical node staging or prophylactic radiotherapy to the regional nodes.

Radiotherapy	Description

Early	- T0 or T1s: limited role
	- T1 or T2 (<4 cm): radiotherapy is an effective option:
	  - Circumcision must be performed prior to treatment
	  - Brachytherapy is preferred
	    - Usually low dose rate interstitial 60 Gy over 4–5 days
	    - Penile preservation rates 85% at 5 years, 70% at 10 years
	    - High dose rate brachytherapy remains investigational
	  - External beam techniques must involve bolus and immobilization:
	    - Usually protracted course over 6–7 weeks
	    - Penile preservation rates 60–65% at 5 years

Advanced	- Treatment volume to include primary and bilateral inguinal nodes ± pelvic lymph nodes - Concurrent chemoradiotherapy using cisplatin is an option - May be given in preoperative setting if initially unresectable
Metastatic	- Palliation of metastatic lesions or uncontrolled regional disease - Usually short fractionation of 20 Gy in five fractions or 30 Gy in ten fractions

Systemic chemotherapy

The best results have been obtained with cisplatin-based chemotherapy. Responses in distant or visceral metastatic disease tend to be of short duration with median overall survival of 6–8 months. The prognosis is better for patients with bulky regional lymph node metastasis (cN2, cN3); among patients treated with paclitaxel + ifosfamide + cisplatin in the neoadjuvant setting, 11 of 30 (37%) survived without recurrence or died of an unrelated cause. This regimen and 5-fluorouracil + cisplatin are the most commonly used regimens in the first line. Topical chemotherapy and imiquimod are effective in the eradication of carcinoma *in situ* of the penis.

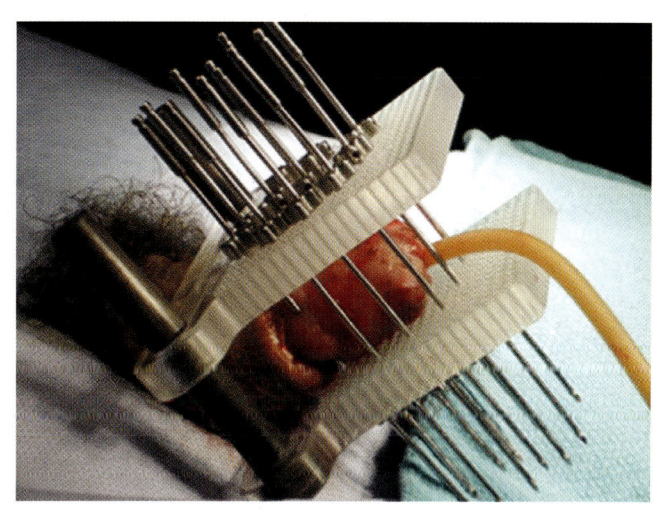

Figure 31.2 Brachytherapy application.

Systemic chemotherapy	Description
Early	- No role

Advanced with regional lymph node metastasis, or unresectable primary	- Data from non-randomized clinical trials and retrospective series suggest improved progression-free and overall survival following lymphadenectomy in patients (cT4, cN2, or cN3) treated neoadjuvantly:
	  - Paclitaxel + ifosfamide + cisplatin:
	    - 10% pathological complete response rate
	    - 37% freedom from recurrence among patients who received chemotherapy
	    - 50% freedom from recurrence among the subset who completed post-chemotherapy ILND and PLND
	- Down-staging of primary tumour and/or lymph nodes may convert unresectable to resectable disease

Metastatic	- Phase II studies of platinum-based chemotherapy show overall response rates of 31–50%:
	  - Paclitaxel + ifosfamide + cisplatin (50%)
	  - Irinotecan + cisplatin (31%)
	  - 5-Fluorouracil + cisplatin (32% in one retrospective series)
	- Median overall survival with cisplatin-based chemotherapy depends upon the extent of metastatic involvement:
	  - Lymph node only (neoadjuvant): 17 months
	  - Lymph node and/or distant metastasis: 6–8 months

Post-treatment assessment

After penile-conserving treatment close follow-up is mandatory as local recurrences can be salvaged by prompt management, usually involving non-penile-sparing surgery. Local recurrences after laser treatment or after brachytherapy or external radiotherapy may occur as late as 10 years after initial treatment. Patients and other healthcare providers should be aware of this risk. Follow-up of the inguinal region is critical for patients with penile cancer. The interval and studies utilized are dependent upon the presence or absence of inguinal metastasis and the pathological characteristics of the primary tumour. Of note, the follow-up is more intense within the first 2 years when inguinal/pelvic recurrence is most common.

Continuing care

Post-therapy care (Fig. 31.3) is directed at the avoidance of short- and long-term complications related to the primary tumour and inguinal nodes. With respect to the primary tumour, voiding pattern and sexual function should be assessed as appropriate. Urethral stricture formation can often be treated with dilation but may require surgical revision. Sexual counselling may be appropriate for patients. Among selected patients, phallic reconstruction may be a viable option to achieve normal voiding and sexual function. Inguinal care is directed at the avoidance of infection with the appropriate antibiotic regimen, preventing seroma formation utilizing closed suction drains and preventing lymphoedema by optimizing surgical technique and early consultation with lymphoedema specialists.

Controversies

- Optimal management of the cN0 inguinal region
- Role of postoperative radiotherapy
- HPV vaccination

Phase III clinical trials

There are no phase III clinical trials.

Areas of research

- Biological relevance of HPV:
  - Prognostic: p16 positivity, a marker for HPV infection was associated with better overall survival in one study
  - Predictive: HPV has not been established as a predictive marker of treatment outcome

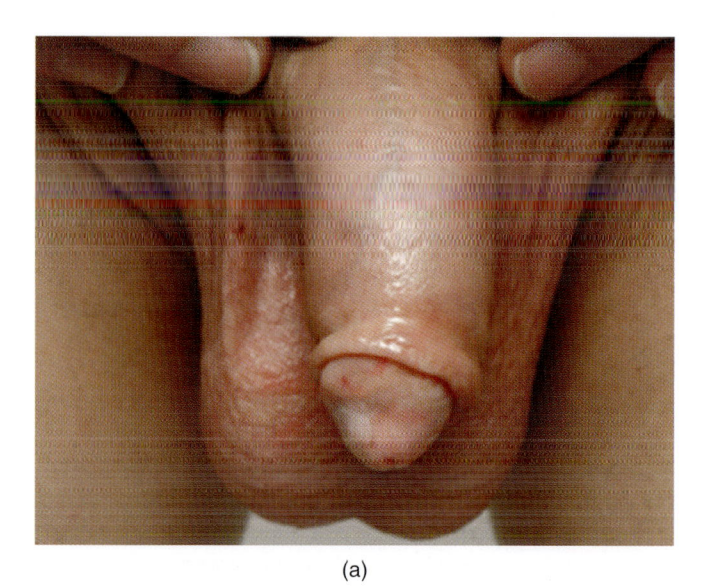

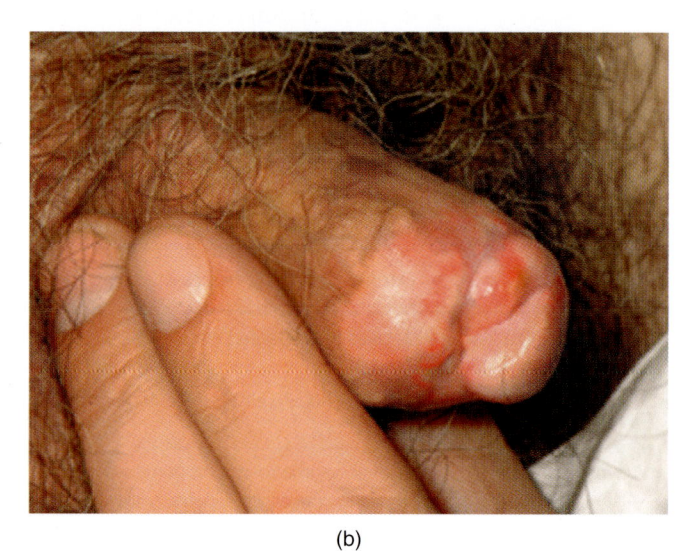

Figure 31.3 (a) 8 years after brachytherapy for a T2 lesion on the right side of the glans (white scar visible). (b) 7 years after brachytherapy for a deeply invasive T3 lesion. Tumour regression left a depressed scar.

- As target for therapy and prevention: vaccination of boys is approved for prevention of viral warts; other therapeutic targeting for penile cancer is investigational
- Penile reconstruction
- Optimal use of neoadjuvant chemotherapy
- Targeted systemic therapy:
  - Case reports show responses to epidermal growth factor receptor (EGFR)-targeted therapy
  - Optimal role has not yet been established
  - No prospective studies
- Chemoradiation as neoadjuvant or definitive therapy:
  - Current standard for vulvar cancer is chemoradiation to pelvic lymph nodes
  - PLND is more commonly used in penile cancer

Recommended reading

Bethune G, Campbell J, Rocker A, Bell D, Rendon R, Merrimen J (2012) Clinical and pathologic factors of prognostic significance in penile squamous cell carcinoma in a North American population. *Urology* 79(5):1092–1097.

Chaux A, Cubilla AL (2012) The role of human papillomavirus infection in the pathogenesis of penile squamous cell carcinomas. *Semin Diagn Pathol* 29(2):67–71.

Crook J, Jezioranski J, Cygler JE (2010) Penile brachytherapy: technical aspects and postimplant issues. *Brachytherapy* 9(2):151–158.

Crook J, Ma C, Grimard L (2009) Radiation therapy in the management of the primary penile tumor: an update. *World J Urol* 27(2):189.

de Crevoisier R, Slimane K, Sanfilippo N et al. (2009) Long-term results of brachytherapy for carcinoma of the penis confined to the glans (N- or NX). *Int J Radiat Oncol Biol Phys* 74(4):1150–1156.

Di Lorenzo G, Buonerba C, Federico P et al. (2012) Cisplatin and 5-fluorouracil in inoperable, stage IV squamous cell carcinoma of the penis. *BJU Int* 110(11 Pt B):E661–666.

Di Lorenzo G, Perdona S, Buonerba C et al. (2013) Cytosolic phosphorylated EGFR is predictive of recurrence in early stage penile cancer patients: a retrospective study. *J Translat Med* 11(1):161.

Graafland NM, Lam W, Leijte JA, Yap T. et al. (2010) Prognostic factors for occult inguinal lymph node involvement in penile carcinoma and assessment of the high-risk EAU subgroup: a two-institution analysis of 342 clinically node-negative patients. *Eur Urol* 58(5):742–747.

Gunia S, Erbersdobler A, Hakenberg OW, Koch S, May M (2012) p16(INK4a) is a marker of good prognosis for primary invasive penile squamous cell carcinoma: a multi-institutional study. *J Urol* 187(3):899–907.

Gunia S, Kakies C, Erbersdobler A, Hakenberg OW, Koch S, May M (2012) Expression of p53, p21 and cyclin D1 in penile cancer: p53 predicts poor prognosis. *J Clin Pathol* 65(3):232–236.

Hegarty PK, Shabbir M, Hughes B et al. (2009) Penile preserving surgery and surgical strategies to maximize penile form and function in penile cancer: recommendations from the United Kingdom experience. *World J Urol* 27(2):179–187.

Heyns CF, Fleshner N, Sangar V, Schlenker B, Yuvaraja TB, van Poppel H (2010) Management of the lymph nodes in penile cancer. *Urology* 76(2 Suppl 1):S43–57.

Leijte JA, Hughes B, Graafland NM et al. (2009) Two-center evaluation of dynamic sentinel node biopsy for squamous cell carcinoma of the penis. *J Clin Oncol* 27(20):3325–3329.

Pagliaro LC, Crook J (2009) Multimodality therapy in penile cancer: when and which treatments? *World J Urol* 27(2):221–225.

Pagliaro LC, Williams DL, Daliani D et al. (2010) Neoadjuvant paclitaxel, ifosfamide, and cisplatin chemotherapy for metastatic penile cancer: a phase II study. *J Clin Oncol* 28(24):3851–3857.

Pettaway CA, Lance RS, Davis JW (2012) Tumors of the penis. In: Kavoussi LR, Novick AC, Partin AW, Peters CA, Wein AJ, eds. *Campbell-Walsh Urology*, 10th edn. Philadelphia: Saunders Elsevier:901–933.

Pizzocaro G, Algaba F, Horenblas S et al. (2010) European Association of Urology (EAU) Guidelines Group on Penile Cancer 2010. EAU penile cancer guidelines 2009. *Eur Urol* 57(6):1002–1012.

Solsona E, Algaba F, Horenblas S, Pizzocaro G, Windahl T (2008) European Association of Urology Guidelines. In: *Guidelines on Penile Cancer*. Arnhem: E.G. Office, Drukkeril Gelderland bv:1–28.

Spiess PE, Hernandez MS, Pettaway CA (2009) Contemporary inguinal lymph node dissection: minimizing complications. *World J Urol* 27(2):205–212.

32 Lymphoma

Richard W. C. Tsang[1] and Michael Crump[2]

[1]Radiation Medicine Program, The Princess Margaret Cancer Centre, Department of Radiation Oncology, University of Toronto, Toronto, ON, Canada
[2]Division of Medical Oncology and Hematology, The Princess Margaret Cancer Centre, University of Toronto, Toronto, ON, Canada

Summary	Key facts
Introduction	**Hodgkin lymphoma** • Most are classical type • Small proportion of nodular lymphocyte-predominant histology, usually presenting at a localized stage **Non-Hodgkin lymphoma** • Many subtypes, but most are of B-cell origin • Broadly divided into aggressive and indolent histologies for treatment purposes • Large geographical variation of individual subtypes of non-Hodgkin lymphoma and varying aetiological agents (e.g. Epstein–Barr virus [EBV] or *Helicobacter pylori*) or predisposing factors (e.g. immunosuppression or autoimmune diseases)
Presentation	• Lymphadenopathy, mass lesion in organs and sometimes constitutional symptoms such as weight loss, fever and night sweats • Standard investigations are computed tomography (CT) of the neck, chest, abdomen and pelvis; fluorodeoxyglucose-positron emission tomography (FDG-PET) scan; complete blood count and blood work for organ function, HIV status, hepatitis serology and bone marrow biopsy
Scenario	**Hodgkin lymphoma** • *Early-stage*: combined brief chemotherapy and radiation therapy with a high cure rate • *Advanced stage*: full courses of chemotherapy with a good cure rate **Non-Hodgkin lymphoma** • *Aggressive histology*: primarily treated with chemotherapy with a moderately high cure rate • *Indolent histology*: usually present in advanced stages and not curable
Trials	• Current phase III trials are testing new drugs with promising activity either alone or in combination with existing regimens, and approaches to individualize treatment based on response assessment (e.g. with FDG-PET scan) during or after a course of chemotherapy

Introduction

Lymphomas are broadly divided into Hodgkin lymphoma and non-Hodgkin lymphoma. This distinction is important because their presentation, biology, prognosis and treatment approaches are different. Hodgkin lymphomas frequently present in lymph nodes and in most cases have an orderly pattern of spread to contiguous lymph node regions, with frequent involvement of the mediastinal and cervical lymph node areas. The non-Hodgkin lymphomas are a very heterogeneous group of disease in terms of aetiology, pathology and molecular genetics, clinical presentation, sites of involvement, the specific treatment required and prognosis.

UICC Manual of Clinical Oncology, Ninth Edition. Edited by Brian O'Sullivan, James D. Brierley, Anil K. D'Cruz, Martin F. Fey, Raphael Pollock, Jan B. Vermorken and Shao Hui Huang. © 2015 UICC. Published 2015 by John Wiley & Sons, Ltd.

Incidence, aetiology and screening

Incidence, aetiology and screening	Description

Incidence	**Hodgkin lymphoma**
	• Global incidence:
	  ▪ Age standardized rate (ASR) per 100,000 for women 0.8 and for men 1.2
	• Death rate:
	  ▪ ASR per 100,000 for women 0.3 and for men 0.5
	
	Non-Hodgkin lymphoma
	• Increasing in incidence.
	• Global Incidence:
	  ▪ ASR per 100,000 for women 4.2 and for men 6.0
	• Death rate:
	  ▪ ASR per 100,000 for women 2.1 and for men 3.3
	• Malignant lymphomas are more common in developed countries
	• Marked geographical variation in many subtypes of non-Hodgkin lymphomas:
	  ▪ Burkitt lymphoma is common in Africa, rare in Westernized countries
	  ▪ Follicular lymphoma is common in North America and Europe, but rare in Latin America and Asia
	  ▪ Adult T-cell leukaemia/lymphoma is endemic in the Caribbean and South Japan, but rare elsewhere

Aetiology and predisposing conditions	• *Immunosuppression or autoimmune diseases:*
	  ▪ Human immunodeficiency virus (HIV) infection
	  ▪ Sjogren syndrome, rheumatoid arthritis
	  ▪ Iatrogenic (after organ transplantation)
	• *Viral agents*: EBV, human T-cell lymphotropic virus [HTLV-1], human herpes virus type 8, hepatitis C
	• *Bacterial infections:*
	  ▪ *H. pylori* in gastric lymphoma
	  ▪ *Chlamydia psittaci* in orbital lymphoma
	  ▪ *Campylobacter jejunii* in α heavy chain disease
	• *Chemical:*
	  ▪ Drugs: alkylating agents, immunosuppressive drugs
	  ▪ Pesticides, e.g. phenoxy herbicides, organophosphates
	  ▪ Other chemicals, e.g. hair dyes

Screening	• Limited use in lymphomas: ▪ For individuals at risk, e.g. iatrogenic immunosuppression or in the presence of HIV infection, a high index of suspicion to biopsy suspicious masses

Presentation

- Usually lymphadenopathy at a peripheral lymph node site such as the neck, axilla or inguinal areas
- Constitutional symptoms of weight loss, fever or night sweats
- If mediastinal mass: chest pain, cough, shortness of breath or superior vena cava obstruction
- If organ infiltration: mass effect (pain) or organ dysfunction; back pain

Diagnostic work-up

Diagnostic work-up	Description

Work-up	• History and physical examination including Waldeyer's ring:
	  ▪ CT head and neck, chest, abdomen and pelvis; FDG-PET scan
	  ▪ Blood work including complete blood count, liver function tests, creatinine, protein, lactate dehydrogenase (LDH), β_2-microglobulin, erythrocyte sedimentation rate (ESR; if Hodgkin lymphoma), HIV serology, hepatitis serology, bone marrow biopsy
	  ▪ If doxorubicin chemotherapy anticipated, cardiac ejection fraction

(continued)

Diagnostic work-up	Description
Tumour markers	• No specific tumour markers, although the LDH and β_2-microglobulin levels reflect tumour burden and activity and may relate to prognosis in non-Hodgkin lymphoma, whereas the ESR is important in a similar fashion for Hodgkin lymphoma • Molecular profiling has gained interest both in accurately diagnosing the subtype of lymphoma and in prognostication, but has limited availability and does not usually affect treatment decisions

HODGKIN LYMPHOMA

Pathology and natural history

Pathology and natural history: Hodgkin lymphoma	Description

Hodgkin lymphoma, nodular lymphocyte predominant (NLPHL)	• Accounts for <5% of Hodgkin lymphoma
	• More common in males
	• Stage I presentation in a peripheral lymph node region (cervical, axillary or inguinal/femoral regions):
	  ▪ Mediastinum rarely involved
	• Characterized by a variant of the Reed–Sternberg cell, known as the L & H cell or popcorn cell:
	  ▪ These cells express B-cell markers (CD20+) and are negative for CD15 and CD30
	• May do well with localized therapy, such as excision and/or radiation therapy
	• Late relapse (beyond 5–10 years) is sometimes seen, but remains treatable
	• Rarely can transform into more aggressive B-cell lymphomas (diffuse large B-cell lymphoma)
	• Prognosis is excellent for localized presentations, either treated with radiation therapy or combined modality therapy, but if advanced stage, prognosis is similar to classical Hodgkin lymphoma

Classical Hodgkin lymphoma (CHL) (including lymphocyte-rich, nodular sclerosis, mixed cellularity, and lymphocyte-depleted subtypes)	• Malignant cell is the Reed–Sternberg (RS) cell:
	  ▪ CD30+, CD15+, CD45– and J chain negative
	• EBV-related proteins are found in approximately 30–50% of cases (higher in developing countries, up to 70–80%)
	• *Lymphocyte-rich CHL*:
	  ▪ Uncommon (about 5% of all Hodgkin lymphoma)
	  ▪ Usually present with localized disease in a peripheral lymph node region
	• *Nodular sclerosis CHL*:
	  ▪ Most common subtype in Westernized countries, e.g. 65–70% in the USA
	  ▪ Only subtype without a male predominance
	  ▪ Nodular growth pattern, with collagen bands and the RS variant called the lacunar cell
	  ▪ High proportion of early-stage disease (I or II) with neck and mediastinal involvement
	• *Mixed cellularity CHL*:
	  ▪ More common in developing countries, where it is associated with prior EBV infection
	  ▪ Frequency increases with age and in HIV infection in Western countries
	  ▪ Presents more often in males, with B symptoms and in advanced stages
	  ▪ Tendency to involve the spleen and bone marrow, with less frequent involvement of the mediastinum
	• *Lymphocyte-depleted CHL*:
	  ▪ Very rarely seen in primary presentation
	  ▪ Some previously reported cases are probably non-Hodgkin lymphoma misdiagnosed as lymphocyte-depleted CHL
	  ▪ Has the worst prognosis although not well characterized due to rarity

Staging and prognostic grouping

Ann Arbor system

The TNM system is impractical for lymphomas and therefore the Ann Arbor staging system is adopted by UICC (Table 32.1). The Ann Arbor system reflects the anatomical extent of disease but by itself is not adequate to prognosticate for the purpose of determining the treatment programme.

Pathological stages (pS) are rarely used as staging laparotomy is no longer a standard practice.

Table 32.1 Ann Arbor stage summary: Hodgkin lymphoma

Stage	Hodgkin lymphoma	Substage
I	Single node region	
	Localized single extralymphatic organ/site	IE
II	Two or more node regions, same side of the diaphragm	
	Localized single extralymphatic organ/site with its regional nodes ± other node regions same side of diaphragm	IIE
III	Node regions both sides of diaphragm	
	+ Localized single extra lymphatic organ/site	IIIE
	Spleen	IIIS
	Both	IIIE + S
IV	Diffuse or multifocal involvement of extralymphatic organ(s) ± regional nodes; isolated extralymphatic organ and non-regional nodes	
All stages divided	Without weight loss/fever/sweats	A
	With weight loss/fever/sweats	B

Prognostic factors

The most important prognostic factors for Stage I/II disease include Ann Arbor stage, tumour bulk (for mediastinal masses, a mediastinal width-to-maximum intrathoracic diameter ratio of over one-third is considered as bulky disease), presence of B symptoms, number of involved nodal regions, ESR and involvement of extranodal organs (E lesions) (Table 32.2). In addition, age and any co-morbidity of the patient need to be taken into account to tailor a suitable treatment programme. Different groups use a variable combination of these factors to classify patients as 'favourable risk', 'unfavourable risk' or 'intermediate risk' to determine the treatment approach, with a more intensive treatment with chemotherapy and radiation therapy for the 'unfavourable' group. Recent evidence showed that FDG-PET scan performed after one to three cycles of chemotherapy to assess early metabolic response is prognostic and this is being incorporated into the treatment algorithm by many groups. An International Prognostic score (IPS) has been developed and validated which incorporate seven parameters:

- Male sex
- Age ≥45 years
- Ann Arbor stage IV
- Haemoglobin <105 g/L
- Serum albumin <40 g/L
- Leucocyte count ≥15 × 10^9/L
- Lymphocyte count <0.6 × 10^9/L (or <8% of leucocyte count).

Patients are stratified into risk groups based on the presence of these seven factors, with scores ranging from 0 to 7. To date, the use of more intensive treatment approaches for patients with higher IPS risk has not led to improved survival. The result of an 'interim' FDG-PET scan following one to two cycles of chemotherapy has also been shown to be prognostic for advanced-stage Hodgkin lymphoma, although the role of modification of the treatment programme based on the PET response is still being investigated in clinical trials.

Treatment philosophy

The treatment intent is almost always curative, and the majority of patients will require chemotherapy (common chemotherapy regimens are listed in Table 32.3). In early-stage Hodgkin lymphoma, the treatment approach has shifted from the use of extended field radiation therapy to the use of combined modality therapy (CMT). For advanced-stage Hodgkin lymphoma, the main treatment is chemotherapy. Current management strives to optimize the therapeutic ratio by giving the minimal therapy necessary to achieve a high level of cure with the initial treatment approach, and to minimize the long-term late effects of therapy, chiefly cardiac disease and second malignancies. Response-adapted strategies using FDG-PET-CT scan results following the first one to three cycles of chemotherapy are under active investigation.

Scenario: Hodgkin lymphoma	Treatment philosophy
Stage I/II nodular lymphocyte predominant Hodgkin lymphoma	• Radiation therapy • Alternative: CMT as in Stage I/II CHL
Stage I/II CHL (early favourable risk; see Box 32.1)	• CMT (brief chemotherapy followed by radiation therapy) • Alternative: chemotherapy alone
Stage I/II (unfavourable or intermediate risk; see Box 32.1)	• CMT (chemotherapy followed by radiation therapy) • Alternative: chemotherapy alone
Stage III/IV or advanced*	• Chemotherapy ± consolidation radiation therapy
Follow-up	• After definitive treatment, imaging with CT scans or PET-CT to determine response in 6–8 weeks • To assess possible late effects of therapy (haematological, cardiac, thyroid, and monitoring for second malignancies)

*The definition of advanced has been applied variably by different investigators, most frequently with selected inclusion of some Stage I/II patients with more than one adverse prognostic factors, e.g. large mediastinal mass, B symptoms. According to the GHSG series of clinical trials, Stage IIB patients with either bulky mediastinal mass or E lesion are considered to be in the advanced category.

Table 32.2 Prognostic factors for Hodgkin lymphoma

Prognostic factors	Tumour related	Host related	Environment related
Essential	Ann Arbor stage Histological subtype Tumour bulk measures: • Number of nodal regions • Extranodal involvement • Size of tumour mass(es), especially in the mediastinum	Age Gender B symptoms Lymphocyte count ESR Anaemia	
Additional	IPS score (as above, also include serum albumin level)		EBV, HIV infections
New and promising	Early metabolic response with FDG-PET scan		

Data from Hasenclever, D. and Diehl, V, 1998. N Engl J Med 339(21):1506-14.

Table 32.3 Common chemotherapy regimens for Hodgkin and non-Hodgkin lymphoma

Hodgkin lymphoma	Indolent non-Hodgkin lymphoma	Histologically aggressive non-Hodgkin lymphoma*	Salvage therapy*
ABVD (doxorubicin + bleomycin + vinblastine + dacarbazine) BEACOPP (bleomycin + etoposide + doxorubicin + cyclophosphamide + vincristine, prednisone + procarbazine) MOPP (nitrogen mustard + vincristine + prednisone + procarbazine)	Rituximab R-CVP (rituximab + cyclophosphamide + vincristine + prednisone) CHOP or R-CHOP (see next column) FCR (fludarabine + cyclophosphamide + rituximab) FCM-(R) (fludarabine + cyclophosphamide + mitoxantrone [rituximab]) Bendamustine + rituximab Tositumomab + ^{131}I-tositumomab (Bexxar™) ^{90}Y-ibritumomab tiuxetan (Zevalin™)	R-CHOP (rituximab + cyclophosphamide + doxorubicin, vincristine + prednisone) CHOEP (CHOP + etoposide) EPOCH (etoposide + vincristine + doxorubicin + cyclophosphamide + prednisone) CODOX-M (cyclophosphamide + doxorubicin + vincristine + methotrexate + leucovorin + intrathecal cytarabine [ara-C] + methotrexate) IVAC (ifosfamide + etoposide + ara-C)	DHAP (dexamethasone + ara-C + cisplatin) ESHAP (etoposide + methyprednisolone + ara-C + cisplatin) ICE (ifosfamide + mesna + caroboplatin + etoposide) GDP (gemcitabine + dexamethasone + cisplatin)

*The addition of ritumaxab is common in these regimens, with the exception of CODOX-M and IVAC.

Box 32.1 Definition of favourable and unfavourable/intermediate risk groups

There are different methods to define favourable and unfavourable risk groups for the purpose of Stage I/II stratification for treatment. A typical widely adopted system used by the German Hodgkin Study Group (GHSG) is:
- *Favourable risk*: none of the following factors present:
  - Large mediastinal mass
  - ESR ≥50 without B symptoms; ESR ≥30 with B symptoms
  - Extranodal disease
  - >2 nodal areas involved
- *Unfavourable/intermediate risk*: if any one or more of these four factors are present

Treatment

Treatment: Hodgkin lymphoma	Description
Nodular lymphocyte-predominant Hodgkin lymphoma	
Stage I/II	• Involved site radiation therapy (ISRT) alone to 30–35 Gy in 1.75–2-Gy fractions • Alternative: CMT with ABVD × 2–4 cycles followed by ISRT 20–30 Gy (as for Stage I/II CHL)

Treatment: Hodgkin lymphoma	Description
Stage III/IV	• Chemotherapy alone (ABVD or equivalent, 6–8 cycles)
Classical Hodgkin lymphoma	
Stage I/II (early favourable risk; see Box 32.1)	• CMT (ABVD × 2 followed by ISRT 20 Gy) • Chemotherapy alone (ABVD × 4–6) if wish to avoid possible late effects of radiation therapy
Stage I/II (unfavourable or intermediate risk; see Box 32.1)	• CMT (ABVD × 4 followed by ISRT 30 Gy) • Chemotherapy alone (ABVD or equivalent × 4–6) if wish to avoid possible late effects of radiation therapy
Stage III/IV or advanced	• Chemotherapy alone (ABVD or equivalent × 6–8), ± consolidation ISRT • Alternative: intensified chemotherapy regimens (e.g. escalated BEACOPP × 6–8)

Controversies

CMT versus chemotherapy alone in Stage I/II Hodgkin lymphoma

While CMT is generally considered to be the standard for early-stage Hodgkin lymphoma, chemotherapy alone, e.g. ABVD × 4–6 cycles, also results in a high cure rate in this patient population. For favourable risk patients and some unfavourable risk patients without a large mediastinal mass, a progression-free rate of approximately 85–90% is expected. In a phase III trial, this was lower than the 92% achieved with subtotal nodal irradiation therapy (± ABVD × 2 cycles), but the 12-year overall survival (OS) rate was slightly higher in the patients treated with chemotherapy alone compared with those treated with the irradiation approach (94% vs 87%). The advantage of management with chemotherapy alone is to avoid the potential long-term deleterious effects of irradiation, chiefly cardiac disease and second malignancies, at the expense of a slightly higher disease relapse rate compared with CMT. Proponents of this approach indicate that relapsing patients can still be cured with salvage therapy such as radiation and/or further chemotherapy and autologous stem cell transplantation. However, CMT as an initial strategy appears to give the best tumour control rate, and proponents of this approach suggest that the radiation volumes and dose required are now much lower than with subtotal nodal irradiation, and that the long-term side effects of irradiation are therefore predicted to be much less than previously observed. Factors that may influence treatment approach include the age of the patient, and whether the disease location requires a large volume of breast tissues (for women) or lung to be within the radiation field. Ongoing clinical trials of the use of response to FDG-PET to identify patients who would benefit from radiation therapy, or those who may have radiation omitted without compromising disease control, will have mature results in the near future.

Optimal chemotherapy regimen in Stage III/IV Hodgkin lymphoma and role of consolidation radiation

ABVD has been regarded for many years as the standard regimen, and gives a 5-year progression-free rate of ~65% and OS of 80–85% for advanced stage Hodgkin lymphoma. Regimens such as MOPP/ABV hybrid or Stanford V were not superior when tested in phase III clinical trials. However, a series of phase III clinical trials from the GHSG have yielded better results with an intensified regimen (BEACOPP). In the GHSG HD15 trial, six cycles of 'escalated' BEACOPP (requires routine granulocyte-colony stimulating factor [G-CSF] support) resulted in a 5-year treatment failure-free rate of 89% and OS of 95%, comparable to eight cycles of the same regimen. However, in another phase III trial comparing ABVD (6–8 cycles) with BEACOPP (four cycles of escalated and four cycles of standard dose), although BEACOPP showed better initial tumour control, this did not translate into eventual benefit in terms of freedom from second progression or OS when salvage therapy with autologous stem cell transplant was taken into account. The 7-year OS for BEACOPP was 89%, which was not statistically different from the 84% for ABVD, when all first- and second-line therapies are taken into account. BEACOPP has a higher degree of toxicity compared with ABVD, chiefly myelosuppression, gonadal toxicity and also a small risk of secondary myelodysplasia and acute myeloid leukaemia. Proponents of BEACOPP argue that the degree of benefit still outweighs the increased toxicity.

The use of consolidation radiation therapy to residual masses or previously bulky site(s) of disease post chemotherapy has been common practice for patients with advanced-stage Hodgkin lymphoma. A phase III trial has shown that patients in complete remission after MOPP-ABV did not benefit from consolidation radiation (24 Gy); however, those with partial remission (defined by CT scan) were irradiated and had high 5-year event-free and OS rates of 79% and 87%, respectively. Currently FDG-PET has emerged as standard practice to determine remission status for patients with residual abnormalities on CT scan at the end of therapy. Based on the GHSG trial HD15 (post BEACOPP chemotherapy), radiation is not required for patients with residual nodal abnormalities of >2.5 cm achieving complete metabolic response by FDG-PET, while those with a positive scan still had an excellent outcome after application of radiation to areas of residual uptake. For those with residual FDG uptake in limited sites, radiation therapy appears to be indicated and results in a 4-year progression-free survival (PFS) of 86%. This may be considered a reasonable alternative to salvage chemotherapy and autologous stem cell transplantation for those with minimal residual abnormalities in a limited site. Similar studies in patients treated with ABVD are awaited.

Role of FDG-PET in assessing early response and to determine the need for subsequent radiation therapy

There is currently considerable clinical trial activity to determine how FDG-PET can assist in the assessment of response following chemotherapy, and help determine the need for subsequent therapy, such as consolidation radiation therapy. Refinement and international agreement on the interpretation of FDG-PET has resulted in the adoption of the five-point Deauville scoring system: 1, no uptake; 2, uptake $\leq$ mediastinal blood pool; 3, uptake > mediastinal blood pool but $\leq$ liver; 4, uptake > liver; 5, markedly increased uptake or development of new lesions. In determining response, a score of 1–2 is considered negative and of 4–5 is considered positive, but a score of 3 remains controversial, although the expert opinion from the 4th International Workshop on PET in Lymphoma considered scores of 1–3 as indicating complete metabolic response (CMR). In clinical trials that consider treatment intensification, a score of 3 may be considered CMR to avoid over-treatment of some patients, while for trials exploring de-escalation of treatment, a score of 3 may be considered an inadequate response to avoid under-treatment.

A phase III trial in favourable risk early-stage Hodgkin lymphoma has been completed in the UK, testing whether radiation therapy offers benefit when PET scan is negative (Deauville score 1–2) after ABVD x three cycles. Preliminary results indicate that if the PET scan is negative and radiation is omitted, the PFS was just over 90%, although the addition of consolidation radiation gave a higher PFS rate of 94.5% (as randomized) and 97% (as treated). In advanced-stage Hodgkin lymphoma, an 'interim' PET scan after ABVD x two cycles has been shown to be extremely prognostic in patients who have gone on to complete ABVD chemotherapy regardless of the PET scan result. Several clinical trials are in progress to determine if the interim PET result can guide the de-escalation of therapy in those with early responses, and intensify the treatment in those with persistent uptake.

Phase III clinical trials

See Table 32.4.

Table 32.4 Phase III clinical trials

Trial reference	Results
Stage I/II Hodgkin lymphoma	
Engert et al. (2010) N Engl J Med 363:640–652	• In favourable risk group (GHSG HD10 trial), ABVD x 2 + radiation therapy (RT) 20 Gy is standard therapy, with 8-year PFS and OS rates of 86.5% and 95.1%, respectively
Eich et al. (2010) J Clin Oncol. 28:4199–4206	• In unfavourable (intermediate) risk group (GHSG HD11 trial), ABVD x 4 + RT 30 Gy is standard therapy, with 5-year PFS and OS rates of 87.2% and 94.3%, respectively
Meyer et al. (2010) N Engl J Med 366:399–3408	• In favourable and some unfavourable Hodgkin lymphoma without large mediastinal mass, ABVD alone for 4–6 cycles resulted in 12-year PFS and OS rates of 87% and 94%, respectively • A radiation approach (subtotal nodal) gave corresponding rates of 92% and 87%, respectively.
Von Tresckow et al. (2012) J Clin Oncol 30(9):907–913	• In unfavourable (intermediate) risk group (GHSG HD14 trial), BEACOPP (escalated dose) x 2 + ABVD x 2 + RT 30 Gy gave better 5-year PFS compared with ABVD x 4 + RT 30 Gy (95.4% vs 89.1%), with similar 5-year OS rates of ~97%
Herbst et al. (2010) Hematologica 95:494–500	• Meta-analysis of five phase III trials totalling 1245 patients comparing chemotherapy alone with CMT showed that adding RT to chemotherapy improves tumour control and overall survival
Raemaekers et al. (2014) J Clin Oncol 32(12):1188–1194	• Early results of the EORTC H10 trial, comparing a standard CMT treatment with a PET-directed approach where after two cycles of chemotherapy PET-negative patients had radiation given or omitted in a randomized setting • Non-irradiated patients had a slightly higher probability of disease progression
Stage III/IV and advanced Hodgkin lymphoma	
Engert et al. (2012) Lancet 379:1791–1799	• In advanced Hodgkin lymphoma (GHSG HD15 trial), high-dose BEACOPP x 6 + PET-guided RT is standard therapy, with 5-year PFS and OS rates of 90.3% and 95.3%, respectively
Viviani et al. (2011) N Engl J Med 365:203–212	• BEACOPP (four cycles standard dose and four cycles higher dose) gave better initial tumour control compared with ABVD (6–8 cycles), but the 7-year eventual tumour control and OS were not significantly different when subsequent salvage therapy was taken into account
Gordon et al. (2013) J Clin Oncol 31:684–691	• For locally-advanced and Stage III/IV Hodgkin lymphoma a comparison of ABVD with Stanford V gave no significant difference in response rates and the 5-year failure-free survival (FFS) was similar (74% for ABVD and 71% for Stanford V), and OS 88% for both
Aleman et al. (2003) N Engl J Med 348:2396–2406	• Involved field radiation therapy did not improve the outcome in patients with complete remission after MOPP-ABV

Refractory and relapsed Hodgkin lymphoma

The treatment approach for refractory and relapsed Hodgkin lymphoma is most often still curative in intent, with combination salvage chemotherapy regimens (e.g. GDP, DHAP, ICE), followed by autologous haematopoietic stem cell transplantation (ASCT), with or without the addition of radiation therapy. An overall 5-year disease-free survival rate of 40–60% can be expected for patients who are transplant eligible. Where transplant is contraindicated, the approach is palliative in intent. Factors that are important to consider in deciding the nature of further therapy are: refractory disease versus the length of the disease-free interval, the relapsed distribution and burden of disease, constitutional symptoms and the previous chemotherapy/radiation regimens. Selected patients with a localized small-volume relapse of the disease in the original site(s), not initially treated with radiation and with response of >1 year may do well with radiation therapy. However, such patients account for only a small proportion of refractory/relapsed patients (16% in GHSG trials). The majority will require salvage chemotherapy regimens to further cytoreduce the disease burden, followed by ASCT. According to the GHSG experience in over 400 relapsed patients, the parameters associated with a poor prognosis are: early relapse (<12-month disease-free interval), Stage III/IV at relapse and anaemia. If all three factors were absent, the 4-year survival was 83%, compared with 27% if all three factors were present. Refractory patients (those with progression of disease within 3 months of initial therapy) have a particularly poor prognosis. The use of FDG-PET following salvage chemotherapy may guide the use of subsequent therapy such as radiation therapy. Additionally, most transplant programmes will maximally utilize radiation therapy for untreated bulky sites of relapse with >5 cm maximum tumour diameter, either before transplant (e.g. at the Memorial Sloan Kettering Cancer Center, using total nodal irradiation to attempt to control all nodal sites), or with involved site techniques post transplant.

Areas of research in Hodgkin lymphoma

- Identification of:
    - Molecular markers of prognosis and developing new targets for therapy

Table 32.5 Mature B-cell and T-cell neoplasm subtypes of non-Hodgkin lymphoma

Mature B-cell neoplasms (note: hairy cell leukaemia and plasma cell neoplasms are excluded)	Mature T-cell neoplasms

• *Chronic lymphocytic leukaemia (CLL)/small lymphocytic lymphoma
• B-cell prolymphocytic leukaemia
• *Lymphoplasmacytic lymphoma (Waldenström macroglobinemia)
• *Splenic B-cell marginal zone lymphoma
• Splenic B-cell lymphoma/leukaemia, unclassifiable
• *Extranodal marginal zone B-cell lymphoma of mucosa-associated lymphoid tissue (MALT lymphoma)
• Nodal marginal zone lymphoma
• *Follicular lymphoma
• Primary cutaneous follicular centre lymphoma
• *Mantle cell lymphoma
• *Diffuse large B-cell lymphoma (DLBCL), not otherwise specified:
   ▪ T-cell/histiocyte-rich large B-cell lymphoma
   ▪ Primary DLBCL of the central nervous system (CNS)
   ▪ Primary cutaneous DLBCL, leg type
   ▪ EBV-positive DLBCL of the elderly
• DLBCL associated with chronic inflammation
• Lymphomatoid granulomatosis
• *Primary mediastinal (thymic) large B-cell lymphoma
• Intravascular large B-cell lymphoma
• Anaplastic lymphoma kinase (ALK)-positive large B-cell lymphoma
• Plasmablastic lymphoma
• Large B-cell lymphoma arising in HHV8-associated multicentric Castleman disease
• Primary effusion lymphoma
• *Burkitt lymphoma
• B-cell lymphoma, unclassifiable, with features intermediate between DLBCL and Burkitt lymphoma
• B-cell lymphoma, unclassifiable, with features intermediate between DLBCL and classical Hodgkin lymphoma
• Heavy chain diseases
	• T-cell prolymphocytic leukaemia
	• T-cell large granular lymphocytic leukaemia
	• Chronic lymphoproliferative disorder of natural killer (NK) cells
	• Aggressive NK cell leukaemia
	• EBV-positive T-cell lymphoproliferative disease of childhood
	• *Adult T-cell leukaemia/lymphoma
	• *Extranodal NK/T-cell lymphoma, nasal type
	• *Enteropathy-associated T-cell lymphoma
	• Hepatosplenic T-cell lymphoma
	• Subcutaneous panniculitis-like T-cell lymphoma
	• *Mycosis fungoides
	• *Sézary syndrome
	• *Primary cutaneous CD30-positive T-cell lymphoproliferative disorders:
	   ▪ Lymphomatoid papulosis
	   ▪ Primary anaplastic large-cell lymphoma
	• Primary cutaneous peripheral T-cell lymphomas, rare subtypes
	• *Peripheral T-cell lymphoma, not otherwise specified
	• *Angioimmunoblastic T-cell lymphoma
	• *Anaplastic large-cell lymphoma, ALK positive
	• *Anaplastic large-cell lymphoma, ALK negative

*Common and more important subtypes. Swerdlow (2008). Reproduced with permission of WHO.

- Effective new drugs, emphasizing targeted therapies and combining targeted drugs (e.g. brentuximab vedotin, a CD30 antibody coupled to the tubulin toxin MMAE) with conventional therapies
- Conduct of clinical trials to tailor treatment approach based on disease characteristics and the response to initial treatment, i.e. interim metabolic response
- Optimize management of survivorship issues including detection, monitoring and treatment of late effects such as fatigue, gonadal dysfunction/reproduction, immune dysfunction, cardiac disease and second malignancies

NON-HODGKIN LYMPHOMA

Pathology and presentation

Table 32.5 lists the mature B-cell and T-cell neoplasm subtypes.

Pathology and presentation: Mature B-cell lymphomas (ranked according to frequency^)	Description
Diffuse large B-cell lymphoma (DLBCL) (31% of non-Hodgkin lymphoma)	• Most common lymphoma • Median age 64 years • Stage I/II in 50% • Lymph nodes involved most frequently, also extranodal sites common (up to 40–50% of patients; head and neck sites, stomach, etc.) • Immunophenotype: CD20+

Follicular lymphoma (22%)	• Second most common non-Hodgkin lymphoma:
	  ▪ Higher incidence in developed Western countries and Europe
	• Median age 59 years
	• Stage I/II in 25–30%
	• Lymph nodes involved most frequently, preferentially peripheral sites (neck, axilla, inguinal) or abdominal adenopathy
	• High incidence of bone marrow involvement
	• Clinically slow growing, occasionally spontaneous regression (or waxing and waning) seen
	• Immunophenotype: CD5–, CD10+, CD23±, CD43–, CD20+
	• Characterized by t(14; 18)(q32; q21), *Bcl-2*
	• Graded as 1, 2 and 3 based on number of large cells seen per high power field:
	  ▪ Grades 1, 2 and 3A considered as *indolent* lymphoma
	  ▪ Grade 3B considered as *aggressive* lymphoma by most clinicians

Small lymphocytic lymphoma/ chronic lymphocytic leukaemia (CLL) (6%)	• Small lymphocytic lymphoma is the tissue manifestation of CLL • CLL is the commonest leukaemia in adults in Western countries: ▪ Rare in the Far East • Median age 65 years • Many patients present asymptomatically with lymphocytosis discovered incidentally • When presenting as lymphoma, considered *indolent* disease and slow growing • Involvement of blood, bone marrow, lymph nodes and spleen are common • Can have infections and infrequently haemolytic anaemia • Immunophenotype: CD5+, CD10–, CD23+, CD20+ • Staged by the Rai or Binet clinical staging systems, which are also prognostic • Genetic markers add important prognostic information at time of treatment, e.g. V_H gene mutation status, FISH analysis for 13q–, 11q–, 17p– (deletion of TP53) • Transformation (known as Richter's transformation) to an aggressive lymphoma occurs in ~1–2% of patients, usually to DLBCL, with a poor prognosis
Mantle cell lymphoma (MCL) (6% of NHL)	• Median age 63 years • Male predominance • Stage I/II in <20% • Considered an *aggressive* lymphoma, but a minority of cases have a slow proliferation rate and are therefore *indolent* in behaviour • Involves lymph nodes, spleen, bone marrow, occasionally blood, and extranodal organs such as the colon (lymphomatous polyposis), orbit or Waldeyer's ring • Immunophenotype: CD5+, CD10±, CD23–, CD43+, cyclin D1+, CD20+

Pathology and presentation: Mature B-cell lymphomas (ranked according to frequency*)	Description
	• Characterized by t(11; 14)(q13; q32), *Bcl-1* • Blastoid variant has a higher proliferation rate and is associated with a poorer prognosis: ▪ Age, performance status and burden of disease as reflected in lymphocyte count, and LDH level are prognostic (see MIPI score; Box 32.2)

Extranodal marginal zone lymphoma, MALT type (5%)	• Median age 60 years
	• MALT lymphoma is an *indolent* lymphoma, presenting in diverse extranodal MALT sites:
	  ▪ Most frequent extranodal sites are: gastrointestinal tract, commonly stomach, also small bowel (known as immunoproliferative small intestinal disease [IPSID]), orbital adnexa, salivary gland or other head and neck tissues, lung, skin, thyroid and breast
	  ▪ Advanced-stage presentations often involve multiple extranodal sites, soft tissues and bone marrow in approximately 25%
	  ▪ Nodal involvement is usually associated with the extranodal site but relatively uncommon overall
	• Stage I/II in 75–90%.
	• Clinically slow growing
	• Associated or preceded by infection or inflammatory condition of the extranodal organ involved, e.g.:
	  ▪ *H. pylori* in stomach MALT
	  ▪ *Chlamydia psittaci* in orbital MALT
	  ▪ Sjögren syndrome in salivary gland MALT
	  ▪ Lymphocytic thyroiditis in thyroid MALT
	• Immunophenotype: CD5−, CD10−, CD23−, CD43±, CD20+
	• Characterized by a number of chromosomal abnormalities: t(11; 18)(q21; q21) (API2-MALT1), t(14; 18)(q32; q21) (IgH-MALT1), t(3; 14)(p14.1; q32), t(1; 14)(p22; q32), +3, and +18:
	  ▪ Translocation t(11; 18)(q21; q21) involving the *MALT1* gene in gastric MALT lymphoma is usually not associated with *H. pylori* infection and rarely responds to *H. pylori* eradication therapy

Primary mediastinal (thymic) large B-cell lymphoma (2%)	• Subtype of DLBCL presenting in the mediastinum with a thymic B-cell origin
	• Median age 37 years
	• Female predominance
	• Stage I/II in 70%
	• An *aggressive* lymphoma:
	  ▪ Frequently presents with bulky disease of >10 cm and invasion of mediastinal structures (pericardium, chest wall, lung), superior vena cava obstruction and pleural effusions; high LDH
	  ▪ In rare Stage III/IV presentations, extranodal organs (kidney, adrenal gland, CNS) may be involved
	• Immunophenotype: CD19+, CD20/22+, CD79a+, CD30+; lacks surface Ig

Marginal zone lymphoma, nodal type (1%)	• Rare marginal zone lymphoma involving lymph nodes only (with no extranodal or splenic disease) • Median age 58 years • Most present in Stage III/IV (75%) • Considered an *indolent* lymphoma • Involves peripheral lymph nodes and bone marrow • Immunophenotype: CD5−, CD10−, CD23−, CD43±, CD20+, *Bcl-2*+
Lymphoplasmacytic lymphoma (1%)	• A type of small B-cell lymphoma with plasmacytic origin/differentiation, but not fulfilling the diagnostic criteria for any of the other indolent B-cell neoplasms • Median age 63 years • Majority Stage IV • An *indolent* lymphoma • Usually involves the bone marrow, spleen and lymph nodes • May have accompanying IgM paraprotein; such cases are designated Waldenstrom's macroglobulinaemia and can have hyperviscosity, and cryoglobulinaemia (particularly when positive for hepatitis C virus) • Immunophenotype: CD20+, CD5−, CD10−, CD138+, surface Ig+: ▪ Nearly all patients have the point mutation L265P in *MYD88*, an adaptor molecule important in NFκB signalling • Transformation to aggressive B-cell lymphoma (DLBCL) can occur but is rare

(continued)

Pathology and presentation: Mature B-cell lymphomas (ranked according to frequency*)	Description

Burkitt lymphoma (<1%)	• Three clinical types: endemic, sporadic and immunodeficiency associated
	  ■ *Endemic*:
	    ○ Occurs endemically in equatorial Africa
	    ○ Most common childhood cancer in that area, usually at age 4–7 years, with a male predominance
	    ○ Frequently present as a jaw tumour
	  ■ *Sporadic*:
	    ○ Seen throughout the world
	    ○ Accounts for ~1% of non-Hodgkin lymphoma in North America and Europe
	    ○ Usually present in extranodal organs, within the abdomen (gastrointestinal tract, ileocaecal area, gonadal area), breast, etc.
	    ○ Predominance in males in mid-30s, but can also affect children
	  ■ EBV genome is present in majority of endemic BL and ~30% of sporadic cases
	  ■ *Immunodeficiency associated*:
	    ○ Usually due to HIV infection, as part of initial presentation of AIDS
	    ○ Lymph nodes and bone marrow frequently involved, in addition to extranodal organs
	• Majority are stage IV:
	  ■ A staging system proposed by Murphy, or modifications of it (largely based on tumour burden), is commonly used clinically
	• Very *aggressive* lymphoma, with short doubling time and rapid proliferation rate
	• Characteristically involves extranodal organs, and propensity for CNS disease at presentation, or subsequently
	• Immunophenotype: CD19/20/22+, CD10+, *Bcl-6*+, *Bcl-2*–, IgM+, Ki-67 99–100%
	• Characterized by 8q24 translocation involving *c-MYC*, most commonly t(8; 14)(q24, q32)

Splenic B-cell marginal zone lymphoma (<1%)	• Rare type of small B-cell neoplasm accounting for a majority of CD5– chronic lymphoid leukaemias • Median age 67 years • Presents as splenomegaly • Majority are Stage IV • An *indolent* lymphoma • Usually involves the spleen and bone marrow; seldom lymph nodes • Characterized by lymphoma cells in the peripheral blood known as villous lymphocytes • Immunophenotype: CD20+, CD5–, CD23–, CD43–, surface IgM+: ■ May be associated with M protein (usually IgM but can be IgA or IgG) and autoimmune haemolytic anaemia
Primary cutaneous follicle centre lymphoma (<1%)	• Median age 58 years • Slight male predominance • Presents as tumour nodules or plaque-like lesions in the skin, erythematous to violaceous: ■ Usually solitary or localized group of lesions on the scalp or trunk, but can also occur on extremities • *Indolent* B-cell lymphoma • Immunophenotype: CD20+, CD792+, *Bcl-6*–, *Bcl-2*– • In contrast to follicular lymphoma, do not show *Bcl-2* rearrangements

Plasmablastic lymphoma (<1%)	• Rare *aggressive* lymphoma with tumour cells expressing plasma cell phenotype
	• Majority present in advanced stages
	• Median age 50 years
	• Usually associated with immunodeficiency, e.g. HIV infection
	• Presentation most frequently as a mass in the oral cavity, but can involve other sites such as the orbit, soft tissues or gastrointestinal tract
	• Immunophenotype: positive for plasma cell markers, e.g. CD138+, CD38+:
	  ■ Can be weakly CD20+
	  ■ EBV+ particularly in the oral cavity site

Pathology and presentation: Mature B-cell lymphomas (ranked according to frequency*)	Description

Other rare B-cell lymphomas (not discussed in detail)	• Clinically *aggressive*:
	  ▪ B-cell prolymphocytic leukaemia
	  ▪ Other subtypes of DLBCL including:
	    ○ T-cell/histiocyte-rich large B-cell lymphoma
	    ○ Primary cutaneous DLBCL, leg type
	    ○ EBV+ DLBCL of the elderly
	  ▪ DLBCL associated with chronic inflammation
	  ▪ Lymphomatoid granulomatosis
	  ▪ Intravascular large B-cell lymphoma
	  ▪ Anaplastic lymphoma kinase (ALK)-positive large B-cell lymphoma
	  ▪ Large B-cell lymphoma arising in HHV8-associated multicentric Castleman disease
	  ▪ Primary effusion lymphoma
	  ▪ B-cell lymphoma, unclassifiable, with features intermediate between DLBCL and Burkitt lymphoma
	  ▪ B-cell lymphoma, unclassifiable, with features intermediate between DLBCL and classical Hodgkin lymphoma
	  ▪ Heavy chain diseases

*As reported by the NHL Classification Project 1998.

Pathology and presentation: Mature T-cell lymphomas (ranked according to frequency*)	Description

Peripheral T-cell lymphoma, not otherwise specified (PTCL-NOS) (6%)	• Heterogeneous group, but represent the most common T-cell lymphomas in Western countries
	• Median age 60 years
	• Male predominance
	• Majority Stage III/IV (70%)
	• Considered an *aggressive* lymphoma
	• Involves lymph nodes, and bone marrow, spleen, skin and other extranodal organs
	• Immunophenotype: CD4+ > CD8+, CD10–, *Bcl-6*–, CD30±, CD56±, characteristically CD20–
	• T-cell receptor genes clonally rearranged in the majority:
	  ▪ Usually complex karyotype
	  ▪ Use of gene expression profiles may be helpful in distinguishing from other types of T-cell lymphomas

Anaplastic large-cell lymphoma ALK+ and ALK– types (2%)	• *Aggressive* T-cell lymphoma, now separated into ALK-positive and ALK-negative cases, because the latter present in older adults and the prognosis is worse
	• Median age 33 years for ALK+ cases (some present in childhood) and 45–50 years for ALK– cases
	• Male predominance
	• Stage III/IV in 60–70%
	• Involves lymph nodes and extranodal organs, not uncommonly skin, lung and soft tissues
	• Immunophenotype: CD30+ (strong), ALK+ for the ALK+ subtype
	• T-cell receptor genes clonally rearranged in the majority:
	  ▪ ALK+ cases:
	    ○ Translocation t(2; 5)(p23; q35) most common, resulting in *ALK–NPM* fusion gene
	    ○ Other partners include *TPM3*, i.e. t(1; 2)(q25; p23)

Primary cutaneous CD30+ T-cell lymphoproliferative disorders (<1%)	• Encompass a spectrum of CD30+ diseases ranging from primary cutaneous anaplastic large cell lymphoma (c-ALCL) to lymphomatoid papulosis, largely a self-healing benign skin condition
	• c-ALCL:
	  ▪ Median age 60 years
	  ▪ Male predominance
	  ▪ Usually solitary skin nodule; multifocal in 20%
	  ▪ Dissemination outside of the skin occurs in 10% of patients, usually to lymph nodes

(continued)

Pathology and presentation: Mature T-cell lymphomas (ranked according to frequency^A)	Description

	- *Lymphomatoid papulosis*:
	  - Median age 45 years
	  - Male predominance
	  - Papules affecting extremities or trunk, evolving in appearance over several weeks, self-healing
	  - Associated with development of other lymphomas, usually c-ALCL, mycosis fungoides or Hodgkin lymphoma
	  - Excellent prognosis, benign course in the majority, with lymphoma developing in <5%

Mycosis fungoides and Sézary syndrome	- Most common primary cutaneous T-cell lymphoma
	- Age usually >60 years when diagnosed
	- Characterized by an evolution of skin patches, then plaques and then tumours, over a course of many years
	- *Indolent* in behaviour
	- Immunophenotype: CD2+, CD3+, TCRβ+, CD4+, CD5+, CD8–
	- Unique staging system has been used clinically, based on degree of skin and/or lymph node involvement
	- Prognosis depends on the extent of disease:
	  - Tumorous stage or those with erythroderma have a worse prognosis
	  - Histological transformation is an unfavourable event
	- *Sézary syndrome*:
	  - Characterized by erythroderma, generalized lymphadenopathy and presence of Sézary cells (with cerebriform nuclei) in the skin, lymph nodes and peripheral blood
	  - Therefore can be viewed as the leukaemic manifestation of mycosis fungoides progression

Angioimmunoblastic T-cell lymphoma (AITL) (2%)	- *Aggressive* lymphoma with polymorphous infiltrates involving lymph nodes - Median age 65 years - Slight male predominance - Characterized by systemic disease (Stage IV in 90%) with generalized lymphadenopathy, and frequent involvement of spleen, liver and bone marrow, and occasionally skin rash, effusions and ascites - Associated immune abnormalities with haemolytic anaemia, hyperimmunoglobinaemia, cold agglutinins, etc. - Morphologically characterized by proliferating arborizing high endothelial venules - Immunophenotype: pan-T-cell markers (CD3+, CD2+, CD4+, CD5+), reactive CD8+ cells
Adult T-cell leukaemia/lymphoma (ATLL) (<1%)	- Peripheral T-cell neoplasm caused by HTLV-1 - Chiefly seen endemically in some regions of the world: Caribbean, Southwest Japan - Median age 62 years - Slight male predominance - Usually disseminated disease, characteristically general lymphadenopathy, peripheral blood and also skin involvement ± other extranodal organs involved (lung, spleen, bone, liver, CNS) - Hypercalcaemia is common - Different clinical forms recognized: smouldering (indolent), chronic and acute - Immunophenotype: CD2+, CD3+, CD5+, CD25+
Enteropathy-associated T-cell lymphoma (EATL) (<1%)	- Uncommon but may be seen in areas of the world where coeliac disease is more common, e.g. northern Europe: - Monomorphic type (type II), accounting for 30% of cases, may be less associated with coeliac disease - *Aggressive* lymphoma, usually involves the jejunum and ileum, presenting as pain, ulceration and/or perforation - Long-standing malabsorption may precede diagnosis of lymphoma, resulting in poor performance status - Immunophenotype: CD3+, CD5–, CD7+, CD8±, CD4–, CD103+; variably CD30+

Pathology and presentation: Mature T-cell lymphomas (ranked according to frequency*)	Description
Extranodal NK/T-cell lymphoma, nasal type (<1%)	• Extranodal lymphoma • Extremely rare in Western countries, but more prevalent in Asia, Mexico and South America • Median age 50 years • Male predominance • Majority present in Stage IE • Clinically *aggressive* and presents with tissue invasion/destruction and necrosis • Frequently presents in the nasal cavity and/or paranasal sinus areas, and Waldeyer's ring: ▪ Rarely involves skin, testis, lymph nodes • Can rapidly disseminate to other extranodal organs such as lung, skin, liver, gastrointestinal tract and bone marrow • Can cause haemophagocytic syndrome • Immunophenotype: CD2+, CD56+, surface CD3−, cytoplasmic CD3ε+ and EBV+
Lymphoblastic lymphoma (2%)	• Although named a lymphoma, not a mature T-cell malignancy, but a precursor T-cell neoplasm more appropriately referred to as T-lymphoblastic leukaemia/lymphoma, biologically behaving as a lymphoblastic leukaemia • Seen in children and young adults • Usually presents as a mediastinal mass with high frequency of bone marrow involvement (when bone marrow blasts are >25%, the disease is defined as leukaemia)

Other rare T-cell lymphomas (not discussed in detail)	• *Indolent clinical course*:
	  ▪ T-cell large granular lymphocytic leukaemia
	  ▪ Chronic lymphoproliferative disorder of NK cells
	• *Clinically aggressive*:
	  ▪ T-cell prolymphocytic leukaemia
	  ▪ Aggressive NK-cell leukaemia
	  ▪ EBV-positive T-cell lymphoproliferative disease of childhood
	  ▪ Hepatosplenic T-cell lymphoma
	  ▪ Subcutaneous panniculitis-like T-cell lymphoma
	  ▪ Primary cutaneous peripheral T-cell lymphomas, rare subtypes

*As reported by the NHL Classification Project 1998.

Staging and prognostic grouping

Ann Arbor system

The Ann Arbor staging classification (as for Hodgkin lymphoma; see Table 32.1) is also used for non-Hodgkin lymphoma. In general, it is important to distinguish localized disease (Stage I/II) from disseminated lymphoma (Stage III/IV). Most clinicians classify the histology into 'indolent' behaviour group, represented most frequently by follicular lymphoma and MALT lymphoma, and 'aggressive' group, represented and typified by DLBCL. Many rare lymphomas follow the paradigm of this 'indolent' or 'aggressive' categorization in determining the treatment approach.

The staging work-up is shown in Fig. 32.1.

Prognostic factors

Tumour burden is an important prognostic factor and some of the parameters used clinically are a surrogate of the tumour burden, reflecting the anatomical extent of the disease (e.g. Ann Arbor stage, LDH level, number of extranodal sites involved, etc.). As in Hodgkin lymphoma, the Ann Arbor system alone is inadequate to predict prognosis for the purpose of determining the treatment programme. Other important parameters include histological type, immunophenotype (B cell vs T cell), tumour bulk, proliferation index (e.g. Ki-67 growth fraction), as well as age and performance status (Table 32.6).

The International Prognostic Index (IPI) was derived from patients with aggressive lymphomas treated with doxorubicin-based chemotherapy in the pre-rituximab era (see Box 32.2). A variation of the IPI (modified IPI [mIPI]) has been used to describe the prognosis for Stage I/II disease (see Box 32.2). For follicular lymphoma, the IPI is less useful and there are two prognostic indices in common usage, the FLIPI and the FLIPI-2 (see Box 32.3). The latter incorporates the importance of an abnormal β_2-microglobulin, bone marrow involvement and also tumour bulk of >6 cm. For mantle cell lymphomas, there is the mantle-IPI (MIPI) based on age, ECOG performance status, LDH and leucocyte count (see Box 32.4).

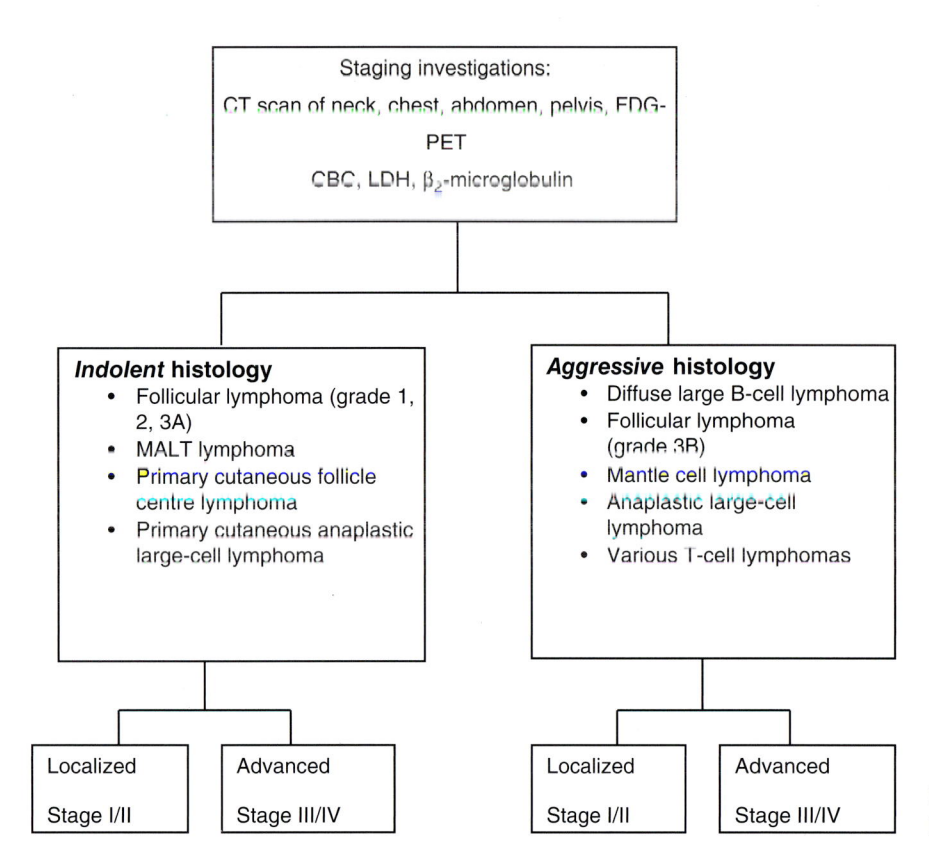

Figure 32.1 Staging of non-Hodgkin lymphoma.

Staging investigations:
CT scan of neck, chest, abdomen, pelvis, FDG-PET
CBC, LDH, β_2-microglobulin

Indolent histology
- Follicular lymphoma (grade 1, 2, 3A)
- MALT lymphoma
- Primary cutaneous follicle centre lymphoma
- Primary cutaneous anaplastic large-cell lymphoma

Aggressive histology
- Diffuse large B-cell lymphoma
- Follicular lymphoma (grade 3B)
- Mantle cell lymphoma
- Anaplastic large-cell lymphoma
- Various T-cell lymphomas

Localized Stage I/II
Advanced Stage III/IV
Localized Stage I/II
Advanced Stage III/IV

Molecular genetics are becoming more important as ancillary tests to help establish the diagnosis and characterize clinical behaviour, particularly in 'grey zone' cases. Gene expression profiling has been used to categorize DLBCL as germinal centre B cell, activated B cell and other (type III), and has been shown to associate with prognosis. While these and other gene expression profiles in other lymphoma subtypes highlight important differences in disease biology, it is still uncertain how these can assist the assignment of treatment, which is still largely based on histology, stage and the traditional clinical and patient factors as outlined above.

In addition, the presenting site of lymphoma for the same histological type, e.g. DLBCL, can have important prognostic implications. DLBCL primarily presenting in the testis, brain and liver has a particularly adverse prognosis, whereas tonsil, gastric and skin DLBCL generally have a better prognosis.

Table 32.6 Prognostic factors for non-Hodgkin lymphoma

Prognostic factors	Tumour related	Host related	Environment related
Essential	Ann Arbor stage Histological subtype Tumour bulk measures: • Extranodal involvement • Size of tumour mass(es), especially in mediastinum • LDH • β_2-microglobulin • Complete blood count (CBC) (haemoglobin, leucocyte count, lymphocyte count) IPI score (aggressive lymphoma; see Box 32.2), or FLIPI score (follicular lymphoma; see Box 32.3)	Age Gender Immune deficiency B symptoms Performance status (ECOG)	None
Additional	Proliferation rate: Ki-67 or S-phase fraction Genetic markers: *Bcl-2*, *c-MYC*, TP53		
New and promising	Microarray gene profiling Early metabolic response on FDG-PET scan		

> **Box 32.2** International Prognostic Index (IPI) for aggressive lymphoma (e.g. DLBCL) and modified IPI for Stage I and II disease
>
> **IPI**
> Score from 0 to 5 with each of the following factors, if present, scoring 1:
> - Age — >60 years
> - LDH — >1 × normal
> - Stage (Ann Arbor) — III or IV
> - Performance status (ECOG) — 2–4
> - EN involvement — >1 site
>
> | Risk groups | |
> |---|---|
> | Low | Score 0–1 |
> | Low–intermediate: | Score 2 |
> | High–intermediate | Score 3 |
> | High: | Score 4–5 |
>
> **Modified IPI (mIPI)**
> Score from 0 to 4, with each of the following factors, if present, scoring 1:
> - Age — >60 years
> - LDH — >1 × normal
> - Stage (Ann Arbor) — II
> - Performance status (ECOG) — 2–4

Data from IPI (1993) and Miller (1998).

Recent reports suggest that an FDG-PET scan performed after one to three cycles of chemotherapy to assess early metabolic response may have prognostic value and this is being tested as a treatment algorithm to modify subsequent treatment (response-adapted approach) by some clinical trial groups.

Treatment philosophy

The treatment intent for most aggressive lymphomas is curative, and the majority of patients will require chemotherapy (see Table 32.3 for common regimens). In early-stage aggressive lymphomas, chemotherapy is followed by radiation therapy. For advanced-stage aggressive lymphomas, the main treatment is chemotherapy. For indolent lymphomas in early stage, most frequently follicular lymphoma, local radiation therapy is the standard approach. Advanced-stage follicular lymphoma is not curable with chemotherapy and therefore, an observation approach is usually adopted, with the use of chemotherapy for patients who meet standard criteria for initiation of therapy (such as reported by the British National Lymphoma Investigation [BNLI] or Groupe d'Etude des Lymphomes Folliculaires [GELF]). The general treatment strategies, using follicular lymphoma as the example for indolent lymphoma, and diffuse large B-cell lymphoma as the example for aggressive lymphomas, are illustrated in Fig. 32.2 for Stage I/II (localized) presentations, and Fig. 32.3 for Stage III/IV (advanced) presentations. Although this approach is practical and adopted by many clinicians, one must be cautious

> **Box 32.3** Follicular Lymphoma IPI (FLIPI) and version 2 (FLIPI-2)
>
> **FLIPI**
> Score from 0 to 5 with each of the following factors, if present, scoring 1:
> - Age — ≥60 years
> - LDH — >1 × normal
> - Stage (Ann Arbor) — III or IV
> - Number of nodal regions* — >4
> - Haemoglobin — <120 g/L
>
> *To determine the number of nodal regions involved by lymphoma, each of the following nodal regions scores 1 (if bilateral score 2):
>
> - Neck (includes all zones 2–5, and preauricular)
> - Axillary
> - Mediastinum (includes lung hilar, retrocrural)
> - Para-aortic (includes common iliac and external iliac)
> - Mesenteric (includes splenic hilar, portal)
> - Inguinal–femoral
>
> | Risk groups | |
> |---|---|
> | Low | Score 0–1 |
> | Intermediate | Score 2 |
> | High | Score 3–5 |
>
> **FLIPI-2**
> Score from 0 to 5 with each of the following factors, if present, scoring 1:
> - Age — >60 years
> - β_2-microglobulin — >1 × normal
> - Bone marrow involvement — Yes
> - Largest node — >6 cm
> - Haemoglobin — <120 g/L
>
> | Risk groups | |
> |---|---|
> | Low | Score 0 |
> | Intermediate | Score 1–2 |
> | High | Score 3–5 |

Data from Solal-Celigny et al. (2004). Blood 104(5):1258–65; Federico et al. (2009) J Clin Oncol 27(27):4555–62

that in specific circumstance what may be regarded as 'indolent' histology for some patients may behave clinically in an aggressive fashion.

> **Box 32.4** Mantle International Prognostic Index (MIPI) for mantle cell lymphoma
>
> Calculated based on age, ECOG performance status, LDH and leucocyte count:
>
> MIPI score = [0.03535 × age (years)] + 0.6978 (if ECOG >1) + [1.367 × $\log_{10}$(LDH/ULN)] + [0.9393 × $\log_{10}$(WBC count in WBC/μL, i.e. 10^{-6} L)]
>
> | Risk groups | |
> |---|---|
> | Low | Score <5.7 |
> | Intermediate | Score 5.7–<6.2 |
> | High | Score ≥6.2 |

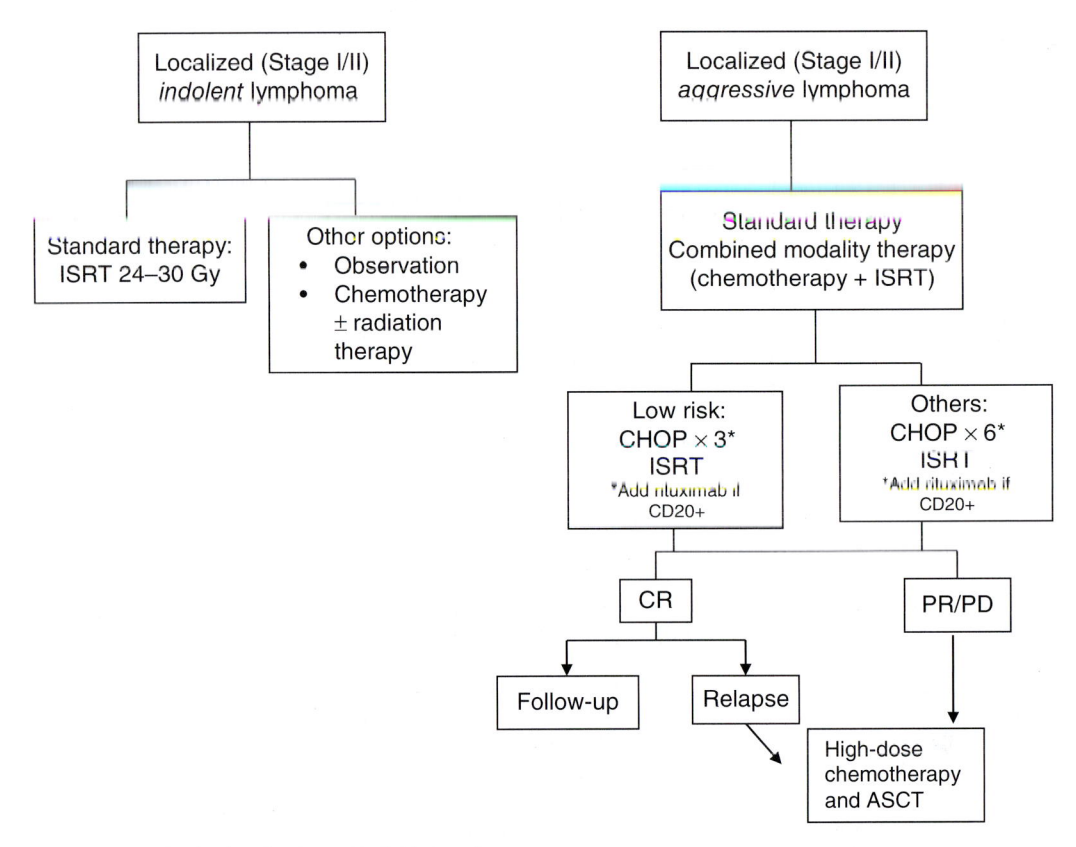

Figure 32.2 Treatment strategies for localized non-Hodgkin lymphoma.
ISRT, involved site radiation therapy; CR, complete remission; PR, partial remission; PD, progressive disease; ASCT, autologous stem cell transplantation.

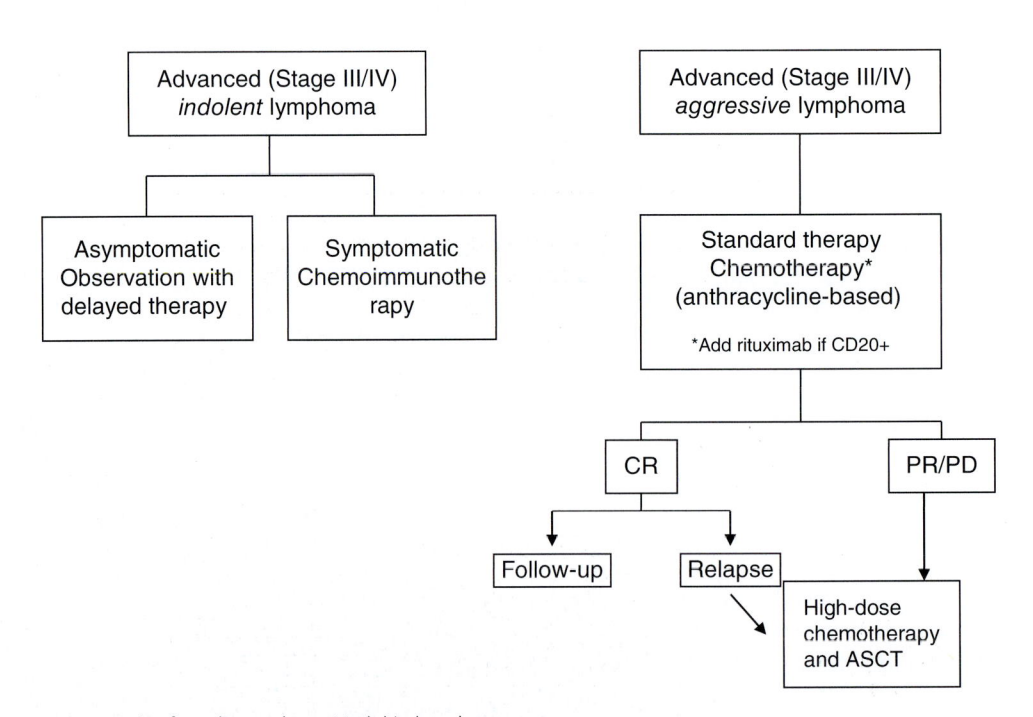

Figure 32.3 Treatment strategies for advanced non-Hodgkin lymphoma.
CR, complete remission; PR, partial remission; PD, progressive disease; ASCT, autologous stem cell transplantation.

Treatment

See Table 32.3.

Treatment: Mature B-cell lymphomas (ranked according to frequency*)	Description

Diffuse large B-cell lymphoma (DLBCL) (31% of non-Hodgkin lymphoma)	• Considered the prototypic aggressive lymphoma, as treatment strategies for other rarer aggressive lymphomas follow a similar approach to DLBCL
	• CD20+: hence addition of rituximab to chemotherapy is standard
	• Subtypes may require a different approach, e.g. primary DLBCL of the CNS require methotrexate-based chemotherapy rather than CHOP
	• 'Dual translocation' cases (involving *Bcl-2* and *c-MYC*) have a poor prognosis
	• *Stage I/II*:
	  ▪ Low-risk non-bulky cases (mIPI 0–1; see Box 32.2): brief chemotherapy (R-CHOP × 3) followed by radiation 35–40 Gy in 1.75–2-Gy fractions
	  ▪ Other Stage I/II: full cycles of chemotherapy (R-CHOP × 6) followed by radiation 30–40 Gy
	  ▪ Option of chemotherapy alone with 4–6 cycles of R-CHOP for non-bulky presentations, or if radiation therapy cannot be safely given
	  ▪ Can expect 5-year FFS of 80% and OS 90%
	• *Stage III/IV*:
	  ▪ Chemotherapy is the mainstay of treatment (R-CHOP × 6–8)
	  ▪ Option of consolidation radiation therapy for sites of residual disease to improve local control
	  ▪ Can expect 5-year FFS of 65–70% and OS 75–80%
	  ▪ IPI (see Box 32.2) or similar prognostic indices are useful to predict outcome
	• Some specific scenarios with a high risk of CNS disease may warrant CNS prophylaxis with high-dose methotrexate ± intrathecal chemotherapy (e.g. primary testis lymphoma)

Follicular lymphoma (22%)	• Considered the prototypic indolent lymphoma, as treatment strategies for other rarer indolent lymphomas follow the approach for follicular carcinoma
	• CD20+: hence addition of rituximab to chemotherapy is standard
	• In advanced stage, considered to be non-curable, hence observation approach if asymptomatic:
	  ▪ Rate of transformation to aggressive lymphoma (DLBCL) of 1–3%/year does not appear to be increased among those managed initially with observation
	• *Stage I/II*:
	  ▪ Involved site radiation therapy (ISRT) to 24–30 Gy
	  ▪ Option of observation or chemotherapy if radiation therapy cannot be safely given
	  ▪ Can expect 10-year FFS of 50% and OS of 70–80%
	• *Stage III/IV*:
	  ▪ 'Watch and wait' if asymptomatic
	  ▪ Others:
	    ○ Chemoimmunotherapy is the mainstay of treatment
	    ○ Options range from mild therapy with a single oral agent (chlorambucil) to multiagent regimens varying in intensity/toxicity
	    ○ Most common regimens are: R-CVP, R-CHOP and bendamustine + rituximab
	    ○ Maintenance rituximab single agent every 2–3 months for 2 years is standard
	    ○ Low-dose radiation therapy, with 4 Gy in two fractions or conventional 20–24 Gy, can be of palliative benefit
	    ○ Can expect 5-year FFS of 50–60% and OS of 80–90%
	• Other treatment options include:
	  ▪ Interferon
	  ▪ Radioimmunotherapy (anti-CD20 based), either with ^{90}Y-ibritumomab or ^{131}I-tositumomab tiuxetan
	  ▪ Patients with multiply relapsing disease can be considered for autologous stem cell transplantation

(continued)

Treatment: Mature B-cell lymphomas (ranked according to frequency*)	Description
Small lymphocytic lymphoma/chronic lymphocytic leukaemia (SLL) (6%)	• CD20+: hence rituximab often added to chemotherapy combinations • Chemotherapy using a variety of regimens: 　▪ Chlorambucil, fludarabine, cyclophosphamide, and bendamustine in combination with rituximab • CD52 antibody alemtuzumab has been used in second-line setting, particularly in patients with TP53 deletion • Very promising results have been seen with the recently approved BTK inhibitor ibrutinib and the PI3 kinase delta inhibitor idelalisib in relapsed and refractory patients • Low-dose RT with 4 Gy in two fractions can be of palliative benefit • Median survival can vary from 15 years (asymptomatic Rai stage 0) to as short as 2 years (for those with anaemia and thrombocytopenia, Rai stage III/IV and 17p– at diagnosis)
Mantle cell lymphoma (MCL) (6% of NHL)	• CD20+: hence addition of rituximab to chemotherapy is standard • *Stage I/II*: 　▪ CMT with R-CHOP × 6 followed by consolidation radiation therapy 30–35 Gy 　▪ High-risk Stage II patients can be treated as for advanced stage • *Stage III/IV*: 　▪ Conventional chemotherapy is not curative, with frequent relapses (median survival 3–5 years) 　▪ No accepted standard regimen and therefore the intensity of the treatment is age/performance status-dependent and risk adapted 　▪ In younger patients achieving remission of disease with chemotherapy with R-CHOP (or equivalent) alternating with ara-C-containing regimens such as DHAP followed by ASCT, or hyper-CVAD, selected patients can expect 3-year FFS of 60–70% and OS of 70–80% 　▪ In older patients or those not candidates for ASCT, combination regimens of bendamustine + rituximab or R-CHOP result in better FFS than R-CVP or FCR, but all are options depending on performance status and co-morbidities 　▪ Novel drugs are under active investigation, e.g. lenalidomide, ibrutinib 　▪ MCL is radiosensitive and radiation therapy can be useful as palliative treatment
Extranodal marginal zone lymphoma, MALT type (5%)	• CD20+: hence addition of rituximab to chemotherapy is standard • *Gastric MALT lymphoma*: 　▪ When associated with *H. pylori* infection, eradication of the organism with established antibiotic regimens is the treatment of choice and is highly successful: 　　○ Complete regression of the lymphoma may take 12–18 months • Similarly, IPSID is known to respond to broad-spectrum antibiotics and there is some evidence of antibiotics eradicating orbital lymphoma and skin lymphoma, but the results are more variable • *Stage I/II (any site, or antibiotic-resistant gastric MALT lymphoma)*: 　▪ Radiation therapy of the involved site 25–30 Gy 　▪ For disease that is surgically resectable without compromising function and with an acceptable cosmetic outcome, surgery may be preferable: 　　○ E.g. localized skin lesions, or hemithyroidectomy for thyroid MALT lymphoma • *Stage III/IV*: 　▪ Conventional chemotherapy is not curative, but is associated with high response rates of ~90% 　▪ Approach is similar to that for advanced-stage follicular lymphoma (see above) • Regardless of stage, MALT lymphoma has a good prognosis: 　▪ Stage I/II patients treated with radiotherapy have a 5-year FFS of 80% and OS of 90–95% 　▪ Stage III/IV patients have similar prognosis, although occasionally transformation to DLBCL can occur and more aggressive treatment is required

Treatment: Mature B-cell lymphomas (ranked according to frequency*)	Description

Primary mediastinal (thymic) large B-cell lymphoma (2%)	• *Stage I/II*:
	    ▪ CMT with R-CHOP × 6 followed by consolidation radiation therapy 30–40 Gy
	    ▪ Cohort data suggest that intensified regimens, such as MACOP-B/VACOP-B, give better results (combined with radiation), and DA-EPOCH alone may also be very effective (without consolidation radiation)
	    ▪ Can expect 5-year FFS and OS of 75–80%
	• *Stage III/IV*:
	    ▪ Chemotherapy is the mainstay of treatment (R-CHOP × 6–8) as for DLBCL
	    ▪ Consolidation radiation therapy for the initially bulky mediastinal site is often useful due to the common finding of residual abnormality post chemotherapy, particularly if there is persistent FDG-PET uptake
	    ▪ Can expect similar prognosis to similarly treated DLBCL cases according to the IPI (see Box 32.2)

Marginal zone lymphoma, nodal type (1%)	• CD20+: hence addition of rituximab to chemotherapy is standard
	• Because of rarity, optimal treatment is not defined but the general approach follows that of indolent lymphomas
	• *Stage I/II*:
	    ▪ Similar approach to localized follicular lymphoma or MALT lymphoma:
	        ○ Radiation therapy 24–30 Gy
	• *Stage III/IV*:
	    ▪ If asymptomatic, 'watch and wait' approach
	    ▪ For symptomatic disease, chemotherapy as for follicular lymphoma/marginal zone lymphoma
	    ▪ 5-year OS of 60–80%, depending on FLIPI prognostic index (see Box 32.3)

Lymphoplasmacytic lymphoma (1%)	• Management approach is similar to that for other indolent lymphomas
	• Asymptomatic patients can be observed
	• Hyperviscosity if present can be treated with plasmapheresis prior to cytoreductive therapy
	• Choice of chemotherapy is largely dictated by the condition of the patient and co-morbidities:
	    ▪ Active agents include rituximab, fludarabine and other nucleoside analogues, alkylating agents chlorambucil and cyclophosphamide, and bendamustine, as single agents or in combinations (CVP or FC)
	• Can expect median survival of 5–10 years:
	    ▪ Prognosis associated with age, performance status and degree of cytopenias

Burkitt lymphoma (<1%)	• Potentially curable with brief intensive combination chemotherapy, with attention to managing tumour lysis syndrome when treatment is initiated:
	    ▪ CNS prophylaxis is required
	    ▪ A typical regimen is CODOX-M-IVAC as proposed by Magrath, consisting of fractionated doses of cyclophosphamide, high-dose IV methotrexate (for CNS effect), incorporation of doxorubicin + ara-C + ifosfamide + etoposide
	• Expected 5-year OS of 50–70%, depending on tumour burden:
	    ▪ High tumour burden (unresected masses >10 cm, high LDH), bone marrow and/or CNS involvement predict for poor prognosis
	    ▪ Children do better than adults

Splenic B-cell marginal zone lymphoma (<1%)	• Splenectomy may improve cytopenias and induce durable remission of the disease • Rituximab in combination with CVP, bendamustine or FC is standard for those requiring systemic therapy, followed by rituximab maintenance • Indolent clinical course expected, although if transformation occurs (to an aggressive lymphoma), the prognosis is less favourable

Primary cutaneous follicle centre lymphoma (<1%)	• Local treatment is highly successful (surgical excision or radiation therapy):
	    ▪ Radiation therapy doses of 24–35 Gy will produce durable remission
	    ▪ Relapse in 20%, usually in skin; extracutaneous sites of relapse in <10%
	• Patients with multifocal skin disease may be observed (if minimally symptomatic)
	• Chemotherapy for symptomatic progression using drugs as for indolent lymphomas (rituximab or combinations)
	• Expected 5-year OS ~95%

(continued)

Treatment: Mature B-cell lymphomas (ranked according to frequency*)	Description
Plasmablastic lymphoma (<1%)	• As for DLBCL, or with more intensive regimens: ▪ Incorporating agents active in plasma cell myeloma (bortezomib) is sometimes attempted but prognosis is usually poor
Other rare B-cell lymphomas	• Treatment approach follows the paradigm of DLBCL

*As reported by the NHL Classification Project 1998.

Treatment: Mature T-cell lymphomas (ranked according to frequency*)	Description

Anaplastic large-cell lymphoma (ALCL) ALK+ and ALK− types (2%)	• *Stage I/II*:
	  ▪ Similar to approach for DLBCL, with CMT
	• *Stage III/IV*:
	  ▪ Combination anthracycline-containing chemotherapy ± etoposide 6–8 cycles (without rituximab)
	• Prognosis is very favourable for the ALK+ subtype:
	  ▪ Best clinical outcomes amongst all non-cutaneous T-cell lymphomas
	  ▪ 5-year OS 70%, compared with 49% for ALK− subtype, based on the ITLP
	  ▪ Children with ALCL ALK+ have an even better prognosis: expected 5-year OS of ~90%
	• Immunoconjugate brentuximab vedotin has excellent clinical activity and is under active investigation as primary treatment (in combination with chemotherapy) and for recurrent/refractory disease

Primary cutaneous CD30+ T-cell lymphoproliferative disorders (<1%)	• *c-ALCL*:
	  ▪ When localized, local radiation therapy (30–40 Gy) is treatment of choice, with favourable outcomes:
	    ○ 5-year FFS and OS of approximately 90%
	  ▪ Even when disseminated, the prognosis is relatively favourable and the clinical course is usually indolent
	• *Lymphomatoid papulosis*:
	  ▪ As the disease is self-remitting and runs a benign course, no cytotoxic treatment is indicated, unless it transforms to a T-cell lymphoma

Mycosis fungoides and Sézary syndrome	• Very early stage with localized patch (uncommon):
	  ▪ Local radiation therapy with good prognosis
	  ▪ Limited skin involvement can be managed with skin-directed topical therapy (topical nitrogen mustard) or psoralen ultraviolet A ray therapy (PUVA)
	• Advanced skin involvement:
	  ▪ Many options:
	    ○ Total body skin electron beam therapy
	    ○ Systemic chemotherapy, with agents such as vorinostat, romedepsin, interferon-α, denileukin difitox, pralatrexate and conventional multiagent chemotherapy (e.g. CHOP)
	  ▪ Treatment is not curative and choice is usually dictated by patient factors such as age, performance status and the clinical aggressiveness of the disease course
	• Aggressive forms of the disease including Sézary syndrome have poor prognosis with 5-year survival of ~15%

Angioimmunoblastic T-cell lymphoma (AITL) (2%)	• Conventional combination chemotherapy (e.g. CHOP) gives response rates of 50–60%, but usually this is not durable • Median survival is a little over a year, 5-year FFS 18% and OS 33%, with patients often succumbing to complications due to infection
Adult T-cell leukaemia/lymphoma (ATLL) (<1%)	• Conventional combination chemotherapy (e.g. CHOP) usually does not result in durable responses • Intensive multiagent regimens are under active investigation and have been associated with better FFS in studies from Asia, but without improvement in OS

Treatment: Mature T-cell lymphomas (ranked according to frequency*)	Description
	• Combination of interferon and zidovudine has resulted in disease response and delay in progression in patients with the acute presentation of ATLL, but is generally not beneficial for those presenting with lymphoma • 5-year OS is 14%, although the less frequent smouldering type can have a better 5-year OS of 60%
Enteropathy-associated T-cell lymphoma (EATL) (<1%)	• Anthracycline-containing chemotherapy, although treatment is generally poorly tolerated by the patient • Prognosis is poor: 5-year FFS of 4% and OS of 20% (median survival 10 months) based on the ITLP

Extranodal NK/T-cell lymphoma, nasal type (<1%)	• Stage I/II:
	  • Radiation therapy (45–55 Gy) alone or combined with radiosensitizing chemotherapy (e.g. cisplatin), followed by combination chemotherapy with ifosfamide + cisplatin + etoposide + dexamethasone
	  • Conventional CHOP chemotherapy is relatively ineffective, with 5-year OS of 35–40%, while initial radiation therapy approaches gave better results
	• Stage III/IV:
	  • Combination chemotherapy, although conventional approaches give dismal results (5-year OS <5%):
	    ◦ More intensive regimens, usually ifosfamide based, with incorporation of L-asparaginase (e.g. the SMILE regimen) may be associated with a better outcome

Lymphoblastic lymphoma (2%)	• Intensive chemotherapy as for acute lymphoblastic leukaemia, including CNS-directed therapy • Prognosis is much worse for adults compared with children

Other rare T-cell lymphomas (not discussed in detail)	• Treatment approach follows the paradigm of other aggressive T-cell lymphomas, e.g. PTCL-NOS, or leukaemias:
	  • T-cell prolymphocytic leukaemia
	  • Aggressive NK-cell leukaemia
	  • EBV-positive T-cell lymphoproliferative disease of childhood
	  • Hepatosplenic T-cell lymphoma
	  • Subcutaneous panniculitis-like T-cell lymphoma
	  • Primary cutaneous peripheral T-cell lymphomas, rare subtypes

*As reported by the NHL Classification Project 1998.

Refractory and relapsed non-Hodgkin lymphoma

The treatment approach for refractory and relapsed aggressive non-Hodgkin lymphoma is most often still curative in intent, with combination salvage chemotherapy regimens (e.g. DHAP, ICE, if CD20+ add rituximab), followed by autologous haematopoietic stem cell transplantation, with or without the addition of radiation therapy. Patients whose disease demonstrates response to the salvage chemotherapy proceed to transplantation. An overall 5-year disease-free survival rate of 40–50% can be expected for patients who are transplant eligible.

Where transplant is contraindicated, the approach is usually palliative in intent. Selected patients with localized small volume relapse of the disease in the original site(s) and not initially treated with radiation may do well with radiation therapy.

For anaplastic large-cell lymphoma with robust positivity for CD30, the use of brentuximab vedotin in salvage therapy regimens may improve the outcome. The use of FDG-PET following salvage chemotherapy may guide the use of subsequent therapy such as radiation therapy.

For indolent lymphomas, typically follicular lymphoma or marginal zone lymphoma, including MALT lymphoma, the treatment of refractory and relapsed disease is based on whether there are symptoms, the goals of therapy, prior disease-free interval, prior exposure to cytotoxic regimens, age, co-morbidity and performance status of the patient. The approach can vary from cautious observation to recommending intensive treatment approaches such as an allogeneic haematopoietic stem cell transplant.

Areas of research

Much effort in the last 10–15 years has been devoted to identifying and characterizing unique disease entities in the category of non-Hodgkin lymphomas. This has led to the

World Health Organization classification (4th edition), which describes these disease entities and the clinicopathological (and molecular, where relevant) characteristics, setting the stage for further work in defining clinical outcomes and improving the treatment strategy for each and every disease entity. The challenge has also been to study the rare disease entities, e.g. some of the T-cell lymphomas. Further progress will be in the following areas.

- Identification of:
  - Molecular signatures of specific lymphoma histologies, relating them to prognosis and clinical outcome, and developing new targets for therapy
  - Effective new drugs and drug combinations, emphasizing targeted therapies and combining targeted drugs with conventional therapies
- Conduct of clinical trials to tailor the treatment approach based on disease characteristics and specific histological types
- Trials to incorporate the response to initial treatment, i.e. interim metabolic response, in an overall strategy to individualize the treatment approach based on early response
- Optimize management of survivorship issues, including detection, monitoring and treatment of late effects such as fatigue, gonadal dysfunction/reproduction, immune dysfunction, cardiac disease and second malignancies.

Recommended reading

NHL in general and B-cell lymphomas

Cheson BD, Pfistner B, Juweid ME et al. (2007) Revised response criteria for malignant lymphoma. *J Clin Oncol* 25:579–586.

Dunleavy K, Pittaluga S, Maeda LS et al. (2013) Dose-adjusted EPOCH-rituximab therapy in primary mediastinal B-cell lymphoma. *N Engl J Med* 368:1408–1416.

Hasenclever D, Diehl V (1998) A prognostic score for advanced Hodgkin's disease. International Prognostic Factors Project on Advanced Hodgkin's Disease. *N Engl J Med* 339(21):1506–1514.

Horning SJ, Weller E, Kim K et al. (2004) Chemotherapy with or without radiotherapy in limited-stage diffuse aggressive non-Hodgkin's lymphoma: Eastern Cooperative Oncology Group study 1484. *J Clin Oncol* 22:3032–3038.

Hoskin PJ, Diez P, Williams M et al. (2013) Recommendations for the use of radiotherapy in nodal lymphoma. *Clin Oncol* 25:49–58.

Lowry L, Smith P, Qian W et al. (2011) Reduced dose radiotherapy for local control in non-Hodgkin lymphoma: a randomised phase III trial. *Radiother Oncol* 100:86–92.

Mead GM, Sydes MR, Walewski J et al. (2002) An international evaluation of CODOX-M alternating with IVAC in adult Burkitt's lymphoma: results of United Kingdom Lymphoma Group LY06 study. *Ann Oncol* 13:1264–1274.

Meignan M, Barrington S, Itti E et al. (2014) Report on the 4th International Workshop on Positron Emission Tomography in Lymphoma held in Menton, France, 3–5 October 2012. *Leuk Lymphoma* 55:31–37.

Miller TP, Dahlberg S, Cassady JR et al. (1998) Chemotherapy alone compared with chemotherapy plus radiotherapy for localized intermediate- and high-grade non-Hodgkin's lymphoma. *N Engl J Med* 339:21–26.

Pfreundschuh M, Trumper L, Osterborg A et al. (2006) CHOP-like chemotherapy plus rituximab versus CHOP-like chemotherapy alone in young patients with good-prognosis diffuse large-B-cell lymphoma: a randomised controlled trial by the MabThera International Trial (MInT) Group. *Lancet Oncol* 7(5):379–391.

Pfreundschuh M, Schubert J, Ziepert M et al. (2008) Six versus eight cycles of bi-weekly CHOP-14 with or without rituximab in elderly patients with aggressive CD20+ B-cell lymphomas: a randomised controlled trial (RICOVER-60). *Lancet Oncol* 9:105–116.

Pfreundschuh M, Ho AD, Cavallin-Stahl E et al. (2008) Prognostic significance of maximum tumour (bulk) diameter in young patients with good-prognosis diffuse large-B-cell lymphoma treated with CHOP-like chemotherapy with or without rituximab: an exploratory analysis of the MabThera International Trial Group (MInT) study. *Lancet Oncol* 9:435–444.

Reyes F, Lepage E, Ganem G et al. (2005) ACVBP versus CHOP plus radiotherapy for localized aggressive lymphoma. *N Engl J Med* 352:1197–1205.

Salles G, Seymour JF, Offner F et al. (2011) Rituximab maintenance for 2 years in patients with high tumour burden follicular lymphoma responding to rituximab plus chemotherapy (PRIMA): a phase 3, randomised controlled trial. *Lancet* 377:42–51.

Specht L, Yahalom J, Illidge T et al. (2014) Modern radiation therapy for Hodgkin lymphoma: field and dose guidelines from the International Lymphoma Radiation Oncology Group (ILROG). *Int J Radiat Oncol Biol Phys* 89(1):49–58.

Swerdlow SH, Campo E, Harris NL et al. (2008) WHO Classification of Tumours of Haematopoietic and Lymphoid tissues. In: Bosman FT, Jaffe ES, Lakhani SR et al., eds. *World Health Organization Classification of Tumours*, 4th edn. Lyon: IARC Press.

Vose JM (2013) Mantle cell lymphoma: 2013 Update on diagnosis, risk-stratification, and clinical management. *Am J Hematol* 88:1082–1088.

Willemze R, Meijer CJ (2000) EORTC classification for primary cutaneous lymphomas: a comparison with the R.E.A.L. Classification and the proposed WHO Classification. *Ann Oncol* 11(Suppl 1):11–15.

Willemze R, Hodak E, Zinzani PL et al. (2013) Primary cutaneous lymphomas: ESMO Clinical Practice Guidelines for diagnosis, treatment and follow-up. *Ann Oncol* 24(Suppl 6):vi149–54.

T-cell lymphomas

Delabie J, Holte H, Vose JM et al. (2011) Enteropathy-associated T-cell lymphoma: clinical and histological findings from the international peripheral T-cell lymphoma project. *Blood* 118:148–155.

Federico M, Rudiger T, Bellei M et al. (2013) Clinicopathologic characteristics of angioimmunoblastic T-cell lymphoma: analysis of the international peripheral T-cell lymphoma project. *J Clin Oncol* 31:240–246.

Iqbal J, Wright G, Wang C et al. (2014) Gene expression signatures delineate biologic and prognostic subgroups in peripheral T-cell lymphoma. *Blood* 123(19):2915–2923.

Schmitz N, Trümper L, Ziepert M et al. (2010) Treatment and prognosis of mature T-cell and NK-cell lymphoma: an analysis of patients with T-cell lymphoma treated in studies of the German High-Grade Non-Hodgkin Lymphoma Study Group. *Blood* 116(18):3418–3425.

Vose J, Armitage J, Weisenburger D et al. (2008) International peripheral T-cell and natural killer/T-cell lymphoma study: pathology findings and clinical outcomes. *J Clin Oncol* 26:4124–4130.

33 Myeloma

J. San Miguel[1], P. Rodríguez-Otero[1], E. M. Ocio[2], B. Paiva[1], N. Gutierrez[2] and M. V. Mateos[2]

[1]Clínica Universidad de Navarra, CIMA, IDISNA, Navarra, Spain
[2]Haematology Department, University Hospital of Salamanca, IBSAL, Salamanca, Spain

Summary	Key facts

Introduction	- Multiple myeloma is a neoplastic haematological disorder characterized by proliferation of clonal plasma cells
	- It accounts for 1% of all cancers and 10% of all haematological malignancies (the second most common one)
	- Myeloma arises in most cases from a premalignant stage termed monoclonal gammopathy of undetermined significance (MGUS):
	  - Present in >3% of the population over the age of 50 years
	  - Eventually goes through an intermediate phase of SMM

Presentation	- Diagnosis of (symptomatic) multiple myeloma requires ≥10% clonal plasma cells in the bone marrow aspirate or a biopsy proven plasmacytoma, monoclonal protein in serum and/or urine, and evidence of end-organ damage (CRAB): hyperCalcaemia (uncommon), Renal impairment (~20–40%), Anaemia (~70%) or Bone lesions (~80%):
	  - In the absence of CRAB, the presence of >60% plasma cells, a free light chain (FLC) ratio of ≥100 or more than one focal lesion on magnetic resonance imaging (MRI) qualify for early myeloma
	- Bone marrow morphological examination, electrophoretic analysis of the monoclonal paraprotein and conventional X-rays remain the 'gold standard' techniques for fast, accurate and cost-effective diagnosis, as well as a detailed medical history, physical examination and routine laboratory testing:
	  - Nevertheless, imaging techniques such as MRI, positron emission tomography-computed tomography (PET-CT) are highly valuable

Scenario	- Symptomatic (active) disease should be treated immediately, whereas smouldering multiple myeloma (SMM) or MGUS requires only clinical observation (with the exception of high-risk smouldering disease that can be included in clinical trials)
	- Treatment modality is mostly related to age:
	  - Patients under 65 years receive induction with novel agents followed by high-dose therapy/autologous stem cell transplantation (HDT/ASCT)
	  - Patients over 65 years (or under 65 if unfit to tolerate HDT/ASCT) usually receive proteasome inhibitors or immunomodulatory drugs (IMiDs) in combination with alkylating agents and corticosteroids
	- Consolidation/maintenance after upfront treatment is commonly used, but not yet standard of care
	- Allogeneic haematopoietic stem cell transplantation (allo-HSCT) may be an option for high-risk patients at early relapse after optimal upfront treatment including ASCT, but within clinical trials

Trials	- Attal et al. (1996) N Engl J Med 335(2):91–97:
	  - High-dose therapy combined with transplantation improved the response rate, event-free survival and overall survival in patients with myeloma
	- San Miguel et al. (2008) N Engl J Med 359(9):906–917:
	  - Bortezomib + melphalan + prednisone was superior to melphalan + prednisone alone in patients with newly diagnosed myeloma who were ineligible for high-dose therapy

(continued)

Summary	Key facts

	• Weber (2007) *N Engl J Med* 357(21):2133–2142; Dimopoulos (2007) *N Engl J Med* 357(21):2123–2132; updated Dimopoulos (2009) *Leukemia* 23(9):1545–1546 (CC-5013-MM009/MM010 trials):
	  ▪ Advantage for lenalidomide + dexamethasone over dexamethasone in terms of response (≥ partial response [PR] 60% vs 22%; complete response [CR] 15% vs 2%), time to progression (TTP) (13.4 vs 4.6 months) and overall survival (OS) (38 vs 32 months, despite a 48% cross-over in the dexamethasone arm)
	• Mateos *et al.* (2013) *N Eng J Med* 369(5):438–447:
	  ▪ In high-risk SMM patients, early treatment with lenalidomide + dexamethasone is associated with a significant delay in TTP to symptomatic disease and longer OS
	• Stewart *et al.* (2015) *N Eng J Med* 372:142–152:
	  ▪ Significant advantage for carfilzomib + lenalidomide + dexamethasone (CRd) vs lenalidomide + dexamethasone (Rd) in terms of response (≥PR 87.1% vs 66.7%), PFS (26.3 vs 17.6 months) and OS (not yet reached)

Introduction

Plasma cell dyscrasias are a heterogeneous group of disorders characterized by deranged proliferation of a single clone of B cells at the last stage of maturation (plasma cells) and usually associated with detectable monoclonal immunoglobulin in serum and/or urine.

This term includes the following entities: monoclonal gammopathies of undetermined significance (MGUS), smouldering multiple myeloma (SMM) (both considered as benign or premalignant disorders), solitary and extramedullary plasmocytomas, multiple myeloma, Waldenström macroglobulinemia, POEMS syndrome (polyneuropathy, organomegaly, endocrinopathy, monoclonal protein, skin changes and primary amyloidosis).

Multiple myeloma is the most frequent malignant, treatment-requiring, plasma cell dyscrasia. Despite recent therapeutic advances that have increased the median survival from 3 years to over 6 years, multiple myeloma continues to be an incurable disease for most patients.

Incidence and aetiology

Incidence and aetiology	Description
Incidence	• Multiple myeloma accounts for 1% of all cancers and approximately 10% of all haematological malignancies: ▪ Each year over 20,000 new cases are diagnosed in the USA • Slightly more common in men than in women • Twice as common in African–Americans compared with Caucasians • Median age at the time of diagnosis is about 65 years

Aetiology	• No well-known direct cause for the development of myeloma:
	  ▪ Increased risk among first-degree relatives and individuals with immune disorders or obesity
	  ▪ Having premalignant MGUS or SMM are the conditions most closely related to the development of active myeloma
	  ▪ Risk factors to predict the malignant transformation have been identified, e.g. serum concentration of the monoclonal protein or the level of (clonal) plasma cells
	• There is the assumption that myeloma always evolves from an asymptomatic premalignant stage of clonal plasma cell proliferation (MGUS); however:
	  ▪ Most MGUS never progress into multiple myeloma
	  ▪ MGUS is present in >3% of the population above the age of 50 years
	  ▪ Progresses to myeloma or related malignancy at a rate of 1% per year
	• MGUS is typically depicted by an excess of one (monoclonal) serum immunoglobulin on routine biochemistry analysis

Pathology

- Plasma cell disorders are characterized by the proliferation of clonal plasma cells in the bone marrow and by the production of monoclonal immunoglobulins
- Myeloma-related organ or tissue impairment (end-organ damage) is a critical aspect in the differentiation of MGUS and SMM from symptomatic treatment-requiring multiple myeloma:
  - End-organ damage attributed to the underlying plasma cell proliferative disorder is defined by at least one of the following criteria:
    ○ Hypercalcaemia: serum calcium >11.5 mg/dL

- Renal insufficiency: serum creatinine >2 mg/dL (creatinine clearance <40 mL/min)
- Anaemia: normochromic, normocytic with a haemoglobin value of >2 g/dL below the lower limit of normal, or a haemoglobin value of <10 g/dL
- Bone lesions: lytic lesions on skeletal radiography, CT or PET-CT

Presentation and natural history

Based on clinical and biological data, a multistep model of disease progression, starting with MGUS and ending with symptomatic myeloma, sometimes with the intermediate entity (SMM), has been proposed. Both MGUS and SMM are considered to be precursors of active multiple myeloma. However, the rate of progression of these two premalignant conditions to symptomatic multiple myeloma differs greatly. Thus, while MGUS evolves to multiple myeloma or a related malignancy at a rate of 1% per year, the cumulative probability of progression to active multiple myeloma in SMM is 10% per year in the first 5 years.

Patients may present with pain (mainly back pain) or fatigue (due to anaemia). In asymptomatic patients the disease is detected on a routine analysis due to an elevated erythrocyte sedimentation rate (ESR) or a serum M component.

Diagnostic work-up

Diagnostic work-up	Description

Assessment of patient profile	• Clinical history and physical examination:
	  ▪ To assess pain, asthenia, co-morbidities (heart, lung, renal, peripheral neuropathy, liver disease), amyloid symptoms and clinical signs of hypercalcaemia
	• Complete blood count and differential:
	  ▪ Look for anaemia – CRAB, neutropenia, thrombocytopenia
	• Chemistry including calcium and creatinine; $\beta 2$-microglobulin and lactate dehydrogenase (LDH):
	  ▪ Look for hypercalcaemia or renal impairment – CRAB
	• Assessment of International Staging System (ISS; see Table 33.1) specifically requires that in addition to $\beta 2$ microglobulin, albumin is measured

Assessment of tumour profile	• Serum protein electrophoresis and immunofixation (to quantify and characterize the monoclonal protein, respectively) plus immunoglobulin quantitation by nephelometry
	• Routine urinalysis on 24-hour urine collection for electrophoresis and immunofixation to identify and quantify Bence Jones proteinuria
	• Measurement of serum free light chains, particularly for the management (diagnosis and follow-up) of non-secretory or oligosecretory patients, and in light chain (AL) amyloidosis
	• Cytogenetics (typically evaluated by fluorescent *in situ* hybridization [FISH] on purified plasma cells) has become one of the most important prognostic factors, and is considered mandatory for all patients with newly diagnosed myeloma:
	  ▪ Presence of t(4; 14), t(14; 16) and/or del(17p), and probably chromosome 1 abnormalities, currently define high-risk disease
	• Immunophenotyping is performed in some centres and determines the degree of clonality from the balance between normal and clonal plasma cells:
	  ▪ Clonal plasma cells are identified by their aberrant phenotypes, which are also informative for MRD monitoring
	  ▪ Associated with higher risk of transformation in patients with MGUS or SMM

Assessment of tumour extent	• Conventional microscopy to quantify and morphologically characterize plasma cell infiltration in the bone marrow aspirate
	• Trephine biopsy is particularly indicated for patients with suspected myeloma and low marrow plasmacytosis
	• Skeletal survey remains the gold standard to evaluate bone disease:
	  ▪ Should include skull, cervical, thoracic and lumbar spine, femura, humeri, chest and pelvis X-ray evaluation
	• Magnetic resonance imaging (MRI):
	  ▪ Considered mandatory in presumed diagnosis of solitary plasmacytoma, for detailed evaluation of a painful skeletal area, where there is suspicion of cord compression and before kyphoplastia
	  ▪ Highly recommended in SMM
	• Computed tomography (CT):
	  ▪ Recommended to evaluate a painful area that appeared normal on X-ray
	  ▪ Low-dose whole-body CT may become a new standard for evaluation of bone disease
	• Positron emission tomography (PET)/CT:
	  ▪ May be informative in the assessment of total marrow involvement and extramedullary disease
	  ▪ Role in myeloma is yet to be fully established; therefore not recommended for routine purposes, unless high LDH or suspected extramedullary disease

(continued)

Diagnostic criteria	Description
Monoclonal gammopathy of undetermined significance (all three criteria must be met)	• Serum monoclonal protein <3 g/dL • Clonal bone marrow plasma cells <10% • Absence of end-organ damage
Smouldering or asymptomatic multiple myeloma (both criteria must be met)	• Serum monoclonal protein (IgG or IgA) ≥3 g/dL and/or clonal bone marrow plasma cells ≥10% • Absence of end-organ damage
Multiple myeloma (all three criteria must be met)	• Clonal bone marrow plasma cells >10% • Presence of serum and/or urinary monoclonal protein (except in patients with non-secretory multiple myeloma) • Evidence of end-organ damage • In the absence of end-organ damage, the presence of >60% PC, a FLC ratio of >100 or more than one focal lesion on MRI qualify a patient for early multiple myeloma treatment
Plasma cell leukaemia	• Most aggressive variant of the human monoclonal gammopathies • Presence of >20% plasma cells in peripheral blood and an absolute plasma cell count of >2 × 10^9/L
Solitary plasmacytoma of bone (all the criteria must be met)	• Single area of bone destruction due to clonal plasma cells • No M-protein in serum and/or urine; if present, should be a small M-component • Bone marrow not consistent with multiple myeloma • Normal skeletal survey and no related organ or tissue impairment (other than a solitary bone lesion)
Extramedullary plasmacytoma	• Plasma cell tumour that arises outside the bone marrow • No M-protein in serum and/or urine, although a small M-component may sometimes be present • Bone marrow not consistent with multiple myeloma • Normal skeletal survey and no related organ or tissue impairment (including bone lesion)

Staging of plasma cell neoplasms

Patients with multiple myeloma may show very variable disease courses, with survival ranging between a few months and more than a decade. The clinical and laboratory staging system originally developed by Salmon and Durie (1975) has been replaced by the International Staging System (ISS) as therapies and their effect on outcome have improved considerably over time (Table 33.1).

Prognostic risk factors (Table 33.2)

The outcome for patients with multiple myeloma is highly heterogeneous with a survival ranging from a few months to >10

Table 33.1 International Staging System (ISS) for multiple myeloma

Stage	Criteria	Median survival (months)
I	Serum β2 microglobulin <3.5 mg/L Serum albumin ≥ 3.5 g/dL	62
II	Neither stage I nor III	44
III	Serum β2-microglobulin >5.5 mg/L	29

Data source: Greipp (2005)

Table 33.2 Prognostic factors for survival for multiple myeloma

Prognostic factors	Tumour related	Host related	Environment related
Essential	t(4; 14) 17p deletions Chromosome 1 abnormalities: 1q gains and 1p deletions International Staging System (ISS): • *Stage I*: β2-microglobulin <3.5 mg/dL and albumin ≥3.5 mg/dL • *Stage III*: β2-microglobulin >5.5 mg/dL) • *Stage II*: the rest	Age Performance status	Response to initial treatment
Additional	t(14; 16) Hypodiploidy LDH	Co-morbidities	
New and promising	DNA copy number abnormalities by SNP arrays		

Data source: Munshi *et al*, (2011). *Blood*, 117, 4696–700. San-Miguel *et al*, (2009). *Cancer J*, 15, 457–64.

years. This heterogeneity relates to specific characteristics of the tumour itself and of the host.

Treatment philosophy

- Fit elderly patients (65–80 years) and young patients with severe co-morbidities:
  - Treatment goal should be to prolong survival and ensure quality of life
- Very elderly patients (>80–85 years):
  - Treatment plan should ensure quality of life and avoid additional costs of expensive treatments
- Young patients (<65 years):
  - Goal of large cooperative groups should be to investigate therapeutic schemes with a cure on the horizon

Treatment

In clinical practice, the first stratification is usually done according to the age of the patient (65–70 years): transplant or non-transplant candidate. A sequential approach is taken:
- Induction therapy
- High-dose chemotherapy plus autologous stem cell transplantation (ASCT)
- Consolidation/maintenance approaches.

Once the patient relapses/progresses from a first or subsequent line of therapy, the goal of therapy should first be defined for the particular patient. To define this and select the most appropriate treatment, several factors should be taken into consideration:
- General condition of the patient
- Type of relapse
- Efficacy and toxicity of previous treatments
- Further options available.

First-line treatment	Description

Patients younger than 65–70 years or transplant candidates	- Sequential approach
	- *Induction therapy*:
	  - Novel agent-based combinations have replaced VAD (vincristine, adriamycin and dexamethasone) or Thalidomide + dexamethasone
	  - Thalidomide in combination with cyclophosphamide + dexamethasone, or doxorubicin + dexamethasone, are possible options (with complete response [CR] rates in the range of 13–16%), but inferior to proteasome inhibitor combinations
	  - Bortezomib-based combinations are the most widely used:
	    ○ Triple-drug combinations based on bortezomib have become a standard:
	      – Bortezomib + thalidomide + dexamethasone (VTD)
	      – Bortezomib + lenalidomide + dexamethasone (VRD)
	      – Bortezomib + cyclophosphamide + dexamethasone (CyBorD)
	      – Bortezomib + adriamycin + dexamethasone (PAD)
	      – All these novel regimens resulted not only in high CR rates (12–30%), but also in a significant prolongation of the progression-free survival (PFS) (median of 56 months for VTD) as compared with the old standard regimens (28 and 35 months for thalidomide + dexamethasone or conventional chemotherapy, respectively)
	    ○ Bortezomib + dexamethasone is not optimal (CR rates of 6%)
	  - Novel proteasome inhibitors, such as carfilzomib or ixazomib, have been evaluated in phase II clinical trials as part of the induction in combination with lenalidomide + dexamethasone with promising efficacy results (26–40% stringent CR):
	    ○ Phase III randomized trials are currently ongoing
	- *High-dose therapy followed by ASCT*:
	  - Melphalan at dose of 200 mg/m² is the gold standard
	  - Melphalan + ASCT upgrades the overall response rates (40–50%) and CR rates after induction with novel agent-based combinations:
	    ○ Thus, induction with novel agents and melphalan + ASCT are complementary strategies rather than alternatives
	  - Optimization of the conditioning regimen is being investigated by adding other drugs, such as busulphan or bortezomib
	- *Post-ASCT strategies*:
	  - *Consolidation therapy*:
	    ○ Administration of two to three cycles of a regimen similar to the one given as induction, with the goal of improving the quality and depth of response
	    ○ VTD (three cycles) has been used as consolidation after tandem ASCT resulting in a 30% upgrade in CR rate (including an increase in molecular remissions: from 3% to 18%)

(continued)

First-line treatment	Description

	- *Maintenance therapy*:
	  ○ Administration of therapy during a prolonged period of time (≥2 years) to maintain the response previously achieved
	  ○ Thalidomide after ASCT extended the PFS in all six randomized trials (HR = 0.65; 95% CI 0.59–0.72), but the overall survival (OS) was improved only in three of them
	  ○ Three trials with lenalidomide maintenance after ASCT showed a significant prolongation of the PFS (41–46 months vs 22–27 months in the placebo arm) and an increase in the OS in one of them
	  ○ Maintenance therapy with single-agent bortezomib is under investigation:
	    – HOVON group has shown that PAD induction and bortezomib maintenance is superior to VAD + thalidomide maintenance in terms of PFS (35 vs 28 months) and OS (61% vs 55% at 5 years)
	    – Spanish group has shown that VT is superior to thalidomide or interferon for PFS but not for OS
	  ○ Maintenance can be associated with side effects (an increase in second primary malignancies has been reported with lenalidomide)
	  ○ None of the drugs evaluated is currently approved for maintenance therapy
	  ○ Treatment decisions for individual patients must balance potential benefits and risks carefully, as a widely agreed-on standard is not established

Patients older than 65–70 years or not candidates for HDT/ASCT	- Gold standard includes the administration of sequential cycles of novel agent-based combinations, usually completed up to between 9 and 12 months
	- MP + thalidomide (MPT) is standard of care:
	  ▪ Superior to melphalan + prednisone (MP) in six randomized trials in terms of CR rates (10% vs 2.5%), PFS (20.4 vs 15 months) and OS (median advantage of 6 months)
	  ▪ Melphalan + prednisone (MP) should no longer be considered the standard of care because the CR rate is very low with the OS not superior to 3 years
	- Other thalidomide-based combinations are available, such as cyclophosphamide + thalidomide + adjusted dose of dexamethasone (CTDa)
	- MP + bortezomib (VMP):
	  ▪ Superior to MP in a large randomized trial, with benefit in CR rate (30% vs 4%), time to progression and OS (median advantage of 13 months)
	  ▪ Common induction regimen, especially outside the USA
	- MP + lenalidomide (MPR):
	  ▪ Superior to MP in a large randomized trial in terms of CR rate (10% vs 3%), but benefit in terms of PFS was observed only for those patients who received maintenance therapy with lenalidomide (31 months)
	  ▪ Median PFS for MPR without maintenance and MP alone was 14 and 13 months, respectively
	  ▪ No differences have been so far observed in OS
	- Lenalidomide + dexamethasone (Ld):
	  ▪ Continuous Ld is superior to MPT, both in terms of PFS (25.5 vs 20.7 months) and OS (at 4 years 59% vs 51%)
	  ▪ If Ld is given for only 18 cycles, it is not superior to MPT (PFS 21.2 months and OS 55% at 4 years)
	- Toxicity profile is an important concern in elderly patients:
	  ▪ MPT: peripheral neuropathy (grade 3–4 15%) and thrombosis (grade 3–4 6%)
	  ▪ VMP: peripheral neuropathy (grade 3–4: 13%) and gastrointestinal toxicity (grade 3–4: 19%)
	  ▪ MPR: myelosuppression (grade 3–4: 90%)
	  ▪ Rd: infections (28%)
	  ▪ Discontinuation rate due to toxicity has been common for all these drug combinations (30–35%)
	- *Optimization of treatment*:
	  ▪ Objective for elderly patients with multiple myeloma is to reduce the toxicity, improve the tolerability and maintain the efficacy
	  ▪ Thalidomide:
	    ○ Reduce the dose to 100 mg/day or even 50 mg/day
	    ○ Antithrombotic prophylaxis required
	    ○ MPT with reduced doses of MP and thalidomide resulted in grade 3–4 peripheral neuropathy rates of 2%: discontinuation rates were low and OS was prolonged compared with MP in a randomized trial of patients older than 75 years

First-line treatment	Description

	- Bortezomib:
	  ○ Change conventional schedule of administration (once instead of twice per week):
	    – Reduced rate of peripheral neuropathy in the Spanish and Italian trials to around 5% (similar figures for subcutaneous administration), as well as the discontinuation rates
	  ○ Change route of administration (subcutaneous instead of intravenous)
	  ○ Use of maintenance with VT or VP prolongs PFS up to approximately 3 years, but the benefit in terms of OS is not yet well established
	- Lenalidomide:
	  ○ Combination of lenalidomide + low-dose dexamethasone (Rd) continuous
	    – Avoids the use of alkylating agent
	    – Resulted in a significant reduction of adverse events: grade 3–4 neutropenia 20%; grade 3–4 infections 9%
	    – One of the new standards of care

Solitary plasmocytoma	• Solitary plasmacytoma of bone and extramedullary plasmacytoma: ■ Involved field radiation to 40–45 Gy in 1.8–2-Gy fractions over 4–5 weeks with excellent local control

Treatment for relapse	Description

Available therapeutic options	• Treatments approved based on randomized phase III trials:
	  ■ Bortezomib
	  ■ Lenalidomide + dexamethasone
	  ■ Thalidomide + dexamethasone
	  ■ Bortezomib + doxil
	  ■ Carfilzomib*
	  ■ Pomalidomide + dexamethasone*
	
	*Approved based on accelerated approval by the FDA
	
	• Most commonly used:
	  ■ Thalidomide + cyclophosphamide + dexamethasone
	  ■ Lenalidomide + dexamethasone (± adriamycin or cyclophosphamide)
	  ■ Pomalidomide + dexamethasone
	  ■ Bortezomib + dexamethasone (± adriamycin or cyclophosphamide)
	  ■ Bortezomib + lenalidomide + dexamethasone
	  ■ Bendamustine + dexamethasone (± bortezomib or lenalidomide)
	• Recent phase III trial with novel agents:
	  ■ Carfilzomib + lenalidomide + dexamethasone has shown superior PFS (26 vs 17 months) and OS over lenalidomide + dexamethasone
	  ■ Panobinostat + bortezomib + dexamethasone has shown superior PFS (12 vs 8 months) over bortezomib + dexamethasone, with no differences in OS
	  ■ Elotuzumab + lenalidomide + dexamethasone has shown superior PFS (19 vs 14 months) over lenalidomide + dexamethasone, with no differences in OS
	• Novel agents under investigation with promising efficacy:
	  ■ Other oral proteasome inhibitors (MLN9708, oprozomib)
	  ■ Anti-CD38 MoAb (daratumumab/SAR650984)
	  ■ Check-point inhibitors (anti-PD1/PDL1)
	  ■ Kinesin spindle protein inhibitor (Filanesid)
	  ■ Deacetylase inhibitors (panobinostat, rocilinostat)
	  ■ XPO-1 inhibitors (Selinexor)
	• *Factors to take into account to select treatment*:
	  ■ Age and general condition of the patient:
	    ○ Candidate for active treatment (see below and Fig. 33.1)
	    ○ Elderly/unfit patients not candidates for aggressive treatment → palliative care:
	      – Oral cyclophosphamide (50 mg/day) + prednisone (30 mg on alternating days)

Treatment for relapse	Description

	• Type of relapse/progression:
	  ○ *Biochemical (asymptomatic) relapse/progression* → no treatment
	    – Alternative: if the patient is receiving maintenance treatment, the dose may be increased or a steroid added
	  ○ *Non-aggressive relapse/progression* → two drug combinations
	  ○ *Aggressive relapse* → three or more drugs combinations
	    – Chemotherapy + novel agents (VDL-PACE-like regimen) can be an option in young patients
	▪ Duration of previous response after ASCT in young patients:
	  ○ *Early relapse* (<1 year post ASCT):
	    – Goal is to 'overcome drug resistance' → combination of non–cross-resistant agents VDL-PACE or VRD or CRD followed by RIC-Allo
	  ○ *Intermediate relapse* (1–3 years post ASCT):
	    – Goal is to 'prolong survival until curative treatments are developed' → sequential novel agent combinations, starting with a different drug from that used in maintenance
	    – If <55 years and suboptimal response → RIC-Allo
	  ○ *Late relapse* (>3 years):
	    – → Re-induction (with the same or an alternative regimen) + second ASCT
	▪ Treatment used upfront and its efficacy
	• *Factors to take into account to select treatment*:
	▪ Patient's characteristics and previous toxicity:
	  ○ Peripheral neuropathy → lenalidomide or pomalidomide
	  ○ Renal impairment → proteasome inhibitors (immunomodulatory drugs [IMiDs] are a second option)
	  ○ Thromboembolic event → proteasome inhibitors (IMiDs are a second option)
	  ○ Low bone marrow reserve → proteasome inhibitors or thalidomide
	  ○ Poor performance status or long distance to hospital → IMiDs (oral administration)

Second and subsequent relapses	• Decisions should be initially based on the general condition of the patient:
	▪ Candidate for active treatment:
	  ○ Alternative drugs to those previously used or select agent with highest previous sensitivity
	  ○ Experimental agents in clinical trials
	▪ Unfit or non-candidate for active treatment:
	  ○ Palliative care, i.e. oral cyclophosphamide (50 mg/day) + prednisone (30 mg on alternating days)
	▪ Radiation therapy:
	  ○ May be used to palliate bone pain, impending cord compression or pathological fracture
	  ○ Small fields to doses of 8 Gy in a single fraction, or 20 Gy in five fractions of 4 Gy, or 30 Gy in ten fractions of 3 Gy are typical

Post-treatment assessments

At the beginning of each cycle and after pre-planned upfront treatment, the following assessments should be made:

- Lab and clinical examination:
  - Haemoglobin, neutrophil and platelet count, creatinine and calcium
  - Pain
  - Peripheral neuropathy
- Quantification of the monoclonal protein:
  - Serum and urine electrophoresis plus immunofixation
  - Quantification of immunoglobulins (nephelometry)
  - 24-hour urine electrophoresis is recommended in light-chain myeloma
  - Serum free light chains for non-secretory or oligosecretory myeloma
- If complete response (CR) is achieved (no monoclonal protein by immunofixation):
  - Bone marrow aspirate or biopsy to confirm CR (≤5% plasma cells)
  - Serum free light-chains plus immunohistochemistry to confirm stringent CR
  - Minimal residual disease (MRD) assessment by multiparameter flow cytometry or allele-specific oligonucleotide (ASO)-polymerase chain reaction (PCR) to confirm immunophenotypic or molecular CR, respectively
  - PET/CT may be useful to evaluate MRD outside the bone marrow but its exact role is yet to be fully established.

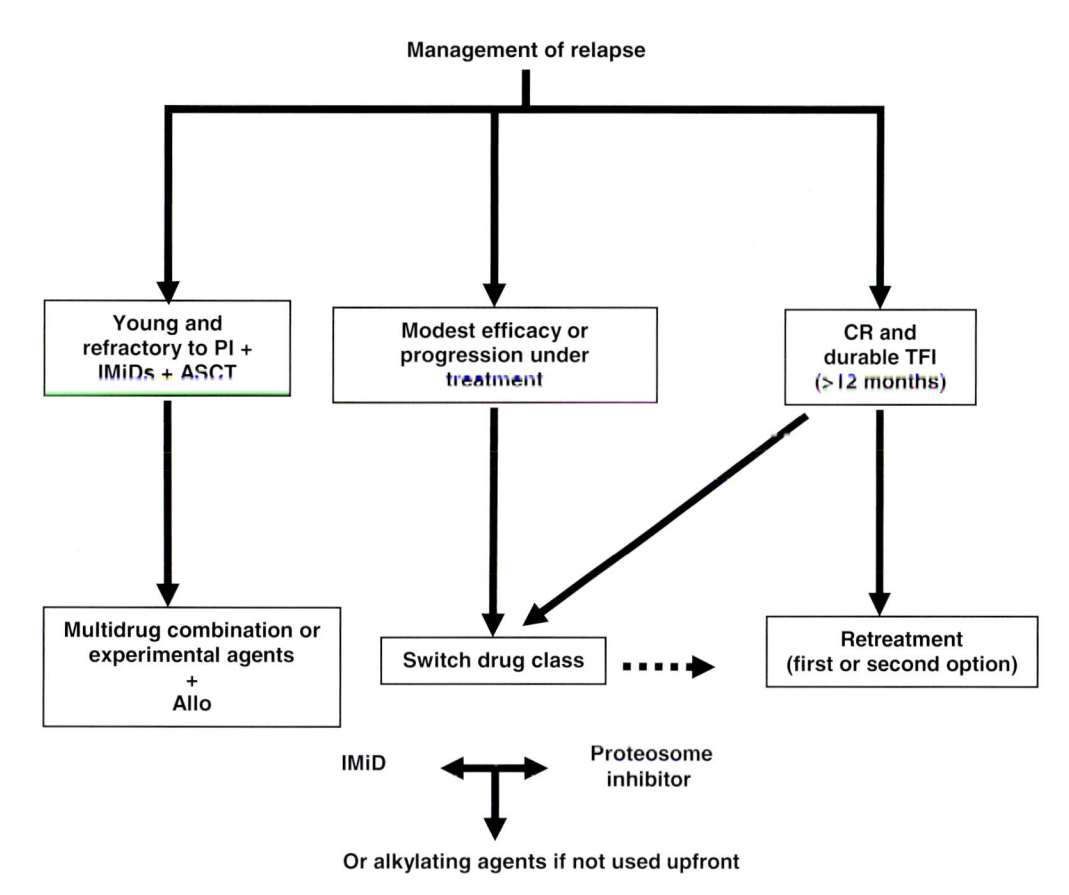

Figure 33.1 Schema for management of relapse. Applies to treatment outside clinical trials. If there is a clinical trial with novel agents available for which the patient is a candidate, this would be the preferred option.
PT, proteasome inhibitor.

controversies

- *New methods of prognostication.* Novel insights into the genomic features of multiple myeloma have led to the publication of molecular classifications and expression signatures with the potential to predict prognostic categories. The crucial step is the translation of genomic signatures into routine clinical diagnostic tools. In fact, although many expectations have been raised with the development of gene expression profiling, it is important to note that so far there is minimal overlap between the different proposed signatures. The ability of each of these signatures to be used in different contexts of treatments and stages remains to be validated.
- *When to start therapy?* If patients present with any multiple myeloma-related (CRAB) symptomatology, or the novel criteria of >60% of plasma cell infiltration or FLC ratio of >100 or more than one focal lesion on MRI, treatment should be started immediately. If they do not present any myeloma-related symptoms, the recommendation is to 'watch and wait' until symptoms emerge. However, under the SMM category, there are different patient populations:
  - Patients at low or intermediate risk of progression to active disease (who will not obtain any benefit from early treatment)
  - Patients at high risk of developing symptomatic multiple myeloma (who are the target for early experimental treatments in well-controlled clinical trials).

Several investigational trials are currently underway to evaluate and consolidate the ability of novel agents to delay the progression from high-risk asymptomatic ('early multiple myeloma') to symptomatic myeloma. The Spanish group has recently shown in a randomized trial that early treatment with lenalidomide + dexamethasone in high-risk SMM patients significantly delays the time to progression to symptomatic disease, translating into a benefit in overall survival as well.

- Patients younger than 65–70 years or transplant candidates:
  - *ASCT in the upfront setting or reserved for relapse?*
    - Several groups are currently evaluating these two approaches and until results are available, ASCT remains the standard of care for young patients
    - An argument in favour of the use of ASCT upfront is that it increases the CR rate and the PFS; moreover, relapses and disease progressions after ASCT are usually sensitive to rescue with novel agents, but it is not known whether ASCT is as effective after prolonged exposure to novel agents

- Single or tandem ASCT?
  - Tandem ASCT was abandoned because three randomized trials did not show any significant benefit in terms of OS and the introduction of novel agents improved the outcome for young multiple myeloma patients. However, recent data indicate that tandem ASCT may overcome the adverse prognosis of high-risk cytogenetics
  - Accordingly, bortezomib-based combinations + tandem ASCT should be considered for patients with high-risk or ultra-high-risk cytogenetic abnormalities, defined by the presence of t(4; 14) and/or del17p plus either ISS stage 3 or high LDH level.
- Patients older than 65–70 years or who are not candidates for HDT-ASCT
  - Is there any role for maintenance therapy?
    - Thalidomide as a single agent is not optimal because most patients need to discontinue it due to toxicity: peripheral neuropathy is a cumulative toxicity leading to discontinuations
    - Bortezomib in combination with thalidomide (VT) or with prednisone (VP) showed promising efficacy results in terms of CR rates (up to 42%), PFS (median of around 37 months) and 5-year OS of approximately 59%. However, the benefit in terms of OS is not yet defined. In an Italian trial, VT as maintenance after a four-drug combination (VMPT) resulted in superior PFS and OS as compared with induction with VMP without maintenance
    - Lenalidomide as maintenance in a randomized trial extended the PFS up to 31 months vs 13 and 14 months for the other two arms (MPR and MP) without maintenance. No differences have so far been observed in terms of OS. In the lenalidomide + dexamethasone (Ld) (FIRST) trial, continuous lenalidomide prolonged PFS as compared to 18 cycles of Ld (25 vs 21 months) with no differences in OS
    - Carfilzomib and ixazomib are being evaluated as part of consolidation or maintenance in different trials.
  - Is there any role for ASCT in elderly patients?
    - In fit patients between the ages of 65 and 70 years, sequential intermediate doses of therapy, i.e. melphalan 100 mg/m² × two courses, followed by peripheral blood stem cell infusion is an attractive option. Results of a phase II trials using PAD as induction, melphalan 100 mg/m² × two courses, and consolidation and maintenance with lenalidomide resulted in a CR rate of 53%, translating into a median PFS of 48 months and overall survival of 83% at 5 years.
  - Are these novel agent-based combinations able to overcome the poor prognosis in the presence of high-risk cytogenetic abnormalities?
    - These combinations (particularly those based on bortezomib) improved the outcome of patients with high-risk features as compared to conventional agents; however, they are unable to completely overcome the poor prognosis with high-risk cytogenetic abnormalities
    - Proteasome inhibitors (bortezomib and carfilzomib) are particularly useful in patients with t(4; 14), while pomalidomide is apparently valuable in patients with deletion 17p
- Is there any role for allogeneic stem cell transplantation in myeloma?
  - Although myeloablative allo-HSCT is a potentially curative treatment, it was not considered as part of the treatment options for myeloma due to the high transplant-related mortality
  - Reduced intensity conditioning (RIC) regimen followed by allo-HSCT has changed the scenario, resulting in a significant reduction of the transplant-related mortality (from 46% to 30%)
  - Allo-HSCT could be offered to young patients relapsing within the first year from ASCT, following an optimized novel agent-based combination as induction
  - It could be also offered to young patients relapsing between 1 and 3 years after autologous stem cell transplantation, if they have high-risk features and can be treated within a clinical trial:
    - Complete response (or at least very good partial response) is mandatory to proceed to allogeneic stem cell transplantation
  - The best way to offer allogeneic transplant for myeloma patients is their inclusion in clinical trials.

Phase III clinical trials

See Table 33.3.

Areas of research

- Biological:
  - Global mutational screening using whole genome- and whole exome-based sequencing strategies
  - Intraclonal heterogeneity and evolution of myeloma cells with potential clinical implications
  - Genome-wide association studies (GWAS) to identify multiple myeloma risk and to predict treatment response
- Clinical:
  - Evaluation of the depth of response: immunophenotypic, molecular and imaging assessments
  - Role of novel agents and mechanisms of action to overcome resistance to first-generation agents
  - Development of biomarkers predicting sensitivity/resistance

Table 33.3 Phase III clinical trials

Trial reference	Results
Attal et al. (1996) N Engl J Med 335(2):91–97	• High-dose therapy combined with transplantation improves the response rate, event-free survival and overall survival in patients with myeloma
Rosiñol et al. (2012) Blood 120(8):1589–1596	• Use of VTD is a highly effective induction regimen prior to ASCT, compared with thalidomide + dexamethasone and conventional chemotherapy • These results have been consolidated in other phase III trials
Fayers et al. (2011) Blood 118(5):1239–1247	• Thalidomide added to MP improves OS and PFS in previously untreated elderly patients with multiple myeloma, extending the median survival time by on average 20%
San Miguel et al. (2008) N Engl J Med 359(9): 906–917	• Bortezomib + melphalan + prednisone was superior to melphalan + prednisone alone in patients with newly diagnosed myeloma who were ineligible for high-dose therapy
Richardson et al. (2005) 352:247–2498; updated Richardson et al. (2007) Blood 110(10):3557–3560	• Advantage for bortezomib over dexamethasone in terms of response (≥PR 43% vs 18%; CR 9% vs 2%), TTP (6.2 vs 3.5 months) and OS (30 vs 24 months)
Fermand et al. (2006) Blood (ASH abstracts) 108:abstract 3563	• Advantage for thalidomide + dexamethasone over dexamethasone alone in terms of response (≥PR 65% vs 28%) and PFS at 1 year (46% vs 31%)
Weber (2007) N Engl J Med 357(21):2133–2142; Dimopoulos (2007) N Engl J Med 357(21): 2123–2132; updated Dimopoulos (2009) Leukemia 23(9):1545–1546	• Advantage for lenalidomide + dexamethasone over dexamethasone alone in terms of response (≥PR 60% vs 22%; CR 15% vs 2%), TTP (13.4 vs 4.6 months) and OS (38 vs 32 months, despite a 48% cross-over in the dexamethasone arm)
Orlowski et al. (2007) J Clin Oncol 25:3892–3901	• Similar responses for the bortezomib + doxil and bortezomib arms (≥PR 44% vs 41%; CR/VGPR 27% vs 19%) • Significant benefit in terms of TTP (9.3 vs 6.5 months) but not in OS
San Miguel et al. (2013) Lancet Oncol 14(11):1055–1066	• Demonstrated the activity of pomalidomide + dexamethasone in patients who had failed lenalidomide + dexamethasone and bortezomib • Significant advantage for pomalidomide + dexamethasone over dexamethasone alone in terms of response (≥PR 21% vs 3%), TTP (3.6 vs 1.8 months) and OS (not reached vs 7.8 months, despite a 29% cross-over in the dexamethasone arm)
Attal et al. (2012) N Eng J Med 266(19):1782–1792	• Showed superiority of lenalidomide maintenance vs placebo after autologous stem cell transplant in terms of PFS (41 vs 23 months), but no differences in OS were found
McCarthy et al. (2012) N Eng J Med 366 (19):1770–1781	• Advantage for lenalidoide maintenance vs placebo after autologous stem cell transplant in terms of PFS (46 vs 27 months) and OS at 3 years (88% vs 80%)
Palumbo et al. (2014) N Eng J Med 371(10): 895–905	• PFS and OS were significantly longer with high-dose melphalan followed by ASCT compared to consolidation with MPR (PFS 34 vs 22.4 months and OS at 3 years 81.6% vs 65.3%) • Advantage for lenalidomide maintenance vs placebo in PFS (41.9 vs 21.6 months), but no differences in OS
Benbouker et al. (2014) N Eng J Med 371(10): 906–917	• Advantage for continuous lenalidomide + dexamethasone (Rd) vs 18 cycles of Rd vs MPT in terms of PFS (25.5 vs 20.7 vs 21.2 months, respectively) and OS at 4 years (59% vs 56% vs 51%; only statistically different for the comparison of continuous Rd vs MPT) in patients with newly diagnosed multiple myeloma not eligible for high-dose therapy
San Miguel et al. (2014) Lancet Oncol 15(11):1195–206	• Addition of panobinostat to bortezomib + dexamethasone showed significant advantage in terms of response (nCR and CR 27.6% vs 15.7%) and PFS (11.9 vs 8.08 months), but not for OS (33.6 vs 30.3 months)
Stewart et al. (2015) N Engl J Med 372:142–152	• Significant advantage for carfilzomib + lenalidomide + dexamethasone (CRd) vs lenalidomide + dexamethasone (Rd) in terms of response (≥PR 87.1% vs 66.7%), PFS (26.3 vs 17.6 months) and OS (not yet reached)

Recommended reading

(2003) Criteria for the classification of monoclonal gammopathies, multiple myeloma and related disorders: a report of the International Myeloma Working Group. *Br J Haematol* 121:749–757.

Cavo M, Rajkumar SV, Palumbo A *et al.* (2011) International Myeloma Working Group consensus approach to the treatment of multiple myeloma patients who are candidates for autologous stem cell transplantation. *Blood* 117:6063–6073.

Dimopoulos M, Kyle R, Fermand JP *et al.* (2011) Consensus recommendations for standard investigative workup: report of the International Myeloma Workshop Consensus Panel 3. *Blood* 117:4701–4705.

Fernandez de Larrea C, Kyle RA, Durie BG (2013) Plasma cell leukemia: consensus statement on diagnostic requirements, response criteria and treatment recommendations by the International Myeloma Working Group. *Leukemia* 27:780–791.

Greipp PR, San MJ, Durie BG *et al.* (2005) International staging system for multiple myeloma. *J Clin Oncol* 23:3412–3420.

Gutierrez NC, Castellanos MV, Martin ML *et al.* (2007) Prognostic and biological implications of genetic abnormalities in multiple myeloma undergoing autologous stem cell transplantation: t(4;14) is the most relevant adverse prognostic factor, whereas RB deletion as a unique abnormality is not associated with adverse prognosis. *Leukemia* 21:143–150.

Kyle RA, Rajkumar SV (2004) Multiple myeloma. *N Engl J Med* 351:1860–1873.

Mateos MV, Oriol A, Martinez-Lopez J *et al.* (2010) Bortezomib, melphalan, and prednisone versus bortezomib, thalidomide, and prednisone as induction therapy followed by maintenance treatment with bortezomib and thalidomide versus bortezomib and prednisone in elderly patients with untreated multiple myeloma: a randomised trial. *Lancet Oncol* 11:934–941.

Mateos MV, Hernández MT, Giraldo P *et al.* (2013) Lenalidomide plus dexamethasone for high-risk smoldering multiple myeloma. *N Eng J Med* 369(5):438–447.

Munshi NC, Anderson KC, Bergsagel PL *et al.* (2011) Consensus recommendations for risk stratification in multiple myeloma: report of the International Myeloma Workshop Consensus Panel 2. *Blood* 117:4696–4700.

Ocio EM, Richardson PG, Rajkumar SV *et al.* (2014) New drugs and novel mechanisms of action in multiple myeloma in 2013: a report from the International Myeloma Working Group (IMWG). *Leukemia* 28(3):525–542.

Paiva B, Gutierrez NC, Rosinol L *et al.* (2012) High-risk cytogenetics and persistent minimal residual disease by multiparameter flow cytometry predict unsustained complete response after autologous stem cell transplantation in multiple myeloma. *Blood* 119:687–691.

Paiva B, Martinez-Lopez J, Vidriales MB *et al.* (2011) Comparison of immunofixation, serum free light chain, and immunophenotyping for response evaluation and prognostication in multiple myeloma. *J Clin Oncol* 29:1627–1633.

Palumbo A, Anderson K (2011) Multiple myeloma. *N Engl J Med* 364:1046–1060.

Perez-Persona E, Vidriales MB, Mateo G *et al.* (2007) New criteria to identify risk of progression in monoclonal gammopathy of uncertain significance and smoldering multiple myeloma based on multiparameter flow cytometry analysis of bone marrow plasma cells. *Blood* 110:2586–2592.

Rajkumar SV, Harousseau JL, Durie B *et al.* (2011) Consensus recommendations for the uniform reporting of clinical trials: report of the International Myeloma Workshop Consensus Panel 1. *Blood* 117:4691–4695.

Rajkumar SV, Dimopoulos MA, Palumbo A *et al.* (2014) International Myeloma Working Group updated criteria for the diagnosis of Multiple Myeloma. *Lancet Oncol* 15(12):e538–548.

San-Miguel JF, Paiva B, Gutiérrez NC (2013) New tools for diagnosis and monitoring of multiple myeloma. *Am Soc Clin Oncol Educ Book* 2013.

San Miguel J (2015) Multiple myeloma: A model for scientific and clinical progress. *Hematology Am Soc Hematol Educ Program* 2015.

34 Leukaemia

Tsila Zuckerman[1] and Jacob M. Rowe[1,2]

[1]Department of Hematology and Bone Marrow Transplantation, Rambam Health Care Campus, Bruce Rappaport Faculty of Medicine, Technion, Israel Institute of Technology, Haifa, Israel
[2]Department of Hematology, Shaare Zedek Medical Center, Jerusalem, Israel

Summary	Key facts

Introduction	**Acute myeloid leukaemia**
	• Most common acute leukaemia in adults:
	  ▪ Annual incidence: 3.7 per 100,000
	• Frequency increases with age:
	  ▪ Median age at diagnosis is 70 years
	
	Acute lymphoblastic leukaemia
	• Age-adjusted incidence rate in the USA is 1.7 per 100,000 individuals per year
	  ▪ Approximately 6070 new cases and 1430 deaths were estimated for 2013 in the USA
	• Most common leukaemia in paediatrics, accounting for up to 80% of paediatric leukaemia (compared to 20% of adult leukaemia)
	• Median age at diagnosis is 14 years with 60% of diagnosed patients being ≤20 years old and only 24% diagnosed at ≥45 years
	
	Chronic myeloid leukaemia
	• Accounts for 15% of adult leukaemias
	• Estimated that 5980 new cases would be diagnosed in the USA in 2014 and 810 would die of the disease
	• Median age is 67 years, but occurs in all age groups
	
	Chronic lymphocytic leukaemia
	• Most common leukaemia in adults in Western countries:
	  ▪ Approximately 30% of all leukaemias in the USA
	  ▪ Estimated that 15,720 new cases would be diagnosed in the USA in 2014
	  ▪ Incidence varies by race and geographical location
	  ▪ Higher incidence among Caucasians as compared with African Americans or Asians
	  ▪ Incidence of CLL is extremely low in Asia
	• Male-to-female ratio of approximately 1.7:1
	• Considered to be mainly a disease of the elderly, with a median age at diagnosis of 70 years

Presentation	**Acute myeloid leukaemia**
	• Marrow failure: anaemia, neutropenia with infections and thrombocytopenia presenting as spontaneous skin or mucosal bleeding
	• Coagulopathy (DIC): may present as bleeding, thrombosis or both
	• Hyperleukocytosis with leukostasis:
	  ▪ Common when white blood cell count (WBC) >100,000/μL
	  ▪ May present as hypoxaemia, retinal haemorrhage and confusion

(continued)

Summary	Key facts
	Acute lymphoblastic leukaemia • Bone marrow (BM) failure: anaemia, neutropenia presenting as fever, thrombocytopenia presenting as skin or mucosal bleeding • Lymphadenopathy in 55% • Splenomegaly in 45% • Bone pain • CNS involvement presenting as headache, confusion, cranial nerve palsy **Chronic myeloid leukaemia** • Three different phases: chronic (CP), accelerated (AP) and blastic (BC) • Most patients are diagnosed with CP, often revealed as an incidental finding during routine blood tests, such as increased WBC with presence of all stages of neutrophil differentiation in peripheral blood (PB) • In symptomatic patients, in AP or BC: fatigue, weight loss, night sweats, abdominal pain and early satiety **Chronic lymphocytic leukaemia** • Majority are asymptomatic at diagnosis and it is an incidental finding • During disease evolution: may present with adenopathy, splenomegaly, BM failure and hypogammaglobulinaemia • Autoimmune phenomena such as autoimmune haemolytic anaemia and idiopathic thrombocytopenia may occur • Richter transformation: transformation to aggressive lymphoma

Scenario	**Acute myeloid leukaemia**
	• Fit patients should be treated with induction therapy (7 + 3)
	• Possible post-induction therapy: chemotherapy, autologous or allogeneic stem cell transplantation:
	   ▪ Treatment decision is based on AML risk and donor availability
	• Unfit patients: supportive treatment or clinical trials
	
	Acute lymphoblastic leukaemia
	• Participation in clinical trials is highly encouraged
	• Treatment is composed of induction and consolidation (BFM protocol) or repeated cycles of chemotherapy (Hyper-CVAD), both followed by prolonged maintenance (for 2.5 years)
	• CNS prophylaxis is mandatory
	• Minimal residual disease (MRD) monitoring is an important risk factor and is mandatory in paediatric trials and is being increasingly used in adults
	• In Ph+ ALL, tyrosine kinase inhibitors (TKIs) should be incorporated with chemotherapy
	   ▪ Elderly or unfit patients may benefit from TKIs and steroids
	• Monoclonal antibodies show promising results when added to chemotherapy
	• Young adults (age 15–39 years): may be best treated with paediatric inspired protocol
	• Allogeneic stem cell transplantation is recommended:
	   ▪ Paediatric patients: ≥CR2, high risk or MRD positive
	   ▪ Adults: recommended in CR1
	• Elderly or unfit patients should be treated with supportive treatment or clinical trials
	
	Chronic myeloid leukaemia
	• Treatment with TKIs (first or second generation):
	   ▪ Careful monitoring of haematological, cytogenetic and molecular response at 3, 6 and 12 months after initiating TKIs is essential to assure adequate response
	   ▪ Inadequate response or failure should promote screening for mutations at the *BCR-ABL* binding site
	• Allogeneic stem cell transplantation reserved for patients with suboptimal response to TKIs
	
	Chronic lymphocytic leukaemia
	• Patients with early disease stage according to Rai or Binnet classification: watch without treatment
	• Patients with advanced or rapidly progressive disease: treat according to their age and performance status
	• Fit patients: treat with combination of rituximab and chemotherapy (fludarabine-based or bendamustine)
	• Relapsed patients: treat with monoclonal antibody (alemtuzumab or ofatumumab) or targeted therapy (ibrutinib)
	• Elderly and less fit patients: treat with chlorambucil

Trials	**Acute myeloid leukaemia**
	• Fernandez *et al.* (2009) *N Engl J Med* 361:1249–1259:
	   ▪ Phase III randomized trial demonstrating that adults aged <60 years benefit from daunorubicin dose intensification in induction in terms of higher complete remission rate and overall survival
	   ▪ Benefit was most prominent in patients with the favourable and intermediate-risk cytogenetics and in those younger than 50 years

Summary	Key facts

	- Löwenberg *et al.* (2009) *N Engl J Med* 361:1235–1248:
	  - Phase III randomized trial showing that adults with AML aged >60 years benefit from daunorubicin dose intensification in induction in terms of higher complete remission rate and no excessive toxicity
	  - Improved event-free survival and overall survival were restricted to patients aged 60–65 years old
	- Patel *et al.* (2012) *N Engl J Med* 366:1079–1089:
	  - Integrated molecular risk profile allowed for a better definition of genetic risk in a large cohort of AML patients tested for 18 genes involved in AML
	  - Specific molecular alterations could predict improved outcome with daunorubicin dose intensification in induction
	- Sanz (2009) *Blood* 113:1875–1891:
	  - Review from the expert panel of the European LeukemiaNet on the diagnosis, treatment, follow-up and specific complications of APL
	- Döhner (2010) *Blood* 115:453–474:
	  - Review from the expert panel of the European LeukemiaNet on the diagnosis, treatment and follow-up of adult AML patients
	
	Acute lymphoblastic leukaemia
	- Goldstone AH *et al.* (2008) *Blood* 111:1827–1833:
	  - Results of the international phase III randomized MRC/ECOG study in adult ALL established allogeneic stem cell transplantation as the treatment of choice in patients in first complete remission
	- Huguet *et al.* (2009) *J Clin Oncol* 27:911–918:
	  - Treatment of adult Ph-negative ALL patients with paediatric intensified protocols demonstrated beneficial response in those aged up to 45 years
	  - In patients older than 45 years, the beneficial effect was offset by increased toxicity
	- Pui *et al.* (2011) *J Clin Oncol* 29:386–391:
	  - Adolescents (aged 15–18 years) with ALL have an inferior outcome as compared with younger patients
	  - Effect of age could have been abolished by the implementation of risk-adjusted intensive chemotherapy
	- Bassan *et al.* (2010) *Blood* 28:3644–3652:
	  - Phase II study demonstrating that addition of imatinib to chemotherapy in Ph-positive ALL patients improved disease-free and overall survival, and decreased relapse rate
	- Advani (2013) *Am Soc Hematol Educ Program* 2013:131–137:
	  - Review describing the new approach to treatment of ALL using four different types of antibodies, including naked antibodies, T-cell engaging bispecific antibodies, immunoconjugates and chimeric antigen receptors
	- Patel *et al.* (2010) *Br J Haematol* 148:80–89:
	  - Detection of minimal residual disease by PCR for immunoglobulin gene rearrangement at the time of chemotherapy and especially after second consolidation could predict for inferior outcome with a significantly higher relapse rate and lower disease-free survival
	
	Chronic myeloid leukaemia
	- Baccarani *et al.* (2013) *Blood* 122:872–884:
	  - Review by the expert panel of the European LeukemiaNet which contains up-to-date recommendations on diagnosis, treatment and follow-up of patients with CML
	- Saglio *et al.* (2010) *N Engl J Med* 362:2251–2259:
	  - Phase III randomized, open-label, multicentre study comparing imatinib to nilotinib as first-line treatment of chronic phase CML
	  - Nilotinib was found to be associated with significantly increased cytogenetic and molecular responses at 12 months and lower progression to accelerated phase or blast crisis
	- Cortes *et al.* (2009) *J Clin Oncol* 27:4754–4759:
	  - Increased imatinib dose (800 mg vs 400 mg) in treatment of newly diagnosed chronic phase CML patients resulted in more rapid reduction of tumour burden as manifested by higher cytogenetic and molecular responses at specific time points
	- Kantarjian *et al.* (2012) *Blood* 119:1123–1129:
	  - Randomized, multicentre phase III trial comparing imatinib to dasatinib as first-line treatment for chronic phase CML
	  - At 24 months, treatment with dasatinib was found to be associated with a similar cytogenetic response, and significantly increased and deeper molecular responses
	- Jabbour *et al.* (2011) *J Clin Oncol* 29:4260–4265:
	  - Patients with chronic phase CML treated with second-generation tyrosine kinase inhibitors have faster and deeper responses as demonstrated by cytogenetic analysis
	  - Hence, the response (optimal versus suboptimal) should be evaluated as early as 3 months from treatment initiation

(continued)

Summary	Key facts

	Chronic lymphocytic leukaemia
	• Knauf *et al.* (2009) *J Clin Oncol* 27(26):4378–4384:
	  ▪ Comparison between bendamustine and chlorambucil in first-line treatment of CLL demonstrated superior complete and partial remission, and improved progression free survival in patients treated with bendamustine
	• Bauer *et al.* (2012) *Cochrane Database Syst Rev* (11):CD008079:
	  ▪ In a meta-analysis the addition of rituximab to chemotherapy demonstrated improved overall survival and progression-free survival as compared to the chemotherapy-only group
	• Hallek *et al.* (2010) *Lancet* 376:1164–1174:
	  ▪ Phase III randomized trial comparing the addition of rituximab to fludaraine and cytoxan in CLL
	  ▪ Addition of rituximab was associated with better overall and progression-free survival
	• Fischer *et al.* (2012) *J Clin Oncol* 30(26):3209–3216:
	  Phase II study of newly-diagnosed CLL patients treated with a combination of rituximab and bendamustine demonstrated the efficacy and safety of this combination as compared to the results in the literature for FCR
	• Byrd *et al.* (2013) *N Engl J Med* 369(1):32–42:
	  ▪ Phase I–II study using ibrutinib, an oral inhibitor of BTK, in relapsed CLL demonstrated high frequency of durable remission, including in patients with high genetic risk CLL

Introduction

Leukaemia is a malignant disease of the haematopoietic system characterized by accumulation of lymphoid or myeloid cells in the bone marrow (BM) and peripheral blood (PB). In *acute* leukaemia, the accumulated cells are undifferentiated or minimally differentiated (termed blast cells) and this is associated with secondary suppression of normal haemopoiesis. In *chronic* leukaemia there is accumulation of mature cells in the blood or bone marrow and, at least initially, there is no suppression of normal haemopoiesis. Acute and chronic leukaemias are broadly divided according to the affected lineage into acute myeloid leukaemia (AML) and chronic myeloid leukaemia (CML) associated with abnormal myelopoiesis, while acute lymphoblastic leukaemia (ALL) and chronic lymphocytic leukaemia (CLL) are associated with abnormal lymphopoiesis. In addition, the clinical presentation and disease course significantly differ between acute and chronic leukaemias. In acute leukaemia the disease onset is abrupt with rapid progression and, unless treated without delay will result in patient death, whereas chronic leukaemia is often an incidental finding with slow progression over time.

With the advance of laboratory techniques and knowledge regarding the biological basis of the leukaemias, acute leukaemias have been further classified into subgroups enabling their categorization into different prognostic entities with an aim to provide tailored (personalized) therapy. The in-depth delineation of the biological processes underlying the chronic leukaemias has revolutionized their treatment and outcome, rendering the diseases (mainly CML) manageable life-long with targeted therapy.

Disease evaluation and classification incorporate an integration of morphology, immunohistochemistry, immunophenotyping, cytogenetic and molecular studies.

ACUTE MYELOID LEUKAEMIA

Acute myeloid leukaemia (AML) is characterized by the accumulation of ≥20% early myeloid progenitors termed 'myeloblasts', accompanied by secondary suppression of normal haemopoiesis. The disease onset is abrupt and unless treated early, can be lethal. The incidence increases with age (median 70 years) and the 5-year survival is 15–25%, a significant improvement since 1998.

Pathogenesis and aetiology

Pathogenesis

AML is a genetically heterogeneous disease characterized by somatic acquisition of genetic and epigenetic alterations in haematopoietic myeloid progenitors that perturb normal mechanisms of self-renewal, proliferation and differentiation.

It results from multistep cooperating mutations in haematopoietic precursors. These mutations are divided into two classes. Class I mutations confer a proliferative and/or survival advantage, usually as a consequence of aberrant activation of signal transduction pathways, such as mutation in fms-like tyrosine kinase 3 (*FLT3*) and RAS signalling pathways. Class II mutations impair haematopoietic differentiation, usually resulting from mutations in transcription factors or transcriptional co-activators important for normal haematopoietic development, such as t(8; 21) and inv(16)/t(16; 16) in the core binding factor (CBF) leukaemias. Additionally, somatic alterations in epigenetic regulators (i.e. genes regulating DNA methylation and post-translational histone modifications) were recently found to be a common event in haematopoietic transformation.

Aetiology

Although largely unknown, some predisposing factors are implicated to be associated with the disease:

- Hereditary:
  - Chromosome aneuploidy: Down syndrome (trisomy 21)
  - Defective DNA repair: Fanconi anaemia, Bloom syndrome, ataxia telangiectasia
  - Congenital neutropenia: Kostmann syndrome
- Ionizing radiation (therapeutic or non-therapeutic)
- Chemicals: benzene, petroleum products, tobacco, chloramphenicol
- Obesity
- Prior cytotoxic therapy:
  - Alkylating agents (chlorambucil): associated with chromosome 5 and 7 aberrations
  - Topoisomerase II inhibitors (anthracyclines, mitoxantrone, epipodophyllotoxins):
    - Often associated with chromosome 11q23 aberrations
    - Typically with a short latency from exposure of 1–3 years

Classification

The French–American–British (FAB) classification introduced in 1976 is based on morphological evaluation and cytochemistry of blasts and their level of differentiation, and divides myeloid leukaemia into seven subcategories (M0–7). Although inaccurate and with almost no prognostic significance, it is commonly used in initial diagnosis. The World Health Organization (WHO) classification of 2008 incorporates morphological, biological (genetic and molecular) and clinical features to categorize cases of AML into unique groups with prognostic implication (see Box 34.1).

The four abnormalities initially included in the subgroup *AML with recurring genetic abnormalities* involve rearrangements of genes (*RUNX1*, *CBFB*, *RARA* and *MLL*) that encode transcription factors and are associated with fairly distinct clinical and morphological features. In recent years, it has become more widely appreciated that multiple genetic lesions, including numerical abnormalities and gene mutations, cooperate to establish the leukaemic process and influence its morphological and clinical characteristics. Hence, two provisional entities of the more common mutated *NPM1* and *FLT3-ITD* (present in about 50% and 30% of normal karyotype AML, respectively) have been added. More than 18 mutations, not all driving mutations, have so far been identified and their integrated influence on prognosis has been studied and will be incorporated in future classification.

AML with myelodysplasia-related changes includes AML that either evolves from previously documented myelodysplastic syndrome (MDS) or myeloproliferative neoplasm (MPN), has specific MDS cytogenetic abnormalities or exhibits dysplasia in ≥50% of cells in two or more lineages. Usually, this AML subtype confers a poor prognosis.

> **Box 34.1** WHO classification of AML
>
> 1. *AML with recurrent genetic abnormalities*:
>   - AML with t(8; 21) (q22; q22); *RUNX1-RUNX1T1*
>   - AML with inv(16) (p13.1q22) or t(16; 16) (p13.1; q22); *CBFB-MYH11*
>   - APL with t(15; 17) (q22; q12); *PML-RARA* (M3)
>   - AML with t(9; 11) (p22; q23); *MLLT3-MLL*
>   - AML with t(6; 9) (p23; q34); *DEK-NUP214*
>   - AML with inv(3) (q21; q26.2) or t(3; 3) (q21; q26.2); *RPN1-EVI1*
>   - AML (megakaryoblastic) with t(1; 22) (p13; q13); *RBM15-MKL1*
>   - Provisional entity: AML with mutated *NPM1*
>   - Provisional entity: AML with mutated *CEBPA*
> 2. *AML with myelodysplasia-related changes*
> 3. *Therapy-related myeloid neoplasm*
> 4. *AML, not otherwise specified*:
>   - AML with minimal differentiation (M0)
>   - AML without maturation (M1)
>   - AML with maturation (M2)
>   - Acute myelomonocytic leukaemia (M4)
>   - Acute monoblastic/monocytic leukaemia (M5)
>   - Acute erythroid leukaemia (M6)
>   - Pure erythroid leukaemia
>   - Erythroleukaemia, erythroid/myeloid
>   - Acute megakaryoblastic leukaemia (M7)
>   - Acute basophilic leukaemia
>   - Acute pan-myelosis with myelofibrosis

Therapy-related AML usually has abnormal cytogenetics and confers a poor prognosis as well.

All cases not included in the former categories fall into the group of *AML not otherwise specified* and are described by morphology only. This is a heterogeneous group which will probably decrease in number with increasing knowledge on leukaemia genetics.

Myeloid sarcoma (also known as granulocytic sarcoma or chloroma) is a rare extramedullary tumour of immature myeloid cells. It is reported in 2.5–9.1% of patients with AML and occurs concomitantly, following or, rarely, antedating the onset of systemic bone marrow leukaemia. It is more common in t(8; 21) AML.

Presentation

The disease is typically characterized by an acute presentation with signs and symptoms related to marrow failure, coagulation disorders and organ infiltration:

- Anaemia: presents as weakness, lethargy, shortness of breath and palpitations
- Neutropenia: associated with fever, infection (usually Gram-negative bacilli or *Staphylococcus*)
- Thrombocytopenia: presents as purpura, menorrhagia, mucosal (epistaxis, gingival) or retinal bleeding

- Gum hypertrophy and skin infiltration (common in M4 and M5 AML)
- Extramedullary sarcoma [M2 with t(8; 21)]
- Hyperleukocytosis with leukostasis:
  - Usually evident when the white blood cell count (WBC) is ≥100,000/μL
  - May present as hypoxaemia, retinal haemorrhage and confusion
- Disseminated intravascular coagulopathy (DIC):
  - May present as haemorrhage or thrombosis
  - Laboratory evaluation demonstrates prolonged prothrombin time (PT) and partial thromboplastin time (PTT), decreased fibrinogen and elevated D-dimer
  - Particularly common in acute promyelocytic leukaemia (APL)
- Central nervous system (CNS) involvement: headache, confusion, cranial nerve palsy:
  - Occurs rarely at presentation and during follow-up in 5% of patients
- Tumour lysis syndrome: a metabolic abnormality occurring either spontaneously or following treatment when high tumour burden is present and may present as hyperphosphataemia, hyperkalaemia, hyperuricaemia, hypocalcaemia and renal dysfunction

Diagnostic work-up

- Complete blood count (CBC) and peripheral blood smear:
  - Usually discloses anaemia and thrombocytopenia with elevated WBC composed mainly of blasts and absence of mature neutrophils:
    - Occasionally, the WBC is also decreased and blasts are not found in the PB; known as aleukaemic leukaemia
  - Blood smear, Giemsa stained, should be carefully inspected for blast cells and morphological features:
    - Presence of Auer rods (clumps of azurophylic granules forming needle-like structures in the blast cytoplasm) should be carefully looked for as it is pathognomonic for AML.
- Immunohistochemistry for myeloperoxidase (MPO), non-specific esterase (NSE) and periodic acid-Schiff (PAS):
  - Presence of ≥3% MPO stain in blasts is diagnostic of AML, but its absence does not preclude the diagnosis
  - NSE and PAS stains are used for monocytic and erythroid leukaemia, respectively
  - Immunostains are not routinely performed nowadays and have been largely replaced by immunophenotyping
- BM aspirate for morphology evaluation, including blast count and search for dysplasia:
  - Biopsy is performed if an aspirate is not possible (dry tap) and it is important to assess the overall cellularity
- Immunophenotype of PB and/or BM:
  - Immunophenotyping with monoclonal antibodies for cell surface antigens, using multiparameter flow cytometry, is employed to determine lineage involvement of a newly diagnosed AML
  - For most markers, >20% of the cells expressing the marker is arbitrarily considered diagnostic, although with sensitive multicoloured technology a much lower percentage is often diagnostic
  - It reliably differentiates AML from ALL and confirms the diagnosis of M0, M6 and M7 AML (Table 34.1)
- Cytogenetic and molecular analysis of BM:
  - Conventional cytogenetic analysis is mandatory, with a minimum of 20 metaphase cells analysed in order to determine normal karyotype
  - Molecular studies for specific gene mutations are recommended in normal-karyotype AML and should include at least polymerase chain reaction (PCR) analysis for: nucleophosmin 1 (*NPM1*), fms-related tyrosine kinase 3 – internal tandem duplication (*FLT3-ITD*), core enhancing binding protein A (*CEBPA*) and t(15; 17) (typical for APL)
    - \>15 other known mutations in AML which have prognostic significance, but currently mostly used in the research setting
    - With advance in molecular techniques, such as whole genome sequencing, it is assumed that allocation of genetic composition for each patient with leukaemia will be less costly and more widely used
- HLA typing at diagnosis and a donor search started according to individual risk
- Fertility consultation:
  - Male patients should be offered the possibility of sperm preservation
  - Fertile female patients should be offered gonadotropin-releasing hormone (GNRH) antagonists to prevent menstrual bleeding during thrombocytopenia, with some evidence supporting gonadal protection with these agents
  - Ovarian cryopreservation is a new option
- Cardiac evaluation in older patients, including echocardiogram

Table 34.1 Tumour markers: Immunophenotyping diagnosis of AML

Precursor stage	CD34, CD38, CD133, HLA-DR
Granulocytic markers	CD13, CD15, CD16, CD33, CD65, anti-MPO
Monocytic markers	NSE, CD11c, CD14, CD64, lysozyme, CD4, CD11b, CD36, NG2 homologue
Megakaryocytic markers	CD41, CD61, CD42
Erythroid marker	Glycophorin A

WHO (2014). Reproduced with permission of WHO.

Differential diagnosis

- Severe sepsis with leukaemoid reaction (pseudo-leukaemia)
- Acute lymphoblastic leukaemia
- CML – blast crisis

Prognostic factors

Factors adversely influencing the likelihood of entering complete remission (CR), the length of CR and curability of AML include:
- Unfavourable cytogenetic and/or molecular markers
- Favourable cytogenetics: CBF with *c-Kit* mutation
- Intermediate cytogenetics with mutated *FLT3, TET2, MLL-PTD, DNMT3A, AXSL1, PHF6*
- Age >60 years
- Not achieving CR after induction therapy
- Performance status and co-morbidities
- WBC >100,000/μL at presentation
- AML post MDS or treatment related
- Minimal residual disease (MRD) positivity post induction (defined by multiparametric flow cytometry or PCR for known translocation/mutated gene)

Chromosome abnormalities, such as translocations, inversions and deletions, are detected in approximately 55% of adult patients with AML. In the last decade, cytogenetic abnormalities at diagnosis were found to be the most powerful predictors of prognosis in patients with AML. Accordingly, three prognostic groups were identified and verified in large cohorts of patients: favourable, intermediate I/II and unfavourable risk. Among patients younger than 65 years treated with standard chemotherapy:
- *Favourable* karyotype: CR rates of 85–90% and 5-year overall survival (OS) of 50–60%
- *Intermediate-risk* cytogenetics: CR rates of 65–75% and 5-year OS of 35–45%
- *Unfavourable-risk* cytogenetics: a CR rate of 45–55% and a 5-year OS of only 10–20%.

Overall, <40% of patients with AML can be cured. Although these risk groups also apply to patients aged >65 years, their outcome in each risk category is inferior, emphasizing the effect of age (and intolerance to intensive treatment) as a significant isolated prognostic factor.

The complex karyotype group is defined as having three or more genetic alterations in at least two metaphases. This is more common with increasing age (>60 years), in therapy-related AML and prior MDS, and is associated with an OS of 10–15%. Monosomal karyotype, defined as two or more monosomies (excluding sex chromosome monosomy), or a single monosomy associated with structural chromosome abnormality (excluding CBF AML) is the subgroup with the worst prognosis and an OS of <5%.

In recent years, molecular markers have been added which enable in particular better segregation of the heterogeneous group of normal karyotype (NK) AML to prognostically-specific subgroups. Among the >20 newly discovered gene mutations in AML, the *NPM1, FLT3-ITD* and *CEBPA* are the more common and have been integrated into prognostic groups as provisional entities. Table 34.2 summarizes the common mutations. Figure 34.1 presents the revised cytogenetic and molecular risk stratification.

Table 34.2 Common mutations in NK-AML

Mutation	Prevalence	Prognosis
NPM1	45–64%	Favourable
Flt3-ITD	28–34%	Unfavourable
CEBPA^{dm}	10–18%	Favourable

Treatment

Treatment is divided into supportive and definitive.

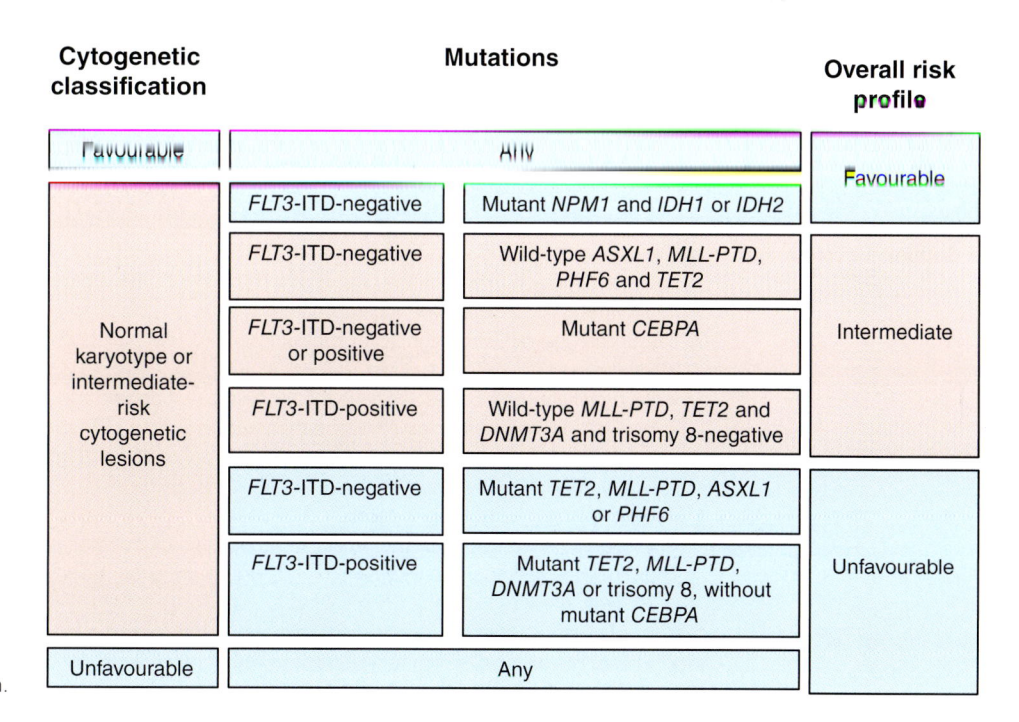

Cytogenetic classification	Mutations		Overall risk profile
Favourable	Any		Favourable
Normal karyotype or intermediate-risk cytogenetic lesions	FLT3-ITD-negative	Mutant *NPM1* and *IDH1* or *IDH2*	
	FLT3-ITD-negative	Wild-type *ASXL1, MLL-PTD, PHF6* and *TET2*	Intermediate
	FLT3-ITD-negative or positive	Mutant *CEBPA*	
	FLT3-ITD-positive	Wild-type *MLL-PTD, TET2* and *DNMT3A* and trisomy 8-negative	
	FLT3-ITD-negative	Mutant *TET2, MLL-PTD, ASXL1* or *PHF6*	Unfavourable
	FLT3-ITD-positive	Mutant *TET2, MLL-PTD, DNMT3A* or trisomy 8, without mutant *CEBPA*	
Unfavourable	Any		

Figure 34.1 Revised risk stratification.

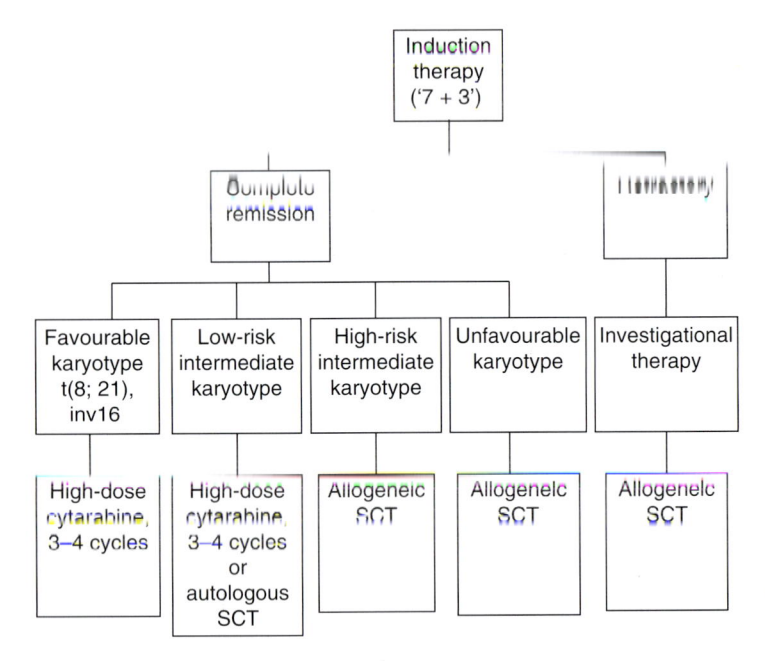

Figure 34.2 Treatment algorithm for AML.
*SCT, stem cell transplantation.

Definitive treatment in patients aged 18–60 years with non-APL AML (Fig. 34.2)

The upper age limit of 60 years is set as an eligibility criterion in most studies of adults. However, the decision on treatment intensity depends not on the chronological age of the patient, but rather on the 'biological age', as reflected by the performance status of the individual.

Treatment of newly diagnosed, fit patients with AML is divided into two phases: induction and post remission. The goal of induction treatment is to induce prompt CR. CR is defined as <5% blasts in BM, absence of extramedullary disease, absolute neutrophil count of >1.0 × 10^9/L, platelet count of >100,000/µL and independence from red blood cell (RBC) transfusion. It is likely that in the future, as more sensitive techniques become standardized, this will be defined by the presence or absence of MRD.

The goal of post-remission therapy is to eradicate residual leukaemic cells, prevent relapse and prolong survival. Various post-remission strategies exist, including repeat cycles of intensive conventional chemotherapy and high-dose chemotherapy followed by either autologous or allogeneic stem cell transplantation. The selection of treatment is based on patient's individual risk stratification as determined by cytogenetic and molecular analyses at diagnosis.

Treatment	Description

Supportive treatment	• Patient instruction and support regarding the disease and treatment course
	• Intensive hydration (aim for urine output of >100 mL/h) to prevent renal failure from tumour lysis
	• Allopurinol is given to prevent hyperuricaemia
	• Rasburicase is given when significant hyperuricaemia already exists or as prophylaxis against the tumour lysis syndrome:
	  ▪ Recombinant urate oxidase enzyme that converts existing uric acid to allantoin
	  ▪ Five to ten times more soluble in urine than uric acid
	• Hydroxyurea at a dose of 50 mg/kg/day is administered to control high WBC of >50,000/µL until the start of chemotherapy
	• RBC and platelet transfusion support:
	  ▪ As per recommendation of the American Association of Blood Banks (AABB), RBC transfusion should be given when haemoglobin (Hb) is <8.0 g/dL, unless the patient has symptomatic anaemia or suffers from coronary disease
	  ▪ Prophylactic platelet transfusion is recommended to maintain a threshold of 5–10 × 10^9/L
	  ▪ Filtered products are recommended for prevention of alloimmunization

Treatment	Description

	- Infection prevention:
	  - AML patients undergoing induction are considered at high risk for both bacterial and fungal infection
	  - According to the National Comprehensive Cancer Network (NCCN) guidelines, antibiotic prophylaxis with fluoroquinolones is optional
	  - Antifungal prophylaxis for *Candida* is highly recommended
	- Febrile neutropenia should be aggressively treated with antipseudomonal β-lactam agents (cefipime, carbapenem) or piperacillin–tazobactam:
	  - Mandatory that cultures are obtained from blood, central line catheters and other sources (sputum, urine, etc.) according to clinical presentation prior to starting antimicrobial therapy
	  - Choice of antibiotics depends on hospital flora and local bacterial susceptibility
	- Leukapheresis for WBC of >100,000/μL or symptoms of leukostasis
	- DIC replacement therapy with fresh frozen plasma, cryoprecipitate and platelet transfusion with a goal of correcting PT and PTT, and keeping fibrinogen >150 mg/dL and platelet count >50,000/μL
	  - Close coagulation monitoring is required
	- Irradiated blood products whenever the option of an allogeneic transplant is considered

Definitive treatment in patients aged 18–60 years with non-APL AML: *Induction therapy*	- '3 + 7' protocol: 3 days of anthracycline (daunorubicin 60 mg/m^2, idarubicin 10–12 mg/m^2 or mitoxantrone 10–12 mg/m^2) and 7 days of IV continuous infusion of cytarabine (100–200 mg/m^2):
	  - No evidence for superiority of idarubicin or mitoxantrone over daunorubicin
	  - Higher doses of daunorubicin (90 mg/m^2) were found to be superior to 45 mg/m^2 without excessive toxicity, especially in patients aged <50 years and with the favourable and intermediate risk disease category
	  - Addition of a third cytotoxic agent (etoposide, fludarabine, thioguanine) or use of high-dose cytarabine in induction failed to demonstrate a superior CR and was associated with increased toxicity
	- Repeat BM aspirate and biopsy at Day 14 from start of induction:
	  - If not in remission, repeat 7 + 3 (daunorubicin 60 mg/m^2, except for patients who originally received 90 mg/m^2, in which case 45 mg/m^2)
	- BM should be repeated at recovery of blood count and examined for morphology, immunophenotype and molecular biology or cytogenetics if a marker was previously identified
	- CR is achieved in 60–80% of patients

Definitive treatment in patients aged 18–60 years with non-APL AML: *Post-remission therapy*	- *Chemotherapy*:
	  - High-dose cytarabine (3 g/m^2 every 12 hours on Days 1, 3 and 5) was found to be superior to intermediate or standard dose (400 mg/m^2 or 100 mg/m^2 continuous IV for 5 days), especially in patients with favourable cytogenetics
	  - Optimal number of cycles is unknown, but three to four cycles are commonly administered
	- *Autologous stem cell transplantation* (SCT) is considered an alternative option for post-remission therapy in patients with favourable and intermediate cytogenetic risk groups:
	  - Outcome is at least as good as after the use of conventional consolidation chemotherapy and is associated with transplant-related mortality of only 1–2%
	- *Allogeneic SCT*:
	  - Most efficacious antileukaemic therapy
	  - Associated with the lowest risk of relapse due mainly to the potent graft-versus-leukaemia (GvL) effect
	  - Found to be most beneficial in patients with intermediate and unfavourable cytogenetics, but due to significant toxicity is limited to patients with good performance status without considerable co-morbidities and having an HLA-matched sibling or unrelated donor:
	    - Recent introduction of reduced intensity and reduced toxicity conditioning, improved supportive care, better HLA matching and use of alternative donors (matched unrelated, cord blood and haplo-identical) has decreased the toxicity of this modality and increased its accessibility to older and less fit patients with an outcome approaching or equivalent to that of sibling transplant

Management of patients aged ≥60 years

Increasing age is associated with a higher incidence of adverse factors associated with decreased ability to tolerate therapy (poor performance status, co-morbidities) and adverse AML-related factors (unfavourable cytogenetics, secondary AML and therapy resistance). However, age by itself should not preclude patients from receiving intensive treatment. Patients are practically divided into those aged 60–74 years and those aged ≥75 years. This is an arbitrary separation which is used in most clinical trials as an inclusion criterion. However, outside of studies, age is just one important factor influencing the selection of therapy. It is the patient's performance status and co-morbidities that influence decision-making regarding treatment choice. CR rates with standard induction therapy in the 60–74-year group are 50% overall and ≤30% for a subset with adverse cytogenetics.

In fit patients, the standard '7 + 3' regimen gives the best results in terms of CR rate and OS. Patients aged ≤65 years benefit from an increased daunorubicin dose of 90 mg/m² for 3 days. Alternative regimens under investigation include the purine analogue clofarabine (30 mg/m² for 5 days). The hypomethylating agent decitabine for 5–10 days has been tried in elderly patients with AML with a CR of 24–47%. Azacytidine was found to prolong survival compared to other low-intensity therapies, not necessarily in association with achievement of CR.

The issue of post-remission therapy is still controversial due to inherent bias in the selection of patients into clinical trials, although recent data from the registries suggest that repeated cycles of modest-dose consolidation are associated with a longer survival compared to lower doses. The introduction of reduced-intensity conditioning allogeneic SCT enables the use of this modality in older patients with reasonable toxicity. The use of matched unrelated donors resulted in a survival comparable to that for matched related donors in this age group in a multicentre German transplant study.

Patients aged ≥75 years old may be offered supportive treatment with hydroxyurea or low-dose cytarabine (20 mg b.i.d. SC for 10 days) to control WBC.

Targeted therapy

Gemtuzumab ozogamicin (GO) consists of a humanized anti-CD33 monoclonal antibody conjugated with calicheamicin, a potent antitumour anthracycline antibiotic. Despite much controversy and early withdrawal from the market, the final results of randomized studies demonstrated improved event-free survival (EFS) and/or OS when GO was combined with induction chemotherapy for patients with newly diagnosed AML with favourable and intermediate-risk cytogenetics, and in patients with APL. This is anticipated to open a new discussion over its use.

Activating mutations in the *FLT3* gene result in increased survival and proliferation of leukaemic blasts, are common in AML and are associated with an adverse prognosis. Therefore, the FLT3 receptor is an appealing target for inhibition. Multiple small inhibitory molecules are currently in development for *FLT3*-mutated *AML*, and agents such as sorafenib are beginning to show promising efficacy when combined with chemotherapy in induction. AC220 is a novel second-generation tyrosine kinase inhibitor (TKI) that is highly selective for both wild-type and mutant *FLT3* and has significant activity against KIT. Studies showed a relatively high CR rate (45%), but acquisition of AC220 resistance is an emerging problem.

Post-treatment assessment

- Complete response (CR) in AML (as well as ALL) is defined as the presence of ≤5% blasts in BM, absence of extramedullary disease, absolute neutrophil count of >1.0 × 10⁹/L, platelet count of >100 × 10⁹/L and freedom from RBC transfusion:
  - CR with incomplete recovery (CRi) is defined as above, but without complete neutrophil and platelet recovery
- BM examination is usually repeated on Days 12–15 from the start of induction therapy:
  - Should include both aspirate and biopsy since aspirate may be difficult to interpret in a severely neutropenic patient
  - If blasts are still present and the marrow is not completely hypocellular, a second course of induction should be given (unless the patient is severely ill and will not tolerate additional chemotherapy and prolonged neutropenia)
  - To be repeated at recovery from induction and to also include flow cytometry, PCR and cytogenetic analysis if one of these tests was positive at diagnosis
  - Not routinely recommended to be repeated during follow-up:
    - Should be reserved for suspicion of relapse, usually presenting as an unexplained drop in blood counts
- Most relapses occur within the first 2 years following therapy

Controversies

- Treatment of elderly AML
- Use of gemtuzumab ozogamicin
- Number of consolidation cycles needed in AML

Areas of research

- Implication of cooperating mutations in the prognosis of an individual patient
- Use of hypomethylating agents
- Incorporation of MRD assessment into risk stratification
- Role of targeted therapy (FLT3-ITD inhibitors)

Acute promyelocytic leukaemia

APL (FAB M3) accounts for about 10–15% of AML cases. Patients tend to be younger (median age 40 years), have low WBC, high incidence of DIC and improved survival compared with other AML types. The disease is associated with a balanced translocation of t(15; 17) (q22; q12), creating a fusion protein, PML-RARA, that interacts with the nuclear repressor protein complex. The formation of this protein complex attracts histone deacetylase, which alters the chromatin confirmation and therefore inhibits transcription.

Treatment

Treatment includes aggressive control of DIC coupled with early initiation of the differentiation agent all-*trans*-retinoic acid (ATRA). ATRA should be started at the initial suspicion of APL, usually based on morphology only without waiting for PCR confirmation, as ATRA can prevent and aid in the treatment of DIC. DIC is managed by checking platelet count, international normalized ratio (INR) and fibrinogen every 8–12 hours, and administering platelets and blood products to maintain a platelet count of >30,000–50,000, an INR of <1.5 and fibrinogen of >150 mg/dL, while avoiding fluid overload.

Prognostic risk factors for APL include a WBC of >10,000/μL at presentation and age >60 years.
- *Low-risk patients*:
  - Induction with high-dose anthracyclines (daunorubicin 50 mg/m^2/day × 4 days) and oral ATRA 45 mg/m^2/day until remission is documented
  - Post-remission therapy consists of repeat cycles of anthracyclines with ATRA
  - Monitoring molecular remission by RT-PCR for PML-RARA is of value only after consolidation, since it is commonly positive post induction and hence should not guide treatment decisions at this point
- *High-risk patients*:
  - Early initiation of chemotherapy in addition to ATRA is important to control DIC
  - Addition of intermediate–high-dose cytosine arabinose (ara-C) in consolidation improves survival
  - Maintenance therapy with ATRA ± chemotherapy is controversial and may not be necessary in low-risk patients:
    - Generally recommended to follow the protocol used in induction and administer maintenance if this was given in the protocol
  - CNS prophylaxis is recommended, especially if high-dose ara-C was not given
  - Arsenic trioxide (ATO) has shown promising results both in induction (with ATRA) and relapse, either as a single agent or combined with ATRA:
    - Plays a special role in patients unable to receive high-dose anthracyclines
  - Differentiation syndrome secondary to ATRA and arsenic trioxide (ATO) may manifest as fluid overload, fever, hypotension, renal failure and congestive heart failure with lung infiltrates on chest X-ray, leading to acute respiratory distress:
    - More common with increase in WBC and necessitates immediate treatment with IV dexacort 10 mg × 2/day and temporary cessation of ATRA or ATO

ACUTE LYMPHOBLASTIC LEUKAEMIA

Acute lymphoblastic leukaemia (ALL) is characterized by accumulation of ≥20% early lymphoid progenitors termed 'lymphoblasts' in the BM and/or PB, occasionally infiltrating lymph nodes, spleen and other solid organs. Bone marrow infiltration is accompanied by secondary suppression of normal haemopoiesis. The disease onset is abrupt and unless treated early, can be lethal. The peak incidence is observed in the paediatric age group (2–4 years) and the incidence rises again in patients >60 years of age.

Pathogenesis and aetiology

ALL is characterized by gross numerical and structural chromosomal abnormalities, including hyperdiploidy, hypodiploidy, translocations t(12; 22), (1;19), (9; 22) and (4; 11), and rearrangements (*MYC*, *MLL*). However, several observations indicate that these lesions alone are insufficient to induce leukaemia and cooperating lesions are required. Many of the genes involved encode proteins with key roles in lymphoid development (e.g. *PAX5*, *IZKF1*), cell cycle regulation and tumour suppression (*CDKN2A/CDKN2B*), lymphoid signalling, transcriptional regulation and co-activation (*ETV1*, *ERG*). It is suggested that the initial event confers self-renewal coupled with mutation, leading to the developmental arrest and secondary cooperative event in cell cycle regulation, tumour suppression and chromatin modification, eventually leading to the establishment of a leukaemic clone.

Aetiology

Although unknown, several predisposing factors have been described:
- Ionizing radiation such as in atomic bomb survivors
- Hereditary syndromes: Down, Bloom, Klinefelter, Fanconi, ataxia telangiectasia and neurofibromatosis
- Viral: association of human T-cell lymphocytic virus 1 (HTLV-1) in T-lymphoblastic leukaemia/lymphoma and Epstein–Barr virus (EBV) in mature B-cell ALL.

Classification

ALL is subdivided into B precursor (75% of cases) and T precursor (25%).

The WHO classification (2008) integrates immunophenotyping with genetic and molecular data, and segregates ALL into B (B-ALL) and T type (T-ALL) with unique genetic alterations (Box 34.2). The term 'lymphoma' is reserved for patients presenting with an extramedullary mass or adenopathy and, arbitrarily, ≤20% blasts in BM.

Presentation

- Acute presentation with signs and symptoms related to marrow failure:
  - Anaemia: presents as weakness, lethargy, shortness of breath and palpitations

Box 34.2 WHO classification of ALL

B-lymphoblastic leukaemia/lymphoma
- B lymphoblastic leukaemia/lymphoma, NOS
- B lymphoblastic leukaemia/lymphoma with recurrent genetic abnormalities
- B-lymphoblastic leukaemia/lymphoma with t(9; 22) (q34; q11.2); *BCR-ABL1*
- B-lymphoblastic leukaemia/lymphoma with t(v; 11q23); *MLL* rearranged
- B-lymphoblastic leukaemia/lymphoma with t(12; 21) (p13; q22); *TEL-AML1* (*ETV6-RUNX1*)
- B-lymphoblastic leukaemia/lymphoma with hyperdiploidy
- B-lymphoblastic leukaemia/lymphoma with hypodiploidy
- B-lymphoblastic leukaemia/lymphoma with t(5; 14) (q31; q32); *IL3-IGH*
- B lymphoblastic leukaemia/lymphoma with t(1; 19) (q23; p13.3); *TCF3-PBX1*

T-lymphoblastic leukaemia/lymphoma

WHO (2014). Reproduced with permission of WHO.

Table 34.3 Immunophenotyping of ALL

Disease classification	Immunophenotype
B lineage ≈75%	HLA-DR+, TdT+, CD19+,
Common B lineage markers	CD22+, CD79a
Pro B	CD10–
Common	CD10+
Pre B	cIgM
Mature B cell	sIgM, c or s kappa or lambda
T lineage ≈25%	c or s CD3+, CD7+
Common T-lineage markers	cCD3+, CD7+, CD5±, CD2–, sCD3, CD1a–
Early T	
Cortical	CD2+, CD5+, CD1a+, sCD3±
Mature	CD2+, CD5+, sCD3+, CD1a–

c, cytoplasmic; s, surface.

- Neutropenia: associated with fever, infection (usually Gram-negative or *Staphylococcus*)
- Thrombocytopenia: presents as purpura, menorrhagia, mucosal (epistaxis, gingival) or retinal bleeding
- Hyperleukocytosis with leukostasis: hypoxaemia, retinal haemorrhage, confusion
- Bone pain: more common in children
- Mediastinal mass with cough and superior vena cava syndrome in T-ALL
- CNS involvement: headache, confusion, cranial nerve palsy:
  - Occurs in 6% of patients at presentation
- Lymphadenopathy (55% of patients)
- Splenomegaly and hepatomegaly (45% of patients)

Diagnostic work-up

- CBC and peripheral blood smear examination:
  - Blasts usually have a large nucleus and scanty and blueish cytoplasm compared to myeloid blasts
- Immunohistochemistry:
  - Usually positive for Tdt (terminal deoxynucleotidyl transferase) in lymphoblasts of both T- and B-cell precursor lineage, but not in mature B-cell ALL
  - Immunostains are not routinely performed nowadays as have largely been replaced by immunophenotyping
- BM aspirate for morphology evaluation, including blast count:
  - Biopsy if dry tap
- Immunophenotyping of PB and/or BM (Table 34.3):
  - Basically, T-lineage ALL is established by the presence of cytoplasmic CD3 and CD7, whereas B-lineage ALL is characterized by the presence of CD1a, CD22 and CD79a, with or without CD10
- Cytogenetic and molecular analysis of BM:
  - Conventional cytogenetic analysis is mandatory, with a minimum of 20 metaphase cells analysed
  - Although less well established compared to AML, the last decade is characterized by increasing knowledge of the importance of both numerical chromosomal changes (hyperdiploid, hypodiploid) and translocations associated with ALL
    - Hyperdiploidy (>50 chromosomes) and hypodiploidy (<44 chromosomes) are associated with good and poor prognosis, respectively
    - Translocation t(9; 22) (q34; q11.2); *BCR-ABL* (2% in children, 40% in older adults) should be looked for in every B-cell ALL, since it has both prognostic and treatment implications
  - More recently, specific gene mutations, such as *IKZF1* mutation, although this has not yet been translated into practical recommendations
- CT chest, abdomen and pelvis for T-ALL
- Testicular examination and lumbar puncture (LP) to evaluate extramedullary disease:
  - LP is best performed after clearing of peripheral blood from blasts
- Fertility consultation:
  - Male patients should be offered the possibility of sperm preservation
  - Fertile female patients should be offered GNRH antagonists to prevent menstrual bleeding during thrombocytopenia, with some evidence supporting gonadal protection with these agents
- Cardiac evaluation in older patients including echocardiogram

Differential diagnosis

- Lymphoma in leukaemic phase
- Infections: EBV, cytomegalovirus (CMV)
- BM failure: aplastic anaemia, megaloblastic anaemia

Prognostic factors

Adverse prognostic factors are:
- Age >35 years
- Elevated WBC at diagnosis (>30,000/μL for B lineage; >100,00/μL for T lineage):
  - Elevated WBC in T-lineage ALL is less important as a prognostic factor than an elevated WBC in B-lineage ALL
- Presence of adverse cytogenetics/molecular aberrations:
  - Numerical changes: hypodiploidy (<44 chromosomes)
  - Chromosomal translocations: Philadelphia chromosome (Ph) [t(9; 22)], t(4; 11), t(8; 14) and complex karyotype
  - Gene mutations: *IKZF1* mutation is present in 15% of paediatric patients, >75% of Ph+ paediatric patients and >50% of adults with ALL, and is associated with poor outcome
- Achieving CR >4 weeks post induction
- Minimal residual disease (MRD):
  - Detection of residual leukaemic clone, using patient-specific immunoglobulin gene rearrangement by PCR, at 16 weeks after induction is associated with poor outcome

Treatment

The initial aim of chemotherapy is to achieve rapid and complete remission (CR). CR is defined as <5% blasts in BM, absence of extramedullary disease, absolute neutrophil count of >1.0 × 10^9/L, platelet count of >100,000/μL and independence from RBC transfusion.

There are different approaches to treatment of adult ALL. The most commonly used is the BFM (British–Frankfurt–Muenster)-like protocol which utilizes alternating multiple agent chemotherapy upfront and includes four treatment phases. Other possible protocols include the M. D. Anderson Hyper-CVAD regimen, mainly used in the USA. Another option is to use an intensive leukaemia regimen such as high-dose cytarabine and mitoxantrone. Overall, there is no significant difference in both CR and long-term outcome between the different protocols.

Treatment: Acute lymphoblastic leukaemia	Description

Supportive treatment	- Patient instruction and support regarding the disease and treatment course
	- Intensive hydration (aim for urine output of >100 mL/hour) to prevent renal failure from tumour lysis
	- Allopurinol or rasburicase to prevent hyperuricaemia
	- RBC and platelet transfusion support:
	  - Prophylactic platelet transfusion is recommended to maintain a threshold of 10 × 10^9/L
	  - Filtered products are recommended for alloimmunization prevention.
	- Antibiotic prophylaxis with quinolones is recommended:
	  - For febrile neutropenia, the use of broad-spectrum antibiotics is recommended
	  - Antifungal (antimould) agents as prophylaxis
	- Leukopheresis for WBC of >100,000/μL or symptoms of leukostasis

Definitive treatment	- BFM (British–Frankfurt–Muenster)-like protocol:
	  1. Remission induction:
	     - Two cycles are administered, each over 4 weeks, including vincristine, dexacort, daunorubicin and L-asparaginase in the first cycle and cytarabine and cyclophosphamide in the second cycle of intensification
	  2. Consolidation:
	     - Five cycles of chemotherapy with the aim to further decrease tumour burden and prevent relapse
	  3. CNS prophylaxis:
	     - Periodic intrathecal chemotherapy, cycles of high-dose methotrexate and cranial irradiation
	     - Cranial irradiation is given to adults not planned for SCT (at a dose of 18–24 cGy over 12 fractions)
	     - Children are precluded from radiation due to cognitive impairment
	     - Continued through all stages of treatment
	     - With this approach, the risk of CNS relapse decreases from 30% to 5%
	  4. Maintenance therapy allows completion of 2.5-year treatment:
	     - Daily 6-mercaptopurine (MP), weekly methotrexate and vincristine + prednisone every 3 months
	- M. D. Anderson Hyper-CVAD regimen:
	  - Cycles of cyclophosphamide + adriamycin + vincristine + prednisone, alternating with high-dose cytarabine + methotrexate
	  - Excludes asparaginase
	  - Administered for a total of eight cycles with maintenance given only to patients with precursor ALL
	- Intensive leukaemia regimen such as high-dose cytarabine + mitoxantrone

Allogeneic stem cell transplantation

Data from large cooperative trials and meta-analysis have demonstrated the beneficial effect of post-remission therapy using allogeneic SCT from matched sibling donors on the OS, implying potent GVL effect. In the largest study to date by the ECOG MRC group, this effect was most prominent in the standard-risk group, while in other studies it was more beneficial in the high-risk category (almost no group except ECOG-MRC studied this in standard-risk ALL). Improved supportive care and use of reduced-intensity SCT in patients aged >60 years were found to be associated with reduced transplant-related mortality while preserving the beneficial effect of transplant. Alternative donors such as matched unrelated, umbilical cord and haploidentical donors are increasingly used in patients lacking a matched sibling, with encouraging results.

Treatment of Ph+ ALL

Presence of the Ph chromosome with t(9, 22); *BCR-ABL* is associated with poor prognosis across all age groups. Its frequency increases with age (~50% of patients are >60 years old). Although never tested prospectively, the addition of the TKI imatinib (400–800 mg/day) in combination with chemotherapy in induction has led to a marked improvement in the treatment outcome of this leukaemia, with a CR rate of 95–100% as compared to <30% in historical controls. This enables more patients to proceed to allogeneic SCT. Dasatinib, a second-generation TKI with a broader kinase inhibition against both tyrosine and Src kinases, has been studied and provided similar results. In older adults, it offers the option of using the less toxic chemotherapy followed by reduced-intensity SCT. The use of imatinib coupled with minimal chemotherapy (vincristine + prednisone only) yielded a high CR rate in older adults. TKIs cannot be employed without further consolidation with SCT due to a high percentage (~80%) of emerging mutations, especially with the use of imatinib. In addition, imatinib has poor penetration capacity to the CNS compared to dasatinib and this should be taken into consideration in treatment planning.

The use of TKIs post allogeneic SCT is controversial and still under investigation, although reported by some authors to be beneficial. There is poor tolerance of the drug post transplant mainly due to a decrease in CBC. In addition, it is unclear which treatment strategy is the best: prophylactic for all patients or pre-emptive as based on periodic PCR analysis.

Additional targeted therapy includes nelarabine, a nucleoside analogue inhibitor, with good results in relapsed/refractory T-ALL.

Monoclonal antibody

CD20 is expressed in 30–40% of B-precursor ALL blasts, 40–50% of older adults and 80–100% of mature B-ALL blasts (Burkitt type). Rituximab, the chimeric monoclonal antibody (MAB) to CD20, was used both in precursor B-ALL harbouring the CD20 and in mature B-ALL. In mature B-ALL, various studies have demonstrated improved outcome (some even up to 30%) when rituximab 375 mg/m² was added, usually for eight cycles given either on Day 1 of each chemotherapy cycle or at the beginning and end of each chemotherapy cycle.

In precursor B-ALL, the German ALL group administered rituximab on Day 1 of induction phase 1 and 2 and on six cycles of consolidation in adults aged <55 years, and found a similar CR rate. However, achievement of MRD negativity was superior in the rituximab group and this translated into better continuous CR and OS in the standard-risk group (defined as a WBC of <30,000/μL and no adverse cytogenetics) and improved MRD and continuous CR in the high-risk group. Similar results were obtained with the addition of rituximab to the hyper-CVAD protocol. The effect of the addition of rituximab on the outcome for older adults (>60 years) is unclear due to excessive infections in the treated group. The use of rituximab in paediatric ALL patients has not been studied.

Another attractive target is CD19, which is expressed during the early stages of B-cell maturation and development. Blinatumomab represents a new approach to targeted therapy. This monoclonal antibody is designed to target both CD19-expressing B cells and CD3-expressing T cells, thereby recruiting cytotoxic T cells to lyse the CD19-expressing blasts. It has shown promising results in MRD-positive ALL patients, with 80% achieving MRD negativity, and in patients with relapsed/refractory disease. It is currently being intensively investigated in first CR and in the refractory/relapsed setting.

Other monoclonal antibodies directed against CD22, CD52 and T cell are under investigation.

ALL in adolescents and young adults

In the paediatric group aged 2–10 years, the long-term outcome is excellent, with 80% of patients achieving a long-term survival. This is in contrast to adults for whom the cure rate is only 30–40%. This may reflect both a different biology of the disease, which is less favourable in adults (more Ph+, less hyperdiploid), and lower tolerability to aggressive therapies in this patient population. The improvement in the paediatric risk group is also attributed to the risk-adapted therapy which incorporates in decision-making such variables as time to response to induction, cytogenetics and molecular markers, and MRD assessment.

Over the last two decades, improvement has been noted in the outcome for adolescents and younger adults (15–19 years old), with a 5-year OS increase from 41% to 62%, while lower rates of improvement have been achieved in patients aged 20–59 years. Despite this improvement in the young adults, it still falls short of the outstanding results in the paediatric group.

The definition of young adults remains debatable and most studies include patients up to 30–35 years. The adolescent group (15–21 years) is at the intersection between paediatrics and adults, and as such receives treatment for either group. Retrospective analysis of the results of the large cooperative group showed improved outcome for this group when treated with paediatric protocols. This is attributed to greater cumulative dosing of the more non-myelosuppressive drugs (steroids, vincristine, L-asparaginase), more intensive CNS prophylaxis and better adherence to the treatment schedule. The results of prospective studies are awaited.

ALL in older adults

According to SEER data, the incidence of ALL beyond age 60 years is increasing and 31% of patients with ALL are in this age group. The Cooperative group studies show a dismal prognosis in this age category, with only 57% of patients achieving CR and a 3-year disease-free survival (DFS) of 18% and an OS of 12%, as compared to 81%, 38% and 38%, respectively, for the group aged 30–59 years. A recent UKALL XII/ECOG 2993 study retrospectively analysing patients with ALL younger or older than 55 years, demonstrated an OS of 37% versus 14%, respectively, which was mainly attributed to a high mortality rate in induction (4% vs 18%) as well as a necessity for dose reduction by 46%. These results imply the need for novel strategies in the management of older patients with ALL.

Minimal residual disease in ALL

Several studies have shown the importance of detecting MRD at different time points and hence it is used as an independent prognostic factor both in paediatric and adult ALL. MRD was found to be important in both the induction and relapse settings, as well as post allogeneic SCT.

Several methods are currently used for MRD detection in ALL and these include PCR for immunoglobulin or T-cell receptor gene rearrangements, PCR for *BCR-ABL* transcripts and multiparametric flow cytometry. The PCR methods are generally very sensitive and have a high degree of standardization, and most current data are based on this technique. However, they are time consuming and expensive. The sensitivity of the flow cytometry method depends on the technique used (3–4 vs 26 colours). While this is a quick, quantitative method, interpretation of results is problematic when the marrow is regenerative or hypoplastic. It also demands an experienced team. Standardization of methods is of paramount importance not only to ensure comparability between different laboratories for the same protocol, but also to compare results of different treatment protocols.

Post-treatment assessment

- Complete response (CR) in ALL (and in AML) is defined as the presence of <5% blasts in BM, absence of extramedullary disease, absolute neutrophil count of >1.0 × 10^9/L, platelet count of >100 ×10^9/L and freedom from RBC transfusion
    - CR with incomplete recovery (Cri) is defined as above, but without complete neutrophil and platelet recovery

- In ALL, follow-up examination should be performed upon completion of phase 1 or 2 of induction:
    - However, most studies incorporate earlier response assessment, since the depth of response is crucial in risk assessment and determination of future therapy
- Outside of clinical studies it is reasonable to repeat BM examination upon completion of each therapeutic cycle:
    - However, it is important to keep in mind that in ALL, late relapses, even following allogenic SCT, are not rare (in contrast, in AML most relapses occur within the first 2 years following therapy)

Controversies

- Paediatric-inspired therapies in adult ALL
- Duration of TKI use in Ph$^+$ ALL

Areas of research

- Refining definition of genetic alterations associated with disease prognosis
- Role of monoclonal antibodies
- Treatment of young adults

CHRONIC MYELOID LEUKAEMIA

Chronic myeloid leukaemia (CML) is a pluripotent stem cell disease with leukocytosis and the presence of t(9; 22); *BCR-ABL*. CML occurs in three different phases: chronic, accelerated and blastic. Without effective therapy, the chronic phase progresses within 3–5 years through an accelerated phase (usually lasting 6 months) into a rapidly fatal acute leukaemia known as the blast crisis.

Pathogenesis and aetiology

Pathogenesis

The immediate cause of CML is the presence of a reciprocal translocation t(9; 22); *BCR-ABL*. In this translocation a large part of the abelson (*ABL*) gene on chromosome 9 is translocated to the breakpoint cluster region (*BCR*) gene on chromosome 22, creating *BCR-ABL*, a hybrid oncogene (p210) coding for the *BCR-ABL* fusion protein. *BCR-ABL* is a constitutively active tyrosine kinase that dysregulates downstream signalling pathways and increases the proliferation and survival of leukaemic cells. The discovery of *BCR-ABL* was a key milestone in understanding CML and designing novel targeted therapies to treat it. The mechanisms of CML evolution to blast crisis are complex and are associated with secondary chromosomal changes that may contribute to the malignant phenotype. These additional clonal cytogenetic aberrations (ACAs), also called major route

ACAs, include duplication of the Ph chromosome, trisomy 8, isochromosome 17q and trisomy 19. These secondary molecular and chromosomal changes promote increased proliferation, enhanced survival, genomic instability and arrest of differentiation, a distinctive feature in blast crisis.

Presentation

Most CML patients are diagnosed with a *chronic phase* (CP), often revealed as an incidental finding during routine blood tests. This phase is characterized by an uncontrolled proliferation of myeloid elements that retain their ability to differentiate, resulting in an abnormal number of mature granulocytes. In symptomatic CML, the symptoms are secondary to increased proliferation and splenomegaly and generally appear gradually. These may include: fatigue, weight loss, non-specific bone pain, sweating, abdominal discomfort and early satiety. Uncommon presenting symptoms may include: acute abdominal pain secondary to splenic infarction, symptoms of leukostasis, and hypermetabolism manifesting as hyperuricemia and gouty arthritis. Physical examination usually detects splenomegaly.

Accelerated phase (AP) is characterized by symptoms of night sweats, fever, weight loss, bone pain, difficulty in controlling counts with therapy and increased basophils and blasts. *Blast crisis* (BC) is essentially acute leukaemia and is characterized as ≥20% blasts. In two-thirds of patients the BC is that of AML and in a third it is of ALL. The WHO definitions of AP and BC are presented in Table 34.4.

Diagnostic work-up

- CBC: leukocytosis (usually $>25 \times 10^9$/L):
  - Differential count reveals granulocytes at all stages of differentiation in peripheral blood with increased basophil count
  - Blasts usually amount to <10% in the chronic phase

Table 34.4 WHO definitions of accelerated phase (AP) and blast crisis (BC)

Criteria for AP	Criteria for BC
Blasts 10–19% in PB or BM	Blasts ≥20% in PB or BM
PB basophils ≥20%	Extramedullary blast proliferation (chloroma)
Persistent thrombocytopenia (<100 $\times 10^9$/L) unrelated to therapy or persistent thrombocytosis (>1000 $\times 10^9$/L) unresponsive to therapy	Large foci or clusters of blasts in BM biopsy
Increased spleen size and increased WBC count unresponsive to therapy	
Cytogenetic evidence of clonal evolution	

- Thrombocytosis occurs in 50% of patients
- Hb can be normal or reduced
- Chemistry: serum LDH is elevated as well as uric acid and serum B12
- BM examination:
  - Reveals hypercellular marrow (75–90% cellularity), increased granulocyte to erythroid ratio (10:1–30:1), increased eosinophils and basophils and a blast count of <10% in CP
  - In 50% of patients, increased reticulin with fibrosis is observed
  - Additional BM tests include cytogenetic and molecular analysis:
    ○ Conventional cytogenetic evaluation should be performed to detect the presence of Ph chromosome at diagnosis
    ○ In addition, it is important to perform cytogenetic analysis in order to detect possible additional chromosomal abnormalities
    ○ If BM aspiration is not feasible, FISH analysis on PB is used to confirm the presence of t(9; 22):
      – FISH is not an acceptable method for follow-up due to lack of the standardization
    ○ Quantitative RT-PCR (QPCR) of BM should also be performed before initiation of treatment and for follow-up:
      – Results are reported as percentage of *BCR-ABL1* transcripts/control gene (usually either *BCR* or *ABL*)
      – Since there are no standard reagents the results are reported as the International Scale (IS), which includes a conversion factor derived from comparison and validation with a reference laboratory; all molecular response criteria and treatment recommendations are based upon IS results
- Sokal and Hasford prognostic scores were developed in the pre-TKI era with the aim of evaluating the length of the chronic phase (Box 34.3):
  - High-risk category remains valid with the use of first- and second-generation of inhibitors
  - More recent European Treatment and Outcome Study (EUTOS) score predicts response in patients treated with imatinib

Treatment

In the pre-targeted therapy era, patients were treated with interferon. Beside significant side effects, the best outcome reported was a cytogenetic response in only 10% of patients. The majority of patients were treated with allogeneic SCT.

Tyrosine kinase inhibitors

The introduction of TKIs in the late 1990s represented a major breakthrough in the treatment of CML. This oral treatment has resulted in significant cytogenetic and molecular responses

Leukaemia

Box 34.3 Risk calculation for CML

Study	Calculation	Risk definition by calculation
Sokal et al. (1984)	Exp [0.116 (age − 43.4)] + 0.0345(spleen size − 7.51) + 0.188[(platelets/700)^2 − 0.563] + 0.0887(% blasts − 2.1)	Low: <0.8 Intermediate: 0.8–1.2 High: >1.2
Hasford et al. (1998)	0.666 when age ≥50 years + (0.042 × spleen) + 1.0956 when platelet count ≥1500 × 10^9/μL + (0.0584 × blast cells) + 0.20399 when basophils >3% + (0.0413 × eosinophil) × 100	Low: ≤ 780 Intermediate: 781–1480 High: >1480
EUTOS	7 × basophils + 4 × spleen size Basophils as percentage measured in PB, spleen measured in cm BCM by manual palpitation All calculations should be made before any treatment	Low ≤87 High >87

Source: NCCN Clinical Practice Guidelines in Oncology: Chronic Myelogenous Leukemia. Version 3.2014. http://www.nccn.org/professionals/physician_gls/pdf/cml.pdf

which translate into essential improvement in DFS and OS. In order to evaluate the efficacy of treatment, response definitions have been determined (Table 34.5)

- First-generation TKI: imatinib
- Second-generation TKIs: nilotinib and dasatinib
- Third-generation TKIs: bosutinib and ponatinib

Chronic phase treatment: TKIs	Description

Imatinib	• Selective *BCR-ABL* TKI
	• Dose: 400 mg/day:
	  ▪ Higher doses (600 mg/day or 800 mg/day) induce a deeper and faster response, with no difference in response at 12 months
	  ▪ Higher dose may be of benefit in high-risk Sokal score CP-CML
	• Major side effects include cytopenia, nausea, rush, fluid retention and hepatic toxicity:
	  ▪ Managed by co-administration of growth factors and temporary drug interruption

Nilotinib	• More potent selective TKI • Dose: 300 mg b.i.d.: ▪ Should be given on an empty stomach (2 hours before and 1 hour after food) • Major side effects: QT prolongation (monitor ECG at baseline, after 7 days of treatment and periodically thereafter), increased risk of vascular events (mainly peripheral arterial occlusive disease), cytopenia, elevated lipase, amylase and hepatic transaminases
Dasatinib	• Potent dual inhibitor of ABL and SRC kinases: ▪ Active against all *BCR-ABL* mutations except T315I • Dose: 100 mg/day • Side effects: cytopenia, nausea, rush, fluid retention, pleura–pericardial effusion and, rarely, pulmonary hypertension

Bosutinib	• Dual *SRC-ABL* TKI:
	  ▪ Active against most of imatinib-resistant mutations except for V299L and T315I
	• Dose: 500 mg daily
	• Promising clinical results in first-, second- and third-line CML treatment:
	  ▪ As first-line treatment, provides complete cytogenetic response (CCyR) significantly earlier than imatinib
	• Relatively safe; major side effects are gastrointestinal ones, rush and cytopenia

Ponatinib	• TKI designed to inhibit *BCR-ABL* with mutations, especially *T315I* • Dose: 45 mg/day • Major side effects: arterial and venous occlusion:

Table 34.5 Definitions of response to treatment in CML

Haematological response – complete (CHR)	Cytogenetic response (CR)	Molecular response (MR)
WBC <10 × 10⁹/L Platelet count <450 × 10⁹/L No immature granulocytes <5% basophils in PB Non-palpable spleen No signs/symptoms related to disease	Complete (CCyR): no Ph+ metaphases Partial: 1–35% Ph+ metaphases Major (complete + partial): 0–35% Ph+ metaphases Minor: >35% Ph+ metaphases	Complete (CMR): no detectable BCR-ABL transcripts by QPCR (IS) (assay sensitivity ≥4.5 or 5 log) Major (MMR): BCR-ABL1; IS ≤0.1%

First-line treatment should be initiated with either imatinib, dasatinib or nilotinib. Although dasatinib and nilotinib demonstrated superior cytogenetic and molecular responses at certain time points and lower rates of disease progression compared to imatinib, the long-term benefit of this has yet to be determined.

Monitoring the response to TKI is fundamental in CML therapy; this aims to prevent disease progression to AP or BC. It is determined by assessing haematological, cytogenetic and molecular responses at 3, 6, 12 and 18 months from initiation of treatment with either first- or second-line TKI as suggested by the European LeukemiaNet recommendations for the management of chronic myeloid leukaemia published in 2013.

Relapse is defined as any sign of loss of response (by haematological or cytogenetic assessment). A 1 log increase in BCR-ABL transcript levels with loss of MMR should promote marrow evaluation for loss of CCyR, but of itself is not defined as relapse.

Resistance to TKIs

Two main groups of resistance mechanisms exist: BCR-ABL-independent mechanisms and BCR-ABL-dependent mechanisms. The latter may result from (1) duplication or over-amplification of the BCR-ABL oncogene that might lead to an elevated ABL kinase activity and (2) mutation at the BCR-ABL binding site. Over 55 types of mutations in the BCR-ABL oncoprotein have been identified. BCR-ABL-independent mechanisms may result from a decrease in the intracellular level of TKIs due to drug efflux, drug influx, drug binding, or drug concentration or activation of alternative signalling pathways downstream of BCR-ABL.

Allogeneic stem cell transplantation

Allogeneic SCT remains the only long-term curative treatment; however, the morbidity and mortality associated with the procedure mean it should be performed only under certain circumstances in the current era of CML therapy:
- Patients who present with BC or progress to AP or BC on therapy
- Patients who failed a second-generation TKI and failed or were unable to receive ponatinib.

Areas of research

- Defining the patient population in which TKI therapy could be safely stopped
- Management of paediatric and adolescent disease
- New biological markers for selection of optimal first-line treatment

CHRONIC LYMPHATIC LEUKAEMIA

Chronic lymphatic leukaemia (CLL) is a neoplastic disease with accumulation of small, mature appearing lymphocytes in the PB, BM, lymph nodes and spleen. It is mainly a disease of the elderly and is characterized by a slowly progressing course, often lasting many years. However, the disease may follow an intermediate or aggressive course.

Pathogenesis and epidemiology

Pathogenesis

CLL is initiated by genetic alteration such as deletion of the long arm of chromosome 13 (13q14) followed by other genetic alterations such as deletion of the long arm of chromosome 11 (11q22.3), deletion of the short arm of chromosome 17 (17p13.1) and trisomy of chromosome 12. In addition, somatic mutations are present such as in TP53. Moreover, the microenvironment has a significant role in promoting CLL cell proliferation and survival through aberrant activation of the B-cell receptor (BCR).

Epidemiology

It is the most common leukaemia in the Western world with an estimated incidence of 4.3 per 100,000. The median age at diagnosis is 72 years and it is very uncommon before 45 years of age. It is more common in men than in women and in Caucasians, and rare in Asians, implicating a possible genetic predisposition. Familial predisposition exists with up to 10% of affected patients having a first- or second-degree relative with the disease.

Presentation

- Majority of patients are asymptomatic at diagnosis:
  - CLL is an incidental finding on blood tests performed for other reasons

- During disease evolution: may present with adenopathy, splenomegaly with associated abdominal pain and early satiety, fatigue due to anaemia, purpura or petechiae due to thrombocytopenia, and recurrent infections due to associated hypogammaglobulinaemia
- Autoimmune phenomena may develop such as Coombs positive autoimmune haemolytic anaemia and idiopathic thrombocytopenia secondary to autoantibodies produced by the abnormal clone
- General symptoms such as fever, weight loss and night sweats are uncommon and usually represent transformation to aggressive lymphoma, termed Richter transformation

Diagnostic work-up

- CBC:
  - >5000/L of mature appearing lymphocytes
  - PB smear discloses the presence of smudge cells
- No need for BM analysis or lymph node biopsy unless diagnosis is unclear or transformation is suspected
- Chemistry: LDH
- Flow cytometry of peripheral blood demonstrates: CD5+, CD23+, CD10−, CD19+, CD20dim, sIgdim, Cycline D1−
- FISH analysis of PB for: trisomy12, del13q, del11q, del17p
- Optional: PCR for immunoglobulin heavy chain mutational status and flow cytometry for Zap70 and CD38
- CT scan of the neck, chest, abdomen and pelvis for evaluation of initial disease and response to therapy in clinical trials; otherwise its role is questionable
- Serum immunoglobulin level
- Virology: hepatitis B, hepatitis C and HIV status

Differential diagnosis
- *Monoclonal B cell lymphocytosis*:
  - This diagnosis is established when there are <5000/L mature lymphocytes in PB and no evidence of adenopathy and/or splenomegaly
  - 1–1% of the individuals with this diagnosis annually transform to CLL requiring therapy
- *Small lymphocytic lymphoma*:
  - Diagnosed when there are <5000/L mature lymphocytes in PB with associated adenopathy and /or splenomegaly
  - Lymph node biopsy confirms the diagnosis
- *Mantle cell lymphoma*
  - This lymphoma may be associated with peripheral lymphocytosis
  - Presence of cycline D1 in FISH analysis or flow cytometry will confirm this diagnosis

Staging and prognostic factors

The median survival in patients with CLL varies according to the Rai and Binet classifications from >12 years for patients at low risk to 8 and 2 years for patients at intermediate and high risk, respectively (Tables 34.6 and 34.7). At early stages of the disease, there is significant variability in time to disease progression. Biological prognostic factors are given in Tables 34.8 and 34.9, and will presumably be used more frequently in the future.

Table 34.6 Rai staging system for CLL

Stage	Description	Risk status
0	Lymphocytosis, lymphocytes in blood >15,000/μL and >40% lymphocytes in the bone marrow	Low
I	Stage 0 with enlarged node(s)	Intermediate
II	Stage 0–I with splenomegaly, hepatomegaly or both	Intermediate
III	Stage 0–II with haemoglobin <11.0 g/dL or haematocrit <33%	High
IV	Stage 0–III with platelets <100,000/μL	High

Source: NCCN Clinical Practice Guidelines in Oncology: Non-Hodgkin's Lymphomas. Version 3.2014.

Table 34.7 Binet staging system for CLL

Stage	Description
A	Haemoglobin ≥10 g/dL and platelets ≥100,000/mm^3 and <3 enlarged areas
B	Haemoglobin ≥10 g/dL and platelets ≥100,000/mm^3 and ≥3 enlarged areas
C	Haemoglobin <10 g/dL and platelets <100,000/mm^3 and any number of enlarged areas

Source: NCCN Clinical Practice Guidelines in Oncology: Non-Hodgkin's Lymphomas. Version 3.2014.

Table 34.8 Immunoglobulin heavy chain variable (IGHV) region gene mutation and surrogates by flow cytometry

	Outcome association	
	Favourable	Unfavourable
DNA sequencing of IGHV	>2% mutation	≤2% mutation
Flow cytometry		
CD38	<30%	≥30%
Zap 70	<20%	≥20%

Source: NCCN Clinical Practice Guidelines in Oncology: Non-Hodgkin's Lymphomas. Version 3.2014.

Table 34.9 Interphase cytogenetics

Unfavourable	Neutral	Favourable
del(11q)	Normal	del(13q) as a sole abnormality
del(17p)	+12	

Source: NCCN Clinical Practice Guidelines in Oncology: Non-Hodgkin's Lymphomas. Version 3.2014.

1ST LINE TREATMENT

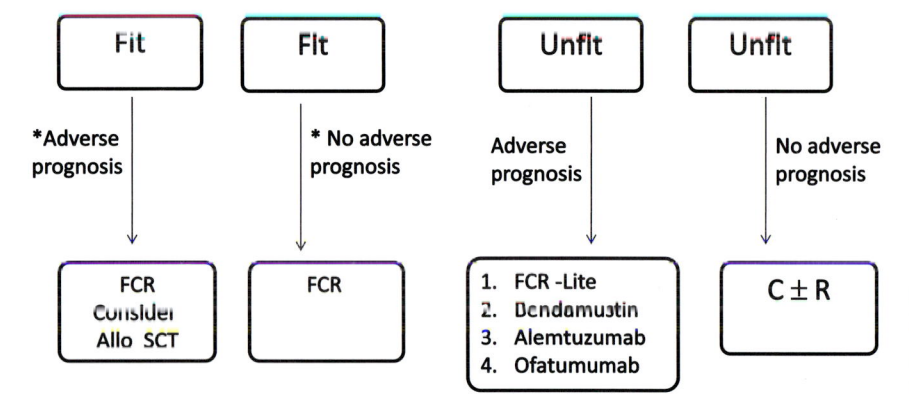

Fit — *Adverse prognosis → FCR Consider Allo SCT

Fit — *No adverse prognosis → FCR

Unfit — Adverse prognosis →
1. FCR-Lite
2. Bendamustin
3. Alemtuzumab
4. Ofatumumab

Unfit — No adverse prognosis → C ± R

Figure 34.3 Treatment algorithm for CLL: first-line therapy.

FRC, fludarabine + cyclophosphamide + rituximab; C ± R, cyclophosphamide ± rituximab.

Treatment

The decision as to when and how to treat depends on patient and disease characteristics. Patient data that need to be taken into consideration for treatment decision-making include: age (< or >70 years) and existing co-morbidities. Disease characteristics include: stage (Rai 0–II or Binet A–B; see Tables 34.6 and 34.7), disease activity (symptomatic disease) and presence of unfavourable markers (deletion 17p–, *TP53* mutation). Early detection of patients with more aggressive disease biology might ultimately result in early onset of the appropriate therapy.

Algorithms for first- and second-line treatment of CLL are presented in Figs 34.3 and 34.4.

2ND LINE TREATMENT

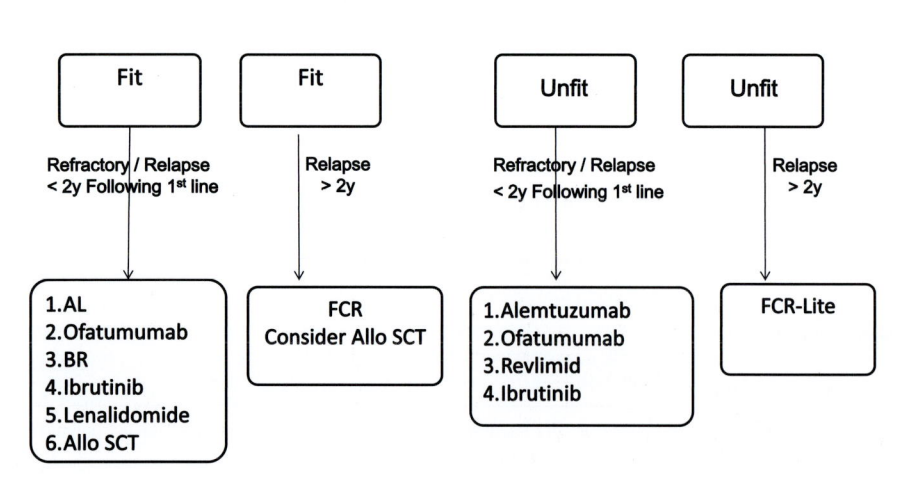

Fit — Refractory / Relapse < 2y Following 1st line →
1. AL
2. Ofatumumab
3. BR
4. Ibrutinib
5. Lenalidomide
6. Allo SCT

Fit — Relapse > 2y → FCR Consider Allo SCT

Unfit — Refractory / Relapse < 2y Following 1st line →
1. Alemtuzumab
2. Ofatumumab
3. Revlimid
4. Ibrutinib

Unfit — Relapse > 2y → FCR-Lite

Figure 34.4 Treatment algorithm for CLL: second-line therapy.

AL, alemtuzumab; BR, bendamustin + rituximab.

Treatment: Chronic lymphatic leukaemia	Description

Supportive treatment	- *Infection prophylaxis*:
	  - In patients with recurrent significant sinopulmonary infections and hypogammaglobulinaemia (IgG <500 mg/dL) monthly IV immunoglobulin 0.3–0.5 g/kg is recommended
	  - In patients receiving fludarabine or alemtuzumab, herpes zoster prophylaxis with acyclovir and *Pneumocystis jirovecii* pneumonia (PCP) prophylaxis should be given concomitantly
	  - Influenza vaccines should be given annually and pneumococcal vaccines should be given every 5 years:
	    - Live vaccines should be avoided in patients treated with fludarabine and alemtuzumab
	- *Immune complications*:
	  - In patients developing autoimmune haemolytic anaemia while on fludarabine, this treatment should be stopped
	  - Otherwise, treat as for patients without CLL
	- *Blood products*: RBC should be irradiated to prevent transfusion-associated graft-versus-host disease

Definitive treatment	- Variety of agents, including single-agent alkylators, combination chemotherapy, immunotherapy and targeted therapy
	- Ankylating agents:
	  - Chlorambucil (CLB) has been used for several decades: disease control with no or very low remission rates and few side effects when used for a short term
	  - Bendamustin (B): significant OR and event-free survival (EFS), but no improvement in OS compared to chlorambucil
	- Purine analogues, mainly fludarabine, generally used in combination with cyclophosphamide (FC): significantly better ORR, CR and EFS compared to chlorambucil
	- Chemoimmunotherapy combinations:
	  - FC + rituximab (FCR), an anti-CD20 antibody: improved not only CR and EFS but also OS
	  - B + R yields similar results
	- Monoclonal antibodies:
	  - Alemtuzumab directed against CD52: activity in refractory or relapsing patients following alkylating agents or purine analogues and in patients with an adverse genetic profile (del17p and del11q)
	  - Ofatumumab, a fully humanized anti-CD20 antibody: response in patients who have relapsed on fludarabine as well as in those with bulky adenopathy (>5 cm)
	- Targeted therapy:
	  - Ibrutinib targets the BTK pathway and phase I–II studies demonstrated a 71% response rate in refractory CLL patients
	  - Several new therapies targeting the BCR signalling pathway are under investigation
	  - Novel agents are under intensive investigation, including the new monoclonal antibody obinutuzumab (GA101) and immunomodulatory drugs, such as revlimid (lenalidomide)
	  - Allogeneic stem cell transplantation is indicated in patients with short-duration response or non-responders to fludarabine-containing regimens, especially in those with poor prognostic features such as del(11q22.3)

Areas of research

- Introduction of novel agents (monoclonal antibodies, targeting BCR and immunomodulatory drugs)
- Determining the role of MRD detection post therapy and maintenance treatment

Recommended reading

Advani AS (2013) New immune strategies for the treatment of acute lymphoblastic leukemia: antibodies and chimeric antigen receptors. *Am Soc Hematol Educ Program* 131–137.

Baccarani M, Deininger MW, Rosti G et al. (2013) European LeukemiaNet recommendations for the management of chronic myeloid leukemia: 2013. *Blood* 122(6):872–884.

Bassan R, Rossi G, Pogliani EM et al. (2010) Chemotherapy-phased imatinib pulses improve long-term outcome of adult patients with Philadelphia chromosome-positive acute lymphoblastic leukemia: Northern Italy Leukemia Group protocol 09/00. *Blood* 28(22):3644–3652

Bauer K, Rancea M, Roloff V et al. (2012) Rituximab, ofatumumab and other monoclonal anti-CD20 antibodies for chronic lymphocytic leukaemia. *Cochrane Database Syst Rev* (11):CD008079.

Byrd JC, Furman RR, Coutre SE et al. (2013) Targeting BTK with ibrutinib in relapsed chronic lymphocytic leukemia. *N Engl J Med* 369(1):32–42.

Cancer Genome Atlas Research Network. (2013) Genomic and epigenomic landscapes of adult de novo acute myeloid leukemia. *N Engl J Med* 368(22):2059–2074.

Cornelissen JJ, Gratwohl A, Schlenk RF et al. (2012) The European LeukemiaNet AML Working Party consensus statement on allogeneic HSCT for patients with AML in remission: an integrated-risk adapted approach. *Nat Rev Clin Oncol* 9(10):579–590.

Cortes JE, Kantarjian HM, Goldberg SL et al. (2009) High dose imatinib in newly diagnosed chronic-phase chronic myeloid leukemia: high rates of rapid cytogenetic and molecular responses. (2009). *J Clin Oncol* 27(28):4754–4759.

Döhner H, Estey EH, Amadori S et al. (2010) Diagnosis and management of acute myeloid leukemia in adults: recommendations from an international expert panel, on behalf of the European LeukemiaNet. *Blood* 115(3):453–474.

Fernandez HF, Sun Z, Yao X et al. (2009) Anthracycline dose intensification in acute myeloid leukemia. *N Engl J Med* 361(13):1249–1259.

Fielding AK (2010) How I treat Philadelphia chromosome-positive acute lymphoblastic leukemia. *Blood* 116(18):3409–3417.

Fischer K, Cramer P, Busch R et al. (2012) Bendamustine in combination with rituximab for previously untreated patients with chronic lymphocytic leukemia: a multicenter phase II trial of the German Chronic Lymphocytic Leukemia Study Group. *J Clin Oncol* 30(26):3209–3216.

Goldstone AH, Richards SM, Lazarus HM et al. (2008) In adults with standard-risk acute lymphoblastic leukemia, the greatest benefit is achieved from a matched sibling allogeneic transplantation in first complete remission, and an autologous transplantation is less effective than conventional consolidation/maintenance chemotherapy in all patients: final results of the International ALL Trial (MRC UKALL XII/ECOG E2993). *Blood* 111(4):1827–1833.

Hallek M, Fischer K, Fingerle-Rowson G et al. (2010) Addition of rituximab to fludarabine and cyclophosphamide in patients with chronic lymphocytic leukaemia: a randomised, open-label, phase 3 trial. *Lancet* 376:1164–1174.

Hoelzer D (2011) Novel antibody-based therapies for acute lymphoblastic leukemia. *Hematol Am Soc Hematol Educ Program*:243–249.

Huguet F, Leguay T, Raffoux E et al. (2009) Pediatric-inspired therapy in adults with Philadelphia chromosome-negative acute lymphoblastic leukemia: the GRAALL-2003 study. *J Clin Oncol* 27(6):911–918.

Jabbour E, Kantarjian HM, O'Brien S et al. (2011) Front-line therapy with second-generation tyrosine kinase inhibitors in patients with early chronic phase chronic myeloid leukemia: what is the optimal response? *J Clin Oncol* 29(32):4260–4265.

Kantarjian HM, Shah NP, Cortes JE et al. (2012) Dasatinib or imatinib in newly diagnosed chronic-phase chronic myeloid leukemia: 2-year follow-up from a randomized phase 3 trial (DASISION) *Blood* 119(5):1123–1129.

Knauf WU, Lissichkov T, Aldaoud A et al. (2009) Phase III randomized study of bendamustine compared with chlorambucil in previously untreated patients with chronic lymphocytic leukemia. (2009). *J Clin Oncol* 27(26):4378–4384.

Löwenberg B, Ossenkoppele GJ, van Putten W et al. (2009) High-dose daunorubicin in older patients with acute myeloid leukemia. *N Engl J Med* 361(13):1235–1248.

Mrózek K, Marcucci G, Nicolet D et al. (2012) Prognostic significance of the European LeukemiaNet standardized system for reporting cytogenetic and molecular alterations in adults with acute myeloid leukemia. *J Clin Oncol* 30(36):4515–4523.

Mullighan CG (2012) The molecular genetic makeup of acute lymphoblastic leukemia. *Hematol Am Soc Hematol Educ Program*:389–396.

Patel B, Rai L, Buck G et al. (2010) Minimal residual disease is a significant predictor of treatment failure in non T lineage adult acute lymphoblastic leukaemia: final results of the international trial UKALL XII/ECOG2993. *Br J Haematol* 148(1):80–89.

Patel JP, Gönen M, Figueroa ME et al. (2012) Prognostic relevance of integrated genetic profiling in acute myeloid leukemia. *N Engl J Med* 366(12):1079–1089.

Pui CH, Pei D, Campana D et al. (2011) Improved prognosis for older adolescents with acute lymphoblastic leukemia. *J Clin Oncol* 29(4):386–391.

Rowe JM, Löwenberg B (2013) Gemtuzumab ozogamicin in acute myeloid leukemia: a remarkable saga about an active drug. *Blood* 121(24):4838–4841.

Rowe JM, Tallman MS (2010) How I treat acute myeloid leukemia. *Blood* 116(17):3147–3156.

Saglio G, Kim DW, Issaragrisil S et al. (2010) Nilotinib versus imatinib for newly diagnosed chronic myeloid leukemia. *N Engl J Med* 362(24):2251–2259.

Sanz MA, Grimwade D, Tallman MS et al. (2009) Management of acute promyelocytic leukemia: recommendations from an expert panel on behalf of the European LeukemiaNet. *Blood* 113(9):1875–1891.

Stock W (2010) Adolescents and young adults with acute lymphoblastic leukemia.(2010). *Hematol Am Soc Hematol Educ Program*:21–29.

The National Comprehensive Cancer Network (NCCN) Guidelines for Acute Myeloid Leukemia (AML), version 2013.

The National Comprehensive Cancer Network (NCCN) Guidelines for Acute Lymphocytic Leukemia (ALL), version 2013.

Vardiman JW, Thiele J, Arber DA et al. (2009) The 2008 revision of the World Health Organization (WHO) classification of myeloid neoplasms and acute leukemia: rationale and important changes. *Blood* 114(5):937–951.

Zuckerman T, Ganzel C, Tallman MS, Rowe JM (2012) How I treat hematologic emergencies in adults with acute leukemia. *Blood* 120(10):1993–2002.

35 Cervix

Lynette Denny[1] and Leon Van Wijk[2]

[1]Department of Obstetrics & Gynaecology, Faculty of Health Sciences, University of Cape Town, and Groote Schuur Hospital, Cape Town, South Africa
[2]Department of Radiation Oncology, Groote Schuur Hospital, Cape Town, South Africa

Summary	Key facts

Introduction	- *Incidence*:
	  - Third most common female cancer diagnosed globally and the fourth most common cause of mortality (after breast, colorectal and lung cancer)
	  - In 2012, just under half a million new cases of cervical cancer were diagnosed globally and approximately 266,000 women died from the disease
	  - Over 85% of cervical cancers were diagnosed in developing countries, where there is a paucity of prevention programmes, national cancer control programmes, access to diagnosis and treatment, and substantial out of pocket expenses for individual women due to lack of free or subsidised health care
	- *Epidemiology*:
	  - Persistent infection of the cervix with high-risk types of human papillomavirus (HR-HPV) is the most important risk factor for the development of cervical cancer and its precursors
	  - Other important risk factors include smoking, long-term oral contraception use, high parity, low socioeconomic status and co-infection with other sexually transmitted diseases (STIs), such as *Chlamydia trachomatis* and human immunodeficiency virus (HIV) or other conditions causing cell-mediated immune deficiency

Presentation	- Most women present with abnormal vaginal bleeding, irregular bleeding, postcoital or peri- or post-menopausal bleeding: - May be associated with an offensive vaginal discharge, pelvic pain, dyspareunia and/or symptoms related to metastatic disease particularly to lung, bone and liver, among other sites - Early invasive cancers are usually asymptomatic and detected through abnormal cervical cancer screening tests and colposcopic examination
Scenario	- *Early-stage disease*: surgery (either conservative or radical) - *Advanced-stage disease*: radiation with or without concurrent chemotherapy - Treatment may be given with curative or palliative intent

Trials	- Creasman *et al.* (1998) *Am J Obstet Gynecol* 178(1 Pt 1):62–65:
	  - Stage IA2 carcinoma of the cervix with 3–5 mm of invasion is at very low risk for lymph node metastases, recurrences or death
	- Jones *et al.* (1993) *Gynecol Oncol* 51(1): 26–32:
	  - Consevative hysterectomy is adequate therapy for patients in whom the diagnosis of early invasive cervical cancer is established by conization with free margins and the depth of invasion is <3 mm
	- Green *et al.* (2001) *Lancet* 358:781–786:
	  - Concomitant chemotherapy and radiotherapy improves overall and progression-free survival, and reduces local and distant recurrence

Anatomy and physiology of the cervix

- Cervix is a fibrous organ lined by squamous and columnar (glandular) cells
- At birth there is an abrupt junction between the squamous and columnar cells – the congenital or original squamocolumnar junction (OSCJ)
- Women are exposed to oestrogen during various stages of their lives:
  - At birth (via maternal oestrogen transmitted through the placenta)
  - At menarche when the hypothalamic–pituitary–ovarian axis matures and girls begin to produce their own oestrogen from the ovaries
  - Throughout reproductive life during the menstrual cycle, for as long as women have functional ovaries
  - During pregnancy when both oestrogen and progestogen are secreted at high levels
- Similar to squamous cells in other parts of the body, squamous cells are constantly exfoliating and being replaced by the basal layer of the cervical/vaginal epithelium
- Squamous cells contain glycogen in the cytoplasm and glandular cells contain mucin:
  - Exposure to oestrogen stimulates the conversion of the glycogen into lactic acid by the resident microorganisms of the vagina, known as the lacto- or doderlein bacilli
  - Lactic acid is responsible for the healthy vagina maintaining a pH of <4.5
  - This acidity, combined with other ill-defined factors, is responsible for converting the exposed columnar epithelia into squamous epithelia, a process known as metaplasia (during which one mature type of epithelium is converted into another type)
  - This ongoing dynamic process is responsible for creating a new SCJ (NSCJ)
- ~90% of cervical cancers originate in the transformation zone (TZ), the area between the original SCJ and the NSCJ
  - This is where the process of metaplasia takes place constantly during the reproductive years, a process which evolves from immature to mature phases (Fig. 35.1)
  - TZ is not usually visible to the naked eye and when the cervix is examined it is the new SCJ that is being visualized
- Blood drainage of the cervix mainly follows the uterine artery to the internal iliac artery (also known as the hypogastric artery):
  - Uterine artery provides the blood supply to the fundus and the body of the uterus, and descends to the cervix and vagina to give branches to those anatomical areas
  - Also a rich anastomosis between the uterine and ovarian arteries (branches of the aorta), the posterior division of the internal iliac artery, the iliolumbar artery, the middle sacral artery, the pudendal and obturator arteries
- Lymphatic drainage of the cervix is into the paracervical and parametrial lymph nodes, as well as the internal, external, obturator and common iliac veins:
  - Obturator lymph nodes are the most medial portion of the external iliac nodal region and play a key role as one of the first sites of lymphatic spread of cervical cancer following paracervical invasion
- Cervix is innervated from the sacral roots (S2–4) crossing through the hypogastric plexuses

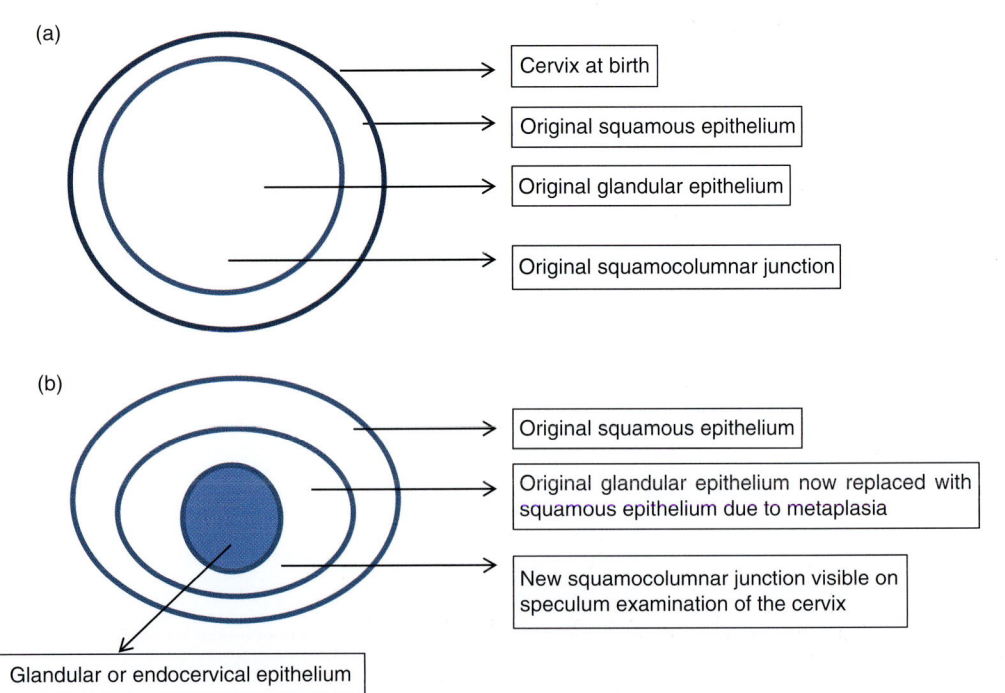

Figure 35.1 Schematic diagram of the cervix (a) at birth and (b) after the onset of the metaplastic process that converts glandular/columnar epithelium into squamous epithelium.

Incidence, aetiology and screening

Incidence, aetiology and screening	Description

Incidence	- In 2012, estimated that globally:
	  - 528,000 women were diagnosed with cervical cancer corresponding to an age-standardized incidence rate (ASIR) of 15.4 per 100 000 women.
	  - 266,000 women died of the disease, with an age-standardized mortality rate (ASMR) of 7.8 per 100,000 women
	  - Majority of the cases diagnosed (445,000; 85%) were in developing countries, as were the deaths (230,000, 87%)

Aetiology	- HPV infection precedes the development of cervical cancer by a number of decades:
	  - Assumed that HPV infection initiates when the virus enters the basal keratinocytes via defects in the epithelium covering the cervix, allowing attachment to the basement membrane
	  - HPV infection is easily and silently transmitted largely through skin-to-skin contact, and infection is usually asymptomatic, in both men and women.
	- Persistent infection of the cervix with HPV is necessary for the development of and progression of precancerous lesions of the cervix, either to higher grades of precancerous disease or to cancer
	- While HPV infection causes cervical cancer, most HPV infections do not lead to cervical cancer:
	  - Approximately 90% of HPV infections resolve within several months of initial infection without any significant clinical consequences for the individual (on average 12 months; range 6–18 months)
	  - Clearance of HPV infection occurs due to activation of the cell-mediated immunity of the body:
	    - Humoral and cell-mediated immune responses to genital HPV types are difficult to detect as infection neither causes lysis of the cell nor has a viraemic phase
	- Cervical cancer progresses slowly over decades from preinvasive cervical intraepithelial neoplasia to invasive cervical cancer, a process that can take 10–30 years
	- Co-factors that increase the risk of cervical cancer include smoking, long-term oral contraception use, high parity, low socioeconomic status, immune suppression (transplant patients, infection with HIV, long term steroid use) and co-infection with other STIs, such as *C. trachomatis*
	- Low-risk types of HPV, such as 6 and 11, are associated with the expression of genital warts as well as low-grade cervical epithelial lesions (LSIL):
	  - While a significant cause of physical, psychosexual and social discomfort, genital warts are not associated with cancer

Screening (see Box 35.1)	- American Association for Cervical Colposcopy and Pathology recommendations for screening are:
	  - Women under the age of 21 years: do not screen regardless of age of onset of sexual activity
	  - Women aged 21–29 years: screen with cytology 3 yearly:
	    - If cytology is normal: HPV DNA testing is not recommended in this age group due to the high number of transient infections and the risk of over-treatment
	  - For women aged 30–65 years:
	    - Cytology alone every 3 years
	    - Cytology + HPV DNA co-testing every 5 years (preferred)
	  - Screening should stop at age 65 years once a woman has had 3 consecutive previously negative Paps and a negative HPV DNA test in the last 5 years
	  - For women who have been treated for high-grade squamous intraepithelial lesion (HSIL) or adenocarcinoma *in situ*: screening should be continued for 20 years, even if that exceeds the threshold of 65 years
	  - Women who have undergone hysterectomy for a prior diagnosis of HSIL or a more severe diagnosis should also continue screening for 20 years
	    - Women who have undergone hysterectomy for reasons unrelated to cervical pathology do not need to be screened
	- Until further long-term information is available, women who have been vaccinated against HPV should follow routine guidelines, particularly as the two types in the vaccines, HPV 16 and 18, only account for 70% of cervical cancers
	- Screening tests such as visual inspection with acetic acid (VIA), in which the cervix is washed with 3–5% acetic acid and inspected with the naked eye and a bright light:
	  - No other screening tests are performed and if the VIA test is positive, the woman is offered immediate ablative treatment with cryotherapy

(continued)

Incidence, aetiology and screening	Description
	- Many advantages:
- Provides immediate treatment to women without resources
- Avoids more accurate yet more expensive screening tests
- Allows for treatment without the costs of out of pocket expenses associated with histopathology
- Equipment required is not expensive and is available in many low resource settings
- Only option for screening in many very poor countries with limited resources and allows for the development of infrastructure to provide services to older women
- Many disadvantages:
- Limited quality control
- Many lesions are missed
- Many women are overtreated

Prevalence of HPV infection

- The WHO HPV centre (www.who.int/hpvcentre) estimated that, based on 436,430 women tested, the global prevalence of HPV infection was 11.4%:
  - Of tested women younger than 25 years, 20.8% (47,275) were infected
  - Next highest proportion of women infected were aged 25–34 years (13.5%; 55,107) followed by women aged 35–44 years (7.9%; 40,182)

- Overall HPV infection rate in all ages in developed regions was 10.3% compared to 14.3% in developing areas (Fig. 35.2):
  - Highest prevalence in women with normal cytology was in the Caribbean (35.4%) (but study tested just over 200 women)
  - In Africa prevalence was 21.3%, in Latin America 17.6%, in North America 12.5% and in Asia 10.9%
- HPV infection is considered to be the most common STI globally and most sexually active adults aged >15 years will be exposed to the virus at some point in their lives:
  - 2-year cumulative incidence rate for infection with HPV in young women reaches 32% (among both women who were virgins and women who had been sexually active at entry to the study)
- Studies have consistently shown higher prevalence of HPV infection, persistent infection with HPV, infection with multiple types of HPV and higher prevalence of cervical cancer precursors in *HIV-infected women*:
  - 68% of one cohort of HIV-positive women were infected with high-risk types of HPV, and 94% of these infections persisted over a 36-month period, with only 6% clearing infections
  - In a South African study of 5595 women aged 35–65 years followed for 36 months, of whom 577 were HIV positive at enrolment:
    - Among the 123 women who subsequently seroconverted, HPV prevalence was 20.3% before seroconversion, 23.6% at seroconversion and 49.1% after seroconversion
    - HIV seroconversion was associated with newly detected HPV infection and increased risk of low-grade cytological abnormalities compared with HIV-negative women

Primary prevention of cervical cancer

- Development of vaccines against certain types of HPV has been a major breakthrough in the options available for the primary prevention of cervical cancer

---

Box 35.1 Factors considered important to ensure the success of cytologically-based screening programmes

- Adequate field facilities with appropriately trained health personnel to perform quality cervical smears
- Wide coverage of the target population (at least 70%) at regular intervals: a minimum of 3–5 years between smears and mechanisms for contacting women on an individual basis, e.g. through personally addressed letters
- An efficient health infrastructure with functioning management and information systems
- A cytology service with built-in quality assurance, ongoing training of cytotechnicians and regular audit of performance of laboratories
- An accessible and functional referral system for colposcopic assessment of women with abnormal smears
- Adequate diagnosis, treatment and follow-up of women with abnormal smears and follow-up of women who have been treated for preinvasive disease of the cervix
- Community understanding and acceptability
- Screening programmes should be planned at national level and be organized to encompass a call and recall system
- A cancer registry should be established to monitor the impact of the screening programmes on cervical cancer incidence and mortality

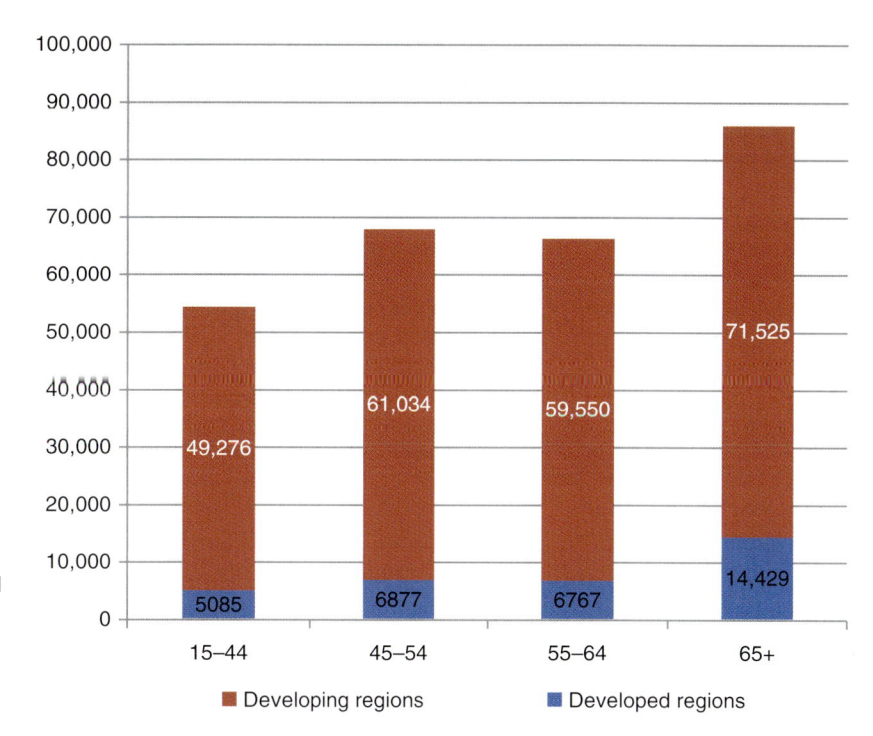

Figure 35.2 Annual number of deaths from cervical cancer by age group in developed and developing regions.

Data source: Globocan (2008) Lyon: IARC. Reproduced with permission of WHO.

- Vaccines use HPV type-specific L1 proteins that self-assemble into virus-like particles (VLPs):
  - L1 VLPs induce high levels of serum neutralizing IgG that are presumed to transudate across the cervical epithelium in high enough concentrations to bind to virus particles and prevent infection
- Monovalent (against HPV 16), bivalent (against HPV 16 and 18) and quadrivalent (against HPV 6, 11, 16 and 18) vaccines have been tested in randomized placebo-controlled trials and shown to be safe, immunogenic and highly efficacious for up to 8 years after vaccination
- Two are commercially available:
  - Bivalent vaccine (Cervarix, GlaxoSmithKline Biologicals, Rixensart, Belgium):
    - Given by intramuscular injection at 0, 1 and 6 months
  - Quadrivalent vaccine (Gardasil, Merck & Co. Inc, West Point, Pennsylvania, USA):
    - Given by intramuscular injection at 0, 2 and 6 months
  - Good evidence from randomized placebo-controlled trials that both offer full protection against types 16 and 18, which are estimated to cause >70% of cervical cancers worldwide and a slightly lower fraction of cervical cancer precursors, as well as preinvasive lesions of the anogenital tract associated with the types present in the vaccines
  - Some data that the immune response to vaccination against types 16 and 18 provides some cross-protection against types 31 and 45, both important in the aetiology of cervical cancer, thus increasing the projected protection from vaccination to 75–80%
  - Quadrivalent vaccine also prevents the development of genital warts caused by types 6 and 11 (both associated with benign disease) and respiratory papillomatosis, a rare condition affecting young children
  - Whether booster doses of either vaccine will be required is not known (long-term follow-up studies are ongoing), but anticipated that both vaccines will be associated with lifelong protection
- Both vaccines are prophylactic and should be administered to individuals prior to infection:
  - Ideally administered to girls (and boys, depending on available resources) prior to the onset of sexual activity, which varies considerably from country to country and in different cultures
  - Vaccination of girls aged 9–12 years with high coverage likely to be the most clinically- and cost-effective strategy for cervical cancer prevention
- *Vaccination in HIV-positive women and men*:
  - Published studies show vaccination in HIV-positive individuals to be immunogenic and safe
  - Efficacy of the vaccines in HIV-positive individuals however remains to be proven
  - Studies with mature data on the ability of vaccination to prevent HPV infection in HIV positive people are awaited

Pathology

Pathology	Description
Preinvasive disease (cervical cancer precursors)	• Persistent infection of the cervix with high-risk types of HPV results in dysplastic changes of the cervical cells. ■ Morphologically represented by an increasing nuclear-to-cytoplasmic ratio associated with nuclear hyperchromasia ■ Changes have been known by a number of terminologies ranging from: 　○ Pap class I–IV 　○ Mild, moderate and severe dyskaryosis 　○ Mild, moderate, severe dysplasia 　○ Cervical intraepithelial neoplasia (CIN) grades 1–3 and carcinoma *in situ* (CIS) 　○ Squamous intraepithelial lesions (SILs) ■ CIN 1 (corresponding to HPV infection or low-grade SIL [LSIL]) involves the lower one-third of the epithelium, whereas CIN 2/3 (corresponding to HSIL) involves two-thirds or more of the epithelium, and full thickness involvement of the epithelium has previously been known as carcinoma *in situ* ■ In 1988, in order to resolve the 'terminology chaos' around cervical cancer precursors, the Bethesda system of reporting cytological abnormalities (see Table 35.1) was introduced and has been widely adopted globally • *LSIL* is common and represents the usually benign cytopathological signs of HPV infection (koilocytosis): ■ Should be regarded as a risk factor for cervical cancer, rather than a true precursor • *High-grade SIL (HSIL)* is rare and represents a truly premalignant condition: ■ Although LSIL can be viewed as an epidemiological exposure or risk factor for cervical cancer, HSIL can be viewed as more closely linked to the cancer outcome • While this conceptual distinction is clinically useful, it is not perfect: ■ A continuum of changes encompassing LSIL and HSIL exists without a clear endpoint: 　○ E.g. At the microscopic level, the characteristic cells of LSIL are abnormal but terminally differentiated; they progress to the surface, produce keratins, die and exfoliate as would normal cells 　○ The gradient from LSIL to HSIL is characterized by increasing nuclear atypia and failure of cellular differentiation in progressively more superficial levels of epithelium, with CIN3 representing full-thickness replacement of the epithelium with undifferentiated, atypical cells
Squamous cell cancer (SCC)	• *Microinvasive carcinoma*: ■ Associated with squamous intraepithelial neoplasia and may arise either from the surface epithelium or from the endocervical glands involved in dysplasia ■ Characterized by small nests of cells that have breached the basement membrane of the surface or endocervical epithelium ■ A desmoplastic reaction to the invading cells is commonly present in the stroma of the cervix ■ FIGO staging requires that the depth of invasion to be measured from the basement membrane of the site of origin, i.e. the tumour size is the distance from the basement membrane to the deepest nest of invading cells ■ Diagnosis almost always requires an excisional procedure of the cervix to enable the pathologist to perform the appropriate measurements, which ultimately impact on treatment ■ Critical information from the pathologist should include: 　○ Depth of invasion and width of the tumour 　○ Presence or absence of lymphovascular space invasion (while important, does not change the staging) 　○ Involvement or not of the endo- and ecto-cervical margins of the excised tissue 　○ Grade of the tumour (which like lymphovascular space invasion does not change the staging of the disease) • *Invasive SCC*: ■ Usually occurs in women aged >40 years, most often between the ages of 50 and 60 years ■ Macroscopically may consist of firm indurated masses, or be ulcerated, fungating or polypoid ■ Microscopic examination reveals irregular, haphazardly infiltrating nests of cells with eosinophilic cytoplasm and enlarged atypical hyperchromatic nuclei: 　○ Atypical mitoses are common as is a desmoplastic reaction around the tumour and the presence of lymphatic or vascular space invasion by tumour cells ■ While invasive SCC is graded, grading does not determine treatment and it is not necessarily correlated with prognosis

Pathology	Description

	- Variants of SCC:
	  - *Basaloid SCC*: locally aggressive tumour composed of basaloid cells resembling those of carcinoma in situ
	  - *Verrucous carcinoma*:
	    - Relatively rare on the cervix
	    - Cervix exhibits papillary excrecences that resemble condyloma accuminatum
	    - Underlying connective tissue displays bulbous nests of squamous epithelium that invade the stroma with a pushing margin, but display little cytological atypia
	    - Tumour invades locally but does not metastasize
	  - *Papillary squamous* and *transitional carcinoma*:
	    - Characterized by superficial papillary architecture with substantial nuclear atypia not seen in verrucous carcinomas
	    - Usually associated with underlying typical SCC and an excisional procedure is necessary to make the diagnosis
	    - Invasive form of these neoplasms is associated with local recurrence and metastases
	  - *Warty carcinoma*:
	    - Rare papillary neoplasm that displays marked condylomatous change, but also has features of routine SCC, usually at the deep margin

Adenocarcinoma	- Accounts for 20–25% of cervical cancers
	- Adenocarcinoma *in situ* is a precursor to invasive adenocarcinoma, and is usually found alongside invasive adenocarcinoma and with squamous dysplasia
	- HPV 18 is more commonly associated with invasive adenocarcinoma than HPV 16
	- Critically important in evaluating a woman with adenocarcinoma is to determine the origin of the cancer: cervix, uterus, ovary or other metastatic sites such as the gastrointestinal tract
	- Microinvasive adenocarcinoma is a recognized entity and classically displays altered endocervical architecture
	- Difficulty in making a histological diagnosis is well known due to the complexity of normal endocervical glands
	- Depth of invasion is measured in the same way as in squamous lesions and similarly staged
	- *Mucinous adenocarcinoma*: several variants:
	  - Endocervical
	  - Intestinal
	  - Signet ring
	  - Villoglandular variants
	  - Endometrioid types
	  - HPV DNA has been detected in all the various types

Adenosquamous carcinoma	- Composed of mucinous and squamous cancers - Unique type: - Neither 'collision' tumours nor poorly differentiated squamous tumours - Tend to be more aggressive than adenocarcinomas
Other subtypes	- *Glassy cell carcinomas*: rare form of poorly differentiated adenosquamous carcinomas - *Adenoid cystic carcinoma*: rare but aggressive malignant neoplasm and patients with advanced-stage disease have a poor prognosis - *Neuroendocrine tumours*: rare aggressive tumours and usually specific immunohistochemistry is required to make the diagnosis. - *Clear cell adenocarcinoma (CCA)*: associated with intrauterine dietheylstilbestrol (DES) exposure, but also occurs in the absence of DES exposure - *Papillary serous carcinoma*: a bimodal distribution, occurring in women aged <40 years and >65 years: - Microscopically, identical to serous tumours of the endometrium, ovary and peritoneum and essential to exclude primary tumours at these sites to ensure that the primary is indeed the cervix

Table 35.1 Bethesda classification of cervical cancer

Category	Specifics
Specimen type	Conventional Liquid based cytology
Adequacy of the specimen	Satisfactory for evaluation: • Presence of sufficient squamous cells, endocervical cells, cells not obscured by blood, debris or inflammatory cells • Reason given Unsatisfactory for evaluation
General categorization	Negative for intraepithelial lesion (NILM) or cancer, or Epithelial cell abnormalities described Other abnormalities
NILM	Organisms: • *Trichomonas vaginalis* • Candida • Bacterial vaginosis • Actinomyces • Herpes simplex • Schistosomiasis • Tuberculosis • Amoebiasis Other: • Reactive cellular changes associated with inflammation, radiation or intrauterine device (IUD) use • Atrophy
Interpretation of epithelial cell abnormalities	• Atypical squamous cells of undetermined significance (ASC-US) • Atypical squamous cells for which a high-grade lesion cannot be excluded (ASC-H) • Low-grade squamous intraepithelial lesion encompassing HPV infection or CIN 1 (mild dysplasia) • High-grade squamous intraepithelial lesion encompassing CIN 2 and CIN3/CIS plus any suggestive of invasive lesions • Squamous cell carcinoma
Interpretation of glandular cell abnormalities	• Atypical cells: endocervical, endometrial or glandular • Atypical cells likely to be cancerous: endocervical or glandular • Adenocarcinoma *in situ*: endocervical • Adenocarcinoma: endocervical, endometrial, extrauterine or NOS (not otherwise specific)
Interpretation of other abnormalities	• Endometrial cells noted in a woman over 40 years of age: • If NILM, further investigation may be warranted
Other cancers	• Metastatic to the cervix: • Type specified, e.g. lymphoma, breast, lung, etc.

Adapted from Bethesda system 2001, National Institutes of Health (www.asccp.org)

Presentation and natural history

Persistent infection of the cervix with certain high-risk types of HPV has been well established as a necessary cause of cervical cancer.

- Identified in nearly all carcinomas of the cervix and relative risk of cervical cancer associated with infection with these is higher than the risk of lung cancer associated with smoking
- Pooled odds ratio from 11 case–control studies (involving 1918 women with histologically confirmed SCC of the cervix and 1928 controls) for cervical cancer associated with the presence of any HPV infection was 158.2 (95% CI 113.4–220.6):
  - Fifteen HPV types were classified as high-risk (types 16, 18, 31, 33, 39, 45, 51, 52, 56, 58, 59, 68, 73 and 82) and were considered carcinogenic
- The International Agency for Research on Cancer (IARC) confirmed that HPV 16, 18, 31, 33, 35, 45, 52 and 58 were most frequently found in cervical cancer:
  - Four less constantly found types (39, 51, 56 and 59) were classified as having sufficient evidence for a causal relationship with cervical cancer
  - HPV 68 was classified as 'probably carcinogenic to humans'
  - HPV 6 and 11 were not classified as carcinogenic

- A meta-analysis of HPV types found in invasive cervical cancers worldwide on a total of 10,058 cases (including SCCs, adenocarcinomas and adenosquamous carcinomas) confirmed HPV 16 (51%) and 18 (16.2%) to be the commonest:
  - >16 other types of HPV were also associated with cervical cancer, of which types 45, 31, 33, 52 and 58 were the most prevalent
- A more recent publication evaluated HPV infection in paraffin-embedded samples of histologically confirmed cases of invasive cancer from 38 countries in Europe, North America, central South America, Africa, Asia and Oceania taken over a 60-year period:
  - 10,575 cases of invasive cervical cancer were included in the study and 85% (n = 8977) were positive for HPV DNA
  - Eight most common types of HPV detected were 16, 18, 31, 33, 35, 45, 52 and 58, and their combined contribution to the 8977 positive cases was 91%
  - HPV types 16, 18 and 45 were the three most common types in each type of cervical cancer (SCC, adenocarcinoma and adenosquamous carcinoma)

Presentation and natural history		Description
Presentation	Local	• Vaginal bleeding • Offensive vaginal discharge • Pelvic pain, dyspareunia, dysuria, difficulty in passing faeces • Polypoid, ulcerative, fungation mass of the cervix
	Metastatic	• Rectovaginal or vesicovaginal fistulae • Symptoms related to liver, bone, lung or other metastases such as shortness of breath, cough, chest pain, bone pain, constitutional symptoms of loss of weight, deep vein thrombosis, lymphoedema
Routes of spread	Local	• By continuity to upper and lower vagina
	Regional	• By contiguity to parametria and to pelvic side walls bilaterally
	Metastatic	• Haematogenously to liver, lung, bone (among many other sites) • Via lymphatics pelvic side wall, inguinal area, para-aortic, mediastinal and supraclavicular lymph nodes

Diagnostic work-up

Colposcopic examination

- Women with an abnormal cervical smear should undergo colposcopic examination:
  - Involves passing a speculum through the vagina to visualize the cervix
  - After the application of 3–5% acetic acid, the cervix is illuminated and magnified
  - Information the colposcopist requires in order to make a diagnosis is given in Table 35.2

HPV DNA testing

- If HPV testing in a woman with atypical squamous cells of undetermined significance (ASCUS) cytology is positive: repeat in a year and if still positive, refer for colposcopy
- If HPV DNA testing in a woman with ASCUS cytology is negative: either rescreen with DNA testing in 5 years or cytology alone in 3 years:
  - If the tests remain positive, refer for colposcopy
- FDA approved tests used for HPV DNA testing include:
  - Hybrid Capture 2 test: detects 13 oncogenic HPV types (16, 18, 31, 33, 35, 39, 45, 51, 52, 56, 58, 59 and 68) using full genome probes complementary to HPV DNA, specific antibodies, signal amplification and chemilluminescent detection
  - Cervista HPV HR test detects 14 high-risk HPV types (as above + 66) using a signal amplification method for detection of specific nucleic acid sequences; uses a primary reaction that occurs on the targeted DNA sequence and a secondary reaction that produces a fluorescent signal

Cone biopsy

Women with any type of Pap abnormality may harbour invasive disease. Women who meet the following criteria should be offered a cone biopsy:
- Abnormal Pap smear but no access to colposcopy ('if you cannot see it, you cannot treat it')
- Marked disparity between cytology and colposcopy, e.g. HSIL Pap but negative colposcopy or a Pap smear suspicious for cancer that is not colposcopically visible
- Any evidence of a glandular abnormality
- Suspicion of microinvasive disease
- Inability to see the entire lesion, i.e. lesion extends into the endocervical canal.

There are a number of techniques for performing a cone biopsy:
- Loop excision under local or general anaesthesia
- Cold knife excision, usually under general anaesthesia
- Laser excision.

Table 35.2 Guide to colposcopic diagnosis

Colposcopic sign	0 points	1 point	2 points
Margin	Condylomatous or micropapillary contour Indistinct borders Flocculated or feathered margins Jagged, angular lesions Satellite lesions, aceto-whitening that extends beyond TZ	Regular lesions with smooth outlines Sharp peripheral margins	Rolled, peeling edges Internal borders between areas of differing appearance
Colour	Shiny, snow-white colour Indistinct aceto-whitening, semitransparent rather than completely opaque	Shiny, off-white Intermediate white	Dull, oyster grey
Vessels	Uniform, fine calibre Randomly arranged with poorly formed patterns Non-dilated capillary loops Ill-defined areas of fine punctation or mosaic	Absence of surface vessels following application acetic acid	Definite punctation or mosaicism Individual vessels dilated, arranged in sharply demarcated, well-defined patterns
Iodine staining	Positive iodine uptake, producing a mahogany brown colour Negative iodine uptake by an area that is recognizable as a low-grade lesion by above criteria (<2/6)	Partial iodine uptake Variegated, tortoise-shell appearance	Negative staining of a lesion, which is a high-grade lesion by the above criteria (≥3/6) Mustard yellow appearance
Score	0–2 benign or HPV or LSIL	3–5 CIN 1 or CIN 2 (LSIL or HSIL)	6–8 CIN 2 or 3 (HSIL)

In health systems that are robust and function well, the colposcopist will identify the most abnormal area of the cervix during the colposcopic examination and biopsy the area. Only once the histology of the lesion is confirmed by the pathologist is the lesion treated.

In many low resource settings, a 'see and treat' option is adopted where the woman is examined colposcopically and if the colposcopist considers the patient to have a high-grade precursor, immediate treatment is offered to avoid the woman having to make multiple visits to the clinic.

Women with glandular lesions

All women with glandular abnormalities on Pap smear should be referred for colposcopic evaluation.
- If a satisfactory colposcopy is possible, i.e. the SCJ is visible and there is no abnormality, it is reasonable to empirically treat women with the syndromic approach for endocervical infection for chlamydia, gonococcus or other organisms
- Pap smear should then be repeated after 6 weeks
- If HPV DNA testing is performed and the test is HPV 18 positive, she should be referred for colposcopy ab initio
- Any glandular lesion suggestive of adenocarcinoma in situ or cancer requires a cone biopsy and urgent referral

Work-up once invasive cancer is diagnosed

This should include where available:
- Histological diagnosis of cervical cancer
- Complete blood count (CBC), electrolytes, creatinine, liver function, calcium, magnesium
- Chest X-ray or computed tomorgraphy (CT) of the chest
- Ultrasound of abdomen to assess hydronephrosis
- CT scan of the abdomen and pelvis
- Magnetic resonance imaging (MRI) of the pelvis
- Examination under anaesthesia (EUA) if necessary to assess primary tumour volume and extent

Staging and prognostic grouping

FIGO and UICC TNM staging
- Staging system for cancer of the cervix includes the UICC TNM and FIGO stages (updated in 2009) (Table 35.3):
  - Main change in the FIGO staging in 2009: division of Stage II into IIA1, which is a clinically visible lesion of ≤4 cm in greatest dimensions, and Stage IIA2, which is a clinically visible lesion of >4 cm in greatest dimension
  - Stage IIB remains as tumour with parametrial extension but not to the pelvic side wall

Table 35.3 UICC TNM categories and FIGO stage, and stage grouping: Cervix

TNM categories and FIGO stage		
TNM	**FIGO stage**	**Findings**
Tx		Primary tumour cannot be assessed
T0		No evidence of primary tumour
Tis	(Excluded from FIGO staging)	Carcinoma *in situ*
T1	I	Cervical cancer confined to cervix (extension to corpus should be disregarded)
T1a	IA	Invasive carcinoma, diagnosed microscopically, with deepest invasion ≤5 mm and the widest diameter ≤7.0 mm
T1a1	IA1	Measured stromal invasion of ≤3.0 mm in depth and extension ≤7 mm
T1a2	IA2	Measured stromal invasion of >3 mm and not >3 mm with an extension of not >7.0 mm
T1b	IB	Clinically visible lesions limited to the cervix uteri or preclinical cancers greater than Stage 1A†
T1b1	IB1	Clinically visible lesion ≤4.0 cm in greatest dimension
T1b2	IB2	Clinically visible lesion >4.0 cm in greatest dimension
T2	IIA	Cervical carcinoma invades beyond the uterus, but not to the pelvic wall or to the lower third of the vagina
T2a	IIA	Without parametrial invasion
T2a1	IIA1	Clinically visible lesion ≤4.0 cm in greatest dimension
T2a2	IIA2	Clinically visible lesion >4.0 cm in greatest dimension
T2b	IIB	With obvious parametrial extension
T3	III	Tumour extends to the pelvic side wall and/or involves lower third of the vagina and/or causes hydronephrosis or non-functioning kidney**
T3a	IIIA	Tumour involves lower third of the vagina, with no extension to the pelvic side wall
T3b	IIIB	Extension to the pelvic wall and/or hydronephrosis or non-functioning kidney
T4	IV	Carcinoma has extended beyond the true pelvis or has involved (biopsy proven) the mucosa of the bladder or rectum. A bullous oedema, as such, does not permit a case to be allotted to Stage IV
T4a	IVA	Spread of the growth to adjacent organs
T4b	IVB	Spread to distant organs

*All macroscopically visible lesions – even with superficial invasion – are allotted to stage 1B carcinomas. Invasion is limited to a measured stromal invasion with a maximal depth of 5.0 mm and a horizontal extension of not >7 mm. Depth of invasion should not be >5 mm taken from the base of the epithelium of the original tissue – squamous or glandular. The depth of invasion should always be reported in millimetres, even in those cases with early (minimal) stromal invasion (1 mm). The involvement of vascular/lymphatic spaces should not change the stage.

**On rectal examination there is no cancer-free space between the tumour and the pelvic side wall. All cases with hydronephrosis or non-functioning kidney are included, unless they are known to be due to another cause.

Stage grouping			
Stage 0*	Tis	N0	M0
Stage I	T1	N0	M0
Stage IA	T1a	N0	M0
Stage IA1	T1a1	N0	M0
Stage IA2	T1a2	N0	M0
Stage IB	T1b	N0	M0
Stage IB1	T1b1	N0	M0
Stage IB2	T1b2	N0	M0
Stage II	T2	N0	M0
Stage IIA	T2a	N0	M0
Stage IIA1	T2a1	N0	M0
Stage IIA2	T2a2	N0	M0
Stage IIB	T2b	N0	M0
Stage III	T3	N0	M0
Stage IIIA	T3a	N0	M0
Stage IIIB	T3b	Any N	M0
	T1, T2, T3	N1	M0
Stage IVA	T4	Any N	M0
Stage IVB	Any T	Any N	M1

N1 Regional; M1 distant metastasis IVB
*FIGO no longer includes stage 0 (Tis).
Sobin (2009). Reproduced with permission of John Wiley & Sons.
Pecorelli (2010). Reproduced with permission of Elsevier.

- FIGO is a clinical staging system: clinical, surgical findings and radiological biopsies of suspected lesions in the liver, lung or lymph nodes cannot be used to modify FIGO clinical staging clinical diagnosis
- Important to note there are other staging systems:
  - American Society for Gynecologic Oncology (SGO) considers negative lymphovascular space invasion and negative margins post cone biopsy as criteria for microinvasive disease
  - SGO does not consider the 7-mm cut-off for lateral spread in the definition of minimally invasive disease and the diagnosis must be made on a cone biopsy or hysterectomy specimen; a punch biopsy is not sufficient

Prognostic factors

See Table 35.4.

Table 35.4 Prognostic risk factors in cervical cancer

Prognostic factors	Tumour related	Host related	Environment related
Essential	Unilateral vs bilateral disease Parametrial invasion Invasion to side wall Size of tumour Lymph node invasion Positive surgical margins	Immunosuppression (i.e. HIV infection) Performance status Morbid obesity	Quality of and availability of anticancer therapies Expertise of healthcare personnel Multidisciplinary teams
Additional	Lymphovascular space invasion Histological type	Anaemia during treatment	Ability to manage co-morbid conditions
New and promising	Tumour hypoxia VEGF, mEGFR, HIF-1α, COX-2 PAI-1 expression SCC-Ag and hsCRP for early detection of recurrence	Serum MyoD1 hypermethylation Persistence of HPV infection following treatment	Adequate laboratory facilities to measure tumour markers

Treatment philosophy

Scenario	Treatment philosophy
Tumours up to stage IB1/IIA <4 cm in diameter	• Only about 5% of all cervical cancer cases presenting at multidisciplinary gynaecological assessment clinics in tertiary hospitals in developing countries • Preferably treated with surgery: 　▪ Surgical procedure and recovery in hospital takes <2 weeks 　▪ Extension of the tumour and completeness of removal can be assessed immediately 　▪ Ovarian function is retained, which is particularly important for premenopausal patients 　▪ Patient keeps a functional, elastic and lubricated vagina 　▪ Most complications are seen within a few days of the procedure 　▪ Surgery is not appropriate for women where the disease has spread beyond the cervix 　▪ Surgery for cervical cancer requires skill and experience: 　　○ Radiotherapy should be considered if there is no qualified surgeon available • Radiation therapy: 　▪ Same high 5-year survival rates as surgery for early disease, but 　▪ Takes about 6 weeks to administer 　▪ Total extent of the tumour cannot be evaluated in the same way as with a surgical specimen 　▪ Sequelae, such as loss of vaginal elasticity (fibrosis), shortening and narrowing (stenosis) and dryness of the vagina, may occur months to years after radiation and may make intercourse painful 　▪ Long-term risk of second malignancies
Stage IB2–IIIB	• About 80% of all cases seen in developing countries are in Stage IB2–IIIB, with cervical tumours and parametrial involvement extending towards or up to the pelvic side walls, with or without obstruction of the ureters: 　▪ These bulky tumours (may measure up to 10 cm in diameter) have a cure rate of 30–75% when treated with radical radiotherapy • Large stage IIA tumours (>4 cm in diameter) are treated like Stage IB2 tumours • Chemotherapy is often added to radiotherapy to improve the overall survival
Stage IVA	• Rectal or, less commonly, bladder invasion accounts for about 10% of cases: 　▪ Only about 5–10% of these can be cured • Fistulae between the involved organs and the vagina are frequent, requiring either anterior or posterior exenteration with diversion surgery • Stage IVB (5% of cases), with distant metastases, is incurable by any currently known means: 　▪ Effective palliative care can be given, particularly for relief of pain and bleeding

Scenario	Treatment philosophy

Metastatic disease	• Treatment of metastatic/recurrent disease should be individualized, taking into account the localization of the disease, prior treatment, general condition of the patient and personal circumstances
	• Chemotherapy, if used, in general has a palliative intent (preferably used in a clinical trial setting)
	• Treatment of women who present *de novo* with metastatic disease needs to be individualized and carefully planned
	• All investigations and interventions should be tailored towards improvement of symptoms and quality of life, e.g.:
	  ▪ Localized radiation to bony metastases or lymph nodes
	  ▪ Chemotherapy for lesions not suitable for local therapies
	  ▪ Nutritional supplementation
	  ▪ Treatment of symptomatic anaemia
	  ▪ Meticulous management of pain syndromes
	  ▪ Surgical diversion procedures if appropriate and patient's performance status is high enough

Recurrent disease	• No standard treatment available for women with recurrent cervical cancer and each case should be carefully investigated and individualized:
	  ▪ Prior treatment has a major impact on future treatments
	• *Locally recurrent disease*:
	  ▪ For women pretreated with surgery or radiation, pelvic exenteration (posterior, central and anterior) has been associated with an approximately 33–50% 5-year survival rate in well-selected patients:
	    ○ Essential to ensure that there is no disease beyond the pelvis and that pelvic lymph nodes are not involved
	    ○ Careful preoperative planning, counselling and imaging is mandatory
	• For women *not* treated with primary or adjuvant radiation at diagnosis, radical radiation is advised for pelvic recurrences that are not amenable to surgical intervention

Treatment

As mentioned above, treatment based on colposcopic diagnosis differs in different resource settings. In well-resourced health systems:
- May be ablative (cryotherapy, cold coagulation, electrocautery or carbon dioxide laser) or excisional (large loop excision of the transformation zone (LLETZ] or loop electrosurgical excision procedure (LEEP])
- LLETZ and LEEP are therapeutic procedures and the following criteria must be met to perform them:
  - Consent from the patient
  - Cytology or other screening test must have been performed and colposcopy must be available
  - Reasonable parity between the screening test and the colposcopic diagnosis, i.e. if the Pap is HSIL and the colposcopy is negative, a diagnostic, not therapeutic, procedure should be performed ('if you cannot see it you cannot treat it')
  - Entire extent of the lesion must be visible – lesions going into the endocervical canal cannot be assessed colposcopically
  - No evidence or suspicion of microinvasion.

In low-resource settings, treatment will depend on resources and may involve either cryotherapy or an excisional procedure.

Surgery

Surgery	Description

Local (conservative and fertility sparing surgery)	• *Cone biopsy*:
	  ▪ May be sufficient treatment for young women wishing to preserve fertility and who fulfil the following criteria:
	    ○ Able to return for regular follow-up
	    ○ Margins of the cone biopsy are free of disease (both dysplasia and invasive cancer) and the dimensions of the tumour do not exceed those of a Stage A1
	    ○ No lymphovascular invasion
	    ○ Cervix is anatomically possible to evaluate in its entirety, i.e. not distorted due to previous surgery during follow-up

(continued)

Surgery	Description
	- *Simple trachelectomy*:
- Cervix is removed up to the isthmus
- Tumour dimensions should not exceed those of Stage A1
- Most surgeons insert a merciline or other form of tape at the same time for prevention of cervical incompetence should the patient fall pregnant
- Frozen section should be performed intraoperatively to ensure the endocervical margin is free of dysplastic or invasive disease
- Similar criteria as for cone biopsy must be fulfilled, i.e. woman wishing to preserve fertility and stage not higher than Stage 1A1
- *Simple hysterectomy* (see Box 35.2):
- Performed for same indications as cone biopsy or simple trachelectomy, i.e. Stage 1A1 disease but in a women for whom fertility is no longer an issue
- May be performed abdominally, laparoscopically or vaginally
Radical surgery	- *Radical trachelectomy*:
- May be performed in women with Stage IA2 or IB1 disease as long as the tumour is <2 cm in diameter
- Cervix is removed up to the isthmus as well as the upper 2 cm of the vagina and parametria:
- Extent of the parametrial dissection is determined by the size of the tumour, access to the parametria and the expertise of the surgeon
- Parametria may be dissected and removed either to where the ureter runs below the uterine artery or to the origin of the uterine artery (which is a branch of the internal iliac artery)
- If the endocervical margin is involved with disease (determined intraoperatively by frozen section), the surgeon should proceed to perform radical surgery either abdominally or laparoscopically:
- Intraoperative frozen section must confirm that the endocervical margin is clear of disease
- Most surgeons insert a mercilene or other form of tape at the same time to prevent cervical incompetence should the patient become pregnant
- Regular follow-up must be possible and the cervix evaluable at each visit
- If lymph node dissection is required, this can be done through the extraperitoneal approach, abdominally or laparoscopically
- *Radical hysterectomy*:
- For early invasive cancers, either Stage B1 or A1
- Surgical removal of the uterus, cervix and surrounding tissues (parametria), including 2 cm of the upper vagina:
- Removal of as much cancer-free tissue from around the tumour as possible is associated with a much better cure rate
- Parametria may be dissected to the origin of the uterine artery (from the internal iliac artery; type 3 hysterectomy) or to the area where the ureter passes under the uterine artery (modified type 2 hysterectomy):
- In the latter, less parametrium is removed
- Procedure can be done through an abdominal incision, laparoscopically or vaginally depending on patient characteristics and the availability of expertise in these procedures
- Ovaries are not routinely removed because cervical cancer rarely spreads to the ovaries, unless the patient is postmenopausal
- If at the time of surgery pelvic lymph nodes are found to be involved, they may be resected and either the hysterectomy abandoned, the pelvis and primary being subsequently treated by radiotherapy, or surgery completed and postoperative pelvic radiation given (see Box 35.3)
- *Bilateral pelvic lymphadenectomy or nodal dissection*:
- Removal of groups of lymph nodes in the pelvis, which are often involved in invasive cervical cancer
- Nodal dissection in addition to radical hysterectomy in women with Stage 1A2, 1B1, IIA1 disease, the desire to preserve ovarian function, vascular invasion, tumour size and radiological evidence of node involvement can be considered in the decision process
- Specific lymph nodes removed are the external, internal, common iliac nodes as well as the obturator lymph nodes:
- Although more debatable, para-aortic nodes may be resected as well if pelvic nodes are involved
- Women with higher stages may be treated with neoadjuvant chemotherapy prior to surgery, a common approach in many South American countries and other areas where radiotherapy is not available
- *Debulking large lymph nodes during surgery*:
- Theoretical advantage is to improve the effectiveness of postoperative radiation
- However, while studies have shown that local control in surgically resected bulky nodes is excellent, this has no impact on distant metastases in node-positive patients and therefore does not translate into overall improved survival

Box 35.2 Invasive carcinoma found incidentally at simple hysterectomy

- Although uncommon in units that routinely screen women prior to surgery, cancer is occasionally incidentally found
- If the lesion is microinvasive (Stage 1A1, no lymphovascular invasion, excision margins clear), then the simple hysterectomy may suffice
- For women with Stage 1A2, laparoscopic or extraperitoneal lymphadenectomy may be subsequently performed to determine lymph node status and the need for adjuvant radiation if the nodes are positive
- For women with higher-stage disease, simple hysterectomy is inadequate treatment and the options include:
  - Whole pelvic radiation with brachytherapy
  - Reoperation and radical parametrectomy, upper colpectomy and bilateral pelvic lymph node dissection and removal of bulky nodes if found in the para-aortic area
- Adjuvant radiation in women who are node negative but have poor prognostic factors related to the primary tumour, such as large primary tumour, deep stromal invasion and lymphovascular invasion

Box 35.3 Node-positive operable cervical cancer: should the hysterectomy be completed?

Around 10–25% of women with Stage B1 and IIA1 cancer of the cervix will have positive lymph nodes with risk factors including:
- Depth of tumour invasion
- Tumour size
- Parametrial involvement
- Lymphovascular space involvement

Data from a number of trials have not shown improved survival by completing the hysterectomy in the face of clinically obvious lymph node involvement or extension of the disease beyond the cervix.

Disadvantages of completing the surgery include:
- Delaying the initiation of radiation therapy
- Adding surgical morbidity
- Using two radical modalities of surgery increases both cost and risk of complications

Radiotherapy

Radiation therapy plays a central role in the treatment of the majority invasive cervical cancers.

- Mainly used for bulkier tumours (Stages IB2 and IIA2–IVB) and cases with extensive involvement of the lymph nodes seen at laparotomy or preoperative imaging
- Also used to manage cancers in patients who are unable to tolerate general anaesthesia due to co-morbid conditions and high anaesthetic risk
- In addition to its curative role, can alleviate symptoms, especially bone pain and vaginal bleeding, and plays an role in palliative care

Radiotherapy	Description

External beam radiotherapy	• Typical clinical target volume would include the primary cervical tumour, uterus, upper vagina only (if the vagina is involved, the whole vagina is included), parametria, presacral and pelvic lymph nodes and ideally is determined using MRI
	• Pelvic doses of 45–50 Gy in 1.8–2-Gy daily fractions over 5 weeks are usual:
	  ■ If the para-aortic nodes are to be treated, doses of 40–45 Gy in 1.8–2-Gy daily fractions over 4–5 weeks may be given
	  ■ Intensity-modulated radiation therapy (IMRT) is avoided in patients with an intact cervix because of the unpredictable movement of the target

Brachytherapy	• Many potentially appropriate brachytherapy prescriptions that depend on:
	  ■ Local availability of brachytherapy techniques and technology
	  ■ Dose rate (low dose rate [LDR], high dose rate [HDR] and pulse dose rate [PDR]), e.g.:
	    ○ LDR dose: 35–40 Gy at 40–70 cGy/h
	    ○ HDR dose: 30 Gy in five 6-Gy fractions beginning in the third or fourth week of external beam radiotherapy
	    ○ PDR dose: 35–40 Gy at 60–80 cGy/h beginning as soon as possible after external beam radiotherapy
	  ■ Dosimetric technique
	• Traditionally prescribed using point A representing the lateral cervix–medial parametrium and point B representing the lateral parametrium and obturator nodes, but this being replaced by 3D image-based treatment planning

Intracavitary therapy alone	• For selected patients with carcinoma *in situ* (CIS), microinvasive or occult invasive lesions, e.g.:
	  ■ 55 Gy at 60–80 cGy/h in one or two applications for CIS
	  ■ 60–65 Gy for Stage IA
	  ■ 75–80 Gy for occult Stage IB1

Systemic therapy and chemoradiation

Concurrent chemotherapy (chemoradiation) has been shown to improve survival, particularly for earlier stage bulky disease.

Women need careful screening for renal function, bone marrow function, and overall nutritional and performance status before chemoradiotherapy is considered and follow-up for these same parameters during treatment are warranted. This requirement for monitoring and safe mixing and administration of chemotherapy may make chemotherapy inappropriate or unsafe in poorly resourced settings. If the facilities, monitoring and screening are not available or the woman has poor renal or bone marrow function or performance status, then radiation alone should be considered.

Indications for postoperative chemoradiation are:
- Positive pelvic node(s)
- Positive or close (≤5 mm) margin
- Parametrial invasion
- Unexpected histological finding of cancer after hysterectomy (except in superficially invasive cancers >3 mm and ≤5 mm, adequate resection margins and no vascular invasion – consider pelvic lymph node dissection)
- Patients at high risk for central recurrence after radical surgery and negative lymph nodes: consider for adjuvant radiotherapy if two of the following are present:
  - Deeply (>10 mm) invasive tumours
  - >4 cm in diameter
  - Lymphovascular space involvement.

Treatment of advanced cervical cancer has incorporated combined chemotherapy and radiation therapy since randomized trials in 1999 showed concurrent cisplatin-based chemotherapy with radiation demonstrated a survival advantage. Cisplatin is included in the WHO's Model List of Essential Medicines and is the most commonly used drug given concurrently with radiation for cervical cancer.

- Cisplatin-based chemotherapy in the setting of recurrent/metastatic disease has palliative utility
- A randomized trial of cisplatin versus an inactive drug (hydroxyurea) suggested a potential, though overall limited, survival benefit
- Individual patients may show an exceptional sensitivity to platinum and, whether treated with single-agent platinum or platinum combinations, may achieve a complete response that can be long-lasting; some may even be cured
- Based on several trials performed in the USA by the Gynecologic Oncology Group (GOG), cisplatin + paclitaxel is being considered as a reference for further study

The alternative drug, carboplatin, has been studied and shown to also improve survival outcomes with greater bone marrow (white blood cell) toxicity than cisplatin, but fewer gastrointestinal symptoms.

Additional combinations of chemotherapy drugs with radiation are being studied to further increase survival advantage without further increasing the toxicity of combined treatment.

Of the more recently developed targeted agents, antiangiogenesis drugs seem to be the most promising. Bevacizumab, a humanized monoclonal antibody directed against vascular endothelial growth factor (VEGF)-A, has been studied the most extensively.

- Adding bevacizumab to cytotoxic doublets (paclitaxel + cisplatin or paclitaxel + topotecan) led to a clear survival benefit (bevacizumab versus no bevacizumab hazard ratio (HR) of death was 0.71; 97% CI 0.54–0.94; one-sided $P = 0.0035$)
- Median progression-free survival was 5.9 months without bevacizumab and 8.2 months with bevacizumab (HR 0.67; 95% CI 0.54–0.82, two-sided $P = 0.00807$)
- Response rate with bevacizumab was higher than without bevacizumab (48% vs 36%, 2-sided $P = 0.0078$)
- Treatment with bevacizumab was associated with more grade 3–4 bleeding (5% vs 1%), thromboembolic events (9% vs 2%) and gastrointestinal fistula (3% vs 0%):
  - Despite the increased toxicity the gain in efficacy was considered clinically relevant, and a major step forward

Suggested follow-up

- After surgery, all women should be examined at 6 weeks to check for postoperative recovery and complications:
  - Women treated with conservative or radical surgery should be followed 6 monthly with colposcopy and cytology for the first 3 years and then yearly for 10–15 years
- Women treated with pelvic radiation should be examined every 3 months, both digitally and with a speculum and careful assessment for central or other recurrences, particularly if the recurrence is amenable to surgical intervention:
  - Role of cytology in the follow-up of women treated with radiation is controversial and is not generally recommended
  - However, if a central recurrence is suspected, histological sampling should be performed, if necessary under anaesthetic to make a firm diagnosis

Special circumstances

HIV-positive women (see also Chapter 59.1)

- HIV-positive women should be screened with cytology (or an alternative screening test) on HIV diagnosis, regardless of age, and if normal repeat screening 3 yearly
- HIV-positive women with abnormal smears (ASCUS or greater) should be sent for colposcopic assessment *de novo*
- If found to have low-grade lesions, yearly follow-up with cytology and colposcopy is recommended until progression to high-grade disease, when women should be offered treatment identical to that for HIV-negative women
- Women with high-grade lesions or any suspicion of cancer should be treated in the same way as HIV-negative women

Table 35.5 Phase III clinical trials

Trial reference	Results
Rose et al. (1999) N Engl J Med 340(15):1144–1153	• Randomized trial of radiotherapy in combination with three concurrent chemotherapy regimens (cisplatinum alone, cisplatinum + fluorouracil + hydroxyurea, and hydroxyurea alone) in women with locally-advanced cervical cancer (n = 526) • Both groups that received cisplatinum had a higher rate of progression-free survival than the group that received hydroxyurea alone
Keys et al. (1999) N Engl J Med 340(15):1154–1161	• Women with bulky Stage 1B cervical cancers were randomly assigned to receive radiotherapy alone or in combination with cisplatinum, followed in all patients by adjuvant hysterectomy • Both progression-free survival and overall survival were significantly higher in the combined therapy group at 4 years
Peters et al. (2000) J Clin Oncol 18(8):1606–1613	• Patients initially treated with radical surgery for Stage IA2, IB and IIA cancer of the cervix and who qualified for adjuvant radiation (positive nodes and/or positive margins and/or positive parametria) were randomized to receive radiation or radiation + chemotherapy (fluorouracil) • Progression-free and overall survival were significantly improved in the patients receiving concurrent chemotherapy

It is well documented that the treatment failure rate for HIV-positive women with preinvasive disease of the cervix is much higher than in HIV negative women, with recurrence of disease reaching up to 50% within 6–12 months of treatment. Close follow-up is therefore advised. In addition, a careful examination of the vulva, the perineum and perianal area is essential as intraepithelial lesions of these areas are commonly found in HIV-positive women, with or without abnormal cervical cytology or cervical disease.

Pregnant women

- Screening women during pregnancy is best done in the first 20 weeks of gestation:
    - Thereafter, the impact of high levels of progestogen make smears harder to interpret and less accurate due to the viscosity of the endocervical mucus
- Cervical cancer in pregnancy is diagnosed by an abnormal cervical smear or due to symptoms such as abnormal vaginal bleeding:
    - All abnormal lesions should be biopsied; this is not associated with increased risk of miscarriage
- Conisation during pregnancy is not recommended unless essential to make a diagnosis:
    - Risk of miscarriage is not known but is considered relatively high, and the decision to do the cone should be taken by a multidisciplinary team
- Options for treatment of pregnant women at <20 weeks of gestation include:
    - Depending on stage, radical surgery with sacrifice of the fetus
    - Primary radical chemoradiation with sacrifice of the fetus
- Options for treatment of pregnant women at >20 weeks of gestation:
    - Neoadjuvant chemotherapy (most SCC are very sensitive to platinum-containing chemotherapy and the fetus is remarkably tolerant of platinum) and surgery delayed until fetal lung maturity (usually by 32–34 weeks of gestation) when a caesarean section with radical surgery can be performed simultaneously
    - Although data are sparse, vaginal delivery is not recommended in pregnant women with cervical cancer
    - Neoadjuvant chemotherapy until fetal lung maturity is reached, delivery by caesarean section and then primary radical chemoradiation post delivery for women with higher stages of disease

Phase III clinical trials

See Table 35.5.

Recommended reading

Alberts DS, Kronmal R, Baker LH et al. (1987) Phase II randomized trial of cisplatin chemotherapy regimens in the treatment of recurrent or metastatic squamous cell cancer of the cervix: Southwest Oncology Group Study. J Clin Oncol 5(11):1791–1795.

Arbyn M, Castellsague X, de Sanjose S et al. (2011) Worldwide burden of cervical cancer in 2008. Ann Oncol 22(12):2675–2686.

Bonomi P, Blessing JA, Stehman FB, Di Saia PJ, Walton L, Major FJ (1985) Randomized trial of three cisplatin dose schedules in squamous cell carcinoma of the cervix: a Gynecologic Oncology Group study. J Clin Oncol 3:1079–1085.

Conely LK, Ellerbrock TV, Bush TJ, Chiasson Ma, Sawo D, Wright TC (2002) HIV-1 infection and risk of vulvovaginal and perianal condylomata acuminate and intraepithelial neoplasia; a prospective cohort study. Lancet 359:108–113.

Creasman WT, Kohler MF (2004) Is lymph vascular space involvement an independent prognostic factor in early cervical cancer? Gynecol Oncol 92:525–529.

Denny L, Boa R, Williamson AL et al. (2008) Human papillomavirus infection and cervical disease in human immunodeficiency virus-1 infected women. Obstet Gynecol 111(6):1380–1387.

De Sanjose S, Quint WGV, Alemany L et al. (2010) Human papillomavirus genotype attribution in invasive cervical cancer: a retrospective cross-sectional worldwide study. Lancet Oncol 11(11):1048–1056.

Hacker NF, Vermorken JB (2014) Cervical cancer. In: Berek JS, Hacker NF, eds. Gynecologic Oncology. Lippincott Williams and Wilkins.

Hakama M, Miller AB, Day NE, eds. (1986) Screening for Cancer of the Uterine Cervix. IARC Scientific Publications no. 76. Lyon: International Agency for Research on Cancer:47–60.

Hakama M, Louhivuori K (1988) A screening programme for cervical cancer that worked. Cancer Surveys 17(3):403–416.

Harper DM, Franco EL, Wheeler CM et al. (2006) Sustained efficacy up to 4.5 years of a bivalent L1 virus-like particle vaccine against human papillomavirus types 16 and 18: follow-up from a randomized control trial. Lancet 367:1247–1255.

Hoogendam JP, Zaal A, Rutten EG et al. (2013) Detection of cervical cancer recurrence during follow-up: A multivariable comparison of 9 frequently investigated serum biomarkers. Gynecol Oncol 131(3):655–660.

Lim K, Small W Jr, Portelance L et al. (2011) Consensus Guidelines for Delineation of Clinical Target Volume for Intensity-Modulated Pelvic Radiotherapy for the Definitive Treatment of Cervix Cancer. Int J Radiat Oncol Biol Phys 79(2):34–55.

Marcus E, Randall ME, Fracasso PM, Toita T, Tejkarati SS, Michael H (2013) Cervix. In: Barakat RR, Berchuck A, Markman M, Randall ME, eds. Principles and Practice of Gynecologic Oncology, 6th edn. Wolters Kluwer/Lippincott, Williams & Wilkins: Chapter 21.

Monk BJ, Tewari KS, Koh WJ (2007) Multimodality therapy for locally advanced cervical carcinoma: state of the art and future directions. J Clin Oncol 25(20):2952–2965.

Monk BJ, Sill MW, McMeekin DS et al. (2009) Phase III trial of four cisplatin containing doublet combinations in stage IVB, recurrent, or persistent cervical carcinoma: a Gynecologic Oncology Group study. J Clin Oncol 27:4649–4655.

Munoz N, Bosch FX, de Sanjose S et al. (2003) Epidemiologic classification of human papillomavirus types associated with cervical cancer. N Engl J Med 348:518–527.

Pötter R, Haie-Meder C, Van Limbergen E et al. (2006) Recommendations from gynaecological (GYN) GEC ESTRO working group (II): concepts and terms in 3D image-based treatment planning in cervix cancer brachytherapy-3D dose volume parameters and aspects of 3D image-based anatomy, radiation physics, radiobiology. Radiother Oncol 78(1):67–77.

Singh DK, Anastos K, Hoover DR et al. (2009) Human papillomavirus infection and cervical cytology in HIV-infected and HIV-uninfected Rwandan women. J Infect Dis 199(12):1851–1861.

Tewari KS, Monk BJ (2005) Gynecologic Oncology Group trials of chemotherapy for metastatic and recurrent cervical cancer. Curr Oncol Rep 7(6):419–434.

The Future II Study Group (2007) Quadrivalent vaccine against human papillomavirus to prevent high-grade cervical lesions. N Engl J Med 356:1915–1927.

Tierney JF, Vale C, Symonds P (2008) Concomitant and neoadjuvant chemotherapy for cervical cancer. Clin Oncol (R Coll Radiol) 20(6):401–416.

Winter WE 3rd, Maxwell GL, Tian C et al. (2004) Association of haemoglobin level with survival in cervical carcinoma patients treat with concurrent cisplatin and radiotherapy: A Gynecologic Group Study. Gynecol Oncol 94(2):495–501.

36 Uterus

Gunnar B. Kristensen[1], Vera M. Abeler[2], Kristina Lindemann[1] and Carien L. Creutzberg[3]

[1]Department of Gynecological Cancer, Oslo University Hospital, The Norwegian Radium Hospital, Oslo, Norway
[2]Department of Pathology, Oslo University Hospital, The Norwegian Radium Hospital, Oslo, Norway
[3]Department of Radiation Oncology, Leiden University Medical Center, Leiden, The Netherlands

Summary	Key facts
Introduction	<ul><li>Uterine cancers are the most common gynaecological cancer in developed countries and fourth most common cancer in women:<ul><li>Rising incidence due to increased obesity rates and ageing of population</li></ul></li><li>Endometrial carcinomas (90%) comprise endometrioid endometrial carcinomas (85%), serous carcinomas (5–7%), clear cell carcinomas (3%) and mucinous carcinomas (2%):<ul><li>Two types:<ul><li>Type 1: associated with oestrogen, with a favourable prognosis</li><li>Type 2: unrelated to oestrogen, often non-endometrioid, with inferior outcome</li></ul></li></ul></li><li>Mixed carcinomas (5%) have epithelial and stromal (homologous or heterologous) components and are considered dedifferentiated epithelial cancers</li><li>Uterine sarcomas (3–5%)</li></ul>
Presentation	<ul><li>Postmenopausal vaginal bleeding</li><li>Rarely symptoms of advanced disease</li><li>Work-up:<ul><li>Vaginal and pelvic examination, cervical cytology</li><li>Vaginal ultrasound to evaluate endometrial thickness</li><li>Endometrial biopsy or (micro)curettage</li><li>Chest X-ray</li><li>Optional: magnetic resonance imaging (MRI) to evaluate depth of invasion</li><li>Optional: computed tomography (CT)/positron emission tomography (PET)-CT if suspected advanced disease</li></ul></li></ul>
Scenario	<ul><li>Surgical treatment with hysterectomy and salpingo-oophorectomy:<ul><li>Laparoscopic procedure is oncologically safe for early-stage disease</li><li>Laparotomy if suspected advanced disease</li><li>Pelvic and para-aortic lymphadenectomy (LA) is controversial; no proven survival benefit, mainly for high-risk disease</li><li>Sentinel node procedure is investigational</li><li>Consider radical hysterectomy if macroscopic cervical invasion</li></ul></li><li>Adjuvant therapy based on stage and risk factors:<ul><li>Radiotherapy (RT) and/or chemotherapy</li></ul></li></ul>

(continued)

UICC Manual of Clinical Oncology, Ninth Edition. Edited by Brian O'Sullivan, James D. Brierley, Anil K. D'Cruz, Martin F. Fey, Raphael Pollock, Jan B. Vermorken and Shao Hui Huang. © 2015 UICC. Published 2015 by John Wiley & Sons, Ltd.

Summary	Key facts

Trials	- ASTEC (Study of Lymphadenectomy and Adjuvant External Beam Radiotherapy in Patients With Endometrial Cancer) and Italian trials: LA versus no LA for Stage I:
	   - LA has no survival benefit, no disease-free survival (DFS) benefit and no difference in relapse patterns
	- PORTEC 1 (Post Operative Radiation Therapy for Endometrial Carcinoma), ASTEC, GOG99 (Gynecological Oncology Group), NRH (Norwegian Radium Hospital) trials: RT versus no RT for intermediate-risk Stage I:
	   - RT significantly decreases vaginal and pelvic recurrence
	   - RT does not provide a survival benefit and should only be used in presence of risk factors
	- PORTEC-2: vaginal brachytherapy (VBT) versus external beam RT (EBRT):
	   - VBT is as effective as EBRT for local control; fewer side effects, better quality of life
	- Nordic Society of Gynecological Oncology (NSGO)/ European Organisation for Research and Treatment of Cancer (EORTC)/Iliade trials: RT alone or RT + chemotherapy for high risk:
	   - Chemotherapy + RT 7% improved progression-free survival (PFS) and cancer-specific survival (CSS); overall survival (OS) not significant
	- GOG122: chemotherapy (AP × 8) versus whole abdominal RT for Stage III–IV:
	   - Chemotherapy group had a slightly better OS; both arms toxic; frequent relapses
	- Japanese Gynecologic Oncology Group (JGOG) and Italian trials: RT versus chemotherapy for Stage I-III:
	   - No difference in OS and relapse-free survival (RFS)

Introduction

Endometrial carcinoma is derived from epithelial cells in the mucosa lining of the endometrial cavity and comprises the subtypes endometrioid endometrial (85–90%), serous (5–7%), clear cell (3%) and mucinous carcinomas (2%).

Mixed carcinomas (5% of all uterine carcinomas) have epithelial and mesenchymal (homologous or heterologous) components and are considered dedifferentiated epithelial carcinomas, especially uterine carcinosarcomas.

Uterine sarcomas (3–5% of all uterine cancers) arise from mesenchymal cells from the endometrial stroma or myometrium. Uterine sarcomas comprise leiomyosarcoma, endometrial stromal sarcomas and undifferentiated sarcomas. They are not dealt with in this chapter.

Type I and type II endometrial carcinomas have been defined based on clinical behaviour and histopathology. Type I are oestrogen-related tumours of the endometrioid type, developing from endometrial hyperplasia and have a good prognosis. Type II are non–oestrogen-related, mainly poorly differentiated endometrioid and non-endometrioid (e.g. serous and clear cell) carcinomas with a worse prognosis, arising from atrophic endometrium.

The clinicopathological differences between type I and type II cancers are paralleled by specific gene alterations, despite some overlap. Genetic mechanisms involved in type I include inactivation of *PTEN*, microsatellite instability, mutations of *KRAS*, *PIK3CA* and the β*1-catenin* gene. Conversely, genetic abnormalities in type II include *TP53* mutation, *HER2/neu* amplification and inactivation of *p16*. In the future we may move towards a classification based on the molecular biological traits driving the malignant behaviour of individual tumours.

Incidence, aetiology and screening

Incidence, aetiology and screening	Description

Incidence	- Great variation worldwide in the age standardized rate (ASR) per 100,000 women of endometrial cancer, with an increasing incidence rate in developed countries:
	   - Global ASR: 8.2 per 100,000 women
	   - ASR in less developed regions: 5.9 per 100,000 women
	   - ASR in developed regions: 13.0 per 100,000 women
	- Death rate:
	   - Global ASR: 1.9 per 100,000 women
	   - ASR in less developed regions: 1.7 per 100,000 women
	   - ASR in developed regions: 2.3 per women

Incidence, aetiology and screening	Description

Aetiology	• *Age*:
	  ▪ Postmenopausal women
	  ▪ Pre- or peri-menopausal women with obesity
	• *Reproductive factors*:
	  ▪ Nulliparity
	  ▪ Polycystic ovary syndrome
	  ▪ Hormone replacement therapy:
	    ○ Unopposed oestrogen use
	    ○ Tamoxifen
	• *Endocrine disorders*:
	  ▪ Obesity
	  ▪ Diabetes mellitus
	• *Hereditary*:
	  ▪ Lynch syndrome

Screening	• Of limited use in cancer of the uterus • Yearly vaginal ultrasound and endometrial biopsy is recommended in women with Lynch syndrome until hysterectomy is performed

Pathology

Pathology	Description

Subtype 1	• Endometrioid adenocarcinoma:
	  ▪ Accounts for 80% of cases
	  ▪ Can have squamous cell differentiation
	• Grade of differentiation is evaluated according to the WHO/FIGO grading system:
	  ▪ Grade 1: <5% non-squamous solid growth
	  ▪ Grade 2: 5–50% non-squamous solid growth
	  ▪ Grade 3: >50% non-squamous solid growth
	  ▪ Increase grade by 1 if marked nuclear atypia

Subtype 2	• Serous carcinoma:
	  ▪ Accounts for 5–7% of cases
	  ▪ Aggressive tumours with a tendency to early spread, including to the abdominal cavity
	• Clear cell carcinoma:
	  ▪ Accounts for about 3% of cases
	  ▪ Often grouped with serous carcinomas but have a different behaviour, may behave more like ovarian clear cell cancers

Other	• Carcinosarcoma:
	  ▪ Accounts for about 3–5% of cases
	  ▪ Dedifferentiated endometrial cancer
	  ▪ Aggressive tumours with a tendency to early spread
	• Undifferentiated carcinomas
	• Squamous cell carcinoma
	• Mucinous carcinoma
	• Sarcomas
	  ▪ Very rare, but aggressive

Natural history and presentation

Endometrial carcinoma occurs mostly in postmenopausal women. The predominant symptom is postmenopausal bleeding, which most often occurs while the tumour is in an early phase. Tumours with type II histology have a more aggressive behaviour and often have metastases to regional lymph nodes at the time of diagnosis. Tumours of serous papillary and clear cell types have a tendency to intraperitoneal spread.

Natural history		Description

Presentation	Local	• Postmenopausal bleeding
		• Thickened endometrium on vaginal ultrasound (>4 mm)
		• Can mimic cervical cancer in case of invasion into the cervix
		• If locally advanced:
		  ▪ Pain
		  ▪ Uraemia

	Metastatic	• Intraperitoneal:
		  ▪ Palpable tumour
		  ▪ Ascites
		• Lung:
		  ▪ Usually asymptomatic
		• Lymph nodes:
		  ▪ Usually asymptomatic
		• Vagina:
		  ▪ Bleeding/discharge
		• Bone:
		  ▪ Rare at time of primary diagnosis
		  ▪ Pain
		  ▪ Palpable tumour (rare)
		• Brain:
		  ▪ Rare at time of primary diagnosis
		  ▪ Cerebral symptoms

Routes of spread	Local	• Invasion into the myometrium (and lymph vessels or blood vessels):
		  ▪ Invasion through the myometrium into surrounding tissue:
		    ○ Parametrium
		    ○ Bladder
		    ○ Rectum
		• Invasion into the uterine cervix:
		  ▪ Cervical mucosa
		  ▪ Cervical stroma

	Regional	• Metastases to pelvic lymph nodes • Metastases to para-aortic lymph nodes
	Metastatic	• Peritoneal cavity • Lung • Bone • Liver • Brain

Diagnostic work-up

Diagnostic work up	Description

Work-up	• Initial work-up of postmenopausal bleeding:
	  ▪ Gynaecological examination with cervical cytology
	  ▪ Transvaginal ultrasound
	  ▪ Endometrial biopsy
	• Further work-up in case of endometrial cancer:
	  ▪ Chest X-ray
	• In case of suspected advanced disease and/or spread of disease:
	  ▪ CT chest/abdomen/pelvis (± PET)
	  ▪ MRI pelvis

Tumour markers	• Tumour markers are not routinely used in endometrial cancer: ▪ Serum CA125 may be increased in case of regional or distant spread

Staging and prognostic risk grouping

UICC TNM staging
See Table 36.1.

Prognostic risk factors
Major prognostic factors for endometrial carcinoma are stage, age, histological type, grade, depth of myometrial invasion and presence of lymphovascular space invasion (LVSI) (Table 36.2). Such clinical and histopathological features predict micrometastatic disease. Pelvic (and para-aortic) lymphadenectomy, if performed, informs about microscopic lymph node dissemination. The use of lymphadenectomy for Stage I endometrial carcinoma is controversial, and is primarily used to tailor adjuvant treatment.

Most patients with endometrial carcinoma are diagnosed at an early stage, due to early symptoms of vaginal bleeding. Based on staging studies and prospective and retrospective data, Stage I endometrial carcinoma has been classified as low risk, intermediate risk or high risk for lymph node metastases and/or early disease spread to the abdominal cavity and to distant sites. The majority of patients have low–intermediate (55%) or high–intermediate (30%) risk features; only 15% have a high-risk profile.

- *Low risk*: endometrioid cell type grade 1–2, with <50% myometrial invasion
- *Intermediate risk*: endometrioid cell type grade 1–2, with ≥50% myometrial invasion or endometrioid cell type grade 3, with <50% myometrial invasion:
  ▪ Often divided into low–intermediate and high–intermediate groups depending on lymphovascular space invasion and age

Table 36.1 UICC TNM categories, with FIGO equivalent, and stage grouping: Endometrial carcinomas and carcinosarcomas

TNM categories		
TNM	**Corpus uteri**	**FIGO**
T1	Confined to corpus (includes endocervical glands)	I
T1a	Tumour limited to endometrium or less than one-half of myometrium	IA
T1b	One-half or more of myometrium	IB
T2	Invades cervix	II
T3 and/or N1	Local or regional as specified below	III
T3a	Serosa/adnexa	IIIA
T3b	Vaginal/parametrial	IIIB
N1, N2	Regional lymph node metastasis	IIIC
T4	Mucosa of bladder/bowel	IVA
M1	Distant metastasis	IVB

Stage grouping			
Stage IA	T1a	N0	M0
Stage IB	T1b	N0	M0
Stage II	T2	N0	M0
Stage IIIA	T3a	N0	M0
Stage IIIB	T3b	N0	M0
Stage IIIC	T1, T2, T3	N1, N2	M0
Stage IIIC1	T1, T2, T3	N1	M0
Stage IIIC2	T1, T2, T3	N2	M0
Stage IVA	T4	Any N	M0
Stage IVB	Any T	Any N	M1

Table 36.2 Prognostic factors for endometrial carcinoma

Prognostic factors	Tumour related	Host related	Environment related
Essential	Depth of myometrial invasion Grade of differentiation Tumour cell type Lymphovascular space invasion		Postsurgical treatment
Additional	Metastasis to lymph nodes Site of distant metastasis	Age Performance status Race Co-morbidities	Extent of resection Postsurgical treatment
New and promising	Molecular profile		

- *High risk*: endometrioid cell type grade 3, with ≥50% myometrial invasion or tumours of serous papillary or clear cell type or carcinosarcoma

Risk and site of relapse according to risk group are:
- *Low risk*: 3% risk of relapse, mainly vaginal
- *Intermediate risk*: 14%, mainly locoregional
- *High risk*: 25%, locoregional and distant.

Rates of endometrial cancer death are 8–10%. Five-year overall survival rates according to stage (FIGO Annual Report 2006) are:
- Stage I: 80–90%
- Stage II: 70–80%
- Stage III: 50–60%
- Stage IV: 20–30%.

Treatment philosophy

Most cases present at an early stage when the goal is cure with minimal morbidity. For many patients, this can be accomplished by surgery with removal of the uterus with adnexae. Patients with a high risk of recurrence are given adjuvant treatment.

For patients with spread to regional lymph nodes, the goal is also cure. For intra-abdominal spread, the goal is long-term survival. This can usually be accomplished by surgery followed by appropriate additional treatment with chemotherapy ± radiation.

For patients with distant metastases, the goal is palliation.

Scenario	Treatment philosophy

Local disease	• Intention is cure
	• *Medically operable*:
	  ▪ Surgery:
	    ○ Hysterectomy with bilateral salpingo-oophorectomy:
	      – Laparotomy or laparoscopic approach
	      – Modified radical hysterectomy in case of macroscopic involvement of the cervix
	    ○ Consider pelvic and para-aortic lymph node dissection in high-risk patients
	    ○ Therapeutic benefit of lymphadenectomy is controversial
	  ▪ Adjuvant treatment:
	    ○ Adjuvant radiotherapy reduces the risk of locoregional relapse in (high)intermediate-risk patients without improving survival
	    ○ Concomitant chemoradiotherapy may improve survival in high-risk patients
	    ○ Role of adjuvant chemotherapy alone is currently under investigation
	    ○ In case of involvement of cervical stroma, consider adjuvant radiotherapy after simple hysterectomy
	• *Medically inoperable*:
	  ▪ Radiotherapy (EBRT and/or intracavitary brachytherapy)
	  ▪ Palliative treatment with hormones or chemotherapy

Regional disease	• Includes spread to adnexa, parametria and regional lymph nodes (pelvic and para-aortic)
	• *Resectable disease*:
	  ▪ Surgical resection, followed by chemotherapy ± radiotherapy
	• *Unresectable disease*:
	  ▪ Consider chemotherapy ± radiotherapy before surgery

Metastatic disease	• *Intra-abdominal metastases*:
	  ▪ Resectable disease:
	    ○ Surgical debulking to no residual tumour, followed by chemotherapy
	  ▪ Unresectable disease:
	    ○ Consider chemotherapy or hormonal therapy ± radiotherapy before surgery
	• *Isolated extra-abdominal metastases*:
	  ▪ Consider hysterectomy and bilateral salpingo-oophorectomy as treatment for primary tumour
	  ▪ Consider surgical resection of metastatic site
	  ▪ Consider radiotherapy for metastases
	  ▪ Consider systemic treatment with chemotherapy
	  ▪ Hormonal treatment may be effective in hormone receptor-positive tumours
	• *Disseminated metastases*:
	  ▪ Palliative hysterectomy and bilateral salpingo-oophorectomy or radiotherapy may be considered
	  ▪ Chemotherapy
	  ▪ Hormonal treatment may be effective in hormone receptor-positive tumours

Recurrent disease	• *Isolated local* (vagina and top of vagina):
	  ▪ Radiotherapy:
	    ○ EBRT and brachytherapy boost (preferably image-guided brachytherapy)
	    ○ Consider brachytherapy alone in case of poor performance status and low-volume disease
	    ○ In case of previous irradiation, consider surgery (± brachytherapy alone in case of low volume disease)
	• *Regional* (regional lymph nodes on pelvic side wall or para-aortic area):
	  ▪ Consider surgical resection/debulking
	  ▪ Radiotherapy (consider intensity-modulated EBRT with simultaneous integrated or stereotactic boost for macroscopic residual disease)
	  ▪ Consider concomitant chemoradiation
	  ▪ Consider chemotherapy
	• *Metastatic*:
	  ▪ Intra-abdominal, including liver:
	    ○ Chemotherapy
	    ○ Hormonal treatment
	  ▪ Lung:
	    ○ Chemotherapy
	    ○ Hormonal treatment
	    ○ In case of a single lesion, surgery or stereotactic radiation may be considered

Scenario	Treatment philosophy

	- Brain:
	    - Radiation (stereotactic or whole-brain RT)
	        - Bone:
	            - Radiation
	            - Chemotherapy
	            - Hormonal treatment

Follow-up	- Goals are to:
	    - Detect potentially curable recurrence at an early stage
	    - Evaluate recovery from treatment
	    - Evaluate and treat complications of treatment
	    - Provide psychological support
	- Majority of recurrences occur during the first 3 years after treatment
	- Recommended schema for follow-up:
	    - First–second year: every 3 months (especially if not previously irradiated)
	    - Third–fifth year: every 6–12 months
	- No proven role for standard follow-up investigations
	- Mandatory: history, focused on review of symptoms; vaginal and pelvic exam
	- Optional: vaginal ultrasound; annual chest X-ray
	- On indication (symptoms, suspicion of recurrence):
	    - Vaginal cytology (only if not irradiated)
	    - Examination under anaesthesia with biopsies
	    - CT of chest, abdomen, pelvis or MRI scan of pelvis

Treatment

Surgery	Description

Early disease	- Hysterectomy and bilateral salpingo-oophorectomy:
	    - Abdominal exploration (check for metastases)
	    - Staging (omentectomy, peritoneal biopsies, pelvic and para-aortic lymphadenectomy) in case of:
	        - Serous papillary histology
	        - Clear cell histology
	        - Undifferentiated histology
	    - Consider pelvic and para-aortic lymphadenectomy in case of:
	        - Endometrioid type grade 3

Advanced non-metastatic disease	- Radical hysterectomy (instead of simple hysterectomy) in case of macroscopic cervix involvement - Pelvic and para-aortic lymphadenectomy or complete debulking of all macroscopically involved lymph nodes in case of suspicion of lymph node metastases on (PET)-CT or MRI scan

Metastatic disease	- *Intra-abdominal metastases*:
	    - Surgical debulking to no residual tumour when possible
	    - Grossly enlarged lymph nodes should be removed
	    - Consider neoadjuvant treatment with chemo(radio)therapy in case of primary unresectable tumour
	- *Isolated extra-abdominal metastases*:
	    - Consider hysterectomy and bilateral salpingo-oophorectomy as treatment for primary tumour
	    - Consider surgical resection of metastatic site
	- *Disseminated metastases*:
	    - Consider surgery or palliative radiotherapy for symptomatic uterine tumour if uncontrolled symptoms under systemic therapy

Radiotherapy

Radiotherapy	Description

Early disease	- *Low-risk and low–intermediate risk:*
	  - No indication for radiotherapy or brachytherapy
	- *(High)–Intermediate risk:*
	  - Vaginal brachytherapy alone
	  - Clinical target volume (CTV): upper third to half (4 cm) of vagina + 3 mm margin
	  - Typical scheme: 21 Gy high dose rate brachytherapy in three fractions of 7 Gy specified at 5 mm from the vaginal surface and vault
	  - Lower dose schema and biologically equivalent low- or pulsed-dose rate schema also effective
	- *High-risk and/or type 2 cancers:*
	  - Pelvic EBRT (consider vaginal brachytherapy alone if fully staged node-negative Stage II endometrioid cancer or early stage serous cancer)
	  - Brachytherapy boost (to vault only) if cervical invasion
	  - Consider concomitant chemoradiotherapy
	- CTV: upper half of the vagina, parametrial tissues, and obturator, internal and external iliac lymph node regions up to the common iliac bifurcation:
	  - CTV includes common iliac regions up to the aortic bifurcation in case of involved (or highly suspicious) lymph nodes
	  - Consider internal target volume (ITV) contouring of the vaginal vault region with a full and an empty bladder
	  - See atlases (Taylor et al.; RTOG) for proper CTV contouring
	- Prescribed dose is typically 45–50 Gy in 1.8–2-Gy fractions
	- Technique: multifield 3D CT-based radiotherapy planning (often four-field box technique is used with or without supplementary fields for dose homogeneity):
	  - Consider intensity-modulated RT (IMRT) if proper quality assurance can be ensured
	- In case of medically inoperable patient:
	  - Consider full curative EBRT + intracavitary brachytherapy
	  - Consider intracavitary brachytherapy alone for poor condition and/or grade 1–2 superficially invasive disease

Advanced non-metastatic disease	- Pelvic EBRT + brachytherapy boost in case of simple hysterectomy and cervical stromal involvement:
	  - Consider brachytherapy alone for low-volume grade 1 disease with minimal endocervical stromal involvement
	- Pelvic and/or para-aortic lymph node metastases:
	  - Pelvic (and para-aortic) EBRT
	- Unresectable primary:
	  - Pelvic external beam radio(chemo)therapy
	  - Followed by surgery if feasible; otherwise boost
	- CTV: upper half of the vagina, parametrial tissues, obturator, internal and external iliac lymph node regions up to the aortic bifurcation (if pelvic nodes +), and up to higher para-aortic levels I–II depending on location of lymph nodes on pathology report and/or on (PET)-CT:
	  - Consider ITV contouring of the vaginal vault region with a full and an empty bladder
	  - See atlases (Taylor *et al.*; RTOG) for proper CTV contouring
	  - Planning target volume (PTV): CTV with 7–10-mm margin
	- Dose prescribed is typically 45–50 Gy in 1.8–2-Gy fractions:
	  - Consider 10–15-Gy boost for macroscopic residual nodal disease or area of extensive nodal involvement
	- Technique: multifield 3D CT-based radiotherapy planning:
	  - Consider IMRT if proper quality assurance can be ensured
	  - Consider (simultaneous integrated) boost for macroscopic residual nodal disease
	  - Consider concomitant chemoradiation and/or adjuvant chemotherapy
	- Brachytherapy boost:
	  - CTV: vaginal vault + 3 mm margin
	  - Typical scheme: 10 Gy high dose rate brachytherapy in two fractions of 5 Gy specified at 5 mm from the vaginal surface and vault
	  - Biologically equivalent low- or pulsed-dose rate schemas can be used

Radiotherapy	Description
Metastatic disease	• Palliative EBRT is very effective for palliation of most symptoms: 　▪ Primary tumour: bleeding, lymphoedema, pain 　▪ Bulky lymph node metastases: lymphoedema, pain 　▪ Bone metastases: pain, neurological symptoms, prevention of fracture 　▪ Brain metastases: neurological symptoms • Typical dose schedules: 　▪ Bulky primary or nodal mass: 30 Gy in ten fractions (if good general condition); otherwise 8–16 Gy in 8-Gy fractions or 20–24 Gy in 4-Gy fractions 　▪ Bone metastases: 8 Gy in one fraction (or 20 Gy in five fractions if risk of fracture) 　▪ Brain metastases: 20 Gy in five fractions 　▪ Consider stereotactic RT in case of single or limited brain metastases

Systemic therapy

Chemotherapy

Doxorubicin + cisplatin (AP), doxorubicin + cisplatin + paclitaxel (TAP), and paclitaxel + carboplatin (TC) are all acceptable regimens for patients with advanced or recurrent endometrial cancer and good performance status.

The TC combination is considered the standard following initial reports of its effectiveness and high tolerability. In a randomized phase III non-inferiority trial (GOG209) in 1300 patients it was found to be as effective as, but less toxic than, the TAP combination (unpublished data). Carboplatin is dosed based on glomerular filtration rate (GFR). GFR can be calculated using a formula (e.g. Cockroft–Gault) or measured. The total dose is calculated using Calvert's formula:

$$\text{Dose (mg)} = \text{AUC (area under the curve)} \cdot (\text{GFR} + 25)$$

It is common to use AUC = 5 or 6. Paclitaxel is usually dosed to 175 mg/m^2 of body surface area. The courses are given intravenously with an interval of 3 weeks. It is usually not needed to give granulocyte colony stimulating factor (G-CSF) support. It is common to give six courses. In case of residual tumour before the start of treatment, a response evaluation should be performed after three and six courses. In the treatment of relapses suspected to be resistant to carboplatin, doxorubicin dosed at 50–60 mg/m^2 given intravenously every 3 weeks can be considered.

Chemotherapy	Description
Early disease	• Chemotherapy ± radiation as adjuvant treatment after surgery in high-risk patients such as those with serous cancers or stage III disease: 　▪ Chemotherapy + radiation seems to be slightly more effective than radiation alone • Effect of chemotherapy alone is still unproven: 　▪ If chemotherapy is given alone, six courses are usual
Advanced non-metastatic disease	• Pelvic and/or para-aortic lymph node metastases: 　▪ Chemotherapy + radiation 　▪ When used alone, six courses of TC are the standard 　▪ When used in combination with radiotherapy: 　　○ Two cycles of cisplatin 50 mg/m^2 in Weeks 1 and 4 of radiotherapy followed by four cycles of TC, or 　　○ 4–6 cycles before or after radiotherapy • Unresectable primary: 　▪ Radiotherapy + chemotherapy (schedule as above), followed by surgery if feasible 　▪ Alternative is hormonal therapy
Metastatic disease	• Choice of chemotherapy will depend on the performance status of the patient: 　▪ Age, performance status, co-morbidity and prognosis are important for the choice of either single-agent or combination chemotherapy or no chemotherapy at all • Targeted therapies only in clinical trials (e.g. multitarget tyrosine kinase inhibitors)

Hormonal therapy

Despite many endometrial cancers being oestrogen and/or progesterone receptor positive, phase III clinical trials and a meta-analysis of adjuvant hormonal therapy have not shown a survival advantage for adjuvant hormonal therapy. However, hormonal therapy can be used with potential good and prolonged responses for patients with grade 1 endometrial cancers and/or those with oestrogen and/or progesterone receptor positivity.

Table 36.3 Phase III clinical trials

Trial name	Results
Local disease: adjuvant radiotherapy	
PORTEC-1 Creutzberg et al. (2000) Lancet 355:1404–1411 GOG-99 Keys et al. (2004) Gynecol Oncol 92:744–751 ASTEC-RT Blake et al. (2009) Lancet 373:137–146 NRH Aalders et al. (1980) Obstet Gynecol 56:419-27	Phase III trials of adjuvant EBRT (46 Gy) versus surgery alone for intermediate-risk Stage I endometrial cancer:<ul><li>RT significantly reduced locoregional recurrence, but trials (including meta-analysis) showed no survival benefit</li><li>More gastrointestinal toxicity with RT</li><li>High–intermediate risk factors defined; no benefit from RT in absence of these risk factors</li><li>GOG-99 (with lymphadenectomy, node negative) showed similar improvement of locoregional control with RT as other trials without lymphadenectomy</li><li>EBRT should only be used in the presence of risk factors and not be used in patients with low-risk disease</li></ul>
PORTEC-2 Nout et al. (2010) Lancet 375:816–823	Phase III trial of postsurgical EBRT versus vaginal brachytherapy (VBT) alone for high–intermediate risk Stage I endometrial cancer:<ul><li>VBT was as effective as EBRT to reduce vaginal recurrence (<2% in both groups)</li><li>Similar overall survival rates</li><li>VBT had significantly fewer side effects and better quality of life</li></ul>
Local disease: lymphadenectomy	
ASTEC ASTEC Study Group et al. (2009) Lancet 373:125–136	Phase III trial of surgery with pelvic lymphadenectomy versus no lymphadenectomy for Stage I endometrial cancer:<ul><li>9% pelvic nodes positive in lymphadenectomy arm</li><li>No overall or relapse-free survival benefit for lymphadenectomy</li><li>More toxicity (lymphoedema), longer operating time with lymphadenectomy</li></ul>
Italian Benedetti Panici et al. (2008) J Natl Cancer Inst 100(23):1707–1716.	Phase III trial of surgery with pelvic (and para-aortic in 30%) lymphadenectomy versus no lymphadenectomy for Stage I endometrial cancer:<ul><li>13% pelvic nodes positive in lymphadenectomy arm</li><li>No overall or relapse-free survival benefit for lymphadenectomy</li><li>Similar patterns of relapse</li></ul>
Adjuvant therapy for locally advanced disease and/or nodal metastases	
NSGO/EORTC/Iliade Hogberg et al. (2010) Eur J Cancer 46:2422–2431	Pooled phase III trials of adjuvant radiotherapy alone versus radiotherapy + four cycles of chemotherapy for endometrial cancer with high-risk features (grade 3 and/or serous cancer and/or deep invasion and/or Stage II–III)<ul><li>Significant 7% higher relapse-free and cancer-specific survival rates with RT + chemotherapy</li><li>Non-significant trend for 7% overall survival difference</li><li>Different regimens (doxorubicin + cisplatin, epirubicin + cisplatin, paclitaxel + doxorubicin + cisplatin, carboplatin + paclitaxel) and different timing: RT then chemotherapy, and chemotherapy then RT used</li></ul>
JGOG Susumu N, Sagae S et al. (2008) Gynecol Oncol 108:226–233 Italian Maggi et al. (2006) Br J Cancer 95(3):266–271	Phase III trials of adjuvant pelvic radiotherapy alone versus chemotherapy alone (three or five cycles of cyclophosphamide + doxorubicin + cisplatin alone for (high)intermediate-risk Stage I or Stage II–III endometrial cancer<ul><li>No survival difference</li></ul>
GOG-122 Randall et al. (1995) J Natl Cancer Inst Monogr 19:13–15	Phase III trial of adjuvant chemotherapy (eight cycles of doxorubicin + cisplatin) versus whole-abdominal radiotherapy for Stage III–IV endometrial cancer (residual disease up to 2 cm allowed):<ul><li>Small survival benefit for chemotherapy; significant toxicity</li><li>High relapse rates in both arms</li></ul>

Progestational agents are the standard hormonal therapy for advanced or metastatic grade 1 or 2 disease, especially for progesterone receptor-positive tumours. Reported response rates range from 15% to 34%, with a median response duration of several months. For progesterone and oestrogen receptor-positive tumours, response rates of up to 77% have been observed, in contrast to 9% for receptor-negative tumours. Progestins should be considered for relatively asymptomatic patients with unknown receptor status and grade 1 or 2 disease. Grade 3 disease is unlikely to respond to hormonal therapy (<10%). Standard doses are megestrol acetate 160 mg/day or medroxyprogesterone acetate 200 mg/day. For patients with disease progression after a response to progestins, tamoxifen or aromatase inhibitors may be considered.

Targeted therapy

Several targetable pathways have been identified in endometrial cancer and the PI3K/AKT/mTOR pathway may be the most promising. The PI3K/AKT/mTOR pathway is of special interest as it has been implicated in conferring resistance to conventional therapies. Therefore, PI3K/AKT/mTOR pathway inhibitors are currently being investigated either alone or in combination with hormonal and/or cytotoxic agents. Other targets of interest are FGFR2, MEK and VEGF. Multi-targeted growth factor tyrosine kinase inhibitors, such as brivanib and pazopanib, are also being studied.

Controversies

- Role and extent of pelvic and para-aortic lymphadenectomy, especially for high-risk disease
- Role of adjuvant brachytherapy in intermediate-risk patients
- Role of adjuvant chemotherapy
- Role of combined chemotherapy and radiotherapy versus chemotherapy alone in high-risk disease
- Frequency and extent of follow-up visits and investigations
- Role of (PET)-CT and MRI in preoperative work-up
- Optimal systemic therapy for advanced disease
- Individualized treatment of recurrent disease

Phase III clinical trials

See Table 36.3.

Areas of research

- *Adjuvant therapy*:
  - Ongoing trials:
    - Adjuvant radiotherapy with chemotherapy versus radiotherapy alone for high-risk disease (PORTEC-3)
    - Adjuvant radiotherapy with chemotherapy versus chemotherapy alone for advanced (Stage III–IV) disease (GOG-258)
    - Adjuvant pelvic radiotherapy versus chemotherapy alone (three cycles) ± brachytherapy for high–intermediate- and high-risk early-stage disease (GOG-249)
    - Adjuvant chemotherapy versus no further treatment for Stage I–II node-negative disease with high–intermediate- or high-risk factors (ENGOT-EN2-DGCG)
    - Adjuvant vaginal brachytherapy alone (two dose levels) versus observation for high–intermediate-risk disease (PORTEC-4)
    - Identification of molecular profiles for subgroups of endometrial cancer in order to tailor treatment
  - Planned trials:
    - Role of lymphadenectomy-directed adjuvant therapy versus uterine factor-based adjuvant therapy in high-risk disease, including role of sentinel node biopsy
- *Follow-up*:
  - Ongoing and planned trials:
    - TOTEM trial: extensive (CA125, CT scans, cytology) versus minimalist (history and vaginal and pelvic exam) follow-up
    - TEACUP and ENDCAT trials: telephone- versus hospital-based follow-up
- *Metastastic disease*:
  - Role of targeted therapies (especially multitarget tyrosine kinase inhibitors)

Recommended reading

Aalders J, Abeler V, Kolstad P, Onsrud M (1980) Postoperative external irradiation and prognostic parameters in stage I endometrial carcinoma: clinical and histopathologic study of 540 patients. *Obstet Gynecol* 56:419–427.

ASTEC/EN.5 Study Group, Blake P, Swart AM et al. (2009) Adjuvant external beam radiotherapy in the treatment of endometrial cancer (MRC ASTEC and NCIC CTG EN.5 randomised trials): pooled trial results, systematic review, and meta-analysis. *Lancet* 373:137–146.

ASTEC Study Group, Kitchener H, Swart AM et al. (2009) Efficacy of systematic pelvic lymphadenectomy in endometrial cancer (MRC ASTEC trial): a randomised study. *Lancet* 373:125–136.

Benedetti Panici P, Basile S et al. (2008) Systematic pelvic lymphadenectomy vs. no lymphadenectomy in early-stage endometrial carcinoma: randomized clinical trial. *J Natl Cancer Inst* 100(23):1707–1716.

Creutzberg CL, van Putten WL, Koper PC et al. (2000) Surgery and postoperative radiotherapy versus surgery alone for patients with stage-1 endometrial carcinoma: multicentre randomised trial. PORTEC Study Group. Post Operative Radiation Therapy in Endometrial Carcinoma. *Lancet* 355:1404–1411.

ESMO guideline. Available at http://www.esmo.org

Hogberg T, Signorelli M, de Oliveira CF et al. (2010) Sequential adjuvant chemotherapy and radiotherapy in endometrial cancer—results from two randomised studies. *Eur J Cancer* 46:2422–2431.

Keys HM, Roberts JA, Brunetto VL et al. (2004) A phase III trial of surgery with or without adjunctive external pelvic radiation therapy in intermediate risk endometrial adenocarcinoma: a Gynecologic Oncology Group study. *Gynecol Oncol* 92:744–751.

Kokka F, Brockbank E, Oram D, Gallagher C, Bryant A (2010) Hormonal therapy in advanced or recurrent endometrial cancer. *Cochrane Database Syst Rev* 12:CD007926.

Kong A, Johnson N, Kitchener HC, Lawrie TA (2012) Adjuvant radiotherapy for stage I endometrial cancer. *Cochrane Database Syst Rev* (3):CD003916.

Maggi R, Lissoni A, Spina F et al. (2006) Adjuvant chemotherapy vs radiotherapy in high-risk endometrial carcinoma: results of a randomised trial. *Br J Cancer* 95(3):266–271.

May K, Bryant A, Dickinson HO, Kehoe S, Morrison J (2010) Lymphadenectomy for the management of endometrial cancer. *Cochrane Database Syst Rev* (1):CD007585.

Miller D, Filiaci V et al. (2012) Randomized phase III noninferiority trial of first line chemotherapy for metastatic or recurrent endometrial carcinoma: A Gynecologic Oncology Group study. *Gynecol Oncol* 125:771–773.

NCNN guideline. Available at http://www.nccn.org

Nout RA, Smit VT, Putter H et al. (2010) Vaginal brachytherapy versus pelvic external beam radiotherapy for patients with endometrial cancer of high-intermediate risk (PORTEC-2): an open-label, non-inferiority, randomised trial. *Lancet* 375:816–823.

Randall ME, Spirtos NM, Dvoretsky P (1995). Whole abdominal radiotherapy versus combination chemotherapy with doxorubicin and cisplatin in advanced endometrial carcinoma (phase III): Gynecologic Oncology Group Study No. 122. *J Natl Cancer Inst Monogr* 19:13–15.

Susumu N, Sagae S, Udagawa Y et al. (2008). Randomized phase III trial of pelvic radiotherapy versus cisplatin-based combined chemotherapy in patients with intermediate- and high-risk endometrial cancer: a Japanese Gynecologic Oncology Group study. *Gynecol Oncol* 108:226–233.

Taylor A, Rockall AG, Powell ME (2007) An atlas of the pelvic lymph node regions to aid radiotherapy target volume definition. *Clin Oncol* 16(7):542–550.

Vale CL, Tierney J, Bull SJ, Symonds PR (2012) Chemotherapy for advanced, recurrent or metastatic endometrial carcinoma. *Cochrane Database Syst Rev* 8:CD003915.

37 Ovary and fallopian tube

Gemma Owens and Henry Kitchener

Faculty Institute for Cancer Sciences, University of Manchester, Manchester Academic Health Science Centre, St Mary's Hospital, Manchester, UK

Summary	Key facts
Introduction	**Ovarian cancer** • Global incidence of 6.3 per 100,000 women • Lifetime risk for developing ovarian cancer is estimated to be 1 in 70 • 90% of malignant ovarian tumours are epithelial **Fallopian tube cancer** • Rare malignancy that accounts for <2% of all gynaecological cancers • Mimic ovarian cancer in their histological and clinical behaviour
Presentation	**Ovarian cancer** • Non-specific symptoms and abdominal/pelvic mass • Initial work-up involves clinical assessment, serum CA125 and pelvic ultrasound • Staging CT chest, abdomen and pelvis is required prior to initiation of primary treatment **Fallopian tube cancer** • Abnormal vaginal bleeding or profuse watery vaginal discharge are the commonest symptoms • Initial work-up and staging investigations is as per ovarian cancer

Scenario	**Ovarian cancer and Fallopian tube cancer**
	• *Local/regional (Stage I/II)*:
	  ▪ Full staging surgery ± adjuvant platinum-based chemotherapy
	  ▪ Fertility-sparing surgery (oophorectomy only) may be considered in young women if confined to the ovary
	• *Metastatic (Stage III/IV)*:
	  ▪ Primary optimal debulking surgery + platinum-based chemotherapy
	  ▪ If primary debulking unlikely to be successful or the patient is not medically fit for surgery, consider primary chemotherapy and then interval-debulking surgery following three cycles:
	    ◊ Follow with a further three cycles of chemotherapy postoperatively

Trials	• Phase III trials, particularly with regards to optimizing chemotherapy have indicated that six cycles of carboplatin + paclitaxel should be standard care with debulking surgery, either initially or after three cycles of neoadjuvant chemotherapy, if optimal surgical primary debulking is considered to be unlikely

OVARIAN CANCER

Incidence, aetiology and screening

Ovarian cancer accounts for more than a third of all cancers of the female genital tract in developed countries. Cancers of the ovary can be derived from coelomic epithelium (epithelial tumours), primitive germ cells of the embryonic gonad (germ cell tumours) or gonadal/stromal tissue (sex cord stromal tumours). More than 90% of all primary ovarian cancers are epithelial ovarian cancers (EOC).

UICC Manual of Clinical Oncology, Ninth Edition. Edited by Brian O'Sullivan, James D. Brierley, Anil K. D'Cruz, Martin F. Fey, Raphael Pollock, Jan B. Vermorken and Shao Hui Huang. © 2015 UICC. Published 2015 by John Wiley & Sons, Ltd.

Incidence, aetiology and screening	Description
Incidence	- Lifetime risk for developing ovarian cancer is estimated to be 1 in 70
- Estimated to be 225,000 new cases of ovarian cancer globally in 2008, accounting for approximately 4% of all cancers diagnosed in women
- Global Incidence: age standardized ratio (ASR) per 100,000 women is 6.3:
- Incidence rates are highest in Europe and North America, and lowest in Africa
- Mortality rate: ASR per 100,000 women is 3.8
Aetiology	- Not completely understood but genetic mutations are known to be responsible, with different mutations being liable for different histotypes
- *Reproductive factors*:
- Ovarian cancer risk is reduced by factors that interrupt ovulation, e.g.:
- Pregnancy and breastfeeding:
- Risk decreases with increased parity
- Risk reduction has also been observed in women who have experienced incomplete pregnancies
- Oral contraceptive pill:
>5 years of use reduces the risk by 15–29%
- Factors that prolong exposure to ovulation such as nulliparity, infertility and early menarche and/or late menopause are associated with an increased risk of developing ovarian cancer
- *Genetic factors*:
- Family history accounts for 5–10% of ovarian cancers
- Women who have a first-degree relative diagnosed with ovarian cancer have a three- to four-fold increased risk of developing ovarian cancer compared to women with no family history
- Susceptibility increases if associated with:
- *BRCA 1* and *2* gene mutations:
- Increased risk of ovarian fallopian tube and peritoneal cancer
- 20–50% increased lifetime risk with *BRCA 1* and 10–20% increased risk with *BRCA 2*
- Typically occurs at an earlier age than sporadic cases.
- Lynch syndrome (hereditary non-polyposis colon cancer [HNPCC]):
- Increases risk of colon, endometrial and ovarian cancer
- Associated ovarian cancers are usually Stage I endometrioid or clear cell tumours
- *Related conditions*:
- Previous cancer:
- Women with a previous history of breast cancer have a two-fold risk of developing ovarian cancer
- If breast cancer was diagnosed before 40 years of age, the risk increases to four-fold
- Endometriosis:
- Women with endometriosis have been shown to have a 30–66% increased risk of ovarian cancer
Screening	- Currently no acceptable population screening test for epithelial ovarian cancer
- Two large population screening studies, PLCO Study (Prostate, Lung, Colorectal, and Ovarian Cancer Screening Trial of the US NIH) and UKCTOCS Study (United Kingdom Collaborative Trial of Ovarian Cancer Screening), have evaluated regular transvaginal ultrasound and serum CA125 testing:
- PLCO study has concluded that simultaneous screening with CA125 and transvaginal ultrasound did not reduce ovarian cancer mortality
- Data are awaited from the UKCTOCS trial to determine whether a reduction in mortality or a stage shift has been demonstrated

Presentation

- *Early disease*:
  - Usually asymptomatic, apart from abdominal distension
- *Advanced disease*:
  - Vague and non-specific; may mimic other conditions
  - Abdominal pain
  - Abdominal distension/bloating
  - Palpable abdominal mass
  - Urinary symptoms, particularly frequency or urgency
  - Nausea
  - Weight loss
  - Abnormal vaginal bleeding

Diagnostic work-up

Diagnostic work-up	Description

Work-up	• Initial investigations:
	  ▪ Clinical assessment including abdominal, vaginal ± rectal examination
	  ▪ Serum CA125
	  ▪ Abdominal and pelvic ultrasound
	  ▪ Calculate risk of malignancy index (RMI) (see Box 37.1)
	• Before surgery or chemotherapy:
	  ▪ Baseline full blood count, renal and liver function
	  ▪ Carcinoembryonic antigen (CEA)
	  ▪ Chest X-ray to detect effusions or lung metastases
	  ▪ Staging computed tomography (CT) chest, abdomen and pelvis
	  ▪ Imaging of bowel if relevant

Tumour markers	• CA125:
	  ▪ Most commonly used blood biomarker
	  ▪ Value is limited as it is 'tumour associated' rather than 'tumour specific'
	  ▪ Elevated in other benign and malignant conditions, including endometriosis, physiological cysts, adenomyosis, fibroids, ovarian hyperstimulation syndrome, pelvic abscesses, chronic diseases such as liver disease, inflammatory bowel disease and renal disease, breast cancer and gastrointestinal malignancies
	  ▪ Unreliable in premenopausal women as levels fluctuate in response to physiological changes during the menstrual cycle
	• Other markers:
	  ▪ In women under 40 years with suspected ovarian cancer, it is advisable to measure alpha-fetoprotein (AFP) and beta-human chorionic gonadotropin (β-hCG) in addition to CA125, to identify those who may have a non-epithelial ovarian cancer

Box 37.1 Risk of malignancy index

RMI is a scoring system which can be used to predict whether an ovarian mass is likely to be malignant. It takes into consideration the ultrasound findings (U), serum CA125 level and patient's menopausal status (M).

$$RMI = U \times M \times CA125$$

where U = 0 if no features present, 1 if one feature present, 3 if two to five features present, and M = 1 if premenopausal and M = 3 if postmenopausal.

Ultrasound features include multiple cysts, solid areas within the cysts, bilateral lesions and the presence of ascites and metastases.

A RMI score of ≥200 gives a sensitivity of 85% and a specificity of >95% for ovarian cancer, and warrants referral to a gynaecological oncology centre.

Pathology and natural history

Ovarian tumours are classified into three major categories according to their cell of origin (Fig. 37.1).

Epithelial ovarian cancers account for 60% of all ovarian tumours and 90% of all primary ovarian cancers are epithelial. These arise from the cells on the surface of the ovaries and are likely to also originate from the fallopian tubes. In the past decade, a number of authors have observed that 35–45% of high-grade serous carcinomas appear to arise from the fimbrial end of the fallopian tube. Epithelial ovarian cancers can be further classified as:
- Serous
- Mucinous
- Endometrioid
- Clear cell
- Transitional cell (Brenner)
- Mixed
- Undifferentiated carcinomas.

Epithelial ovarian cancers form pelvic masses that metastasize early within the peritoneal cavity, yet present late, and less often metastasize to extraperitoneal sites.

Non-epithelial ovarian cancers include germ cell tumours and sex-cord stromal tumours. *Germ cell tumours* are a heterogeneous group of several histologically distinct types, which have a variety of clinical presentations. They make up approximately 10% of all ovarian tumours. These tumours are derived from the primitive ovarian germ cells and occur mainly in young women. *Sex-cord stromal tumours* constitute approximately 7% of ovarian malignancies. There is a spectrum of phenotype from relatively benign to malignant tumours. They can occur at any age.

Epithelial tumours
Derived from coelomic epithelium
- Serous
- Mucinous
- Endometrioid
- Clear cell
- Brenner

Germ cell tumours
Derived from primitive germ cells of the embryonic gonad
- Dysgerminoma
- Endodermal sinus tumour
- Mature/immature teratoma

Sex cord stromal tumours
Gonadal/stromal origin
- Granulosa cell tumours
- Sertoli-leydig tumours

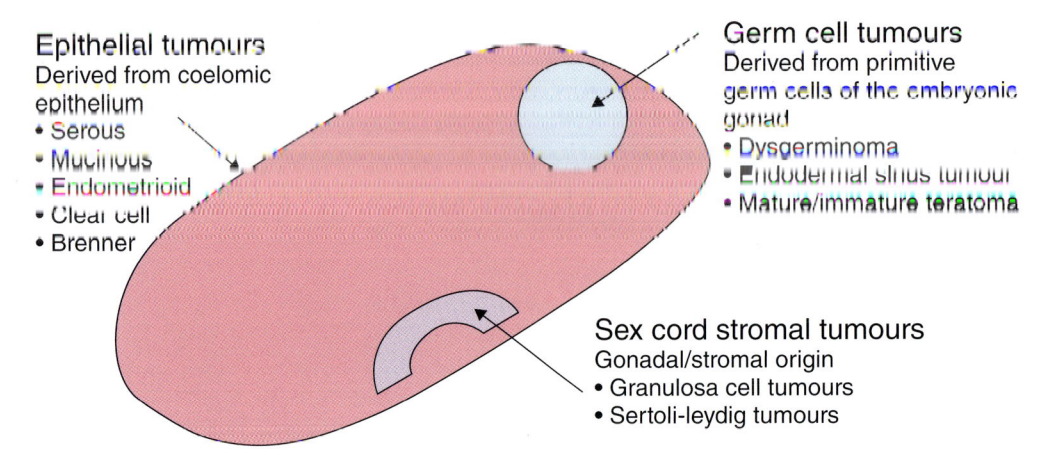

Figure 37.1 Pathological types of ovarian carcinoma.

Pathology and natural history	Description
Epithelial ovarian cancers	
Primary peritoneal tumours	• Refers to a malignancy arising in the epithelium lining the peritoneal cavity • Often clinically and histologically identical to metastatic epithelial ovarian cancer • Diagnosed when disseminated peritoneal ovarian cancer is seen in the absence of an obvious ovarian mass
Borderline tumours	• Tumours of low malignant potential with no stromal invasion • Most common in premenopausal women, between 30 and 50 years of age • 15% of all epithelial tumours of the ovary • Confined to the ovary for a long period of time • Can be associated with extraovarian disease with invasive or non-invasive peritoneal and omental implants • Invasive implants are associated with a worse prognosis • Prognosis is very good with a 10-year survival of 85–95%, but recurrences can occur up to 30 years after initial presentation, particularly in women with invasive implants
Germ cell tumours	
Dysgerminomas	• Most common type of malignant germ cell tumour (approximately 50%) • Median age at presentation is 17 years • Serum lactate dehydrogenase (LDH) has been reported to be elevated in dysgerminomas and may be a useful tumour marker • Histologically similar to seminoma of the testis • Usually presents with a pelvic mass, but endocrine and menstrual disorders may be the initial presenting features • Unilateral tumours in 85% • May metastasize early to the para-aortic nodes
Endodermal sinus tumours	• Uncommon tumours (approximately 1% of all ovarian malignancies) • Median age at presentation is 19 years • Usually unilateral solid tumours • Microscopically, the most characteristic feature is the Schiller–Duval body (a papillary structure with a central Hood vessel) • Rapidly growing • 90% of recurrences occur within the first year • AFP may be elevated and serves as a useful diagnostic biomarker and predictor of tumour recurrence

Teratomas	• *Mature cystic teratoma (dermoid cyst)*:
	  ▪ Account for 15–20% of all ovarian tumours
	  ▪ Usually benign; malignant tumour is found in <1% of cases
	  ▪ Contains elements from all germ cell layers, e.g. hair, cartilage, bone, thyroid and neural tissue

	• *Immature teratoma*:
	   ■ Malignant tumours
	   ■ Occur in children and adolescents
	   ■ Almost always unilateral
	   ■ AFP can be a useful tumour marker	

Other	• *Embryonal carcinomas and choriocarcinomas*:
	   ■ Rare tumours
	   ■ Both produce hCG and can cause precocious puberty
	• *Mixed germ cell tumours*:
	   ■ Account for approximately 8% of all malignant germ cell tumours
	   ■ Dysgerminoma is the most common constituent, often in combination with endodermal sinus tumour
	   ■ Prognosis is largely dependent on the components and the proportion of the tumour occupied by the malignant component	

Sex-cord stromal tumours		
Granulosa cell tumours	• 70% of sex-cord stromal tumours • Juvenile and adult types • Average age of presentation is 52 years • Characterized histologically by Call–Exner bodies • Secrete oestrogens; therefore can lead to precocious puberty in young girls and menorrhagia or postmenopausal bleeding in older women secondary to uterine endometrial hyperplasia • Secrete inhibin, which can be used as a tumour marker • 95% are unilateral • Low grade malignancy characterized by a long natural history with a significant capacity to recur many years after an apparent clinical cure: ■ Patients need long-term follow-up • Prognosis is generally good with an overall 5-year survival rate of 80%; recurrence is however associated with a high mortality	
Sertoli–Leydig tumours	• Rare and usually benign • Contain Sertoli cells and/or Leydig cells and originate from specialized gonadal stroma cells • Secrete androgens • May present with signs of virilization: oligomenorrhoea, breast atrophy, acne, hirsuitism, clitoromegaly and male pattern balding • Treatment includes surgery, chemotherapy and rarely, radiotherapy	
Metastatic ovarian cancer		
Secondary ovarian tumours	• 10% of ovarian tumours are secondary • Commonly originate from the gastrointestinal tract ('Krukenberg tumour'), endometrium and breast	Local

Route of spread	• Direct spread to the uterus and fallopian tubes
	• Via the peritoneum to pelvic/abdominal organs and the omentum
	• Lymphatic drainage via:
	   ■ Utero-ovarian, infundibulopelvic and round ligament pathways
	   ■ External iliac accessory pathway into the external iliac, common iliac, hypogastric, lateral sacral, para-aortic and, occasionally, the inguinal lymph nodes
	• Haematogenous spread to the liver, lungs and other organs
	• Extraperitoneal and extrapleural sites are uncommon
		Regional
		
		Metastatic

Staging and prognostic grouping

FIGO classification
The international staging rules are based on the International Federation of Gynecology and Obstetrics (FIGO) classification (Table 37.1). FIGO stage is based on findings from surgical exploration.

UICC TNM staging
See Table 37.2.

Prognostic factors
Multiple factors, including age, grade, FIGO stage, presence of residual disease, CA125, performance status, presence or absence of ascites and histological subtype, have all been

Table 37.1 FIGO staging classification for ovarian, fallopian tube and peritoneal cancer

I	Tumour confined to ovaries or fallopian tube(s)
IA	Tumour limited to one ovary (capsule intact) or fallopian tube; no tumour on ovarian or fallopian tube surface; no malignant cells in the ascites or peritoneal washings
IB	Tumour limited to both ovaries (capsules intact) or fallopian tubes; no tumour on ovarian or fallopian tube surface; no malignant cells in the ascites or peritoneal washings
IC	Tumour limited to one or both ovaries or fallopian tubes, with any of the following: IC1: Surgical spill intraoperatively IC2: Capsule ruptured before surgery or tumour on ovarian or fallopian tube surface IC3: Malignant cells present in the ascites or peritoneal washings
II	Tumour involving one or both ovaries or fallopian tubes with pelvic extension (below pelvic brim) or peritoneal cancer
IIA	Extension and/or implants on the uterus and/or fallopian tubes and/or ovaries
IIB	Extension to other pelvic intraperitoneal tissues
III	Tumour involving one or both ovaries, or fallopian tubes, or primary peritoneal cancer, with histologically or cytologically confirmed peritoneal implants outside the pelvis and/or metastasis to the retroperitoneal lymph nodes
IIIA	Metastasis to the retroperitoneal lymph nodes with or without microscopic peritoneal involvement beyond the pelvis
IIIA(i)	Positive retroperitoneal lymph nodes only (cytologically or histologically proven)
IIIA(ii)	Metastasis >10 mm in greatest dimension
IIIA2	Microscopic extrapelvic (above the pelvic brim) peritoneal involvement with or without positive retroperitoneal lymph nodes
IIIB	Macroscopic peritoneal metastases beyond the pelvic brim <2 cm in greatest dimension, with or without positive retroperitoneal lymph nodes.
IIIC	Macroscopic peritoneal metastases beyond the pelvic brim >2 cm in greatest dimension, with or without positive retroperitoneal lymph nodes
IV	Distant metastases excluding peritoneal metastases
IVA	Pleural effusion with positive cytology
IVB	Metastases to extra-abdominal organs (including inguinal lymph nodes and lymph nodes outside of the abdominal cavity

Source: Mutch, Prat (2014), reproduced with permission of Elsevier.

Table 37.2 UICC TNM categories, with FIGO equivalent, and stage grouping: Ovary

TNM categories		
TNM	Ovary	FIGO
T1	Limited to the ovaries	I
T1a	One ovary, capsule intact	IA
T1b	Both ovaries, capsule intact	IB
T1c	Capsule ruptured, tumour on surface, malignant cells in ascites or peritoneal washings	IC
T2	Pelvic extension	II
T2a	Uterus, tube(s)	IIA
T2b	Other pelvic tissues	IIB
T2c	Malignant cells in ascites or peritoneal washings	IIC
T3 and/or N1	Peritoneal metastasis beyond pelvis and/or regional lymph node metastasis	III
T3a	Microscopic peritoneal metastasis	IIIA
T3b	Macroscopic peritoneal metastasis ≤2 cm	IIIB
T3c and/or N1	Peritoneal metastasis >2 cm regional lymph node metastasis	IIIC
M1	Distant metastasis (excludes peritoneal metastasis)	IV

Stage grouping			
Stage IA	T1a	N0	M0
Stage IB	T1b	N0	M0
Stage IC	T1c	N0	M0
Stage IIA	T2a	N0	M0
Stage IIB	T2b	N0	M0
Stage IIC	T2c	N0	M0
Stage IIIA	T3a	N0	M0
Stage IIIB	T3b	N0	M0
Stage IIIC	T3c	N0	M0
	Any T	N1	M0
Stage IV	Any T	Any N	M1

reported as prognostic factors for women with ovarian cancer (Table 37.3). Advanced disease at diagnosis, macroscopic residual disease (>2 cm) following cytoreductive surgery and platinum-resistant ovarian tumours have the worst prognosis.

Table 37.3 Prognostic risk factor for epithelial ovarian cancer

Prognostic factors	Tumour related	Host related	Environment related
Essential	Histological type Grade Surgical stage Residual disease	Age Co-morbidities Performance status	Maximum diameter of residual disease after optimal debulking
Additional	Nodal involvement Site of metastasis DNA ploidy CA125	BRCA 1 Genetic predisposition	Type of chemotherapy CA125 fall Ultra-radical surgery
New and promising	Molecular profile Cellular proliferative activity Tumour angiogenesis markers p53 expression Expression of human kallikrein (hK) genes, particularly hKs 6-10-11		Interval debulking surgery (IDS) Neoadjuvant chemotherapy

Data from NCCN, ESMO, NICE, ASCO+I40.

Improved prognosis is associated with the following factors:
- Early stage at diagnosis
- Small tumour volume before surgery
- No residual disease following surgery
- Low-grade, well-differentiated tumours
- Absence of ascites
- Good American Society of Anesthesiologists (ASA) performance status
- Serous or endometrioid tumours
- Platinum sensitivity.

Estimated 5-year survival rates for patients by FIGO stage are:
- Stage I: 80–90%
- Stage II: 60–75%
- Stage IIIA: 35–60%
- Stage IIIC: 20–25%
- Stage IV: <15%.

Treatment philosophy: Epithelial ovarian cancer

The goals of surgery for ovarian cancer are to remove all tumour tissue and to accurately stage the cancer. Primary surgery for ovarian cancer involves a total abdominal hysterectomy with bilateral salpingo-oophorectomy, omentectomy, peritoneal washings and peritoneal biopsies. Optimal debulking is sometimes not possible and bulk residual tumour deposits (>2 cm) are associated with a poorer prognosis. Patients with advanced disease should undergo aggressive primary cytoreductive surgery unless successful debulking is unlikely, in which case primary chemotherapy with interval-debulking surgery may be more appropriate. Primary surgery is always followed by chemotherapy unless the disease is well-differentiated Stage IA or IB.

Variant epithelial ovarian cancer	Treatment philosophy
Primary peritoneal tumour	• Treatment involves primary platinum-based chemotherapy • Role of surgery has not been proven; however, in daily practice treated as ovarian carcinoma
Borderline tumour	• No evidence to support initial adjuvant chemotherapy; however, if recurrence occurs, chemotherapy should be offered
Local and regional disease	• Full staging surgery ± adjuvant chemotherapy: ▪ In women of reproductive years with well-differentiated disease confined to one ovary, fertility-sparing surgery can be considered after appropriate counselling • Optimal tumour debulking to no residual disease
Metastatic disease	• Primary optimal debulking surgery + chemotherapy • If patient is unsuitable for primary debulking surgery, primary chemotherapy and interval-debulking surgery following the third cycle can be offered, followed by three further cycles of chemotherapy
Recurrent disease	• Options include second-line chemotherapy, surgery, novel agents, clinical trials and palliation • If relapse occurs >6 months following completion of platinum-based chemotherapy, then retreat with platinum-based chemotherapy • If platinum-resistant, various cytotoxic and non-cytotoxic agents can be used, preferably in trials • Often regarded as palliation as prognosis is poor despite further treatment

(continued)

Scenario: Epithelial ovarian cancer	Treatment philosophy

Follow-up	• Aims to identify disease recurrence, and provide psychological support and reassurance
	• Follow up for a minimum of 5 years following treatment
	• Visits should be every 3–6 months in Years 1 and 2, then 6–12 monthly in Years 3–5
	• At each review, patients should be asked about symptoms and a pelvic examination undertaken:
	   ▪ Gynecologic Cancer InterGroup trial OVO5/EORTC 55955 suggested that routine CA125 monitoring had no impact on survival
	   ▪ However, CA125 monitoring can be part of specific research projects and should be measured also if there is suspicion of relapse or at the patient's request

Treatment: Epithelial ovarian cancer

Surgery

Surgical management of ovarian cancer can be divided into:
- Primary cytoreduction or debulking surgery
- Interval and secondary cytoreduction
- Palliative and salvage surgery.

Surgery: Epithelial ovarian cancer	Description

Staging laparotomy and cytoreduction	• Standard primary management.
	• Aims to:
	  ▪ Establish the diagnosis
	  ▪ Enable accurate staging
	  ▪ Undertake maximal debulking
	• Procedure should involve:
	  ▪ Vertical midline incision
	  ▪ Retrieval of peritoneal fluid or washings for cytology
	  ▪ Careful inspection and palpation of all peritoneal surfaces to determine the extent of any macroscopic disease
	  ▪ Infracolic omentectomy
	  ▪ Biopsy or resection of any suspicious lesions or adhesions
	  ▪ Biopsy of the pelvic and abdominal peritoneum
	  ▪ Oophorectomy or abdominal hysterectomy and bilateral salpingo-oopherectomy (depending on stage; see below)
	  ▪ Retroperitoneal lymph node assessment by palpation of the pelvic and para-aortic nodes, and sampling of any enlarged lymph nodes or random sampling if no lymph nodes are enlarged
	• *Early disease*:
	  ▪ Standard management involves staging surgery as outlined above
	  ▪ If the tumour appears to be confined to one ovary and the women wishes to preserve fertility, unilateral oophorectomy can be considered:
	    ○ Risk of recurrence in the remaining ovary needs to be discussed with the woman
	  ▪ Assessment and sampling of lymph nodes should be considered in order to ensure optimal staging
	  ▪ Overall relapse rate of 11% has been quoted in the literature, but this is less likely in fully-staged women
	• *Advanced disease*:
	  ▪ *Primary cytoreductive surgery*:
	    ○ Total abdominal hysterectomy, bilateral salpingo-oophorectomy, infracolic omentectomy and tumour debulking should be performed at laparotomy
	    ○ Aim to leave no residual disease at the time of closing the abdomen
	    ○ Supracolic omentectomy should be performed even if there is no obvious tumour on the omentum
	    ○ May require bowel resection to achieve complete debulking
	    ○ Routine pelvic and para-aortic lymphadenectomy may not improve outcome:
	      – However, enlarged lymph nodes should be removed as part of the cytoreductive procedure
	  ▪ *Interval debulking surgery*:
	    ○ In selected patients who may not be good candidates for initial surgery, three to four cycles of neoadjuvant chemotherapy may be given initially, followed by interval debulking surgery and further chemotherapy

Surgery: Epithelial ovarian cancer	Description
	○ Histological confirmation of diagnosis is required prior to commencing neoadjuvant chemotherapy, usually by ultrasound-guided biopsy ○ Indications include: – Unfit for surgery due to significant co-morbidities, poor performance status and presence of large pleural effusions or gross ascites – Fixed bulky disease outside of the abdomen – Extensive mesenteric involvement – Coeliac axis disease – Optimal debulking at laparotomy appears unlikely
Second-look laparotomy or laparoscopy	• Refers to an operation undertaken after completion of chemotherapy to assess response to chemotherapy • No longer recommended in the routine management of women with ovarian cancer as no survival benefit has been shown
Prophylactic surgery	• Prophylactic risk-reducing surgery is recommended for *BRCA 1* and *2* carriers once their family is complete • Usually involves laparoscopic bilateral salpingo-oophorectomy • *HNPCC* carriers can also be considered for hysterectomy in addition to bilateral salpingo-oophorectomy in view of the risk of developing endometrial cancer • Does not completely eliminate the risk of developing cancer as there is a small risk of developing primary peritoneal cancer in the absence of the ovaries

Systemic therapy

Prior to commencing chemotherapy, baseline investigations should be conducted, including a full blood count, urea and electrolytes, liver function tests, CA125, chest X-ray and CT of the abdomen and pelvis.

Systemic therapy: Epithelial ovarian cancer	Description
Adjuvant chemotherapy	
Low-risk disease (Stage IA or IB grade 1)	• Does not require chemotherapy following surgery
High-risk disease (Stage IC or grade 2 or 3, and Stages II–IV)	• Chemotherapy should be offered following surgery, in the form of six cycles of carboplatin + paclitaxel • Should be started no later than 8 weeks after primary surgery • Docetaxel can be used in place of paclitaxel if drug hypersensitivity occurs or pre-existing neuropathy • Women who have had suboptimal surgery for apparent Stage I disease: ▪ Reviewed by a medical oncologist to discuss the risks and benefits of adjuvant chemotherapy, or ▪ Consider for reoperation by a well-trained gynaecological oncologist
Neoadjuvant chemotherapy (induction chemotherapy)	
	• Refers to chemotherapy given prior to interval debulking surgery (see above) • Three cycles of neoadjuvant chemotherapy, followed by radiological assessment of response to chemotherapy ▪ If there is evidence of a response to chemotherapy (objective tumour reduction or stable disease with CA125 response), interval debulking surgery should proceed, followed by a further three cycles of chemotherapy ▪ If there has been no response to chemotherapy, different chemotherapy should be administered • Histological confirmation of diagnosis is required prior to commencing neoadjuvant treatment
Other treatment modalities	
	• Bevacizumab (Avastin), a vascular endothelial growth factor (VEGF) antagonist has been shown to improve progression-free survival in combination with carboplatin and paclitaxel in recent phase III clinical trials (ICON7 and GOG218)

Table 37.4 Common chemotherapy regimens

Drugs	Dose and route	Cycle
Intravenous		
Paclitaxel + carboplatin*	175 mg/m² IV over 3 hours 80 mg/m² IV over 3 hours	Every 3 weeks × 6 Days 1, 8 and 15
Paclitaxel + cisplatin	135 mg/m² IV infusion over 24 hours 75 mg/m² IV	Every 3 weeks × 6
Intraperitoneal		
Paclitaxel + Cisplatin + Paclitaxel	135 mg/m² as a 24-hour infusion IV 75–100 mg/m² IP 60 mg/m² IP	Day 1 every 3 weeks × 6 Day 2 Day 8
Alternative drugs		
Docetaxel (IV)	75 mg/m²	Every 3 weeks

*Single-agent carboplatin can be an option for very selective patients.
Source: Berek et al. (2012), with permission of Elsevier.

Common chemotherapy regimens are given in Table 37.4.

The use of combined paclitaxel + carboplatin as primary chemotherapy for advanced ovarian cancer is based on the findings of the GOGIII/OV10 and AGO#/GOG158 trials. While it might be argued that single-agent carboplatin is safer and better-tolerated, that is an over-simplification, as the platelet-sparing effect of paclitaxel can facilitate cumulative dosing with carboplatin.

Intraperitoneal chemotherapy has been shown to improve survival in patients with optimally debulked advanced disease compared to intravenous chemotherapy in several studies. Despite this consistent finding, intraperitoneal chemotherapy is still not widely accepted due to the additional adverse effects and the logistic implications.

Evaluating chemotherapy response

- Serum CA125 should be measured at regular intervals during chemotherapy as the CA125 level correlates with objective tumour response
- CT scans should be repeated after six cycles of chemotherapy unless there is clinical evidence of progressive disease, such as rising or static CA125 levels or persistent ascites, in which case the repeat CT scan should be performed earlier
- In women whose CA125 levels are normal at baseline, a CT scan should be performed after three cycles of chemotherapy to assess response to treatment

Treatment philosophy: Non-epithelial ovarian cancers

Scenario: Non-epithelial ovarian cancers	Treatment philosophy

Germ cell tumours	• Very responsive to platinum-based chemotherapy (recommended regimens are given in Table 37.5)
	• Dysgerminomas are also radiosensitive (with a 5-year survival rate of >90%)
	• Surgery is generally conservative, i.e. laparotomy, with careful evaluation of extent of disease, biopsies of all suspicious areas and limited cytoreduction:
	  ▪ Particularly important in women for whom fertility preservation matters
	• *Endodermal sinus tumours*:
	  ▪ Prognosis has improved with the use of multiple chemotherapeutic agents
	• *Immature teratomas*:
	  ▪ Standard treatment involves surgery and chemotherapy

Sex-cord stromal tumours	• Metastatic, cytoreductive surgery is the mainstay of treatment:
	  ▪ If patient is young and disease is confined to one ovary, conservative surgery should be performed
	• Platinum-based chemotherapy (as per epithelial ovarian cancer) is advised for patients with advanced or recurrent disease
	• No evidence to support adjuvant chemotherapy in patients with Stage I disease:
	  ▪ Adjuvant therapy is required if the disease is beyond stage IB or if poorly differentiated

Table 37.5 Recommended chemotherapy regimens for germ cell tumours

Chemotherapy	Dose and route	Cycle
Intravenous		
Etoposide +	100 mg/m^2/day IV for 5 days	Every 3 weeks × 3
Cisplatin ±	20 mg/m^2/day IV for 5 days	Every 3 weeks × 3
Bleomycin	30,000 IU IV/IM on Days 1, 8 and 15	For 12 weeks

Source: Berek et al. (2012), with permission of Elsevier.

Treatment: Recurrent disease

Many women with advanced disease will unfortunately relapse following initial treatment. Recurrent disease can be very difficult to treat due to acquired resistance to platinum-based chemotherapy; hence, the mainstay of treatment for relapsed disease with platinum-resistant tumours is palliation, although other experimental regimens can be used.

Treatment: Recurrent disease	Description
Chemotherapy	• Choice of second-line chemotherapy is determined by the level of platinum sensitivity • If relapse occurs >6 months following initial chemotherapy, platinum-based combination chemotherapy should be offered (i.e. carboplatin + pegylated liposomal doxorubicin [PLD], carboplatin + paclitaxel or carboplatin + gemcitabine) • If relapse occurs within 6 months of initial chemotherapy, chemotherapy with PLD, gemcitabine, weekly paclitaxel or topotecan can be offered; however, the prognosis is poor

Secondary cytoreductive surgery	• No randomized controlled trials to evaluate this
	• Aggressive surgical debulking is recommended for the following patients:
	   ▪ Good prospects for complete excision
	   ▪ Good performance status
	   ▪ Solitary or limited number of sites of recurrence
	   ▪ No ascites
	   ▪ Prolonged disease-free survival (>12 months)
	• A large retrospective study of surgery in women with recurrent disease found that complete resection was associated with a significantly longer survival than those with macroscopic residual disease
	• A phase III trial to evaluate the exact role of surgery in recurrent disease is ongoing

Radiotherapy	• Can sometimes be offered for palliation, e.g. to reduce pain caused by lymphadenopathy or metastatic bone disease
Novel agents	• Antiangiogenic drugs, e.g. bevacizumab • Poly(ADP-ribose) polymerase (PARP) inhibitors
Other options	• Hormonal treatments, e.g. tamoxifen, aromatase inhibitors and gonadotropin-releasing hormone analogues • Recruitment to clinical trials • Palliative care

Phase III clinical trials

See Table 37.6.

Table 37.6 Phase III clinical trials

Trial name	Summary
Early-stage disease	

ACTION and ICON-1	• Two largest randomized clinical trials on early ovarian cancer conducted to determine whether adjuvant platinum-based chemotherapy would improve overall survival (OS) and recurrence-free survival in women with early-stage ovarian cancer:
	  ▪ 'Adjuvant Chemo Therapy in Ovarian Neoplasm' trial (ACTION; n=448)
	  ▪ International Collaboration in Ovarian Neoplasm trial (ICON-1; n = 477)
	• Combined analysis showed a statistically significant improvement in overall and recurrence-free survival at 5 years (82% vs 74% and 76% vs 65%, respectively)
	• In a separate analysis of the ACTION trial, however, it became clear that adjuvant chemotherapy only improved OS and disease-free survival (DFS) significantly in inadequately staged patients, underlining the importance of the completeness of surgical staging

Advanced disease and metastatic disease	
GOG111 and GOG158	• Established the use of carboplatin + paclitaxel as the standard chemotherapy regimen for women with advanced ovarian cancer • GOG111 showed an improvement in PFS and OS in women with Stage III/IV disease who received cisplatin + paclitaxel compared to women who received cisplatin + cyclophosphamide • GOG158 then compared cisplatin (75 mg/m^2) + paclitaxel (135 mg/m^2 over 24 hours) to an outpatient regimen of carboplatin (AUC = 7.5) + paclitaxel 175 mg/m^2 over 3 hours: ▪ Although there was no difference in PFS or OS between the regimens, the latter regimen was associated with reduced toxicity and easier administration

ICON-7 and GOG182	• Two randomized phase III trials aimed at showing a PFS benefit of bevacizumab (a VEGF inhibitor) combined with first-line paclitaxel + carboplatin, followed by maintenance bevacizumab in women with ovarian cancer:
	  ▪ Different dosages of bevacizumab were used in these trials: 7.5 mg/kg body weight in ICON-7 and 15 mg/kg body weight in GOG-182
	• Bevacizumab increased PFS to 2 and 4 months, respectively, as compared to standard treatment alone:
	  ▪ ICON-7 showed that the benefit was greatest among patients at high risk for progression, with PFS of 14.5 months with standard therapy alone and 18.1 months with standard therapy + bevacizumab

JGOG3016	• Compared a conventional regimen of paclitaxel + carboplatin given every 3 weeks with a dose-dense weekly paclitaxel regimen in women with advanced (Stage II–IV) epithelial ovarian cancer • Median PFS was significantly longer in the dose-dense paclitaxel treatment group compared with the conventional treatment group (28 months vs 17.2 months) • OS at 3 years was higher in the dose-dense treatment arm compared with the conventional treatment arm (72.1% vs 65.1%)
GOG172	• Compared conventional adjuvant treatment with intravenous paclitaxel and cisplatin against intravenous paclitaxel + intraperitoneal cisplatin and placlitaxel in patients with Stage III ovarian cancer • Intraperitoneal regimen was associated with an improved PFS (18.3 vs 23.8 months) and OS (49.7 vs 65.6 months)
EORTC 55971	• Women with bulky Stage IIIC or IV ovarian cancer were randomized to receive either primary debulking surgery followed by platinum-based chemotherapy or neoadjuvant chemotherapy followed by interval debulking surgery and further chemotherapy • Neoadjuvant chemotherapy followed by interval debulking surgery was not inferior to primary debulking surgery followed by chemotherapy for women with far-advanced Stage IIIC and IV ovarian cancer
Recurrent disease	
ICON-4/AGO-OVAR-2.2	• International, multicentre, randomized trials between 1996 and 2002, which recruited 802 patients with platinum-sensitive ovarian cancer who relapsed >6 months following treatment • Investigated paclitaxel + platinum chemotherapy against conventional platinum-based chemotherapy as a second-line treatment (first-line at relapse) • Paclitaxel + platinum chemotherapy improved survival and PFS among patients with relapsed platinum-sensitive ovarian cancer compared with conventional platinum-based chemotherapy: ▪ Absolute difference in 2-year survival of 7% and 1-year PFS of 10% between the paclitaxel and conventional treatment groups

Areas of research

- *Current trials*:
  - AGO-OVAR OP4 ('Desktop'): randomized controlled trial comparing the efficacy of cytoreductive surgery followed by chemotherapy versus chemotherapy alone for recurrent platinum-sensitive ovarian cancer
  - ICON-8: randomized three-arm phase III trial designed to evaluate the safety and efficacy of dose-dense, dose-fractionated carboplatin and paclitaxel chemotherapy in the treatment of patients with ovarian cancer
  - GOF0212: randomized three-arm trial comparing the effectiveness of paclitaxel, polyglutamate paclitaxel and observation only in managing patients with Stage III or IV ovarian cancer
  - ICON-6: three-arm, double-blind placebo-controlled randomized trial designed to assess the safety and efficacy of cediranib (an inhibitor of VEGFR-1, -2 and -3) in combination with platinum-based chemotherapy in patients with relapsed ovarian, fallopian tube or epithelial cancer:
    - Patients were randomized in a 2:3:3 ratio to receive six or fewer cycles of platinum based chemotherapy with either (1) placebo, (2) cediranib 20 mg/day during chemotherapy followed by placebo for up to 18 months (concurrent), or (3) cediranib 20 mg/day followed by maintenance cediranib (concurrent + maintenance)
    - This trial has now closed but results have yet to be reported
- Other areas of research:
  - Identification of genetic and molecular pathways of pathogenesis
  - Identification of molecular markers of prognosis
  - Use of targeted agents, particularly poly(ADP-ribose) polymerase (PARP) inhibitors
  - Molecular profiling and risk prediction studies

CANCER OF THE FALLOPIAN TUBE

Introduction

Primary fallopian tube cancer is a rare and aggressive gynaecological malignancy that accounts for <2% of cancers of the reproductive tract. The most common age of onset is between 40 and 65 years. The true incidence of fallopian tube cancer is likely to have been underestimated as it is often misdiagnosed as ovarian cancer. Cancers of the fallopian tube mimic ovarian cancer in their histological and clinical behaviour. Overall 5-year survival rates for women with primary fallopian tube cancer are estimated to be 33–40%. Surgical treatment and chemotherapy regimens are similar to those used for epithelial ovarian cancer, but the prognosis remains worse than for other gynaecological cancers.

Incidence, aetiology and screening

Incidence, aetiology and screening	Description

Incidence	- Rare malignancy: 0.1–1.8% of all gynaecological cancers
	- Mean age at diagnosis is 55 years
	- Mean incidence is 3.6 per million women per annum.
	  - Higher incidence in Caucasian women
	  - Bilateral disease is rare and represents <25% of cases

Aetiology	- Thought to be similar to that of ovarian cancer
	- *Reproductive factors*:
	  - Use of the oral contraceptive pill and multiparity may significantly reduce the risk of fallopian tube cancer
	  - No consistent correlation has been established between cancer of the fallopian tube and age, ethnicity, pelvic inflammatory disease, infertility or endometriosis
	- *Genetic factors*:
	  - Evidence suggests that *BRCA 1* and *2* carriers have a greater lifetime risk of tubal cancer than the general population
	- Low- and high-grade serous carcinomas of the pelvis that were originally thought to arise from the ovary may originate from the fimbrial (distal) end of the fallopian tube

Screening	- Fallopian tube cancer is a rare disease and cannot be screened for

Pathology and natural history

Primary fallopian tube carcinoma is usually diagnosed by histopathological examination. The histological subtypes are:
- Serous
- Endometrioid (predominant type; >90% of fallopian tube cancers are papillary serous adenocarcinomas)
- Mixed
- Undifferentiated
- Transitional
- Mucinous
- Clear cell.

Pathological diagnosis can be difficult due to the close proximity of the fallopian tubes to the ovaries and uterus.

Ovarian, endometrial, breast and gastrointestinal primaries frequently metastasize to the fallopian tubes. Primary fallopian tube cancer spreads by transluminal migration, haematogenous dissemination, lymphatic and transcoelomic spread. The median part of the fallopian tube drains via the para-aortic lymph nodes, while the distal part of the tube drains into the pelvic nodes.

Presentation

- Abnormal vaginal bleeding or profuse watery vaginal discharge are the commonest symptoms
- May present with abdominal distension, pressure or vague history of lower abdominal pain
- 'Laztko's triad of symptoms' has been reported in approximately 15% of patients: intermittent profuse vaginal discharge, colicky pain relieved by discharge and an abdominal or pelvic mass
- Clinical examination may reveal an adnexal mass in 60% of cases

Diagnostic work up

Correct preoperative diagnosis is made in only 0.3% of cases as cancer of the fallopian tubes is not routinely suspected.

Diagnostic work-up	Description

Work-up	• Ultrasound may identify an adnexal mass:
	  ▪ Cancer of the fallopian tube should be considered if an unexplained solid adnexal mass is seen in association with normal ovaries
	  ▪ Ultrasound features include a sausage-shaped cystic mass or a multilocular mass with a cogwheel appearance in the adnexa, and areas of neovascularization within the fallopian tube when using colour Doppler
	• CT or magnetic resonance imaging (MRI) can help characterize adnexal masses further and distinguish them from ovarian masses
	• Tubal cancers may be diagnosed incidentally from a routine cervical smear if abnormal glandular cells are identified in the absence of an endometrial or cervical primary

Tumour markers	• Serum CA125 is raised in a significant percentage of cases

Table 37.7 UICC TNM categories, with FIGO equivalent, and stage grouping: Fallopian tube cancer

TNM categories		
TNM	Fallopian tube	FIGO
Tis	Carcinoma *in situ*	
T1	Limited to tube(s)	I
T1a	One tube; serosa intact	IA
T1b	Both tubes; serosa intact	IB
T1c	Serosa involved; malignant cells in ascites or peritoneal washings	IC
T2	Pelvic extension	II
T2a	Uterus and/or ovaries	IIA
T2b	Other pelvic structures	IIB
T2c	Malignant cells in ascites or peritoneal washings	IIC
T3 and/or N1	Peritoneal metastasis outside the pelvis and/or regional lymph node metastasis	III
T3a	Microscopic peritoneal metastasis	IIIA
T3b	Macroscopic peritoneal metastasis ≤2 cm	IIIB
T3c and/or N1	Peritoneal metastasis >2 cm and/or regional lymph node metastasis	IIIC
M1	Distant metastasis (excludes peritoneal metastasis)	IV

Staging and prognostic risk grouping

FIGO classification

The FIGO staging criteria is the most commonly used staging system (as for staging of the ovary; see Table 37.1). More than 50% of patients present with Stage I or II disease, 40% with Stage III disease and 10% with Stage IV disease. Primary fallopian tube cancer is often diagnosed at an earlier stage compared with ovarian cancer.

UICC TNM staging

See Table 37.7.

Stage grouping			
Stage 0	Tis	N0	M0
Stage IA	T1a	N0	M0
Stage IB	T1b	N0	M0
Stage IC	T1c	N0	M0
Stage IIA	T2a	N0	M0
Stage IIB	T2b	N0	M0
Stage IIC	T2c	N0	M0
Stage IIIA	T3a	N0	M0
Stage IIIB	T3b	N0	M0
Stage IIIC	T3c	N0	M0
	Any T	N1	M0
Stage IV	Any T	Any N	M1

Table 37.8 Prognostic factors for cancer of the fallopian tube

Prognostic factors	Tumour related	Host related	Environment related
Essential	Histological type Stage Residual disease	Age Co-morbidities Performance status	Maximum diameter of residual disease after optimal debulking
Additional	Grade Lymph node status Presence of ostial closure Fimbrial lesion DNA ploidy		Type of chemotherapy
New and promising	HER2/neu expression	p53 expression	

Prognostic factors

Prognostic factors for women with primary fallopian tube cancer are shown in Table 37.8.

Treatment philosophy

Full staging surgery, i.e. total abdominal hysterectomy with bilateral salpingo-oophorectomy, infracolic omentectomy, peritoneal washings and peritoneal biopsies is the primary treatment of choice for primary fallopian tube cancer. Patients with advanced disease should undergo aggressive primary cytoreductive surgery unless the patient and multidisciplinary team decide that primary chemotherapy with interval debulking surgery would be more appropriate.

Scenario	Treatment philosophy
Local and regional disease	• Full staging surgery ± adjuvant chemotherapy • Fertility-sparing surgery can be considered after appropriate counselling in women of reproductive years with well differentiated disease confined to one fallopian tube
Metastatic disease	• Primary optimal debulking surgery + chemotherapy • If patient is unsuitable for primary debulking surgery, primary chemotherapy and interval-debulking surgery following the third cycle can be offered, if appropriate
Recurrent disease	• Very poor prognosis • Further surgical treatment may be considered • No effective second-line or salvage chemotherapy is currently available: ▪ In daily practice, as for ovarian carcinoma
Follow-up	• As per ovarian cancer

Treatment

Surgery

Surgery	Description

Early disease	• Should involve full staging surgery:
	  ▪ A midline laparotomy
	  ▪ Peritoneal washings
	  ▪ Careful evaluation of the peritoneal cavity to determine extent of disease
	  ▪ Total abdominal hysterectomy and bilateral salpingo-oophorectomy
	  ▪ Infracolic omentectomy
	  ▪ Palpation of the pelvic and para-aortic nodes, and sampling of any enlarged lymph nodes or random sampling if no lymph nodes are enlarged
	• Alternatively, a unilateral salpingo-oophorectomy may be considered if isolated to the fallopian tube and patient wishes to conserve fertility

Advanced disease	• Standard management for advanced disease involves optimal debulking surgery/primary cytoreductive surgery with the aim of minimal residual disease at closure of the abdomen: • If optimal debulking is unlikely to be achieved, interval-debulking surgery is preferable (i.e. surgery attempted after three to four cycles of chemotherapy)

Radiotherapy

Radiotherapy was previously used as adjuvant therapy for tubal cancer; however, it has become redundant because of its high rate of complications and poor efficacy when compared with chemotherapy. However, patients with serosal involvement with patent ostia and no overt residual disease or positive peritoneal cytology with no gross residual disease could be considered for adjuvant radiotherapy if chemotherapy is contraindicated or declined.

Systemic therapy

Systemic therapy	Description
Early disease	• All women should be considered for platinum-based chemotherapy ± paclitaxel, with the exception of women where histology confirms a Stage IA or IB adenocarcinoma
Advanced disease	• All women undergoing primary cytoreductive surgery should be offered adjuvant platinum/paclitaxel-based chemotherapy • Primary chemotherapy is an alternative if primary surgery is not appropriate ▪ Following the third cycle of chemotherapy, the patient should be re-evaluated and subsequently considered for interval debulking surgery, if possible

Recommended reading

Alberta Health Services (2013) Epithelial ovarian, fallopian tube, and primary peritoneal cancer (Clinical Practice Guideline Gyne-005). Available from http://www.albertahealthservices.ca/hp/if-hp-cancer-guide-gync005-epithelialovarian.pdf

Armstrong DK, Bundy B, Wenzel L et al. (2006). Intraperitoneal cisplatin and paclitaxel in ovarian cancer. N Engl J Med 354(1):34–43.

Berek JS, Crum C, Friedlander M (2012) FIGO Cancer Report 2012 – Cancer of the ovary, fallopian tube, and peritoneum. Int J Gynecol Obstet 119(Suppl 2):S118–S129.

Burger RA, Brady MF, Bookman MA et al. (2011) Incorporation of bevacizumab in the primary treatment of ovarian cancer. N Engl J Med 365:2473–2483.

Colombo N, Peiretti M, Parma G et al. (2010) Newly diagnosed and relapsed epithelial ovarian carcinoma: ESMO Clinical Practice Guidelines for diagnosis, treatment and follow-up. Ann Oncol 21(Suppl 5):v23–v30.

Elattar A, Bryant A, Winter-Roach BA, Hatem M, Naik R (2011) Optimal primary surgical treatment for advanced epithelial ovarian cancer. Cochrane Database Syst Rev (8):CD007565.

Galaal K, Naik R, Bristow RE, Patel A, Bryant A, Dickinson HO (2010) Cytoreductive surgery plus chemotherapy versus chemotherapy alone for recurrent epithelial ovarian cancer. Cochrane Database Syst Rev (6):CD007822.

Hennessy BT, Coleman RL, Markman M (2009) Ovarian cancer. Lancet 374:1371–1382.

Jaaback K, Johnson N, Lawrie TA (2011) Intraperitoneal chemotherapy for the initial management of primary epithelial ovarian cancer. Cochrane Database Syst Rev (11):CD005340.

Katsumata N, Yasuda M, Takahashi F et al. (2009) Dose-dense paclitaxel once a week in combination with carboplatin every 3 weeks for advanced ovarian cancer: a phase 3, open-label, randomized controlled trial. Lancet 374:1331–1338.

Mutch DG, Prat J (2014) FIGO staging for ovarian, fallopian tube and peritoneal cancer. Gynecol Oncol 133(3):401–404.

National Comprehensive Cancer Network. (2013) NCCN Ovarian Cancer Guidelines. Available from http://www.nccn.org/professionals/physician_gls/f_guidelines.asp

National Institute for Health and Clinical Excellence (2011) Recognition and initial management of ovarian cancer (Clinical guideline 122). Available from www.nice.org.uk/CG122

Parmar MK, Ledermann JA, Colombo N et al. (2003) Paclitaxel plus platinum-based chemotherapy versus conventional platinum-based chemotherapy in women with relapsed ovarian cancer: the ICON4/AGO-OVAR-2.2 trial. Lancet 361:2099–2106.

Perren TJ, Swart AM, Pfisterer J et al. (2011) A phase 3 trial of bevacizumab in ovarian cancer. N Engl J Med 365(26):484–496.

Rustin GJS, van der Burg ME, Griffin CL et al. (2010) Early versus delayed treatment of relapsed ovarian cancer (MRC OV05/ERTC 55955): A randomised trial. Lancet 376:1155–1163.

Tanglitgamol S, Manusirivithaya S, Laopaiboon M, Lumbiganon P, Bryant A (2013) Interval debulking surgery for advanced epithelial ovarian cancer. Cochrane Database Syst Rev (4):CD006014.

Vergote I, Tropé CG, Amant F et al. (2010) Neoadjuvant chemotherapy or primary surgery in Stage IIIC and IV ovarian cancer. N Engl J Med 363:943–953.

Vergote I, Amant F, Kristensen G, Ehlen T, Reed NS, Casado A (2011) Primary surgery or neoadjuvant chemotherapy followed by interval debulking surgery in advanced ovarian cancer. Eur J Cancer 47(Suppl 3):S88–92.

Winter-Roach BA, Kitchener HC, Lawrie TA (2012) Adjuvant (post-surgery) chemotherapy for early stage epithelial ovarian cancer. Cochrane Database Syst Rev (3):CD004706.

38 Vulva

M. H. M. Oonk[1], E. Pras[2] and A. G. J. van der Zee[1]

[1]Department of Gynecological Oncology, University Medical Center Groningen, University of Groningen, Groningen, The Netherlands
[2]Department of Radiotherapy, University Medical Center Groningen, University of Groningen, Groningen, The Netherlands

Summary	Key facts
Introduction	- Incidence: 2.3 per 100,000 women per year - Occurs especially in elderly women - About 90% is squamous cell cancer of the vulva: - Less frequent are melanoma, basal cell cancer and adenocarcinoma - Patients with vulvar intraepithelial neoplasia (VIN) or lichen sclerosis (LS) have a 5–10% chance of developing vulvar cancer - Human papillomavirus (HPV) is associated with the development of vulvar cancer in approximately 20%

Presentation	- Complaints: itching, vulvar lump, vulvar pain
	- Physical examination: vulvar lump, enlarged inguinofemoral lymph nodes
	- Usual work-up: CT for diagnosing lymph node metastases, chest X-ray to exclude metastases:
	  - CT/MRI/ultrasound for diagnosing lymph node metastases
	  - Chest X-ray to exclude lung metastases
	  - When indicated rectoscopy/urethracystoscopy
	- Final diagnosis by punch biopsy

Scenario	- *Microinvasive cancer*:
	  - Wide local excision
	- *Early-stage disease*:
	  - Wide local excision in combination with inguinofemoral lymphadenectomy, when possible preceded by a sentinel lymph node procedure
	    ○ Sentinel lymph node procedure in case of unifocal tumour <4 cm and no suspicious groin nodes
	    ○ Only when experienced multidisciplinary team is available
	- Radiotherapy:
	  - Adjuvant in case of more than one lymph node metastasis or extranodal tumour growth
	  - Primary (if feasible in combination with chemotherapy) for locally advanced disease

Trials	- Very limited number of randomized controlled trials
	- Levenback et al. (2012) *J Clin Oncol* 30:3786–3791:
	  - Sentinel node biopsy is a reasonable alternative to inguinofemoral lymphadenectomy in women with squamous cell carcinoma of the vulva, especially for tumours of <4 cm
	- Van der Zee et al. (2008) *J Clin Oncol* 26:884–889:
	  - In patients with early-stage vulvar disease (unifocal squamous cell carcinomas, <4 cm and no suspicious nodes at palpation) and a negative sentinel node, the groin recurrence rate is low, survival excellent and treatment-related morbidity minimal
	- Stehman et al. (1992) *Int J Radiat Oncol Biol Phys* 24:289–296:
	  - Radiotherapy on inguinofemoral lymph nodes for patients with vulvar cancer and clinically non-suspicious groins was significantly inferior to inguinofemoral lympadenectomy
	- Homesley et al. (1986) *Obstet Gynecol* 68:733–740:
	  - Addition of groin and pelvic irradiation therapy after radical vulvectomy and inguinal lymphadenectomy was superior to pelvic node dissection in patients with positive groin lymph nodes

UICC Manual of Clinical Oncology, Ninth Edition. Edited by Brian O'Sullivan, James D. Brierley, Anil K. D'Cruz, Martin F. Fey, Raphael Pollock, Jan B. Vermorken and Shao Hui Huang. © 2015 UICC. Published 2015 by John Wiley & Sons, Ltd.

Incidence, aetiology and screening

Vulvar cancer is a rare gynaecological malignancy predominantly occurring in elderly women. It represents approximately 5% of all malignancies of the female genital tract. Squamous cell cancers are the most frequent histology. Less frequent are melanomas, basal cell cancers, sarcomas and adenocarcinomas. There is evidence for two separate pathways leading to vulvar cancer. The first and most common pathway (80%) leads to squamous cell cancer in a background of lichen sclerosis and/or differentiated VIN. This type occurs in older women and is not caused by high-risk human papillomavirus (HPV). The second pathway is related to high-risk HPV infection (predominantly 16 or 18) and the presence of usual VIN. This type predominantly affects younger women and the immune system is associated with progression to invasive disease. Smoking is very prevalent in this group of vulvar cancer patients.

Incidence, aetiology and screening	Description

Incidence	• 2.3 per 100,000 women per year:
	  ■ Disease of older women:
	    ○ 54% are >70 years
	    ○ Only 15% are <50 years

Aetiology	• Risk factors:
	  ■ Cigarette smoking
	  ■ Vulvar dystrophy (e.g. LS)
	  ■ Vulvar or cervical (intraepithelial) neoplasia
	  ■ HPV infection
	  ■ Immunodeficiency syndromes
	  ■ Northern European ancestry
	• Premalignant vulvar disease:
	  ■ Differentiated VIN: related to lichen sclerosis, HPV negative
	  ■ Usual VIN: related to HPV infection and smoking

Screening	• No screening • Patients with LS are advised to use a potent steroid weekly to keep the disease minimally active: ■ Yearly check-up is advised because of 5–10% chance of developing invasive cancer • Cervical smear in HPV-/usual VIN-related vulvar cancer

Pathology

Pathology	Description
Squamous cell cancer	• Most common vulvar malignancy (90%) • 5-year survival in patients with negative nodes is approximately 90%, and for patients with lymph node metastases approximately 50%

Melanoma	• Second most common vulvar malignancy
	• Postmenopausal Caucasian women
	• Pigmented lesion
	• Three types:
	  ■ Superficial spreading melanoma:
	    ○ Remains superficial
	  ■ Mucosal lentiginous melanoma:
	    ○ Remains superficial
	  ■ Nodular melanoma:
	    ○ Tends to penetrate deeply and metastasize widely
	• Prognosis is poor for nodular melanoma:
	  ■ Mean 5-year survival 22–54%
	  ■ Survival in case of invasion of <1 mm is excellent

Basal cell cancer	• 2–4% of all vulvar cancers • 'Rodent ulcer' with rolled edges, usually situated on the anterior labia majora • Lymphogenic metastases are very rare: no indication for groin treatment • Excellent prognosis
Adenocarcinomas	• Arise in a Bartholin gland or occur in association with Paget disease • Prognosis by stage is similar to that for squamous cell carcinomas

Natural history and presentation

Generally, patients with vulvar cancer are in their sixth or seventh decade of life and present with a vulvar lump or mass, and there is often a long history of pruritus. Less common symptoms include vulvar bleeding, discharge or dysuria. Occasionally an inguinal metastatic mass is the presenting symptom. Distant metastases are rare at the time of presentation.

Natural history		Description
Presentation	Local	• Vulvar lump or mass • (History of) Pruritis • History of VIN/LS • Discharge or bleeding • Pain • Complaints with voiding/defaecation • Inguinal lump
	Metastatic	• Inguinal mass • Coughing
Routes of spread	Local	• Direct extension to anal sphincter/urethra/vagina

Natural history	Description

Regional	• Lymphatic embolization:
	  ▪ Inguinofemoral lymph node
	    ○ Ipsilateral in tumours of >1 cm from the midline
	    ○ Bilateral in tumours within 1 cm of the midline
	• 30% of patients with inguinofemoral lymph node metastases also have positive pelvic nodes

Metastatic	• Haematogenous spread is uncommon: ▪ Lungs, liver, bone

Diagnostic work-up

Diagnostic work-up	Description

Work-up	• Punch biopsy for histology
	• Tumour characteristics that guide treatment:
	  ▪ Diameter of tumour
	  ▪ Depth of invasion
	  ▪ Distance from clitoris/urethra/anus
	  ▪ Midline or lateralized tumour
	  ▪ Unifocal or multifocal tumour
	• In case of palpable lymph nodes: fine needle aspiration cytology
	• Computed tomography (CT), magnetic resonance imaging (MRI) or ultrasound for lymph node metastases in the groin/iliacal area
	• CT thorax/chest X-ray for distant metastases
	• When tumour invades the anus/rectum or urethra/bladder: rectoscopy or urethracystoscopy

Tumour markers	• No tumour markers for vulvar cancer

Staging and prognostic grouping

UICC TNM staging

See Table 38.1.

Prognostic factors

The most important prognostic factor for survival in vulvar cancer patients is the status of the inguinofemoral lymph nodes (Table 38.2). Number and size of lymph node metastases, and the presence of extranodal tumour growth, have major influence on prognosis. Prognosis for patients without lymph node metastases

Table 38.1 UICC TNM categories and stage grouping: Vulva

TNM categories, including corresponding FIGO classification		
TN	Vulva	FIGO
T1	Confined to vulva/perineum	I
T1a	≤2 cm with stromal invasion ≤1.0 mm	IA
T1b	>2 cm or stromal invasion >1.0 mm	IB
T2	Lower urethra/vagina/anus	II
T3	Upper urethra/vagina, bladder rectal/mucosa, fixed to pelvic bone	IIA
N1a	1–2 nodes <5 mm	IIIA
N1b	1 node ≥5 mm	IIIA
N2a	≥3 nodes <5 mm	IIIB
N2b	≥2 nodes ≥5 mm	IIIB
N2c	Extracapsular spread	IIIC
N3	Fixed or ulcerated	IVA
M1	Distant metastasis	IVB

Stage grouping			
Stage 0*	Tis	N0	M0
Stage I	T1	N0	M0
Stage IA	T1a	N0	M0
Stage IB	T1b	N0	M0
Stage II	T2	N0	M0
Stage IIIA	T1, T2	N1a, N1b	M0
Stage IIIB	T1, T2	N2a, N2b	M0
Stage IIIC	T1, T2	N2c	M0
Stage IVA	T1, T2	N3	M0
	T3	Any N	M0
Stage IVB	Any T	Any N	M1

*FIGO no longer includes stage 0 (Tis).

Table 38.2 Prognostic risk factors for cancer of the vulva

Prognostic factors	Tumour related	Host related	Environment related
Essential	Lymph node metastases: • Number • Size • Extracapsular tumour growth		Experience of treating centre/concentration of care for vulvar cancer patients in tertiary referral centres
Additional	FIGO stage Depth of invasion Diameter of primary tumour Histological type	Age Smoking Adjacent dermatosis (LS, VIN) Immune status	Surgical margins
New and promising	EGFR status p53 over-expression P16INK4a level Microvessel density	HPV status Pretreatment haemoglobin level	

is excellent with 5-year survival rates of approximately 90%; this drops to approximately 50% when lymph node metastases are present. Metastases of <2 mm in diameter carry a significantly better prognosis than metastases of >2 mm in diameter.

For local control, surgical excision margins are related to the occurrence of local recurrent disease. Pathological margins of ≤8 mm are thought to be related to a higher risk of local recurrence.

Treatment philosophy

The aim of modern vulvar cancer treatment is to minimize treatment-related morbidity, without compromising survival rates. Surgery is the first choice in the treatment of patients with vulvar cancer.

Scenario	Treatment philosophy
Local disease	• Wide local excision with surgical margins of 1–2 cm • For preservation of important structures (clitoris/anus/urethra), a narrower excision may be an option in combination with postoperative radiotherapy on the vulva • Primary radio(chemo)therapy

Regional disease	• No imaging techniques provide adequate information on lymph node status
	• Inguinofemoral lymphadenectomy is performed to determine whether or not there are lymph node metastases:
	  ▪ Sentinel node procedure is an alternative in selected patients (see below):
	    ○ Performed with combined technique (radioactive tracer and blue dye)
	    ○ Only in centres with an experienced multidisciplinary team

Metastatic	• No curative options exist when distant metastases are present at first presentation • Treatment is aimed at relief of complaints

Recurrent	• Local recurrence:
	  ▪ Wide local excision of vulvar tumour
	  ▪ In case of depth of invasion of >1 mm and no lymphadenectomy previously: uni- or bi-lateral (depending on relation with midline) inguinofemoral lymphadenectomy
	  ▪ Good prognosis: 3-year survival 67%
	• Groin recurrence:
	  ▪ Combination of radiotherapy/chemotherapy/surgery
	  ▪ Difficult to treat
	  ▪ Poor prognosis
	• Distant metastases:
	  ▪ Chemotherapy (e.g. cisplatin, mitomycin C, bleomycin, cyclophosphamide)
	  ▪ Response rates are low
	  ▪ Poor prognosis

Scenario	Treatment philosophy

Follow-up	• Lifelong follow-up is advised at gradually increasing intervals:
	  ▪ Risk of groin recurrence especially in first 2 years
	  ▪ Risk of local recurrence: lifelong

Treatment

Surgery

Radical vulvectomy with inguinofemoral lymphadenectomy *en bloc* replaced simple local excision in the second half of the last century and became the standard of care for a prolonged period of time (Fig. 38.1). The rationale for this approach was the assumption that the prognosis is better after elective inguinofemoral lymphadenectomy compared to surveillance of the groins, despite the fact that only 20–30% of patients will have lymph node metastases. However, the morbidity of this treatment was very high. Wound breakdown and infections, and lymphoedema were of great concern and often prolonged hospitalization. Since then, many modifications to surgery have been proposed in the treatment of patients with vulvar cancer, in order to reduce the complication rate. Inguinofemoral lymphadenectomy through separate groin incisions (Fig. 38.2), replacement of radical vulvectomy by wide local excision, abandonment of bilateral inguinofemoral lymphadenectomy in clearly lateralized tumours, and abandonment of inguinofemoral lymphadenectomy in microinvasive tumours (depth of invasion <1 mm).

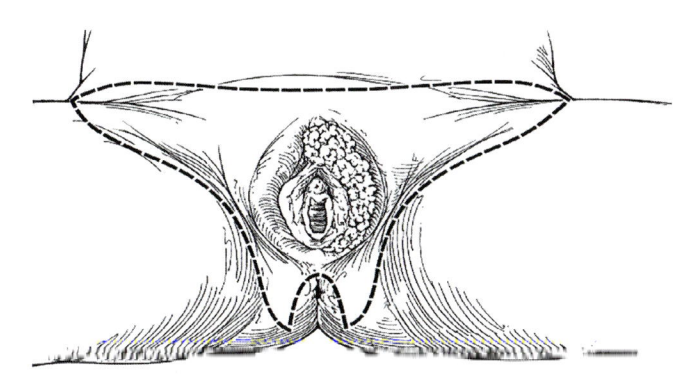

Standard treatment consists of a wide local excision with margins of at least 1–2 cm, combined with an inguinofemoral lymphadenectomy in case of a depth of invasion of >1 mm. When a tumour is clearly lateralized (medial margin not within 1 cm of the midline), only ipsilateral inguinofemoral lymphadenectomy is required. In all other cases, bilateral inguinofemoral lymphadenectomy should be performed.

Recently, the sentinel lymph node procedure (Fig. 38.3) has been introduced in the treatment of early-stage vulvar cancer. The GROningen INternational Study on Sentinel nodes in Vulvar cancer (GROINSS-V) showed that it is safe to omit inguinofemoral lymphadenectomy in patients with a negative sentinel node. Patients eligible for the sentinel node procedure should have unifocal vulvar disease with a diameter of <4 cm and no suspicious groin nodes on palpation. Preoperative imaging is recommended to rule out gross nodal involvement (which may obstruct lymph flow and thereby cause bypassing of the sentinel node). The GOG-173 study recently confirmed the accuracy of the sentinel node procedure in early-stage vulvar cancer, especially when performed in patients with tumours of <4 cm. This procedure should only be performed by an experienced multidisciplinary team in high-volume gynaecological cancer centres, as failures can occur at each stage of this multidisciplinary procedure.

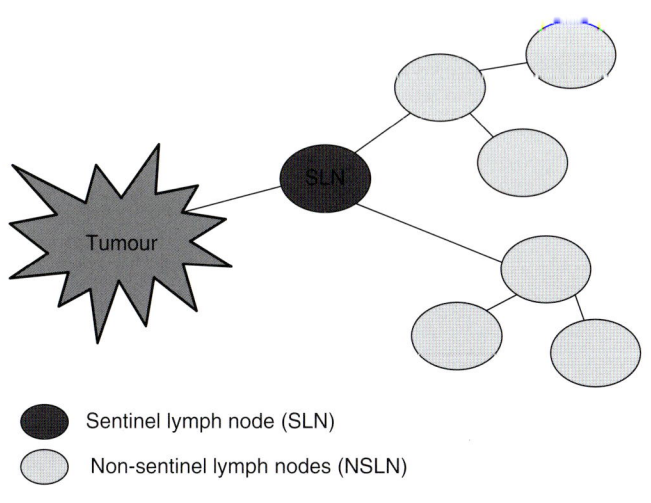

Figure 38.1 Radical vulvectomy with bilateral inguinofemoral lymphadenectomy *en bloc*.

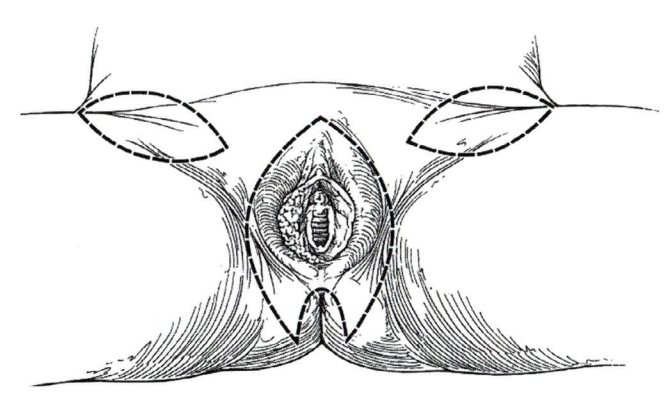

Figure 38.2 Radical vulvectomy with bilateral inguinofemoral lymphadenectomy through separate incisions.

Figure 38.3 Concept of the sentinel lymph node procedure.

Surgery	Description
Early disease	• Wide local excision: 　▪ Surgical margin of 1–2 cm • Inguinofemoral lymphadenectomy: 　▪ Unilateral in clearly lateralized disease (medial margin not within 1 cm of the midline) 　▪ All others: bilateral • Sentinel lymph node procedure in selected patients: 　▪ Unifocal tumours <4 cm 　▪ No suspicious nodes on palpation and imaging 　▪ Experienced multidisciplinary team
Advanced non-metastatic	• Wide local excision when possible • When tumour involves anus/rectum/rectovaginal septum/proximal urethra: 　▪ Pelvic exenteration combined with radical vulvectomy and bilateral inguinofemoral lymphadenectomy, or 　▪ (Chemo)radiation with the aim of sphincter-preserving surgery for salvage • Preoperative (chemo)radiation for down-sizing and planned surgery
Metastatic	• For inguinofemoral lymph node metastases: 　▪ By separate incisions

Radiotherapy

Radiotherapy is indicated after wide local excision and inguinofemoral lymphadenectomy in case of more than one lymph node metastases or when extranodal tumour growth is present. Primary radiotherapy of up to 60–65 Gy on the vulvar tumour, in order to preserve clitoral or anal sphincter function, is also possible but less attractive because of the morbidity associated with vulvar radiation. This should be balanced against the morbidity of a stoma.

Radiotherapy	Description
Early local disease	• *Primary tumour*: 　▪ For preservation of clitoral function/anal sphincter function: 　　○ Treatment volume/doses: 60–65 Gy in daily 1.8–2-Gy fractions, usually with concurrent weekly cisplatin (40 mg/m^2) • Radiotherapy to the groins is not an alternative to inguinofemoral lymphadenectomy (higher groin recurrence rate) • *Postoperative radiotherapy*: 　▪ Positive or close margin (<8 mm) 　▪ Extranodal extension or more than one inguinal node involved

Radiotherapy	Description
Advanced local disease	• Radiotherapy alone or combined with chemotherapy: 　▪ 65–70 Gy with radiotherapy alone 　▪ 63–65 Gy when combined with chemotherapy: 　　○ 45 Gy in 1.8-Gy fractions to the primary and nodal region 　　○ Boost to 54 Gy in 1.8-Gy fractions to high-risk area 　　○ Boost to 63 Gy in 1.8-Gy fractions to gross disease 　▪ Primary tumour clinical target volume (CTV) includes the gross disease and subclinical extension 　▪ Lymph node CTV includes the superficial and deep inguinofemoral lymph nodes, and the internal and external iliac lymph nodes • Salvage surgery is an option when residual tumour is present at 8–10 weeks after primary (chemo)radiotherapy
Metastatic disease	• Radiotherapy for inguinofemoral lymph node metastases: 　▪ After inguinofemoral lymphadenectomy: 45–50 Gy in 25 fractions over a period of 5 weeks: 　　○ In case of more than one lymph node metastases 　　○ In case of extranodal tumour growth • Radiotherapy for distant metastases: 　▪ In case of complaints/for pain relief

Systemic therapy

Systemic therapy	Description
Early	• No role in early-stage disease
Advanced non-metastatic disease	• In case of non-resectable local disease, neoadjuvant chemoradiation is an option: 　▪ Often with cisplatin (40 mg/m^2) • Drugs that have been applied are mitomycin C, 5-fluorouracil and cisplatin • No standard protocol
Metastatic disease	• Active agents are cisplatin, methotrexate, cyclophosphamide, bleomycin and mitomycin C • Response rates are low

Table 38.3 Phase III clinical trials

Trial reference	Results
Primary treatment	

Stehman et al. (1992) Int J Radiat Oncol Biol Phys 24:389–396	• Aim: to determine if groin radiation is superior to and less morbid than groin dissection
	  ▪ GOG randomized trial in 58 vulvar cancer patients with clinically non-suspicious inguinal nodes
	  ▪ Study was prematurely closed when interim monitoring revealed an excessive number of groin recurrences in the radiation group
	• Radiotherapy on inguinofemoral lymph nodes for vulvar cancer patients with clinically non-suspicious groins was significantly inferior to groin dissection

Judson et al. (2004) Gynecol Oncol 95:226–230	• Aim: to determine whether transposition of the sartorius muscle improves postoperative morbidity in women with squamous cell vulvar cancer undergoing inguinofemoral lymphadenectomy: ▪ 61 patients were included, 28 were randomized for sartorius transposition, and 33 without • No differences in postoperative morbidity, including wound cellulitis, wound breakdown, lymphoedema and rehospitalization • Sartorius transposition after inguinofemoral lymphadenectomy does not reduce postoperative wound morbidity
Carlson et al. (2008) Gynecol Oncol 110:76–82	• Aim: to evaluate vapour heated (VH) fibrin sealant's influence on lower extremity lymphoedema after inguinal lymphadenectomy in vulvar cancer patients: ▪ 137 patients were randomized; 67 to the sutured closure arm and 70 to the VH fibrin sealant arm (VH fibrin sealant sprayed into the groin, followed by suture closure) • No difference in incidence of grade 2–3 lymphoedema • VH fibrin sealant did not reduce leg lymphoedema and may increase the risk for complications in the vulvar wound
Manci et al. (2009) Ann Surg Oncol 16:721–728	• Aim: to analyse whether different groin incisions (above and below the inguinal ligament) reduce groin wound complications and whether number of removed lymph nodes is the same: ▪ 62 patients were randomized • No differences in short- and long-term complication rate • There was no difference in chronic lymphoedema, number of nodes removed or hospital stay
Adjuvant treatment	
Homesley et al. (1986) Obstet Gynecol 68:733–740	• Aim: to compare radiation therapy and pelvic node dissection in vulvar cancer patients with positive groin nodes • Randomized prospective study in 114 patients • 2-year survival rates were 68% for the radiation therapy group and 54% for the pelvic node dissection group • Most dramatic survival advantage for patients with clinically suspicious or fixed ulcerated groin nodes and for those with two or more positive groin nodes • Addition of groin and pelvic irradiation therapy after radical vulvectomy and inguinal lymphadenectomy was superior to pelvic node dissection
Kunos et al. (2009) Obstet Gynecol 114:537–546	• Long-term follow-up of the randomized controlled trial by Homesley et al. (1986) • Radiation after radical vulvectomy and inguinal lymphadenectomy significantly reduced local relapses and decreased cancer-related deaths • Late toxicities remained similar after radiation or pelvic node dissection

Controversies

- Wide local excision and inguinofemoral lymphadenectomy:
  - What excision margins are sufficient in wide local excision in order to reduce local recurrent disease?
  - Management during or after inguinofemoral lymphadenectomy in order to reduce treatment-related morbidity
- Implementation of the sentinel node procedure in early-stage vulvar cancer:
  - Learning curve and exposure rate: how many patients should be treated in a centre to allow safe implementation of the sentinel node procedure?
  - Preoperative imaging: what is the best imaging technique to rule out gross nodal involvement?

Phase III clinical trials

As vulvar cancer is rare, there is a scarcity of randomized controlled trials (Table 38.3).

Areas of research

- New treatment strategies for patients with (sentinel) lymph node metastases
- Significance of sentinel node micrometastases in vulvar cancer patients
- Further reduction of treatment-related morbidity in patients with early-stage disease
- Development of better treatment strategies in advanced disease

Recommended reading

De Hullu JA, Hollema H, Lolkema S et al. (2002) Vulvar carcinoma. The price of less radical surgery. *Cancer* 95:2331–2338.

Gadducci A, Tana R, Barsotti C, Guerrieri ME, Genazzani AR (2012) Clinico-pathological and biological prognostic variables in squamous cell carcinoma of the vulva. *Crit Rev Oncol Hematol* 83:71–83.

Homesley HD, Bundy BN, Sedlis A, Adcock L (1986) Radiation therapy versus pelvic node resection for carcinoma of the vulva with positive groin nodes. *Obstet Gynecol* 68:733–740.

Levenback CF, Ali S, Coleman RL et al. (2012) Lymphatic mapping and sentinel lymph node biopsy in women with squamous cell carcinoma of the vulva: a gynecologic oncology group study. *J Clin Oncol* 30:3786–3791.

Oonk MH, van Hemel BM, Hollema H et al. (2010) Size of sentinel node metastasis and chances of non-sentinel node involvement and survival in early-stage vulvar: results form GROINSS-V, a multicentre observational study. *Lancet Oncol* 11.646–652.

Sharma DN (2012) Radiation in vulvar cancer. *Curr Opin Obstet Gynecol* 24:24–30.

Shylasree TS, Bryant A, Howells RE (2011) Chemoradiation for advanced primary vulvar cancer. *Cochrane Database Syst Rev* (4):CD003752.

Stehman FB, Bundy BN, Thomas G et al. (1992) Groin dissection versus groin radiation in carcinoma of the vulva: a Gynecologic Oncology Group study. *Int J Radiat Oncol Biol Phys* 24:289–296.

Van der Zee AGJ, Oonk MH, De Hullu JA et al. (2008) Sentinel-node dissection is safe in the treatment of early stage vulvar cancer. *J Clin Oncol* 26:884–889.

Woelber L, Kock L, Gieseking F et al. (2011) Clinical management of primary vulvar cancer. *Eur J Cancer* 47:2315–2321.

39 General principles of head and neck cancer management

Mitali Dandekar[1], Anil K. D'Cruz[1], Shao Hui Huang[2], Brian O'Sullivan[2] and Jan B. Vermorken[3]

[1]Department of Head and Neck Surgical Oncology, Tata Memorial Centre, Mumbai, India
[2]Department of Radiation Oncology, The Princess Margret Cancer Centre, University of Toronto, Toronto, Canada
[3]Department of Medical Oncology, Antwerp University Hospital, Edegem, Belgium

Summary	Key facts

Introduction	• Head and neck cancer is the sixth most common cancer in both genders globally
	• Risk factors include:
	  ▪ Tobacco, areca nut and alcohol
	  ▪ Dental hygiene for oral cavity cancer
	  ▪ Human papillomavirus (HPV) as a cause for oropharyngeal cancers in the Western world (populations without traditional habits associated with the disease)
	  ▪ Epstein–Barr virus (EBV) for nasopharyngeal cancer, which is common in East Asia and the Mediterranean

Treatment philosophy	• A multidisciplinary approach is required for successful management of head and neck cancers
	• Surgery and radiotherapy (RT) are both effective local treatment modalities:
	  ▪ Treatment decisions are based on optimization of oncological and functional outcomes
	  ▪ Surgery represents the mainstay of treatment in oral cavity and many paranasal sinus cancers
	    ○ Adjuvant radiotherapy ± chemotherapy is frequently used for some paranasal sinus tumours to further enhance disease control in selected cases
	    ○ Preoperative radiotherapy ± chemotherapy may be used for some sinonasal tumours to maximize protection of critical structures (e.g. optic apparatus and brain)
	  ▪ Definitive radiation with or without chemotherapy is the preferred primary treatment for oro- and laryngo-pharyngeal cancers, and is ordinarily the only curative option for nasopharyngeal cancer
	• Rehabilitation is important since the treatment of these cancers has implications for cosmesis, speech and swallowing

Introduction

Head and neck cancers are a heterogeneous group of disorders and the term is usually applied to mucosal squamous cell carcinomas of the upper aerodigestive tract (ICD coding C00–C14, C30–32). Although there may be some peculiarities with respect to epidemiology, biology, presentation, work-up and treatment of these cancers, the main features and broad principles of management are fundamentally the same. Preservation of anatomical form and function is imperative, as well as disease control. This chapter attempts to bring together these issues and primarily covers the general principles of management and follow-up of squamous cell carcinoma of the oral cavity, oropharynx, larynx and hypopharynx, nasopharynx and paranasal sinuses. Anatomical site-specific details are covered in Chapters 40–46.

UICC Manual of Clinical Oncology, Ninth Edition. Edited by Brian O'Sullivan, James D. Brierley, Anil K. D'Cruz, Martin F. Fey, Raphael Pollock, Jan B. Vermorken and Shao Hui Huang. © 2015 UICC. Published 2015 by John Wiley & Sons, Ltd.

Incidence, aetiology and screening

Incidence, aetiology and screening	Description
Incidence	- Head and neck cancers account for 4.8% of all malignancies - Mortality from head and neck cancers is 4.6% - Male-to-female ratio is 2.7:1
Aetiology	- Tobacco (both smoked and smokeless) and alcohol are the most important risk factors, with a synergistic effect when consumed together - Areca nut is known to be an independent risk factor in oral cancers - High-risk human papillomavirus (HPV) type (mostly subtype 16) has a proven causative role in oropharyngeal cancers - Epstein–Barr virus (EBV) is known to be associated with nasopharyngeal cancers - Exposure to nickel, leather and wood dust has an established role in nasal and paranasal sinus cancers. - In particular, this accounts for adenocarcinomas - Plummer–Vinson syndrome is associated with post-cricoid cancer - Hereditary conditions like Fanconi anaemia, Li-Fraumeni syndrome, xeroderma pigmentosum and ataxia telangiectasia are associated with cancers in the head and neck
Screening	- No evidence for population-based screening in head and neck cancers - Some evidence for recommending screening for oral cancers in individuals with high-risk habits (alcohol and tobacco) - HPV vaccination in teenage males and females is a topic of discussion in countries where there is a high risk for HPV-related oropharyngeal cancer

Pathology

The majority of head and neck cancers are squamous cell carcinomas. The World Health Organization (WHO; 2005) histological classification of these carcinomas is:
- Verrucous carcinoma
- Basaloid squamous cell carcinoma
- Papillary squamous cell carcinoma
- Spindle cell or sarcomatoid variant (often misleadingly termed 'carcino-sarcoma')
- Acantholytic squamous cell carcinoma
- Adenosquamous carcinoma
- Carcinoma cuniculatum.

Other carcinomas, (e.g. mucoepidermoid and adenoid cystic carcinoma) may also arise from minor salivary glands in these locations.

Natural history

Smoking-related head and neck cancers often develop in preneoplastic fields of genetically altered cells. The majority of the evidence is from oral lesions, which are easily accessible and more extensively studied. Dysplastic changes in the surrounding mucosa may predispose to local recurrences and second primary tumours despite adequate treatment of the primary lesion. HPV-related oropharyngeal cancer does not have the same field effect.

Second primary cancers occur at the rate of approximately 1% per year. Incidence varies from 6–25%. Most of these tumours occur either in the head and neck region or in the lung. They can occur as simultaneous (diagnosed at the time of the index cancer), synchronous (within 6 months of the diagnosis of the index cancer) or metachronous (6 months after diagnosis of the index cancer) primary tumours.

Morphological changes for smoking-related head and neck cancer have been genetically characterized:
- Dysplasia: loss of heterozygosity at chromosomes 3p, 9p and 17p
- Carcinoma: alterations at 11q, 4q and chromosome 8.

The *TP53* mutation is common in smoking-related head and neck cancer but rare in HPV-related oropharyngeal cancers. The epidermal growth factor receptor (*EGFR*) gene also plays a role in the carcinogenesis of head and neck squamous cell carcinoma.

Diagnostic work-up

Diagnostic work-up	Description
Assessment of patient profile	• Disease-related information: 　▪ Addictions: tobacco, alcohol, areca nut 　▪ Irritation: sharp teeth and ill-fitting dentures • Familial cancer syndromes: Fanconi anaemia, ataxia telangiectasia, xeroderma pigmentosum, etc. • History of previous malignancy in upper aerodigestive system • Medical history and co-morbidities • General assessment of performance status: 　▪ Commonly used performance assessment scales are the Karnofsky score and the Eastern Cooperative Oncology Group(ECOG) score, also termed the WHO or Zubrod score • Investigations for fitness for cancer-directed treatment
Assessment of tumour profile	• Biopsy of lesion • Fine needle aspiration cytology (FNAC), particularly for nodes • Image-guided biopsy if lesion is deep seated • Assessment of HPV status, generally by the surrogate marker p16 expression, is considered a prerequisite in oropharyngeal cancers
Assessment of tumour extent	• Clinicoradiological evaluation for operability: 　▪ Criteria for inoperability: 　　○ Involvement of skull base 　　○ Encasement of internal carotid artery 　　○ Infiltration of prevertebral fascia • *Examination for extent of disease*: 　▪ Endoscopy to map mucosal extent of disease and for biopsy 　▪ Evaluation under anaesthesia indicated in cases where flexible fibre-optic endoscopy and clinical evaluation is inadequate • *Imaging for extent of disease*: 　▪ Computed tomography (CT) scan preferred: 　　○ For better cortical bone and cartilage delineation 　　○ May be superior for anatomical delineation of neck nodes 　　○ Indicated in gingivobuccal complex cancers, laryngeal and hypopharyngeal cancers 　　○ *Limitations*: assessment of perineural spread, dural involvement and marrow infiltration 　▪ Magnetic resonance imaging (MRI) preferred: 　　○ For better soft tissue delineation, including anatomical delineation of retropharyngeal lymph nodes 　　○ Indicated in tongue, and oropharyngeal cancers, and especially in nasopharyngeal cancer 　　○ Paranasal sinuses for assessment of dural and intraorbital involvement: differentiation of secretions from tumour 　　○ Medullary bone and perineural spread 　　○ Assessment of early cartilage erosion makes it occasionally necessary in laryngeal and hypopharyngeal cancers 　　○ *Limitation*: tends to overestimate cortical erosion • Ultrasound (US): 　　○ High sensitivity/specificity (with guided FNAC) for evaluation of cervical lymphadenopathy 　　○ Best evaluated with a 5–10-MHz linear transducer 　▪ Barium swallow: 　　○ To determine oesophageal involvement in hypopharyngeal cancers • *Imaging for metastatic disease*: 　▪ CT-positron emission tomography (PET): 　　○ Locally-advanced disease: N2, N3 nodes, advanced T stage, hypopharyngeal cancers which have a high propensity for distant metastasis 　　○ Unknown primary with cervical metastasis 　▪ Contrast-enhanced CT (CE-CT) chest: 　　○ Incidence of synchronous tumours (both second primary and metastatic) is up to 15% in locally-advanced cancers 　　○ Chest is the commonest site for synchronous tumours in head and neck cancer patients; hence, a CE-CT thorax may be indicated, particularly in smokers and if CT-PET is unavailable

Table 39.1 Histological parameters for head and neck cancers

Essential	Desirable	Optional	New/promising
Size	Grade	Patterns of invasion	HPV status in other sites
Adjacent structure involvement: bone/skin	Perineural invasion	Stromal response	EGFR expression
Surgical cut margins	Lymphovascular invasion	Characteristics of tumour (endophytic, exophytic and ulcerative)	Bcl-2 oncogene
Nodal metastasis: size, number and level	Tumour thickness		Disruptive *TP53* mutations
Extracapsular extension	Type of squamous cell carcinoma		*NOTCH1*
HPV status in oropharyngeal cancers			

Synoptic reporting of pathological specimens

Histopathology should include the histological parameters listed in Table 39.1 which have a bearing on adjuvant therapy and prognosis.

Treatment philosophy (see Fig. 39.1)

Curative intent
Non-metastatic HNC (Stage I–IVB) (except for those unable to tolerate standard treatment due to co-morbidity or poor performance status)

Palliative intent
Metastatic HNC (Stage IVC) or non-metastatic but unable to tolerate standard treatment

Early stage (I/II)
- Single modality (surgery/RT)
- Surgery preferred in oral cavity, paranasal sinuses
- Laser surgery is a suitable alternative in earl glottic cancers
- Robotic surgeries have an emerging role in early oropharyngeal cancers
- RT preferred in oropharynx, nasopharynx larynx, and hypopharynx
- Surgery/radiotherapy in glottic cancers

Advanced stage (III/IVA/IVB)
- Multimodality
- Oral cavity, paranasal sinuses: surgery with PORT with/without concurrent chemotherapy
- Oropharynx, nasopharynx: CCRT with/without salvage surgery
- Larynx/hypopharynx: CCRT or ICT followed by RT/CCRT if deemed suitable for organ preservation; alternatively surgery with PORT with/without concurrent chemotherapy
- Bioradiotherapy with cetuximab is another treatment option

Metastatic with good performance status
- Local treatment first (RT/CCRT) for local control, followed by systemic therapy; or systemic therapy first followed by local treatment, as indicated
- Chemotherapy with/without targeted therapy (cetuximab)
- Oligometastases can be treated aggressively as some may be curable, especially in HPV-related oropharyngeal cancer and EBV-related nasopharyngeal cancer

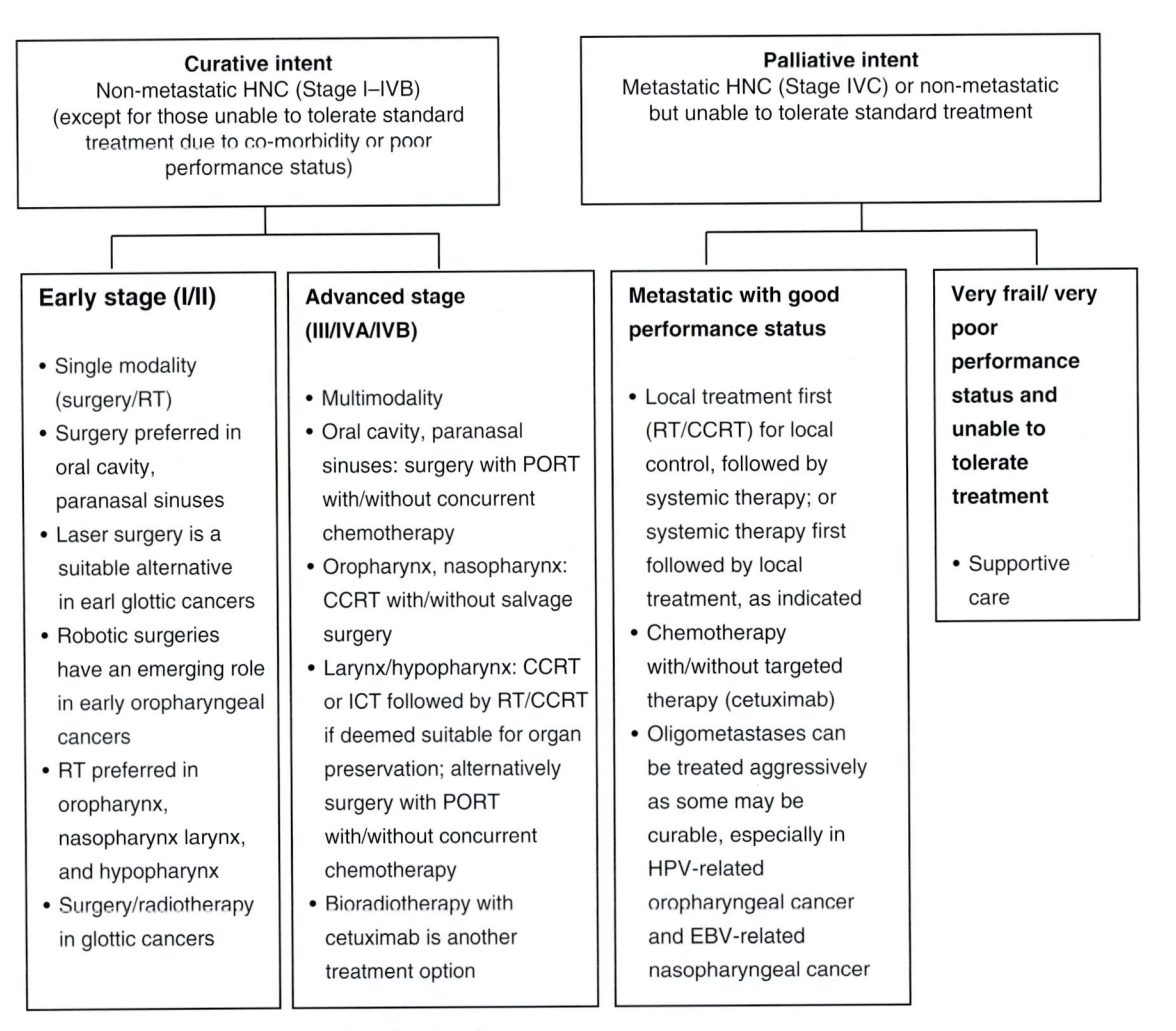

Very frail/ very poor performance status and unable to tolerate treatment
- Supportive care

Figure 39.1 Algorithm for the management of head and neck cancer
HNC, head and neck cancer; RT, radiotherapy; PORT, postoperative radiotherapy; CCRT, concurrent chemoradiotherapy; ICT, induction chemotherapy; EBV, Epstein–Barr virus; HPV, human papillomavirus.

Scenario	Treatment philosophy
Non-metastatic head and neck cancers (Stages I–IVB)	• Goal of treatment is to achieve maximum cure rates with minimum morbidity • Since head and neck cancers have implications for speech and swallowing, an attempt is made at organ preservation: ▪ Non-surgical protocols showing similar cure rates as surgery

Stage I/II (early): single modality treatment (either surgery or radiotherapy)	• Surgery is preferred to radiotherapy as a single modality in:
	  ▪ Sites where surgery is not morbid (cosmetically and functionally), e.g. oral cancers
	  ▪ Accessible lesions
	  ▪ Lesions involving or close to bone to minimize radiotherapy-related bone damage
	  ▪ Young patients (to keep radiotherapy in reserve in case of a second primary)
	• Radiotherapy is preferred over surgery as a single modality when:
	  ▪ There is impairment of function/cosmesis with surgery, e.g. base of tongue
	  ▪ Surgery is technically difficult with high morbidity and poor results, e.g. nasopharynx
	  ▪ There is a high risk for surgery
	• Radiotherapy can be external, brachytherapy or combined external beam with brachytherapy

Stage III/IVA (advanced): multimodality treatment	• Options:
	  ▪ Surgery followed by adjuvant post-operative radiotherapy (PORT) or postoperative chemo-radiotherapy (POCRT)
	  ▪ Definitive radiotherapy (RT) or concurrent chemo-radiotherapy (CCRT) [ordinarily using platinum-based chemotoxic agent(s)]
	  ▪ Bioradiotherapy with cetuximab in case CCRT is not feasible, followed by planned (when indicated) or salvage surgery (in case of relapse)
	• Primary surgery is preferred in oral and paranasal sinuses due to involvement/proximity of bone
	• Primary chemoradiotherapy (CRT) is preferred in lesions suitable for organ preservation in the laryngopharynx, oropharynx and nasopharynx

Stage IVB	• Primary CRT when surgery is not possible
Stage IVC	• Palliative treatment for symptom control
Metastatic head and neck cancer (Stage IVC)	• Goal is to achieve optimum palliation depending on the performance status of the patient

Treatment principles

Treatment for head and neck cancer includes surgery, radiotherapy and chemotherapy, as sole modalities or as combined modalities.

Principles of surgical resection

- *Primary disease*:
  - En bloc resection
  - Third dimension (base of tumour) should be carefully considered
  - Adequate margins in all dimensions (clear margin >5 mm)
    - Frozen section confirmation for margins may be assessed if this facility is available
  - In laser resection, piecemeal resection has been described as a technique to facilitate adequate resection (bisecting tumour to reach normal tissue)
- *Management of neck*:
  - Minimum extent of neck dissection is a selective neck dissection (SND), with levels dependent on the site and the draining lymph nodes, e.g.:
    - SND (level I–III) in the oral cavity and oropharynx
    - Level II–IV in the larynx and hypopharynx
  - In clinically involved neck disease (cN+), modified radical neck dissection (Level I–V) is performed
  - Radical neck dissection is rarely indicated:
    - Internal jugular vein (IJV), sternocleidomastoid muscle or spinal accessory nerve is sacrificed only when involved by tumour
  - Contralateral neck should be addressed when the probability of contralateral metastases is high, e.g.:
    - Tumours crossing or reaching the midline
    - Large tumours of the tongue, larynx and hypopharynx
- Reconstruction options:
  - Small defects are closed with local flaps
  - Free flaps are preferred over pedicled flaps
  - Bone is best reconstructed with bone
  - *Mucosal defects*:
    - Primary closure/local flap/split thickness skin grafting (STSG)/ healing by secondary intention according to the site involved
    - Pedicled flap may be considered in repairing a pharyngeal mucosal defect
  - *Soft tissue loss*:
    - Free flap (free radial artery forearm flap, anterolateral thigh flap, lateral arm flap)/pedicled flap, e.g. pectoralis major myocutaneous (PMMC) flap
  - *Skeletal defects*:
    - Free fibula/scapula/iliac crest
    - PMMC flap can be considered in select posterior mandibular defects

- Repair with an obturator may be considered for palatal defects, with the exception of those crossing the midline or extending superiorly up to the orbital floor
- External skin defects:
  - Local flaps/forehead flap
  - Deltopectoral flap/PMMC
  - Free flaps

Principles of radiotherapy

Radiotherapy can be used as definitive treatment instead of surgery for organ preservation or as an adjuvant treatment with or without chemotherapy to enhance disease control following surgery. There are two types of radiotherapy: external beam radiotherapy (EBRT) and brachytherapy. The term 'radiotherapy' usually refers to EBRT.

Definitive radiotherapy

Definitive radiotherapy is widely used in the management of head and neck cancer where surgical resection may result in significant functional or cosmetic deficit, especially in cancers of the oropharynx, larynx and hypopharynx. In cancer of the nasopharynx, radiotherapy is the only curative local treatment to eradicate disease, and is used in all stages of presentations with the exception of distant metastasis. For locally-advanced head and neck cancer, it is often combined with concurrent chemotherapy to offer a better chance of cure.

Typical definitive radiotherapy dose schedules and volume constraints are given in Tables 39.2 and 39.3.

Table 39.2 Typical definitive radiotherapy schedules

Radiotherapy regimen	Systemic therapy
60–70 Gy in 30–35 fractions in 5–6 weeks (six fractions per week), RT alone	None
60 Gy in 25 fractions over 5 weeks (five fractions per week), RT alone	None
65-66 Gy in 30 fractions over 6 weeks (five fractions per week), RT alone	None
72 Gy in 60 fractions b.i.d. over 6 weeks (ten fractions per week), RT alone	None
64 Gy in 40 fractions b.i.d. (at least 6 hours apart) over 4 weeks (ten fractions per week), RT alone	None
70 Gy in 35 fractions over 7 weeks (five fractions per week) ± chemotherapy	Cisplatin: • High-dose (preferable): 100 mg/m^2 IV on Days 1, 22 and 43 of radiotherapy • Weekly cisplatin (30–40 mg/m^2 weekly) is acceptable if concerns about tolerance of high-dose cisplatin • Cumulative dose of 200 mg/m^2 should be achieved
70 Gy in 35 fractions over 6 weeks (six fractions per week) ± cetuximab	Cetuximab: • 400 mg/m^2 loading dose over 120 minutes, 1 week prior to commencing radiotherapy, then 250 mg/m^2 weekly during radiotherapy • Only indicated where there are contraindications to cisplatin-based chemotherapy

Table 39.3 Typical dose volume constraints for organ at risk for radiotherapy planning

Region of interest	Dose to be reported (Gy)	Tolerance (2 Gy/fraction)
Spinal cord	0.1 cm^3	≤45 Gy
Brainstem	0.1 cm^3	≤50 Gy
Mandible	0.1 cm^3	≤70 Gy
Optic chiasm	Maximum dose	≤52 Gy
Optic nerve	Maximum dose	≤45 Gy
Parotid gland	Mean dose	<26 Gy
Submandibular gland	Mean dose	<39 Gy
Larynx	Mean dose	<45 Gy
Brachial plexus	Maximum dose	≤63 Gy

Adjuvant radiotherapy

Indications
- *Postoperative radiotherapy alone*:
  - Primary:
    - Large primary: T3/T4
    - High-grade tumour
    - Close resection margins
  - Lymph nodes:
    - Involved neck lymph nodes (node positivity)
  - Relative indications:
    - Thick tumour/deep infiltration
    - Perineural invasion (PNI)
    - Lymphovascular invasion (LVI)
    - Early nodal metastasis (N1 disease)
- *Postoperative CRT*:
  - Microscopically positive resection margins
  - Lymph node extracapsular extension (ECE) to adjacent soft tissues

Adjuvant therapy regimen
- *Postoperative radiotherapy alone*:
  - Primary and involved nodal disease: 56–60 Gy in 28–30 2-Gy fractions over 6 weeks, using reducing fields (at least 57.6 Gy)
  - Sites of high risk like ECE, residual disease, positive tumour margins: 4–10-Gy dose augmentation ('boost') depending on the initial dose chosen (up to 66–70 Gy)
- *Postoperative radiotherapy combined with* chemotherapy:
  - Cisplatin 100 mg/m^2 IV every 3 weeks × 3 (Days 1, 22 and 43 during RT) (level I evidence).
  - 40 mg/m^2 weekly with hydration and antiemetic prophylaxis
  - Cumulative dose of 200 mg/m^2 should be achieved (level IIB evidence).
- Commencing postoperative radiotherapy as soon as possible (within 6 weeks after surgery) is optimal, and requires careful planning and multidisciplinary collaboration
- Overall treatment time (OTT) is optimally ≤100 days and/or radiation treatment time (RTT) is <8 weeks (prolonged RTT is associated with inferior overall survival)

Principles of brachytherapy (see also Chapter 10)

Interstitial brachytherapy (BRT) represents an alternative to EBRT for selected head and neck cancers. It can be applied as a definitive treatment for early disease; as a complementary treatment in combination with surgery; as a local 'boost' in combination with EBRT to enhance the local dose to the immediate tumour region; or as a salvage option for small burden persistent or recurrent disease. However, no randomized trials have been performed so far and the GEC-ESTRO recommendations have been established through expert panel consensus.

Lesions suitable for brachytherapy are:
- Accessible lesions

> **Box 39.1** Example BRT schedules
> - T1–2N0:
>   - Radical BRT: 60–70 Gy LDR with iridium-192 or equivalent doses with fractionated HDR
> - T1–3N0–1:
>   - External RT: 56–60 Gy in 28–30 fractions over 6 weeks
>   - 'Boost' with BRT: LDR iridium-192: 15–20 Gy
>   - HDR: one approach is 14 Gy in four fractions (4, 3, 3 and 4 Gy) over 2 days

- Small (preferably<3 cm), superficial lesions
- Lesions away from bone
- N0 nodal status.

In general, low dose rate (LDR) should deliver a high total dose for local control (60–70 Gy) while maintaining the dose rate between 0.3 and 0.6 Gy/hour in order to minimize late side effects. With high dose rate (HDR), a smaller dose per fraction (3–4 Gy) with a higher number of fractions is required. PDR offers the biological advantages of LDR brachytherapy with the technological advantages of the HDR after-loading method. Daytime PDR schedules have been introduced by some to avoid hospitalization and to reduce overall treatment costs. Example BRT schedules are given in Box 39.1.

Principles of systemic therapy

Systemic therapy includes chemotherapy and biotherapy (targeted agents, such as epithelial growth factor receptor [EGFR] inhibitor). In the curative setting, systemic therapy is generally used combined with radiotherapy to intensify treatment for locally-advanced head and neck cancer. In the palliative setting, it is the main treatment modality.

A schedule for chemotherapy, if indicated, is given in Box 39.2.

Post-treatment assessment

- Indicated in locoregionally advanced disease and especially to determine whether surgery (especially neck dissection) is needed for patients initially treated by radiotherapy or CRT

> **Box 39.2** Schedule for chemotherapy
> - Cisplatin-based regimen: three-drug chemotherapy (taxane + platinum + 5-fluorouracil [5-FU] [TPF]) is superior to two-drug chemotherapy (platinum +5-FU [PF])
> - TPF (TAX 324): docetaxel 75 mg/m^2 + cisplatin 100 mg/m^2 + 5-FU 1000 mg/m^2/day × 4
> - TPF (TAX 323): docetaxel 75 mg/m^2 + cisplatin 75 mg/m^2 + 5-FU 750 mg/m^2/day × 5 (+ antibiotic prophylaxis)
> - Both TPF regimens are repeated every 3 weeks
> - Docetaxel in the TPF regimens can be replaced by paclitaxel 175 mg/m^2 (3-hour infusion)

- CT-PET scan is the imaging modality of choice due to its high negative predictive value of up to 95%
  - To be considered 10–12 weeks after treatment completion to avoid false positive results
- Alternatively, CE-CT scan or MRI depending on the site of origin and nature of the disease

Follow up

The majority of recurrences occur in the first 24 months; hence meticulous follow-up is warranted in the first 2 years:
- Every 2–3 months or more frequently in first 2 years
- Every 4–6 months or more frequently for the third year
- Every 6 months or more frequently for Years 4–5
- Annually after 5 years.
- *At every follow-up visit*:
  - Thorough head and neck examination for locoregional control, second primary tumour and late sequelae of treatment
  - Investigation specific to symptoms and positive clinical findings
- *Annually*:
  - Serum T3, T4 and thyroid-stimulating hormone (TSH) for all patients receiving radiotherapy
  - Chest X-ray is advisable in smokers and in patients at risk for distant metastases

Treatment for recurrence or metastatic disease:

Scenario: Recurrence	Treatment philosophy

Biopsy-proven local and/or regional recurrence	• Resectable: salvage surgery ± postoperative re-irradiation
	• Unresectable: re-irradiation (small fraction size, b.i.d.) ± systemic therapy:
	  ▪ Optimizing re-irradiation regimens
	    ○ Longer interval since previous radiation (preferably >1 year)
	    ○ Use of high-precision radiotherapy (e.g. intensity-modulated RT [IMRT]/image-guided [IGRT], stereotactic RT)
	    ○ Small clinical target volume surrounding gross disease
	    ○ Total dose preferably to be ≥60 Gy for disease control
	    ○ Small fraction size (1.1–1.5 Gy/fraction), twice daily with ≥6 hours apart to minimize risk of severe late toxicity
	    ○ Continuous course to avoid tumour repopulation
	    ○ Short course stereotactic RT (30–40 Gy in 3–5 fractions, once daily) may be suitable for some patients

Distant metastasis	• Cure is generally not possible, except for EBV-related nasopharyngeal cancer or HPV-related oropharyngeal cancer with oligometastasis:
	  ▪ Palliative measures for symptom control, including best supportive care (BSC) with or without systemic treatment (and on indication, irradiation) depending on the general condition of the patient
	  ▪ Consider surgery for single lung metastasis or a second (lung) primary
	• Palliative systemic therapy for recurrent/metastatic disease:
	  ▪ Adding cetuximab, the first clinically available EGFR-directed monoclonal antibody, to a standard chemotherapy regimen (platinum + 5-fluorouracil) leads to survival benefit and should be considered in patients with an adequate performance status (i.e. Karnofsky performance score >70)

Continuing care

- Abstinence from tobacco/alcohol
- Oral hygiene
- Shoulder physiotherapy in all cases of neck dissections
- Bite guide prosthesis following mandibulectomy
- Jaw stretching exercises to prevent postoperative trismus
- Swallowing and speech rehabilitation
- Assessment of quality of life (QoL):
  - Global QoL: University of Washington QoL questionnaire, European Organization for Research and Treatment of Cancer Quality of Life Questionnaire (EORTC QLQ)-H&N35, Functional Assessment of Cancer Therapy – Head and Neck (FACT-H&N)
  - Site-specific QoL questionnaires:
    - Voice: Voice-Related Quality Of Life (V-RQOL), Voice Handicap Index (VHI)
    - Swallowing: Sydney Swallow Questionnaire, M. D. Anderson Dysphagia Inventory
- Assessment of toxicity:
  - CRT-related toxicity should be graded and documented according to the Common Terminology Criteria of Adverse Events (CTCAE) or RTOG/EORTC

Recommended reading

Barnes L, Eveson JW, Reichart P, Sidransky D, eds. (2005) *World Health Organization Classification of Tumours. Pathology and Genetics of Head and Neck Tumours.* Lyon: IARC Press.

Bernier J, Cooper JS, Pajak TF *et al.* (2005) Defining risk levels in locally advanced head and neck cancers: a comparative analysis of concurrent postoperative radiation plus chemotherapy trials of the EORTC (#22931) and RTOG (# 9501). *Head Neck* 27(10):843–850.

Bjordal K, Hammerlid E, Ahlner-Elmqvist M *et al.* (1999) Quality of life in head and neck cancer patients: Validation of the European Organization for Research and Treatment of Cancer Quality of Life Questionnaire H&N35. *J Clin Oncol* 17(3):1008–1019.

Bonner JA, Harari PM, Giralt J *et al.* (2006) Radiotherapy plus cetuximab for squamous-cell carcinoma of the head and neck. *N Engl J Med* 354(6):567–578.

Chen AY, Frankowski R, Bishop-Leone J *et al.* (2001) The development and validation of a dysphagia-specific quality-of-life questionnaire for patients with head and neck cancer. The M. D. Anderson Dysphagia Inventory. *Arch Otolaryngol Head Neck Surg* 127:870–876.

CTCAE version 4. URL: http://www.hrc.govt.nz/sites/default/files/CTCAE%20manual%20-%20DMCC.pdf

Leemans CR, Braakhuis BJM, Brakenhoff RH (2011) The molecular biology of head and neck cancer. *Nat Rev Cancer* 11:9–22.

Lorch JH, Goloubeva O, Haddad RI *et al.* (2011) Induction chemotherapy with cisplatin and fluorouracil alone or in combination with docetaxel in locally advanced squamous-cell cancer of the head and neck: long-term results of the TAX 324 randomised phase 3 trial. *Lancet Oncol* 12(2):153–159.

Mazeron JJ, Ardiet JM, Haie-Meder C *et al.* (2009) GEC-ESTRO recommendations for brachytherapy for head and neck squamous cell carcinomas. *Radiother Oncol* 91(2):150–156.

Peters LJ, Goepfert H, Ang KK *et al.* (1993) Evaluation of the dose for postoperative radiation therapy of head and neck cancer: first report of a prospective randomized trial. *Int J Radiat Oncol Biol Phys* 26(1):3–11.

Pignon JP, Bourhis J, Domenge C, Designe L (2000) Chemotherapy added to locoregional treatment for head and neck squamous-cell carcinoma: three meta-analyses of updated individual data. MACH-NC Collaborative Group. Meta-Analysis of Chemotherapy on Head and Neck Cancer. *Lancet* 355:949–955.

Pignon JP, le Maitre A, Maillard E, Bourhis J (2009) Meta-analysis of chemotherapy in head and neck cancer (MACH-NC): an update on 93 randomised trials and 17,346 patients. *Radiother Oncol* 92(1):4–14.

Sher DJ, Posner MR, Tishler RB *et al.* (2011) Relationship between radiation treatment time and overall survival after induction chemotherapy for locally advanced head and neck carcinoma: a subset analysis of TAX 324. *Int J Radiat Oncol Biol Phys* 81(5):e813–e818.

Vermorken JB, Remener E, van Herpen C *et al.* (2007) Cisplatin, fluorouracil, and docetaxel in unresectable head and neck cancer. *N Engl J Med* 357:1695–1704.

40 Nasopharynx

Anna W.M. Lee[1], W.T. Ng[2], Quynh Thu Le[3], Anthony T.C. Chan[4], Jimmy Y.W. Chan[5] and Henry C.K. Sze[4]

[1] Center of Clinical Oncology, The University of Hong Kong-Shenzhen Hospital, China
[2] Department of Clinical Oncology, Pamela Youde Nethersole Eastern Hospital, Hong Kong, China
[3] Department of Radiation Oncology, Stanford University Medical Center, Stanford, CA, USA
[4] Department of Clinical Oncology, Chinese University of Hong Kong, Hong Kong, China
[5] Department of Otolaryngology, University of Hong Kong, Hong Kong, China

Summary	Key facts
Introduction	- Nasopharyngeal carcinoma (NPC) has a distinct racial and geographical distribution - Aetiology is multifactorial (including inherited genetic predisposition and environmental factors): - Consistent association of Epstein–Barr virus (EBV) with non-keratinizing carcinoma suggests an oncogenic role in pathogenesis
Presentation	- Most common presenting symptom is a painless enlarging upper neck mass - Nasal: discharge, bleeding, obstruction - Aural: tinnitus, impaired hearing - Headache - Symptoms and signs of cranial nerve palsy (especially V and VI) - Systemic symptoms and signs of distant metastasis - Rarely dermatomyositis (as a paraneoplastic syndrome)

Scenario	- *Primary treatment*:
	  - Radiotherapy (RT) is the primary modality; the intensity-modulated (IMRT) technique is preferred:
	    - Stage I: definitive RT alone
	    - Stage II:
	      – RT + concurrent cisplatin
	      – RT alone may be considered for low-risk subgroups
	    - Stage III–IVB:
	      – RT + cisplatin-based concurrent ± adjuvant chemotherapy
	      – RT + induction–concurrent chemotherapy can be considered especially for Stage IVA–B
	    - Stage IVC: individualized
	- *Treatment of recurrence*:
	  - Salvage surgery for early local recurrence and/or cervical nodal relapse
	  - Re-irradiation if inoperable

Trials	- Intergroup-0099 Study; Al-Sarraf et al. (1998) *J Clin Oncol* 16(4):1310–1317:
	  - First randomized trial to demonstrate survival benefit of concurrent chemoradiotherapy (CRT) as compared to RT alone in advanced disease
	- Peng et al. (2012) *Radiother Oncol* 104(3):286–293:
	  - First randomized trial to confirm superiority of IMRT as compared to conventional 2D-RT
	- Li et al. (2013) *Cancer* 119(17):3170–3176:
	  - First randomized trial to show that selective upper neck irradiation is safe for node-negative NPC
	- Chen et al. (2012) *Lancet Oncol* 13:163–171:
	  - First randomized trial to evaluate the value of adding adjuvant chemotherapy after concurrent CRT (caveat: immature data)
	- Chen et al. (2011) *Natl Cancer Inst* 103:1–10:
	  - First randomized trial to demonstrate the benefit of concurrent CRT as compared to RT alone in Stage II (caveat: based on 2D-RT and suboptimal metastatic work-up)

UICC Manual of Clinical Oncology, Ninth Edition. Edited by Brian O'Sullivan, James D. Brierley, Anil K. D'Cruz, Martin F. Fey, Raphael Pollock, Jan B. Vermorken and Shao Hui Huang. © 2015 UICC. Published 2015 by John Wiley & Sons, Ltd.

Incidence, aetiology and surveillance

Nasopharyngeal carcinoma (NPC) has a distinct racial and geographical distribution, with 80% of patients coming from Asia. The incidence is highest among Southern Chinese and intermediate among Eskimos and populations in certain regions in North Africa. Incidence in high-risk populations starts to rise after 30 years of age, peaks at 40–60 years and declines thereafter. The peculiar epidemiological patterns suggest a multifactorial aetiology that includes both inherited genetic predisposition and environmental factors.

Incidence, aetiology and surveillance	Description

Incidence	• World age-standardized rate (ASR): 1.2 per 100,000:
	  ▪ >86,000 new cases of NPC in 2012
	• Distinct geographical and racial distribution
	  ▪ 80% of patients come from Asia
	  ▪ ASR in developed countries ≤0.5
	  ▪ ASR in Southern China ≥20 per 100,000 male population
	• Chinese descendants who have migrated to Western countries show progressively lower risk, but still retain a higher risk than the indigenous populations
	• Male-to-female ratio is 2–3:1
	• Age distribution:
	  ▪ Peak incidence at 40–60-years old in high-risk regions
	  ▪ Bimodal peaks at 15–25 and 50–59 years old in low-risk regions
	• Familial aggregation in diverse populations

Aetiology	• Multifactorial:
	  ▪ *Inherited genetic predisposition*:
	    ○ Specific haplotypes in human leucocyte antigen (HLA) and deoxyribonucleic acid (DNA) repair genetic polymorphisms may play pivotal roles in conferring differential risks of NPC
	  ▪ *Environmental factors*:
	    ○ EBV: probable oncogenic role for non-keratinizing carcinoma
	    ○ Carcinogens in traditional Southern Chinese food, particularly volatile nitrosamines in preserved salted fish
	    ○ Cigarette smoking, especially for keratinizing carcinoma

Screening	• EBV serology and/or DNA provide sensitive tools for screening of non-keratinizing carcinoma • Generally recommended for high-risk cohorts (family members of patients): ▪ Annual screening by EBV serology and nasopharyngoscopy can improve early detection No level I evidence to confirm cost-effectiveness of screening

Pathology

The World Health Organization classification system (2005) should be used to avoid confusing terms. Carcinoma of the nasopharynx is classified into non-keratinizing, keratinizing and basaloid type. The majority of patients, particularly those in high-risk regions, have the non-keratinizing type, which is almost invariably associated with EBV, irrespective of ethnic background. This type is further sub-classified into undifferentiated and differentiated subtypes; it is generally considered that this distinction has little clinical and prognostic significance. Other histological types are very rare.

Pathology	Description

Non-keratinizing carcinoma	• Most common histology: frequency varies from ≥95% of NPC in high-risk regions to 75% in low-risk regions
	• Microscopic features:
	  ▪ Solid sheets, irregular islands and trabeculae of tumour cells, intermingled with lymphocytes and plasma cells; no keratinization
	• Immunohistochemistry: almost invariably positive for EBV-encoded RNA (EBER) staining
	• Sub-classification:
	  ▪ Undifferentiated subtype (≥90% of non-keratinizing carcinoma):
	    ○ Syncytial-appearing large tumour cells with indistinct cell borders, round-to-ovoid vesicular nuclei and large central nucleoli
	  ▪ Differentiated subtype (<5% of non-keratinizing carcinoma):
	    ○ Cellular stratification and pavementing, often with a plexiform growth
	    ○ Slightly smaller tumour cells show fairly well-defined cell borders, more chromatin-rich nuclei, less prominent nucleoli and lower nuclear-to-cytoplasmic ratio

(continued)

Pathology	Description

Keratinizing carcinoma	• Frequency varies from <5% of NPC in high-risk regions to 25% in low-risk regions
	• Microscopic features:
	  ▪ Typical squamous differentiation with intercellular bridge and/or keratinization
	  ▪ Irregular islands of tumour cells with distinct cell borders, occasional keratin pearl formation, abundant desmoplastic stroma infiltrated by lymphocytes, plasma cells, neutrophils and eosinophils:
	    ○ Tumour cells are polygonal, stratified, with eosinophilic glassy cytoplasm
	• Immunohistochemistry:
	  ▪ Variable results on EBV detection: almost always positive in endemic areas, but only positive in a proportion of cases in low-risk regions

Basaloid squamous cell carcinoma	• Very rare
	• Microscopic features:
	  ▪ Small basaloid cells with hyperchromatic nuclei without nucleoli and scanty cytoplasm; closely packed, growing in a solid pattern with a lobular configuration
	  ▪ Squamous cells

Other	• Very rare
	• Various histology:
	  ▪ Adenocarcinoma
	  ▪ Salivary gland-type carcinoma
	  ▪ Soft tissue neoplasms
	  ▪ Haematolymphoid tumours
	  ▪ Tumours of bone and cartilage
	  ▪ Benign epithelial tumours

Presentation and natural history

NPC is a highly malignant cancer with extensive local infiltration, early lymphatic spread and a high predisposition for haematogenous dissemination.

Presentation and natural history		Description

Presentation		• Usually asymptomatic in the early stage
		• Most common presenting symptom is a painless, enlarging upper neck mass
		• Blood-stained post-nasal secretion, nasal bleeding/obstruction
		• Aural (tinnitus, impaired hearing, pain, discharge)
		• If locally advanced:
		  ▪ Headache
		  ▪ Facial numbness, diplopia
		  ▪ Trismus
		  ▪ Slurring of speech, swallowing difficulty
		• Systemic (weight loss or sign of distant metastasis)
		• Rarely dermatomyositis (as a paraneoplastic syndrome)

Routes of spread	Local	• *Anterior extension*:
		  ▪ Nasal fossa
		• *Lateral extension*:
		  ▪ Parapharyngeal and carotid spaces, pterygoid muscles
		• *Anterolateral extension*:
		  ▪ Pterygoid process, pterygomaxillary fissure, maxillary sinus, infratemporal fossa
		• *Posterior extension*:
		  ▪ Prevertebral muscles
		  ▪ C1–2 vertebrae
		• *Inferior extension*:
		  ▪ Oropharynx, hypopharynx

Presentation and natural history		Description

		• *Superior extension*:
		  ▪ Bone invasion at skull base (commonest basisphenoid, clivus), sphenoid and ethmoid sinuses
		  ▪ Direct infiltration or perineural spread via basal foramina (commonest foramen lacerum and ovale), cranial nerves (commonest fifth and sixth), intracranial extension (commonest cavernous sinus)

	Regional	• ≥85% of cases have lymphatic involvement at diagnosis, often bilateral involvement
		• Orderly spread from upper neck downward towards the clavicle:
		  ▪ Skip metastasis is rare (between 0.5% and 8% in different studies)
		• Three main routes of spread:
		  ▪ Retropharyngeal node of Rouvière
		  ▪ Deep anterior cervical chain
		  ▪ Posterior cervical chain
		• Frequency of nodal involvement at different radiological levels:
		  ▪ First echelon: level II (70%), lateral retropharyngeal (69%)
		  ▪ Second echelon: levels III (45%), V (27%) and IV (11%)
		  ▪ Third echelon: level IB (3%), supraclavicular (3%), level VI (2%) and parotid (1%)

	Metastatic	• ≤10% of patients present with gross metastasis • ≥20% of patients with advanced locoregional diseases subsequently develop distant metastasis • Commonest sites of metastases: bone, lung, liver, distant lymph node

Diagnostic work-up

Diagnostic work-up	Description

Work-up	• History and physical exam including cranial nerve examination
	• Nasopharyngoscopy and biopsy
	• Staging after confirmation of diagnosis:
	  ▪ Magnetic resonance imaging (MRI) of nasopharynx, base of skull and neck
	  ▪ Computed tomography (CT) if MRI is contraindicated or unaffordable
	  ▪ Complete blood cell count, serum biochemistry (including liver function tests)
	  ▪ Chest X-ray
	  ▪ Full metastatic work-up if Stage III–IV, suspicious clinical sign or biochemical abnormality:
	    ○ Positron emission tomography (PET)-CT is preferred
	    ○ Alternatively, CT chest and upper abdomen, isotope bone scan

Tumour markers	• Plasma/serum load of EBV-DNA: both pre- and post-treatment copies are useful for prognostication and early detection of disease relapse (particularly distant metastasis). • Serum EBV serology IgA antiviral capsid antigen: useful for screening and diagnosis, but doubtful value for prognostication and post-treatment monitoring

Staging and prognostic grouping

UICC TNM staging

The TNM staging at presentation is unanimously the most important prognostic factor (Table 40.1).

Prognostic factors

Among patients with distant metastases, those with oligometastasis (particularly lung alone) have a better prognosis than those with other sites of metastasis (Table 40.2). Histologically, non-keratinizing carcinoma has a better prognosis than the keratinizing type. There is increasing evidence that the gross tumour volume (GTV) and EBV-DNA are independent prognostic factors valuable for supplementing the TNM staging. Female patients have a better prognosis than male patients. Elderly patients, particularly those with multiple co-morbidities, have a poor prognosis. Attempts to improve prognostic accuracy are important for developing personalized medicine with treatment tailored to individual risk.

Treatment philosophy

Definitive radiation therapy (RT) is the primary treatment modality because NPC is a radiosensitive tumour and its anatomical location makes surgical resection technically difficult. Early cancers (Stage I) are treated with RT alone with excellent outcome. A combined modality treatment strategy with the addition of concurrent chemotherapy using cisplatin is universally recommended for Stage III–IVB. There are variations in the major guidelines regarding whether adjuvant chemotherapy

Table 40.1 UICC TNM categories and stage grouping: Nasopharynx

TNM categories	
T1	Nasopharynx, oropharynx or nasal cavity
T2	Parapharyngeal extension
T3	Bony structures of skull base/paranasal sinuses
T4	Intracranial, cranial nerves, hypopharynx, orbit, infratemporal fossa/masticator space
N1	Unilateral cervical, unilateral or bilateral retropharyngeal lymph nodes, above supraclavicular fossa, ≤6 cm
N2	Bilateral cervical above supraclavicular fossa, ≤6 cm
N3a	>6 cm
N3b	Supraclavicular fossa
M1	Distant metastasis

Stage grouping			
Stage 0	Tis	N0	M0
Stage I	T1	N0	M0
Stage II	T1	N1	M0
	T2	N0, N1	M0
Stage III	T1, T2	N2	M0
	T3	N0, N1, N2	M0
Stage IVA	T4	N0, N1, N2	M0
Stage IVB	Any T	N3	M0
Stage IVC	Any T	Any N	M1

Table 40.2 Prognostic factors for nasopharyngeal carcinoma

Prognostic factors	Tumour related	Host related	Environment related
Essential	Presenting stage Histological type	Age Performance status Co-morbidities	Facilities for staging work-up (MRI, PET-CT) Facilities for high-quality radiotherapy (conformal techniques and precision) Appropriate addition of chemotherapy Expertise in radiotherapy and chemotherapy
Additional	EBV-DNA Gross tumour volume Site of metastases	LDH	Optimization of radiotherapy dose fractionation Optimization of chemotherapy sequence and drugs
New and promising	Biomarkers Gene signatures		Advances in diagnostic and therapeutic technology

Data sources: Chan (2012), NCCN (2014).

using cisplatin-based combinations should be further added. Induction–concurrent chemotherapy is currently being evaluated in randomized trials. This strategy may be considered particularly for Stage IVA–B because upfront use of a potent combination at full dose may be more effective for eradicating micrometastasis, and shrinkage of locoregional disease may help in attaining a wider margin for RT. CRT is generally recommended for Stage II, but it is also questioned whether low-risk patients can be safely treated by RT alone and be spared unnecessary chemotherapy. Treatment for Stage IVC should be individualized: radical treatment should be considered for those with oligometastasis and good performance status. All patients should be closely monitored because early detection of recurrence significantly affects the chance of survival. Aggressive salvage should be considered for patients with local/regional recurrence or oligometastasis whenever possible. Patients should be followed up for life to ensure proper management of late toxicities (if any).

Scenario	Treatment philosophy
Local disease (Stage I)	• Definitive RT alone
Regional disease (Stage II–IVB)	• *Stage II*: 　▪ RT + concurrent chemotherapy 　▪ RT alone may be considered for non-bulky disease and low EBV-DNA • *Stage III–IVB* (variation in major guidelines): 　▪ RT + concurrent chemotherapy (universal acceptance) 　▪ Addition of adjuvant chemotherapy (advocated in NCCN guideline) 　▪ Addition of induction chemotherapy to concurrent chemoradiotherapy may be considered particularly for Stages IVA–B

Scenario	Treatment philosophy

Metastatic disease (Stage IVC)	• Individualized:
	  ▪ Oligometastasis and good performance status:
	    ○ Induction and concurrent chemotherapy, definitive RT to nasopharyngeal and cervical regions, plus surgery/high-dose RT to metastasis
	  ▪ Extensive metastasis: palliative chemotherapy ± RT to symptomatic sites

Recurrent disease (see Chapter 39)	• *Local and/or regional*:
	  ▪ Salvage surgery
	  ▪ Re-irradiation if salvage surgery is not feasible
	  ▪ Addition of induction and/or concurrent chemotherapy may be considered
	• *Distant*:
	  ▪ Oligometastasis and good performance status:
	    ○ Chemotherapy and surgery/high-dose RT to metastasis
	  ▪ Extensive metastasis:
	    ○ Palliative chemotherapy ± RT to symptomatic sites
	• Patients encouraged to participate in clinical trials to test new drugs

Follow-up	• History, physical exam and nasopharyngoscopy 6–8 weeks post-RT:
	  ▪ Additional boost dose may be considered if residual local/regional disease detected
	• History, physical exam, nasopharyngoscopy and imaging exam (MRI, PET-CT) 12–16 weeks post RT:
	  ▪ Consider surgery if feasible for persistent disease
	• Regular follow-up for patients with documented complete remission:
	  ▪ History, physical exam and nasopharyngoscopy:
	    ○ Every 2–3 months for the first 3 years
	    ○ Every 4–6 months for Years 4 and 5
	    ○ Every 6 months for Years 6–10
	    ○ Annually thereafter
	  ▪ Follow-up past 5 years is recommended because recurrence can occur much later than in other head and neck cancers
	  ▪ Chest radiograph and MRI annually for at least first 3 years is preferred
	  ▪ Metastatic surveillance if suspicious signs
	• Plasma/serum EBV-DNA is a useful additional tool for post-treatment surveillance, particularly for distant metastases:
	  ▪ Full metastatic follow-up should be performed if persistent/progressive elevation

Treatment

Surgery

Surgery	Description
Primary treatment	Surgery has little role other than in biopsy for diagnosis

Early local recurrence	• Small and superficial tumour in the nasopharynx (rT1) can be resected via the endoscopic approach, or by transoral robotic surgery:
	  ▪ *Endoscopic approach*:
	    ○ *En bloc* resection of tumour using electric knife with an adjustable angle of knife point or laser
	    ○ Particularly useful for tumours located at the roof or posterior wall of the nasopharynx
	    ○ For tumours arising from the lateral wall, endoscopic access is facilitated by removing the medial wall of the maxillary sinus
	  ▪ *Transoral robotic surgery*:
	    ○ 360° motion of the instruments provides excellent access to cutting and suturing tissue
	    ○ Tumour is visualized using a 0° 8-mm dual channel camera introduced transorally
	    ○ Tumour is removed using a 5-mm Maryland grasping forceps mounted on the left robotic arm and 8-mm scissors with monopolar diathermy mounted on the right robotic arm
	    ○ Particularly useful for tumours with minimal parapharyngeal invasion

(continued)

Surgery	Description

Advanced local recurrence	• Different approaches have been advocated, with choice of option based on location of the recurrence and expertise
	• For tumours that extend across the midline or invade the parapharyngeal space, an open approach is indicated
	• *Maxillary swing approach* (one of the approaches with extensive data):
	  ▪ Particularly useful for tumours with parapharyngeal extension
	  ▪ A temporalis muscle or microvascular free flap is needed if the petrosal internal carotid artery is exposed during the operation
	• *Two-stage operation* for a more advanced tumour encasing the petrosal internal carotid artery (ICA) or eroding the skull base:
	  ▪ First stage: extracranial–intracranial vascular bypass
	  ▪ Second stage: tumour, including the petrosal ICA and the skull base around the carotid canal, is removed *en bloc* via a combined craniofacial approach

Regional recurrence (see Chapter 39)	• Surgical resection is the treatment of choice for operable nodal recurrence:
	  ▪ For retropharyngeal nodal recurrence: maxillary swing approach
	  ▪ For other cervical nodal recurrence: modified radical neck dissection is preferred:
	    ○ *Note*: Radical neck dissection is not recommended routinely unless structures are involved
	  ▪ For nodal recurrence with macroscopic extracapsular spread: extended radical neck dissection with removal of the overlying skin followed, preferably, by insertion of afterloading tubes for brachytherapy

Metastases (see Chapter 39)	• Individualized: ▪ Oligometastasis and good performance status: resection of metastasis may be considered

Radiotherapy

Radiotherapy	Description

Early disease	• RT is the primary treatment modality:
	  ▪ IMRT is preferred
	• Patient set up in supine position, immobilized by thermoplastic head and neck (including shoulder) mask
	• Fusion of MRI and PET-CT with planning contrast-enhanced CT for target delineation
	• Clinical target volume (CTV):
	  ▪ CTV_1: gross tumour volume (GTV) with 2–5-mm margin (some centres also include whole nasopharynx)
	  ▪ CTV_2: CTV_1 with 5-mm margin + high-risk subclinical sites:
	    ○ Local: entire nasopharynx (if not covered in CTV_1), parapharyngeal spaces, posterior third of the nasal cavity/maxillary sinuses, pterygoid fossae, lower half of the sphenoid sinus, skull base, anterior half of clivus
	    ○ Nodal: bilateral retropharyngeal, levels Ib, II, III and Va
	  ▪ CTV_3: lower nodal levels IV, Vb and supraclavicular fossa
	    ○ Selective sparing of Ib and lower nodes for node-negative neck
	    ○ Differential margin at areas adjacent to critical normal structures
	      – Planning target volume (PTV) – CTV with 3–5-mm additional margin
	• Planning organ at risk volume (PRV):
	  ▪ 3–5 mm for spinal cord
	  ▪ 1–3 mm for other critical organs at risk (OAR)
	• Dose prescription:
	  ▪ CTV_1: 70 Gy in 33–35 fractions (avoid large fractional dose)
	  ▪ CTV_2: 60 Gy (equivalent)
	  ▪ CTV_3: 50 Gy (equivalent)
	• Planning priority and dose constraint for OAR (see Box 40.1)

Radiotherapy	Description
Advanced non-metastatic disease	• RT same as for early disease except increase CTV$_2$ if T3–4 to cover entire sphenoid sinus, whole clivus, cavernous sinus • Chemotherapy in concurrence with RT is recommended (see below)
Metastatic disease	• Individualized: 　▪ Stage IVC with oligometastasis and good performance: definitive RT as above + chemotherapy and surgery/high-dose RT to metastasis 　▪ Stereotactic ablative radiotherapy may be considered for suitable cases 　▪ Extensive metastases: palliative RT

Box 40.1 Intensity-modulated radiation therapy for nasopharyngeal carcinoma: examples of specification on planning priorities and dose constraints for organs at risk

Organ at risk	RTOG 0615	PYNEH Ideal	PYNEH Acceptable
Priority 1: Critical organs at risk (OAR) and gross tumour volumes (GTV)			
Spinal cord	≤1% V >50 Gy	≤45 Gy	≤1 mL >50 Gy
Brainstem	≤1% V >60 Gy	≤54 Gy	≤1% V >60 Gy
Optic chiasm	≤54 Gy	≤54 Gy	≤60 Gy
Optic nerves	≤54 Gy	(Priority 2)	
Brachial plexus	≤66 Gy	(Priority 3)	
Mandible/temporomandibular joint	≤70 Gy, ≤1 mL >75 Gy	(Priority 3)	
GTV-T and GTV-N	–	Minimal ≥68.6 Gy	Minimal ≥66.5 Gy
Priority 2: Other critical OAR and planning tumour volumes (PTV)			
Optic nerves	(Priority 1)	≤54 Gy	≤60 Gy
Temporal lobes	–	1 mL <65 Gy	≤72 Gy
PTV	95% V ≥100% D, 99% V ≥93% D	100% V ≥95% D	95% V ≥100% D, 99% V ≥93% D
(PTV_70)	<20% V ≥77 Gy, <5% V ≥80 Gy	<10% V ≥75 Gy	<20% V ≥77 Gy
Priority 3: Organs with intermediate importance			
Brachial plexus	(Priority 1)	≤66 Gy	≤1 mL >66 Gy
Mandible/temporomandibular joint	(Priority 1)	≤1 mL >70 Gy	≤1 mL >75 Gy
Parotid glands (at least one gland)	Mean <26 Gy, ≥50% V <30 Gy	Mean <26 Gy	≥50% V <30 Gy
Pituitary	–	≤60 Gy	≤65 Gy
Lens	(Priority 4)	≤6 Gy	≤10 Gy
Eyeball	(Priority 4)	≤50 Gy	Mean <35 Gy
Priority 4: Organs with less importance			
Lens	≤25 Gy	(Priority 3)	
Eyeballs	≤50 Gy	(Priority 3)	
Cochlea	≤5% V ≥55 Gy	Mean <50 Gy	≤55 Gy
Glottic larynx	Mean <45 Gy		Mean <45 Gy
Postcricoid pharynx, oesophagus (within field)	Mean <45 Gy		Mean <45 Gy
Oral cavity (excluding PTV)	Mean <40 Gy	Mean <40 Gy	Mean <50 Gy

*RTOG 0615, Radiation Therapy Oncology Group 0615 Study; PYNEH, Pamela Youde Nethersole Eastern Hospital; V, volume; D, prescribed radiotherapy dose in Gy.

Systemic therapy

Systemic therapy	Description
Early disease	• *Stage I*: not indicated • *Stage II*: concurrent chemotherapy using cisplatin 30 mg/m² in 1 L of normal saline, intravenous infusion (IVI) over 2 hours, weekly starting on the first day of RT • *Good-risk Stage II* (non-bulky and low EBV-DNA, with thorough metastatic work-up, irradiated by conformal/IMRT) – may be spared

Advanced non-metastatic disease	• Variation in major guidelines
	• Concurrent chemotherapy: two common schemes:
	  ▪ Cisplatin 30–40 mg/m² IV infusion weekly
	  ▪ Cisplatin 100 mg/m² IV infusion every 3 weeks
	• Concurrent–adjuvant chemotherapy (Intergroup-0099 regimen advocated in NCCN guideline):
	  ▪ *Concurrent phase*: cisplatin 100 mg/m² IV infusion every 3 weeks or cisplatin 30–40 mg/m² IV infusion weekly
	  ▪ *Adjuvant phase*: cisplatin 80 mg/m² IV infusion + 5-fluorouracil (5-FU) 1000 mg/m²/day IV infusion for 96 hours, every 4 weeks for three cycles
	• Induction–concurrent chemotherapy (can be considered particularly for Stage IVA–B:
	  ▪ *Induction phase*: various regimens have been used:
	    ○ Cisplatin 100 mg/m² IV infusion and 5-FU 1000 mg/m²/day IV infusion for 120 hours, every 3 weeks for three cycles
	    ○ TPF regimen (docetaxel + cisplatin + 5-FU) has also been explored recently in clinical trials, but more definitive results are still awaited
	  ▪ *Concurrent phase*: cisplatin either 100 mg/m² IV infusion every 3 weeks or 30–40 mg/m² IV infusion weekly

Metastatic disease	• *Platinum-based doublets*:
	  ▪ Platinum compounds (cisplatin, carboplatin) + fluorouracil/capecitabine, gemcitabine, taxanes (paclitaxel, docetaxel), bleomycin, ifosfamide, anthracyclines, irinotecan and/or vinorelbine
	• *Platinum-based triplets*:
	  ▪ Less commonly used due to higher toxicity rate
	  ▪ Options include paclitaxel + cisplatin + 5-FU; carboplatin + paclitaxel + gemcitabine ± maintenance chemotherapy using 5-FU
	• Molecular targeted therapy:
	  ▪ About 10% response rate only
	  ▪ No current role outside clinical trials
	• Immunotherapy (including adoptive immunotherapy against EBV antigen and EBV vaccine):
	  ▪ Experimental; no current role outside clinical trials

Controversies

While there is universal agreement that Stage I patients should be treated with definitive RT alone and concurrent cisplatin-based CRT is recommended for patients with Stage III–IVB disease, major controversies remain.

Need for adjuvant chemotherapy for all Stage II patients

The NCCN guidelines recommend inclusion of Stage II patients because the Intergroup-0099 Study designed for Stage III–IV (according to the AJCC/UICC staging system, 4th edition) had included 17 patients with Stage II (according to the current 7th edition). This raised concerns because many centres could achieve satisfactory results for Stage II non-keratinizing carcinoma by RT alone even when using the 2D-RT technique.

The randomized trial by Chen QY et al. (2011) showed that the CRT group had significantly better results than the RT alone group: 5-year overall survival (OS) (95% vs 86%) and distant failure-free rate (D-FFR) (95% vs 84%). However, the patients were treated by 2D-RT and staged by conventional metastatic work-up (chest radiography, abdominal sonography, bone scan).

The question remains whether the magnitude of benefit will be substantially smaller for patients irradiated by the modern conformal/IMRT technique and more accurate metastatic work-up by PET-CT. Further studies on risk-stratification by additional prognostic factors (including tumour volume and EBV-DNA copies) are warranted to spare patients unnecessary treatment and associated toxicities.

Value of adjuvant chemotherapy in addition to concurrent chemotherapy

The Intergroup-0099 Study using concurrent + adjuvant chemotherapy was the first trial to achieve significant benefit in both progression-free survival (PFS) and OS. Three subsequent trials confirmed that this regimen could improve PFS ± OS. An exploratory study showed that patients who had received two or more cycles of adjuvant chemotherapy had significantly better D-FFR. However, the adjuvant phase was generally poorly tolerated and meta-analyses on trials testing adjuvant chemotherapy *per se* showed little benefit.

Hence, there are variations in major guidelines regarding whether concurrent–adjuvant chemotherapy or concurrent chemotherapy alone is the standard recommendation. The preliminary results of the randomized trial by Chen L et al. (2012) showed that the concurrent–adjuvant CRT group had similar 2-year results as compared to the concurrent CRT group. However, longer follow-up is needed to confirm the results because, though statistically insignificant, the actuarial curves and hazard ratio for failure-free rate and D-FFR show trends in favour of the concurrent + adjuvant group. A large scale meta-analysis based on updated data of 4798 patients from 19 trials showed that there was a significant benefit in favour of CT regarding OS (absolute benefit at 5 years 6.4%). There was a significant interaction between treatment effect on OS and the timing of CT ($P = 0.01$); in favour of concomitant with adjuvant CT (HR 0.65; 95% CI 0.56–0.76) or concomitant without adjuvant CT (HR 0.79; 95% CI 0.68–0.92), compared to induction CT (HR 0.96, 95% CI 0.80–1.16]) or adjuvant CT (HR 0.93; (5% CI 0.70–1.24).

Possibility of further improvement by changing to an induction–concurrent sequence

This strategy is theoretically beneficial for NPC because upfront use of potent chemotherapy combinations at full dose may be more effective for eradicating micrometastasis, and shrinkage of locoregional disease may help in attaining a wider margin for RT. All single-arm phase II studies have shown encouraging results, but two randomized phase II trials showed conflicting results. Five randomized phase III trials are on-going to evaluate this strategy.

Benefit of accelerated fractionation for non-keratinizing NPC

Prolongation of overall treatment time is detrimental, but the benefit of acceleration has not been fully studied. One randomized phase III trial on patients treated with RT alone showed that the group with altered fractionation (78 Gy in 60 fractions over 6 weeks) and significantly better 5-year local failure-free rate (L-FFR) and OS than the conventional fractionation group (70 Gy in 35 fractions over 7 weeks). The altered fractionation group had higher acute toxicities, but the incidence rates of late neurological damage were similar. However, the applicability in the modern era is questionable as the management during the study period was suboptimal by modern standards (patients were staged by CT, irradiated by 2D-RT and none had chemotherapy). The NPC-9902 Trial suggested that concurrent–adjuvant chemotherapy + accelerated fractionation could achieve significantly better PFS than conventional RT alone, but further validation is needed. This issue is one of the study objectives of the ongoing NPC-0501 Trial.

Phase III clinical trials

See Table 40.3.

Table 40.3 Phase III clinical trials

Trial reference	Results
Radiotherapy	
Peng et al (2012) *Radiother Oncol* 104(3):286–293	• Comparison of outcomes and toxicities for IMRT vs conventional 2D-RT for the treatment of NPC • IMRT was significantly better than 2D-RT in 5-year local control rate (91% vs 85%) and overall survival (OS) (80% vs 67%) • Nodal control rate (N-FFR) was similar (92% vs 93%) • Distant control rate (D-FFR) was not reported • Subgroup analyses showed that the greatest improvement was for T4, N2 and Stage III • IMRT group had significantly lower radiation-induced toxicities than the 2D-RT group, but temporal necrosis rate was still worrisome (13% vs 21%)
Li et al. (2013) *Cancer* 119(17):3170–3176	• Comparing of prophylactic upper (UNI) versus whole-neck irradiation (WNI) in the treatment of patients with node-negative NPC • With a median follow-up of 39 months, no patient in either group had nodal relapse • Both groups had similar 3-year relapse-free survival, D-FFR and OS (90% in the UNI group vs 87% in the WNI group)
Pow et al. (2006) *Int J Radiat Oncol Biol Phys* 66(4):981–991	• Comparison of xerostomia and quality of life after IMRT vs 2D-RT for early-stage NPC • At 12 months post-RT, the IMRT group had significantly better recovery of stimulated salivary flow than the 2D-RT group: the proportion of patients with recovery to above 25% of baseline was 83% vs 10% for parotid flow, and 50% vs 5% for whole salivary flow • IMRT group showed consistent improvement in xerostomia-related symptoms, and attained significantly higher subscale scores on quality of life (for role-physical, bodily pain and physical function)

(continued)

Table 40.3 (Continued)

Trial reference	Results
Adjuvant systemic therapy	
Intergroup Study 0099 Al-Sarraf et al. (1998) *J Clin Oncol* 16(4):1310–1317	• Comparison of CRT vs RT alone in patients with advanced NPC • First trial to demonstrate significant survival from the addition of chemotherapy to RT for NPC • When compared with RT alone, the CRT group (using concurrent cisplatin + adjuvant cisplatin and 5-FU) had significantly better 3-year PFS (69% vs 24%) and OS (78% vs 47%) • Further follow-up showed sustained improvement (5-year OS: 67% vs 37%)
Chen L et al. (2012) *Lancet Oncol* 13:163–171	• Comparison of concurrent CRT + adjuvant chemotherapy vs concurrent CRT alone in patients with locoregionally advanced NPC • No significant difference in failure-free rate between concurrent CRT + adjuvant chemotherapy group and the concurrent CRT-only group: 86% vs 84% at 2 years (hazard ratio 0.74; 95% CI 0.49–1.10; $P = 0.13$) • Corresponding D-FFR was 88% vs 86% (hazard ratio 0.71; 95% CI 0.48–1.10; $P = 0.12$) • Caution is needed in interpretation: longer follow-up is needed to confirm the results because, although statistically insignificant, the concurrent + adjuvant group showed a favourable trend for the above endpoints
Chen QY et al. (2011) *Natl Cancer Inst* 103:1–10	• Comparison of concurrent CRT vs RT alone in Stage II NPC • CRT group had significantly better results than the RT alone group: 5-year OS (95% vs 86%); PFS (88% vs 78%) and D-FFR (95% vs 84%). • No significant difference in 5-year locoregional FFR (93% vs 91%) • CRT group had significantly more acute toxicities, but the late toxicity rate did not increase statistically significantly • Caution is needed in interpretation: some centres achieved better results by RT alone for Stage II (particularly for those cases without adverse prognostic factors)

Areas of research

- Optimizing the timing or the sequencing of systemic chemotherapy with concurrent CRT. Presently, several trials are ongoing to test whether changing the sequence of chemotherapy can decrease distant metastasis and improve OS:
  - Induction–concurrent vs concurrent–adjuvant CRT: NPC-0501 by Hong Kong NPC Study Group
  - Induction–concurrent vs concurrent CRT: NPC2006 by GORTEC, NCT01245959 by Sun Yat-Sen University, NCT00201396 by Taiwan Cooperative Oncology Group
- Biomarker-driven personalized therapy:
  - NPC-0502 Trial by Hong Kong NPC Study Group is randomizing patients with persistently detectable EBV-DNA after concurrent CRT to adjuvant chemotherapy with gemcitabine + cisplatin vs observation
  - RTOG will be testing the concept that post-CRT EBV-DNA level can be used in risk stratification to select patients who may benefit from adjuvant chemotherapy
- Identifying the optimal radiation fractionation:
  - NPC-0501 Trial by Hong Kong NPC Study Group is also trying to evaluate the benefit of accelerated RT fractionation compared to conventional fractionation
  - Impact of large fractional dose (simultaneous boost in IMRT) on therapeutic ratio
  - Value of dose escalation for selected high-risk patients
- Development of new technology and more accurate knowledge of tolerance dose for the optimization of therapeutic ratio
- Development of novel systemic therapy with greater potency and fewer toxicities
- More accurate prognostication by improvement of TNM staging, biomarkers and gene signature for development of personalized medicine
- Prevention and early detection

Recommended reading

Al-Sarraf M, LeBlanc M, Giri PG et al. (1998) Chemoradiotherapy versus radiotherapy in patients with advanced nasopharyngeal cancer: phase III randomized Intergroup study 0099. *J Clin Oncol* 16(4):1310–1317.

Baujat B, Audry H, Bourhis J et al. (2006) Chemotherapy in locally advanced nasopharyngeal carcinoma: an individual patient data meta-analysis of eight randomized trials and 1753 patients. *Int J Radiat Oncol Biol Phys* 64:47–56.

Chan AT, Leung SF, Ngan RK et al. (2005) Overall survival after concurrent cisplatin-radiotherapy compared with radiotherapy alone in locoregionally advanced nasopharyngeal carcinoma. *J Natl Cancer Inst* 97:536–539.

Chan ATC, Gregoire V, Lefebvre JL et al. (2012) Nasopharyngeal cancer: EHNS-ESMO-ESTRO Clinical Practice Guidelines for diagnosis, treatment and follow-up. *Ann Oncol* 23(Suppl 7):vii83–85.

Chen L, Hu CS, Chen XZ et al. (2012). Concurrent chemoradiotherapy plus adjuvant chemotherapy versus concurrent chemoradiotherapy alone in patients with locoregionally advanced nasopharyngeal carcinoma: a phase 3 multicenter randomized controlled trial. *Lancet Oncol* 13:163–171.

Chen QY, Wen YF, Guo L et al. (2011) Concurrent chemoradiotherapy vs. radiotherapy alone in stage ii nasopharyngeal carcinoma: Phase III randomized trial. *Natl Cancer Inst* 103:1–10.

Lee AWM, Tung SY, Chua DT et al. (2010) Randomized trial of radiotherapy plus concurrent-adjuvant chemotherapy vs. radiotherapy alone for regionally advanced nasopharyngeal carcinoma. *J Natl Cancer Inst* 102:1188–1198.

Lee AWM, Fee WE Jr, Ng WT *et al.* (2012) Nasopharyngeal carcinoma: salvage of local recurrence (review article). *Oral Oncol* 48:768–774.

Lee AWM, Lin JC, Ng WT (2012) Current management of nasopharyngeal cancer. *Semin Radiat Oncol* 22:233–244.

Lee AWM, Ng WT, Chan LK *et al.* (2012) The strength/weakness of the AJCC/UICC staging system (7th edition) for nasopharyngeal cancer and suggestions for future improvement. *Oral Oncol* 48:1007–1013.

Lee N, Harris J, Garden AS *et al.* (2009) Intensity-modulated radiation therapy with or without chemotherapy for nasopharyngeal carcinoma: radiation therapy oncology group phase II trial 0225. *J Clin Oncol* 27:3684–3690.

Lee N, Zhang Q, Pfister DG *et al.* (2012) Phase II study of the addition of bevacizumab to standard chemoradiation for loco-regionally advanced nasopharyngeal carcinoma: Radiation Therapy Oncology Group (RTOG) Trial 0615. *Lancet Oncol* 13:172–180.

Li JG, Yuan X, Zhang LL *et al.* (2013) A randomized clinical trial comparing prophylactic upper versus whole-neck irradiation in the treatment of patients with node-negative nasopharyngeal carcinoma. *Cancer* 119(17):3170–3176.

Lin JC, Wang WY, Chen KY *et al.* (2004) Quantification of plasma Epstein-Barr virus DNA in patients with advanced nasopharyngeal carcinoma. *N Engl J Med* 350:2461–2470.

Lo YM, Chan LY, Lo KW *et al.* (1999) Quantitative analysis of cell-free Epstein-Barr virus DNA in plasma of patients with nasopharyngeal carcinoma. *Cancer Res* 59:1188–1191.

NCCN Treatment guidelines in Oncology: Head and Neck Cancers. Version 2.2013 NCCN.org

Pan ZQ, He XY, Guo XM *et al.* (2012) A Phase III study of late course accelerated hyperfractionated radiotherapy versus conventionally fractionated radiotherapy in patients with nasopharyngeal carcinoma. *Am J Clin Oncol* 35:600–605.

Peng G, Wang T, Yang KY *et al.* (2012) A prospective, randomized study comparing outcomes and toxicities of intensity-modulated radiotherapy vs. conventional two-dimensional radiotherapy for the treatment of nasopharyngeal carcinoma. *Radiother Oncol* 104(3):286–293.

Pow HN, Kwong LW, McMillan S *et al.* (2006) Xerostomia and quality of life after intensity-modulated radiotherapy vs. conventional radiotherapy for early-stage nasopharyngeal carcinoma: initial report on a randomized controlled clinical trial. *Int J Radiat Oncol Biol Phys* 66(4):981–991.

41 Oral cavity

Richa Vaish[1], Mitali Dandekar[1], Jai Prakash Agarwal[2], Kumar Prabhash[3] and Anil K. D'Cruz[1]

[1]Department of Head and Neck Surgical Oncology, Tata Memorial Centre, Mumbai, India
[2]Department of Radiation Oncology, Tata Memorial Centre, Mumbai, India
[3]Department of Medical Oncology, Tata Memorial Centre, Mumbai, India

Summary	Key facts
Introduction	- Global health problem - Main aetiological factors include tobacco (smoked and smokeless) and alcohol - Squamous cell carcinoma (SCC) is the most common histological subtype - Affects multiple subsites that comprise the oral cavity: - Lip, buccal mucosa, oral tongue, floor of mouth, upper alveolus, lower alveolus, retromolar trigone and hard palate - Although each subsite has distinct features, the broad principles of management remain the same
Presentation	- Commonly presents as a non-healing ulcer, exophytic mass, patch, growth, facial swelling, pain that can refer to the ear, ankyloglossia, neck nodes, spontaneous loosening of teeth - Buccal cancers usually cause fewer symptoms and hence patients present late compared to tongue cancers

Scenario	- *Early cancers*: single-modality treatment
	- *Locally-advanced cancers*: warrant a multimodality approach
	- *Locally-advanced resectable disease*:
	  - Surgery is the initial treatment of choice (excepting some superficial T3 lesion on lip, retromolar trigone and buccal mucosa/gingiva where aesthetic/functional considerations may warrant alternative strategies, e.g. radiotherapy)
	  - Postoperative radiotherapy ± chemotherapy should be considered for cases with adverse pathological features
	- *Locally-advanced unresectable disease*:
	  - Definitive radiotherapy with concurrent chemotherapy may be appropriate for selected cases where cure is still possible
	  - Induction chemotherapy may be considered for selected cases
	  - Patients unable to tolerate intensified treatment: palliative treatment whenever appropriate
	- *Metastatic disease*: palliative treatment whenever appropriate

Trials	- RTOG 9501; Cooper *et al.* (2004) *N Engl J Med* 350:1937–1944:
	  - Postoperative adjuvant chemoradiotherapy improves local and regional control rates and disease-free survival in high-risk postoperative head and neck cancer patients
	- EORTC 22931; Bernier *et al.* (2004) *N Engl J Med.* 350:1945–1952
	  - Postoperative concurrent chemoradiotherapy is better than radiotherapy alone in patients with locally-advanced head and neck cancers
	- Sankaranarayanan *et al.* (2005) *Lancet* 365:1927–1933:
	  - Visual screening of the oral cavity can reduce mortality only in individuals at high-risk for oral cancers
	- Zhong *et al.* (2013) *J Clin Oncol* 31(6):744–751:
	  - In resectable Stage III or IVA oral SCC, taxane + platinum + 5-fluorouracil (TPF) induction chemotherapy does not improve survival compared to upfront surgery
	- Pignon *et al.* (2009) *Radiother Oncol* 92:4–14 (meta-analysis):
	  - Concurrent chemoradiotherapy is the best way to combine chemotherapy with radiotherapy in head and neck cancer

UICC Manual of Clinical Oncology, Ninth Edition. Edited by Brian O'Sullivan, James D. Brierley, Anil K. D'Cruz, Martin F. Fey, Raphael Pollock, Jan B. Vermorken and Shao Hui Huang. © 2015 UICC. Published 2015 by John Wiley & Sons, Ltd.

Introduction

Oral cancers are a heterogeneous group of cancers that affect multiple subsites. This chapter focuses on the predominant histological subtype: squamous cell carcinoma (SCC). Although each subsite has distinct features, the broad principles of management remain the same. The various subsites included in oral cavity cancers are the following:
- Lip: comprising of the external and inner upper and lower lip as well as the commissure
- Tongue: anterior two thirds of the tongue comprising of the dorsum, lateral borders and ventral surface posteriorly limited by circumvallate papillae
- Gum: including upper and lower alveolar mucosa
- Floor of mouth: including the anterior, lateral and unspecified floor of the mouth
- Palate: includes the hard palate
- Buccal mucosa: comprising the buccal mucosa of the cheek and the vestibule of the mouth as well as the retromolar area.

Incidence, aetiology and screening

Oral cancer is a global health problem. There is a wide geographical variation in its incidence, with approximately two-thirds of cases occurring in the developing countries of South-East Asia, Central and Eastern Europe, and Northern America. Tobacco, areca nut and alcohol are the main aetiological factors. Gingivo buccal cancers (alveolar ridge, buccal mucosa and retromolar cancer) are the predominantly involved subsites in the South-East Asian subcontinent, while tongue and floor of mouth cancers are more common in the Western world due to difference in the type of tobacco consumption. The age group between 55 and 64 years has the highest incidence in the Western world, while it presents a decade earlier in developing countries.

Incidence, aetiology and screening	Description

Incidence	- Oral cavity cancer is the tenth most common cancer amongst men:
	  - The age-standardized rate (ASR) of oral cancer worldwide is about 4 per 100,000
	  - Affects around 300,000 individuals every year globally
	  - South Central Asia has the highest incidence of 73,350 cases in men
	  - Other regions of high incidence are Eastern Asia, Northern America, Central and Eastern Europe
	- Incidence steadily increases after 40 years of age
	- Oral cavity cancer is aggressive compared to other head and neck subsites:
	  - Mortality: ASR is 2.7 per 100,000 for males worldwide (98,000 cases in men)
	- Male-to-female ratio is 2:1
	- More common in low socioeconomic group because of limited access to health education and health services, prone to substance abuse, poor oral hygiene and malnutrition

Aetiology	- Tobacco (smokeless and smoked):
	  - Most important aetiological agent
	  - Polyaromatic hydrocarbons, acrolein and nitrosamines are the main carcinogens in tobacco
	- Alcohol:
	  - Synergistic effect with tobacco
	  - Metabolism of alcohol produces acetaldehyde which acts as the carcinogen
	  - Other mechanisms proposed are inhibition of DNA methylation
	- Areca nut:
	  - Proven independent risk factor
	  - Common in the Asian subcontinent
	  - Relative risk in those who use areca nut alone is around 58.4%
	- Betel quid with or without tobacco:
	  - Betel quid is the combination of areca nut, slaked lime and tobacco rolled in betel leaves; commonly used in South-East Asia
	  - Slaked lime potentiates the carcinogenic effect of areca nut and tobacco
	  - Commonly associated with gingivobuccal sulcus cancers and usually occurs at the site where the quid is lodged
	- Human papillomavirus (HPV):
	  - Individual studies have detected HPV DNA in up to 25% of oral cavity cancers
	  - Remains unclear whether or not there is a causal association for oral cavity cancers
	- Solar radiation
	- Poor oral hygiene:
	  - Sharp tooth/ill-defined dentures causing constant irritation lead to cancer over a period of time

(continued)

Incidence, aetiology and screening	Description

Screening and early detection	- Lack of robust evidence to recommend its routine use in the general population
	- Some benefits in high-risk individuals (tobacco and/or alcohol habits)
	- A number of ancillary methods have been described to aid early detection:
	  - Toluidine blue supravital staining, brush cytology, light-based techniques, autofluorescence, etc.
	  - Benefits only seen in isolated reports
	  - Systematic review of published data does not justify routine use in clinical practice

Pathology

Squamous cell carcinoma (SCC) is the predominant cancer in the oral cavity (90%). Salivary gland and bone tumours, soft tissue sarcomas and melanomas are the other tumours that can occur in this region.

Histopathological subtypes	Description
Conventional squamous cell carcinoma/epidermoid carcinoma	- Arise either from normal epithelium or areas of epithelial dysplasia - Histopathological examination shows keratinization with keratin pearl formation, invasive growth pattern and squamous differentiation - Classified as well, moderately and poorly differentiated - High propensity for regional metastasis: - Most common site of distant metastasis is to the lung

Verrucous carcinoma/ Ackerman tumour	- Exophytic, warty, slow growing variant
	- Well-differentiated carcinoma with marked keratinization
	- Mitosis and DNA synthesis is confined to the basal layer; hence establishing diagnosis is often difficult on histology:
	  - Deep knife biopsy is helpful
	  - Clinical and radiological findings are used to establish diagnosis in difficult cases
	- Up to 20% harbour foci of conventional SCC:
	  - Chances of recurrence are higher in the presence of SCC
	- Low propensity to neck metastasis

Basaloid squamous cell carcinoma	- Aggressive high-grade variant - Has both a basaloid and a squamous component - Presents as a mass with central ulceration and submucosal induration
Papillary squamous cell carcinoma	- Exophytic, papillary growth - Usually pedunculated with a thin stalk, but can also be sessile with a broad base - Histopathological examination shows papillae with a thin fibrovascular core under the cover of neoplastic, immature basaloid or pleomorphic cells - Rarely metastasizes distantly - Associated with a good prognosis

Spindle cell carcinoma	- Presents as polypoidal mass with or without ulceration
	- Biphasic tumour comprising an SCC and a malignant spindle cell component of epithelial origin:
	  - Spindle cell component forms the majority of the tumour on histology
	  - Metastatic nodes have either an SCC or a spindle cell component with SCC, but never a spindle cell component alone
	- Low propensity to distant metastasis

Acantholytic squamous cell carcinoma	- Uncommon and more aggressive variant - Histopathologically, SCC with acantholysis showing a pseudoglandular pattern - Pseudolumina is filled with acantholytic or dyskeratotic cells

Histopathological subtypes	Description
Adenosquamous carcinoma	• Rare aggressive variant • Ulcerated exophytic or polypoidal mass with ill-defined mucosal induration • Characterized by the presence of both SCC and adenocarcinoma: ■ Histopathological examination shows the presence of distinct SCC and adenocarcinoma with mucin • High prevalence of aneuploidy
Carcinoma cuniculatum	• Rare variant • Histopathological examination shows broad processes of stratified squamous epithelium with keratin cores and presence of keratin in crypts

Presentation

- Non-healing ulcer, exophytic mass, a white/red patch, mucosal thickening, referred ear pain, ankyloglossia, neck nodes, spontaneous loosening of teeth, overlying skin ulceration and oedema of the hemiface
- Buccal cancers usually cause fewer symptoms and hence patients present late compared to tongue cancers

Natural history

Oral carcinogenesis is a complex multistep process that occurs on exposure to known carcinogens. Established genetic changes, none of which has a role in early detection, described in oral carcinogenesis:

- Loss of heterozygosity of 9p, 3p and 17p are the earliest changes and are associated with dysplasia
- 11q, 13q and 14q are later changes leading to carcinoma *in situ*
- Loss of 6p, chromosome 8 and 4q are the last changes to occur and result in invasion.

Molecular changes are characterized by loss of cadherins leading to metastasis.

Of clinical relevance is the fact that well-established clinical premalignant conditions make oral cancers amenable to prevention and early detection. Histologically these premalignant conditions go through the stages of hyperplasia, mild, moderate and severe dysplasia, carcinoma *in situ* and lastly frank invasive malignancy. The changes from normal mucosa to invasive carcinoma occur over the period of many years.

The World Health Organization (WHO) (2005) recommends the term *potentially malignant disorders* in preference to 'premalignant lesions'. These include potentially malignant lesions and potentially malignant conditions.

Presentation and natural history	Description

Potentially malignant disorders/premalignant lesions	• *Potentially malignant lesions* include:
	  ■ Leukoplakia:
	    ○ White patch usually diagnosed by exclusion of other known conditions
	    ○ Malignant transformation rate of 0.3–17% (average 4–5%)
	    ○ Can be homogenous or non-homogenous in appearance:
	      – Non-homogenous leukoplakia is more ominous and can be speckled or nodular.
	  ■ Erythroplakia:
	    ○ Fiery red patch.
	    ○ Can be smooth, granular or ulcerated
	    ○ High malignant transformation rate
	    ○ Distinguished from other conditions such as erosive lichen planus, which are bilateral and multiple
	• *Potentially malignant conditions* include:
	  ■ Lichen planus:
	    ○ Malignant potential is debatable
	    ○ Malignant transformation <1%
	  ■ Oral submucous fibrosis (OSMF):
	    ○ Unique to South-East Asia
	    ○ Symptoms: intolerance to spices and trismus; clinically characterized by fibrotic bands affecting cheeks, faucial pillars and lips
	    ○ Chronic, progressive and irreversible; characterized by atrophy and fibrosis of the epithelium

(continued)

Presentation and natural history	Description
	<ul><li><ul><li>Arecoline, arecaidine, guvacine and guacoline present in areca nut have a proven causal role</li><li>Malignant transformation rate approximately 0.5% annually.</li><li>Usually treated symptomatically</li></ul></li><li>Actinic cheilitis:<ul><li>Ulcerative crust-forming lesion usually affecting the lower lip</li><li>Seen in elderly men with prolonged exposure to sunlight</li></ul></li><li>Other conditions:<ul><li>Xeroderma pigmentosum, Fanconi anaemia and immunodeficiency related to solid organ transplant and HIV have been reported to be associated with head and neck cancers in general</li></ul></li><li>Given the widely variable transformation rate, it is important to treat only those lesions that are at a high risk for malignancy, including:<ul><li>Non-homogenous consistency</li><li>Erythroleukoplakia</li><li>Severe dysplasia</li><li>Idiopathic (absence of habits)</li><li>Female gender</li><li>High risk sites on hard palate, floor of mouth, dorsum of tongue</li><li>Size >200 mm^2</li></ul></li><li>Isolated reports of retinoids, beta-carotene, green tea and non-steroidal anti-inflammatory drugs showing benefits as chemopreventive agents in reversing potentially malignant lesions</li><li>No level I evidence to support chemoprevention and therefore high-risk lesions are better excised</li><li>Low-risk lesions can be observed with encouragement to alter habits</li></ul>
Routes of spread	*Local spread in mandible:*<ul><li>Understanding the routes of spread into the mandible is important in making a decision on mandibular preservation:<ul><li>It was initially believed that the lymphatics of the oral cavity passed through the mandible *en route* to the cervical nodes, necessitating a mandibulectomy in all cases that were surgically treated</li><li>Marchetta refuted this theory by demonstrating that the mandible was involved by direct extension</li><li>Current belief is that the preferred route of entry is at the point of abutment of the tumour with the mandible</li><li>Alternative route of spread is from the occlusal surface of the mandible, particularly for tumours involving the retromolar region and the edentulous mandible in view of the decreased vertical height of the mandible</li></ul></li><li>Preferential spread along the inferior alveolar nerve, once considered significant, is no longer valid and the nerve does not need to be traced back to its origin at the skull base</li><li>In an irradiated mandible, periosteal integrity is compromised, resulting in multiple routes of tumour entry</li><li>Larger tumours may similarly invade the mandible through multiple routes</li></ul>*Regional:*<ul><li>Specific subsites of the oral cavity follow a well-studied, predictable pattern of nodal metastasis:<ul><li>*Buccal and lower alveolar cancers*: level IB (submaxillary group) is the first echelon of nodal spread</li><li>*Tongue*: level II (subdigastric/jugulodigastric group) forms the first echelon followed by the mid-jugular nodes:<ul><li>Potential metastasis to level III or IV without level II involvement may occur and should be accounted for in surgical or radiotherapy treatment volumes</li></ul></li><li>*Floor of the mouth*: level IB is most commonly involved because of the anterior location of these tumours; level II may also be involved</li><li>*Retromolar trigone*: levels IB and II are most commonly involved</li><li>*Lip*: first echelon is level IA (submental group) in case of the middle third of the lip and level IB in case of the lateral one-third on either side</li><li>Level V (posterior cervical nodes) is rarely involved in oral cavity cancers</li><li>Level IIB (submuscular recess) rarely shows isolated metastasis:<ul><li>Metastasis to this level occurs secondary to level IIA involvement</li><li>Highest incidence in the tongue and retromolar trigone</li></ul></li></ul></li></ul>

Diagnostic work-up

Diagnostic work-up	Description
Assessment of patient profile	• Disease-related information (onset and duration) of pain, difficulty in swallowing, movement of tongue, trismus, alteration in speech, dental history • Premalignant lesions/conditions • History of habits and addictions • Medical history/co-morbidities • Performance status/nutrition status • Details of prior treatment

Assessment of tumour profile	• *Biopsy*:
	  ▪ To establish the diagnosis of carcinoma and the histological subtype
	  ▪ Difficult to ascertain grade and other histological prognostic factors on biopsy
	  ▪ Punch biopsy from most representative area, avoiding obviously necrotic areas
	  ▪ Incisional biopsy for submucosal lesions/patch/verrucous lesions when punch biopsy is not feasible or non-contributory
	• *Scrape cytology*:
	  ▪ Acts as an adjunct and not a substitute for formal biopsy:
	    ○ A negative scrape cytology with strong clinical suspicion warrants biopsy
	  ▪ At present no role for ancillary diagnostic tools/molecular techniques (brush biopsy, toludine blue, autofluorescence) though there is an emerging interest

Assessment of tumour extent	• Location
	• Size
	• Extent and involvement of adjoining structures
	• Ankyloglossia
	• Trismus/infratemporal fossa involvement
	• Hypoglossal nerve palsy
	• Mandible involvement/proximity to the mandible
	• Overlying skin involvement
	• Cervical adenopathy
	• Examination under anaesthesia is occasionally helpful in case of:
	  ▪ Painful lesion
	  ▪ Posterior extension of the lesion to the oropharynx
	  ▪ Trismus
	  ▪ Recurrent cases

Imaging	• *Helical computed tomography (CT) and multidetector CT*:
	  ▪ Preferred investigation in cancers of the buccal mucosa, alveolus, retromolar trigone and hard palate
	  ▪ Good delineation of local spread, bone involvement and metastatic nodes
	  ▪ CT is the most specific modality for mandibular erosion with high positive predictive value and low negative predictive value
	  ▪ Limitation:
	    ○ Inferior soft tissue characterization
	    ○ For imaging the tongue only when MRI not available
	• *Magnetic resonance imaging (MRI; multiplanar and gadolinium enhanced)*:
	  ▪ Preferred investigation for lesions of the tongue and floor of the mouth
	  ▪ Superior soft tissue characterization provides useful information for extent, including tumour thickness
	  ▪ High negative predictive value, but tends to overestimate bone involvement as signal intensity cannot differentiate between inflammation and invasion
	• *Positron emission tomography (PET)-CT*:
	  ▪ Not recommended for routine imaging
	  ▪ Optional role for evaluating distant metastases in advanced disease, particularly with large (N2/N3) and low-level neck nodes and in the post-treatment setting
	• *Ultrasonography (US) with or without guided fine needle aspiration (FNA)*:
	  ▪ Cost-effective investigation in evaluating the neck for metastatic nodes
	  ▪ Addition of FNA of the node adds to the specificity of US
	  ▪ Ideally performed with a 5–10-MHz linear transducer for better accuracy
	  ▪ Limitation: operator dependent

(continued)

Diagnostic work-up	Description

	• Orthopantomogram (OPG):
	  ▪ Not usually done today with the availability of multidetector CT and MRI
	  ▪ Low specificity and sensitivity due to high incidence of periodontitis and odontogenic infections
	  ▪ Requires at least 30% mineral loss before erosion can be detected
	  ▪ Limitations in:
	    ○ Midline lesion
	    ○ Early lesion
	  ▪ Useful for planning dental prophylaxis prior to radiotherapy

Staging and prognostic grouping

UICC TNM staging
See Table 41.1.

Table 41.1 UICC TNM categories and stage grouping: Lip and oral cavity

TNM categories	
T1	≤2 cm
T2	>2–4 cm
T3	>4 cm
T4a	*Lip*: through cortical bone, inferior alveolar nerve, floor of mouth, skin *Oral cavity*: through cortical bone, deep/ extrinsic muscle of tongue, maxillary sinus, skin of face
T4b	Masticator space, pterygoid plates, skull base, internal carotid artery
N1	Ipsilateral single ≤3 cm
N2	(a) Ipsilateral single >3–6 cm (b) Ipsilateral multiple ≤6 cm (c) Bilateral, contralateral ≥6 cm
N3	>6 cm
M1	Distant metastasis

Stage grouping			
Stage 0	Tis	N0	M0
Stage I	T1	N0	M0
Stage II	T2	N0	M0
Stage III	T3	N0	M0
	T1, T2, T3	N1	M0
Stage IVA	T1, T2, T3	N2	M0
	T4a	N0, N1, N2	M0
Stage IVB	Any T	N3	M0
	T4b	Any N	M0
Stage IVC	Any T	Any N	M1

Prognostic factors (see Table 41.2)

TNM staging is the most important prognostic factor. However there are other host- and environment-related factors as well as certain tumour factors that additionally may be beneficial. Various molecular markers and quality of life factors hold promise for the future.

Individual histopathological factors that have implications for prognosis are classified as essential, desirable and optional (Table 41.3; see Box 41.1).

Treatment philosophy

Treatment of oral cavity cancer includes single-modality surgery, radiotherapy (external beam radiotherapy [EBRT] and/or brachytherapy) for early disease (Stage I/II)) or various combinations of these modalities with or without systemic therapy (chemotherapy and/or target agents). Treatment selection is based on considerations of disease control, anticipated functional and cosmetic outcomes, and availability of resources and expertise.

More advanced lesions (Stage III/IV) are generally treated with surgery ± postoperative radiotherapy/chemoradiotherapy if resectable (excepting some superficial T3 lesions on the lip, retromolar trigone and buccal mucosa/gingiva where aesthetic/functional considerations may warrant alternative strategies, e.g. radiotherapy). Toxicity considerations, especially in the presence of bone invasion (e.g. osteoradionecrosis) may influence the treatment decision. Definitive radiotherapy with or without systemic therapy remains a valid option for unresectable disease, high operative risk or very advanced disease where surgical resection may result in significant morbidity (e.g. oral tongue cancer requiring near total glossectomy). There is no proven role in routine practice, at present, for neoadjuvant treatment prior to surgery in patients with resectable disease.

The treatment algorithm or carcinoma of the oral cavity is summarized in Fig. 41.1.

Table 41.2 Prognostic factors for carcinoma of the oral cavity

Prognostic factors	Tumour related	Host related	Environment related
Essential	T category N category Extracapsular extension (ECE) Surgical resection margin	Performance status Addictions (tobacco/areca nut/alcohol)	Dose of radiotherapy/chemoradiotherapy
Additional	Tumour volume Hypoxia	Age Co-morbidity	Overall treatment/radiation treatment time Interval from surgery to start of postoperative radiotherapy
New and promising	EGFR expression *TP53* mutation *Bcl-2* *ERCC1*	Swallowing-related quality of life Global quality of life	

Table 41.3 Adverse histopathological features (see also Box 41.1)

Essential	Desirable	Optional
Size Involvement of adjacent structure bone/skin Surgical resection margins* Nodal metastasis: size, number and level, extracapsular extension (ECE)	Grade Perineural invasion Lymphovascular invasion Tumour thickness Type of SCC	Patterns of invasion Stromal response Characteristics of tumour: endophytic, exophytic and ulcerative

---

Box 41.1 Adverse histopathological features

- *Size/adjacent structure involvement*:
  - Integral part of the TNM staging and necessitates the need for postoperative adjuvant radiotherapy if >4 cm (T3) in any dimension or involves adjacent structures like bone and skin (T4)
- *Surgical margins*:
  - Known to impact on locoregional control
  - Minimum resection margin of 0.5 cm is considered to be adequate
  - In the presence of microscopically involved margins, some advocate revision surgery:
    - However, the role of revision surgery in this setting is contentious
    - Hence, it is important to ensure adequate margins at primary surgery
  - Tumour shrinkage of up to 30% is expected after excision and this should be factored in at the time of surgery
- *Nodal metastasis*:
  - One of the strongest prognostic factors: known to decrease survival by up to 50%
  - While nodal metastasis strongly dictates the use of adjuvant therapy, its role in a single N1 metastasis is debatable, particularly for early stage disease with low-risk features
  - Risk of distant metastasis is influenced by the N category rather than by the T category of the cancer
  - Low level nodal involvement carries a poor prognosis
- *Extracapsular extension/spread (ECE or ECS)*:
  - Known to further worsen the outcome associated with nodal metastasis
  - Probability of ECE is proportional to the size of the lymph node
  - ECE can either be gross (clinical – matted nodes, restricted mobility, adjoining structure involvement), radiological (crenated, fuzzy margins, perinodal soft tissue stranding) or microscopic:
    - Microscopic ECE could be present even in small nodes and should be meticulously sought
- *Grade*:
  - Most widely used, easy-to-follow grading system is that described by Broder (grades I–IV from well differentiated to undifferentiated)
  - Vast majority of oral tumours (60%) are moderately differentiated
  - Poorly differentiated tumours are known to be more aggressive with a worse outcome
- *Perineural invasion (PNI)*:
  - Characterized by tumour invasion and spread along nerve sheaths; usually refers to involvement of small nerves in the vicinity of the tumour:
    - Detected in 5–50% of tumours on routine haematoxylin and eosin staining
  - Shown in multiple reports to predict increased incidence of local recurrence, regional metastasis and decreased survival

- *Lymphovascular invasion (LVI)*:
  - Characterized by tumour that involves either a lymphatic or a blood vessel
  - Seen in approximately 30% of cases
  - LVI, like PNI, predicts poor prognosis, although it has not been as extensively reported as the latter
- *Tumour thickness/depth of invasion*:
  - Tumour thickness and depth of invasion are not interchangeable terms: former is the distance between the tumour surface and the deepest extent; latter is measured from the adjacent mucosal basement membrane and is the deepest extent of the tumour
  - Depth of invasion is a strong predictor of cervical nodal metastasis:
    - ≥4 mm is associated with a higher incidence of nodal metastasis
- *Patterns of invasion*:
  - Based on tumour–host relationship, four patterns:
    1. Broad front with pushing margins
    2. Invasive front with infiltrating margins
    3. Small groups or cords of infiltrating cells (n >15)
    4. Marked and widespread cellular dissociation into small groups of cells (n <15) and/or into single cells corresponding to extensive and deep infiltration
  - Types 3 and 4 are non-cohesive and associated with a poorer prognosis
- *Type of SCC*:
  - Verrucous and spindle cell variants have a better prognosis compared to basaloid and adenosquamous variants.
- *Stromal invasion*:
  - Varying reports on the prognostic implications of the lymphocytic infiltration at the advancing tumour front
  - Not a commonly used prognostic indicator

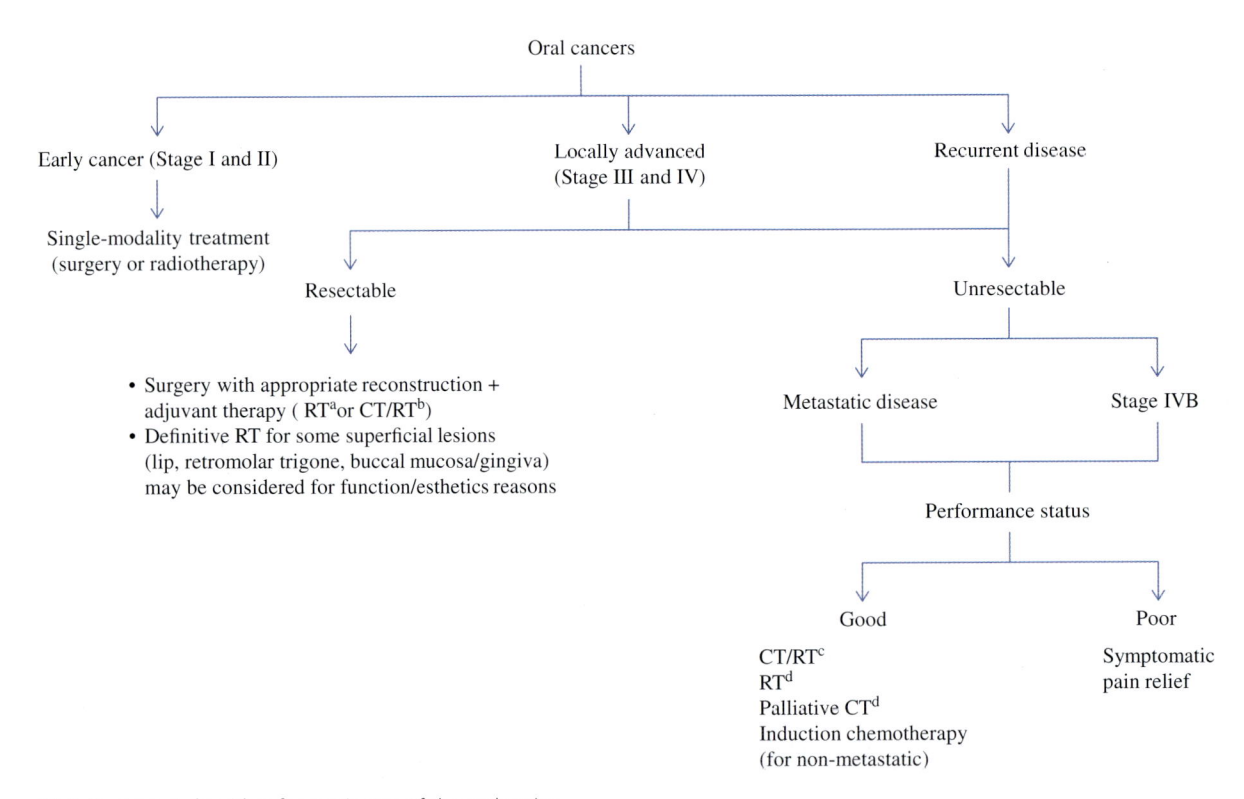

Figure 41.1 Treatment algorithm for carcinoma of the oral cavity

[a] T3/4 disease, N2/3 nodal disease or low-level node (optional in N1 disease), perineural invasion, lymphovascular emboli, high grade, close margins.
[b] Microscopically involved margins and/or extracapsular spread.
[c] Most durable palliation.
[d] When chemoradiotherapy not feasible.
RT, radiotherapy; CT, chemotherapy.

Scenario	Treatment philosophy

Resectable disease	• Primary surgery with or without postoperative radiotherapy is preferred:
	• *Primary:*
	  ▪ A minimum tumour-free resection margin of 0.5 cm: margins to be adequate on mucosa, soft tissue and bone
	  ▪ Appropriate reconstruction for restoration of form and function: local, axial or microvascular-free tissue transfer
	• *Neck:*
	  ▪ *cN0 neck*:
	    ◦ Elective neck treatment is warranted in:
	      – T3/T4 disease
	      – Approach to primary via cheek flap
	      – Tumour thickness >4 mm
	      – Factors for poor prognosis: high grade, perineural invasion, lymphovascular invasion
	      – Poor patient follow-up
	      – Nodal involvement suspected on imaging
	    ◦ Procedure is supraomohyoid dissection (SOHD): clearance of level I, II and III
	  ▪ *cN+ neck*:
	    ◦ Modified radical neck dissection (MND) (level I–V clearance):
	      – All non-lymphatic structures (spinal accessory nerve, internal jugular vein and sternocleidomastoid) to be preserved unless involved by the tumour
	    ◦ Radical neck dissection (RND):
	      – Rarely performed
	      – Done only when large N3 nodal disease involves internal jugular vein, spinal accessory nerve and sternocleidomatoid muscle
	  ▪ *Special considerations*:
	    ◦ Extended SOHD (level IV clearance):
	      – Advocated by some in tongue/floor of mouth cancer (increased incidence of skip metastasis)
	    ◦ SOHD (sparing IIB) to decrease morbidity of shoulder dysfunction by avoiding dissection of the accessory nerve when level IIA is negative for metastasis
	    ◦ Level V:
	      – Rarely involved in oral cancers (<1%)
	      – Dissection recommended when involved or other multiple nodes are positive at other levels
	    ◦ Bilateral neck:
	      – Lesions approaching or crossing the midline
	• *Preservation of mandible during surgery:*
	  ▪ Marginal mandibulectomy:
	    ◦ Tumour close to mandible to achieve adequate margins
	    ◦ Superficial bony erosion
	  ▪ Contraindications to marginal mandibulectomy:
	    ◦ Inadequate clearance of disease/paramandibular disease
	    ◦ Prior radiotherapy (relative contraindication)
	    ◦ Inability to achieve adequate remnant/edentulism resulting in pipestem mandible
	• *Reconstruction:*
	  ▪ As appropriate (see Box 41.2)
	• *Indication for adjuvant radiotherapy:*
	  ▪ *Primary*:
	    ◦ Large primary: T3/T4
	    ◦ High-grade tumour
	    ◦ Lymphovascular and perineural invasion
	    ◦ Close margin
	  ▪ *Lymph nodes*:
	    ◦ Node positivity
	• *Indication for adjuvant chemoradiotherapy:*
	  ▪ Positive margins
	  ▪ Extracapsular extension (ECE)

Scenario	Treatment philosophy

Unresectable non-metastatic disease	• Definitive radiotherapy (70 Gy in 35 fractions over 7 weeks) with concurrent chemotherapy (CRT)
	• Induction chemotherapy may be considered for patients with unresectable tumours where clear surgical margins or resection with acceptable morbidity may not be possible with upfront surgery:
	   ▪ Reassessment is required to address suitability for either surgery or concurrent chemoradiotherapy
	   ▪ Interval between the end of neoadjuvant chemotherapy and potential local treatment should be as short as reasonably achievable
	• If patient is unable to tolerate intensified CRT treatment:
	   ▪ Palliative treatment (radiotherapy or systemic therapy) for symptom relief
	• If patient is unable to tolerate any treatment:
	   ▪ Best supportive care

Metastatic disease	• *Good performance status*:
	   ▪ Systemic therapy (chemotherapy or target agents)
	   ▪ Palliative radiotherapy can be given to control local symptoms or pain relief
	• *Poor performance status*: best supportive care (BSC)

Recurrent disease	• *Salvage surgery*:
	   ▪ Best option if feasible
	   ▪ Considerations before curative intent treatment:
	      ○ Performance status
	      ○ Stage of initial (early stage is better salvaged) and recurrent disease
	      ○ Disease-free interval (longer duration has better prognosis; preferably >1 year)
	      ○ Previous adjuvant treatment (radiotherapy or chemoradiotherapy) (lower salvage possibility)
	   ▪ *Re-irradiation for unresectable disease*:
	   ▪ Re-irradiation with or without systemic agents
	   ▪ Optimizing re-irradiation regimens (see Chapter 39)

Box 41.2 Reconstruction

- *Mucosal defects*:
  - Small defect: primary closure/local flap/split thickness skin grafting:
    - Some lesions can be left to granulate secondarily
  - Large defect: preferably replaced with like tissue, i.e. bone with bone, soft tissue with soft tissue and mucosa with skin
- *Soft tissue loss*:
  - Pedicled flaps, e.g. pectoralis major myocutaneous flap (PMMC), or
  - Free tissue transfer, e.g. free radial artery forearm flap (FRAFF), anterolateral thigh flap (ALT), lateral arm flap
- *Skeletal defects ± soft tissue and skin loss*:
  - Free tissue transfer preferred to pedicled flap in view of better functional outcome and quality of life
  - Flaps used: scapula, iliac bone, radius, fibula
  - Preferred: free fibula (long bone segment, multiple osteotomies possible due to segmental blood supply, minimal donor site morbidity, large skin paddle, ease of harvest)
  - Bone replacement not essential in posterior mandibular defects
- *Skin defects* can be covered with:
  - Local flaps /forehead flap
  - Deltopectoral flap/PMMC
  - Free flaps
- *Lip reconstruction*:
  - Less than one-third defect: primary closure
  - One-third to two-thirds defect: Abbe, Abbe Estlander, Karapandzic flap
  - Greater than two-thirds defect: Gilles fan flap, reverse Karapandzic flap, nasolabial flap
  - Total lip resection: free tissue transfer (FRAFF with palmaris longus muscle)

General principles	Description

Early disease	- Single modality therapy
	- Surgery or radiotherapy:
	  - Surgery is preferred because it is simple, low cost, not associated with significant functional or cosmetic deficit, and can be repeated
	  - Also preferred in young patients (who are prone to a second primary) and in those with submucous fibrosis (who tolerate radiotherapy poorly)
	  - Brachytherapy can be used in early disease:
	    - Accessible
	    - Small (preferably <3 cm)
	    - Away from bone
	    - N0 status
	    - Superficial

Locally-advanced resectable disease	- Surgery followed by adjuvant radiotherapy or chemoradiotherapy: - Surgery must ensure adequate clearance (tumour-free margins) as well as appropriate reconstruction to minimize morbidity and ensure acceptable quality of life
Locally-advanced unresectable disease	- Cancers involving the masticator space, encasement of the carotid artery or prevertebral muscle are classified as Stage IVB and are ordinarily considered unresectable - In some situations, Stage IVB cancers may respond to neoadjuvant chemotherapy or radiotherapy, and may be amenable to curative surgery - Patient with good performance status: concurrent chemoradiotherapy is the standard therapy for the proportion of patients for whom cure may still be possible - Patient with poor performance status and cannot tolerate intensified (chemo-)radiotherapy: palliative treatment may be considered for symptom control including pain relief
Metastatic disease	- Governed by the patient's predominant symptoms - Palliative radiotherapy may be given to control locoregional symptoms - Skeletal metastasis: palliative radiotherapy to the involved site - Visceral metastasis: considered for chemotherapy - Best supportive care (BSC) in all cases, irrespective of whether or not anticancer therapy is given: - BSC or BSC + chemotherapy depending on the general condition of the patient
Recurrent disease/ second primary (see Chapter 39)	- Evaluation for recurrent disease/second primary is done as for the index cancer - Best option: surgical salvage ± radiotherapy or chemoradiotherapy whenever feasible - If unresectable: re-irradiation with tight target volume to spare normal tissue as much as possible may be considered

Treatment

The treatment plan as applicable to each subsite in the oral cavity is given below. This should be read in conjunction with the treatment philosophy and general principles above as only site-specific details of each modality are highlighted here.

Surgery

Surgery	Description

Lip	- *T1–2 tumours*:
	  - Wide excision:
	    - Excision to be planned appropriately to ensure adequate reconstruction and oral competence (V-shaped excision for small lesions to facilitate exposure)
	  - Oral competence is a concern when treating lip lesions:
	    - A strong indication to consider radiotherapy in early lesions when excision will be functionally disabling or with aesthetic concern
	- *T3–4 tumours*:
	  - Composite resection of lip ± adjoining structures if involved (with/without mandible or skin) with appropriate reconstruction

(continued)

Surgery	Description

Buccal mucosa	• *T1–2 tumours:*
	  ▪ Wide excision ± marginal mandibulectomy for margins
	• *T3–4 tumours:*
	  ▪ Composite resection of the buccal mucosa ± adjoining structures if involved (with/without mandible or upper alveolus or overlying skin) with reconstruction

Oral tongue and floor of mouth	• *T1–2 tumours:*
	  ▪ Wide excision glossectomy/hemiglossectomy
	• *T3–4 tumours:*
	  ▪ Anterior two-thirds/total glossectomy with/without oblique marginal mandibulectomy/segmental/hemimandibular resection to achieve tumour-free margins.
	• Access: mandibular swing/pull-through technique
	• In all the above subsites, decision for marginal/segmental mandibulectomy should be made as per the guidelines

Lower alveolus and retromolar trigone (RMT)	• *Mandible uninvolved or minimally involved:*
	  ▪ Wide excision with marginal mandibulectomy (caution to be exercised in RMT disease, edentulous mandible, paramandibular disease, post radiotherapy cases)
	• *Mandible grossly involved:*
	  ▪ Wide excision (cheek flap) with segmental/hemi-mandible resection

Upper alveolus and hard palate	• *Maxillary antrum not involved:*
	  ▪ Upper alveolectomy/partial maxillectomy
	  ▪ Radical radiotherapy/brachytherapy for selected early T1–2 hard palate lesions
	  ▪ In the presence of submucosal disease with normal overlying mucosa, possibility of minor salivary gland tumours should be strongly suspected
	• *Maxillary antrum involved:*
	  ▪ Orbital floor-preserving total maxillectomy with reconstruction

Management of neck
- N0: observe or SOHD (as highlighted in Scenario)
- N+: MND/RND
- Lip lesions show a low propensity to neck node metastasis, particularly superficial lesions
- Midline and large lesions necessitate bilateral dissection:
  - Usually the case in lip lesions
  - Upper lip may drain to the preparotid lymph nodes:
    - Appropriate clinicoradiological evaluation of this region is essential

Radiotherapy
EBRT with or without chemotherapy is generally employed in three clinical scenarios:

- Adjuvant to primary surgery to enhance locoregional control for cases with unfavourable pathological features
- Primary treatment for cases unable to tolerate or unsuited for surgery
- Salvage treatment in the persistent or recurrent disease setting.

Primary radiotherapy is preferred to surgery as a single modality in the following situations:
- Severe impairment of function/cosmesis with surgery (large, superficial lip lesions)
- Surgery is technically difficult (e.g. Stage IVB) with high morbidity and poor results
- Patient refuses surgery
- High risk of operation due to co-morbidities.

Radiotherapy	Description
Tumours suitable for brachytherapy	
T1–2N0	• Radical brachytherapy (BRT): ▪ 60–70 Gy low dose rate iridium-192 or equivalent doses with fractionated high dose rate

T1–3N0–1	• EBRT:
	  ▪ 56–60 Gy in 28–30 fractions over 6 weeks
	  ▪ + Boost BRT:
	    ○ Low dose rate iridium-192: 15–20 Gy or
	    ○ High dose rate: 14 Gy in four fractions over 2 days (4, 3, 3, 4 Gy)

Radiotherapy	Description
Tumours not suitable for brachytherapy	

Stage I–II	• EBRT alone:
	  ▪ 66–70 Gy in 33–35 fractions over 6–7 weeks
	  ▪ Generally bilateral neck RT is administrated, but unilateral RT may be considered for very lateralized primary lesions, especially in buccal mucosa/gingiva, retromolar trigone, lip and lateral tongue (>1.0 cm from midline) with:
	    ○ N0–1 disease
	    ○ N0–2b (small volume N2b) where imaging of the contralateral neck is unequivocally negative (i.e. no suspicion of nodal involvement)

Stage III–IV	• Concomitant chemoradiotherapy:
	  ▪ 66–70 Gy in 33–35 fractions over 6–7 weeks + concomitant cisplatin 30–40 mg/m^2 for 6–7 weeks or 3-weekly cisplatinum, 100mg/m^2 × three cycles
	  or
	• Commonly used altered fractionated radiotherapy regimens:
	  ▪ 64 Gy in 40 fractions over 4 weeks (twice daily 6 hours apart, ten fractions/week)
	  ▪ 65 Gy in 30 fractions over 6 weeks (daily, five fractions/week)
	  ▪ 72 Gy in 60 fractions over 6 weeks (twice daily 6 hours apart, ten fractions/week)
	  ▪ 60 Gy in 25 fractions over 5 weeks (daily, five fractions/week)

Adjuvant setting	• Primary and involved nodal disease:
	  ▪ 60 Gy in 30 fractions over 6 weeks
	• Site of residual disease, positive resection margins, presence of ECE:
	  ▪ 66–70 Gy in 33–35 fractions over 6.5–7 weeks
	• Uninvolved nodal stations:
	  ▪ 45–50 Gy
	• Note: if there is a small local or regional recurrence immediately after surgery, a focal boost dose to 70 Gy in 33–35 fractions to the small recurrent area and 60–66 Gy in 30–33 fractions to the remaining area could be used to enhance disease control after postoperative radiotherapy

Systemic therapy

Postoperative concurrent cisplatinum-based chemoradiotherapy has been shown to improve locoregional control and survival for patients with high-risk pathological features (e.g. positive resection margin and ECE) in clinical trials. Currently, its role is under evaluation for intermediate-risk patients following surgery (PNI, LVI, close margin, T3 or T4a tumour, T2 with >5 mm thickness, single lymph node of >3 cm or two or more lymph nodes of <6 cm without ECE).

Systemic therapy	Description

Chemotherapy	• Chemotherapy is not a definitive treatment for oral cavity cancers and should never be given if the initial lesion is resectable
	• Chemotherapy can be given as:
	  ▪ Concurrent chemoradiotherapy
	  ▪ Induction/neoadjuvant chemotherapy
	  ▪ Chemotherapy for recurrent/metastatic disease

Concurrent chemoradiotherapy	• Adjuvant treatment in resectable cancer:
	  ▪ Extracapsular spread
	  ▪ Positive (<1 mm) margin
	• Definitive treatment in advanced (unresectable) cancer:
	  ▪ If the patient can tolerate chemotherapy/radiotherapy, palliation is more durable than other modalities of treatment
	• Dose:
	  ▪ 100 mg/m^2 cisplatin administered on Days 1, 22, and possibly Day 43 of radiation as concurrent chemotherapy every 3 weeks, or
	  ▪ Weekly dose of cisplatin between 30–40 mg/m^2 with concurrent radiation
	  ▪ Minimum total cumulative dose of cisplatin of 200 mg/m^2 over the entire course is recommended
	  ▪ Should the patient be unsuitable for above, incorporation of cetuximab is acceptable; however, level I evidence for this in oral cancers is lacking
	• Antiemetics and hydration should be used prophylactically

(continued)

Systemic therapy	Description

Induction/ neoadjuvant chemotherapy	• Limited role in patients who are likely to have a positive margin if offered surgery as the initial treatment
	• Induction chemotherapy with cisplatinum-based regimen (docetaxel or paclitaxel + cisplatinum and 5-flurouracil [5-FU])
	  ■ Three drugs preferred over two drugs
	  ■ Followed by definitive treatment with surgery or chemoradiotherapy
	  ■ Dose (every 3 weeks):
	    ○ Docetaxel: 75 mg/m^2
	    ○ Cisplatin: 75 or 100 mg/m^2
	    ○ 5-FU: 750 mg/m^2/day for 5 days when given with the lower cisplatin dose or at 1000 mg/m^2/day for 4 days if combined with the higher cisplatin dose
	  ■ Reassessment after two to three cycles

Biotherapy	• Targeted agents, in particular epidermal growth factor receptor (EGFR) inhibitors (cetuximab is the only approved drug with level I evidence, although other EGFR inhibitors, such as nimotuzumab, have been used in some regions of the world without level I evidence), have a potential role in head and neck cancers • However, benefit of adding cetuximab to radiation for the treatment of locoregionally advanced SCC head and neck cancer has been shown primarily in cancers of the oropharynx and laryngopharynx • Role in oral cavity cancers has not been adequately studied in phase III randomized trials
Palliative setting	• Platinum-based chemotherapy has been the cornerstone for patients with good performance status (ECOG 0-1) • Can be combined with cetuximab (400 mg/m^2 initially followed by 250 mg/m^2/week until disease progression) • Combined use of cetuximab + platinum/5-FU leads to better overall survival, progression-free survival, response rate and disease control rate, with an acceptable toxicity profile and no negative effect on quality of life • Patients with compromised performance status/co-morbidities can be offered single-agent chemotherapy or BSC only: ■ Preferred single agents are cisplatin, carboplatin, methotrexate, paclitaxel, docetaxel or 5-FU

Post-treatment assessment, follow-up and continuing care

Ninety per cent of locoregional recurrence occurs in the first 24 months. Follow up recommendations are:
- Every 2–3 months for first 2 years
- Every 4–6 months for next 3 years
- Annually thereafter

Post-treatment assessment, follow-up and continuing care	Description
Assessment of disease status and sequelae of treatment	• Thorough examination of oral cavity and neck for locoregional control • Upper aerodigestive tract evaluation for second primary cancer • Examination of treated area for late sequelae of treatment

Investigation post treatment	• Thyroid function evaluation annually particularly for those receiving postoperative radiotherapy
	• Baseline imaging:
	  ■ CT/MRI optional at follow up – provides baseline post treatment status
	• Routine CT/MRI scans are not recommended at each visit:
	  ■ Evaluation only for suspected locoregional recurrence to assess the extent and suitability for salvage
	• CT-PET scan for suspected, non-accessible recurrences and to rule out distant metastasis:
	  ■ Recommended 12 weeks after the completion of adjuvant treatment to prevent false-positive results
	• Image-guided biopsies for deep-seated suspected recurrences
	• Appropriate imaging to rule out second primary cancer based on symptoms/clinical findings, e.g. barium swallow, endoscopy (oesophagus), chest X-ray/CT scan (lung)

Post-treatment assessment, follow-up and continuing care	Description
Rehabilitation	• Abstinence from tobacco/alcohol • Oral/dental hygiene: fluoride gel application • Shoulder physiotherapy particularly in cases of neck dissections • Bite guide prosthesis/guided palatal plate following mandibulectomy to prevent jaw deviation • Jaw stretching exercises to prevent postoperative trismus • Swallowing and speech rehabilitation

Controversies

Management of clinically node-negative neck in early oral cancers

For tumours amenable to per oral excision, the controversy regarding neck dissection persists. Four small studies addressing this issue have been published followed by a meta-analysis of them. Although the meta-analysis suggested a survival benefit with elective neck dissection, its routine indication is still questionable due to certain limitations and a single study influencing the result towards the neck dissection arm. The role of sentinel node biopsy is still investigational.

Extent of therapeutic neck dissection

A randomized controlled trial demonstrated equal control rates in patients undergoing a selective neck dissection in the presence of cervical metastasis as compared to a modified radical neck dissection. Prospective studies suggest the presence of level IIB metastasis in <5% of neck dissections, the majority of which occur in the presence of level IIA metastasis and in tongue cancers. Isolated level IIB metastases account for <1%. Similarly, metastasis to level V occurs in up to 5% of neck dissections. The evidence favours a therapeutic level I-IV dissection for node positive necks, thus safeguarding the spinal accessory nerve at levels IIB and V.

Role of neoadjuvant chemotherapy in advanced cancers

Randomized controlled trials on the use of neoadjuvant chemotherapy in resectable advanced oral cancers neither demonstrate improvement in locoregional control nor any survival benefit. There is however, scope for organ preservation. In unresectable cases, a randomized trial has shown a survival benefit in patients receiving platinum-based neoadjuvant chemotherapy. Oral cavity cancer represented 17% of the study population in this trial (TAX 323).

Extent of adjuvant therapy in advanced cancers

Two large trials on the role of chemotherapy in addition to radiotherapy for adjuvant treatment in high-risk cases suggest a significant benefit for those with microscopically-positive resection margins and extracapsular spread in nodal metastasis. An individual patient data meta-analysis determined a benefit of chemoradiotherapy over radiotherapy alone. A meta-analysis on the various modalities of radiotherapy demonstrated altered fractionation radiotherapy to be more efficacious than plain radiotherapy. However, the most suitable method of adjuvant treatment for the intermediate-risk group (T3-4 cancers, high-grade tumours, multiple positive lymph nodes, low level nodes in oral cancers, perineural invasion, lymphovascular invasion, individually and in combination) remains to be established.

Phase III clinical trials

See Table 41.4.

Areas of research

Screening

Oral cavity cancer is a major public health problem in certain parts of the world (South-East Asia), with the majority presenting at a late stage. The only study with mortality as an endpoint demonstrated the benefit of screening in high-risk individuals (tobacco and alcohol habits). This study was powered for the entire cohort and the high-risk finding was on a subset analysis. A trial adequately designed to statistically demonstrate benefit in high-risk individuals would help in early detection of cancers in high incidence areas.

Early detection

Isolated publications show the benefit of a number of diagnostic tools in early detection: optical examination, autofluorescence, spectroscopy, brush cytology, salivary diagnostics, etc. None is accepted in routine clinical use. Establishing the role of diagnostic tools in early detection is an area of research.

Table 41.4 Phase III clinical trials

Trial reference	Results
Neck dissection	
Fasunla et al. (2011) Oral Oncol 47(5):320–324	• Disease-specific death rate is reduced by elective neck dissection in comparison to observation
(1998) Am J Surg 176(5):422–427	• Recurrence and survival rates are similar in supraomohyoid and modified radical classical neck dissection in node-negative T2–4 oral squamous cell carcinomas
Adjuvant therapy	
Cooper et al. (2004) N Engl J Med 350:1937–1944	• Postoperative adjuvant chemoradiotherapy improves local and regional control rates and disease-free survival in postoperative high-risk head and neck cancer patients
Bernier et al. (2004) N Engl J Med 350:1945–1952	• Postoperative concurrent chemoradiotherapy is better than radiotherapy alone in patients with locally-advanced head and neck cancers
Screening	
Sankaranarayanan et al. (2005) Lancet 365:1927–1933	• Visual screening of the oral cavity can reduce mortality in individuals at high risk for oral cancers
Chemotherapy	
Zhong et al. (2013) J Clin Oncol 31(6):744–751	• In patients with resectable Stage III or IVA oral SCC, TPF induction chemotherapy does not improve survival compared with upfront surgery
Zorat et al. (2004) J Natl Cancer Inst 96:1714–1717	• Neoadjuvant chemotherapy improves overall survival in patients with unresectable advanced head and neck cancer, but not in patients with resectable disease
Licitra et al. (2003) J Clin Oncol 21:327–333	• Neoadjuvant chemotherapy reduces the number of patients requiring mandibulectomy and/or postoperative radiotherapy with no benefit in overall survival
MACH-NC Collaborative Group (2000 and 2009) Lancet 355:949–955; Radiother Oncol 92:4–14 (meta-analysis)	• Concurrent chemoradiotherapy is the best approach to combine chemotherapy with radiotherapy
Blanchard et al. (2013) J Clin Oncol 31:2854–2860 (individual patient data meta-analysis)	• Three-drug induction chemotherapy (TPF) is superior to two-drug (PF) for survival and locoregional control

Chemoprevention

As for early detection, isolated publications show the benefit of chemopreventive agents (retinoids, beta-carotene, green tea, etc.) in the reversal of premalignant lesions of the oral cavity. Although some of these studies were randomized, numbers were too small to draw meaningful conclusions. A meta-analysis of the published literature also did not demonstrate a benefit of their use in the reversal of leukoplakia. The search for novel agents and establishing their role in chemoprevention is a potential area for research.

Adjuvant treatment in cases with intermediate-risk factors on histology

Oral cavity cancers are known to be associated with poor outcomes. Researchers have attempted to improve results with aggressive multidisciplinary treatment. This comes at the price of increased toxicity. The role of adjuvant chemoradiotherapy is well established for close, positive margins/extracapsular spread. The role of intensified treatment for other high-risk factors (lymphovascular invasion, perineural invasion, larger and deeper tumours) needs to be established.

Tumour biology

A few studies have shown conflicting results at the molecular level regarding differences associated with geography, ethnicity, carcinogen type and exposure. Larger and well-matched molecular epidemiology studies are required to validate differences, if any.

Other

- Role of neoadjuvant chemotherapy in organ preservation and locally-advanced oral cancer
- Margins after neoadjuvant chemotherapy and adjuvant therapy

Recommended reading:

Bernier J, Domenge C, Ozsahin M et al. (2004) Postoperative irradiation with or without concomitant chemotherapy for locally advanced head and neck cancer. *N Engl J Med* 350:1945–1952.

Blanchard P, Bourhis J, Lacas B et al. (2013) Taxane-cisplatin-fluorouracil as induction chemotherapy in locally advanced head and neck cancers: an individual patient data meta-analysis of the meta-analysis of chemotherapy in head and neck cancer group. *J Clin Oncol* 31:2854–2860.

Brennan J, Mao L, Ruban RHH et al. (1995) Molecular assessment of histopathological staging in squamous-cell carcinoma of the head and neck. *N Engl J Med* 332:429–435.

Cooper JS, Pajak TF, Forastiere AA et al. (2004) Postoperative concurrent radiotherapy and chemotherapy for high-risk squamous cell carcinoma of the head and neck. *N Engl J Med*. 350:1937–1944.

Huang SH, Hwang D, Lockwood G, O'Sullivan B (2009) Predictive value of tumor thickness for cervical lymph-node involvement in squamous cell carcinoma of the oral cavity: a meta-analysis of reported studies. *Cancer* 115(7):1489–1497.

Licitra L, Grandi C, Guzzo M et al. (2003) Primary chemotherapy in resectable oral cavity squamous cell cancer: a randomized controlled trial. *J Clin Oncol* 21:327–333.

Leusink FKJ, van Es RJJ, de Bree R et al. (2012) Novel diagnostic modalities for assessment of the clinically node-negative neck in oral squamous-cell carcinoma. *Lancet Oncol* 13:e554–556.

NCCN Treatment guidelines in Oncology: Head Neck Cancer Version 1.2013. Available at NCCN.org

Pignon JP, Bourhis J, Domenge C, Designe L (2000) Chemotherapy added to locoregional treatment for head and neck squamous-cell carcinoma: three meta-analyses of updated individual data. MACH-NC Collaborative Group. Meta-Analysis of Chemotherapy on Head and Neck Cancer. *Lancet* 355:949–955.

Pignon JP, le Maitre A, Maillard E et al. (2009) Meta-analysis of chemotherapy in head and neck cancer (MACH-NC): An update on 93 randomised trials and 17,346 patients. *Radiother Oncol* 92:4–14.

Sankaranarayanan R, Ramadas K, Thomas G et al. (2005) Effect of screening on oral cancer mortality in Kerala, India: a cluster-randomised controlled trial. *Lancet* 365:1927–1933.

Zhong LP, Zhang CP, Ren GX et al. (2013) Randomised phase III trial of induction chemotherapy with docetaxel, cisplatin and fluorouracil followed by surgery versus up-front surgery in locally advanced resectable oral squamous cell carcinoma. *J Clin Oncol* 31(6):744–751.

Zorat PL, Paccagnella A, Cavaniglia G et al. (2004) Randomised phase III trial of neoadjuvant chemotherapy in head and neck cancer: 10-year follow-up. *J Natl Cancer Inst* 96:1714–1717.

42 Larynx and hypopharynx

Jai Prakash Agarwal[1], Tejpal Gupta[1], Rahul Krishnatry[1], Amit Joshi[2] and Mitali Dandekar[3]

[1]Department of Radiation Oncology, Tata Memorial Centre, Mumbai, India
[2]Department of Medical Oncology, Tata Memorial Centre, Mumbai, India
[3]Department of Head and Neck Surgical Oncology, Tata Memorial Centre, Mumbai, India

Summary	Key facts
Introduction	• Common cancer in the head and neck region • Squamous cell cancer is the most common type: ▪ Glottis is the most common; post cricoid is the least common • Tobacco and alcohol use are the most important causes
Presentation	• Commonly present with symptoms of voice change, dysphagia and neck swelling • Baseline quality of voice and swallowing function is important for post-treatment assessment and rehabilitation • Computed tomography (CT) neck and chest is suggested in locally-advanced tumours
Scenario	• Early tumours are managed with either radiotherapy (RT) alone or organ-preserving surgery • Chemoradiotherapy (CRT) is the treatment of choice for locally-advanced tumours confined to the laryngeal framework • Hypopharyngeal tumours have poor outcomes due to early lymph node and distant metastasis • Role of induction therapy is still not fully defined

Trials	• Veterans Affairs Laryngeal Cancer Study Group; Wolf *et al.* (1991) *N Engl J Med* 324:1685–1690:
	  ▪ Induction chemotherapy with definitive RT was an equivalent option to surgery
	• RTOG 91-11; Forastiere *et al.* (2013) *J Clin Oncol* 31(7):845–852:
	  ▪ Chemoradiation was the best modality for organ preservation
	• MACH-NC meta-analysis of chemotherapy on head and neck cancer; Pignon *et al.* (2009) *Radiother Oncol* 92(1):4–14:
	  ▪ Concurrent CRT was the best way to combine chemotherapy with RT
	• MARCH meta-analysis of hyperfractionated or accelerated RT in head and neck cancer; Bourhis *et al.* (2006) *Lancet* 368:843–854:
	  ▪ Increased intensity using altered fractionation (hyperfractionated or accelerated) RT was more effective than conventional fractionation RT
	• DAHANCA 5; Overgaard *et al.* (1998) *Radiother Oncol* 46(2):135–146
	  ▪ Hypoxic sensitizer in addition to RT improved outcomes for supraglottic and pharyngeal cancer compared to RT alone
	• DAHANCA 6 & 7; Overgaard *et al.* (2010) *Lancet Oncol* 11(6):553–560:
	  ▪ A six-fraction weekly RT regimen improved local control and voice preservation compared to a five-fraction weekly schedule
	• EORTC trial 24891; Lefebvre *et al.* (2012) *Ann Oncol* 23(10):2708–2714:
	  ▪ Laryngeal preservation in hypopharyngeal cancers with induction chemotherapy and definitive RT

Introduction

Traditionally, carcinomas of the larynx and hypopharynx are considered together because of anatomical and physiological similarities. Due to their close anatomical proximity, cancers from one site frequently involve the other. Treatment and anatomical preservation can thus have implications for both sites. There are, however, important differences. Hypopharyngeal tumours have a much higher rate of submucosal and lymphatic spread, and distant metastasis, and

UICC Manual of Clinical Oncology, Ninth Edition. Edited by Brian O'Sullivan, James D. Brierley, Anil K. D'Cruz, Martin F. Fey, Raphael Pollock, Jan B. Vermorken and Shao Hui Huang. © 2015 UICC. Published 2015 by John Wiley & Sons, Ltd.

commonly present with advanced disease, thus leading to poorer outcomes.

Anatomically the larynx is divided into three subsites: the supraglottis, glottis and subglottis. The supraglottis includes the suprahyoid epiglottis (including the tip, lingual and laryngeal surfaces), laryngeal aspect of the aryepiglottic fold, arytenoid, infrahyoid epiglottis and ventribular bands (false cords). The glottis includes vocal cord, anterior and posterior commissure.

The hypopharynx is the part of pharynx lying posterior to the larynx and extends from the oropharynx above to the oesophageal inlet below, is cone shaped and consists of three regions or subsites: the paired pyriform sinuses, the lateral and posterior pharyngeal wall, and the post-cricoid area.

Incidence, aetiology and prevention

Incidence, aetiology and prevention	Description
Incidence	- One of the most common head and neck cancer sites - Second only to oral cavity cancer among all upper aerodigestive tract cancers in most cancer registries - Decreasing incidence from 5 per 100,000 in 1975 to 3.07 per 100,000 in 2009 - Incidence of >7 per 100,000 in South America and Eurasia - >60% of patients are older than 60 years - More common in males (5–6 times) and African–Americans (4:3) - Hypopharyngeal tumours are less common than laryngeal tumours

Aetiology	- Tobacco and alcohol are the two most important risk factors and have a synergistic effect:
	  - Cigarette, cigar and pipe smoking: 2–25 times increase in risk
	  - Moderate to heavy alcohol consumption: 1.5–2 times increase in risk
	  - Tobacco smoking is the most important risk factor for glottic cancer
	  - Alcohol is more prominent for supraglottic and hypopharyngeal cancer
	  - Continuation of smoking and/or alcohol during and or after treatment is associated with poorer outcomes
	- Diet:
	  - Higher incidence among patients with vitamin and nutrient deficient diets
	  - Hypopharyngeal cancer: association with Plummer Vinson syndrome; characterized by iron-deficiency anaemia, koilonychia, oesophageal webs, dysphagia and weight loss
	- Association with genetic conditions:
	  - Fanconi anaemia and dyskeratosis congenita
	- Field cancerization:
	  - Synchronous (7%) and metachronous malignancies (10–20%) in the aerodigestive tract
	  - More commonly with hypopharyngeal cancer
	- Occupation/industrial chemicals:
	  - Sulphuric acid mist, nickel or wood dust, asbestos, mustard gas exposure
	- Gastroesophageal reflux disease (GERD):
	  - Chronic irritation can be an important factor in non-smokers
	- Human papillomavirus (HPV):
	  - Common types 16 and 18

Screening and prevention	- Currently no role for screening
	- Primary prevention:
	  - Public awareness: smoking/alcohol cessation
	    - 35% decrease in the incidence of cancers with smoking and alcohol cessation over 25 years
	- Chemoprevention: investigational

Pathology

Pathology	Description
Carcinoma *in situ*	- Squamous cell carcinoma that does not breach the lamina propria - Commonly seen in vocal cords
Squamous cell carcinomas (SCC)	- >95% of cases - Variants:

(continued)

Pathology	Description

	- Verrucous carcinoma:
	  - Most common variant; 4% of all laryngeal cancers
	  - Slow growing tumours
	  - Gross warty appearance
	- SCC with spindle cell features: benign reactionary process with little clinical significance
	- Basaloid SCC and lymphoepithelioma of non–nasopharyngeal origin are uncommon
	- HPV may account for some non–smoking-related lesions

Others	- Small cell carcinoma, primary lymphoma, sarcoma, etc. are rarely seen: - Treatment is dictated by histology as in other sites

Presentation and natural history

The initial presentation varies depending on the regions involved. Multiple subsites may be involved in advanced cases because the regions are in close proximity. The glottis is the most common subsite (mostly involving the anterior one-third of the vocal cord), the supraglottis is involved in one-third of cases and the subglottis is the least commonly involved subsite (<2%).

Glottic carcinoma usually presents early with change in voice quality. In contrast, hoarseness or change in voice is not typical in early supraglottic/pyriform tumours.

Subglottic cancers are rare and often present late with either lymph node involvement or stridor. Pyriform sinus cancers present at an advanced stage due to non-specific complaints in early stages. Mild dysphagia, odynophagia, foreign body sensation and lump in the throat are common early symptoms. Otalgia due to referred pain may also be an early symptom.

Supraglottic and pyriform regions are rich in lymphatics and cervical adenopathy is common even with small primaries. In contrast, the glottis is devoid of lymphatics and hence lymph node involvement is unlikely in early stages. Retropharyngeal nodes may be involved in hypopharyngeal tumours, especially in those involving the posterior pharyngeal wall. Distant metastasis is common in hypopharyngeal tumours, with the lung being the most common site, and rare in glottic cancers (<5%).

Natural history and presentation		Description

Presentation	Local	- *Early laryngeal cancer:*
		  - Hoarseness
		  - Change in voice quality
		- *Early hypopharyngeal cancer:*
		  - Dysphagia
		  - Cervical lymph nodes
		- *Advanced laryngeal and/or hypopharyngeal cancer:*
		  - Hoarseness
		  - Dysphagia
		  - Cervical lymphadenopathy
		  - Weight loss
		  - Pain: local or referred to the ear
		  - Stridor

	Regional	- Glottic larynx: extremely rare in tumours confined to the glottis (T1 is ~0%; T2 is ~2%) - Bilateral lymph nodes are common with supraglottic and hypopharyngeal tumours - Hypopharyngeal tumours more commonly manifest with neck nodes, especially in the lower and central neck (levels III, IV and VI) - Retropharyngeal lymph node involvement is common in post-pharyngeal wall tumours, similar to nasopharyngeal cancer
	Metastatic	- Distant metastasis is common, particularly with hypopharyngeal tumours - Symptoms depend on site of metastasis, e.g. chronic dry cough for lung metastasis, bone pain for bone metastasis, etc.
Routes of spread	Local	- Most common pattern of spread; primarily mucosal - Submucosal spread is commonly associated with hypopharyngeal tumours occurring up to 2 cm from the visible tumour edge - Pre-epiglottic fat involvement is a marker for poor prognosis

Larynx and hypopharynx

Natural history and presentation	Description
	- Advanced lesions may eventually cause fixation of the larynx due to involvement of cricoarytenoid muscle or joint
- Spread to cartilages:
- Initially causes sclerosis
- Additional growth causes cartilage erosion
- Further growth results in destruction and penetration of the cartilages (and precludes laryngeal-preservation strategies)
- Perineural spread is uncommon
Regional	- Likelihood of lymph node involvement varies greatly with the extent of the primary tumour
- Bilateral lymph node involvement is common
- Jugulodigastric (level II) node is usually the first echelon
- Level IV, retropharyngeal and central compartment metastases is more common in hypopharyngeal cancers
Metastatic	- One of the most common head and neck cancer sites to develop metastases is the hypopharynx (10–20%); the least common is the glottis
- Most common metastatic site is the lung followed by the liver and bone

Diagnostic work-up

The pretreatment evaluation of patient includes assessment of performance status or fitness for therapy, disease confirmation and extent, baseline functional status for follow-up assessment of therapy efficacy and rehabilitation planning.

Diagnostic work-up	Description
Assessment of patient profile	- Age, gender, socioeconomic status
- Nutritional status, weight loss, co-morbidities
- History of continued lifestyle habits like tobacco and alcohol
- Assessment of tumour HPV status, and prior aerodigestive system malignancies and anticancer therapies (e.g. primary RT or chemotherapy)
- Quality of life assessment including voice function, hearing, swallowing and thyroid function:
- Voice quality and swallowing function assessment are important prior to organ-preservation treatment
- Dental assessment and fluoride prophylaxis:
- If extraction is done, a 7–10-day interval may be necessary for healing of the dental wound before the start of RT treatment
- Routine haematological indices and biochemistry
Assessment of tumour profile	- Histological proof of malignancy, type and grade
- Investigational, e.g. Ki-67 or tumour HPV status may assist in investigation protocols

Diagnostic work-up	Description
Assessment of tumour extent	- Physical examination for local tumour extent including laryngeal crepitus and evaluation of the neck for involved lymph nodes
- Fibre-optic/rigid endoscopy for extent of local tumour
- Pan-endoscopy of other primaries in head and neck/thoracic sites; important in laryngo-hypopharyngeal tumours to rule out synchronous malignancies in the upper aerodigestive tract
- Stroboscopy may be considered for early glottic lesions
- CT scan for local extent, cartilage involvement, neck and retropharyngeal nodes:
- Pretreatment tumour volume is a useful prognostic marker
- MRI is best at identifying subtle cartilage involvement and base of tongue infiltration:
- Gross cartilage involvement precludes organ preservation
- Chest X-ray: to rule out aspiration pneumonia when suspected:
- CT thorax is preferred to detect lung metastasis
- FDG-positron emission tomography (PET)-CT: to detect distant metastases and synchronous, second primary tumours (if available)
- Biopsy for confirmation
Tumour markers	- *TP53*, VEGF, cyclin D1 amplification, EGFR, *Bcl-2*

Staging and prognostic grouping

UICC TNM staging

See Table 42.1.

Table 42.1 UICC TNM categories and stage grouping: Larynx

TNM categories	
Larynx	
Supraglottis	
T1	One subsite, normal mobility
T2	Mucosa of more than one adjacent subsite of the supraglottis or glottis or adjacent region outside the supraglottis; without fixation
T3	Cord fixation or invades post-cricoid area, pre-epiglottic tissues, paraglottic space, thyroid cartilage erosion
T4a	Through thyroid cartilage; trachea, soft tissues of neck: deep/extrinsic muscle of tongue, strap muscles, thyroid, oesophagus
T4b	Prevertebral space, mediastinal structures, carotid artery
Glottis	
T1	Limited to vocal cord(s), normal mobility
	(a) one cord
	(b) both cords
T2	Supraglottis, subglottis, impaired cord mobility
T3	Cord fixation, paraglottic space, thyroid cartilage erosion
T4a	Through thyroid cartilage; trachea, soft tissues of neck: deep/extrinsic muscle of tongue, strap muscles, thyroid, oesophagus
T4b	Prevertebral space, mediastinal structures, carotid artery
Subglottis	
T1	Limited to subglottis
T2	Extends to vocal cord(s) with normal/impaired mobility
T3	Cord fixation
T4a	Through cricoid or thyroid cartilage; trachea, deep/extrinsic muscle of tongue, strap muscles, thyroid, oesophagus
T4b	Prevertebral space, mediastinal structures, carotid artery
Hypopharynx	
T1	<2 cm and limited to one subsite
T2	>2–4 cm or more than one subsite
T3	>4 cm or with hemilarynx fixation, extension to oesophagus
T4a	Thyroid/cricoid cartilage, hyoid bone, thyroid gland, central compartment soft tissue
T4b	Prevertebral fascia, carotid artery, mediastinal structures
All sites	
N1	Ipsilateral single ≤3 cm
N2	(a) Ipsilateral single >3–6 cm
	(b) Ipsilateral multiple ≤6 cm
	(c) Bilateral, contralateral ≤6 cm
N3	>6 cm
M1	Distant metastasis

Stage grouping			
Stage 0	Tis	N0	M0
Stage I	T1	N0	M0
Stage II	T2	N0	M0
Stage III	T1, T2	N1	M0
	T3	N0, N1	M0
Stage IVA	T1, T2, T3,	N2	M0
	T4a	N0, N1, N2	M0
Stage IVB	T4b	Any N	M0
	Any T	N3	M0
Stage IVC	Any T	Any N	M1

Prognostic factors

Traditionally, most robust data exist for correlation of extent of the primary lesion and neck disease as major determinants of outcomes in terms of local control and survival (Table 42.2). This includes fundamental staging parameters of T category, N category and overall stage group, and are essential factors. Similarly, large meta-analysis have confirmed correlation between age of >70 years (host factors), tobacco and alcohol use (environmental), and worse outcomes.

Recent trials in organ preservation have shown that functional outcomes are more appropriate endpoints to predict quality of life in survivors than mere anatomical preservation or control rates.

Treatment philosophy

The ultimate goal of treatment remains cure with best possible functional organ preservation. With this goal in mind, treatment options are strategized. For better understanding, laryngeal and hypopharyngeal cancers can be considered according to the subsites of glottis, supraglottis and hypopharynx, and subcategories according to TNM staging.

Localized tumours with no metastasis are usually divided into early or locally advanced (resectable or unresectable). The philosophy of treatment for early cancers is to achieve cure

Table 42.2 Prognostic factors for survival for laryngeal and hypopharyngeal carcinoma

Prognostic factors	Tumour related	Host related	Environment related
Essential	T, N, M categories Extracapsular extension	Co-morbidities Age >70 years Performance status	Able to provide standard treatment (resources) Treatment quality Resection margins
Additional	Regions/subsites involved Low neck nodes Tumour volume Vocal cord impairment Tracheostomy	Gender Laryngeal function	Nutrition Social/environmental (e.g. anatomical station) Overall treatment time
New and promising	Tumour markers: TP53, VEGF, cyclin D1 amplification, EGFR, Bcl-2 Tumour HPV status Chemoresistance genes	Baseline quality of life	Optical imaging New sensitizers in photodynamic therapy

with minimum morbidity. Both RT and conservative surgery are equally good options for disease control, with the choice dependent on other factors such as availability of resources (expertise, equipment, pharmaceutical and human resources), patient preferences, associated morbidity and chance of functional preservation or recovery. The impact of treatment complications on a patient's future socioeconomical rehabilitation needs to be considered. Planned use of combined modality treatment is discouraged as the toxicity of the two modalities is additive.

In locally-advanced cancers, the cornerstone of treatment is organ and function preservation (comprehensive organ preservation) whenever achievable with multimodality treatment. Non-surgical organ preservation is the initial treatment of choice. For unresectable patients, alternative approaches are considered, including definitive RT ± chemotherapy or initial treatment to render them resectable. In metastatic and unresectable patients with poor response to initial treatment, the goal is to provide palliation of major symptoms either with modalities or best supportive care (BSC) as feasible and suitable.

Scenario	Treatment philosophy
Carcinoma *in situ*	• Managed conservatively with minimally invasive surgery, vocal cord stripping or microlaryngeal laser surgery (Table 42.3) • Radiotherapy (RT) is an option particularly with multiple recurrences after surgery

Early local disease only	• Cure with functional organ preservation using single-modality treatment
	  ▪ Endoscopic surgery (Tables 42.3 and 42.4) alone, or
	  ▪ Definitive radiotherapy alone

Locoregional disease	• Resectable:
	  ▪ Cure with functional organ preservation whenever feasible using multimodality therapy (concurrent or sequential chemoradiotherapy [CRT]) or altered fractionated RT in selected cases
	• Unresectable:
	  ▪ Organ preservation approach with intensified treatment such as concurrent or sequential CRT or altered fractionation RT if performance status is suitable
	  ▪ Palliation in patients with poor performance status who cannot tolerate attempts to achieve locoregional control

Metastatic disease	• Palliation/BSC

Recurrent disease/second primary	• *Recurrent disease:*
	  ▪ Surgical salvage/(re)irradiation, whichever is appropriate or feasible
	  ▪ Palliation in patients unsuited for curative approaches
	• *Second primary:*
	  ▪ Treat wherever feasible using approaches with intention of cure

Table 42.3 Types of endoscopic cordectomy: European Laryngological Society Working Committee (1999)

Type of cordectomy	Extent
Type I	Subepithelial cordectomy
Type II	Sublingamental cordectomy
Type III	Transmuscular cordectomy
Type IV	Total cordectomy
Type V	Extended cordectomy: • Va: with anterior cordectomy • Vb: with arytenoids • Vc: with subglottis • Vd: with ventricle

Table 42.4 Types of endoscopic supraglottic laryngectomy: European Laryngological Society Working Committee (2009)

Type of supraglottic laryngectomy	Extent
Type I	Limited excision of small size superficial lesions of free edge of epiglottis, aryepiglottic fold, arytenoids, ventricular fold or any other part of the supraglottis
Type II	Medial supraglottic laryngectomy without resection of pre-epiglottic space: • Type IIa: superior hemi-epiglottectomy • Type IIb: total epiglottectomy
Type III	Medial supraglottic laryngectomy with resection of pre-epiglottic space: • Type IIIa: without ventricular fold excision • Type IIIb: with ventricular fold excision
Type IV	Lateral supraglottic laryngectomy: • Type IVa: with ventricular fold excision • Type IVb: with arytenoid excision

Treatment principles

Treatment principles	Description

Laser surgery versus radiotherapy in early glottic cancer	• *Advantage of laser:*
	  ▪ Treatment completed in a single modality setting:
	  ▪ RT is reserved for recurrent cancers
	• *Advantages of RT:*
	  ▪ Expertise of laser may not be available in all centres
	  ▪ Trend towards better voice quality with RT

Advanced laryngopharyngeal cancers	• Organ preservation strategies to be adopted whenever feasible using CRT/altered fractionation/RT with or without hypoxic sensitizers/targeted therapy
	• Relative contraindications to organ preservation strategies:
	  ▪ Gross cartilage erosion and extra-laryngeal disease
	  ▪ Dysfunctional larynx

Surgical principles for laryngopharyngeal cancers	• *Conservative laryngeal surgery:*
	  ▪ At least one functioning cricoarytenoid unit is a prerequisite for conservative surgery
	  ▪ Cricoid cartilage erosion precludes conservative laryngeal surgery
	• *Surgical resection margins for which withholding adjuvant RT may be considered:*
	  ▪ At least 5 mm in laryngeal cancers
	  ▪ In hypopharyngeal cancers, due to their propensity for submucosal spread of up to 10–20 mm (predominantly inferior extent followed by lateral and superior), surgical margins should be adequately wide (up to 2 cm)

Treatment principles	Description

	• *Reconstruction:*
	  ▪ Pharyngeal reconstruction is indicated in total laryngopharyngectomy:
	  ▪ Options depend on the extent of lower resection:
	    ○ If total pharyngectomy only: free jejunum, folded PMMC, folded FRAFF
	    ○ If total pharyngectomy with oesophagectomy: gastric pull up
	  ▪ Pharyngeal augmentation is indicated in cases of total laryngectomy with partial pharyngectomy when the residual pharyngeal wall is inadequate for primary closure (residual unstretched pharyngeal mucosa of approximately <3 cm):
	    ○ Patch pectoralis major myocutaneous flap (PMMC)
	    ○ Free flap: free radial artery forearm flap (FRAFF), anterolateral thigh flap (ALT)
	• *Voice rehabilitation:*
	  ▪ Tracheoesophageal speech gives the best voice outcome after total laryngectomy:
	    ○ Tracheoesophageal puncture is preferably performed at primary surgery; otherwise as a secondary procedure
	  ▪ Other options:
	    ○ Oesophageal speech
	    ○ Electrolarynx

Treatment

Glottic cancer

Treatment: Glottic cancer	Description

Carcinoma *in situ*	- *Primary treatment options:*
	  - Voice preserving surgery (preferred), or
	  - Radical RT
	- *Surgery:*
	  - Endoscopic resection: generally with laser excision
	- *Radiotherapy:*
	  - Small field to include the entire glottis with superior–inferior 2-cm margins
	  - Commonly used RT schedules:
	  - 50 Gy in 20 fractions over 4 weeks; 2.55 Gy/fraction, five fractions per week
	  - 60–66 Gy in 30–33 fractions over 6–6.5 weeks; 2 Gy/fraction, five fractions per week

Early disease: T1–2N0	- *Primary treatment options:*
	  - Endoscopic resection (laser/surgery) (see Table 42.3), or
	  - Radical RT
	- *Surgery:*
	  - For T1 disease without anterior commissure involvement:
	    - Endoscopic resection; generally laser excision
	  - Role of conservative open surgery is diminished with advent of laser; may be used in selected cases
	- *Radiotherapy:*
	  - For T1–2 disease:
	    - Small field including whole glottis with superior–inferior 2-cm margins
	    - Altered fractionation schedules, especially in T2 diseases
	  - Commonly used RT schedules:
	    - 66–70 Gy in 33–35 fractions over 5.5–6 weeks; 2 Gy/fraction, six fractions per week
	    - RTOG 9512 protocol: 79.2 Gy in 66 fractions over 6.5 weeks; 1.2 Gy/fraction, b.i.d., ten fractions per week

Early disease: T3N0	- *Primary treatment options:*
	  - Concurrent CRT (preferred)
	  - Surgery
	- *Concurrent CRT:*
	  - Primary tumour with involved nodes to a dose of 66–70 Gy with conventional fractionation
	  - Elective nodal volume including bilateral levels II, III, IV and V to a dose of 45–50 Gy with conventional fractionation
	  - Concomitant chemotherapy with cisplatin 100 mg/m^2 three times weekly, or
	  - Weekly cisplatin 30–50 mg/m^2 to a minimal cumulative dose of 200 mg/m^2, or
	  - Carboplatin + 5-fluorouracil (5-FU) or, with lower evidence, single-agent carboplatin or taxanes
	- *Alternative treatment:*
	  - Altered fractionation RT
	  - Commonly used RT schedules:
	    - Hyperfractionation (radiobiologically preferred) to 81.6 Gy in 68 fractions over 7 weeks, 1.2 Gy/fraction, b.i.d. with an interval of at least 6 hours; concomitant boost to a dose of 72 Gy over 6 weeks using 1.8-Gy/fraction for total volume and a 1.5-Gy boost in the last 12 fractions (more pragmatic) with or without chemotherapy
	    - Accelerated RT:
	  - 66–70 Gy in 6 days over 6 weeks or 64 Gy in 40 fractions over 4 weeks; 1.6 Gy/fraction, b.i.d., or
	  - 70 Gy in 35 fractions over 6 weeks; 2.0 Gy/fraction, six fractions per week
	- *Surgery:*
	  - Total laryngectomy with bilateral selective neck dissection (level II–IV)
	  - Voice conservative procedures to be considered in place of total laryngectomy whenever feasible, e.g. supracricoid laryngectomy

(continued)

Treatment: Glottic cancer	Description
Locally-advanced resectable disease: T3–4aN+	• *Primary treatment options:* 　■ CRT (preferred option), or 　■ Surgery or 　■ Induction chemotherapy • *Chemoradiotherapy:* 　■ As for early disease: T3N0 • *Surgery:* 　■ As for early disease: T3N0 • *Induction chemotherapy:* 　■ Complete or partial response: radical (chemo)radiotherapy as for early disease: T3N0 　■ Stable or progression of disease: salvaged with surgery as for early disease: T3N0
Locally-advanced unresectable: T4bAny N	• *Primary treatment options:* 　■ *Performance status 0–2*: 　　○ Radical CRT (preferred option) 　　○ Induction chemotherapy (investigational) for good performance status; followed by response assessment 　• Partial response: concurrent CRT/radical RT 　• Progressive disease/stable disease: palliative treatment/BSC 　　■ *Performance status 3*: 　　　○ BSC in poor performance status • *Chemoradiotherapy:* 　■ As for early disease: T3N0 • *Induction chemotherapy:* 　■ DCF: docetaxel (D) + cisplatin (C) + 5-FU (F), 3-weekly, two to three cycles 　■ Other drugs used in the triple regimen are paclitaxel instead of docetaxel (T), and carboplatin instead of cisplatin
Metastatic disease	• *Primary treatment options:* 　■ Palliative RT for locoregional control wherever suitable: 　　○ 'QUAD SHOT': 14 Gy in four fractions over 2 days, b.i.d., with optional repeat of up to two cycles at 1-month intervals 　　○ Palliative local RT with weekly 6–8 Gy/fraction, 30 Gy in ten fractions daily or short fractionation 　■ Palliative chemotherapy or BSC in poor performance status • *Palliative chemotherapy:* 　■ PS 0–1: platinum + 5-FU + cetuximab; alternatives are platinum doublets with 5-FU or a taxane 　■ PS 2: single-agent chemotherapy, e.g. methotrexate (40–60 mg/m^2 given weekly) 　■ Meteronomic chemotherapy: oral methotrexate 15.5 mg/m^2 weekly and celecoxib 200 mg b.i.d. or similar regimens (investigational) 　■ Patients with performance status of 3 or less should receive only BSC 　■ In all circumstances participation in trials should be recommended

Supraglottic cancer

Treatment: Supraglottic cancer	Description
Early cancer: T1–3N0	• *Primary treatment:* 　■ Laser or open surgery + neck dissection, or 　■ Radical RT (preferred option) • *Surgery:* 　■ Endoscopic resection + selective neck dissection; simultaneous or sequential (see Table 42.4) 　■ Open conservative laryngeal surgery (supracricoid/supraglottic laryngectomy) • *Radiotherapy:* 　■ Primary tumour with involved nodes to a dose of 66–70 Gy with conventional fractionation 　■ Uninvolved nodes including bilateral levels II, III, IV and V to a dose of 45–50 Gy with conventional fractionation 　■ Altered fractionation: 　　○ Hyperfractionation to 81.6 Gy over 7 weeks; 1.2 Gy/fraction b.i.d. with a 6-hour interval; concomitant boost to a dose of 72 Gy over 6 weeks; 1.8 Gy/fraction for total volume and a 1.5-Gy boost in the last 12 fractions 　■ Accelerated RT: 　　○ 66–70 Gy, 6 days a week for 6 weeks

Treatment: Supraglottic cancer	Description

Locally-advanced resectable disease: T3Any N+	• *Primary treatment:*
	  ▪ Radical chemoradiation (preferred), or
	  ▪ Surgery, or
	  ▪ Induction chemotherapy
	• *Chemoradiotherapy:*
	  ▪ RT as for early cancer: T1–3N0
	  ▪ Concomitant chemotherapy with cisplatin 100 mg/m^2 3-weekly:
	    ○ Weekly cisplatin, carboplatin, taxanes are other options
	• *Surgery:*
	  ▪ Total laryngectomy with bilateral selective neck dissection (modified neck dissection if node positive)
	  ▪ Conservative open procedure whenever feasible
	• *Induction chemotherapy:*
	  ▪ Complete or partial response: consider radical (chemo)radiotherapy as for early cancer: T1–3N0
	  ▪ Stable or progression of disease salvaged with surgery as above
	• In all circumstances participation in trials should be recommended

Locally-advanced resectable disease, T4aAny N	• *Primary treatment:*
	  ▪ Surgery (preferred option for gross cartilage involvement or exolaryngeal spread), or
	  ▪ Radical chemoradiation, or
	  ▪ Induction chemotherapy (investigational)

Locally-advanced unresectable disease: T4bAny N	• *Primary treatment:*
	  ▪ Concurrent CRT
	  ▪ Induction chemotherapy (investigational) for good performance status; followed by response assessment:
	    ○ Partial response: concurrent CRT/radical RT
	    ○ Progressive disease: palliative treatment
	  ▪ Palliative radiotherapy/chemotherapy or BSC in poor performance status

Metastatic	• *Primary treatment:*
	  ▪ Palliative chemotherapy or BSC in poor performance status
	• *Palliative RT for locoregional control:*
	  ▪ 'QUAD SHOT': 14 Gy in four fractions over 2 days, b.i.d., with optional repeat of up to two cycles at 1-month intervals
	  ▪ Palliative local RT with weekly 6–8 Gy/fraction; 30 Gy in ten fractions daily or short fractionation
	• *Palliative chemotherapy:*
	  ▪ PS 0-1: platinum + 5-FU + cetuximab; alternatives are platinum doublets with 5-FU or a taxane
	  ▪ PS 2: single-agent chemotherapy could be used with methotrexate as the reference drug (40–60 mg/m^2 weekly)
	  ▪ PS 3: BSC

Hypopharynx

Treatment: Hypopharynx	Description

Early cancer: T1–2N0	• *Primary treatment:*
	  ▪ Radical RT (preferred option), or
	  ▪ Surgery
	• *Radiotherapy:*
	  ▪ Primary tumour with involved nodes to a dose of 66–70 Gy with conventional fractionation.
	  ▪ Uninvolved nodes including bilateral levels II, III, IV and V to dose of 45–50 Gy with conventional fractionation
	  ▪ Altered fractionation:
	    ○ Hyperfractionation (preferred) to 81.6 Gy over 7 weeks; 1.2 Gy/fraction b.i.d. with a 6-hour interval; concomitant boost to a dose of 72 Gy in 6 weeks using 1.8 Gy/fraction for total volume and 1.5 Gy boost in last 12 fractions
	  ▪ Accelerated RT: 66–70 Gy, 6 days a week for 6 weeks
	• *Surgery:*
	• Partial pharyngectomy (open/endoscopic) with bilateral level II–IV neck dissection (modified neck dissection depending on nodal stage on frozen section)

(continued)

Treatment: Hypopharynx	Description

Locally-advanced resectable disease: T1N+, T2–3Any N	• *Primary treatment:*
	  ▪ Radical chemoradiation (preferred option), or
	  ▪ Surgery (preferred for dysfunctional larynx), or
	  ▪ Induction chemotherapy
	• *Radiation:* as for supraglottic cancer except:
	  ▪ Retropharyngeal nodes coverage important in post-pharyngeal wall tumours
	  ▪ Levels IV and VI nodes are covered
	  ▪ Upper oesophagus involvement should be ruled out
	• *Surgery:*
	  ▪ Laryngopharyngectomy with ipsilateral modified neck dissection and contralateral level II–IV
	• *Induction chemotherapy:*
	  ▪ As for supraglottic larynx

Locally-advanced resectable: T4aN1	• *Primary treatment:*
	  ▪ Surgery (preferred option particularly for gross cartilage involvement and/or exolaryngeal spread), or
	  ▪ Radical chemoradiation, or
	  ▪ Induction chemotherapy (investigational)
	• Locally-advanced resectable disease: T1N+, T2–3Any N

Locally-advanced unresectable: T4bAny N	• *Primary treatment:*
	  ▪ Concurrent CRT
	  ▪ Induction chemotherapy (investigational) for good performance status; followed by response assessment:
	    ○ Partial response: concurrent CRT/radical RT
	    ○ Progressive disease: palliative treatment
	• Palliative radiotherapy/chemotherapy or BSC in poor performance status:
	  ▪ As for supraglottic larynx

Metastatic disease	• *Primary treatment:*
	  ▪ Palliative chemotherapy or BSC in poor performance status:
	    ○ As for supraglottic larynx

Adjuvant treatment for postoperative high- and intermediate-risk features

Adjuvant treatment by risk stratification		Description

Intermediate	Multiple lymph nodes (LNs) involved, or Vascular/lymphatic/perineural invasion, or pT3/pT4	• *Radiotherapy:*
		  ▪ Interval between surgery and adjuvant treatment should ideally be <6 weeks
		  ▪ Include the whole surgical bed with bilateral neck nodes
		  ▪ Primary and involved nodes: 60–66 Gy with conventional fractionation
		  ▪ Uninvolved nodes: 50–60 Gy with conventional fractionation
		  ▪ Overall treatment time: 100 days

High risk	Extracapsular nodal spread, or Positive resection margin	• *Chemoradiotherapy:*
		  ▪ As above, plus
		  ▪ Concomitant cisplatin based chemotherapy to a dose of 100 mg/m² 3-weekly
		  ▪ Other chemotherapy options are weekly carboplatin + 5-FU or weekly platinum regimens

Model for neck dissection in post radical chemoradiation patients

This is described in Table 42.5.

Table 42.5 Model for node dissection

	Investigations	Timing	Treatment	Timing
Initial N0–1	Clinically suspected residual disease, addressed with one of the following: • PET-CT • CT or MRI • US neck	8–12 weeks	If negative, observe only If borderline, observe closely or selective neck dissection If residual disease, selective or comprehensive neck dissection	8–12 weeks
Initial N2–3	Clinically residual disease, addressed with one of the following: • PET-CT (preferred choice): 　▪ High negative predictive value • CT or MRI • US neck	8–12 weeks	If negative, observe only If borderline, observe closely or selective neck dissection If residual disease, selective or comprehensive neck dissection There is an emerging role for super-selective neck dissection (SSND), which addresses nodal level at risk only Decreasing role for planned neck dissection (PND) with advent of PET-CT follow-up surveillance	8–12 weeks
Isolated neck recurrence	Clinical examination negative for local recurrence or second primary • PET-CT • CT or MRI • US neck-guided FNA, if required	NA	Comprehensive neck dissection (preferred option) There is an emerging role for super-selective neck dissection (SSND), which addresses nodal level at risk only Re-irradiation with concurrent chemotherapy (if unresectable and patient suitable for re-irradiation) Palliative chemotherapy/targeted therapy or BSC when not suitable for either surgery or radiation	NA

Salvage for recurrence or second primary

Salvage for recurrence or second primary	Description
Previous surgery only	• *Previous laser surgery:* 　▪ Recurrent disease is managed using principles for primary disease as described earlier • *Previous radical surgery:* 　▪ Repeat surgery (preferred option) 　▪ If unresectable, but good general condition: 　　○ Radical chemoradiation, or 　　○ Induction chemotherapy followed by (chemo)radiotherapy 　▪ If resectable and in a poor general condition: 　　○ Palliative therapy or BSC • *Following surgery for recurrence:* 　▪ Adjuvant postoperative RT ± chemotherapy may be considered according to risk factors • *Poor general condition:* 　▪ Palliative radiation/chemotherapy or BSC as tolerated to achieve best symptomatic control
Previous radiotherapy (see Chapter 39)	• Salvage surgery (preferred option) • If unresectable: 　▪ Chemo-re-irradiation can be considered if: 　　○ Performance status 0–2 　　○ Second primary after 2 years and in low-dose region; <2-year higher chances of toxicity 　　○ Recurrence after 2 years; those with a recurrence within 2 years are unlikely to respond and show more toxicity 　　○ No grade 2 or more late toxicity

Salvage for recurrence or second primary	Description
	• Caveats: 　◦ Use most conformal RT with minimal margins and reduce dose to spine and 　◦ Limit on maximum dose to spine at a total dose of ≤100 Gy biological effective dose (BED) combined 　◦ Carotid blow out 　◦ Radical dose to gross tumour of 60–70 Gy in 1.8–2 Gy/fraction with concurrent cisplatin/cisplatin + 5-FU/taxanes • Re-irradiation alone without chemotherapy may be considered in selected patients with performance status 2, age >70 years and contraindication for chemotherapy • Palliative radiation/chemotherapy/targeted therapy or BSC if above criteria not fulfilled

Follow-up and continuing care

Eighty percent of recurrences in laryngeal and hypopharyngeal tumours occur within 2–3 years, either locoregionally or at distant sites. Localized glottic cancers may recur as late as 5 years or beyond. Thereafter, the risk of second primary cancers due to field cancerization increases, so careful follow-up is warranted. This justifies relatively close follow-up in the first few years after treatment. First follow-up is usually planned at 12 weeks with imaging study (CT, MRI or PET-CT) in patients with initial large neck nodes (N2–3). The focus is assessment of the response to organ preservation therapy and plan for neck dissection when residual disease is suspected.

In addition to survivorship, issues related to functional rehabilitation and return to pre-disease normal daily life (e.g. return to work) are crucial. They form a very important aspect of intervention and should be anticipated and instituted prior to treatment and continued indefinitely. Suggested guidelines are given in Table 42.6.

Important remaining aspects in aftercare are:
- Monitoring and reporting of late effects
- Comprehensive rehabilitation
- Prevention and treatment for aspiration pneumonia
- Nutrition.

Controversies

Radiotherapy versus surgery in early glottic cancer

Although vast numbers of retrospective single-institute series report similar cure rates with both RT and surgery (hemilaryngectomy or cordectomy or laser), only one true comparative study (laser surgery vs RT) and two RT fractionation studies have

Table 42.6 Guidelines for follow-up and continuing care

Time frames	Frequency	Work-up	Specific issues	Intervention
First 2 years	2–3 monthly	Clinical exam, quality of life, nutritional assessment, functional status of voice, swallowing and laryngeal oedema	Locoregional or distant recurrences, stoma care, etc. Assessment of voice prosthesis Quality of life, nutritional assessment, functional status of voice, swallowing, employment	Investigate with appropriate method to identify recurrence or second primary Rehabilitation, vocational training, re-employment To address specific issue related to voice prosthesis (leaking prosthesis blocked valve) consider change of prosthesis at regular intervals
	At 8–12 weeks	CT, MRI or PET-CT	Pretreatment N2/N3 nodes	Neck node dissection if residual
	6 monthly	Thyroid function Dental evaluation	Hypothyroidism Xerostomia and caries	Thyroxine if required Scaling and fluoride paste application
2–5 years	3–6 monthly	Clinical examination with judicious application of schema above	Judicious application of schema above	Judicious application of schema above
	Yearly	Thyroid function Dental evaluation as above Metastasis	As above Chest X-ray	As above
After 5 years	Yearly	As above	As above	As above

been reported. The local control rates with RT range from 85% to 95% for T1 and from 65% to 80% for T2, and ultimate control rates after salvage surgery for recurrences are >95% (T1) and 90% (T2). Unfortunately, many studies comparing voice quality between post-laser excision and RT have presented conflicting conclusions. A recent meta-analysis in >7600 patients suggested a trend toward improved voice quality with RT compared to transoral laser excision, and this is confirmed by a recent randomized trial. Usually, the final decision for optimum primary treatment is based on the preferences and expertise of the attending physicians, patient choices, cord mobility at presentation and anticipated voice quality after therapy. Irradiation is still the preferred initial treatment, with surgery reserved for salvage after RT failure at most centres.

Role of neoadjuvant/induction chemotherapy in locally-advanced patients

Induction chemotherapy is an attractive alternative treatment for larynx preservation. It is based on the hypothesis that a chemosensitive patient will also be radiosensitive, and it enables resectable patients to preserve their larynx if they respond to induction chemotherapy treatment. An added benefit for patients fail to respond to chemotherapy is an early salvage surgical procedure, which is easier to perform after chemotherapy alone than after chemoradiation.

Until now most randomized studies have failed to show overall survival or laryngectomy-free survival benefit with the use of cisplatin + 5-FU-based induction chemotherapy over concurrent chemoradiation. A MACH-NC meta-analysis of randomized controlled trials (1965–2011) showed a cumulative benefit of 6% for overall survival (non-significant) and 7% for distant metastasis rate ($P = 0.05$) for all head and neck cancer patients with use of induction chemotherapy. In a subsite analysis specifically for laryngeal preservation, no significant improvement in survival was found ($P = 0.47$). A recent 10-year updated report for RTOG 91-11, a trial comparing three cycles of PF induction chemotherapy followed by RT versus concomitant cisplatin-based CRT versus single-modality RT, showed a separation of survival curves beyond 4.5 years in favour of induction chemotherapy. This was caused by a higher number of deaths unrelated to laryngeal cancer despite the absence of a documented increase in late toxicities in the concomitant group. It is postulated that this may be due to associated co-morbidities not specific to the treatment or random event unrelated to treatment. Interestingly, however, delayed functional decline could have led to the chronic toxicities, including aspiration pneumonia and associated cardiopulmonary compromise. So, better documentation of late toxicities can be proposed and newer modalities of radiation like intensity-modulated RT (IMRT) may provide a solution in future trials.

Also, it is now known from various phase III studies that TPF is superior to PF for laryneal preservation. With the advent of various newer agents like cetuximab in induction and concurrent settings, new trials are required. In a recent phase II TREMPLIN trial using TPF induction chemotherapy followed either by concurrent cisplatin-based chemoradiotherapy or concurrent cetuximab + RT, neither showed superiority in terms of overall survival. Yet, more failures occurred in the cetuximab + RT arm, which could be salvaged by the surgery. Therefore, more studies are needed. Ultimately, induction with the best available regimen (TPF) followed by RT should be compared with best available concurrent chemoradiotherapy (RT + high-dose cisplatin × 3) with an adequate assessment of organ function, toxicity and quality of life. Guidelines for future neoadjuvant trial designs have been proposed (Box 42.1).

Neck dissection in neck node positive patients undergoing organ preservation treatment

The presence of neck node involvement has been associated with poor outcomes in terms of both locoregional and distant recurrences. Various approaches are described in the literature to address involved neck nodes, including pre-RT neck dissection, post-RT planned or post-RT response assessment-based neck dissection. There is often controversy also relating to the extent and timing of neck dissection. The optimal management of the node-positive neck remains undetermined.

The primary justification for post-RT planned neck dissection is the high chance of residual neck disease (25%) for a bulky initial presentation (N2/3) treated with radical chemoradiation in spite of a complete clinical response. This is further complicated by challenges related to early identification of nodal disease in post-RT necks due to fibrosis, accurate clinical follow-up and poor outcomes in spite of post-salvage neck surgery. The implication of viable tumour cells on histopathology in post-RT nodes is another controversy.

The ideal investigation to ascertain residual disease and decide about further treatment post CRT is still undefined.

Box 42.1 Criteria for modern neoadjuvant chemotherapy trials

Inclusion
T4, advanced nodal stages, laryngeal dysfunction, age >70 years, hypopharynx primary

Assessments
Voice quality, intelligible speech, swallowing, aspiration, salivary function, quality of life, socioeconomic impact

Endpoints
Laryngo-oesophageal dysfunction standard definition development

Lab to clinic implications
Targeted agents to increase tumour control and to decrease toxicity

Timing has different meaning for different investigations, ranging from viability to clonogenic capacity of residual tumour cells (ultrasound [US], FNA cytology or PET). If these are performed earlier than the time needed for regression, false-positive results may occur. Alternatively, undue delay in identification may compromise outcomes.

Clinical assessment at 8–12 weeks post CRT has been suggested; this is when the acute effects of treatment will have subsided but is before fibrosis sets in. In initial N1 and N2 disease, when physical examination of the neck shows no cervical adenopathy, observation with close follow-up may be more appropriate. When clinical examination is ambiguous, or if an N3 node was present at initial presentation but there is a complete clinical response, CT, MRI, PET-CT or neck US at 8–12 weeks can be planned. If clinically suspected residual nodal disease is present, a planned neck dissection is advisable. Imaging may also facilitate the determination of the extent of nodal disease.

Early nodal disease after residual disease in post CRT (4–12 weeks) has some potential advantages in improving regional control and survival. However, the benefit of surgery in patients with a complete clinical response after CRT is undetermined. Most retrospective single-institution reviews are limited by inadequate statistical power to detect a survival advantage for this subset of patients. The morbidity of a potentially unnecessary procedure cannot be ignored. Moreover false-negative patient selection for observation can lead to persistence or progression of disease in the neck and delayed salvage ND. This has been associated with an increased frequency and severity of post surgical complications and outcomes. A 'window' between acute and chronic CRT treatment effects on normal tissues (8–12 weeks) has been suggested to minimize the surgery-related complications.

The gold standard surgical procedure for treatment of residual or recurrent cervical lymph nodes following CRT is radical neck dissection (RND) or modified radical neck dissection (MRND). However, considerable debate regarding the use of selective neck dissection (SND) or super-selective neck dissection (SSND; confined to one or two contiguous neck node levels when there is a single positive neck node level) prevails. Post nodal disease, risk stratification and adapted treatment strategies have not been adequately investigated.

Phase III clinical trials

See Table 42.7.

Table 42.7 Phase III clinical trials

Trial name	Results
Local disease	
RTOG 91-11 Forastiere et al. (2013) J Clin Oncol 31(7):845–852	• Concurrent chemoradiation was the best option to spare the larynx in patients with advanced laryngeal cancer, but was associated with a higher incidence of unexplained non-cancer-related death at long-term follow-up • Trend for better survival with the induction regimen
IAEA-ACC study Overgaard et al. (2010) Lancet Oncol 11(6):553–560	• Accelerated RT was more effective than conventional fractionation
DAHANCA 5 Overgaard et al. (1998) Radiother Oncol 46(2):135–146	• Hypoxic sensitizer in addition to RT improved outcomes compared to RT alone
DAHANCA 6 & 7 Overgaard et al. (2010) Lancet Oncol 11(6):553–560	• A six fraction-weekly RT regimen improved local control and voice preservation but not regional control compared to a five fraction-weekly schedule
EORTC 24891 Lefebvre et al. (2012) Ann Oncol 23(10):2708–2714	• Laryngeal preservation in hypopharyngeal cancers with induction chemotherapy
Adjuvant systemic therapy	
MACH-NC Collaborative Group (meta-analysis) Pignon et al. (2009) Radiother Oncol 92(1):4–14	• Concurrent chemotherapy was the best form of adjuvant chemotherapy
PARADIGM Haddad et al. (2013) Lancet Oncol 14(3):257–264	• Upfront chemoradiation remains the standard of care over induction chemotherapy followed by chemoradiation
Combined analysis of EORTC (22931) and RTOG (9501) Bernier et al. (2005) Head Neck 27(10):843–850	• Improving outcomes with postoperative adjuvant chemoradiation

Trial name	Results
Advanced disease and metastatic disease	
ECOG 5397 Burtness et al. (2005) *J Clin Oncol* 23(34):8646–8654.	• Addition of cetuximab to cisplatin significantly improved response rate
QUAD SHOT (phase II) Corry et al. (2005) *Radiother Oncol* 77(2):137–142	• Palliative RT treatment had minimal toxicity and a good response rate, which impacted positively on patients' quality of life
EXTREME trial Vermorken et al. (2014) *Ann Oncol* 25(4):801–807	• Addition of cetuximab to two-drug chemotherapy (platinum + 5-FU) resulted in significant improvement in overall survival compared to chemotherapy alone in the recurrent/metastatic setting

Areas of research

Aspects of treatment that are being evaluated include:
- *Chemoprevention*:
  - Identify newer and more effective agents
- *Prognostification*:
  - Comprehensive prognostic scoring criteria
  - Inclusion of factors like age, co-morbidity, pretreatment quality of life scores, other functional scores
  - Development of comprehensive scores of co-morbidity assessment
  - Importance of HPV-positive laryngeal cancer
- *Modification of existing modalities*:
  - Surgery:
    - Microlaryngeal surgeries, sequencing of neck dissection in advanced nodal stages, surgical voice restoration techniques
  - Radiation:
    - Altered fractionation, IMRT to spare dysphagia/aspiration-related structures (DARS), role of adaptive treatments, re-irradiation with high-precision techniques
    - Combination with more potent and newer chemotherapy agents in concurrent and neoadjuvant settings for improved functional organ preservation
  - Chemotherapy:
    - Taxane-based neoadjuvant chemotherapy with newer target agents for improved organ preservation rates and palliation in metastatic or advanced unresectable cases
- *Newer modalities/agents*:
  - Exploration of newer targets and individualized therapies with identification of chemo-radioresistance-like mutations on chromosome 3q, 7p and 11q
  - Newer agents like small-molecule epidermal growth factor receptor (EGFR) tyrosine kinase inhibitors, PI3K/Akt/mTOR inhibitors, vascular endothelial growth factor (VEGF) receptor inhibitors and proteasome inhibitors
- *Post treatment care*:
  - Comprehensive team management with development of techniques to objectively assess functional outcomes and improve them.

Recommended reading

Aaltonen LM, Rautianimen N, Sallman J et al. (2014) Voice quality after treatment of early vocal cord cancer: a randomized trial comparing laser surgery with radiation therapy. *Int J Radiat Oncol Biol Phys* 90(2):255–260

Agarwal JP, Baccher GK, Waghmare CM et al. (2009) Factors affecting the quality of voice in the early glottic cancer treated with radiotherapy. *Radiother Oncol* 90(2):177–182.

Ang KK et al. (2005) *Radiotherapy for Head and Neck Cancers: Indications and Techniques*, 3rd edn. Philadelphia: Lippincott Williams & Wilkins.

Bernier J, Cooper JS, Pajak TF et al. (2005) Defining risk levels in locally advanced head and neck cancers: a comparative analysis of concurrent postoperative radiation plus chemotherapy trials of the EORTC (#22931) and RTOG (# 9501). *Head Neck* 27(10):843–850.

Bourhis J, Overgaard J, Audry H et al. (2006). Hyperfractionated or accelerated radiotherapy in head and neck cancer: a meta-analysis. *Lancet* 368:843–854.

Burtness B, Goldwasser MA, Flood W, Mattar B, Forastiere AA; Eastern Cooperative Oncology Group (2005) Phase III randomized trial of cisplatin plus placebo compared with cisplatin plus cetuximab in metastatic/recurrent head and neck cancer: an Eastern Cooperative Oncology Group study. *J Clin Oncol* 23(34):8646–8654.

Cooper JS, Zhang Q, Pajak TF et al. (2012) Long-term follow-up of the RTOG 9501/intergroup phase III trial: postoperative concurrent radiation therapy and chemotherapy in high risk squamous cell carcinoma of the head and neck. *Int J Radiat Oncol Biol Phys* 84(5):1198–1205.

Corry J, Peters LJ, Costa ID et al. (2005) The 'QUAD SHOT'–a phase II study of palliative radiotherapy for incurable head and neck cancer. *Radiother Oncol* 77(2):137–142.

Dawson LA, Myers LL, Bradford CR et al. (2001) Conformal re-irradiation of recurrent and new primary head-and-neck cancer. *Int J Radiat Oncol Biol Phys* 50(2):377.

De Crevoisier R, Domenge C, Wibault P et al. (2001) Full dose reirradiation combined with chemotherapy after salvage surgery in head and neck carcinoma. *Cancer* 91(11):2071.

Forastiere AA, Zhang Q, Weber RS et al. (2013) Long-term results of RTOG 91-11: a comparison of three nonsurgical treatment strategies to preserve the larynx in patients with locally advanced larynx cancer. *J Clin Oncol* 31(7):845–852.

Gupta T, Chopra S, Agarwal JP et al. (2009) Squamous cell carcinoma of the hypopharynx: single-institution outcome analysis of a large cohort of patients treated with primary non-surgical approaches. *Acta Oncol* 48(4):541–548

Haddad R, O'Neill A, Rabinowits G et al. (2013) Induction chemotherapy followed by concurrent chemoradiotherapy (sequential chemoradiotherapy) versus concurrent chemoradiotherapy alone in locally advanced head and neck cancer (PARADIGM): a randomised phase 3 trial. *Lancet Oncol* 14(3):257–264.

Higgins KM, Shah MD, Ogaick MJ, Enepekides D (2009) Treatment of early-stage glottic cancer: meta-analysis comparison of laser excision versus radiotherapy. *J Otolaryngol Head Neck Surg* 38(6):603–612.

Laskar SG, Baijal G, Murthy V et al. (2012) Hypofractionated radiotherapy for T1N0M0 glottic cancer: retrospective analysis of two different cohorts of dose-fractionation schedules from a single institution. *Clin Oncol* 24(10):e180–e186.

Lefebvre JL, Ang KK; Larynx Preservation Consensus Panel (2009) Larynx Preservation Consensus Panel Larynx preservation clinical trial design: Key issues and recommendations—A consensus panel summary. *Head Neck* 31:429–441.

Lefebvre JL, Andry G, Chevalier D et al. (2012) Laryngeal preservation with induction chemotherapy for hypopharyngeal squamous cell carcinoma: 10-year results of EORTC trial 24891. *Ann Oncol* 23(10):2708–2714.

Lefebvre JL, Pointreau Y, Rolland F et al. (2013) Induction chemotherapy followed by either chemoradiotherapy or bioradiotherapy for larynx preservation: the TREMPLIN randomized phase II study. *J Clin Oncol* 31(7):853–859.

NCCN Treatment guidelines in Oncology: Head Neck Cancer Version 1.2013 NCCN.org

Overgaard J, Mohanti BK, Begum N et al. (2010) Five versus six fractions of radiotherapy per week for squamous-cell carcinoma of the head and neck (IAEA-ACC study): a randomised, multicentre trial. *Lancet Oncol* 11(6):553–560.

Pignon JP, le Maître A, Maillard E, Bourhis J; MACH-NC Collaborative Group (2009) Meta-analysis of chemotherapy in head and neck cancer (MACH-NC): an update on 93 randomised trials and 17,346 patients. *Radiother Oncol* 92(1):4–14.

Trotti A, Zhang Q, Bentzen S et al. (2014) Randomized trial of hyperfrationation versus conventional fractionation in T2 squamous cell carcinoma of the vocal cord (RTOG 9512). *Int J Radiat Oncol Biol Phys* 89(5):959–962.

Wolf G et al. (1991) Induction chemotherapy plus radiation compared with surgery plus radiation in patients with advanced laryngeal cancer: The Department of Veterans Affairs Laryngeal Cancer Study Group. *N Engl J Med* 324:1685–1690.

Yamazaki H, Nishiyama K, Tanaka E, Koizumi M, Chatani M (2006) Radiotherapy for early glottis carcinoma (T1N0M0) results of prospective randomized study of radiation fraction size and overall treatment time. *Int J Radiat Oncol Biol Phys* 61(1):77–82.

43 Oropharynx

Shao Hui Huang[1], Hisham Mehanna[2], Jan B. Vermorken[3], and Brian O'Sullivan[1]

[1]Department of Radiation Oncology, The Princess Margaret Cancer Centre, University of Toronto, ON, Canada
[2]Institute of Head and Neck Studies and Education, School of Cancer Sciences, University of Birmingham, Birmingham, UK
[3]Department of Medical Oncology, Antwerp University Hospital, Edegem, Belgium

Summary	Key facts

Introduction	- *Incidence*:
	  - 22nd most common cancer globally
	  - Declining incidence in smoking-related cancers in this site
	  - Rising incidence in HPV-related cancer, especially in the Western world
	  - >90% are squamous cell carcinoma
	- *Risk factors*:
	  - Tobacco use and heavy alcohol intake:
	    - A synergistic effect exists between tobacco and alcohol
	  - High-risk human papillomavirus (HPV) infection, especially types 16 and 18
	    - Mostly involving tonsil or base of tongue

Presentation	- *HPV negative*:
	  - Relatively older age (median ~65 years)
	  - Males more frequently affected
	  - Local symptoms, including sore throat, dysphagia, odynophagia, otalgia
	- *HPV positive*:
	  - Relatively younger age (median 55 years)
	  - Males much more frequently affected (about 85%)
	  - ~Two-thirds present with asymptomatic neck mass, associated with a discrete/small primary
	  - Minimal local symptoms (e.g. pain), even with a large primary
	  - Cystic lymph node appearance is common on imaging (generally CT)

Scenario	- Stage I–II (T1–2N0):
	  - Primary radiotherapy (RT) or transoral surgery and neck dissection
	  - Well-lateralized tumours: RT to primary and ipsilateral neck only
	- Stage III–IV:
	  - Concurrent chemoradiotherapy (CCRT) or bioradiotherapy (BRT):
	    - Platinum-based cytotoxic agents
	    - Cetuximab when CCRT is contraindicated
	  - Altered fractionation RT alone for:
	    - N0 status or small nodal (N1) volume disease or ≤3 nodes
	    - Medically unfit for chemotherapy or if chemotherapy is declined
	    - Elderly (>70 years) or frail patient
	- Induction chemotherapy followed by CCRT, BRT or RT alone is an option that can be considered in individual cases with locoregionally very advanced disease

---

UICC Manual of Clinical Oncology, Ninth Edition. Edited by Brian O'Sullivan, James D. Brierley, Anil K. D'Cruz, Martin F. Fey, Raphael Pollock, Jan B. Vermorken and Shao Hui Huang. © 2015 UICC. Published 2015 by John Wiley & Sons, Ltd.

Summary	Key facts

Trials	• Calais et al. (1999) J Natl Cancer Inst 91(24):2081–2086 (OPC specific):
	  ▪ RT versus CRT for advanced-stage oropharyngeal carcinoma
	  ▪ CCRT improved overall survival, disease-free survival and locoregional control
	• MACH-NC meta-analysis; Pignon et al. (2009) Radiother Oncol 92(1):1–11 (not OPC specific):
	  ▪ Concurrent chemotherapy with radiation conveys a modest survival advantage (6.5% at 5-years) compared to traditional standard fractionation RT alone
	  ▪ Overall impact of chemotherapy is 4.5%
	• MARCH meta-analysis; Bourhis et al. (2006) Lancet 368:843–854 (not OPC specific):
	  ▪ Intensification by hyperfractionation RT alone with augmented dose conveys a modest survival advantage (8%) compared to traditional standard fractionation RT alone
	  ▪ Overall impact of altered fractionation provides a 3.4% survival benefit
	• TAX 323; Vermorken et al. (2007) N Engl J Med 357(17):1695–1704 (not OPC specific):
	  ▪ TPF induction is superior in terms of survival to PF induction regimens, followed by RT alone, for unresectable head and neck cancer
	• TAX 324; Posner et al. (2007) N Engl J Med 357(17):1705–1715 (not OPC specific):
	  ▪ TPF induction is superior in terms of survival to PF induction regimens, followed by concurrent chemoradiotherapy

Introduction

Oropharyngeal cancer (OPC) comprises those cancers arising from the mucosal surfaces of the oropharynx, including base of the tongue and vallecula as the anterior border of the oropharynx; posterior oropharyngeal wall; tonsil region and lateral oropharyngeal wall as the lateral border; soft palate and uvula as the superior border (Box 43.1).

Over 90% of OPC is squamous cell carcinoma (SCC), which is the focus of this chapter. Minor salivary gland tumours, lymphomas (and other haematolymphoid tumours) and mesenchymal tumours also occur in the oropharynx, but require separate consideration and will not be covered in this chapter

Incidence, aetiology and screening

Oropharyngeal SCC can be caused by two distinct carcinogenic processes: tobacco use with synergistic effect from heavy alcohol intake; and persistent high-risk human papillomavirus (HPV) infection, especially HPV subtype 16. Smoking-related (HPV-negative) and HPV-related (HPV-positive) OPC exhibit different clinical behaviours. There may be a subset of OPC in which both HPV and smoking contribute to the aetiogenesis.

Box 43.1 Anatomical borders of the oropharynx

- Anterior wall:
  - Base of tongue
  - Vallecula
- Lateral wall:
  - Tonsillar fossa
  - Anterior faucial pillar
  - Posterior faucial pillar (rare with more adverse prognosis)
  - Glossotonsillar sulcus
  - Lateral oropharyngeal wall
- Posterior wall
- Superior wall:
  - Soft palate
  - Uvula
- Inferior limit is the axial plane of the vallecula or superior border of the hyoid bone

Incidence, aetiology and screening	Smoking related (HPV-negative)	HPV related (HPV-positive)
Incidence	• ~52% of OPC worldwide • Prevalence expected to decline, especially in developed countries; attributed to smoking cessation	• ~48% of OPC worldwide • Significant variation by geographical regions: ▪ Prevalence has increased significantly in Europe and North America over time • >95% caused by HPV subtype 16; remainder caused by HPV subtype 18, 31, 33, 35, 52 and 58

Incidence, aetiology and screening	Smoking related (HPV-negative)	HPV related (HPV-positive)

Aetiology	• Smoking (tobacco use)
	• Excessive alcohol consumption:
	  ▪ Synergistic effect with tobacco use
		• Persistent high-risk HPV infection (>95% is HPV 16 subtype)
		• Suggested routes of viral transmission include:
		  ▪ Oral sex
		  ▪ High number of sexual partners
		  ▪ Indirect sexual contact is possible
		  ▪ Vertical transmission (mother-to-child) is also plausible and may explain very young patient affliction

Screening and prevention	• Screening: currently no role • Smoking cessation	• Screening: currently no role • Modification of sexual behaviour • HPV vaccine: ▪ Vaccination in teenage males and females is a topic of discussion in countries at high risk for HPV-related OPC

Pathology

- *Smoking related (HPV-negative)*:
  - Well-to-moderately differentiated, keratinizing morphology
- *HPV related (HPV-positive)*:
  - More likely to be poorly differentiated, non-keratinizing or basaloid morphology

Histological diagnosis should generally be established by tissue biopsy of the primary tumour. Rarely, in persons unfit for open biopsy and in whom biopsies under local anaesthesia have not been successful, a positive cancer diagnosis from fine needle aspiration (FNA) of involved nodes may be acceptable but generally does not reliably confirm HPV association. Establishing the diagnosis for HPV-related OPC can also be challenging if the primary is very small with minimal mucosal changes. A superficial biopsy may miss small viable tumour foci within the tonsil crypt and a tonsillectomy may miss a tumour arising within the tonsil pillar.

Over 90% of OPC is SCC. Variants such as papillary SCC, spindle cell (sarcomatoid) SCC and others may occur. Conventional HPV-negative OPC generally has well-to-moderately differentiated keratinizing morphology, while HPV-positive OPC is characterized by poorly differentiated non-keratinizing or basaloid morphology. However, to determine whether the tumour is an HPV-driven tumour, specific HPV testing is required. Many HPV testing methods exist but currently there is no consensus regarding the optimal method. The methods given in Table 43.1 can be used for detection of HPV-positive tumours, of which p16 staining is generally accepted as a reliable surrogate marker for HPV-driven OPC, which also carries a better cost profile than other testing methods.

Table 43.1 Commonly used HPV testing methods

Type of tumour sample	Tumour markers	Comments
Tumour tissue (formalin-fixed paraffin-embedded [FFPE], or fresh frozen)	HPV DNA (e.g. viral E6 and E7) by polymerase chain reaction (PCR) or in situ hybridization (ISH)	High sensitivity Presence of HPV DNA in tumour may not always indicate the tumour is driven by HPV and may miss some HPV subtype if this subtype is not included in the testing probe
	HPV RNA (e.g. viral E6 and E7 mRNA) by PCR or ISH	Generally considered to be the gold standard of HPV detection High sensitivity and specificity: definitive evidence of viral integration
	p16 over-expression by IHC staining	Commonly used as a surrogate marker for HPV-driven OPC Less costly, easy to conduct High sensitivity but low specificity; agnostic to HPV subtype which is an advantage compared to HPV subtype specific testing method when one takes clinical situation into account Some rare tumour histologies, such as neuroendocrine tumour, can also result in p16 expression
Cell blocks from fine needle aspiration (FNA)	p16 over-expression by ISH staining	Requires enough tumour cells Less reliable than p16 staining on FFPE Reagent is important to minimize degradation: • Avoid alcohol fixation • Prepare cell blocks from unfixed cells in saline and then fix in formalin

Presentation and natural history

The natural history of smoking-related OPC appears to differ from that of HPV-related OPC. An asymptomatic neck mass at presentation without obvious oropharyngeal lesions ('unknown primary') is common in HPV-positive disease, while local symptoms are typical in HPV-negative disease. An HPV-positive nodal mass is often of cystic appearance (30–50%; may be mistaken for a 'brachial cleft cyst' carcinoma), and also has a soft or 'spongy' feeling on palpation (may be mistaken for 'lymphoma').

Presentation and natural history		Smoking related (HPV-negative)	HPV related (HPV-positive)

Presentation	Local	• Usually a visible local mucosal mass:
		  ▪ May occur in any oropharyngeal mucosal subsite
		• Associated with local symptoms: odynophagia, dysphagia, otalgia
			• Likely discrete small primary lesion (mostly T1-2); soft or 'spongy' feeling on palpation:
			  ▪ Arising 'deep' from basal cell layer of crypt with minimal mucosal changes, or growing outward as a exophytic lesion
			  ▪ Predominantly in tonsil or base of tongue
			• Paucity of local symptoms, even in those with a larger primary tumour
			• Multicentric synchronous primaries may occur in a small proportion of patients (e.g. contralateral tonsil or other head and neck region outside of the oropharynx)

	Regional	• Large palpable lymph nodes are surprisingly infrequent and usually associated with large primary tumours • Often necrotic or conglomerate; unlikely to be cystic	• About two-thirds present with an asymptomatic neck mass without an obvious oropharyngeal primary ('unknown primary') • Gross lymph node involvement is frequent, even in small (T1–2) primary lesions • Often the first sign prompting patients to seek medical attention • Cystic lymph nodes are frequent and present in ~50% cases
	Metastatic	• ~1% present with lung metastasis • Not curable, resulting in death within 2 years of manifestation of distant metastasis	• ~0.5% present with metastatic lesions, mainly in lung; may also present in other organs, such as liver and bone • Long-term survival is possible for selected patients with single-organ metastasis
Routes of spread	Local	• Superior to nasopharynx • Inferior to hypopharynx • Lateral to para-oropharyngeal space • Anterior to deep/extrinsic muscle of oral tongue • Posterior to paraspinal soft tissue	• As for HPV-negative OPC • Discontiguous but adjacent lesion seems to occur sometimes
	Regional	• Level II lymph node involvement is most common, followed by level III lymph node region • Level I and IV lymph node involvement is uncommon • Retropharyngeal lymph node involvement occurs in about 10% of cases	• As for HPV-negative OPC, except lymph node involvement is more common at presentation compared to HPV-negative disease with the same T category
	Distant	• Lung is the most common first distant metastatic site	• Lung is the most common (>0%) first distant metastatic site • Two distant metastasis phenotypes exist: aggressive 'disseminating' phenotype (to multiple organ and unusual sites) and slow growing 'indolent' phenotype

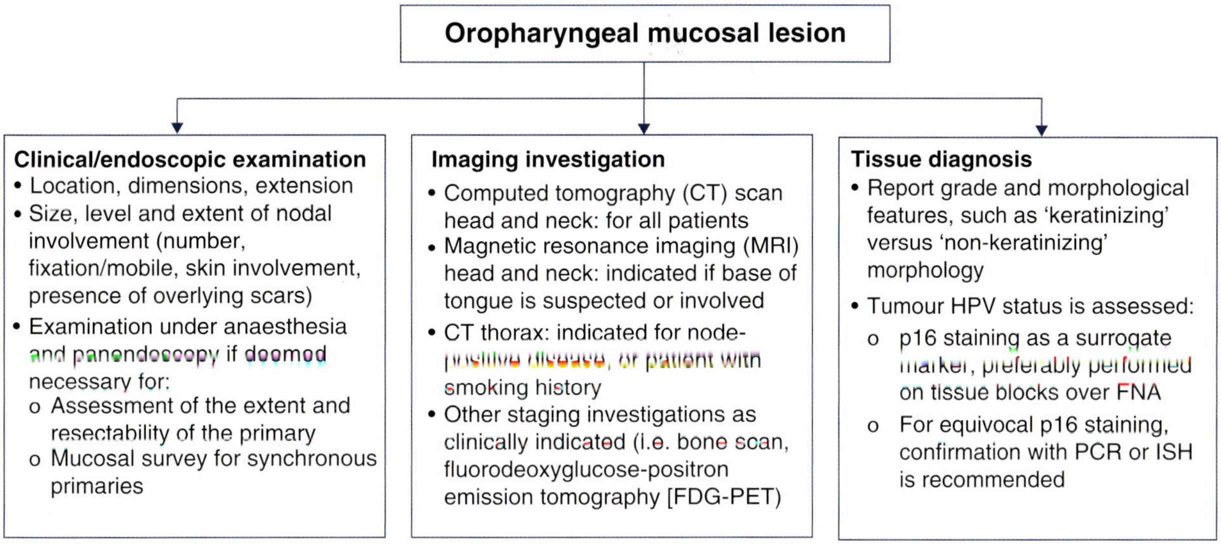

```
┌─────────────────────────────────┐
│   Oropharyngeal mucosal lesion  │
└─────────────────────────────────┘
         │         │         │
         ▼         ▼         ▼
```

Clinical/endoscopic examination
- Location, dimensions, extension
- Size, level and extent of nodal involvement (number, fixation/mobile, skin involvement, presence of overlying scars)
- Examination under anaesthesia and panendoscopy if deemed necessary for:
  o Assessment of the extent and resectability of the primary
  o Mucosal survey for synchronous primaries

Imaging investigation
- Computed tomography (CT) scan head and neck: for all patients
- Magnetic resonance imaging (MRI) head and neck: indicated if base of tongue is suspected or involved
- CT thorax: indicated for node-positive disease, or patient with smoking history
- Other staging investigations as clinically indicated (i.e. bone scan, fluorodeoxyglucose-positron emission tomography [FDG-PET]

Tissue diagnosis
- Report grade and morphological features, such as 'keratinizing' versus 'non-keratinizing' morphology
- Tumour HPV status is assessed:
  o p16 staining as a surrogate marker, preferably performed on tissue blocks over FNA
  o For equivocal p16 staining, confirmation with PCR or ISH is recommended

Figure 43.1 Diagnosis and staging procedures

Diagnostic work-up

Recommended procedures for diagnosis and staging are shown in Fig. 43.1.

Tumour markers	Smoking related (HPV-negative)	HPV related (HPV-positive)
Marker expression	• Almost all over-express EGFR • p16 inactivation • *TP53* mutation	• HPV E6 and E7 expression in tumour • HPV DNA in tumour (>95% are HPV subtype 16) • p16 over-expression (surrogate marker) • Wild-type *TP53*

Stage and prognostic grouping

UICC TNM staging

The classification of OPC is based on tumour category (T), node category (N) and metastasis (M) category according to physical examination, endoscopy and imaging findings (Table 43.2). Currently, there is no HPV-positive OPC-specific TNM staging system, although emerging evidence suggests a separate TNM staging may be indicated.

Prognostic factors

Tumour HPV status is the most important factor in determining survival of OPC (Table 43.3). Patients with HPV-positive tumour have superior survival outcomes compared to patients with regular HPV-negative (smoking-related) tumour regardless of treatment modalities. T and N category also predict survival. However, the prognostic value of T and N in HPV-positive versus HPV-negative tumours may be different. Hypoxia plays an important role in HPV-negative tumours, but has less influence in HPV-positive tumours. Not surprisingly, life-time smoking burden (i.e. smoking pack-years) also has an impact on survival.

Treatment philosophy: Non-metastatic oropharyngeal cancer (M0) (Fig. 43.2)

For non-metastatic OPC, the goal of treatment is cure for both HPV-positive and HPV-negative patient. No difference in treatment selection recommendation currently exists, although several de-intensification options for selected HPV-positive patients are currently being considered in clinical trials. Stage I–II disease can be treated by either primary radiotherapy or primary surgery. Of patients with T1–2N0 disease, 10–30% may harbour occult neck disease; therefore, neck dissection

Table 43.2 UICC TNM categories and stage grouping

TNM categories	
T1	≤2 cm
T2	>2–4 cm
T3	>4 cm
T4a	Larynx, deep/extrinsic muscle of tongue, medial pterygoid, hard palate, mandible
T4b	Lateral pterygoid muscle, pterygoid plates, lateral nasopharynx, skull base, carotid artery
N1	Ipsilateral single ≤3 cm
N2	(a) Ipsilateral single >3–6 cm
	(b) Ipsilateral multiple ≤6 cm
	(c) Bilateral, contralateral ≤6 cm
N3	>6 cm
M1	Distant metastasis.

Stage grouping			
Stage 0	Tis	N0	M0
Stage I	T1	N0	M0
Stage II	T2	N0	M0
Stage III	T3	N0	M0
	T1, T2, T3	N1	M0
Stage IVA	T1, T2, T3	N2	M0
	T4a	N0, N1, N2	M0
Stage IVB	T4b	Any N	M0
	Any T	N3	M0
Stage IVC	Any T	Any N	M1

or elective neck irradiation should be considered even in early-stage disease. Treatment of Stage III–IV is generally considered to be by organ-preservation approaches with a preference for concurrent chemoradiotherapy (CCRT), with surgery reserved for salvage of residual or recurrent disease. Hypoxia modification agents show promising results in HPV-negative OPC with more hypoxic features, but are less effective for HPV-positive tumours.

General principles
- Oropharyngeal function/organ preservation without compromising disease control should be considered:
  - Primary radiotherapy is the most common treatment modality
- Transoral resection and neck dissection ± postoperative radiotherapy are gaining popularity for early stage (I and II) disease
- Chemotherapy should generally be considered for advanced stage (III and IV) disease, especially where there is extensive nodal involvement:
  - Chemotherapy should be given concurrently with radiotherapy to augment local regional control and eradicate occult distant metastases
  - Induction chemotherapy in addition to CCRT has been tested in head and neck cancer patients in the clinical trial setting, but so far studies have been inadequate in size or performance and are not therefore conclusive; however, subset analysis suggested that the most beneficial survival effect was achieved in patients with

Table 43.3 Prognostic risk factors for survival of OPC

Prognostic factors	Tumour related	Host related	Environment related
Essential	HPV status (including p16) T category N category	Smoking, especially during radiotherapy Performance status	Quality of treating facility (staging workup and expertise in multidisciplinary management)
Additional	Number of involved nodes Level of involved nodes Tumour volume Hypoxia	Co-morbidities Age	Ability to receive standard treatment: • Radiation dose • Overall treatment time • Quality of radiotherapy
New and promising	EGFR expression TP53 mutation Bcl-2 ERCC1	Health-related quality of life	

```
┌─────────────────────────────────────────────────────────┐
│         Non-metastatic oropharyngeal carcinoma          │
└─────────────────────────────────────────────────────────┘
              │              │              │
              ▼              ▼              ▼
      ┌──────────────┐ ┌──────────────┐ ┌──────────────────┐
      │  Stage I–II  │ │ Stage III,   │ │ Advanced Stage IV│
      │              │ │ early Stage IV│ │    (T4N2c–3)    │
      └──────────────┘ └──────────────┘ └──────────────────┘
```

Stage I–II

RT alone:
- Primary + elective neck
- RT neck volume:
  - Bilateral level 2–4
  - Unilateral level 2–4 if primary lateralized ≥1 cm from midline

Transoral surgery:
- Resection of primary + ipsilateral neck dissection (level 2–4, possible level 1)

Stage III, early Stage IV

RT ± systemic agents:
- Chemoradiotherapy, or
- Accelerated radiotherapy ± cetuximab
- RT dose: full dose to 'gross' target area; moderate dose to 'elective' areas
- RT volume: include lateral retropharyngeal node region

Advanced Stage IV (T4N2c–3)

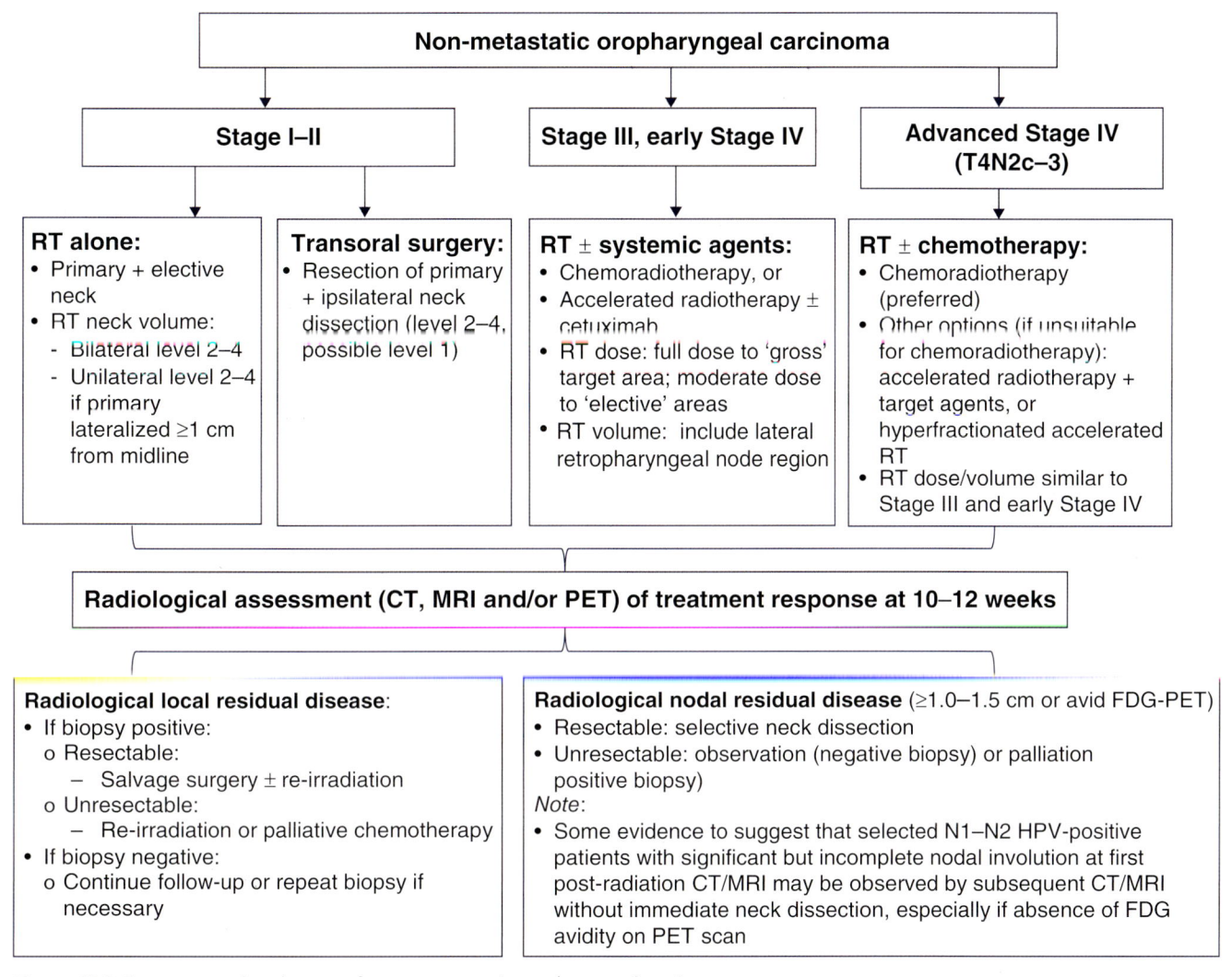

RT ± chemotherapy:
- Chemoradiotherapy (preferred)
- Other options (if unsuitable for chemoradiotherapy): accelerated radiotherapy + target agents, or hyperfractionated accelerated RT
- RT dose/volume similar to Stage III and early Stage IV

Radiological assessment (CT, MRI and/or PET) of treatment response at 10–12 weeks

Radiological local residual disease:
- If biopsy positive:
  - Resectable:
    - Salvage surgery ± re-irradiation
  - Unresectable:
    - Re-irradiation or palliative chemotherapy
- If biopsy negative:
  - Continue follow-up or repeat biopsy if necessary

Radiological nodal residual disease (≥1.0–1.5 cm or avid FDG-PET)
- Resectable: selective neck dissection
- Unresectable: observation (negative biopsy) or palliation positive biopsy)

Note:
- Some evidence to suggest that selected N1–N2 HPV-positive patients with significant but incomplete nodal involution at first post-radiation CT/MRI may be observed by subsequent CT/MRI without immediate neck dissection, especially if absence of FDG avidity on PET scan

Figure 43.2 Treatment options by stage for non-metastatic oropharyngeal carcinomas

OPC and those with N2c/N3 neck disease. Recent meta-analysis data suggest an impact on distant failure on mucosal head and neck cancer overall (not stratified by tumour HPV status), which needs to be confirmed in HPV-positive and HPV-negative OPC subsets
- Oropharyngeal primaries *always* require elective treatment of cervical lymph node regions at risk of involvement:
  - Location of overt nodal disease may influence the extent of elective nodal treatment
  - Minimum radiotherapy extent of the elective neck should include ipsilateral levels II–IV in the clinical N0 situation
  - Gross involvement of any nodal region ordinarily mandates:
    - Radical radiotherapy to 70 Gy in 35 fractions or equivalent doses (± chemotherapy or altered fractionation) is delivered to 'gross' target areas discerned by imaging, with the 'elective' microscopic moderate doses prescribed to the remaining neck regions judged to also be at risk
    - Inclusion of adjacent lymph node echelons and, if treated with radiotherapy, generally extending the microscopic elective dose volumes to the lateral retropharyngeal node region at the base of the skull on the side of nodal involvement, since failure at this site is very problematic
    - Inclusion of ipsilateral level IB and level V is questionable as the risk of involvement is very low (<5%) even with ipsilateral pathologically proven neck disease
  - Bilateral neck irradiation (usually with elective dose intended for microscopic disease excepting regions with overt nodal disease) is generally required for the following situations, especially in tumours originating in the midline region of the oropharynx:
    - Lesions involving the posterior pharyngeal wall (where bilateral retropharyngeal nodes should also be treated)
    - Posterior tonsillar pillar lesions should be treated in the same way as the posterior pharyngeal wall

- Carcinomas arising in the soft palate/uvula generally warrant elective irradiation of both sides of the neck, including the retropharyngeal nodes
- Central base of tongue and vallecular tumours are treated similarly to bilateral nodal regions, but the retropharyngeal nodes may be omitted in N0 presentations
- Although lateralized tonsillar lesions may be treated with ipsilateral radiotherapy approaches, those with medial extension (within 1 cm of the midline on the palate and/or base of tongue) generally require bilateral elective radiotherapy for microscopic disease
- Unilateral neck radiotherapy may be considered for:
  - N0–1 disease with a small and well-lateralized tonsil and ≤1 cm of mucosal involvement of the base of the tongue or soft palate
  - N0–2b (small volume N2b) where imaging of the contralateral neck is unequivocally negative (i.e. no suspicion of nodal involvement)
- Role of post-radiotherapy neck dissection is evolving for patient with N2–3 disease:
  - Radiological complete response: post radiotherapy neck dissection can likely be avoided
  - Radiological incomplete response in the neck: post-radiotherapy neck dissection is advisable for HPV-negative patients or N3 HPV-positive patients, but may be avoided for selected HPV-positive patients with N2 disease with a significant lymph node involution; such patients must undergo continued rigorous imaging surveillance with the goal of avoidance of surgery

Scenario: Non-metastatic OPC (M0)	Description
Stage I–II (T1–2N0)	<ul><li>Primary radiotherapy or primary surgery should be equally effective; the choice depends on local resources and expertise</li><li>Elective neck management by radiation or neck dissection should be undertaken since the risk of occult neck disease remains between 10% and 30%</li><li>If treated with primary radiotherapy:<ul><li>Dose/fractionation schedule: 70 Gy in 35 fractions (or equivalent) over 7 weeks (five fractions/week) is typical</li><li>Neck volumes:<ul><li>Minimum volumes should include ipsilateral levels II–IV</li><li>Bilateral treatment to the neck is generally required</li><li>Unilateral neck treatment may be appropriate for well-lateralized (≥1 cm to the midline) tumours, including tonsillar cancers or very small (T1) palatal and lateral pharyngeal wall cancers</li></ul></li></ul></li><li>If treated with primary surgery:<ul><li>Transoral surgery is preferable to open surgery for functional preservation</li><li>Neck dissection:<ul><li>Should include ipsilateral level II–IV</li><li>Inclusion of level I is debatable</li><li>Level IIB can be omitted if there is no disease in level IIA</li><li>Contralateral neck dissection should also be considered for tumours arising at or very near (<1 cm) the midline in the soft palate and posterior pharyngeal wall, if elective radiotherapy is contraindicated, taking into account potential long-term sequelae of bilateral neck dissections, such as lymphoedema</li></ul></li><li>Postoperative CCRT should be included for tumours with involved surgical margins or nodal disease with extracapsular extension (ECE), though emerging evidence suggests ECE is not prognostic for HPV-positive disease provided adjuvant radiotherapy alone is also used</li><li>Postoperative radiotherapy should be considered for tumours with adverse features, such as close or positive surgical resection margin, tumour thickness >4 mm, presence of lymphovascular invasion and/or perineural invasion</li></ul></li></ul>
Stage III and IV	<ul><li>Organ-preservation strategy with treatment intensification is favoured</li><li>Surgery is usually reserved for salvage of treatment failure after primary radiotherapy</li><li>*Stage III and early Stage IV with minimal nodal disease (T1–2N1–2a or T3N0–2aM0)*:<ul><li>May be treated with either intensive altered fractionation radiotherapy or CCRT, though the latter is more usual</li></ul></li></ul>

Scenario: Non-metastatic OPC (M0)	Description

	- *Advanced Stage IV (T4 or Any'T'N2b–3M0)*:
	  - CCRT is preferred over altered fractionation radiotherapy ± epidermal growth factor receptor (EGFR) inhibitor due to the increased risk of distant metastasis with advanced nodal disease:
	    - Induction chemotherapy may play a role in very advanced disease because of its potential impact to reduce risk of distant metastasis
	  - Typical radiotherapy regimens with associated concurrent systemic treatments are given in Table 43.4
	  - If treated with primary surgery:
	    - Resection of the primary tumour should be followed by reconstruction as necessary
	    - Those patients who have a clinically node-positive neck should have a modified radical or selective level I–IV neck dissection
	    - Ipsilateral neck dissection may be performed if the tumour is well lateralized
	    - Contralateral neck dissection should be considered when tumours encroach on the midline
	    - Adjuvant CCRT or radiotherapy alone should be considered in all cases with adverse risk factors (as given for Stage I–II)

Table 43.4 Radiotherapy regimens with associated concurrent systemic treatments for advanced Stage IV disease

Radiotherapy regimen	Systemic therapy
70 Gy in 35 fractions over 7 weeks (five fractions/week) + chemotherapy	Cisplatin: - High-dose (preferable): 100 mg/m² IV on Days 1, 22 and 43 of radiotherapy - Weekly cisplatin (40 mg/m²) is acceptable if concerns about treatment tolerance of high-dose cisplatin
70 Gy in 35 fractions over 6 weeks (six fractions/week) ± cetuximab	Cetuximab: - 400 mg/m² loading dose over 120 minutes in week prior to commencing radiotherapy, then - 250 mg/m² weekly during radiotherapy
64 Gy in 40 fractions over 4 weeks (b.i.d. 6 hours apart, ten fractions/week), RT alone	None
65–66 Gy in 30 fractions over 6 weeks (five fractions/week), RT alone	None
7.2 Gy in 60 fractions (1.2 per fraction) over 6 weeks (b.i.d. 6 hours apart, ten fractions/week), RT alone	None
60 Gy in 25 fractions over 5 weeks (five fractions/week), RT alone	None

Assessment of treatment response and indication for post-irradiation neck dissection: Non-metastatic oropharyngeal cancer (M0) (Fig. 43.2)

The initial post-radiation imaging evaluation should be performed no earlier than 10–12 weeks after radiotherapy to avoid high false-positive rates. This is especially important for HPV-positive patients as the gross lymph node(s) are commonly cystic with a somewhat slower regression rate. The imaging modalities generally include CT, MRI and/or PET. The role of FDG-PET is unclear, but it may be useful for selected patients who have not achieved a clinical or CT/MRI-based radiological complete response, since absence of FDG avidity is generally indicative of disease sterilization. This is currently being investigated in a phase III trial.

If physical examination and imaging suggest residual disease at the primary site, a biopsy is performed to confirm residual disease. If the primary site is cleared of residual disease yet residual disease at the cervical nodal basin is suggested from imaging/clinical evaluation (≥1.0–1.5 cm), then the following approaches can be considered:
- FNA:
  - If positive: neck dissection
  - If negative: observation
- Selective neck dissection for radiological residual nodal disease or nodal progression
- Surveillance: there is some evidence suggesting a role for surveillance of selected HPV-positive N2 patients with radiological residual disease if there is significant lymph node involution and a negative PET scan, as long as they can undergo repeated imaging assessments

Follow-up and continuing care: Non-metastatic oropharyngeal cancer (M0)

Follow-up should be carried out in a multidisciplinary setting and is recommended at the following frequency:
- 10–12 weeks post treatment to assess treatment response to radiotherapy in case neck dissection is required
- Every 3 months or more frequently for 2 years
- Every 4 months or more frequently in Year 3
- Every 6 months or more frequently for Years 4 and 5
- Annually for Years 6–10, especially for patient with HPV-positive disease, due to the possibility of late-onset distant metastasis

Investigation includes:
- Physical examination
- Fibre-optic endoscopy
- Post-treatment baseline imaging within 6 months of treatment:
  - CT or MRI (if indicated) of primary and neck (if treated):
    - Further re-imaging may be indicated as needed
  - CT chest as clinically indicated, especially for patients with a smoking history
  - Thyroid-stimulating hormone (TSH) every 6–12 months if neck has been irradiated
- Pharynx function (speech/swallowing) evaluation, if indicated
- Dental assessment where applicable
- Audiometry or ophthalmology where applicable.

Important aspects in the follow-up and continuing care include:
- Late toxicity monitoring and reporting, such as:
  - Swallowing dysfunction, especially 'silent' aspiration, and potential pneumonia
  - Osteoradionecrosis, especially in those who continue to smoke who appear at greatest risk
  - Hypothyroidism
  - Xerostomia
  - Soft tissue fibrosis (neck, pharynx, etc.)
- Comprehensive rehabilitation:
  - Nutritional support
  - Psychosocial support
- Monitor for potential second primaries.

Metastatic oropharyngeal cancer (M1)

Less than 1% of oropharyngeal cancer patients have detectable distant metastasis (M1) at initial presentation. For HPV-negative patient with metastatic disease, the goal of treatment is mainly symptom management (reducing pain and mass effect) and supportive care (maintaining nutrition and airway) as cure is considered unrealistic. However, for HPV-positive patient with limited distant metastatic disease, 'cure' may be possible and aggressive treatment for local as well as metastatic disease should be considered. For HPV-positive patient with a 'disseminating' phenotype and multiple organ metastases, supportive care and symptom management is important (similar to the HPV-negative patient).

Treatment for disease recurrence

Patterns of treatment failure are given in Table 43.5.

Biopsy of any lesion(s) suspicious for local and/or regional recurrence is recommended as clinically indicated.

Scenario: Recurrence	Treatment philosophy
Biopsy-proven local and/or regional recurrence	- Perform imaging (preferably PET-CT) to rule out distant metastasis - Resectable: salvage surgery should be deployed whenever possible ± postoperative re-irradiation - Unresectable: re-irradiation (small fraction size, twice daily (b.i.d.), 6 hour apart ± systemic therapy: - If surgery or re-irradiation is not possible, systemic therapy may be considered - Re-irradiation: most options use smaller fraction size to minimize risk of severe late toxicity - Optimization of re-irradiation regimens (see Chapter 39)

Distant metastasis	- HPV-negative OPC with metastatic disease:
	  - Cure is not usually possible
	  - Palliative measures for symptom control, including best supportive care (BSC) with or without systemic treatment (and on indication, irradiation) depending on the general condition of the patient
	  - Consider surgery for single lung metastasis or a second (lung) primary
	- HPV-positive OPC with single-organ, limited metastatic disease:
	  - Cure is possible in selected cases with oligometastases; salvage treatment should be deployed whenever appropriate, including local ablative treatment (surgical resection or high-dose radiotherapy), usually with stereotactic technique ± chemotherapy for metastatic disease
	  - HPV-positive patient with 'disseminating' metastatic disease: cure is not possible; goal for treatment is symptom control and supportive care
	- Palliative systemic therapy for recurrent/metastatic disease:
	  - Adding cetuximab, the first clinically available EGFR-directed monoclonal antibody, to a standard chemotherapy regimen (platinum + 5-fluorouracil) leads to survival benefit and should be considered in patients with an adequate performance status (i.e. Karnofsky performance score >70)

Table 43.5 Pattern of treatment failure

Site of failure	HPV-negative	HPV-positive
Locoregional	Predominant mode of failure	Infrequent
Distant	Often associated with locoregional failure Lung is the most common site, followed by bone and liver Patients with metastatic disease are generally considered incurable	Most common mode of failure Mostly without local or regional failure Two types of distant metastasis: • *Disseminating phenotype*: to multiple organs and unusual sites • *Indolent phenotype*: may be curable with salvage procedures (surgery, chemotherapy or radiotherapy)

Controversies

Various treatment de-intensification strategies for HPV-positive patients are currently under investigation, but it remains unclear which strategies will apply for particular subgroups of patient with this disease. Treatment intensification for HPV-negative patients is approaching a maximum threshold, but the results remain unsatisfactory. Further optimization of treatment strategies is required.

The role of induction chemotherapy is also under investigation in the clinical trial setting.

Post-radiation neck management is evolving, especially in this era of rising incidence of HPV-positive cancer. The role of PET-CT in post-radiation treatment assessment and selection of neck dissection is still debatable, and is under evaluation in a clinical trial.

Phase III clinical trials

See Table 43.6.

Table 43.6 Phase III clinical trials

Trial name	Results
Advanced-stage disease	
GORTEC 94-01 Calais *et al.* (1999) *J Natl Cancer Inst* 91(24):2081–2086 (OPC specific)	• CCRT versus radiotherapy alone: ▪ CCRT improved overall survival, disease-free survival and locoregional control
NCT 00004227 (not OPC specific) Bonner *et al.* (2006) *N Engl J Med* 354(6):567–78	• Cetuximab + RT versus RT alone: ▪ Improves locoregional control and reduces mortality without increasing the common toxic effects associated with radiotherapy to the head and neck cancer • *Note*: trial was not OPC specific; OPC patients made up 56% of the experimental arm (RT + cetuximab) and 63% of control arm (RT alone)
TAX 323 (NCT00003888) (not OPC specific) Vermorken *et al.* (2007) *N Engl J Med* 357(17):1695–1704	• TPF (docetaxel + cisplatin + 5-fluorouracil [5-FU]) versus PF (cisplatin + 5-FU) as induction chemotherapy for unresectable head and neck SCC: ▪ Longer overall survival (OS) with TPF: median OS 19 versus 15 months (HR 0.73; $P = 0.02$) • *Note*: trial was not OPC specific; OPC patients made up 46.4% of the PF arm and 45.4% of the TPF arm
TAX 324 (NCT00273546) (not OPC specific) Posner *et al.* (2007) *N Engl J Med* 357(17):1705–1715	• TPF versus PF as induction chemotherapy + chemoradiotherapy for resectable and unresectable head and neck SCC: ▪ Longer OS with TPF: median OS 71 versus 34 months (HR 0.70; $P = 0.006$) • *Note*: trial was not OPC specific; OPC patients made up 53% of the PF arm and 52% of the TPF arm
Recurrent or metastatic disease	
EXTREME trial (NCT00122460) (not OPC specific) Vermorken *et al.* (2008) *N Engl J Med* 259:1116–1127	• As compared with platinum-based chemotherapy + 5-FU alone, cetuximab + platinum + 5-FU chemotherapy improved OS when given as first-line treatment in patients with recurrent or metastatic head and neck SCC • *Note*: trial was not OPC specific; OPC patients made up 36% of the experimental arm (cetuximab + chemotherapy) and 31% of the control arm (chemotherapy only)

SPECTRUM trial (NCT00460265) (not OPC specific)
Vermorken, *et al.* (2013) *Lancet Oncol* 14(8):697–710
	• Panitumumab in addition to chemotherapy improved survival in HPV-negative but not HPV-positive patients with recurrent and/or metastatic head and neck cancer
	  ▪ HPV-negative: median OS 12 versus 9 months ($P = 0.02$)
	  ▪ HPV-positive: median OS 11 versus 12 months ($P = 0.88$)
	• *Note*: trial was not OPC specific

Areas of research

- Treatment de-intensification for low-risk HPV-positive OPC patients:
  - Less toxicity with equivalent disease control [e.g. current ongoing NRG HN-002 Trial (NCT02254278), and ECOG 3311 Trial (NCT01898494)]
- Optimization of treatment to reduce risk of distant metastasis for high-risk HPV-positive OPC patients:
  - Higher disease control with acceptable toxicity
- Treatment modification to enhance disease control for HPV-negative OPC patients by hypoxia modification and other novel agents
- Role of sequential therapy for HPV-positive and HPV-negative OPC patients
- Detection of biomarkers for better treatment selection
- Role of targeted therapy (hypoxia, EGFR, p53 target therapy, etc.) for HPV-negative patients
- Reducing treatment toxicity:
  - Radiation: adaptive radiotherapy, swallowing-sparing radiotherapy
- Prevention for HPV-positive OPC:
  - Primary prevention: vaccination for boys in addition to girls
  - Secondary prevention: early detection and treatment of preclinical disease

Recommended readings

Ang KK, Harris J, Wheeler R et al. (2010) Human papillomavirus and survival of patients with oropharyngeal cancer. N Engl J Med 363(1):24–35.

Bourhis J, Overgaard J, Audry H et al. (2006) Hyperfractionated or accelerated radiotherapy in head and neck cancer: a meta-analysis. Lancet 368:843–854.

Calais G, Alfonsi M, Bardet E et al. (1999) Randomized trial of radiation therapy versus concomitant chemotherapy and radiation therapy for advanced stage oropharynx carcinoma. J Natl Cancer Inst 91(24):2081–2086.

Huang SH, Xu W, Waldron J, et al. (2015) Refining American Joint Committee on Cancer/Union for International Cancer Control TNM Stage and Prognostic Groups for Human Papillomavirus-Related Oropharyngeal Carcinomas. J Clin Oncol. 33(8):836-45.

Mehanna H, Beech T, Nicholson T, El-Hariry I, McConkey C, Paleri V, Roberts S (2013) Prevalence of human papillomavirus in oropharyngeal and nonoropharyngeal head and neck cancer-systematic review and meta-analysis of trends by time and region. Head Neck 35(5):747–755.

O'Sullivan B, Huang SH, Siu LL et al. (2013) Deintensification candidate subgroups in human papillomavirus-related oropharyngeal cancer according to minimal risk of distant metastasis. J Clin Oncol 31(5):543–550.

Pignon JP, Bourhis J, Domenge C, Designé L (2000) Chemotherapy added to locoregional treatment for head and neck squamous-cell carcinoma: three meta-analyses of updated individual data. MACH-NC Collaborative Group. Meta-Analysis of Chemotherapy on Head and Neck Cancer. Lancet 355:949–955.

Pignon JP, le Maître A, Maillard E, Bourhis J; MACH-NC Collaborative Group (2009) Meta-analysis of chemotherapy in head and neck cancer (MACH-NC): an update on 93 randomised trials and 17,346 patients. Radiother Oncol 92(1):4–14.

44 Major salivary glands

Devendra Chaukar[1], Abhishek D. Vaidya[1,2], Rohan Walvekar[3], Sarbani Ghosh Laskar[4] and Kumar Prabhash[5]

[1]Department of Head and Neck Surgical Oncology, Tata Memorial Centre, Mumbai, India
[2]Department of Surgical Oncology, DMIMS, Sawangi-Wardha, India
[3]Department of Otolaryngology – Head & Neck Surgery, Louisiana State University, New Orleans, USA
[4]Department of Radiation Oncology, Tata Memorial Centre, Mumbai, India
[5]Department of Medical Oncology, Tata Memorial Centre, Mumbai, India

Summary	Key facts

Introduction	- Major salivary gland tumours show a wide variety of clinical, pathological and biological diversity
	- Comprise 3–5% of head and neck cancers:
	  - 70% arise in the parotid; majority of these (80%) are benign
	  - 10% arise from the submandibular gland; half of these are malignant
	  - Only 1% originate in the sublingual glands, 85% of these are malignant
	  - Remainder arise from minor salivary glands; usually malignant (not discussed in this chapter)

Presentation	- Majority present as a painless, mobile mass
	- Constant pain, fixity to overlying skin or surrounding structures, nerve involvement and presence of neck nodes are indicators of malignancy
	- Fine needle aspiration cytology (FNA) should be considered for all patients with salivary gland tumours:
	  - Core biopsy may be considered where FNA is equivocal
	- Ultrasonography (USG) is a useful, economical and easy method of preliminary imaging:
	  - May not provide details about deep lobe of parotid
	  - Specificity, sensitivity and accuracy are operator dependent
	- Magnetic resonance imaging (MRI) is the optimum imaging to provide accurate delineation of disease, local extension and relationship to neurovascular structures
	- Computed tomography (CT) scan is complementary in selected cases with bone or skull base erosion

Scenario	- Surgery is the mainstay of treatment when feasible:
	  - Benign parotid tumours: superficial parotidectomy:
	    - When the tumour extends to involve the deep lobe, total parotidectomy with preservation of the facial nerve is recommended
	  - Malignant parotid tumours: usually warrant total parotidectomy
	    - Extent of surgical resection is based on the extent of disease at presentation
	  - Submandibular gland tumours: submandibular gland excision:
	    - Excision of additional structures for malignant tumours, depending on the extent of disease involvement
	- Adjuvant radiotherapy has a well-defined role in high-risk salivary gland malignancies
	- Unresectable tumours are usually treated with radiotherapy
	- Chemotherapy has a limited role, currently limited to palliative treatment of unresectable, recurrent and metastatic disease
	- Role of targeted therapy is under investigation:
	  - For unresectable tumours is currently mainly limited to the clinical trial setting

Trials	- Paucity of well-designed phase III clinical trials - Laramore et al. (1993) Int J Radiat Oncol Biol Phys 27(2):235–240: - RTOG-MRC randomized trial comparing neutron versus photon irradiation for inoperable salivary gland tumours (stopped earlier than planned for ethical reasons).

(continued)

Summary	Key facts
	- Significantly improved locoregional control rate and a borderline improvement in survival in the neutron group
	- Bph et al. (2007) Br J Surg 94(9):1081-1087:
	- Small randomized study comparing partial parotidectomy with superficial/total parotidectomy in selected benign tumours
	- Partial parotidectomy was as safe as and less morbid than more extensive procedures

Introduction

Major salivary gland tumours comprise only about 3–5% of all head and neck malignancies. However, their importance lies in the diverse clinical and biological presentation. Their behaviour and resulting clinical management are highly dependent on the pathology and grade of tumour. This makes investigation and management of these tumours challenging.

Of all the salivary gland tumours, about 85% arise from the major salivary glands (parotid, submandibular, sublingual glands). The majority of these arise in the parotid (73%) and are usually benign (80–85%). About 11% arise from the submandibular gland, of which about 40% are malignant. Sublingual salivary gland tumours are rare, comprising <1%, but most of these are malignant. Rarely, the parotid may be the site of haematolymphoid tumours, or of secondary deposits from other malignancies.

Incidence, aetiology and screening

Incidence, aetiology and screening	Description

Incidence	- Estimated incidence rate of 11.95 per 100,000 person-years and incidence of 0.9 per 100,000 persons: Incidence tends to increase with age
	- Overall incidence is higher in Caucasians compared to African–Americans
	- Median age of presentation depends upon individual pathology of tumours:
	  - Acinic cell carcinoma (ACC; peak incidence in third decade) and mucoepidermoid carcinoma (MEC; mean age of presentation is about 40 years) tend to occur earlier as compared to squamous cell and small cell carcinomas:
	  - Peak incidence for adenoid cystic carcinoma is at 50–60 years
	  - Adenocarcinoma NOS is most commonly seen in elderly males
	  - Mean age at presentation for malignant mixed tumours: carcinosarcoma is 58 years; carcinoma ex pleomorphic adenoma sixth to seventh decades, approximately one decade older than the peak age for pleomorphic adenomas
	  - Peak incidence for salivary duct carcinoma is in the sixth decade
	- MEC is slightly more common in women; ACC shows no gender predilection; male-to-female ratio for salivary duct carcinoma is 4:1

Aetiology	- Exact aetiology is unknown
	- Most cases are idiopathic
	- Known or proposed aetiological factors:
	  - *Ionizing radiation*:
	    - Higher incidence of both benign and malignant salivary tumours in atomic bomb survivors
	    - Therapeutic radiation to scalp or head and neck may also increase the risk
	    - Dose–response effect
	    - Latency to tumour development is 10 years for malignant and 20 years for benign tumours
	  - *Viral*:
	    - Epstein–Barr virus (EBV) consistently associated with lymphoepithelial carcinoma of the salivary gland in Asians
	    - No evidence for an aetiological role of EBV in other salivary tumours
	  - *Environmental factors*:
	    - Smoking is associated with Warthin tumour
	    - Occupational exposure to silica dust may increase risk
	    - Increased risk among rubber workers exposed to nitrosamines
	  - *Genetic factors*:
	    - E.g. translocation t(6; 9) in adenoid cystic carcinoma (ACC), t(11; 19) in MEC

Screening	- Due to its rarity and no established familial aetiology, currently no described role for screening in salivary gland cancers

> **Box 44.1** WHO Classification of salivary gland tumours
>
> **Malignant epithelial tumours**
> Acinic cell carcinoma
> Mucoepidermoid carcinoma
> Adenoid cystic carcinoma
> Polymorphous low-grade adenocarcinoma
> Epithelial–myoepithelial carcinoma
> Clear cell carcinoma, not otherwise specified
> Basal cell adenocarcinoma
> Sebaceous carcinoma
> Sebaceous lymphadenocarcinoma
> Papillary cystadenocarcinoma
> Low-grade cribriform cystadenocarcinoma
> Mucinous adenocarcinoma
> Oncocytic carcinoma
> Salivary duct carcinoma
> Adenocarcinoma, not otherwise specified
> Myoepithelial carcinoma
> Carcinoma ex pleomorphic adenoma
> Carcinosarcoma
> Metastasizing pleomorphic adenoma
> Squamous cell carcinoma
> Small cell carcinoma
> Large cell carcinoma
> Lymphoepithelial carcinoma
>
> **Benign epithelial tumours**
> Pleomorphic adenoma
> Myoepithelioma (myoepithelial adenoma)
> Basal cell adenoma
> Warthin tumour (adenolymphoma)
> Oncocytoma (oncocytic adenoma)
> Canalicular adenoma
> Sebaceous adenoma
> Ductal papilloma:
> - Inverted ductal papilloma
> - Intraductal papilloma
> - Sialadenoma papilliferum
>
> Cystadenoma:
> - Papillary cystadenoma
> - Mucinous cystadenoma
>
> **Non-epithelial tumours**
>
> **Haematolymphoid tumours**
>
> **Secondary tumour**
>
> **Unclassified tumours**
>
> **Tumour-like lesions**
> Sialadenosis
> Oncocytosis
> Necrotizing sialometaplasia
> Benign lymphoepithelial lesion
> Salivary gland cysts
> Kuttner tumour
> Cystic lymphoid hyperplasia of AIDS

Pathology and natural history

Salivary gland tumours arise from the progenitor cells in the ductal system of the glands. There are two theories of histogenesis: bicellular and multicellular.

According to the multicellular theory, each tumour type originates from a specific cell type within the salivary gland unit. Accordingly, Warthin tumours arise from striated ductal cells, acinic cell tumours from acinar cells, and pleomorphic tumours from the intercalated duct and myoepithelial cells. In contrast, according to the bicellular reserve cell theory, all tumour types originate from one of the two pluripotential cell populations: cells of the excretory duct (squamous cell carcinoma and MEC) or cells of the intercalated duct (pleomorphic adenoma and oncocytic tumours).

Tumours arising from the main ducts are mainly epithelial and highly malignant, while those developing from the terminal ducts have both epithelial and myoepithelial components, and behave less aggressively.

The World Health Organization (WHO) classification of salivary gland tumours is given in Box 44.1.

Pleomorphic adenomas account for the vast majority of benign tumours. Among the malignant tumours, the most common (75%) are: MEC, ACC and adenocarcinoma. The frequency distribution of these malignant tumours is given in Table 44.1.

Table 44.1 Distribution of histopathology of salivary gland tumours

Diagnosis	Frequency
Mucoepidermoid carcinoma	34%
Adenoid cystic carcinoma	22%
Adenocarcinoma	18%
Malignant mixed tumours	13%
Acinic cell carcinoma	7%
Other	6%

Pathology and natural history	Description
Pleomorphic adenoma	- According to the bicellular theory, this tumour originates from an uncommitted reserve cell of the intercalated duct
- Accounts for 75% of all benign tumours
- 90% of pleomorphic adenomas in the parotid arise from the superficial lobe:
- May extend in a 'dumbbell' fashion across the stylomandibular tunnel
- Gross examination:
- Solitary, firm, round tumour with characteristically bosselated cut surface, variegated consistency, whitish–grey colour
- On microscopy:
- Epithelial components in the form of ducts, nests or solid sheets, and myoepithelial cells that appear spindled with a chondroid background
- Thin capsule which may be incomplete, resulting in satellite nodules or pseudopodia:
- Responsible for the high rate of local recurrence following inadequate surgery
- Recurrences occur over several years and are often multicentric
- Malignant transformation is rare:
- Seen most commonly in long-standing tumours
- Risk is 1.5% over 5 years and about 10% over >15 years
Mucoepidermoid carcinoma (MEC)	- Most common malignant tumour of the major salivary glands in adults and children
- Slightly more common in women
- Mean age of presentation is about 45 years, but may occur at all ages
- Slow-growing mass
- Gross examination:
- Both solid and cystic components, with mucinous material within cysts, giving a somewhat bluish colour
- On microscopy:
- Three cell types: mucous, squamoid and intermediate, with a mixture of cystic and solid architecture
- Histological grading correlates well with behaviour and prognosis:
- Low-grade lesions have a larger cystic component with little cytological atypia and low mitotic activity
- High-grade lesions have a larger solid component with squamoid/intermediate cells, cytological atypia, mitotic activity and necrosis
- Low-grade MEC has a low incidence of metastases, and rarely causes death
- Location of tumour also predicts clinical behaviour:
- MEC of the submandibular gland are more aggressive than those of the parotid glands
- Cervical nodes are seen in about 50% of cases
Adenoid cystic carcinomas (ACC)	- More commonly seen in the minor salivary glands
- In the major salivary glands, equally common in submandibular and parotid glands
- Peak incidence: 50–60 years of age
- Gross examination:
- Tan, firm and well-circumscribed, but unencapsulated tumour
- On microscopy:
- Three growth patterns: tubular, cribriform ('Swiss cheese'-like) and solid
- Three grades have been described:
- Grade I (tubular with or without some cribriform areas)
- Grade II (cribriform with no tubular areas and <30% solid areas)
- Grade III (cribriform with >30% solid areas)
- Prognosis is worse for higher grades
- Immunohistochemistry (IHC):
- c-Kit positivity may help in diagnosis
- Cervical lymph nodes are seen at presentation in about 25%
- Characterized by an infiltrative growth pattern and relentless course; recurrences can occur over a prolonged period of time:
- Perineural invasion seen in about 75% of cases; carries worse prognosis when a major nerve trunk is involved
- Distant metastases are seen at presentation in about 25%
- Long-term surveillance is mandatory after treatment in view of tendency for late recurrences and metastases

Pathology and natural history	Description

Adenocarcinoma NOS	• Shows ductal differentiation but lacks the histological features that define other types of salivary carcinoma
	• Found equally in the major and minor salivary glands
	• Usually seen in elderly males
	• May exhibit considerable heterogeneity in pathology and behaviour:
	  ▪ Three grades described: low, intermediate and high
	• Prognosis is worse than for most other salivary gland carcinomas:
	  ▪ 15-year survival rates are about 41%, 34% and 28% for low-, intermediate- and high-grade tumours, respectively

Acinic cell carcinoma	• 90% are seen in the parotid
	• Second most common paediatric salivary gland tumour
	• Low-grade malignancy
	• Shows cellular differentiation akin to the normal salivary acini
	• Seen in all ages, with peak incidence in the third decade
	• Slow growing mass
	• Gross examination:
	  ▪ Well-circumscribed, rubbery, solid mass.
	• On microscopy:
	  ▪ Four histological patterns: solid/lobular, microcystic, papillary–cystic and follicular
	  ▪ Two classical features are presence of acinic cells and a dense lymphoid infiltrate with germinal centres
	• May have protracted course with recurrences and metastases over several years:
	  ▪ Recurrence after resection may occur in up to a third of cases
	  ▪ Nodal and distant recurrences are seen in 10–15%
	• Survival is approximately 80% at 5 years and 70% at 10 years

Malignant mixed tumours	• Three entities: true malignant mixed tumour (carcinosarcoma), carcinoma ex pleomorphic adenoma and metastasizing mixed tumour
	• *Carcinosarcoma*:
	  ▪ Accounts for only 1% of all salivary gland malignancies
	  ▪ 70% arise in the parotid gland, 15% in the submandibular gland and 15% in the palate
	  ▪ Consists of distinct carcinomatous and sarcomatous components
	  ▪ Mean age of presentation is 58 years
	  ▪ Gross examination:
	    ○ Mass may be circumscribed or ill defined, tan–white with haemorrhage and necrosis
	  ▪ On microscopy:
	    ○ Mixture of the two components (carcinoma and sarcoma), but the amounts of each can vary widely
	    ○ Carcinoma component is usually in the form of high-grade salivary duct carcinoma or undifferentiated carcinoma
	    ○ Sarcomatous component is usually a chondrosarcoma
	  ▪ Metastases are common, and occur to lung and bones
	  ▪ Tumours are aggressive, and 66% of patients die of recurrence or metastases within 30 months
	• *Carcinoma ex pleomorphic adenoma*:
	  ▪ Defined as a pleomorphic adenoma in which, or with which, a carcinoma is present
	  ▪ Accounts for >95% of malignant mixed tumours
	  ▪ Most common in parotid gland, followed by submandibular gland and sublingual gland
	  ▪ Peak incidence in sixth to seventh decades, approximately one decade older than the peak age for pleomorphic adenomas
	  ▪ Classic history is of rapid growth in a long-standing mass
	  ▪ Gross examination:
	    ○ Tan–yellow, firm mass with ill-defined, infiltrative borders
	  ▪ On microscopy:
	    ○ Proportions of the two components may vary
	  ▪ Prognosis depends on the type of carcinoma within the mixed tumour
	  ▪ For prognostication, classified as: non-invasive (intracapsular), minimally invasive (<1.5 mm beyond the capsule) or invasive (>1.5 mm):
	    ○ High-grade tumours have a 5-year survival rate of about 25–65% and 0–38% at 20 years

(continued)

Pathology and natural history	Description

Salivary duct carcinoma	- One of the most aggressive primary salivary gland tumours
	- Accounts for <10%
	- Males are more commonly affected (4:1)
	- Peak age of incidence is in the sixth decade
	- 70–90% of cases arise in the parotid
	- Rapidly growing mass, often with skin involvement and facial nerve paralysis
	- Gross examination:
	  - Ill-defined, grey–white with areas of haemorrhage and necrosis
	- On microscopy:
	  - Similar to breast ductal carcinomas
	  - Often central comedo-type necrosis
	- IHC is often positive for carcinoembryogenic antigen (CEA), androgen receptors and sometimes HER2/neu
	- 30–40% develop local recurrence and about 50–75% develop distant metastases:
	  - 40–50% die of disease within 4 years

Presentation

- Most common presentation is mass in the parotid region; usually painless:
    - Features suspicious of malignancy are:
        - Constant pain in the mass
        - Presence of facial nerve paresis or paralysis
        - Fixity of the mass to the overlying skin or underlying structures
        - Presence of neck nodes
- Less commonly, the tumour may arise in the submandibular region, and may present as a painless, mobile mass:
    - Features suspicious of malignancy are:
        - Fixity of the submandibular mass to the skin or mandible
        - Presence of tongue wasting or deviation
        - Loss of sensation in the tongue

Natural history

Natural history		Description

Presentation	Local	**Parotid tumours**
		- *Benign tumours:*
		  - Usually present as a slow growing, painless mass
		  - Usually arises from the 'tail' of the superficial lobe, and produces a bulge below or in front of the ear lobule
		  - Obliteration of the retroauricular sulcus and lifting up of the lobule are characteristic features of a parotid mass
		- *Malignant tumours:*
		  - Rapidly growing
		  - Pain may be the presenting feature in about 10%
		  - Progressive facial nerve involvement
		  - Fixity to skin or to the underlying structure is another feature of malignancy
		  - Cervical nodes may be palpable
		- *Deep lobe involvement:*
		  - Tumours (benign or malignant) of the deep lobe may extend to the parapharyngeal space:
		    - Produce oropharyngeal bulge
		    - May be Eustachian tube blockade or palatal bulge
		    - Extension to post-styloid compartment (usually malignant) may cause lower cranial neuropathies leading to loss of gag reflex, aspiration, hoarseness, dysphagia and atrophy/paresis of tongue
		
		Submandibular gland tumours
		- *Benign tumours:*
		  - Present as non-tender, mobile, well-delineated masses
		
		Malignant tumours:
		  - Mass may be painful
		  - Involvement of overlying skin or fixity to the mandible indicating local extension

Natural history		Description
		▪ Numbness of the tongue (lingual nerve involvement) ▪ Weakness/atrophy of the ipsilateral hemi-tongue (hypoglossal nerve involvement) ▪ Neck nodes may be present
	Metastatic	• *Nodal metastases:* ▪ Most commonly seen in high-grade MEC, undifferentiated carcinoma, squamous cell carcinoma, adenocarcinoma NOS and salivary duct carcinoma ▪ Size (>4 cm) is an important predictive factor for nodal metastases ▪ Grade may be more important than stage for prediction of nodal metastases ▪ Incidence ranges from 15% to 60% at presentation • *Distant metastases:* ▪ Most commonly seen in ACC, salivary duct carcinoma, malignant mixed tumours and high-grade MEC
Routes of spread	Local	**Parotid tumours** • May extend to structures in the vicinity: facial nerve, skin, underlying masseter or mandible • May extend medially to deep lobe, and thence to the parapharyngeal space in the prestyloid compartment • Spread to post-styloid compartment may lead to involvement of the lower cranial nerves IX–XII • May extend posteromedially into infratemporal fossa and involve pterygoid muscles causing trismus **Submandibular tumours** • Deep extension may occur to involve the hypoglossal or the lingual nerve • Superficial extension may occur to involve the marginal mandibular nerve or skin • Superior extension may involve the mandible and floor of mouth • Inferior extension may involve the hyoid
	Regional	• Nodal metastases from the parotid gland travel to intraparotid nodes and thence to the upper deep jugular nodes (levels II–III) • Additional lymphatic drainage is to adjacent levels, including the posterior triangle or level V • Lymphatic spread from the submandibular gland occurs to upper deep cervical nodes
	Metastatic	• Distant metastases occur mainly to the lungs • Skeletal metastases may occur in a small fraction

Diagnostic work-up

Diagnostic work-up	Description

Work-up	• *Fine needle aspiration:*
	▪ Role in the evaluation of salivary gland tumours is controversial:
	  ○ Some perform it routinely while others find it rarely necessary
	▪ It is safe, simple to perform, inexpensive and has minimal morbidity; with high overall sensitivity and specificity
	▪ Preoperative FNA is recommended, since it can change the clinical approach in up to 35% of patients:
	  ○ Allows better preoperative counselling of patients regarding nature of the tumour, likely extent of resection, management of facial nerve and likelihood of the need for neck dissection
	▪ Ultrasound guidance may increase accuracy of FNA in non-palpable tumours or those with a highly heterogeneous architecture
	• *Core biopsy:*
	▪ Relatively new technique for pathological diagnosis of salivary gland cancers
	▪ More invasive: requires local anaesthesia
	▪ May be considered where an initial FNA is either inconclusive or equivocal
	▪ May be used to increase sample adequacy in certain conditions like lymphoma

(continued)

Diagnostic work-up	Description

	• *Ultrasound:*
	   ■ Advantage: inexpensive, non-invasive, simple to perform, ideal for differentiation between a cyst and tumour
	   ■ Not comprehensive enough for assessing deep lobe of parotid or parapharyngeal space
	   ■ Specificity, sensitivity and accuracy are operator dependent
	• *MRI:*
	   ■ Accurately delineates interface between tumour and normal salivary gland
	   ■ Provides accurate delineation of location and extent of tumour, and relation to major neurovascular structures
	   ■ Identifies perineural extension and intracranial extension
	   ■ Provides better diagnosis and visualization of parapharyngeal extension
	• *CT scan:*
	   ■ Advantage: less expensive and more readily available than MRI
	   ■ Better for suspected mandible involvement and involvement of the skull base
	   ■ Similar to MRI for identification of neck nodes
	• *Positron emission tomography (PET) scan:*
	   ■ PET-CT scan: role is under investigation
	   ■ May be used for metastatic work-up in high-grade or locally-advanced tumours with suspicion of distant metastases
	   ■ PET may also have a role in uncommon histologies such as lymphomas, or in cases of intraparotid lymph nodes with FNA diagnosis of squamous carcinoma to rule out a head and neck primary

Tumour markers	• Currently no tumour markers recommended for diagnostic purpose in salivary gland tumours • Several prognostic markers are being investigated, e.g. c-Kit, HER2, Ki-67, p53, Bcl-2, c-ErbB2, androgen receptors

Stage and prognostic grouping

UICC TNM staging
See Table 44.2.

Prognostic factors
Being comprised of a diverse group of entities, the outcomes vary greatly among major salivary gland tumours. The 10-year disease-free survival of salivary gland tumours ranges from 47% to 74%; and the 10-year overall survival is around 50%.

Several studies have identified clinical, histological and molecular variables predicting clinical outcome and survival (Table 44.3).

Clinical variables
- T stage: T3–4 tumours have a higher incidence of occult metastases and extraglandular involvement, and tend to have a worse outcome
- Site of primary: tumours of the submandibular and sublingual glands are more likely to metastasize, and prognosis for these is worse than for those of the parotid gland

Table 44.2 UICC categories and stage grouping: Salivary glands

TNM categories	
T1	≤2 cm, without extraparenchymal extension
T2	>2–4 cm, without extraparenchymal extension
T3	>4 cm and/or extraparenchymal extension
T4a	Skin, mandible, ear canal, facial nerve
T4b	Skull, pterygoid plates, carotid artery
N1	Ipsilateral single ≤3 cm
N2	(a) Ipsilateral single >3–6 cm (b) Ipsilateral multiple ≤6 cm (c) Bilateral, contralateral ≤6 cm
N3	>6 cm
M1	Distant metastasis

Stage grouping			
Stage I	T1	N0	M0
Stage II	T2	N0	M0
Stage III	T3	N0	M0
	T1, T2, T3	N1	M0
Stage IVA	T4a	N0, N1	M0
	T1, T2, T3, T4a	N2	M0
Stage IVB	T4b	Any N	M0
	Any T	N3	M0
Stage IVC	Any T	Any N	M1

Table 44.3 Prognostic factors for salivary gland tumour survival

Prognostic factors	Tumour related	Host related	Environment related
Essential	Histological grade Tumour size Local invasion Perineural invasion	Age	Resection margins and residual disease (R0/R1/R2)
Additional	Nodal metastases	Facial palsy, pain	Adjuvant radiotherapy
New and promising	Molecular markers (c-Kit, Ki-67, HER2, EGFR, VEGF, androgen receptors)		Neutron vs photon radiotherapy

Table 44.4 Molecular markers in salivary gland cancers

Pathology	EGFR	HER2	c-Kit	VEGF	Androgen
Mucoepidermoid carcinoma	40%	25–35%	Rare	50%	Rare
Adenocarcinoma/salivary duct carcinoma	30–40%	20–30%	Rare	85%	15–40%
Adenoid cystic carcinoma	20%	Rare	80–90%	85%	Rare

EGFR, epithelial growth factor receptor; VEGF, vascular endothelial growth factor.

- Age: patients >50 years of age have a worse outcome
- Presenting features: presentation with pain and facial paralysis indicates advanced disease and portends a worse outcome

Pathological variables
- Grade: high-grade MEC, high-grade ACC, salivary duct carcinomas, squamous carcinomas and malignant mixed tumours have worse prognosis:
  - Suggested that grade may be more important than stage for prognostification
- Local invasion: perineural invasion and bone/skull base involvement decrease the disease-free and overall survival
- Resection margins: a positive resection margin leads to an increased chance of recurrence

Molecular markers
Several molecular markers have been identified (Table 44.4), which in specific tumour types are associated with a worse outlook:
- High expression of Ki-67 in MEC is associated with a higher tumour grade and shorter disease-free survival
- MEC with low p27 expression have a worse prognosis
- Tumours with translocation t(11; 9) have a better prognosis
- HER2/neu overexpression is characterized by a shorter disease-free survival in salivary duct carcinoma and MEC.

Philosophy of treatment (Fig. 44.1)

Surgery is the mainstay of treatment for resectable, non-metastatic salivary gland tumours. The goal of surgery is complete extirpation of tumour, while avoiding unnecessary morbidity. Surgical approach and the extent of resection depend upon the location and spread of tumour. Neck dissection is done in all cases where there is clinical or radiographic evidence of lymph node metastasis, and even in node-negative neck in certain high-risk scenarios (grade and size). Adjuvant radiotherapy is recommended in the presence of high-risk features, such as intermediate- or high-grade tumours, and compromised surgical margins. Adjuvant chemoradiotherapy may also be considered, although its efficacy in this setting is limited.

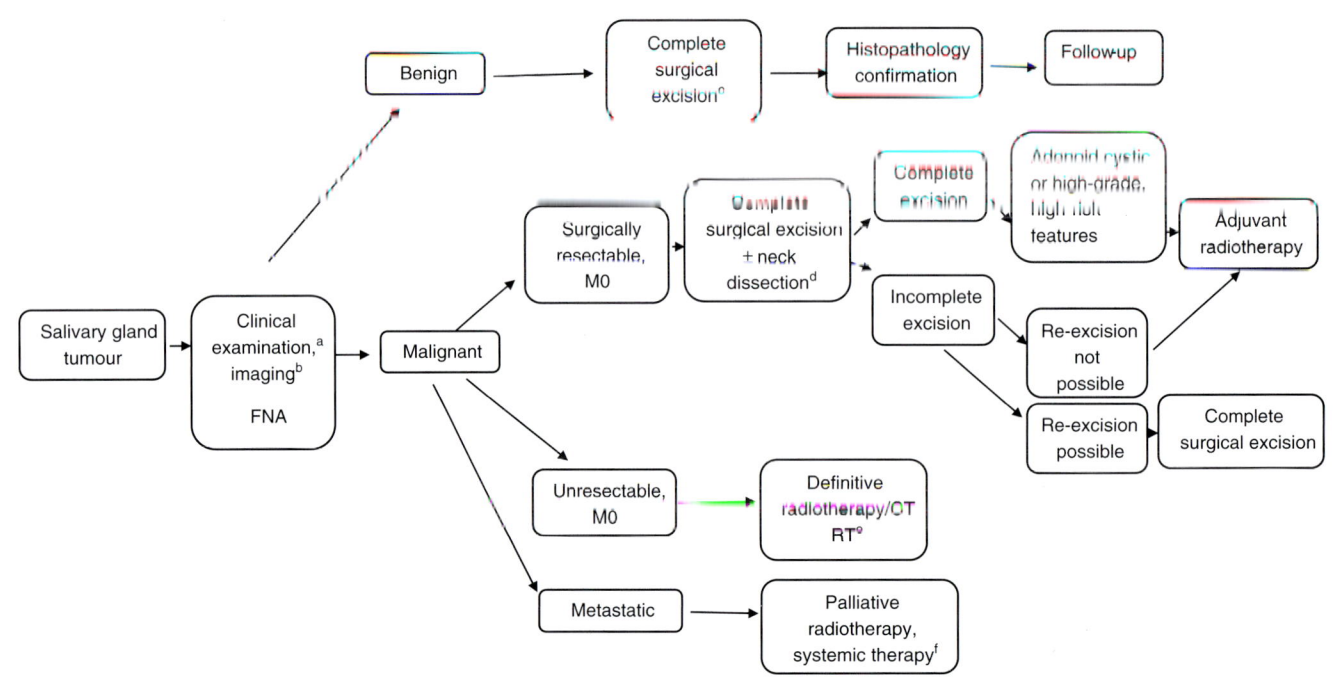

Figure 44.1 Management guidelines for salivary gland tumours.

[a] Clinically benign: mobile, slow growing, painless, no palsy, no neck nodes.
[b] Imaging modality may be Ultrasonography for superficial lesions, or MRI for deeply situated, extensive or recurrent lesions.
[c] Superficial or total parotidectomy depending upon location of tumour; partial parotidectomy in selected cases with small tumours restricted to the tail of the parotid; ensure no capsular breach or spillage.
[d] Excision should ensure oncologically safe margins: neck dissection for N+, suspicious nodes, high-grade tumours, tumours >4 cm.
[e] Chemoradiation (CTRT): this indication is not well established.
[f] Limited evidence for systemic therapy; role of targeted therapy still in research/trial setting; very limited role of metastasectomy in highly selected cases (see text).

Scenario	Treatment philosophy
Local disease	**Parotid gland** • Minimum surgery for benign tumour is a superficial parotidectomy • 'Partial' or 'extracapsular' parotidectomy may be indicated in selected benign cases • Total parotidectomy is done for primary deep lobe tumours, superficial lobe tumours extending to the deep lobe, and metastatic intraparotid node, high-grade malignancies • Every attempt is made to preserve the facial nerve, except when there is preoperative facial paresis/palsy, or when the nerve is encased by tumour and the tumour cannot be separated from the facial nerve at surgery **Submandibular gland** • Complete excision of the gland along with associated fibrofatty tissue at level IB • Surgery may be extended to excise the neighbouring structures depending upon extent of disease

Regional nodal metastases	• Node-positive (N+) neck:
	  ▪ A comprehensive (levels I–V) neck dissection is recommended
	• Node-negative (N0 neck):
	  ▪ No clear consensus
	  ▪ Elective neck dissection may be done for locally advanced (T3/4), high-grade tumours or submandibular gland primaries
	  ▪ Alternative is sampling of level II neck at frozen section, which will guide further neck dissection
	• Adjuvant radiotherapy should be considered in N+ necks

Metastatic disease	• Metastatic disease is usually treated with radiotherapy or systemic therapy • Role of metastasectomy has to be individualized, and depends upon nature of distant metastases, disease-free interval, control of primary and patient's performance status: ▪ For selected metachronous metastases (such as limited unilateral pulmonary metastases), metastasectomy may be considered, but only if the primary is controlled, if complete resection of metastases is possible and if the patient is fit to undergo the extended procedure

Scenario	Treatment philosophy

Recurrent disease	- Locoregional recurrence:
	  - Where resectable, surgery is preferred:
	    - Surgery in these situations has a high risk for facial nerve damage
	  - If the recurrence is unresectable, irradiation should be considered
	  - Where neither surgery nor irradiation is feasible (e.g. previously irradiated), systemic chemotherapy may be considered:
	    - Chemotherapy has only modest benefit and a limited role in salivary gland cancers
	- Metastatic disease on follow-up:
	  - As described above for metachronous metastases

Follow-up	- Follow-up should be 3 monthly for the first 2 years, 6 monthly until Year 5 and yearly thereafter - Long-term follow-up is mandatory, especially in certain tumour types like ACC, since these have a protracted course, with long-term recurrences and metastases - Follow-up examination should include thorough clinical examination, and a chest radiograph as metastases tend to be silent - More advanced imaging may be prompted by suspicion of a recurrence

Treatment

Surgery

Surgery	Description

Early	**Benign parotid tumours**
	- *Superficial parotidectomy*:
	  - Procedure of choice for benign parotid tumours restricted to the superficial lobe
	  - Implies *en masse* removal of all the parotid tissue lateral to the plane of the facial nerve and its branches
	  - Important to avoid enucleation and excision biopsy, which greatly increases the likelihood of recurrence (up to 80%) and nerve damage
	- *'Partial parotidectomy' and 'extracapsular dissection (ECD)'*:
	  - Preserve uninvolved parotid parenchyma and obviate the need for more extensive facial nerve dissection:
	    - Partial parotidectomy implies removing the tumour completely, taking care to avoid capsular rupture or nerve damage, with about 0.5–1-cm tumour-free margins
	    - In ECD, the plane of dissection is in a compartment of loose areolar tissue approximately 2–3 mm from the tumour
	  - Partial parotidectomy and ECD require very careful and stringent case selection:
	    - Only done in benign tumours limited to the superficial lobe; preferably small pleomorphic adenomas in the tail of the parotid
	    - In properly selected benign tumours, these techniques are as safe as and less morbid than superficial parotidectomy
	- *Total conservative (nerve sparing) parotidectomy*:
	  - Implies complete excision of the parotid preserving the facial nerve
	  - Done for a benign neoplasm when the tumour arises from or involves the deep lobe
	  - Isolated deep lobe parotidectomy may be done for selected purely deep lobe tumours, presenting as a parapharyngeal mass
	
	Malignant parotid tumours
	- In small, early (T1–2), low-grade malignant tumour that is well encapsulated and restricted to the superficial lobe, a superficial parotidectomy is sufficient:
	  - Care should be taken to obtain an adequate cuff of tissue all around the tumour
	- Total parotidectomy is done for:
	  - High-grade malignant tumours
	  - T3–4 tumours
	  - Tumours with extraparenchymal spread
	  - Indication of metastasis to intraglandular or cervical lymph nodes
	  - Any primary malignancy originating within deep lobe itself

(continued)

Surgery	Description
	Submandibular gland tumour • Complete excision of the gland along with level IB lymph node-bearing tissue (submandibular lymph-nodal tissue, bounded above by inferior border of mandible, and anteriorly and posteriorly by the bellies of digastric muscle) is recommended • Care is taken to preserve the adjacent neural structures if these are not involved

Advanced non-metastatic	**Parotid tumours**
	• Locally-advanced parotid tumours are those which have involvement of the facial nerve or extraparenchymal extension into skin, cartilage, soft tissue or bone
	• Total parotidectomy is the usual procedure:
	  ▪ Extent of surgery will depend on the extent of disease
	• Facial nerve sacrifice should be done if there is preoperative weakness or palsy:
	  ▪ Even if the preoperative function is normal, the facial nerve or its branch may require sacrifice if there is intraoperative evidence of gross invasion or microscopic infiltration
	  ▪ If facial nerve has to be sampled, to rule out tumour involvement, the most suspicious branch or communicating branch between two branches may be selected
	• If nerve sacrifice is to be done, clear surgical margins at both the proximal and distal nerve stump must be ensured to rule out any perineural spread:
	  ▪ Mastoidectomy and exploration of the intratemporal part of the facial nerve may be required to achieve a negative proximal margin
	• If the facial nerve is sacrificed, the type of repair depends on the remnant stump available and the extent of the defect:
	  ▪ If the proximal and distal cut stumps of the nerve remnant can be approximated, then immediate neurorrhaphy may be done
	  ▪ If the cut proximal and distal stumps are distant, a cable graft (greater auricular or sural nerve) may be employed
	  ▪ Commonly, the entire distal parts of the nerve divisions/branches are sacrificed, so that there is no distal stump remaining; in such cases, nerve repair is not feasible:
	    ○ If immediate nerve repair is not done, a delayed secondary facial reanimation procedures (static or dynamic) may be considered
	• Whether the secondary reanimation procedure employed is dynamic or static depends upon the status of the nerve and its target motor unit, assessed by nerve conduction studies and electromyography:
	  ▪ If the nerve function and the target motor unit (facial muscles) are functional, dynamic reanimation is done:
	    ○ Dynamic procedures include hypoglossal–facial or facial–facial cross-over (when the proximal stump is not available), interposition grafts and regional muscle transfers
	  ▪ If the electrophysiological studies show 'silence', static procedures are done:
	    ○ Static procedures include gold eyelid implants, fascial slings, brow lift, etc.
	• If there is extension beyond the parotid, the surgery may extend to involve resection of the skin or masseter, mandibulectomy, mastoidectomy, resection of the temporal bone or of the contents of infratemporal fossa:
	  ▪ Such radical parotidectomy defects usually require reconstruction with pedicled flaps or free tissue transfer
	
	Submandibular gland tumours
	• Advanced tumours of the submandibular gland require *en bloc* resection of the involved gland and any involved structures in the submandibular triangle (hypoglossal or lingual nerves, digastric or mylohyoid muscles)
	• Resection may also extend to the floor of the mouth and mandible
	• When dealing with ACC, it is advisable to get a frozen section from the parasympathetic secretory branch of the lingual nerve, to rule out perineural invasion
	• Any preoperative affliction or intraoperative thickening of the hypoglossal and lingual nerves warrants their excision
	• Frozen section may be employed to ensure negative margins
	
	Sublingual gland tumours
	• Surgery involves wide local excision and level II neck dissection
	• To achieve margins, adjacent structures may need to be resected, e.g. tongue, mylohyoid muscle, mandible, lingual nerve
	• Excision usually requires a combined transoral and transcervical approach
	• In more advanced tumours, a lip-split incision may be taken and cheek flap elevated to allow access for a composite resection, including marginal mandibulectomy
	• For tumours with bone involvement, a segmental mandibulectomy may be required

Metastatic	• Role for metastasectomy in highly selected cases with pulmonary oligometastases, where the performance status is good, the primary is controlled or controllable, and the metastases can be totally excised

Neck dissection

Neck dissection may be divided in two settings: node positive (N+) and node negative (N0) neck:
- *N+ neck:*
  - When there is a clinical or imaging indication of cervical nodal metastasis, a neck dissection is warranted
  - Recommended to perform a comprehensive modified radical neck dissection (levels I–IV)
- *N0 neck:*
  - Lack of consensus regarding the optimal treatment
  - Several retrospective studies have identified risk factors that may increase the risk of nodal metastases, and therefore warrant neck dissections in salivary gland tumours:
    - T3, T4 tumours
    - Submandibular primary site
    - Size >4 cm
    - High grade
    - Extraparenchymal spread
    - Certain pathological types: undifferentiated carcinoma, squamous cell carcinoma, high-grade MEC, adenocarcinoma NOS, carcinoma ex pleomorphic adenoma and salivary duct carcinoma

It has been suggested that grade may be more important than stage for nodal spread; hence, all high-grade tumours must undergo an elective neck dissection, even when clinically N0.

When an elective neck dissection is performed in an N0 neck, a selective dissection is usually employed. For parotid tumours, a selective neck dissection covering levels I–IV should be done. For submandibular tumours, a selective neck dissection of levels I–III should be done.

Radiotherapy

Salivary neoplasms are relatively radioresistant. However, radiotherapy (RT) may be employed in two distinct settings to treat salivary gland tumours:
- Adjuvant setting
- For unresectable disease.

Radiotherapy	Description
Early/resectable tumours	No role as definitive management

Adjuvant setting	- Although there are no mature data from randomized controlled trials, several retrospective studies have consistently demonstrated benefit of adjuvant RT in selected salivary gland cancers to achieve better locoregional control; these form the basis for the use of RT in the adjuvant setting
	- *Indications*:
	  - High-risk pathology:
	    - Adenocarcinoma
	    - Salivary duct carcinoma
	    - High-grade MEC
	    - Adenoid cystic carcinoma
	    - Carcinoma ex pleomorphic adenoma
	    - Other high-grade tumours
	  - Positive margins
	  - Positive lymph nodes
	  - Nerve involvement (microscopic or major nerve)
	  - T3–4 category (relative indication)
	  - Close margins (<0.5 cm) (relative indication)
	  - Bone involvement
	  - Recurrent disease
	  - Perineural spread
	  - Recurrent pleomorphic adenoma
	- Dose: usually 60 Gy in 30 fractions over 6 weeks
	- Additional boost of 6 Gy (i.e. 66 Gy in 33 fractions over 6.5 weeks) is given to sites with close (<1 mm) or positive margins or extracapsular nodal extension
	- Primary tumour volume (PTV): tumour bed and the involved lymph node bed
	- Clinical target volume (CTV):
	  - Deep lobe in those undergoing superficial parotidectomy
	  - Parapharyngeal space and infratemporal fossa in those with deep lobe involvement
	- Elective regions: 60 Gy in 33 fractions (postoperative bed) and 54–56 Gy in 30–33 fractions (undissected regions considered to be at risk)
	- Ipsilateral cervical lymph nodes are treated when involved
	- For involvement of a major (named) nerve, coverage of the course of the nerve to the skull base should be considered

(continued)

Radiotherapy	Description

Definitive RT for unresectable disease	• Important role in the management of locally-advanced, unresectable or recurrent salivary gland cancer when surgery is not feasible
	• In such scenarios, RT can achieve tumour shrinkage and good symptom palliation
	• Several methods of radiation enhancement have been studied to improve control rates:
	  ■ Fast neutron therapy was deemed promising compared with traditional photon or electron beam therapy.
	    ○ Phase III study (RTOG-MRC) showed that neutron therapy significantly improved local control compared with photon therapy
	    ○ Overall survival was unchanged; distant metastases were lower in the neutron arm
	    ○ Severe late side effects were noted in long-term survivors; this coupled with the scarcity of neutron radiation facilities has led to this therapy not being further explored
	• Treatment volumes are similar to those described for the adjuvant setting
	• Total dose about 70 Gy in 35 fractions over 7 weeks, in conventional fractionation

Elective neck irradiation	• In N0 necks, elective neck irradiation for large or high-grade or advanced tumours • Dose: 50–54 Gy, in conventional fractionation • Targeted nodal levels are I–IV

Systemic therapy

Systemic therapy in salivary gland cancers is restricted mainly to metastatic and recurrent unresectable tumours. Several agents have been studied, but most reported studies have been small, non randomized and with few subjects. This has made the assessment of the efficacy of chemotherapeutic agents difficult. Further complicating assessment is the fact that salivary gland tumours comprise a heterogeneous group, resulting in mixed populations.

The most commonly used agent is cisplatin and its regimens. These have shown only modest response rates. Other agents used are carboplatin, epirubicin, cyclophosphamide, doxorubicin (adriamycin), mitoxantrone, paclitaxel, 5-fluorouracil, vinorelbine, methotrexate and bleomycin. In a meta-analysis, patients treated with either platinum- or anthracycline (e.g. mitoxantrone)-based chemotherapy showed an increase in their median survival. Available data suggest that these two agents may have a useful role in palliative and definitive multimodality treatment of salivary gland malignancies prone to distant metastases, but this needs to be further explored.

Adjuvant chemoradiotherapy is widely used in head and neck cancers. Though there are a few reports of studies employing adjuvant chemoradiotherapy in salivary gland tumours, this indication has not been well established. Trials evaluating the utility of adjuvant chemoradiotherapy are currently underway.

Systemic therapy	Description
Early	• No role
Advanced, non-Metastatic	• Chemoradiotherapy may have some role in the adjuvant setting, but this is still being explored
Metastatic	• Several agents have been used in metastatic salivary gland cancers: ■ Agents that may have some role in the palliation of metastatic salivary tumours are cisplatin and anthracycline, but this is not well established

Targeted therapy

In recent years, several molecular markers and potential targets have been identified in the different types of salivary gland tumours. Subsequently, a large number of phase II trials evaluating the utility of specific targeted therapies in the metastatic and recurrent settings were launched. Unfortunately, response rates were poor (Table 44.5). This may probably be attributed to the fact that though salivary gland tumours over-express these molecular targets, there usually is no mutation in the driver genes. Currently, the use of targeted therapies in salivary gland tumours is restricted to the trial setting.

Controversies

- Neck dissection in N0 necks in salivary gland tumours
- Appropriate method of improving the effectiveness of radiotherapy in the definitive setting
- Role of extracapsular dissection for the management of benign parotid tumours, mainly pleomorphic adenoma

Phase III clinical trials

There is a paucity of clinical trials in salivary gland cancer (Table 44.6).

Table 44.5 Phase II trials of targeted therapy for salivary gland malignancies

Target	Sample size	Drug	Response rate (%)	Stable disease (%)
HER2	14	Trastuzumab	8	Not reported
EGFR	28	Gefitinib	0	67
c-Kit	16	Imatinib	0	60
c-Kit	10	Imatinib	0	20
HER2/EGFR	36	Lapatinib	0	64
EGFR	30	Cetuximab	0	80

From: Adelstein DJ, Shlomo AK, Adel KE. (2012) *Semin Radiat Oncol* 22(3):245–253.

Table 44.6 Phase III clinical trials

Trial name	Result
RTOG-MRC trial Laramore et al. (1993) *Int J Radiat Oncol Biol Phys* 27(2):235–240	Fast neutron radiotherapy led to better locoregional control as compared to photon base radiotherapy in recurrent salivary gland tumours

Areas of research

- RTOG 1008:
  - Randomized phase II study is ongoing of adjuvant concurrent radiation and chemotherapy versus radiation alone in resected high-risk malignant salivary gland tumours
- Identification of:
  - Genetic and molecular pathways of pathogenesis
  - Molecular markers of prognosis
- Better elucidation of pathological prognostic markers and immunohistochemistry
- Development of improved radiation strategies for unresectable tumours
- Development of targeted therapies for advanced disease

Recommended reading

Adelstein DJ, Koyfman SA, El-Naggar AK, Hanna EY. (2012) Biology and management of salivary gland cancers. *Semin Radiat Oncol* 22(3):245–253.

Day TA, Deveikis J, Gillespie MB et al. (2004) Salivary gland neoplasms. *Curr Treat Options Oncol* 5(1):11–26.

Ferlito A, Rinaldo A, Shaha AR, Pellitteri PK, Bradley PJ (2004) Management of malignant sublingual salivary gland tumors. *Oral Oncol* 40(1):2–5.

Laramore GE, Krall JM, Griffin TW et al. (1993) Neutron versus photon irradiation for unresectable salivary gland tumors: final report of an RTOG-MRC randomized clinical trial. Radiation Therapy Oncology Group. Medical Research Council. *Int J Radiat Oncol Biol Phys* 27(2):235–240.

Laskar SG, Murthy V, Wadasadawala T et al. (2011) Mucoepidermoid carcinoma of the parotid gland: Factors affecting outcome. *Head Neck* 33(4):497–503.

Laurie SA, Ho AL, Fury MG et al. (2011) Systemic therapy in the management of metastatic or locally recurrent adenoid cystic carcinoma of the salivary glands: a systematic review. *Lancet Oncol* 12(8):815–824.

Roh JL, Kim HS, Park CI (2007) Randomized clinical trial comparing partial parotidectomy versus superficial or total parotidectomy. *Br J Surg* 94(9):1081–1087.

Spiro RH (1986) Salivary neoplasms: overview of a 35-year experience with 2,807 patients. *Head Neck Surg* 8:177–184.

Terhaard CH, Lubsen H, Rasch CR et al. (2005) The role of radiotherapy in the treatment of malignant salivary gland tumors. Dutch Head and Neck Oncology Cooperative Group. *Int J Radiat Oncol Biol Phys* 61(1):103–111.

Theriault C, Fitzpatrick PJ (1986) Malignant parotid tumors: prognostic factors and optimum treatment. *Am J Clin Oncol* 9:510–516.

Witt RL (2004) Surgery for major salivary gland cancer. *Oncol Clin North Am* 13(1):113–127.

45 Nasal cavity and paranasal sinus

Prathamesh S. Pai[1], Sarbani Ghosh Laskar[2], Shubhada Kane[3], K. Thomas Robbins[4], Piero Nicolai[5] and Lisa Licitra[6]

[1]Department of Head & Neck Surgical Oncology, Tata Memorial Centre, Mumbai, India
[2]Department of Radiation Oncology, Tata Memorial Centre, Mumbai, India
[3]Department of Pathology, Tata Memorial Centre, Mumbai, India
[4]Simmons Cancer Institute at SIU, Springfield, IL, USA
[5]Department of Otorhinolaryngology, University of Brescia, Brescia, Italy
[6]Head and Neck Cancer Medical Oncology Unit, Fondazione IRCCS "Istituto Nazionale dei Tumouri", Milan, Italy

Summary	Key facts
Introduction	- Rare tumours - Maxillary sinus is the most common site followed by nasal cavity and ethmoid sinus - Frontal and sphenoid sinuses are rare epicentres - Varied histology - Advanced stage at presentation - Lack of level I evidence in management
Presentation	- Nasal obstruction - Epistaxis - Anosmia - Proptosis - Headache
Scenario	- Histology and site dictate the management - Locoregional treatment with surgery when feasible and followed by radiotherapy is mainstay of treatment - Minimally invasive surgery has an emerging role in selected cases - Chemotherapy in locally-advanced disease may improve local control rates - Highly conformal radiotherapy is mandatory - Outcomes for tumours in the nasal cavity exceed those that arise from the sinuses
Trials	- Paucity of prospective trials in paranasal sinus cancer

Introduction

Tumours of the nose and paranasal sinuses are unique, rare and often diagnosed at late stages. The sheer number of different pathologies seen in this region makes standardization of guidelines exceedingly difficult. The key to a suitable treatment plan is to identify the right tumour histology and subsites involved. Rarity, lack of an adequate literature and the wide array of histology make it difficult to recommend evidence-based treatment guidelines.

Incidence and aetiology

Incidence and aetiology	Description
Incidence	- Nasal cavity and paranasal sinus cancers are rare (<3% of all head and neck cancers) - Maxillary sinus is the most common site, followed by the nasal cavity and ethmoid sinuses - Frontal and sphenoid sinuses are rarely involved - Inverted papilloma presents in the fifth and sixth decades - Squamous cell carcinoma: peak incidence in the sixth and seventh decades: - Male predilection 2:1 - Esthesio-neuroblastoma: bimodal age distribution in second and sixth decades

Aetiology	- Occupations:
	    - Wood dust (strongly associated with adenocarcinomas)
	    - Nickel
	    - Dusts from textiles
	    - Formaldehyde, chromium, and other chemicals used in leather tanning and textile industry
	    - Flour (baking and flour milling)
	    - Mustard gas
	    - Radium (dial painters)
	- Air pollution
	- Tobacco smoke (strongly associated with squamous cell carcinoma)
	- Viruses
	    - Human papillomavirus (HPV) may be involved in the malignant transformation from inverted papilloma (associated with squamous cell carcinoma)
	    - Epstein–Barr virus (EBV) infection is possibly associated with sinonasal tract lymphomas

Screening and prevention	- Currently no role

Pathology

Sinonasal malignant tumours are varied, complex and rare. The many overlapping histopathological features make diagnosis of these tumours challenging. Limited tissue availability in biopsy samples further complicates the matter.

Sinonasal tumours are unique in that, unlike other head and neck sites, they show diverse differentiation ranging from epithelial and mesenchymal to neuroectodermal and haematolymphoid. There is also a higher probability of having a non-squamous carcinoma with unique biological behaviour. Some have a very good outcomes, such as adenocarcinomas and esthesio-neuroblastomas. Some have a higher chance of distant metastasis, such as melanomas, small cell neuroendocrine tumours and sinonasal undifferentiated carcinoma. Some round cell tumours such as embryonal rhabdomyosarcoma, lymphoma or plasmacytoma require non-surgical protocols. Hence, it is vital to attain a histological diagnosis before further management.

A systematic approach with the use of ancillary techniques such as immunohistochemistry, cytogenetics and molecular pathology help in the differential diagnosis.

Pathology	Description

Inverted papilloma	- Benign, locally aggressive papillary tumour with potential malignant transformation to squamous cell carcinoma in 11% of patients:
	    - Malignant transformation associated with HPV 16 and in the presence of aneuploidy
	- Usually arises from the lateral nasal wall
	- HPV types 6 and 11 seen
	- Increased p53 expression and decreased CD44 expression associated with malignancy
	- Differential diagnosis:
	    - Nasal polyps with squamous metaplasia
	    - Inverted ductal papilloma
	    - Invasive carcinoma

(continued)

Pathology	Description
Squamous cell carcinoma (SCC)	• Most common of the malignant tumours (50%) • Variants seen in 5% • SCC involving the nasal cavity are mostly well-differentiated and keratinizing • SCC involving sinuses are mostly moderately or poorly differentiated and of the non-keratinizing type • Cervical lymph node metastasis develops in up to 20% of patients and can involve the retropharyngeal lymph nodes

Adenoid cystic carcinoma (ACC) and minor salivary gland tumours	• Second in incidence to SCC
	• Most common cancer of salivary origin
	• More common than primary non-salivary adenocarcinoma
	• More frequent in the maxillary sinus (60%) than in the nasal cavity (25%):
	  ▪ Tubular (grade I)
	  ▪ Cribriform (grade II)
	  ▪ Solid (grade III)
	• Differential diagnosis according to grade:
	  ▪ Grade I: cellular pleomorphic adenoma
	  ▪ Grade III: basaloid variant of SCC
	• Perineural spread, soft tissue and bone infiltration and sub-periosteal permeation are common features
	• Mucoepidermoid carcinoma, acinic cell carcinoma, clear cell carcinoma and myoepithelial carcinoma are other types of minor salivary gland tumours which are rarely encountered in the sinonasal region

Adenocarcinoma intestinal and non-intestinal types	• Third most common of the malignant tumours
	• Sub-classified into:
	  ▪ *Intestinal types (ITACs)*: typing and grading has prognostic significance
	    ○ Papillary (grade I)
	    ○ Colonic (grade II/ III), common
	    ○ Solid (grade III)
	    ○ Mucinous
	    ○ Mixed
	    ○ ITACs show diffuse immunopositivity with intestinal markers, e.g. CK20,CDX-2, MUC2 and villin
	  ▪ *Non-intestinal types (non-ITACs)*:
	    ○ High grade
	    ○ Low grade, more common
	    ○ Differential diagnosis of low-grade adenocarcinoma includes:
	      – Respiratory epithelial adenomatoid hamartoma
	      – Salivary gland adenoma
	      – Seromucous adenocarcinoma
	      – Low-grade adenocarcinoma of salivary gland origin like ACC grade I
	    ○ Differential diagnosis of high-grade adenocarcinoma includes:
	      – High-grade tumours like sinonasal undifferentiated carcinoma (SNUC) and sinonasal neuroendocrine carcinoma (SNEC)

Neuroendocrine tumours	**Esthesio-neuroblastoma (ENB)**
	• Arising from the olfactory epithelium in upper nasal cavity, ethmoid and cribriform plate
	• Cervical lymph node metastasis in <5%
	• Presence of sustentacular cells at the periphery of nests marked by S-100
	• Hyams' grading (I–IV) system based on:
	  ▪ Degree of differentiation
	  ▪ Presence of neurofibrillary stroma
	  ▪ Mitotic figures and necrosis indicate higher grade correlates with poor prognosis
	
	Sinonasal undifferentiated carcinoma (SNUC)
	• Locally aggressive tumour of uncertain histogenesis with high propensity for distant metastasis
	• Distinguishing features:
	  ▪ Lack of differentiating features on histology, but always exhibit high grade morphology:
	    ○ Lack of neurofibrillary stroma
	  ▪ Lack of diffuse positivity with neuroendocrine markers
	  ▪ Immune positivity with epithelial markers are the distinguishing features
	    ○ Tumour cells show immune positivity for epithelial markers like panCK, CK7, CK8, CK19 and EMA, but not CK5/6 and CK14

Pathology	Description
	• Differential diagnosis includes NEC and nasopharyngeal undifferentiated carcinoma with round cell morphology like high grade olfactory neuroblastoma **Neuroendocrine carcinoma (NEC)** **Small cell carcinoma (SmCC)** • Rare tumour originating in the nasal cavity with extension into the maxillary and ethmoid sinus • Resembles small cell carcinoma of the lungs • Morphologically is poorly differentiated with no specific diagnostic features • Shows immune positivity with epithelial and neuroendocrine markers (NSE, synaptophysin, chromogranin, CD56)
Malignant mucosal melanoma	• Rare • 80% occur in the nose and 20% in the paranasal sinuses • Metastasis can present early • S-100, Melan-A and HMB-45 immunohistochemistry is confirmatory, especially in case of Amelanotic melanoma.
Lymphomas and related conditions	• Non-Hodgkin lymphoma (NHL) • Diffuse large B cell type, T-cell/natural killer cell lymphoma (NKTCL), plasmacytoma

Presentation

In view of their rarity and the non-specificity of symptoms during the early stages, tumours of the nose and paranasal sinuses are often diagnosed at an advanced stage. Unilateral nasal symptoms, such as obstruction, should alert the physician to rule out malignancy. Inflammatory polyps frequently co-exist with malignant tumours. Endoscopic examination therefore, is strongly recommended to obtain appropriate visualization and to guide biopsy.

- *Nasal cavity (usually unilateral)*:
  - Nasal obstruction
  - Anosmia
  - Swelling
  - Bleeding
  - Purulent nasal discharge
  - Foul smell
  - Post-nasal discharge
- *Orbit*:
  - Epiphora
  - Proptosis
  - Pain
  - Congestion
  - Diplopia
- *Cranial nerves*:
  - Anosmia
  - Numbness of lip, cheek and teeth
  - Impaired eye movement
  - Diminished vision
  - Palatal anaesthesia
  - Dryness of eye
- *Oral cavity*:
  - Growth over palate and gums
  - Loosening of teeth
  - Trismus
- *Nasopharynx*:
  - Blockage of ears
- *Others*:
  - Brain:
    - Headache
    - Altered consciousness/behaviour
  - Lymph node metastasis:
    - Cervical nodes enlargement
  - Systemic spread:
    - Loss of weight
    - Cough and expectoration
    - Bone pain

Diagnostic work-up

- *Medical history*:
  - Thorough history to document symptoms, to correlate with anatomical involvement and identify either environmental or genetic causes
- *Clinical examination (tumour extent)*:
  - External nasal examination: anterior nares and external osteocartilaginous framework
  - Oral examination: palate, teeth, gingivobuccal sulcus, mouth opening
  - Diagnostic nasal endoscopy: floor and lateral wall of the nose, nasal septum, inferior and middle meatus, olfactory groove and nasopharynx
  - Ophthalmic examination: vision, ocular movements
  - Cranial nerves: II, III, IV, V and VI
  - Neck: cervical nodes (levels I–IV)
- *Imaging (preferably prior to biopsy)*:
  - Computed tomography (CT) scan (with bone algorithm and contrast enhanced):
    - Multidetector scanner with thin sections

Table 45.1 UICC TNM categories and stage grouping: Nasal cavity and paranasal sinus

TNM categories	
Maxillary sinus	
T1	Mucosa
T2	Bone erosion/destruction, hard palate, middle nasal meatus
T3	Posterior bony wall maxillary sinus, subcutaneous tissues, floor/medial wall of orbit, pterygoid fossa, ethmoid sinus
T4a	Anterior orbit, cheek skin, pterygoid plates, infratemporal fossa, cribriform plate, sphenoid/frontal sinus
T4b	Orbital apex, dura, brain, middle cranial fossa, cranial nerves other than V2, nasopharynx, clivus
Nasal cavity and ethmoid sinus	
T1	One subsite
T2	Two subsites or adjacent nasoethmoidal site
T3	Medial wall/floor orbit, maxillary sinus, palate, cribriform plate
T4a	Anterior orbit, skin of nose/cheek, anterior cranial fossa (minimal), pterygoid plates, sphenoid/frontal sinuses
T4b	Orbital apex, dura, brain, middle cranial fossa, cranial nerves other than V2, nasopharynx, clivus
All sites	
N1	Ipsilateral single ≤3 cm
N2	(a) Ipsilateral single >3–6 cm
	(b) Ipsilateral multiple ≥6 cm
	(c) Bilateral, contralateral ≥6 cm
N3	>6 cm
M1	Distant metastasis

Stage grouping			
Stage 0	Tis	N0	M0
Stage I	T1	N0	M0
Stage II	T2	N0	M0
Stage III	T3	N0	M0
	T1, T2, T3	N1	M0
Stage IVA	T1, T2, T3	N2	M0
	T4a	N0, N1, N2	M0
Stage IVB	T4b	Any N	M0
	Any T	N3	M0
Stage IVC	Any T	Any N	M1

- Reformatting in coronal and sagittal plane
- Assessment of orbit, ptergyopalatine fossa, infratemporal fossa, skull base, nasopharynx and/or premaxillary soft tissue involvement
- Identification of metastatic nodes including retropharyngeal nodes
- Magnetic resonance imaging (MRI) (contrast enhanced):
  - Non-ionizing imaging
  - Multiplanar capability
  - Better delineation of vascular structures and cerebrospinal fluid (CSF)
  - To differentiate inflammatory changes from tumour
  - To get better delineation of periorbita, orbit, dura, brain and/or cavernous sinus involvement
  - To assess perineural spread
- Positron emission tomography (PET):
  - 18-Fluorodeoxyglucose and CT fusion scan (when available)
  - To rule out distant metastasis:
    – Advanced-stage tumours
    – High-grade malignancies
    – Multiple low-level neck nodes
    – Patients symptomatic for distant metastasis
    – Follow-up imaging in non-surgical treatment options
- *Biopsy tumour profile*:
  - Transnasal endoscopic biopsy for intranasal mass
  - Transoral biopsy for obvious mass
  - Transmaxillary biopsy when indicated
  - Immunohistochemical studies are frequently required

Staging and prognostic grouping

UICC TNM staging
See Table 45.1.

Kadish staging for esthesioneuroblastoma
Group A: lesions are limited to the nasal cavity
Group B: lesions involve the nasal cavity and paranasal sinuses
Group C: lesions extend beyond the nasal cavity and paranasal sinuses
Group D: for tumours with regional (cervical lymph node) or distant metastasis

Prognostic factors
See Table 45.2.

Table 45.2 Prognostic factors for paranasal sinus tumours

Prognostic factors	Tumour related	Host related	Environment related
Essential	T category N category M category		
Additional	Histotype	Age Gender Performance status	Radiation dose Overall treatment time Surgical margins
New and promising			High precision optimal dose radiation Concurrent cytotoxic or biological therapies Ideal integration with advanced surgical techniques

Prognosis in terms of recurrence rate (RR) and overall survival (OS):

- *Inverted papilloma*:
  - RR 12–20%
  - Usually occur within the first 3 years following inadequate excision and do not indicate malignant transformation
- *Squamous cell carcinoma*:
  - RR 30%
  - 5-year OS 60–64%
- *Adenoid cystic carcinoma*:
  - Known for its relentless growth and multiple local recurrences
  - Delayed recurrences, especially at distant sites, can occur even after 10 years, necessitating prolonged follow-up
  - 5-year OS 35% and 10-year OS 10%
  - Grading is prognostic
- *Adenocarcinoma intestinal types*:
  - ITACs are locally aggressive tumours with frequent local failure and infrequent cervical nodal or distal metastasis
  - 5-year OS 70%
- *Neuroendocrine tumours*:
  - Esthesio-neuroblastoma:
    - 5-year OS 60–80%
  - Sinonasal undifferentiated carcinoma:
    - Cervical nodal metastasis and distal metastasis are known to occur
    - 5-year OS
      - Concurrent chemoradiation (CCRT): 43–63%
      - Surgery 20%
      - A combination of the three modalities probably provides greater survival benefit
  - Small cell neuroendocrine carcinoma:
    - Aggressive tumour with high incidence of local recurrence and distal metastasis
    - 5-year OS <30% without CCRT; 60–65% with CCRT
- *Malignant mucosal melanoma*:
  - 5-year OS 20–35%
  - Distant metastasis (often at disease onset) rate is 40%
- *Lymphomas and related conditions*:
  - NKTCL 5-year OS 70%
  - NHL 5-year OS 80%

Outcomes for tumours in the nasal cavity exceed those that arise from the sinuses.

Treatment philosophy

In the nasal cavity and paranasal sinuses the treatment is essentially similar to that in other head and neck subsites. Cure is the primary goal with preservation of important structures whilst maintaining quality of life. Treatment should be individualized based on location and extent of disease, patient performance status, histopathological subtypes of tumour and availability of local expertise. Treatment decision should also take into account patients' preference once informed of their options.

In general, early-stage tumours are better managed by surgery, while primary radiotherapy (RT) is considered for patients unsuitable for surgery. For advanced tumours, a combined modality approach of surgery followed by RT or CRT is advised. Inoperable tumours are managed by CRT or RT alone. Distant metastasis is managed with palliative intent with either chemotherapy or palliative RT to symptomatic sites or best supportive care (BSC) in those with poor performance status.

The sinonasal tumours arise in the vicinity of important structures and management is guided by their involvement. The ability to achieve adequate surgical clearance dictates decision-making. Tumours which are subcranial, free of the anterior facial skeleton or the nasal floor are suitable for endonasal resection. Tumours with minimal transcranial spread with minimal midline involvement are suitable for endonasal craniectomy, while those with transcranial spread and involving the brain with lateral extension are suitable for either craniofacial surgery or a combined cranio-endoscopic approach. Involvement of the pterygopalatine/infratemporal fossa is a relative contraindication for surgery. Bilateral optic nerve involvement, internal carotid encasement and extensive dural enhancement and brain involvement are contraindications for surgery and have extremely poor outcomes.

In selected cases, preoperative moderate-dose radiotherapy ± chemotherapy to a surgically unperturbed target area can be considered to protect the intraorbital contents and/or remaining optic apparatus, followed by definitive surgery.

For anteriorly located tumours of the nasal cavity or vestibule, definitive high dose radiotherapy ± chemotherapy can be considered to improve cosmetic outcomes, while surgery is reserved for salvage,

Scenario	Description
Stage I and II	• Single modality: ▪ Surgery or radiotherapy (RT)

Stage III and IVa	• Combined modality:
	  ▪ Surgery + (chemo)RT
	  ▪ Concomitant chemoradiotherapy (CCRT)

Stage IVb	• When performance status is 0–1:
	  ▪ CCRT
	  ▪ Surgery only in favourable histologies (adenoid cystic carcinoma, low-grade adenocarcinoma), in case of dura involvement or in selected cases of limited extent to the brain and/or nasopharynx
	• When performance status is ≥2:
	  ▪ Palliative RT
	  ▪ Best supportive care (BSC)

Treatment

Treatment of the primary

Treatment of the primary sinonasal tumours	Description

T1/2	• *Surgery*:
	  ▪ Approaches: midfacial degloving, lateral rhinotomy, craniofacial resection, and endoscopic transnasal access in suitable cases:
	    ○ *Nasal cavity and ethmoid sinus*: medial maxillectomy with ethmoidectomy ± postoperative RT
	    ○ *Maxillary sinus*: inferior maxillectomy/orbit floor-sparing maxillectomy ± postoperative RT
	    ○ Tumours of the frontoethmosphenoid complex or nasal cavity and/or maxillary antrum and orbit with secondary extension to the skull base may require craniofacial resection
	    ○ Endoscopic transnasal approaches may be used in selected cases
	• *Radiotherapy*:
	  ▪ Inoperable patients (unsuitable for anaesthesia or who refuse surgery)
	  ▪ Anteriorly located tumours of nasal cavity or vestibule for which surgical resection would result in significant cosmetic defect: definitive RT may be considered with surgery for salvage

T3/4a	• *Surgery*:
	  ▪ *Nasal cavity and ethmoid sinus*: maxillo-ethmoidectomy or craniofacial resection + postoperative (chemo)RT
	  ▪ *Maxillary sinus*: maxillectomy or craniofacial resection + postoperative RT
	  ▪ To protect intraorbital contents and/or remaining optic apparatus or brain, preoperative modest dose (50 Gy in 25 fractions over 5 weeks) RT ± chemotherapy may be delivered to a surgically unperturbed target area:
	    ○ This may be combined with a small volume simultaneous in-field boost to a higher dose where surgical margins are anticipated to be compromised
	• *Radiotherapy*:
	  ▪ CCRT is an option in patients with good performance status, especially for radio- and chemo-responsive histotypes like SNUC, SmSCC, SNEC and high-grade ENB
	  ▪ RT alone or neoadjuvant chemotherapy followed by CRT with the same selection criteria as above

T4b	• Role of resection is debatable; only to be considered for favourable histotypes • CCRT is an option in patients with good performance status, especially for radio- and chemo-responsive histotypes like SNUC, SmSCC, SNEC and high grade ENB • RT alone or neoadjuvant chemotherapy followed by CRT with the same selection criteria as above • In patients for whom curative treatment is not appropriate due to extent of the primary cancer, poor performance status or the presence of distant metastasis, palliative RT may be offered

Treatment of the neck
The incidence of nodal metastasis is low due to the paucity of lymphatics in the paranasal sinuses. Nodal metastasis occurs in larger tumours, aggressive histologies and when adjacent structures are involved.
- For patients treated with primary surgery:
  - N0 neck: observation
  - N+: ipsilateral appropriate neck dissection and adjuvant (chemo)RT, according to histopathology
- For cN+ patients treated with primary RT:
  - High dose (60–70 Gy) to all gross lymph nodes and microscopic dose (50 Gy) to elective neck regions

Surgery
Contraindications
- Extensive brain invasion
- Cavernous sinus and/or internal carotid artery involvement
- Bilateral orbital involvement
- *Relative contraindications*:
  - Extensive skin involvement
  - Infra temporal fossa extension
  - Pterygopalatine fossa involvement

Management of the orbit
Clinicoradiological assessment of orbit involvement is of utmost important. Survival is reduced when the apex of the orbit is grossly involved, while invasion of the anterior part does not have the same negative impact on prognosis.
- Gross intraconal spread: orbital clearance
- Suspicion for periorbita involvement: intraoperative evaluation of the periorbital; fat for frozen section
- Periobita is free: orbital content is preserved

Management of intracranial spread
Survival drops by 50% when the tumour involves the dura and the brain
- Extensive brain involvement: neoadjuvant chemotherapy + RT, CCRT or RT alone
- Minimal brain involvement: excision of involved brain if in non-eloquent area + (chemo)RT
- Dura involved: dura resection with wide margins and repair + chemo(RT)
- Dura not involved or in contact with the tumour: subcranial resection preserving the dura + RT

Endoscopic endonasal surgery
Tumour excision is planned according to the site of origin and the extent, using a one- or two-nostril technique. Resection, which is intended to achieve free margins as in external techniques, is performed in a multibloc fashion, starting from the inner part of the nasal cavity and progressing to the peripheral structures (e.g. periorbita, dura and brain), which can be spared or included as a last layer, according to the situation. Recent advances in surgical instrumentation, the refinement of powered instrumentation and navigation systems, and the development of a philosophy which uses the nasal cavities as a corridor to access adjacent anatomical areas have contributed to the rapid expansion of the indications for endoscopic surgery. Indications are:
- T1–2 tumours of the nasal cavity and ethmoid sinus
- Selected T3, T4a and T4b tumours of the nasal cavity and ethmoid sinus.
  Contraindications are:
- Erosion of the nasal bones
- Erosion of the floor of the nasal cavity
- Involvement of the bony walls of the maxillary sinus (except the medial one)
- Extensive involvement of the frontal sinus
- Invasion of the orbit and/or nasolacrimal system
- Extensive involvement of the nasopharynx
- Dural invasion lateral to the meridian of the orbit
- Gross brain invasion.
  Endoscopic approaches are:
- Endonasal endoscopic resection without craniectomy: complete transnasal clearance of tumours not reaching the anterior skull base
- Endonasal endoscopic resection with craniectomy: complete transnasal clearance of tumours reaching or involving the anterior skull base
- Cranioendoscopic resection: transnasal resection combined with subfrontal craniotomy.

The local control rate with endoscopic resection in studies from Italy and the USA is ~85%, with 5-year disease-specific survival (DSS) of 59–87%. These data compare well with the results of the International Collaborative Study from 17 centres using the external technique: local control of 45.8% and 5-year DSS of 48.3%.

Postoperative CSF leak and intraoperative haemorrhage are the most feared complications. Their occurrence has been significantly decreased by refinement in duraplasty techniques and the introduction of new tissue sealants, respectively. Morbidity in endonasal series is negligible, with CSF leak and meningitis occurring in around 4% and 0.7% of patients, respectively. These figures are extremely favourable when compared to those for anterior craniofacial resection (central nervous system [CNS] complication rate of around 12% and a mortality of 4.5%).

Management of cranionasal separation
- Conventional coronal approach: primary dural repair or patch repair with temporalis fascia or fascia lata, followed by a vascularized pericranial flap
- Endonasal endoscopic approach: multilayered dural repair with collagen matrix or fascia lata inlay beneath the dura, fascia lata overlay of the dura, followed by a nasosepatal (Hadad–Bassagasteguy) flap (if available)

- Craniofacial resection with orbital clearance or extensive soft tissue and bony resection: free flap (anterolateral thigh flap or rectus abdominus flap) to give a cranionasal separation, defect filling and provision of a skin lining when required

- Extensive skin and soft tissue defect/more than half of the palate/orbital clearance/skull base reconstruction: microvascular free flap.

Reconstruction
Post maxillo-ethmoidectomy reconstruction
Defects can be classified according to the Brown and Shaw classification. Planning the adequate reconstruction depends on the palate and the maxillary defect with overlying soft tissues:
- If the palatal defect is less than one-third, an obturator is recommended:
  - Temporary obturator for 2–3 months
  - Interim for 3 months until contracture occurs
  - Final maxillary prosthesis after 3 months

Floor of the orbit reconstruction and support
- Periorbita preserved:
  - No support is required if the bony defect is confined to the infraorbital nerve
  - If the entire floor is removed: titanium mesh covered with vascularized tissue
- Periorbita resected:
  - Fascia lata repair of the defect
  - Temporalis muscle flap for support
  - Free vascularized flap if soft tissue/bone reconstruction is required

Radiotherapy

Radiotherapy	Description

Definitive RT ± chemotherapy (see Table 45.3)	• Indications:
	  ▪ Unsuited for primary surgical resection (disease extent or high operation risk)
	  ▪ Cosmetic considerations (anteriorly located tumours of nasal cavity or vestibule)
	  ▪ Patient preference
	• Dose:
	  ▪ Definitive RT ± concurrent chemotherapy
	  ▪ RT 66–70 Gy in 33–35 fractions over 6.5–7 weeks
	• Clinical target volumes (CTV):
	  ▪ Primary tumour and involved lymph nodes (including potential local subclinical infiltration)
	  ▪ Treatment of potential subclinical lymph node regions is inconsistent:
	    ○ High-risk lymph nodes may be treated in some institutions
	• Important prognostic factors affecting local control include:
	  ▪ Histology
	  ▪ T4b disease
	  ▪ Brain invasion
	  ▪ Infratemporal fossa involvement

Preoperative RT (see Table 45.3) ± **chemotherapy**	• Indications:
	  ▪ For tumours in extreme proximity to critical structures where protection of intraorbital contents and/or orbital apparatus or critical structures are in question with upfront surgery:
	    ○ To protect intraobital contents and/or optic apparatus or brain requiring larger volumes and higher doses in the postoperative setting
	• Dose: 50 Gy in 25 fractions over 5 weeks

Postoperative RT (see Table 45.3) ± **chemotherapy**	• Indications:
	  ▪ Cases with adverse histopathological features:
	    ○ T3–4 tumours
	    ○ Involvement of adjacent structures like bone, dura and brain
	    ○ Compromised surgical margins
	    ○ Presence of lymphovascular invasion, perineural invasion
	    ○ Positive lymph nodes with or without extracapsular spread
	• Dose:
	  ▪ Negative margins: 56–60 Gy in 28–30 fractions over 5.5–6 weeks
	  ▪ Positive margins: 64–66 Gy in 32–33 fractions over 6.5 weeks

Table 45.3 Definitive and adjuvant radiotherapy regimens

Target volume and dose	Description
Definitive radiotherapy	
Gross tumour volume (GTV) 66–70 Gy in 33–35 fractions	All visible disease based on recent pretreatment imaging
Clinical tumour volume (CTV) 1 66–70 Gy in 33–35 fractions	GTV + 0.5 – 1 cm margin depending on the epicentre of the disease and histology
CTV 2 60 Gy in 30 fractions	CTV 1 + adjacent sinus mucosa (approx. CTV 1 + 1 – 1.5 cm, editing from the adjacent, uninvolved organs at risk [OAR])
CTV 3 50 Gy in 25 fractions	Elective nodal regions, e.g. level IB and 2A in squamous carcinoma of the maxillary antrum with skin involvement, and undifferentiated carcinoma Nerve tracts for tumours with perineural extension of tumour like ACC in to skull base, pterygomaxillary fissure, infratemporal fossa
Adjuvant radiotherapy	
CTV 1 66–70 Gy in 33–35 fractions	Any residual disease, i.e. suspected site of positive margin, residual disease, gross extracapsular extension at node
CTV 2 60 Gy in 30 fractions	CTV 1 + all preoperative disease in surgical bed + 1–1.5 cm (editing from the adjacent, uninvolved OAR)
CTV3 50 Gy in 25 fractions	As for definitive radiotherapy
Neoadjuvant radiotherapy	
CTV 1 50 Gy in 25 fractions	To encompass primary and nodal GTV + 0.5 – 1 cm margin cN+ lymph node may receive simultaneous in-field boost (e.g. 60 Gy in 25 fractions) to obviate subsequent resection in small volume nodal disease

Proton/heavy ion therapy
- Equivalent doses to photon therapy:
- Meta-analysis by Ramaekers et al. suggests proton therapy to be superior for the endpoints of disease-free and overall survival
- Main advantage of protons over photons is the ability to reduce radiation-induced late sequelae such as optic neuropathy and temporal lobe necrosis

Sequelae of radiotherapy
- Visual impairment
- Unilateral blindness (30%)
- Bilateral blindness (10%)
- Dry eye syndrome
- Hypothalamic–pituitary axis suppression
- Necrosis of irradiated brain
- Osteoradionecrosis

Systemic therapy in epithelial tumours

Advanced and high-grade tumours can benefit from neoadjuvant chemotherapy for two to three cycles. The treatment schedule is mainly based on cisplatin combined with different drugs depending upon histotype: combination with 5-fluorouracil (5-FU) for ITAC; VP-16 for sinonasal tumours with an neuroendocrine component; doxorubicin for salivary gland tumours; and taxanes and 5-FU for squamous histotype.

Systemic therapy	Description
Intravenous chemotherapy	- Intravenous infusion - Neoadjuvant in specific high-grade tumour histotypes - Cisplatin-based polychemotherapy depending on histotype

Intra-arterial chemotherapy	- Simultaneous surgery, radiotherapy and regional chemotherapy
	- Trimodality therapy (Sato):
	  - Surgical debulking
	  - Daily debridement of residual tumour
	  - RT 1.2 Gy in six fractions over 9 days
	  - Five intra-arterial infusions of 5-FU (250 mg daily) and broxuridine (BUdR) (500 mg daily)
	  - 5-year OS of 76% (but just 45 cases)
	- RadPlat therapy (Samant):
	  - Rapid intra-arterial cisplatin 150 mg/m²
	  - Systemic sodium thiosulfate IV
	  - RT 50 Gy; 2 Gy every 5 weeks)
	  - Followed by planned organ-sparing surgery
	  - 5-year OS 53% (median follow up of 53 months)
	- RadPlat therapy (Homma):
	  - Rapid intra-arterial cisplatin 100–120 mg/m²
	  - Systemic sodium thiosulfate IV
	  - RT 65–70 Gy over 6 weeks
	  - Surgery for residual disease
	  - 5-year OS 69.3% (median follow-up of 4.6 years)
	  - Higher incidence of ocular and visual problems

Topical chemotherapy	- For ethmoid adenocarcinomas (Knegt):
	  - Transmaxillary surgical debulking
	  - Repeated topical chemotherapy (5-FU) and necrotomy
	  - RT for recurrence
	  - 5-year DFS 87%

Follow-up

Regular follow-up should be as usual for all head and neck malignancies. Surveillance needs to be integrated with endoscopic examination.
- 2–6 weeks post radiotherapy
- Every 3 months or more frequently for 2 years
- Every 4 months or more frequently for third year
- Every 6 months or more frequently for Years 4–5
- Annually for Years 6–10

Investigations and assessment

- Fibre-optic nasoendoscopy
- Imaging:
  - Baseline post-treatment imaging (MRI preferred) 2–3 months after completion of treatment with subsequent follow-up examination under anaesthesia (EUA)/biopsy of any suspicious residual abnormalities:
    - Patients with resolving abnormalities should have repeat imaging within 2–3 months to ensure these are either stable or continuing to regress
  - Follow-up imaging with MRI recommended annually for at least 2 years, thereafter when symptomatic
  - In cases where the cavity is closed by a free flap, surveillance with MRI is recommended
  - PET-CT to evaluate response following CCRT, preferably after 3 months
- Pharyngeal function (speech/swallow) as indicated
- Dental assessment where applicable
- Audiometry where applicable
- Ophthalmology review as applicable

Treatment for recurrence and metastatic disease

See Chapter 39.

Controversies

- Endoscopic resection in advanced-stage tumours
- Orbit preservation with periorbital involvement

Phase III clinical trials

There are no phase III trials due to the low incidence of nose and paranasal sinus malignancies. However, a systematic review of treatment over four decades offers the best available evidence for current management guidelines, whilst the International Collaborative Study from 17 worldwide institutes provides evidence for outcomes expected from surgery and adjuvant therapy for advanced tumours.

Areas of research

- Cytogenetic refinement in salivary gland tumours
- Role of HPV in epithelial tumours
- Histology-driven neoadjuvant chemotherapy
- Role of proton therapy and carbon-ion therapy
- Gene signature and genome sequencing

Recommended reading

Brown JS, Shaw RJ (2010) Reconstruction of the maxilla and midface: introducing a new classification. *Lancet Oncol* 11(10):1001–1008.

Cantù G, Bimbi G, Miceli R et al. (2008) Lymph node metastases in malignant tumours of the paranasal sinuses: prognostic value and treatment. *Arch Otolaryngol Head Neck Surg* 134(2):170–177.

Dulguerov P, Jacobsen MS, Allal AS, Lehmann W, Calcaterra T (2001) Nasal and paranasal sinus carcinoma: are we making progress? A series of 220 patients and a systematic review. *Cancer* 92(12):3012–3029.

Ganly I, Patel SG, Singh B (2005) Craniofacial resection for malignant paranasal sinus tumours: Report of an International Collaborative Study. *Head Neck* 27(7):575–584.

Hanna E, DeMonte F, Ibrahim S, Roberts D, Levine N, Kupferman M (2009) Endoscopic resection of sinonasal cancers with and without craniotomy: oncologic results. *Arch Otolaryngol Head Neck Surg* 135(12):1219–1224.

Nicolai P, Battaglia P, Bignami M et al. (2008) Endoscopic surgery for malignant tumours of the sinonasal tract and adjacent skull base: a 10-year experience. *Am J Rhinol* 22(3):308–316.

Ramaekers BL, Pijls-Johannesma M, Joore MA et al. (2011) Systematic review and meta-analysis of radiotherapy in various head and neck cancers: Comparing photons, carbon ions and protons. *Cancer Treat Rev* 37:185–201.

Robbins KT, Homma A (2008) Intra-arterial chemotherapy for head and neck cancer: experiences from three continents. *Surg Oncol Clin North Am* 17(4):919–933.

Robbins KT, Ferlito A, Silver CE (2011) Contemporary management of sinonasal cancer. *Head Neck* 33(9):1352–1365.

Rosenthal DI, Barker JL Jr, El-Naggar AK et al. (2004) Sinonasal malignancies with neuroendocrine differentiation: patterns of failure according to histologic phenotype. *Cancer* 101(11):2567–2573.

Suárez C, Ferlito A, Lund VJ et al. (2008) Management of the orbit in malignant sinonasal tumours. *Head Neck* 30(2):242–250.

46 Head and neck unknown primary

Sarbani Ghosh Laskar[1], Naveen B. Mummudi[2], Vedang Murthy[1] and Gouri Pantvaidya[3]

[1]Department of Radiation Oncology, Tata Memorial Centre, Mumbai, India
[2]Department of Radiation Oncology, Christian Medical College, Vellore, Tamil Nadu, India
[3]Department of Head & Neck Surgical Oncology, Tata Memorial Centre, Mumbai, India

Summary	Description
Introduction	<ul><li>Carcinoma of unknown primary metastasizing to the neck nodes accounts for 2–4% of head and neck cancers</li><li>Outcome is favourable compared with stage-matched patients with a known head and neck primary</li><li>Oropharynx is the commonest site for an occult primary</li><li>Most common histology is squamous cell carcinoma (SCC) (two-thirds of cases)</li></ul>
Presentation	<ul><li>A painless neck mass is the most common presentation</li><li>Unilateral involvement is more common than bilateral</li><li>Most frequently involved nodal station is level II, followed by level III</li><li>Metastases in the upper and middle neck are associated with a primary in the head and neck, whereas the lower neck is more likely to have primaries below the clavicle</li><li>At presentation, distant metastases are found in <20% of patients</li></ul>
Scenario	<ul><li>Primary radiotherapy (RT) is often used to address both neck disease and potential pharyngeal and/or laryngeal mucosal sites of primary disease:<ul><li>Ordinarily, potential mucosal candidate sites are included in an electively irradiated volume in addition to the required lymph node volume</li><li>In patients with fair skin and a long history of sun exposure (e.g. living in Australia or similar location), the skin of the head and neck may be the most likely primary site</li><li>Principles of nodal irradiation should be followed, including those governing RT alone or used as adjuvant with surgery to the neck</li></ul></li><li>cN1 disease: can be managed with either primary surgery ± postoperative RT ± chemotherapy<ul><li>pN1 disease without adverse features may not need further adjuvant RT if the decision is made to withhold treatment to candidate mucosal sites following a meticulous work-up which did not disclose a potential mucosal primary site of disease and especially when circumstantial evidence suggests the primary site is the skin</li></ul></li><li>cN2/3 disease: preference is to treat with definitive RT ± chemotherapy:<ul><li>Post-radiation neck dissection can be performed for residual disease</li></ul></li></ul>
Trials	<ul><li>No published phase III trials specific for head and neck unknown primary</li></ul>

Introduction

Carcinoma of unknown primary (CUP) is a heterogeneous clinical syndrome, defined as the histological diagnosis of metastatic malignant tumour without the detection of a primary despite standard clinical, laboratory and radiological evaluation. Discussion in this chapter is restricted to CUP with metastases to the neck nodes.

UICC Manual of Clinical Oncology, Ninth Edition. Edited by Brian O'Sullivan, James D. Brierley, Anil K. D'Cruz, Martin F. Fey, Raphael Pollock, Jan B. Vermorken and Shao Hui Huang. © 2015 UICC. Published 2015 by John Wiley & Sons, Ltd.

Incidence, aetiology and screening

Incidence, aetiology and screening	Description

Incidence	• Seventh to eighth most frequently occurring cancer in the world and the fourth commonest cause of cancer death in both males and females
	• Annual age-adjusted incidence per 100,000 population in the USA is 7–12 cases
	• Median age for occurrence is around 60 years
	• Marginally more frequent in males
	• Cervical nodal metastasis from an unknown primary site is an uncommon presentation of carcinoma of the head and neck, accounting for 2–4% of all cases
	• Patients in areas where nasopharyngeal carcinoma (NPC) is endemic are more likely to have an occult nasopharyngeal cancer, whereas the vast majority of occult primary cancers detected in the North America are found in the tonsillar fossa or the base of the tongue (mostly HPV-related tumour, especially in non- or light smokers)
	• Fair skinned patients from regions associated with heavy sun exposure (e.g. Australia and the southern USA) have a high risk of having an occult cutaneous primary
	• Primary may eventually manifest itself in around 20–30% of patients:
	   ▪ In those not treated with RT, the oropharynx is the most common site
	   ▪ Actuarial risk of emergence of primary carcinoma in the head-and neck after RT was <10% at 2 years, <15% at 5 years and up to 20% at 10 years

Aetiology	• Risk factors are similar to those seen in squamous cell carcinoma (SCC) of head and neck with a known primary, including tobacco and alcohol use, and sun exposure for skin cancers • Increasing role of human papillomavirus (HPV) and Epstein–Barr virus (EBV) in the aetiology of oropharyngeal (OPC) and nasopharyngeal carcinoma (NPC), respectively: ▪ Since 2000 the prevalence of HPV has significantly increased in North America and Europe; in the USA, HPV-associated OPC accounts for 50–70% of all cases compared with 40% in the previous decade

Pathology

The most frequent histology is SCC (two-thirds of cases), particularly when the upper neck (level II) is involved; followed by adenocarcinoma, undifferentiated carcinoma and other malignancies, including lymphoma and melanoma.

Natural history

It is proposed that angiogenic incompetence of the primary tumour leads to marked apoptosis and cell turnover, resulting in a phenotype with metastatic potential soon after transformation. The primary tumour may remain small and escape clinical detection (also, present imaging modalities are unable to detect small primaries), may exfoliate for mechanical reasons or may involute and disappear after metastasizing as a result of the body's defences or growth inhibition by factors secreted by metastases.

Presentation

- Median age is around 57–60 years (range 30–80 years)
- Median interval between the first symptom and diagnosis and/or referral to the oncology clinic is in the range of 3–4 months
- Male preponderance (almost 80%) and a history of chronic tobacco or alcohol use is usually present
- A painless neck mass is the most common clinical presentation
- Upper aerodigestive tract-related symptoms such as sore throat, otalgia, odynophagia, hoarseness of voice, dysphagia, epistaxis, etc. should be noted
- Unilateral lymph node involvement is more common; bilateral adenopathy is present in about 10% of patients
- Apparent prevalence of ≥N2 cases (median nodal size of 5 cm; range 2–14 cm)
- Most frequently involved nodal station is level II, followed by level III
- Site of lymph nodes could be useful in predicting the possible primary tumour site (Table 46.1):
  - Metastases in the upper and middle neck (levels I, II, III and V) are associated with a primary in the head and neck
  - Lower neck (level IV/supraclavicular fossa) involvement is often associated with primaries below the clavicle

Diagnostic work-up

The order of the initial evaluation is:
1 Complete history and clinical examination is mandatory:
   - Examination under anaesthesia, targeted selected biopsies of candidate sites and tonsillectomy are recommended

Table 46.1 Neck nodal levels

Neck nodes involved	First echelon drainage site
Level I (submental, submandibular nodes)	Floor of mouth, lips, anterior tongue
Level II (jugulodigastric/upper jugular nodes)	Nasopharynx, oropharynx, tongue, larynx, hypopharynx
Level III (middle jugular nodes)	Supraglottic larynx, pyriform sinus, post-cricoid region
Level IV (inferior jugular nodes)	Hypopharynx, subglottic larynx, thyroid, oesophagus, primaries below the clavicle
Level V (posterior triangle)	Nasopharynx, thyroid, primaries below the clavicle (lung, breast, bowel, testis, etc.)

2 Imaging studies should be done prior to any procedure:
- Contrast-enhanced computed tomography (CECT) or magnetic resonance imaging (MRI) face and neck
- CT thorax and abdomen
- Bone scan if the histopathology is undifferentiated/EBV positive
- Fluorodeoxyglucose (FDG)-positron emission tomography (PET)-CECT scan is the preferred modality whenever available:
  - Facilitates directed biopsies from a suspicious site but is not a substitute for mucosal examination
  - Detects 25% of primary tumours not detected with other modalities

3 Tissue diagnosis:
- Immunohistochemistry (IHC) studies:
  - Specific IHC markers aid in identifying the primary site
  - Emerging role of testing for HPV DNA and EBV RNA

4 Pan-endoscopy and directed biopsies

5 Molecular studies, when available, for predictive and prognostic information:
- Micro RNA profiling, microsatellite analysis and image cytometry are investigational methods

Diagnostic work up	Description

History and physical examination	• Personal history can provide clues to the origin of the primary:
	  ▪ Habitual smoking and alcohol consumption may suggest a primary tumour outside the nasopharynx
	  ▪ Multiple partners and orogenital contact may suggest a primary tumour within the oropharynx
	• History of previous malignancy or radiation
	• History of skin lesion is important, especially for melanoma and SCC
	• Accurate physical examination of the neck and a thorough evaluation of the upper aerodigestive tract mucosa with nasopharyngo-laryngoscopy, oesophagoscopy and bronchoscopy
	• Careful examination of the skin, thyroid, breasts, abdomen and other lymph node regions:
	  ▪ Other examinations, such as digital rectal examination and per vaginal examination, depending on history and location of the lymph node
	• Examination under anaesthesia and selected biopsies of candidate sites or directed biopsies from suspicious sites:
	  ▪ Selected biopsies from possible sites of the primary, including base of tongue, tonsil, pyriform sinus and nasopharynx can be performed, but may not be undertaken in all institutions as the yield is variable, especially in areas like the base of the tongue

Tissue diagnosis	• Fine needle aspiration (FNA) is commonly used as a first step to establish histology, but may be unreliable to address diagnostic tumour markers • Core biopsy (such as Tru cut) or an excisional biopsy following positive FNA is useful for IHC (e.g. p16 staining) and molecular biomarker studies (e.g. HPV, EBV, lymphomas, melanoma, etc.), which is helpful for identifying potential source of primary tumours • Specific IHC markers in addition to routine haematoxylin and eosin staining can aid in establishing the histological type of the metastasis and should be interpreted together with the morphological characteristics and clinical presentation: ▪ Especially relevant given the current HPV pandemic in the West and EBV prevalence in endemic regions
Immunohistochemistry and molecular markers (see Tables 46.2 and 46.3)	• Various markers have been studied and proposed, depending on the location of the lymph node and the initial histology • Detection of HPV DNA using polymerase chain reaction (PCR) and/or HPV 16 status using in situ hybridization in the node is strongly associated with a primary in the oropharynx; presence of cystic metastases further strengthens the relation • Detection of EBV with in situ hybridization in poorly differentiated SCC or undifferentiated metastatic lymph nodes may be suggestive of a nasopharyngeal tumour and should be considered in younger patients and in endemic areas: ▪ Reported sensitivity and specificity rates for EBV in core biopsy samples are close to 90%

Diagnostic work up	Description
	• Sensitivity and specificity for circulating EBV DNA with real time PCR in serum for detection of NPC is 96% and 93%, respectively • *In situ* hybridization for small EBV-encoded RNA is more sensitive and specific than PCR in detecting EBV • Circulating EBV DNA levels may also be used subsequently for monitoring treatment response and outcomes in NPC • Microsatellite analysis and image cytometry are experimental molecular genetic modalities, but emerging data show their promise in identifying the primary tumour when this remains clinically obscure: ■ Early reports show that each primary site in the head and neck has a distinct microRNA fingerprint; thus, micro RNA expression profiling analysis may help predict the site of origin of the metastatic disease

Role of tonsillectomy	• Tonsillar fossa is often found to harbour occult primary cancers metastatic to the cervical lymph nodes:
	    ■ Significantly higher likelihood of finding occult tumours with a tonsillectomy than a deep tonsil biopsy as the lesion may be submucosal or deep in the crypts
	    ■ Tonsillectomy is better than conventional imaging for detection of a small primary and can detect a primary in 20–40% of cases
	• Ipsilateral (I/L) or bilateral (B/L) tonsillectomy maybe performed as part of the standard diagnostic evaluation if there is no evidence of a primary site on physical and radiographic examinations:
	    ■ I/L tonsillectomy is sufficient with a single node involving the level IB/II/III areas
	    ■ B/L tonsillectomy is usually indicated in the presence of bilateral level II cervical nodes
	• However, role of routine tonsillectomy in the FDG-PET-CECT era is controversial and there are very little data evaluating the two

Imaging	• *Conventional radiological imaging*:
	    ■ Preferably performed before any invasive diagnostic procedure, such as biopsies or tonsillectomy
	    ■ CECT scan, apart from being a simple and cost-effective modality, provides excellent spatial resolution, improved detection of the extent and invasiveness of the tumour, and demonstrates deep-seated tumours that cannot be visualized directly
	    ■ Study should extend from the skull base to the thoracic inlet
	• MRI with gadolinium contrast has superior soft tissue resolution compared to CT imaging, and is essential in evaluating the nasopharynx or oropharynx
	• *Functional imaging*:
	    ■ Role of FDG-PET-CECT:
	        ○ Detects approximately 25–37% of primary tumours not detected with other modalities
	        ○ No better than conventional imaging for local disease staging
	        ○ Significant false-positive/false-negative rates: sensitivity of 84–88% and specificity of 75–84%
	        ○ To be done when complete head and neck examination (including pan-endoscopy) and neuroradiological review of CT/MRI fail to detect occult primary
	        ○ Prebiopsy PET increases the specificity and positive predictive value (PPV); also facilitates directed biopsies
	        ○ Negative PET does not eliminate the need for a careful endoscopy and biopsy of suspicious/high-risk sites as false-negative rates are seen in up to 16% of cases
	    ■ From a study comparing the rate in detecting the primary with various imaging modalities: CT 9.6%; MRI 0.0%; PET 14.6%; FDG-PET-CECT 44.2%; FDG-PET-CECT + pan-endoscopy + directed biopsies ± tonsillectomy 59.6%
	    ■ Narrowband imaging with magnified endoscopy has shown promise in detecting superficial or flat primary lesions

Table 46.2 Key screening antibodies

	CAM 5.2	EMA	S-100	LCA	PLAP
Carcinoma	+	+	±	–	±
Melanoma	–	–	+	–	–
Lymphoma/leukaemia	–	–	–	+	–
Non-seminomatous germ cell tumour (NSGGCT)	+	–	–	–	+
Germ cell tumour (GCT)	–	–	–	–	+

Table 46.3 Characteristic IHC markers

Tumour type	Markers
Carcinoma: • Squamous cell carcinoma • Adenocarcinoma	Cytokeratins CK5/6, p63, p16, EBER
Thyroid	TTF-1, thyroglobulin
Lung	TTF-1, CK7/20
Breast	GCDFP-15, mammoglobulin, ER
Neuroendocrine	Chromogranin, synaptophysin, PGP 9.5
Others	CDX2, CK7/20
Lymphoma	CLA, ALK1, CD30, CD43
Melanoma	S-100, HMB 45, melan-A
Sarcoma	Vimentin, actin, desmin, MyoD1, myogenin, S-100, CD34, CD99

TTF-1, thyroid transcription factor 1; GCDFP-15, gross cystic disease fluid protein 15; ER, oestrogen receptor; CLA, common leucocyte antigen; ALK1, anaplastic lymphoma kinase protein; HMB, human melanoma black-antimelanoma antibody; PGP 9.5, protein gene product 9.5.

TNM Categories (likely nasopharynx)	
T0	Unknown primary
N1	Unilateral cervical, unilateral or bilateral retropharyngeal lymph nodes, above supraclavicular fossa, ≤6 cm
N2	Bilateral cervical above supraclavicular fossa, ≤6 cm
N3a	>6 cm
N3b	Supraclavicular fossa
M1	Distant metastasis

TNM Category (likely oropharynx, hypopharynx, larynx)	
T0	Unknown primary
N1	Ipsilateral single ≤3 cm
N2	(a) Ipsilateral single >3–6 cm
	(b) Ipsilateral multiple ≤6 cm
	(c) Bilateral, contralateral ≥6 cm
N3	>6 cm
M1	Distant metastasis

Staging and prognostic grouping

UICC TNM staging

Staging of unknown primary is according to the clinical suspicion of the primary tumour with the T- category classified as T0 while the N-category and stage grouping are based on the clinical suspicion of the corresponding primary site of origin.

For example:
- Features suggesting nasopharyngeal primary (from endemic regions, elevated blood EBV DNA titre, poorly differentiated/undifferentiated carcinoma histology, non-smoker), the preferred N-category to be used is that of nasopharyngeal cancer in line with the TNM categories and stage grouping for that site.
- For a smoker with squamous cell carcinoma when smoking-related oro- or hypo-pharyngeal or larynx mucosal primary is suspected, the N-category to be used and stage grouping follows the criteria of oropharynx, hypopharynx, and larynx cancer staging

Table 46.1 UICC TNM stage grouping (likely nasopharynx)

Stage grouping			
Stage II	T0	N1	M0
Stage III	T0	N2	M0
Stage IVB	T0	N3	M0
Stage IVC	T0	Any N	M1

Stage grouping (likely oropharynx, hypopharynx, larynx)			
Stage III	T0	N1	M0
Stage IVA	T0	N2	M0
Stage IVB	T0	N3	M0
Stage IVC	T0	Any N	M1

Table 46.4 Prognostic factors for head and neck unknown primary

Prognostic factors	Tumour related	Host related	Environment related
Essential	Histology N category and number of nodes Extracapsular extension Presence or absence of metastatic disease $p16^{INK4A}$/HPV status, or EBV DNA status	Immunosuppression (especially skin cancer)	
Additional	Tumour differentiation Location of nodal disease (above vs below clavicle)	Gender Haemoglobin level Smoking history	Subsequent discovery of primary Overall treatment time
New and Promising	TP53 Surviving nuclear expression		

Prognostic factors

See Table 46.4.

- Favourable outcome compared with CUP in general as well with stage-matched patients with a known primary in the head and neck
- Most important factor for treatment outcome and survival is the nodal stage; patients with N1 and N2 disease have a significantly better prognosis compared with N3 patients:
  - Five-year survival based on N catgegory: N1 60.8%, all N2 51.1%, N2a 63.6%, N2b 42.5%, N2c 37.5% and N3 26.3%
- Patients without extracapsular extension (ECE) have a superior 5-year disease-specific survival compared to those with ECE (81.5% vs 56.9%)
- Other important factors for treatment outcome are gender (females fare better), haemoglobin levels (higher is better) and tumour differentiation
- Patients with a p16-positive tumour are also found to have a significantly higher 5-year overall and disease-free survival, and a better prognosis due to the absence of field cancerization and the presence of an intact apoptotic response

Treatment philosophy

The rationale for the treatment of patients with CUP has been extrapolated from the corresponding management of the neck in known head and neck primaries with cervical nodal metastases (Fig. 46.1).
- Primary radiotherapy (RT) is often used to address both neck disease and potential mucosal (pharynx and larynx) sites of primary disease:
  - Ordinarily, potential mucosal candidate sites are included in an elective irradiated volume in addition to the required lymph node volume
- Irradiation of potential mucosal candidate sites may be withheld in the following settings following meticulous work-up which did not disclose a potential mucosal primary sites of disease:
  - Non-smoking patient with keratinizing carcinoma with negative test for EBV and HPV on the lymph node biopsy (i.e. unlikely from nasopharynx or oropharynx)
  - Likely skin primary (i.e. fair skinned, atypical lymph node sites, such as intraparotid, or occipital lymph node)
  - Palliative radiotherapy (e.g. extensive nodal disease where cure is unlikely; frail patients)
- Principles of nodal irradiation should be followed including those governing radiotherapy alone or used as adjuvant with surgery to the neck
- cN1 disease can be managed with either primary surgery ± postoperative RT ± chemotherapy:
  - pN1 disease without adverse features may not need further adjuvant radiotherapy if the decision is made to withhold treatment to candidate mucosal sites following meticulous work-up which did not disclose a potential mucosal primary site of disease
- cN2/3 disease: preference is to treat with definitive RT ± chemotherapy
- Patients with a probable skin primary should have irradiation target volumes designed according to relevant routes of spread:
  - In addition to unilateral regional node regions to all or parts of levels I–V, some situations may require treatment of preauricular nodes, parotid nodes or facial nodes that are not typically included in the target areas for a mucosal CUP
  - Widespread nature of the skin of the face, scalp and neck makes it impossible to define a potential primary site irradiaton volume in most cases
- Patients should be actively monitored for post-surgical and post-RT morbidities

Scenario	Treatment philosophy
Early-stage disease	• Radical RT alone or Neck dissection +/- adjuvant therapy depending on surgico-pathological findings and risk stratification
Locally-advanced disease	• Definitive RT with or without concurrent chemotherapy • Salvage neck dissection for residual disease
Metastatic disease	• Palliative RT alone • Palliative chemotherapy • Best supportive care (BSC)

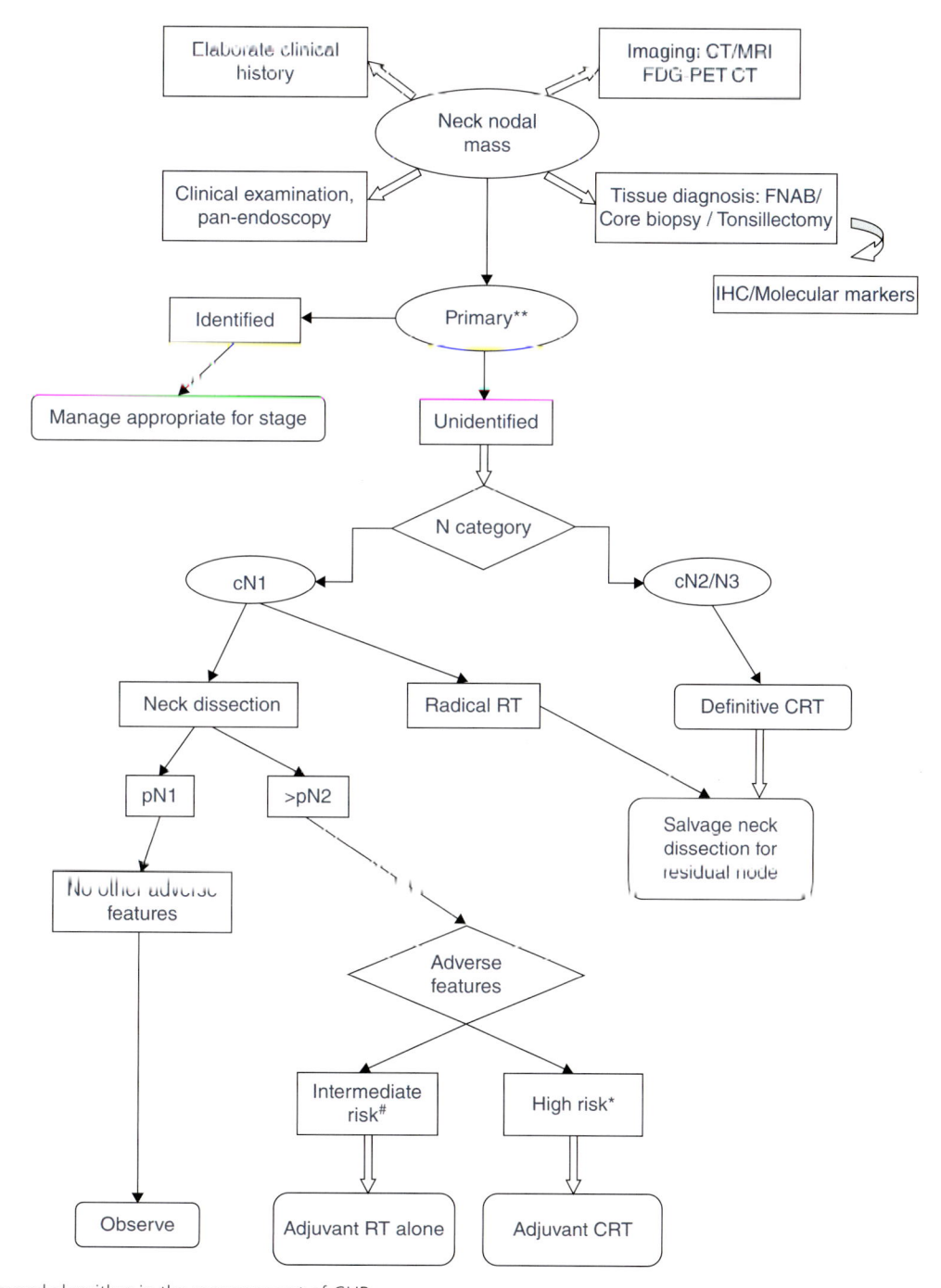

Figure 46.1 Proposed algorithm in the management of CUP.

**Ordinarily, potential mucosal candidate sites are included in an elective irradiated volume in addition to the required lymph node volume, with potential exceptions (see Treatment philosophy).

Treatment

Surgery
Patients with Stage N1 neck disease with no extracapsular extension can be managed by surgery alone.

Extent of neck dissection
The type of neck dissection should be tailored according to disease extent; controversy exists regarding the extent of neck dissection.
- A modified neck dissection (including levels I–V) rather than a selective neck dissection (levels II–V) is performed in some centres due to a putative concern about level 1B involvement in OPC, a common occult primary; however recent evidence has contradicted this.
- Radical neck dissection is warranted only in the presence of large neck nodes with extracapsular invasion into non-lymphatic structures
- Super-selective neck dissection has also been tried in patients when nodal disease is confined to one level; however, this is not yet considered standard practice
- Patients with pathological Stage N2 or higher neck disease or extracapsular extension should be considered for postoperative adjuvant therapy:
  - Surgery + postoperative RT (PORT) ± chemotherapy: resectable disease with intermediate-/high-risk factors on histopathology:
    - B/L nodes
    - Multiple positive nodes
    - Lower level nodes
    - Extracapsular extension
- Extracapsular extension is a predictor of neck recurrence, control of disease above the clavicles, cause specific survival and overall survival.

Complications post surgery
Overall complication rates after neck dissection in patients with unknown primary are comparable to those in patients with known primary cancers.

Radiotherapy
Conventional RT techniques using two parallel, opposed fields and a low anterior neck field have been associated with significant long-term morbidity. Intensity-modulated (IMRT) has the potential to give excellent coverage to the pharyngeal mucosa, and at the same time spare the major salivary glands and reduce dose to the swallowing apparatus, thus increasing the therapeutic ratio. IMRT results in comparable overall survival, locoregional control and disease-specific survival with conventional three-field head and neck irradiation.

Radiotherapy	Description
Definitive radiotherapy	- If excisional biopsy alone: definitive external beam RT (EBRT) - Patients with Stage N1 neck disease with no extracapsular extension can be managed by RT alone

Adjuvant radiotherapy	- Stage N2a–c and N3 disease should be treated with definitive chemoradiation (CRT):
	  - Planned neck dissection following RT if persistent disease:
	    - Some institutions consider planned neck dissection standard after definitive RT for N2/N3 disease
	  - Use of PET-CT post treatment (10–12 weeks) can guide subsequent management of the neck after definitive treatment
	- Controversy exists also regarding the timing of RT:
	  - *Advantages of preoperative RT:*
	    - Avoids delay in initiating RT due to surgical complications
	    - Tumour cells are in a better oxygenated state, thus reducing radioresistance due to hypoxia
	  - *Advantage of postoperative RT:*
	    - Provides accurate pathological evaluation of the dissection specimen and better delineation of disease extent, enabling tailoring of the RT portals

Treatment volume (see Tables 46.5 and 46.6)	- Treatment should be individualized based on risk factors and patient characteristics:
	  - Prophylactic mucosal irradiation volume may be tailored according to the risk factors
	  - *Features suggesting NPC as the primary*:
	    - Lymphoepithelioma/undifferentiated carcinoma
	    - Younger age (<40 years)
	    - Non-smoker
	    - Asian, Inuit, Polynesian ancestry, Mediterranean littoral, including North Africa
	    - Isolated or dominant level V disease; retropharyngeal (RPN) lymph node disease
	    - EBV positive

Radiotherapy	Description

	- *Features suggesting skin carcinoma as the primary*:
	  ○ Squamous cell histology
	  ○ Non-smoker/no history of excess alcohol consumption
	  ○ Fair complexion (e.g. Northern European ancestry)
	  ○ Sun exposure with actinic changes/history of skin SCC
	  ○ Immunocompromised
	  ○ Periparotid/parotid involvement
	- *Features suggesting HPV-positive OPC as the primary*:
	  ○ Squamous cell histology, especially basaloid subtype
	  ○ Non-smoker/no history of excess alcohol consumption
	  ○ History of marijuana use
	  ○ Cystic nodal disease
	- Although there is no consensus regarding the RT treatment volume, in principle both the conservative and comprehensive approaches are valid and acceptable:
	  - *Comprehensive approach*:
	    ○ Extensive prophylactic irradiation of all potential mucosal sites, as well as on both sides of the neck
	    ○ Achieves effective neck control
	    ○ Reduced incidence of subsequent emergence of mucosal primary
	    ○ High morbidity: xerostomia, dysphagia and aspiration, osteoradionecrosis
	  - *Conservative approach*:
	    ○ Limited field of irradiation to I/L neck only after thorough work-up to detect the primary tumour
	    ○ Especially relevant for patients at high risk for skin cancer
	    ○ Not suited for those at high risk for NPC or HPV-related OPC
	    ○ Limited field of irradiation to potential mucosal sites according to risk factors may be considered:
	      – High possibility for HPV-positive OPC: nasopharyngeal mucosa may be spared
	      – High possibility for skin carcinoma: contralateral mucosal sites and neck may be spared
	      – For adenocarcinoma histology, a submandibular or submental node (low probability of a primary along the pharyngeal axis)
	- Increased incidence of subsequent emergence of mucosal primary
	- Strong suggestion of nasopharyngeal primary: hypopharynx can be omitted from treatment
	- Subsequent salvage treatment possible
	- Marked reduction in morbidity
	- No differences in terms of overall survival between bilateral and unilateral neck radiotherapy

Palliative therapy	- In patients with poor performance status and/or a Stage N3 nodal mass, the nodal mass alone may be treated with conservative portals using *en face* electron or photon beams
	- Doses can be escalated or de-escalated depending on clinical response and the patient's performance status
	- Limited target volume to address involved sites without elective radiation to additional/contralateral nodal regions or potential mucosal sites
	- Common dose fractionation schedules include:
	  - 30 Gy in ten fractions (daily)
	  - 20 Gy in five fractions
	  - 32 Gy in eight fractions (bi-weekly)
	- In case of tumour bleeding, a single fraction of haemostatic RT can be delivered to a dose of 6–8 Gy, in addition to other supportive care

Table 46.5 Suggested radical RT volumes

Risk levels	Comprehensive	Conservative	Dose
High	Involved level	Involved level	66–70 Gy in 33–35 fractions
Intermediate	Ipsilateral adjacent level	–	60 Gy in 30 fractions
Low	Bilateral uninvolved levels and potential mucosal sites	± Ipsilateral adjacent level	50 Gy in 25 fractions

Table 46.6 Suggested postoperative RT volumes

Risk levels	Comprehensive	Conservative	Dose
High	Involved level	Involved level	60 Gy in 30 fractions
Low	Bilateral uninvolved levels and potential mucosal sites	± Ipsilateral adjacent level	50 Gy in 25 fractions

Complications post radiotherapy
- Acute: mucositis, dermatitis, xerostomia
- Chronic: hypothyroidism, dysphagia, xerostomia, aspiration pneumonia, oedema

Systemic therapy
- Concurrent platinum agent (cisplatin) with RT in locally-advanced disease, providing renal parameters, serum creatinine and/or creatinine clearance are adequate, and there are no contraindications for chemotherapy:
  - Concurrent monotherapy with cisplatin is used most often
  - In case of contraindications to cisplatin, carboplatin + 5-fluorouracil or, with lower level of evidence, single-agent carboplatin or paclitaxel or docetaxel or cetuximab could be used concurrently
- Induction chemotherapy in Stage N3 disease may be considered to decrease nodal volume, followed by definitive CRT
- Palliative chemotherapy may be attempted for disseminated disease

Follow-up
- Essential in surveillance for recurrence and also for prompt identification of post-treatment complications
- Dental evaluation and periodic monitoring of thyroid function
- Clinical evaluation and nasopharyngo-laryngoscopy every 2 months in the first year, every 3–4 months for next 2 years, and every 6 months thereafter up to 5 years and yearly after
- PET-CT once a year (optional)
- Additional exams can be performed at the discretion of the physician and are usually directed by clinical findings and the patient's symptoms

Controversies
- There is debate on the optimal treatment modality for early-stage nodal disease:
  - Either surgery alone or RT alone may be used
  - Surgery may be preferred in some institutions over RT alone as the histopathology of the resected specimen is useful in prognostication and also in deciding about appropriate adjuvant therapy
- Extent of neck dissection (modified radical versus selective) is contentious; intent of treatment, patient's performance status condition and co-morbidities should be kept in mind when selecting the procedure
- Adjuvant therapy in early-stage nodal disease, post neck dissection, can be avoided in the absence of high-risk pathological features, although there is a paucity of randomized data or high-level evidence for this
- Studies comparing the involved field and elective neck irradiation have not shown any advantage for more extensive RT; however, the majority of these studies are single-institution and retrospective:
  - Even in patients receiving extensive nodal and mucosal irradiation, distant metastases are a frequent site of failure
- There is paucity of data evaluating the role of adjuvant chemotherapy in minimizing systemic failure

Important studies
See Table 46.7.

Table 46.7 Important studies in head and neck unknown primary carcinoma

Study	Results
Rusthoven et al. (2004) Cancer 101(11):2641–2649	• Review of 16 studies evaluating the role of FDG-PET-CT in the detection of an unknown primary tumour • Overall sensitivity, specificity and accuracy rates of FDG-PET-CT in detecting unknown primary tumours were 88.3%, 74.9% and 78.8%, respectively • FDG-PET detected 24.5% of primary tumours and 27% of regional or distant metastases that were not apparent after conventional work-up • However, FDG-PET had low specificity for tonsillar tumours and low sensitivity for base of tongue cancer

Study	Results
Balaker et al. (2012) Laryngoscope 122(6):1279–1282	• Systematic review of 18 studies evaluating different treatment modalities and survival outcome in patients with cancer of unknown primary • Initial clinical stage at time of diagnosis significantly influenced the survival outcome • No significant 5-year survival difference was seen between patients treated with RT or CRT alone when compared to patients who also received surgical treatment • Presence of extracapsular extension portended a worse disease-specific survival
Grau et al. (2000) Radiother Oncol 55(2):121–129	• CUP patients have clinical features and a prognosis similar to that for those with other head and neck malignancies • Radiation to the bilateral neck and the putative mucosal sites in the entire pharyngeal axis and larynx resulted in significantly less locoregional failures compared with patients treated with ipsilateral techniques, but no survival benefit • Nodal stage is an important parameter for neck control along with haemoglobin level, gender and overall treatment time
EORTC-24001	• Phase III randomized, open-label, multicentre study • Patients were stratified according to disease stage (N1–2a vs N2b–3), radiation technique (2D vs 3D conformal vs IMRT), and randomized to undergo selective irradiation of the ipsilateral level of the neck once daily on 5 days a week for 6 weeks, or extensive irradiation of the neck (nasopharyngeal, oropharyngeal, hypopharyngeal and laryngeal mucosa, and ipsilateral neck node areas on both sides of the neck) once daily on 5 days a week for 6 weeks • Trial was completed in July 2014 (600 patients were accrued) • Results are yet available
Nieder et al. (2001) Int J Radiat Oncol Biol Phys 50:727–733	• Meta-analysis of published literature before 2000 • CT or MRI with pan-endoscopy with or without blind biopsies remains the standard work-up of patients presenting with cervical nodal metastasis with no detectable primary tumour on physical examination • In selected patients, especially those with pN1 with no extracapsular extension, surgery alone was sufficient and adjuvant therapy could be avoided • Actuarial risk of emergence of primary after comprehensive RT was <10% at 2 years, <15% at 5 years and up to 20% at 10 years • Some single-institution studies suggested that unilateral irradiation of cervical nodes is not associated with reduced disease-free or overall survival rates or higher mucosal primary emergence rates

Recommended reading

Davis KS, Byrd JK, Mehta V et al. (2014) Occult primary head and neck squamous cell carcinoma: utility of discovering primary lesions. Otolaryngol Head Neck Surg 151(2):272–278.

Gani C, Weinmann M, Bamberg M et al. (2013) Cervical squamous cell lymph node metastases from an unknown primary site: survival and patterns of recurrence after radiotherapy. Clinical Med Insights Oncol 7:173–180.

Golfinopoulos V, Pentheroudakis G, Salanti G, Nearchou AD, Ioannidis JPA, Pavlidis N (2009) Comparative survival with diverse chemotherapy regimens for cancer of unknown primary site: Multiple-treatments meta-analysis. Cancer Treat Rev 35:570–573.

Keller LM, Galloway TJ, Holdbrook T et al. (2014) P16 status, pathologic and clinical characteristics, biomolecular signature, and long-term outcomes in head and neck squamous cell carcinomas of unknown primary: HPV-associated SCC of unknown primary. Head Neck 36(12):1677–1684.

Lee J, Hahn S, Kim D-W et al. (2013) Evaluation of survival benefits by platinums and taxanes for an unfavourable subset of carcinoma of unknown primary: a systematic review and meta analysis. Br J Cancer 108:39–48.

Nieder C, Gregoire V, Ang KK (2001) Cervical lymph node metastases from occult squamous cell carcinoma: cut down a tree to get an apple? Int J Radiat Oncol Biol Phys 50:727–733.

Reddy SP, Marks JE (1997) Metastatic carcinoma in the cervical lymph nodes from an unknown primary site: results of bilateral neck plus mucosal irradiation vs. ipsilateral neck irradiation. Int J Radiat Oncol Biol Phys 37:797–802.

Sivars L, Näsman A, Tertipis N et al. (2014) Human papillomavirus and p53 expression in cancer of unknown primary in the head and neck region in relation to clinical outcome. Cancer Med 3:376–384.

Strojan P, Ferlito A, Langendijk JA et al. (2013) Contemporary management of lymph node metastases from an unknown primary to the neck: II. a review of therapeutic options. Head Neck 35:286–293.

Strojan P, Ferlito A, Medina JE (2013) Contemporary management of lymph node metastases from an unknown primary to the neck: I. A review of diagnostic approaches. Head Neck 35:123–132.

Troussier I, Barry B, Baglin AC et al. (2013) Target volumes in cervical lymphadenopathies of unknown primary: Toward a customized selective approach? On Behalf Of REFCOR. *Cancer/Radiothérapie* 17:686–694.

Weir L, Keane T, Cummings B et al. (1995) Radiation treatment of cervical lymph node metastases from an unknown primary: an analysis of outcome by treatment volume and other prognostic factors. *Radiother Oncol* 35:206–211.

Yasui T, Morii F, Yamamoto Y et al. (2014) Human papillomavirus and cystic node metastasis in oropharyngeal cancer and cancer of unknown primary origin. *PLoS ONE* 9, e95364.

47 Pituitary

Sherise D. Ferguson and Ian E. McCutcheon

Department of Neurosurgery, University of Texas M. D. Anderson Cancer Center, Houston, TX, USA

Summary	Key facts

Introduction	• Most are benign adenomas
	• Typically arise from the anterior lobe of the pituitary gland
	• Radiographically classified by size (≥1 cm)
	• Can be non-functional or functional (secreting):
	  ▪ Secreted hormones: adrenocorticotropic hormone (ACTH), growth hormone (GH), prolactin (PRL), thyroid-stimulating hormone (TSH) and luteinizing/follicle-stimulating hormone (LH/FSH)
	  ▪ Non-functional tumours include those producing LH and/or FSH, and null cell adenomas which make no hormones at all
	  ▪ Prolactinomas are the most common functional adenomas
	• Pituitary carcinomas are extremely rare and have a very poor prognosis

Presentation	• Visual changes from mass effect on optic apparatus
	• Headache
	• Endocrine disturbances
	• Apoplexy (rare)
	• May present as an incidental finding
	• Initial evaluation of pituitary lesions should include:
	  ▪ Magnetic resonance imaging (MRI) of sella with and without contrast (dynamic contrast MR is important for microadenomas)
	  ▪ Endocrinological evaluation
	  ▪ Ophthalmology evaluation (visual field testing)

Scenario	• Surgery is the initial treatment of choice for all pituitary tumours *except* prolactinomas • Surgery may require an endonasal trans-sphenoidal or transcranial approach depending on tumour characteristics • Medical therapy is tried for cases of refractory or recurrent disease in secretory tumours • Radiotherapy is third-line treatment
Trials	• Limited phase III clinical trials available

Introduction

Pituitary tumours are relatively common among the general population. They comprise 10–15% of all intracranial tumours and typically arise from the anterior portion of the gland (adenohypophysis). Pituitary adenomas can be categorized as functional (secreting an excess of hormones) or non-functional (secreting no hormones at all [null cell adenoma] or one or both gonadotropins [clinically non-functional adenoma]). These tumours manifest with neurological symptoms from local mass effect, such as visual disturbances, headaches and cranial nerve palsies, or with a variety of clinical symptoms based on the hormone(s) that they secrete. Surgery is typically the first line of treatment, except for prolactin-secreting tumours which usually respond to medical therapies.

UICC Manual of Clinical Oncology, Ninth Edition. Edited by Brian O'Sullivan, James D. Brierley, Anil K. D'Cruz, Martin F. Fey, Raphael Pollock, Jan B. Vermorken and Shao Hui Huang. © 2015 UICC. Published 2015 by John Wiley & Sons, Ltd.

Incidence, aetiology and screening

Incidence, aetiology and screening	Description
Incidence	- Constitute 10–15% of intracranial tumours - Population incidence: 74–94 per 100,000 - Estimated prevalence: ~22.5% in imaging studies (range 1–40%) and ~14.4% in postmortem studies (range 1–35%) - Overall prevalence of 16.7% - More common in adults: - 2% of adenomas are in children

Aetiology	- 95% of adenomas are sporadic
	- 5% associated with an inherited genetic syndrome:
	   - Multiple endocrine neoplasia (MEN) 1:
	      - Most commonly recognized genetic cause of pituitary tumours (3% of cases)
	      - Autosomal dominant inheritance
	      - Inactivating mutation in tumour suppressor gene *MEN 1*
	      - Characterized by parathyroid, enteropancreatic endocrine and pituitary tumours
	      - Pituitary adenomas occur in 20–30% of patients
	      - Most common associated adenoma is prolactinoma (60% of associated cases)
	      - GH-secreting adenomas ~10%; non-functional adenomas ~15%; ACTH-secreting adenomas ~5%
	      - 85% are macroadenomas at presentation
	      - MEN 1 pituitary tumours are more aggressive than their sporadic counterparts
	   - Familial isolated pituitary adenoma (FIPA):
	      - Autosomal dominant inheritance
	      - Mutations in the aryl hydrocarbon receptor-interacting protein (*AIP*) gene
	      - Account for 2% of pituitary tumours
	      - Prolactinomas and GH-secreting adenomas are the most common
	   - Carney complex:
	      - Autosomal dominant inheritance
	      - Characterized by endocrine hyperactivity, atrial myxomas, skin pigmentation, schwannomas and pituitary tumours (in 10%).
	      - Most common are GH-secreting adenomas
	   - McCune–Albright syndrome
	   - MEN 4

Screening	- Limited usefulness for pituitary tumours - Recommended for members of families with a known genetic syndrome predisposing to pituitary tumourigenesis

Pathology and natural history

Pathology and natural history	Description

GH-secreting tumours (acromegaly)	- Annual incidence is 3–4 per million
	- Prevalence is 40–70 cases per million
	- 9–13% of secreting tumours
	- GH elevation is caused by a pituitary tumour >98% of the time
	- 70% are macroadenomas at diagnosis
	- Neoplastic cells are similar to non-neoplastic somatotroph cells
	- Densely granulated and sparsely granulated are pathological variants:
	   - *Densely granulated* variant is classically described as acidophil adenoma composed of well-differentiated somatotrophs:
	      - Slower growth rates, lower rate of recurrence and overall better prognosis
	   - *Sparsely granulated* tumours consist of less differentiated cells:
	      - Prevalent in younger patients and grow more rapidly
	- ~40% of GH-secreting adenomas co-secrete other pituitary hormones, especially prolactin and thyrotropin

Pathology and natural history	Description

Prolactin-secreting tumours (prolactinomas)	- Estimated prevalence ranges from 6–10 per 100,000 to ~50 per 100,000
	- Most common secreting adenoma (51–66% of functional tumours)
	- 30% of all adenomas
	- Arise from neoplastic transformation of pituitary lactotrophs:
	  - Dot-like paranuclear prolactin immunoreactivity, referred to as the 'Golgi pattern', is a diagnostic feature of prolactinomas
	- Hyperprolactinaemia disrupts normal reproductive function by impeding:
	  - Pulsatile gonadotropin secretion
	  - Hypothalamic sex steroid feedback
	  - Gonadal steroidogenesis
	- Some tumours secrete both GH and prolactin

ACTH-secreting tumours (Cushing disease)	- 2–6% of secreting tumours
	- 50% of patients have a tumour of <5 mm in diameter
	- 10% of tumours become large enough to produce mass effect
	- Classic basophilic adenoma:
	  - Adenomas are derived from anterior pituitary corticotrophs
	  - Neoplastic corticotroph hypersecretion of ACTH leads to excessive production of cortisol from the adrenal cortex
	  - As tumour cells are resistant to negative feedback from resultant hypercortisolism, they continue to produce excessive ACTH
	
	Cushing syndrome
	- Hyperadrenalism (any cause)
	- Most common cause is iatrogenic (exogenous steroids)
	
	Cushing disease
	- ACTH-secreting adenomas:
	  - Most common cause of endogenous hypercortisolism
	- Comprise 80% of all cases of Cushing syndrome
	- Mortality rate is four times that of the general population

Thyrotroph (TSH)-secreting tumours	- Rare: 0.5–1% of pituitary tumours
	- Chromophobic adenoma cells:
	  - Periodic acid-Schiff (PAS) stain reveals positive cytoplasmic granules corresponding to lysosomes
	  - Immunostaining is positive for α- and β-TSH subunits
	- Thyrotroph adenomas secrete excess TSH
	- Cause secondary (central) hyperthyroidism
	- Many are aggressive and invasive, with a higher likelihood of recurrence after surgery

True LH/FSH-secreting tumours	- 1% of all pituitary tumours - Adenoma is composed of gonadotroph cells producing FSH and/or LH
Nonsecreting adenomas (Null-cell or inefficient gonadotropin secreting)	- 40% of pituitary tumours

Pituitary carcinomas	- Very rare: 0.2% of pituitary tumours
	- ~200 cases reported in the USA and ~4616 cases globally
	- Patients typically have pre-existing pituitary adenoma that transforms to malignant tumour over time
	- Increased number of mitotic figures, increased microvascular density, increased MIB-1 (Ki-67) and mutant p53 staining
	- Majority are functional (88%)
	- 42% prolactin-secreting and 33% ACTH-secreting
	- Hallmark is distant metastasis (without metastasis even locally aggressive pituitary tumours are *not* deemed carcinomas):
	  - Reported to metastasize to the cerebral cortex, cerebellum, spinal cord, leptomeninges, cervical lymph nodes, liver, ovaries and bone
	- Associated with poor prognosis:
	  - Patients with systemic metastases have a median survival of 12 months
	  - Patients with metastases confined to the central nervous system (CNS) have a median survival of ~2.6 years

Presentation

- *Endocrine disturbance:*
  - Hormone over-secretion: ~65% of adenomas secrete an active hormone
  - Under-production of pituitary hormones: caused by compression of the normal pituitary by large mass
  - GH–insulin-like growth factor (IGF)-1 axis is most sensitive to compression, followed by the pituitary–gonadal axis causing low levels of serum testosterone (in men)
- *Mass effect:*
  - More common with non-secreting tumours because of delayed detection:
    - Among functional tumours, prolactinomas are most likely to cause mass effect
    - ACTH-secreting tumours are least likely to cause mass effect
  - Optic chiasm compression: bitemporal upper quadrantanopia or hemianopia
  - Third ventricle compression: obstructive hydrocephalus and increased intracranial pressure
  - Cavernous sinus compression (including rare occlusion of cavernous sinus): cranial nerve palsies (III, IV, V and VI), ophthalmoplegia, facial numbness and proptosis
- *Stalk effect:*
  - Prolactin rises when intrasellar pressure increases (e.g. from tumour) and this distorts the gland/stalk and impedes flow of tonic inhibitory dopamine from the hypothalamus to the pituitary
  - As dopamine inhibits prolactin release by lactotrophs, reduction of dopamine flow to the gland causes serum prolactin to rise ('stalk effect'):
    - Serum prolactin level with prolactinoma: >75 ng/mL
    - Serum prolactin level with non-prolactinoma sufficiently large to cause 'stalk effect': ≤100 ng/ml
- *Apoplexy:*
  - Uncommon presentation
  - Urgent condition due to intratumoural infarction, necrosis or haemorrhage
  - Causes rapid swelling/expansion of the pituitary tumour and thus compression of surrounding neural structures
  - Presents with sudden onset of symptoms including: headaches, visual changes, altered mental status and pituitary insufficiency (from acute pituitary or hypothalamic injury)
  - Hypothalamic involvement may produce hypotension, diabetes insipidus, cardiac or respiratory disturbances
  - Lateral extension can lead to cranial nerve palsies
  - All types of pituitary tumour are at similar risk for developing apoplexy, with the exception of Cushing disease where it is rarely seen
  - 50% of apoplexy cases occur in patients *without* a previous diagnosis of a pituitary tumour
  - Occurs more commonly in men than in women
  - Reported predisposing factors: head trauma, bromocriptine therapy, anticoagulation, pregnancy, recent surgery, radiation therapy and hypertension
- Incidental: most common with microadenomas
- Headaches
- Cerebrospinal fluid (CSF) rhinorrhoea: rare presentation of invasive tumours

Presentation	Description

GH-secreting tumours	• No gender predilection
	• Elevated GH is clinically associated with gigantism or acromegaly depending on patient's age
	
	Acromegaly
	• Characterized by progressive enlargement of skeletal bones, soft tissue, connective tissue and viscera:
	  ▪ GH-induced swelling of soft tissue is due to increased deposition of glycosaminoglycan in the dermis and GH-induced sodium and water retention
	  ▪ Disproportionate enlargement of the distal skeleton, particularly hands and feet (increased ring and shoe size)
	  ▪ Overgrowth of skull, facial bones and cartilage produce characteristic features:
	    ○ Increased prominence of nose, ears, lips and nasolabial folds
	    ○ Deep furrows in scalp and forehead
	    ○ Jaw protrusion (prognathism) from mandible growth
	    ○ Frontal bossing due to frontal sinus enlargement
	• Complications:
	  ▪ Airway obstruction: tongue, pharyngeal and upper airway soft tissue growth
	  ▪ Peripheral neuropathies: e.g. carpal tunnel syndrome due to median nerve compression by soft tissue
	  ▪ Hyperglycaemia/diabetes mellitus (25%):
	    ○ GH increases hepatic glucose output and decreases peripheral glucose use
	  ▪ Hypertension (30%) and cardiac hypertrophy:
	    ○ GH has action at renal level promoting retention and subsequent volume expansion
	  ▪ Sleep apnoea (50%)

Presentation	Description
	■ Colonic polyps and colon cancer (twice the risk of the general population): 　○ Colonoscopy and echocardiography should be performed at time of diagnosis 　○ Cardiovascular disease is the most common cause of death 　○ Thyroid and colon cancers are the most common cancers associated with acromegaly 　○ Overall: patients have two- to three-fold the expected mortality rate **Gigantism (rare)** • Usually presents in adolescence. • Elevated GH in children before closure of epiphyseal plates in long bones
Prolactin-secreting tumours (prolactinomas)	• Highest frequency in women aged 20–50 years, at which point the ratio between the sexes is estimated to be 10:1 • Most common pituitary adenoma in children and adolescents: 　■ 50% of paediatric pituitary tumours are prolactinomas • Presentation varies with gender 　■ Men: impotence and decreased libido 　■ Women: secondary amenorrhea (25%) and galactorrhoea (50–80%): 　　○ Primary amenorrhea in approximately 5% of cases 　■ Both sexes: infertility and bone loss 　■ 90% of tumours in women are microadenomas versus 60% in men 　■ Women are usually diagnosed earlier due to more pronounced symptomatology and hence present with smaller tumours
Prolactin-secreting tumours (prolactinomas)	■ Kind tumor more common in women • Rare in children • Can become large and locally invasive: 　■ Giant macroprolactinomas have a predilection for young adults • Symptoms of hypercortisolism are broad and systemic: 　■ Weight gain (most common symptom): 　　○ Excess cortisol is related to changes in adipocyte function 　　○ 50% generalized 　　○ 50% centripetal fat deposition (truncal pattern, sparing extremities) 　　○ 'Moon faces': widened faces due to fat deposition in the preauricular area, temporal fossa, cheeks 　　○ Increased supraclavicular and dorsocervical fat pads ('buffalo hump') 　■ Bone loss (osteopenia/osteoporosis) 　　○ Glucocorticoids inhibit intestinal calcium absorption, increase resorption of osteoclasts and impair osteoblast function 　■ Muscle atrophy: 　　○ Cortisol promotes catabolism of muscle and inhibits muscle protein synthesis 　■ Skin changes: 　　○ Glucocorticoids can cause atrophy of the epidermis 　　○ Easy bruising 　　○ Poor wound healing 　　○ Purple striae (flank, breasts and abdomen) 　■ Hypertension: 　　○ Elevated cortisol can lead to increased plasma and extracellular volume via stimulation of the renin–angiotensin system 　■ Amenorrhoea and decreased libido: 　　○ Due to inhibition of gonadotropin-releasing hormone resulting in hypogonadism 　■ Excessive hair growth in women 　■ Hyperglycaemia and hypokalaemic acidosis 　■ Psychiatric symptoms, i.e. anxiety, emotional liability
Thyrotroph (TSH)-secreting tumours	• Female predilection • Symptoms: goitre, weight loss, anxiety, heat intolerance, hypoglycaemia, tremors, palpitations
True LH/FSH-secreting tumours	• Usually do not produce a clinical syndrome (inefficient hormone secretion)

(continued)

Presentation	Description
Non-secreting adenomas (Null-cell or inefficient gonadotropin secreting)	• Often present with compression effects of tumour • Can be found incidentally
Pituitary carcinomas	• Can present at any age, but usually in the third to fifth decade of life • No sex predominance has been reported

Diagnostic work-up

Diagnostic work-up	Description

Imaging (Figs. 47.1, 47.2, 47.3 and 47.4)	• CT scan may be useful initially for revealing haemorrhage
	• MRI with and without contrast:
	  ▪ Thin (≤3 mm) slices through pituitary are preferred
	  ▪ Dynamic post-contrast MR is useful for detecting small differentially enhancing microadenomas
	  ▪ Used to evaluate gland and assess parasellar and suprasellar extension:
	    ○ Microadenoma: <1 cm and confined to gland
	    ○ Macroadenoma: >1 cm and can extend outside of sella
	    ○ 50% of tumours are <5 mm at time of diagnosis (many are found incidentally)
	    ○ Hypointense lesion when compared to normal gland on post-contrast T1 images

Other	• Endocrine panel:
	  ▪ Routine screening: prolactin, TSH, L-thyroxine, LH, FSH
	  ▪ IGF-1 (surrogate for GH):
	    ○ GH levels are less useful because GH is secreted in a pulsatile fashion during the day, while IGF-1 is released continuously
	  ▪ Cortisol, ACTH (typically collected at 8 AM)
	• Ophthalmological evaluation

Tumour markers	• Adenomas with >3% Ki-67 labelling index may display aggressive behaviour

Diagnostic considerations

Prolactin-secreting tumours

A serum prolactin level of >100 ng/mL suggests a prolactinoma (prolactin levels correlate inexactly with tumour size). Microprolactinomas can cause lower levels of prolactin, and some hormonally inefficient ('silent') tumours provoke levels only slightly above normal. One should note that the differential diagnosis of hyperprolactinaemia is broad and includes: pregnancy, postpartum state, psychiatric drugs (phenothiazines and especially, risperdal), birth control pills, antidepressants (SSRIs) and primary hyperthyroidism.

Intermediate or mildly elevated prolactin levels (25–99 ng/mL) may be caused by the *stalk effect*. This is the result of compression of the pituitary stalk by the mass effect of a large tumour.

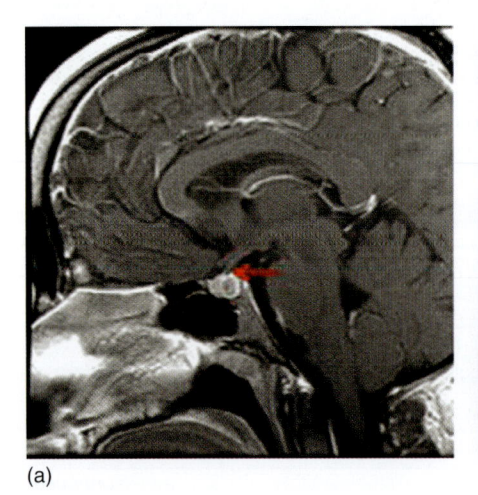

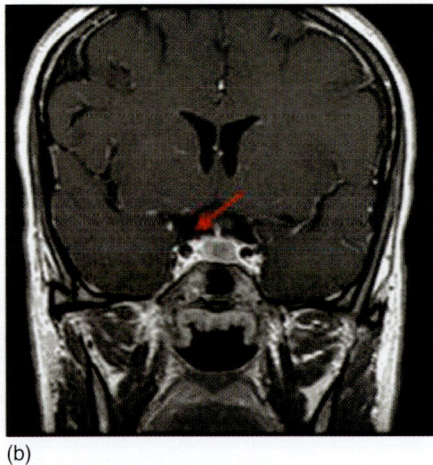

Figure 47.1 MRI of brain (post-contrast, (a) sagittal and (b) coronal sections) showing a microadenoma occupying the left side of the gland.

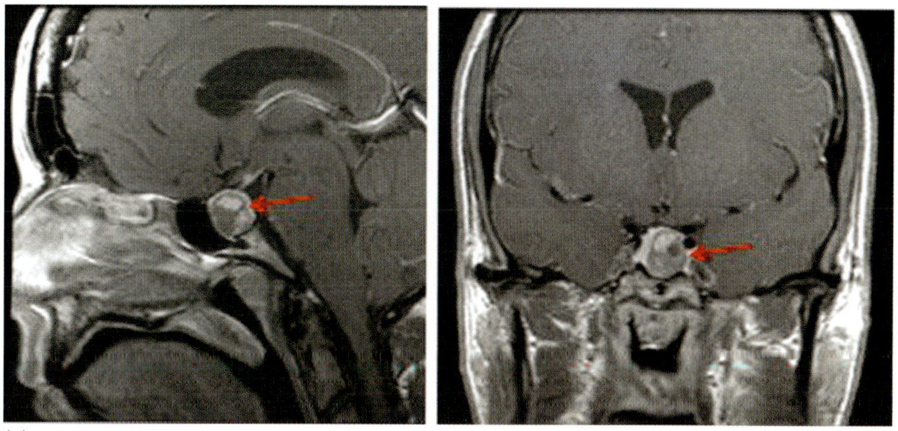

Figure 47.2 MRI of the brain (post-contrast, (a) sagittal and (b) coronal sections) showing a macroadenoma occupying the left side of the gland. This tumour has ballooned the sellar floor, and extends into the suprasellar cistern without compressing the optic apparatus.

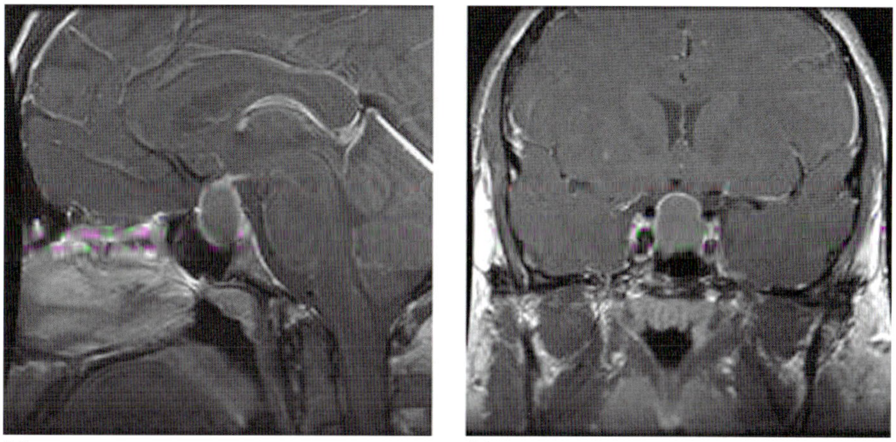

Figure 47.3 MRI of brain (post-contrast, (a) sagittal and (b) coronal sections) showing a macroadenoma with suprasellar extension. The tumour is hypointense and the thin hyperintense rim represents the severely compressed pituitary gland. Here the suprasellar extension does compress the optic nerves and chiasm.

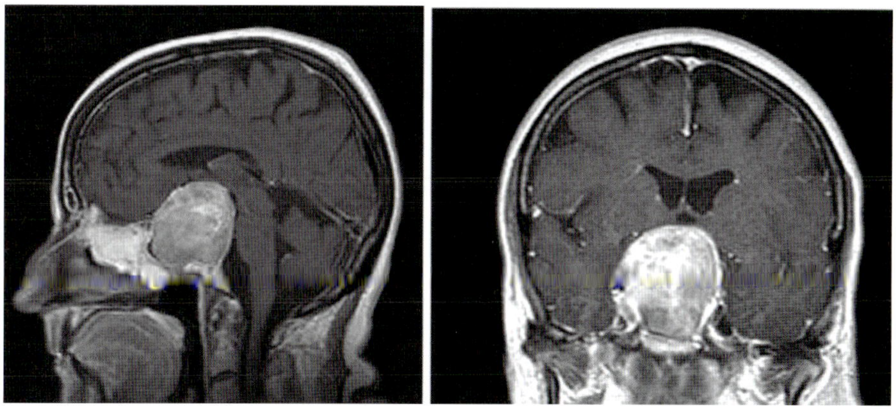

Figure 47.4 MRI of brain (post-contrast, (a) sagittal and (b) coronal sections) showing a very large (i.e. 'giant') macroadenoma with suprasellar extension, invasion of the sphenoid sinus, intrusion into the third ventricle and involvement of both cavernous sinuses. The thin hyperintense stripe on the left edge of the tumour represents the compressed normal gland. This patient has severe visual field deficits and pan-hypopituitarism.

Compression compromises the flow of dopamine through the portal–hypophyseal system, which in turn interferes with dopamine's tonic inhibition of prolactin production.

An unexpectedly low prolactin level, particularly in the face of a large invasive adenoma, is called the *hook effect*. This effect occurs when extremely high levels of prolactin overwhelm the capacity of the radioimmunoassay for prolactin. The assay utilizes a detection antibody that binds to prolactin, and the complex thus formed binds to a capture antibody that immobilizes the hormone and allows detection. When high levels of prolactin are in the circulation (very large or invasive tumours), these binding sites become saturated, causing a falsely low prolactin reading. This effect can be overcome by serum dilution of the sample.

ACTH-secreting tumours

There are several steps in the diagnosis of Cushing disease (ACTH-secreting pituitary tumour) (Fig. 47.5).

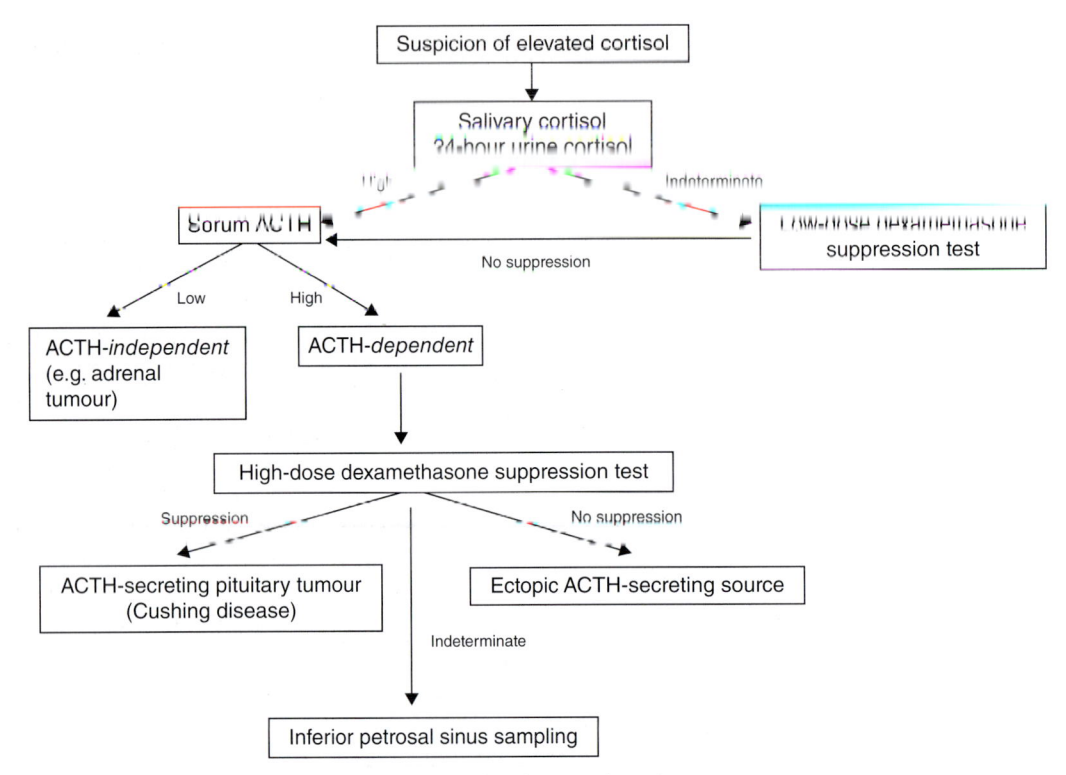

Figure 47.5 Algorithm for diagnostic work-up of hypercortisolism (Cushing syndrome).

Determination of hypercortisolism (Cushing syndrome)

The first step is confirmation of hypercortisolism. This can be accomplished with an 11 PM salivary cortisol, 8 AM serum cortisol and/or a 24-hour urine free cortisol (UFC). If these are indeterminate, one can perform an overnight low-dose dexamethasone suppression test, in which the patient is given 1 mg of dexamethasone at 11 PM and a serum cortisol is drawn the next morning at 8 AM. If cortisol remains high (i.e. is not suppressed by dexamethasone), then Cushing syndrome is probably present.

Differentiating ACTH-dependent and ACTH-independent hypercortisolism

After hypercortisolism is identified, its source has to be determined; whether hypercortisolism is ACTH-dependent (from the pituitary) or -independent (from an extrapituitary source). This can be accomplished with a serum ACTH level. ACTH levels of >20 ng/mL indicate ACTH-dependent hypercortisolism, such as occurs in patients with an ectopic ACTH-secreting tumour (e.g. small cell carcinoma of the lung, carcinoid tumour, phaeochromocytoma or medullary thyroid cancer) or ACTH-secreting pituitary adenoma (Cushing disease). An ACTH level of <5 ng/mL indicates ACTH-independent hypercortisolism (e.g. from an adrenal tumour). This should be followed up with an abdominal CT or MRI to confirm diagnosis.

Pituitary adenoma (Cushing disease) versus ectopic ACTH source

A high-dose dexamethasone test is used to indicate whether ACTH is being secreted by an ectopic source or by a secreting pituitary adenoma. Dexamethasone 8 mg is administered at 11 PM and cortisol is measured the next morning at 8 AM. High-dose dexamethasone will not suppress an ectopic ACTH source but will suppress a pituitary ACTH source. In 95% of patients with Cushing disease, cortisol levels are reduced to <50% of baseline.

If the high-dose dexamethasone test is equivocal, a corticotropin (CRH) stimulation test can be helpful. Cushing disease responds to the administration of CRH with an increase in plasma ACTH. Ectopic ACTH secreting tumours do not.

The last line for definitive diagnosis is bilateral inferior petrosal sinus sampling. The inferior petrosal sinus drains the pituitary gland and carries pituitary-produced ACTH; hence this test is a reliable way to rule out ectopic ACTH production, with a reported sensitivity of 92–96%. It is used as a last resort because it is expensive and invasive. Complications of this procedure include: thromboembolism, sixth nerve palsy, haematoma formation (3–4%) and brainstem injury (0.2%).

GH-secreting tumours

Acromegaly is diagnosed by an elevated IGF-1 level compared with the age- and sex-adjusted normal range, and a failure to suppress GH in response to an oral glucose tolerance test (OGTT). Unlike normal subjects, those with acromegaly do not suppress GH secretion to very low levels with a glucose load. A post-OGTT GH level of <1.0 mg/L is the cut-off level used for diagnosis.

Staging

Similar to other CNS lesions, no TNM (tumour, node, metastases)-based staging system exists for pituitary tumours. As stated above, these tumours are mainly classified based on size (greater or less than 1 cm) and functional status. The Hardy classification further characterizes these tumours based on extension and invasion (Table 47.1).

Treatment philosophy

The goals of treatment are:
- Suppression of excessive hormone secretion (in functional tumours)
- Removal of tumour mass effect
- Preservation of pituitary function
- Prevention of disease recurrence or progression

Table 47.1 Hardy classification of pituitary tumours

Extension	Invasion/spread
0: None	I: Sella normal or focally expanded; tumour <10 mm
A: Expanding into suprasellar cistern	II: Sella enlarged; tumour ≥10 mm
B: Anterior recesses of third ventricle obliterated	III: Localized perforation of sellar floor
C: Floor of third ventricle grossly displaced	IV: Diffuse destruction of sellar floor
D: Intracranial (intradural) extension	V: Spread via CSF or blood-borne
E: Into or beneath cavernous sinus (extradural)	

Scenario	Treatment philosophy

Primary disease	• Surgical resection is first line treatment for most pituitary tumours.
	  ▪ Obtains definitive pathological diagnosis
	  ▪ Accomplishes immediate relief of compressive symptoms
	  ▪ Trans-sphenoidal is preferred due to lower surgical morbidity (see below)
	• Medical therapy is first-line treatment of prolactinomas

Refractory or recurrent disease	• Medical therapy:
	  ▪ Second-line therapy for GH-, ACTH-, TSH- and LH/FSH-secreting tumours in cases of subtotal resection or tumour recurrence
	• Conventional radiotherapy:
	  ▪ Generally third-line treatment for surgically or medically refractory disease
	  ▪ Shown to prevent progression of both residual and recurrent disease
	  ▪ Long-term control as high as 80–94% at 10 years
	  ▪ Generally delivered in fractionated doses of 1.6–1.8 Gy 4–5 times per week over a 5–6-week period: 45–50 Gy in total
	  ▪ Most common complication is delayed hypopituitarism, occurring in up to 80%
	• Stereotactic radiosurgery (SRS):
	  ▪ Also reserved for recurrent or residual lesions
	  ▪ Little data supporting upfront use, but can be considered in elderly patients or those in poor medical condition and who are not surgical candidates
	  ▪ Hormonal remission observed in 40–50% of cases of secreting adenomas
	  ▪ Decrease or stabilization of tumour volume in 66–100%
	  ▪ Mean delay to remission for secreting tumours is 13–144 months
	  ▪ Outcome predictors: low target volume and low initial hormone levels
	  ▪ Dosage:
	    ○ 12–18 Gy for non-functional adenomas
	    ○ 15–30 Gy for functional adenomas
	  ▪ Hypopituitarism is the most common adverse event: 20–40% of cases
	  ▪ Cranial neuropathies are rare (optic nerve most common: <5% of cases)

Follow-up	• Initial MRI follow-up after surgery is 3–4 months to assess extent of resection • Because of risk of recurrence (especially in Cushing disease), follow-up MRI and hormonal testing are recommended • Patients receiving medical therapy should be assessed by MRI 3–6 months after starting treatment

Pituitary surgery: Trans-sphenoidal versus transcranial

Surgery is the primary treatment for most subtypes of pituitary tumours *except* prolactinomas. An endonasal *trans-sphenoidal approach* is recommended as the primary surgical approach because it carries a lower morbidity than transcranial surgery (open craniotomy). The complications of trans-sphenoidal surgery are relatively rare and include:
- CSF rhinorrhoea (3–5%)
- Internal carotid artery injury (rare)

- Nasal septum perforation (8%)
- Visual complications (1%)
- Infection (meningitis)
- Hormonal disturbance:
  - Most commonly diabetes insipidus resulting from damage to the pituitary stalk or posterior pituitary gland:
    - Can be permanent (3%) or transient
    - Onset is typically within 24 hours postoperatively
    - Can be treated with oral or intravenous desmopressin (DDAVP); a synthetic replacement for vasopressin.

The most common endocrinological complication is diabetes insipidus.

A *transcranial approach* is required in 1–4% of pituitary tumour cases. The indications for this approach include:
- Large tumours with parasellar extension (e.g. into the cavernous sinus or middle fossa)
- Inaccessible suprasellar extension (typically lateral)
- Fibrous tumour consistency (unfortunately this is difficult to predict preoperatively)
- Unfavourable carotid anatomy (tortuous course and/or medial deviation)
- Presence of a parasellar aneurysm
- Carotid (or other) artery encasement by tumour
- Previous failed trans-sphenoidal approach.

Intuitively, transcranial approaches carry a higher complication rate compared to trans-sphenoidal surgery, including a higher incidence of infection, postoperative haematoma formation and frontal lobe injury.

In selected patients with pituitary tumours, intraoperative imaging (usually by MRI) can enhance the degree of tumour removal. Such systems allow an MRI to be obtained during surgery without breaking the sterility of the operative field. In this way, resectable residual tumour can be detected, and ultimately, the completeness of the removal can be confirmed before the operation ends. The utility of such systems varies with the surgeon's skill and experience; more experienced pituitary surgeons are more likely to achieve complete resection without such adjunctive technology. We reserve the use of intraoperative MRI in pituitary surgery for patients with the greatest chance of having postoperative residual tumour: those with complex macroadenomas and particularly those undergoing reoperation and in whom post-surgical fibrosis can obscure tissue planes.

Radiotherapy: Conventional versus stereotactic radiosurgery

In the treatment algorithm for pituitary tumours, radiotherapy is mainly reserved for surgically or medically refractory disease, surgically inaccessible tumours and disease recurrence. Conventional radiotherapy is a predefined cumulative radiation dose divided into dose fractions. Fractionated treatment involves daily delivery of small doses of radiation. The drawbacks of conventional radiotherapy include hypopituitarism (reported in up to 80% within 5 years of irradiation), cognitive decline and development of radiation-induced tumours.

Stereotactic radiosurgery (SRS) is high-dose radiation delivered as a single fraction. The radiation source is typically radioactive isotope cobalt-60 housed in the (Gamma Knife®) machine. Patients are held in place by a stereotactic head frame which is attached to the scalp and skull with pins. Due to the high conformity and anatomical selectivity of dose delivery, this apparatus can aim multiple narrow beams of radiation to a desired intracranial target with minimal risk of damage to the surrounding brain. Treatment can be accomplished in a single outpatient session. Although this procedure also carries a risk of hypopituitarism, the cognitive disturbance associated with conventional radiotherapy can be avoided.

Treatment: Specific tumour types

GH-secreting tumours

Treatment: GH-secreting tumours	Description
Surgery	
Early disease	- Provides rapid reduction in serum GH levels - Improves efficiency of subsequent medical therapy - Microadenoma resection: normalization of IGF-1 in 75–95% of cases - Macroadenoma resection: normalization of IGF-1 in 40–68% of cases - Visual field defects improve in 70% of patients; do not change in 25–30% and rarely worsen (<2%) - Predictors of surgical outcome: tumour size, extrasellar growth, dural invasion and preoperative GH level - Long-term recurrence rate is 3–10% - 40–60% cannot be controlled by surgery alone (e.g. when cavernous sinus invasion is present) and will require additional treatment - Subtotal resection (surgical debulking) may improve response to medical therapy

Treatment: GH-secreting tumours	Description
Refractory or recurrent disease	• Repeat surgery has a long-term cure rate of 60% • Lower preoperative GH levels are associated with a greater chance of biochemical remission
Medical therapy	
Early disease	• Medical treatment before surgery is not contraindicated, but there is currently insufficient evidence to make conclusions regarding its effect on patient outcome

Refractory or recurrent disease	• Indicated for cases not cured by surgery or when the patient cannot medically tolerate surgery or when tumour recurs:
	  ■ Three classes of drugs available for treatment of acromegaly: somatostatin receptor ligands (SRL); dopamine (DA) agonists (D2 agonists); GH receptor antagonists
	  ■ Somatostatin analogues (octreotide):
	    ○ Bind to somatostatin receptors and subsequently reduce pituitary GH secretion, decrease plasma IGF-1 levels and suppresses tumour cell proliferation
	    ○ Can be used as initial therapy or if no response to DA agonists
	    ○ Decreases tumour volume in 30% of patients
	    ○ ~70% of patients show a decrease in GH levels; IGF-1 is decreased in 93%
	    ○ ~66% of patients normalize IGF-1 level and 50–66% normalize GH level
	    ○ Octreotide dosage: start at 50–100 μg SQ every 8 hours
	    ○ Average dose required 100–200 μg every 8 hours
	    ○ Side-effects:
	      – Generally well tolerated
	      – Nausea (most common), diarrhoea and abdominal pain
	      – Biliary tract abnormalities such as biliary sludge and cholelithiasis can occur
	  ■ Dopamine agonists (bromocriptine, cabergoline, pergolide)
	    ○ Bromocriptine: decreases GH in 54% of cases
	    ○ Tumour volume is decreased in <20% of cases
	    ○ Can be used alone or as an adjunct to somatostatin analogue therapy
	    ○ Most effective in patients with tumours that co-secrete prolactin or TSH
	    ○ Bromocriptine dosage: 10–15 mg/day
	    ○ Side effects: nausea, headaches, fatigue, depression, hypotension
	  ■ GH antagonists (i.e. pegvisomant):
	    ○ Considered for failure of above treatments
	    ○ Competes with GH for binding, thus prevents hepatic receptor signalling and decreases IGF-1 production
	    ○ Treatment normalizes IGF-1 in 97% of patients
	    ○ No reduction in tumour volume has been reported
	    ○ Pegvisomant dosage: 5–40 mg/day SQ
	    ○ Side effects: carries risk of liver function abnormalities in 25% of cases

Conventional radiation	
Early disease	• No role
Refractory or recurrent disease	• Third-line treatment • Lowers GH levels and normalizes IGF-1 in 60% of patients • Patients with lower GH levels tend to have a better response • Optimal dose range 45–50.4 Gy in 1.8-Gy daily fractions • Maximal response achieved 10–15 years after treatment • Hypopituitarism in 50% of patients; risk of visual defects in 5%
Stereotactic radiosurgery	
Early disease	• Limited data on upfront SRS
Refractory or recurrent disease	• Remission rates of 42–60% at follow-up • Time to remission ranges from 3 to 10 years • 2% risk of recurrence • Median margin dose: 22 Gy with range of 14–35 Gy • Hypopituitarism in 16% of cases

Prolactin-secreting tumours

Treatment: Prolactin-secreting tumours	Description
Surgery	
Early disease	• Only secreting tumour where surgery is *not* the first-line of treatment

Refractory or recurrent disease	• Indications for surgery:
	  ▪ Intolerance to side effects of dopamine agonists
	  ▪ Persistent hyperprolactinaemia, progressive tumour enlargement and/or persistent tumour mass effect despite maximal medical therapy
	  ▪ Patients who are dependent on antipsychotic medications (DA agonists can precipitate psychotic episodes)
	  ▪ Acute neurological progression (worsening of vision)
	• Outcomes correlate with tumour size and preoperative serum prolactin level
	  ▪ Microadenoma: remission rate 82% if preoperative prolactin level <200 ng/mL; 50% if level >200 ng/mL
	  ▪ Macroadenoma: remission rate ranges from 15% to 52%
	  ▪ Overall surgical remission rate: 42%
	• If surgery is not curative, tumour cytoreduction may increase response to subsequent medical therapy
	• 7–50% of surgically resected prolactinomas recur

Medical therapy	

Early disease	• First line of therapy
	• Achieves resolution of visual field defects in 67% of cases
	• Resolution of amenorrhoea in 78% of cases and return of fertility in 53%
	• Resolution of galactorrhoea in 86% of cases
	• Of the dopamine agonists (i.e. bromocriptine, cabergoline, pergolide), bromocriptine is most commonly used:
	• Bromocriptine:
	  ▪ Binds to D2 receptors on lactotrophs, inhibits prolactin synthesis and release, and induces cell necrosis
	  ▪ Reduces tumour size in 6–8 weeks in 75% of patients
	  ▪ 80–90% of patients have normalization of prolactin level in a few weeks
	  ▪ 1% of tumours continue to grow while on bromocriptine
	  ▪ Chance of normalizing serum level with bromocriptine is very low if prolactin is >500 ng/mL
	  ▪ Dosage:
	    ○ Start with 1.25 mg PO each evening (q.h.s.)
	    ○ Add 2.5 mg/day as necessary based on prolactin levels
	  ▪ Side effects: nausea, vomiting, postural hypotension, headache and dizziness; 5–10% of patients cannot tolerate side effects
	• Cabergoline (selective D2 agonist):
	  ▪ Achieves normalization of prolactin level in 86% of patients
	  ▪ Tumour size reduction in 70–90% of cases
	  ▪ Dosage: 0.25 mg PO twice weekly and increase by 0.25 mg every 4 weeks as needed to control prolactin level
	  ▪ Side effects: headache and gastrointestinal symptoms (less than with bromocriptine); 4% of patients cannot tolerate side effects
	  ▪ Contraindications: uncontrolled hypertension, eclampsia or pre-eclampsia

Refractory or recurrent disease	• Persistent hyperprolactinemia occurs in 25% of patients treated with bromocriptine and 10–15% of those treated with cabergoline:
	  ▪ Mechanism of DA agonist resistance is associated with decrease in D_2 receptor gene transcription, resulting in a decrease in the number of D_2 receptors on the cell membrane
	• Options include:
	  ▪ Switching to alternative dopamine agonist
	  ▪ Raising conventional dosage
	  ▪ Experimental therapy (temozolomide)

Conventional radiation	
Early disease	• No role

Treatment: Prolactin-secreting tumours	Description
Refractory or recurrent disease	• Reserved for medically and surgically refractory disease • Normalization with radiation alone occurs in 25–50% • Combined with medical therapy gives 80–100% remission • Dose 45–54 Gy in 1.8-Gy daily fractions • Time to response: 1–10 years
Stereotactic radiosurgery	
Early disease	• Limited data on upfront SRS
Refractory or recurrent disease	• Remission rate 26–43% after failed medical or surgical therapy • Time to remission 13–28 months • No long-term recurrence data published • Margin dose 15–49 Gy with a median of 24 Gy • Hypopituitarism in 14.8% of cases

ACTH-secreting tumours

Treatment: ACTH-secreting tumours	Description
Surgery	
Early disease	• Initial treatment of choice • Remission rate: 86–98% for microadenomas • Lower remission rates are noted in patients with macroadenomas (31–83%) or invasive adenomas (22–65%) • Recurrence rate: 3–17% • Median interval before disease recurrence ranges from 2.3 to 7.2 years after surgery and can be as late as 10 years after surgery

Refractory or recurrent disease	• Repeat trans-sphenoidal surgery:
	  ▪ Reported remission rate after repeat trans-sphenoidal surgery is ~60%
	  ▪ Odds of failure to achieve remission after repeat surgery are 3.7 times those of patients undergoing first time surgery
	• Other pituitary surgical options include:
	  ▪ Hemihypophysectomy (on side of tumour)
	  ▪ Total hypophysectomy
	• Bilateral adrenalectomy:
	  ▪ Reserved for non-resectable adenoma, failed medical therapy and life-threatening Cushing disease
	  ▪ Corrects hypercortisolism in 96–100% of cases
	  ▪ Lifelong gluco- and mineralocorticoid replacement needed
	  ▪ Up to 30% develop Nelson syndrome (triad: hyperpigmentation, elevated ACTH and progression of unresected pituitary tumour)
	    ○ Nelson syndrome may be less likely in patients with prior irradiation of the sella

Medical therapy	
Early disease	• No role

Refractory or recurrent disease	• Reserved for surgically refractory disease
	• Ketoconazole:
	  ▪ Blocks adrenal steroid synthesis by inhibiting several steroidogenic enzymes
	  ▪ Decreases cortisol levels in 70–80% of patients
	  ▪ Dosage:
	    ○ Start 200 mg PO
	    ○ Adjustment based on 24-hour urine free cortisol
	    ○ Usual maintenance dose: 400–1200 mg/day

(continued)

Treatment: ACTH-secreting tumours	Description
	<ul><li>Side effects: elevated liver enzymes, gastrointestinal discomfort and oedema:<ul><li>Hepatotoxicity in 1 per 15,000 patients</li></ul></li><li>Metyrapone:<ul><li>Inhibits 11-β-hydroxylase (involved in final steps of steroid synthesis)</li><li>Normalizes plasma cortisol level in 75% of patients</li><li>Dosage: 750–6000 mg/day divided t.i.d.</li><li>Side effects: lethargy, ataxia, primary adrenal insufficiency, hirsutism</li></ul></li><li>Mitotane:<ul><li>Inhibits several steps in glucocorticoid synthesis</li><li>Remission in approximately 83%</li><li>Unfortunately, relapse rate of 60% has been reported when drug is discontinued</li><li>Dosage:<ul><li>Start with 250–500 mg PO q.h.s.</li><li>Usual dose: 4–12 g/day t.i.d.–q.i.d.</li></ul></li><li>Side effects: anorexia, gastrointestinal problems, cognitive issues, adrenal insufficiency, hypercholesterolemia</li></ul></li></ul>
Conventional radiation	
Early disease	• No role
Refractory or recurrent disease	• Remission rate of 53–83% with conventional radiotherapy • Time to remission range: 18–42 months • Recurrence rate: 0–17% • Dose range: 40–50.5 Gy
Stereotactic surgery	
Early disease	• Limited data on upfront SRS
Refractory or recurrent disease	• Remission rate 35–83% after failed surgery (with additional medical therapy, 85–100%) • Time to remission ranges from 7.5 to 33 months • Recurrence rate: 10–20% • Time to recurrence is typically 24–40 months • Dose range: 15–35 Gy (median 24 Gy) • Hypopituitarism: 24.3%; neurological deficit 3%

TSH-secreting tumours

Treatment: TSH-secreting tumours	Description
Surgery	
Early disease	• First-line treatment: surgical cure rate 38% • Can be invasive (parasellar) and hence difficult to remove
Refractory or recurrent disease	• No outcome data on the utility of repeat surgery due to rarity
Medical therapy	
Early disease	• Hyperthyroid symptoms can be managed with beta-blockers and perhaps low-dose antithyroid medications
Refractory or recurrent disease	• Used for persistent TSH hypersecretion following resection • Octreotide useful in controlling TSH over-secretion in 80–90% of cases • Tumour shrinkage achieved in 33% of patients • Octreotide dosage (less than for acromegaly): 50–100 µg SQ every 8 hours and titrated to T_3 and T_4 levels
Conventional radiation	
Early disease	• No role

Treatment: TSH-secreting tumours	Description
Refractory or recurrent disease	• Second-line therapy in case of failed surgical resection
Stereotactic surgery	
Early disease	• Minimal role
Refractory or recurrent disease	• Limited data available due to rarity

Non-functional pituitary adenomas

Treatment: Non-functional pituitary adenomas	
Surgery	
Early disease	• Non-symptomatic tumours do not necessarily require surgery: ▪ Patients with asymptomatic microadenomas are typically observed with imaging to evaluate for further growth • Surgery indicated for patients with symptoms of mass effect • Following surgery, visual deficits improve in 60–88% of patients, with normalization in 30–50%
Refractory or recurrent disease	• Re-operation can be performed for recurrent disease to address symptoms of mass effect
Medical therapy	
Early disease	• No role
Refractory or recurrent disease	• Somatostatin analogues and dopamine agonists have been shown to be effective • No placebo-controlled long-term studies are available
Conventional radiation	
Early disease	• No role
Refractory or recurrent disease	• Reserved for aggressive tumours, significant post-surgical residual mass or tumour recurrence • Up to 100% control rate has been reported
Stereotactic surgery	
Early disease	• Limited data for use as primary treatment modality
Refractory or recurrent disease	• Achieves tumour control in 50–80% of patients • Dose range: 12–20 Gy, with a median of 16 Gy • New cranial nerve deficit reported in ~14% of cases • Hypopituitarism reported in ~ 20%

Pituitary carcinoma

Treatment: Pituitary carcinoma	Description
Surgery	
Early disease	• Gross total resection is rarely achieved due to tumour's invasive nature • Role mainly palliative and for confirmation of diagnosis
Refractory or recurrent disease	• Repeated surgeries can be performed to remove secondary metastatic lesions • Limited data on outcome for repeated surgical resection

(continued)

Treatment: Pituitary carcinoma	Description
Medical therapy	
Early disease	• Limited role

Refractory or recurrent disease	• Dopamine agonists can offer palliation in the treatment of metastatic prolactin-producing tumours
	• Pituitary carcinomas will typically often overcome dopamine agonist suppression
	• Limited success of chemotherapy trials (carmustine, hydroxyurea, 5-fluorouracil)
	• Temozolomide (most promising):
	  ▪ First used to treat a prolactin-secreting carcinoma
	  ▪ Induces a tumoural and/or hormonal response in 60% of treated cases (based on data from 15 temozolomide-treated secretory pituitary carcinomas)

Conventional radiation	
Early disease	• Can be considered for surgically inaccessible disease
Refractory or recurrent disease	• Radiation is a common adjuvant therapy used after tumour resection • Sellar and parasellar regions are initially treated by fractionated radiation therapy • Doses range: 45–55 Gy • Does not appear to change disease outcome
Metastasis	• Whole-brain radiation or SRS for intracranial metastasis

Table 47.2 Phase III clinical trials

Trial reference	Results
Lombardi G et al. (2009) J Endocrinol Invest 32(3):202–209	• Efficacy shown of the new long-acting formulation of lanreotide (Autogel) in somatostatin analogue-naïve patients with acromegaly

Phase III clinical trials

See Table 47.2.

Areas of research

- Identification of epigenetic changes contributing to tumour pathogenesis
- Characterization of specific tumour-associated growth factors
- Development of targeted therapies and cell markers that predict pituitary tumour drug responsiveness
- Extended trans-sphenoidal techniques for resection of tumour with suprasellar and parasellar extension

Recommended reading

Castinetti F, Régis J, Dufour H, Brue T (2010) Role of stereotactic radiosurgery in the management of pituitary adenomas. Nat Rev Endocrinol 6:214–223.

Colao A, Savastano S (2011) Medical treatment of prolactinomas. Nat Rev Endocrinol 7:267–278.

Ding D et al. (2014) Treatment paradigms for pituitary adenomas: defining the roles of radiosurgery and radiation therapy. J Neurooncol 117(3):445–457.

Ezzat S, Asa SL, Couldwell WT et al. (2004) The prevalence of pituitary adenomas: a systematic review. Cancer 101:613–619.

Ghostine S, Ghostine MS, Johnson WD (2004) Radiation therapy in the treatment of pituitary tumors. Neurosurg Focus 24(5):E8.

Greenberg MS (2010) Handbook of Neurosurgery. New York: Thieme Medical Publishers.

Gross BA, Mindea SA, Pick AJ, Chandler JP, Batjer HH (2007) Medical management of Cushing disease. Neurosurg Focus 23(3):E10.

Heane AP (2011) Clinical review: Pituitary carcinoma: difficult diagnosis and treatment. J Clin Endocrinol Metab 96:3649–3660

Kontogeorgos G (2005) Classification and pathology of pituitary tumors. Endocrine 28:27–35.

Kelly DF (2007) Transsphenoidal surgery for Cushing's disease: a review of success rates, remission predictors, management of failed surgery, and Nelson's Syndrome. Neurosurg Focus 23(3):E5.

McCutcheon IE (2013) Pituitary adenomas: Surgery and radiotherapy in the age of molecular diagnostics and pathology. Curr Probl Cancer 37:6–37.

Melmed S, Colao A, Barkan A et al. (2009) Acromegaly Consensus Group. Guidelines for acromegaly management: an update. J Clin Endocrinol Metab 94:1509–1517.

Melmed S, Casanueva FF, Hoffman AR et al. (2011) Diagnosis and treatment of hyperprolactinemia: an Endocrine Society clinical practice guideline; Endocrine Society. J Clin Endocrinol Metab 96:273–288.

Molitch ME (2013) Management of medically refractory prolactinoma. J Neurooncol 117(3):421–428.

Nomikos P, Buchfelder M, Fahlbusch R (2001) Current management of prolactinomas. J Neurooncol 54:139–150.

Ragel BT, Couldwell WT (2004) Pituitary carcinoma: a review of the literature. *Neurosurg Focus* 16(4):E7.

Sherlock M, Woods C, Sheppard MC *et al*. (2011) Medical therapy in acromegaly. *Nat Rev Endocrinol* 7: 291–300.

Tritos NA, Biller BM, Swearingen B (2011) Management of Cushing disease. *Nat Rev Endocrinol* 7: 279–289.

Verrees M, Arafah BM, Selman WR (2004) Pituitary tumor apoplexy: characteristics, treatment, and outcomes. *Neurosurg Focus* 16(4):E6.

Yamada S, Fukuhara N, Oyama K, Takeshita A, Takeuchi Y (2010) Repeat transsphenoidal surgery for the treatment of remaining or recurring pituitary tumors in acromegaly. *Neurosurgery* 67:949–956.

48 Thyroid

James D. Brierley[1], David P. Goldstein[2] and Monika K. Krzyzanowska[3]

[1]Department of Radiation Oncology, The Princess Margaret Cancer Centre, University of Toronto, Toronto, ON, Canada
[2]Head and Neck Surgical Oncology and Reconstructive Microsurgery, Department of Otolaryngology–Head & Neck Surgery, Department of Surgical Oncology, The Princess Margaret Cancer Centre, University of Toronto, Toronto, ON, Canada
[3]Department of Medical Oncology & Hematology, The Princess Margaret Cancer Centre, Department of Medicine, University of Toronto, Toronto, ON, Canada

Summary	Key facts
Introduction	<ul><li>Papillary and follicular (differentiated thyroid cancer [DTC]), insular and anaplastic thyroid cancers derive from the follicular cells of the thyroid</li><li>Medullary thyroid cancer (MTC) derives from C cells</li><li>Papillary thyroid cancer (PTC) incidence is rising</li></ul>
Presentation	<ul><li>For a mass in the thyroid, the usual work-up is cervical ultrasound and fine needle aspiration</li><li>CT neck and chest if symptomatic or locally advanced</li><li>More extensive investigations for anaplastic thyroid cancer and MTC</li></ul>
Scenario	<ul><li>Local disease: initial treatment is thyroidectomy (lobectomy is sufficient for early DTC)</li><li>Radioactive iodine (RAI) for intermediate-risk and metastatic DTC</li><li>Anaplastic cancer resection of microscopic residual, hyperfractionated external bean radiotherapy (RT) or chemoradiotherapy (CRT) if resected or unresected and good performance status</li><li>Limited role for chemotherapy</li></ul>
Trials	<ul><li>Paucity of phase III trials in thyroid cancer</li></ul>

Introduction

Cancers of the thyroid can derive from thyroid follicular cells (papillary, follicular, insular and anaplastic thyroid cancers), or from C cells (medullary thyroid cancers [MTC]). Papillary and follicular cancers are often grouped together as well-differentiated thyroid cancer (DTC) in distinction from insular and anaplastic cancers which are poorly differentiated. Rarely, tumours can arise from interstitial cells of the thyroid, such as lymphoma (see Chapter 32) and sarcomas. Very rarely tumours from other organs may metastasize to the thyroid.

Incidence, aetiology and screening

Incidence, aetiology and screening	Description
Incidence	<ul><li>DTC is increasing across the world:<ul><li>Age standardized ratio (ASR) per 100,000 for women 4.7 and for men 1.5</li></ul></li><li>Death ASR per 100,000 for women 0.6 and for men 0.3</li><li>In North America PTC accounts for 3% of all cancers in women and 1% in men, but <0.3% of all deaths</li><li>Geographical variation: high in Hawaii and low in Poland</li><li>Medullary cancer 5–10% of all thyroid cancers</li></ul>

UICC Manual of Clinical Oncology, Ninth Edition. Edited by Brian O'Sullivan, James D. Brierley, Anil K. D'Cruz, Martin F. Fey, Raphael Pollock, Jan B. Vermorken and Shao Hui Huang. © 2015 UICC. Published 2015 by John Wiley & Sons, Ltd.

Incidence, aetiology and screening	Description

Aetiology	- DTC family history:
	  - Rare
	  - Cowden and Gardener syndrome
	- Radiation:
	  - Therapeutic, especially in childhood
	  - Accidental, e.g. Chernobyl
	- MTC:
	  - 20–25% familial or associated with multiple endocrine neoplasia (MEN 2A and 2B)

Screening	- Limited use in DTC:
	  - If significant family history, a thyroid ultrasound scan may be performed but there is no consensus on this
	- MTC:
	  - *RET* oncogene (see below):
	    - 90% of patients with the *RET* oncogene develop cancer
	  - Prophylactic thyroidectomy prevents development:
	    - Age at which this should be performed varies depending on the mutation, but for MEN 2B it should be performed in the first year of life

Data source: GLOBOCAN (2008).

Pathology and natural history

Pathology and natural history	Description

Papillary	- Most common type (80% of all thyroid cancers)
	- Female-to-male ratio: 3:1
	- Median age at presentation 45–50 years
	- Characteristic nuclear features include enlargement, crowding, overlap and a hyperchromatic with either finely dispersed chromatin (ground glass) or a clear (orphan Annie) appearance
	- Most common histological variant is follicular variant of PTC
	- Unfavourable histology: tall cell, hobnail cell, columnar cell change in a significant part of the tumour (>30%), solid growth (>30%), widely invasive growth, angioinvasive growth, any dedifferentiation and intrathyroidal psammomatous dissemination
	- *RET/PTC* gene rearrangements in 20–50%
	- Microscopic lymph node involvement is frequent (50–70%), especially to the central nodes (parathyroid or paratracheal)
	- Distant spread is rare (lung commonest, then bone)
	- Excellent prognosis especially in the young:
	  - Older patient has poorer prognosis and tumour is less likely to be iodine avid
	  - 5-year survival:
	    - Confined to the thyroid: 99%
	    - Regional nodal involvement: 96%
	    - Distant metastases: 60%

Follicular	- Can be difficult to differentiate from benign adenoma - Identification of malignancy is dependent on invasion into surrounding normal thyroid tissue (i.e. capsular invasion) or blood vessels - *RAS* mutations in 40–50% - Lymph node involvement is infrequent (10–15%) - Significant risk of distant spread - Intermediate prognosis, especially for poorly differentiated tumours

Hürthle cell	- Hürthle cells can be found in benign thyroid conditions (i.e. lymphocytic thyroiditis or follicular adenoma) or in papillary or follicular carcinoma
	- Pure Hürthle cell carcinoma is a follicular carcinoma:
	  - Typically not iodine avid
	  - Poorer outcome

(continued)

Pathology and natural history	Description
Insular	- Poorly differentiated carcinomas of follicular cell origin - Part of a continuum from differentiated to anaplastic thyroid cancer - Aggressive, locoregional and distant spread - Not iodine avid - Poor prognosis

Anaplastic	- Older patients; median age 65 years
	- Female-to-male ratio: 3:2
	- High mitotic rate, areas of necrosis, can be small round cells
	- Immunohistochemistry is essential for differentiation from non-Hodgkin lymphoma.
	- Mutations of the *p53* tumour suppressor gene is common
	- 20% co-exist with well-differentiated tumour
	- Extrathyroid extension in up to 90% of cases
	- Metastases at presentation in 30–50%:
	   - Lung is the commonest site but can be to any part of the body
	- Cure is usually only possible if incidentally found after surgery for differentiated thyroid cancer
	- Survival:
	   - Median 3–5 months
	   - 1 year <20%

Medullary	- Derived from C cells
	- Amyloid deposits are found in the majority
	- Lymph node metastasis is frequent (50–60% at presentation)
	- Distant metastases (liver, lung, bone) in 25% at presentation
	- Survival:
	   - Localized 10-year survival 90–95%
	   - Regional 60–65%
	   - Distant 40%
	- Hereditary cases (20–25%):
	   - Have germline *RET* oncogene mutation
	   - Have C cell hyperplasia in the same thyroid gland:
	      - Familial MTC
	      - MEN 2A syndrome (phaeochromocytoma and hyperparathyroidism)
	      - MEN 2B syndrome (phaeochromocytoma, mucosal and/or gastrointestinal ganglioneuromas, marfanoid body habitus)
	   - Prognosis varies depending on type of mutation

Presentation

- Usually as an asymptomatic mass in the thyroid
- If locally advanced:
  - Pain
  - Hoarseness (recurrent laryngeal involvement)
  - Oesophageal or tracheal obstruction
- Palpable lateral cervical node(s)
- If rapidly expanding, suspect anaplastic thyroid cancer or lymphoma
- Rarely presents as metastases to bone or lung, and biopsy of metastases diagnoses thyroid primary

Diagnostic work-up

Diagnostic work-up	Description

Work-up	- Initial work-up of the thyroid mass (Figs. 48.1 and 48.2):
	   - Ultrasound and fine needle aspiration cytology
	- If clinical presentation suggesting locally-advanced disease or nodal metastases (e.g. vocal cord paralysis, airway involvement):
	   - Computed tomography (CT) head and neck
	- If anaplastic or medullary carcinoma, also image chest and abdomen to assess for distant metastases:
	   - CT, liver ultrasound, bone scan, positron emission tomography (PET) (if available for anaplastic carcinoma)

(continued)

Diagnostic work-up	Description

Tumour markers	• *Differentiated thyroid cancer:*
	  ▪ Thyroglobulin:
	     ○ No role in diagnosis
	     ○ Value only after thyroidectomy for follow-up
	• *Anaplastic thyroid cancer:*
	  ▪ None
	• *Medullary thyroid cancer:*
	  ▪ Calcitonin (may fall if tumour is dedifferentiated)
	  ▪ Carcinoembryonic antigen (CEA)

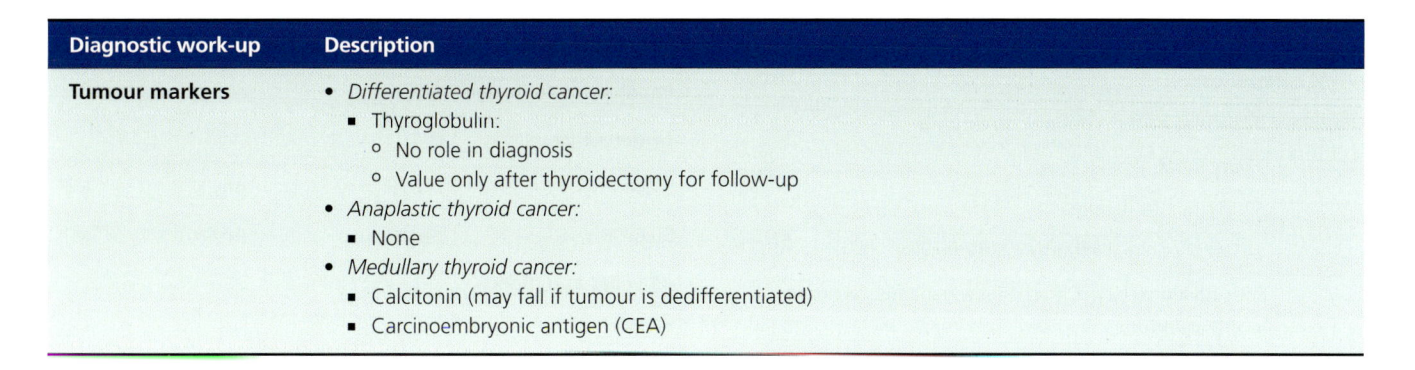

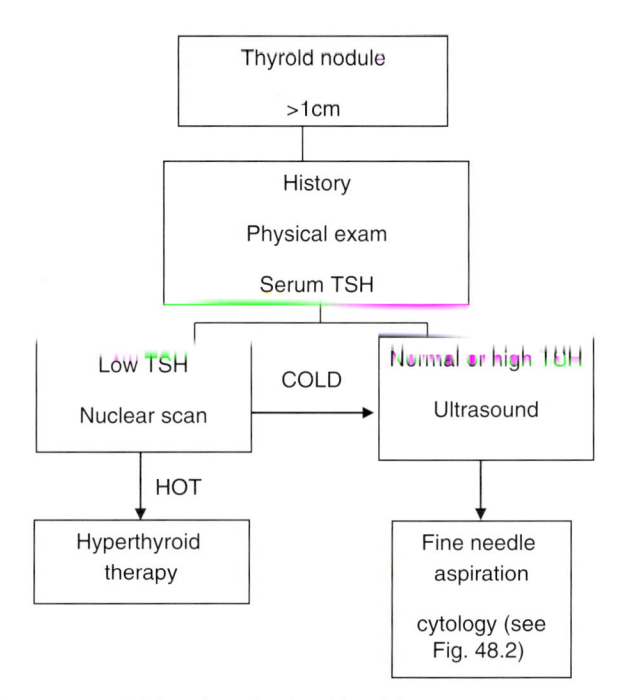

Figure 48.1 Initial work-up for thyroid nodule.

Staging and prognostic grouping

UICC TNM staging
Separate stage groupings are recommended for papillary and follicular (differentiated), medullary and anaplastic (undifferentiated) carcinomas (Table 48.1).

TNM stage grouping in differentiated thyroid cancer is unlike that for other sites as it incorporates age. Patients under the age of 45 years without distant metastatic disease are classified as Stage I; if there is distant metastatic disease, they are classified as Stage II.

Anaplastic thyroid cancer staging is also different as all patients are classified as Stage IV due to the very poor prognosis.

Group classification
Although there are numerous published risk group classifications, the most widely used is the MACIS score that was developed to predict survival. It depends on metastases (M), age (A), completeness of resection (C), extrathyroid invasion (I) and size (S). Electronic MACIS calculators are available online.

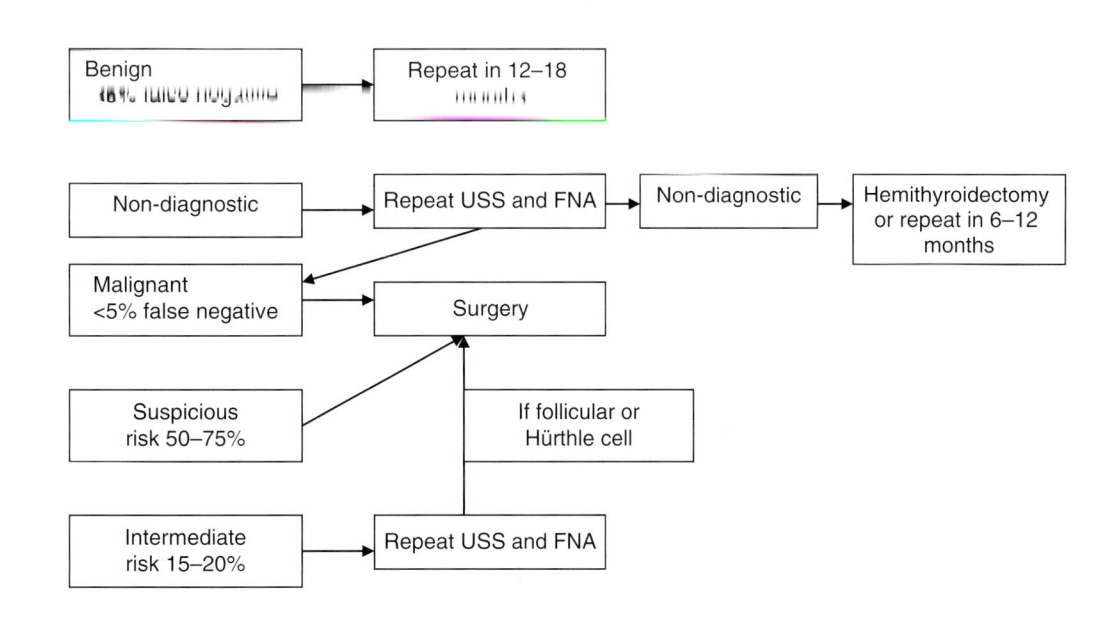

Figure 48.2 Results of fine needle aspirate.

Table 48.1 UICC TNM categories and stage grouping: Thyroid gland

TNM categories	
Papillary, follicular and medullary carcinoma	
T1	≤2 cm, intrathyroidal
T2	>2–4 cm, intrathyroidal
T3	>4 cm or minimal extrathyroidal extension
T4a	Subcutaneous, larynx, trachea, oesophagus, recurrent laryngeal nerve
T4b	Prevertebral fascia, mediastinal vessels, carotid artery
Anaplastic/undifferentiated carcinoma	
T4a	Tumour limited to thyroid
T4b	Tumour beyond thyroid capsule
All types	
N1a	Level VI
N1b	Other regional
M1	Distant metastasis

Stage grouping			
Papillary or follicular			
Under 45 years			
Stage I	Any T	Any N	M0
Stage II	Any T	Any N	M1
45 years and older			
Stage I	T1a, T1b	N0	M0
Stage II	T2	N0	M0
Stage III	T3	N0	M0
	T1, T2, T3	N1a	M0
Stage IVA	T1, T2, T3	N1b	M0
	T4a	N0, N1	M0
Stage IVB	T4b	Any N	M0
Stage IVC	Any T	Any N	M1
Medullary			
Stage I	T1a, T1b	N0	M0
Stage II	T2, T3	N0	M0
Stage III	T1, T2, T3	N1a	M0
Stage IVA	T1, T2, T3	N1b	M0
	T4a	Any N	M0
Stage IVB	T4b	Any N	M0
Stage IVC	Any T	Any N	M1
Anaplastic			
Stage IVA	T4a	Any N	M0
Stage IVB	T4b	Any N	M0
Stage IVC	Any T	Any N	M1

Prognostic factors for follicular-derived tumours

Age is the most important prognostic factor in determining survival and recurrence, with older patients having a worse prognosis than younger patients (Table 48.2). Older patients also tend to have other high-risk factors. A high thyroglobulin at the time of initial iodine therapy and within 12 months of initial therapy are risk factors for subsequent recurrence. *RET/PTC* rearrangements are common in paediatric radiation-induced PTC and are associated with a high rate of lymph node metastases. *BRAF V600E* mutation has been associated with an increased risk of recurrence and death. *RAS* mutations have been found in well-differentiated thyroid carcinomas, which are prone to metastatic spread and dedifferentiation, but are also seen in tumours with an indolent course. Age, tumour size, histology, macroscopic residual disease, five or more lymph node metastases or metastatic nodes of ≥3 nodes with extracapsular extension are all prognostic factors for local recurrence.

Table 48.2 Prognostic factors for survival in differentiated thyroid carcinoma of follicular cell derivation

Prognostic factors	Tumour related	Host related	Environment related
Essential	Extrathyroid extension (T category) M category Post-treatment thyroglobulin	Age	Residual disease: R0, 1 or 2
Additional	N category Site of metastases *BRAF V600E* mutation	Gender	Extent of resection. Iodine ablation Endemic goitre
New and promising	Molecular profile		

Data from Cooper DS *et al* (2009) for the American Thyroid Association (ATA). Guidelines Taskforce on Thyroid Nodules and Differentiated Thyroid Cancer: Revised American Thyroid Association management guidelines for patients with thyroid nodules and differentiated thyroid cancer. Thyroid 19:1167-1214; and NCCN Treatment guidelines in Oncology: Thyroid Carcinoma Version 3.2012 NCCN.org.

DIFFERENTIAL THYROID CANCER

Treatment philosophy

Given the generally excellent prognosis of patients with DTC, the goal of treatment is cure with minimal morbidity. Unfortunately, given the natural history of anaplastic cancer, for these patients the goal is rarely cure but rather palliative to maintain quality of life for as long as possible; this often requires control of the disease in the neck and management of tracheal and oesophageal obstruction. Although DTC and anaplastic thyroid cancer are part of the same spectrum, their management is very different and will be discussed separately, as will that of MTC.

Scenario: Differentiated thyroid cancer	Treatment philosophy
Local disease only	• Lobectomy and isthmusectomy (see Box 48.1) • Total thyroidectomy with or without radioactive iodine (RAI) (see Box 48.1)

Regional nodal metastases present	• Central neck dissection (CND; prelaryngeal, pretracheal and paratracheal):
	  ▪ Prophylactic CND is controversial
	• Lateral neck dissection only when clinical or radiographic evidence of lateral neck nodal metastases is present:
	  ▪ No role for prophylactic lateral neck dissection
	• Postoperative radioactive iodine to be considered

Metastatic disease on presentation	• Total thyroidectomy if RAI treatment is planned:
	  ▪ For young patients with lung metastasis the 10-year survival is 100%
	  ▪ If over 40 years, this falls to 20%
	  ▪ Complete response rate from RAI:
	    ○ 50% for lung metastases
	    ○ 10% for bone metastases
	• Patients who present with solitary bone metastases may benefit from resection if possible
	• If not, external beam radiotherapy (EBRT) is of benefit:
	  ▪ A high dose such as 50 Gy in 25 fractions may be given to young patients to maximize long-term control

Recurrent thyroid cancer	• *Locoregional disease:*
	  ▪ Surgery
	  ▪ RAI may be given after surgical resection even if it has been given previously:
	    ○ If the first dose ablated residual thyroid tissue, there may not have been sufficient RAI to treat residual cancer, so a second, this time therapeutic, dose may be of benefit
	  ▪ EBRT to the cervical nodal region may reduce the risk of further recurrence if there is repeated recurrence after failure of repeated RAI
	• *Metastatic disease on follow-up:*
	  ▪ Initial therapy should be RAI after thyroidectomy if not already performed
	  ▪ If there is further progression, EBRT may be considered for bone metastases and occasionally for lung metastases (for bronchial obstruction or haemoptysis) from a localized lesion
	  ▪ Role of chemotherapy is limited

Follow-up	• *After hemithyroidectomy or thyroidectomy without RAI ablation:*
	  ▪ Cervical ultrasound scan and thyroid-stimulating hormone (TSH) measurement
	  ▪ Serum thyroglobulin (TG) is of limited value after a hemithyroidectomy, but if low after a total thyroidectomy, it may be a useful tumour marker
	• *After RAI ablation:*
	  ▪ TG should be very low or undetectable (range depends on methodology of measurement)
	  ▪ Approximately 6 months to a year after ablation, an ultrasound scan should be performed:
	    ○ If negative, a stimulated TG is often recommended either by withdrawal of thyroxine or with recombinant TSH (thyrotropin alpha [Thyrogen®]) stimulation
	  ▪ Whole-body iodine scan may be performed at the same time
	  ▪ If TG is high and if there is residual uptake on the whole-body scan, surgery with or without postoperative RAI should be considered for surgically resectable disease based on further imaging studies (i.e. ultrasound or cross-sectional imaging)
	  ▪ If surgical salvage is not indicated, further RAI may be given
	  ▪ If thyroglobulin is elevated but the iodine scan is negative, an ^{18}FDG-PET scan may identify surgically salvageable disease

Box 48.1 Rational for lobectomy/isthmusectomy and total thyroidectomy

Lobectomy and isthmusetomy	Total thyroidectomy
Diagnosis of nodule with uncertain cytology	Diagnosis and treatment of microscopic multifocality in contralateral lobe
Reduced surgical complications of hypoparathyroidism and recurrent laryngeal nerve	Required for administration of RAI
Reduced need for lifelong thyroid replacement therapy	RAI can treat residual or metastatic disease
Curative in low-risk cancers	Ablation with surgery and RAI facilitates follow-up with thyroglobulin

Treatment

Surgery

Surgery: Differentiated thyroid cancer	Description
Early disease	• Total thyroidectomy: 　▪ Potential complications or sequalae: 　　○ Recurrent laryngeal nerve palsy 　　○ Permanent hypoparathyroidism 　　○ Long-term thyroid replacement therapy • Hemithyroidectomy and isthmusectomy: 　▪ Sufficient in low-risk patients 　▪ Especially if performed initially for diagnosis
Advanced non-metastatic disease	• Total thyroidectomy • Central compartment node dissection (prelaryngeal, pretracheal and paratracheal): 　▪ Therapeutic if known node involved 　▪ Prophylactic if primary >4 cm or extrathyroid extension • Functional lateral compartment node dissection if known lateral nodal involvement • When extrathyroid extension is present, complete resection with tumour-free margins should be sought, but must be balanced against potential morbidity: 　▪ Tumour debulking leaving gross residual disease should be avoided 　▪ Dissection from the laryngeal nerve, trachea or oesophagus leaving microscopic disease may be acceptable in certain circumstances and in such cases RAI and EBRT may be required
Metastatic disease	• Total thyroidectomy to facilitate subsequent RAI administration

Radiotherapy

Radiotherapy: Differentiated thyroid cancer	Description
Early	• No role
Advanced non-metastatic disease	• In older patients (at least 50+ years) with a significant risk of local recurrence in the neck, either gross residual disease or posterior extrathyroid extension into the tracheoesophageal groove: 　▪ RAI alone may be insufficient 　▪ RT has been shown to improve both local control and survival in appropriately selected cases 　▪ Anterior extension into the strap muscles is adequately treated by *en bloc* resection and RT is not required

Radiotherapy: Differentiated thyroid cancer	Description

	• The American Thyroid Association (ATA) guidelines state that 'The use of external beam irradiation to treat the primary tumor should be considered in patients over age 45 with grossly visible extrathyroidal extension at the time of surgery and a high likelihood of microscopic residual disease'
	• Clinical target volume (CTV):
	   ▪ CTV I: gross or microscopic residual tumour with 0.5 cm margin
	   ▪ CTV II: thyroid bed and level III, IV, VI and partial V nodes from the hyoid to the aortic arch
	   ▪ If recurrent regional nodes or extracapsular extent, regional node volume can be enlarged to include levels II, III, IV, V and VI, and the superior mediastinum, unilaterally or bilaterally as required
	• Typical prescribed dose:
	   ▪ CTV I: 60–70 Gy in 30–35 fractions
	   ▪ CTV II: 50–56 Gy in 25–35 fractions

Metastatic disease	• For symptomatic bone and lung metastases, short-course palliative radiation may be beneficial

Systemic therapy

Systemic therapy: Differentiated thyroid cancer	Description
Early disease	• No role
Advanced non-metastatic disease	• See below

Metastatic disease	• DTC has not been considered a chemosensitive disease
	• Appropriate selection of patients to be treated with systemic treatment is essential:
	   ▪ Considerations include symptoms, burden of disease and rate of progression
	• Until recently, doxorubicin has been the most widely used systemic agent in patients with radio-iodine refractory advanced DTC with response rates of only 20–40%. This is changing as a result of publication of two large phase III trials of oral targeted agents:
	   ▪ In the DECISION trial, treatment with sorafenib versus placebo showed improvement in progression-free survival in patients with progressive disease (10.8 vs 5.8 months).
	   ▪ In the SELECT trial of lenvatinib versus placebo improvements in progression free survival (18.3 vs 3.6 months) and response rate (64.8 vs 1.5 %) were reported.
	   ▪ As yet, no difference in overall survival has been shown with either agent.
	   ▪ Both agents were associated with significant but manageable toxicity.

TSH suppression

Traditionally, TSH suppression has been used in all patients with thyroid cancer.
- *Low- and intermediate-risk disease*:
  ▪ Ensure the TSH is in the lower range of normal; just below normal is sufficient
- *High-risk or metastatic disease*:
  ○ Sufficient thyroxine to render the TSH undetectable may be of benefit in patients with high-risk or metastatic disease

Radioactive iodine

Tri-iodothyroxine, the main biologically active product of the thyroid gland, has a high iodine content and circulating iodine is selectively taken up by thyroid tissue. Consequently, RAI is also selectively taken up by both normal and differentiated malignant cells of the thyroid tissue. The usual radionucleotide used in the management of thyroid cancer is ^{131}I which has a half-life of 8 days. The primary emissions of ^{131}I decay are beta particles (maximal energy of 606 keV) and gamma rays (364 keV). The beta particles are therapeutic while the gamma rays, with the aid of a gamma camera, can diagnose metastatic disease from identifying where the iodine has been taken up. The appropriate dose may be calculated using absorbed dose calculations; however, in most centres empiric doses are often given.

Treatment: RAI	Description

Early disease	• RAI for ablation of remnant thyroid tissue:
	  ▪ In patients at low risk of recurrence, RAI may be given to ablate residual thyroid tissue
	  ▪ Enables follow up with thyroglobulin
	  ▪ Potentially treats any residual microscopic multifocal disease
	  ▪ Identifies metastatic disease
	  ▪ 1110 MBq (30 mCi) is sufficient, but probably unnecessary in low-risk thyroid cancer (confined to the thyroid without any poor histological features)
	  ▪ Benefit is controversial (see below)

Advanced non-metastatic disease	• RAI as adjuvant:
	  ▪ In patients at risk of recurrence, RAI results in a lower recurrence rate
	  ▪ Does not improve survival because of the high rate of salvage with surgery and radioactive iodine
	  ▪ ≥45 years and ≥4 cm, or
	  ▪ Extratrathyroid extension, or
	  ▪ Lymph node involvement
	  ▪ Dose is usually empiric (1110–4600 MBq [30–125 mCi])
	  ▪ Some centres measure absorbed dose
	• RAI as therapy:
	  ▪ If residual disease after resection

Metastatic disease	• RAI as therapy:
	  ▪ Can be curative
	  ▪ If metastases take up RAI, repeated doses may be given providing there is evidence of continued response and no evidence of marrow toxicity or any other significant toxicity
	  ▪ Dose is usually empiric (5550–7400 MBq [150–200 mCi])
	  ▪ Some centres measure absorbed dose

Requirements for RAI therapy are:
- Total thyroidectomy and dissection of all nodal metastases noted on clinical and/or radiographic examination
- Low iodine diet 1–2 weeks before
- High TSH:
  - Thyroid hormone withdrawal
  - Recombinant TSH (Thyrogen®)
- Radiation safety and isolation:
  ○ Reduce family members and others exposure to gamma radiation

Side effects of RAI are listed in Table 48.3.

Table 48.3 Side effects of RAI therapy

Early	Late (possibly dose dependent)
Thyroiditis (8%)	Dry mouth >3 years after treatment (15%)
Nausea/vomiting (5%)	Tear duct problems >3 years after treatment (3%)
Sialadenitis (2%)	Early menopause
Change in taste or smell (10%)	Temporary oligospermia
Dry mouth (30%)	Leukaemia (<0.4%)
Emotional stress/isolation	Other second malignancy (GI, salivary gland, kidney, bone) (1%)

Controversies

RAI in early disease

Several guidelines in the past recommended total thyroidectomy and RAI for all patients with tumours >1–1.5 cm, but several large series have questioned the benefit of this approach in patients with low-risk disease. Although in the majority of cases toxicity is minimal, it can occasionally be significant (see Table 48.3); therefore RAI should be avoided if possible. There is no consensus on how to define low-risk disease: even the age cut-off for poorer outcome, traditionally set at 45 years, is being questioned; 50–60 years may be more appropriate. In addition, no randomized controlled study has been performed looking into the utility of RAI. Guidelines are currently being revised recommending more conservative use of RAI. RAI probably has no benefit in young patients with tumours of <4 cm, providing they have no gross extrathyroid extension, lymphovascular invasion or lateral cervical lymph nodes. Patients with microscopic central nodal involvement probably also do not benefit from RAI. If RAI is required for ablation, 1110 MBq (30 mCi) is adequate.

Lobectomy and isthmusectomy or total thyroidectomy for early disease

A study of over 50,000 patients with PTC found that total thyroidectomy significantly improved recurrence and survival rates for all patients with tumours of >1.0–2.0 cm. However, in a single institutional study of nearly 900 patients with tumours of <4 cm, there was no difference in survival or recurrence rates between patients treated by lobectomy or total thyroidectomy. Lobectomy may be sufficient for young patients with tumours of <4 cm confined to the thyroid without adverse pathological features, especially if a lobectomy and isthmusectomy has been performed for diagnosis. If after a lobectomy RAI is required, a completion thyroidectomy is necessary.

Value of prophylactic central compartment node dissection

There is no controversy regarding the indication for central compartment node dissection in patients with radiographic evidence of nodal metastases on imaging or clinically detectable nodal metastases at the time of surgery. Central neck dissection is also indicated in patients with high-risk differentiated thyroid cancers.

The main controversy is the role of prophylactic neck dissection in patients with low-risk well-differentiated thyroid cancers in whom there is no clinical or radiographic evidence of central compartment nodal metastases. The ATA guidelines state that prophylactic central neck dissection may be performed in patients with PTC with clinically uninvolved nodes, especially for advanced (T3 or T4) tumours. However, this is a grade C recommendation. The reason for the controversy is that the long-term benefit of removing occult microscopic nodal metastases remains unclear. Data on the benefit of the procedure in terms of reduction of risk for recurrent cancer are inconclusive, with some studies demonstrating a benefit and others no benefit. There is also a potential increased risk of hypoparathyroidism and recurrent laryngeal nerve injury with comprehensive central neck dissections, particularly when performed by low-volume surgeons. While the routine use of prophylactic central neck dissection may not be routinely warranted at present in low-risk patients with low-risk tumors, in accordance with the ATA guidelines it may be considered in patients with more advanced tumours (i.e. T3 or T4) or tumours with aggressive histologies that may be at greater risk of nodal metastases and progression of these metastases.

Extent of TSH suppression

Traditionally, TSH suppression has been used in all patients with thyroid cancer; however, TSH suppression is associated with an increased risk of osteoporosis in postmenopausal women, atrial fibrillation and exacerbation of any pre-existing angina. There is no evidence of a benefit to TSH suppression in low-risk patients, but TSH suppression may improve outcome in high-risk patients. The ATA recommends initial TSH suppression to below 0.1 mU/L for high- and intermediate-risk thyroid cancer patients, and maintenance of the TSH at or slightly below the lower limit of normal (0.1–0.5 mU/L) in low-risk patients.

ANAPLASTIC THYROID CANCER

Treatment philosophy

The majority of patients, even those without metastases, have a short survival and a limited expectation for cure. It is important therefore that any discussion of the treatment plan includes a frank discussion of the expected risks and benefits of active therapy compared to best supportive care. The patient's quality of life is of primary importance.

While long-term survival is rare in patients who have extrathyroid extension at the time of diagnosis, population-based data suggest that the best outcome is achieved with a multimodality approach including surgery and radiotherapy with or without concurrent chemotherapy. Radiation may be given to control local and regional neck disease and prevent the devastating effect of progressive disease. Chemotherapy has a limited role.

Scenario: Anaplastic thyroid cancer	Treatment philosophy
Local disease	• Thyroidectomy: ▪ If tumour confined to the thyroid, the role of additional therapy is uncertain

Regional disease	• Thyroidectomy:
	  ▪ No role for extirpative surgery (i.e. laryngectomy, pharyngo-laryngectomy); quality of life should be maintained
	  ▪ Postoperative radiotherapy or chemoradiotherapy
	• If unresectable: radical or palliative radiation

Metastatic disease	• Palliation is important
	• Radiation:
	  ▪ May prevent uncontrolled neck disease
	  ▪ May palliate localized metastases
	• Limited role for chemotherapy

Treatment

Surgery

Surgery: Anaplastic thyroid cancer	Description
Early disease	• Thyroidectomy
Advanced non-metastatic disease	• If there is extrathyroid extension, resection to negative margins (R0) or microscopic residual disease (R1) • No role for debulking leaving gross residual disease (R2) • No role for extirpative surgery; quality of life should be maintained • Tracheostomy should be avoided if possible
Metastatic disease	• No role

Radiotherapy

Radiotherapy: Anaplastic thyroid cancer	Description
Early disease	• Probably no role if no extrathyroid extension

Advanced non-metastatic disease	• A response rate of 80% to radiation has been reported, with suggestion of a dose response
	• CTV:
	  ▪ Due to the increased toxicity of large volumes and the general poor prognosis of patients, there is controversy over the extent of the volume to be treated: to keep volume small and encompassing the gross tumour volume (GTV) with a 1–2 cm margin; or to include all or selected regional nodes
	  ▪ CTV I: GTV with a 0.5–1-cm margin
	  ▪ CTV II: nodes levels II, III, IV, V, VI and the superior mediastinum
	• Radiation may be hyperfractionated or conventional fractionated:
	  ▪ 60 Gy in 40 fractions b.i.d. over 4 weeks to CTV I, 46 Gy in 40 fractions to CTV II
	  ▪ 60–70 Gy in 30–35 fractions to CTV I, 50–56 Gy in 25–35 fractions to CTV II
	  ▪ Concurrent radiation with a taxane, doxorubicin or platins, either singly or in combination, should be considered with conventional fractionation
	• Best results in terms of local control have been reported using combination radiation, chemotherapy and surgery with a local control rate of 60% but a 2-year survival of only 9%
	• Post thyroidectomy or if a resection is not possible, definitive radiation therapy with or without concurrent chemotherapy if:
	  ▪ Good performance status
	  ▪ No evidence of metastatic disease
	  ▪ Patient wishes an aggressive approach
	• If poor performance status or an aggressive approach is not wanted, radiotherapy as for metastatic disease may be given

Metastatic disease	• Dose and fractionation should be tailored to performance status and extent of disease:
	  ▪ 40 Gy in ten fractions delivered as a split course (20 Gy in five fractions and repeated 4–6 weeks later depending on response and performance status)
	  ▪ 30 Gy in ten fractions
	  ▪ 50 Gy in 20 fractions
	• Palliative radiation may be required for bone and lung metastases
	• If metastases is limited, an aggressive approach to the neck to ensure long-term local control as for advanced non-metastatic disease may be considered

Systemic therapy

Systemic therapy: Anaplastic thyroid cancer	Description
Early	• No role
Advanced non-metastatic disease	• Taxanes or platins in combination with radiotherapy, e.g.: 　▪ Paclitaxel 30–60 mg/m^2 IV weekly 　▪ Paclitaxel (50 mg/m^2) + carboplatin (AUC 2 mg/mL) IV weekly 　▪ Cisplatin 25 mg/m^2 IV weekly
Metastatic disease	• Response rate is poor 　▪ Taxanes (paclitaxel or docetaxel), doxorubicin and, perhaps, also the platins have the highest response rate • Overall outcome is very poor with a median time to progression of 6–8 weeks • Example regimens: 　▪ Paclitaxel (135–175 mg/m^2) + carboplatin (AUC 5–6 mg/mL) IV every 3–4 weeks 　▪ Paclitaxel 60–90 mg/m^2 IV weekly or 135–200 mg/m^2 IV every 3–4 weeks 　▪ Doxorubicin 60–75 mg/m^2 IV every 3 weeks or 20 mg/m^2 IV weekly
Support	• Especially for patients undergoing chemoradiation, sepsis is a major concern and pre-emptive use of granulocyte-colony stimulating growth factor (G-CSF) may be required

Radioactive iodine and TSH suppression
Neither has any role in anaplastic thyroid cancer.

MEDULLARY THYROID CANCER

Treatment philosophy

In patients with localized MTC, thyroidectomy may be curative. The extent of surgery should depend upon the extent of disease, with at least a total thyroidectomy and central compartment neck dissection being performed. Lateral neck dissection is indicated depending on the size of the primary and if lateral nodes are present.

Patients with distant metastases may have a prolonged survival; therefore, total thyroidectomy with central neck dissection ± lateral neck dissection should be considered in selected patients to achieve locoregional control of neck disease. The roles of EBRT and chemotherapy are limited. The former may be considered where resection is performed, but there is a risk of microscopic residual disease due to the preservation of structures such as the trachea, recurrent laryngeal nerve or oesophagus. In the setting of metastatic disease, morbidity from surgery must be taken into consideration when making treatment decisions. In carriers of the *RET* oncogene, prophylactic thyroidectomy prevents the development of MTC, but screening needs to be continued for other manifestations of MEN 2 depending on the specific mutation.

Scenario: Medullary thyroid cancer	Treatment philosophy
Local disease	• Thyroidectomy: 　▪ If lobectomy is performed and incidental MTC is found without C cell hyperplasia and calcitonin, normal completion thyroidectomy may not be necessary
Regional disease	• Total thyroidectomy with neck node dissection for cure • If extensive neck disease, microscopic distant metastases are highly likely and surgery is unlikely to be curative, but is of value to maintain control of neck disease • If residual disease or high risk of local regional recurrence, EBRT may be of benefit
Metastatic disease	• Cure is not possible but there is still a role for surgery to control cervical disease: 　▪ Extirpative surgery is not warranted
Recurrent disease	• Reoperation may result in cure in some patients with regional recurrence, although the majority will not achieve biochemical cure

(continued)

Scenario: Medullary thyroid cancer	Treatment philosophy

Follow-up	• Serum calcitonin level is generally proportional to the volume of persistent or recurrent MTC and is a good predictor of outcome
	• Doubling time of calcitonin:
	    ▪ ≤6 months: 5-year survival 25%
	    ▪ >6–24 months: 5-year survival 92%, but 37% at 10 years
	• If undetectable after surgery, recurrence is rare and long-term surveillance with annual calcitonin and possibly baseline ultrasound is appropriate
	• If elevated, staging investigations should be performed
	• Once the doubling time has been established, calcitonin should be repeated every ¼ of the doubling time or on an annual basis whichever is shorter
	• If the calcitonin increases by >20–25%, staging investigation should be repeated with the aim of detecting potentially resectable cervical disease

Treatment

Surgery

Surgery: Medullary thyroid cancer	Description
Early disease	• Total or near total thyroidectomy and central neck node dissection is recommended
Advanced non-metastatic disease	• Thyroidectomy and lateral node dissection should be performed if preoperative imaging suggests lateral nodal involvement or extrathyroid extension

Radiotherapy

Radiotherapy: Medullary thyroid cancer	Description
Early disease	• No role

Advanced non-metastatic disease	• Reduces local recurrence, but does not improve survival after surgery in patients with gross extrathyroid extension, nodal extracapsular extension or significant lymphadenopathy
	• CTV:
	    ▪ CTV I: gross or microscopic residual disease with 0.5–1-cm margin
	    ▪ CTV II: node levels II, III, IV, V, VI and the superior mediastinum
	• Typical prescribed dose:
	    ▪ CTV I: 60–66 Gy in 30–33 fractions
	    ▪ CTV II: 50–56 Gy in 25–33 fractions
	• Intensity-modulated radiotherapy (IMRT) technique if available

Metastatic disease	• Short-course palliative radiation if symptomatic

Systemic therapy

Systemic therapy: Medullary thyroid cancer	Description
Early disease	• No role

Metastatic disease	• Not a chemosensitive disease:
	    ▪ Response rates of 20% with doxorubicin
	• Molecular targeted agents may be effective:
	    ▪ Drugs that inhibit RET and other tyrosine kinase receptors:
	        ○ About 30% response rate
	        ○ Stability of disease for 24 weeks in about 50–75%
	• In a phase III study, vandetanib (300 mg PO daily) resulted in an 11-month prolongation of progression-free survival compared to placebo, but with increased side effects:
	    ▪ Rash
	    ▪ Diarrhoea
	    ▪ QT interval prolongation
	• In another phase III study, cabozantinib (140 mg PO daily) improved progression-free survival in patients with progressive, advanced MTC compared to placebo

Table 48.4 Phase III clinical trials

Trial reference	Results
Differential thyroid cancer:	
Mallick et al. (2012) N Engl J Med 366(18):1674–1685	• No significant difference in rate of thyroid remnant ablation with 30 mCi and 100 mCi
Schlumberger M et al. (2015) N Engl J Med 372:621–30	• Lenvatinib versus placebo in radioiodine-refractory thyroid cancer
Brose MS, et al (2014) Lancet 384:319–28	• Sorafenib significantly improved progression-free survival compared with placebo in patients with progressive radioactive iodine-refractory differentiated thyroid cancer
Medullary thyroid cancer:	
Wells et al. (2012) J Clin Oncol 30:134–141	• Vandetanib resulted in prolongation of progression free survival, and improved objective response rate, disease control rate and biochemical response compared to placebo
Elisei R, et al. (2013) J Clin Oncol 31:3639–46	• Cabozantinib (140 mg per day) achieved a statistically significant improvement of PFS in patients with progressive metastatic MTC

Hypercalcitoneamia

Hypercalcitonineamia is associated with diarrhoea. Treatment is with:
- Antimotility agents such as imodium
- Somatostatin analogues may be effective:
  - Do not appear to have previously reported tumour static effect

Phase III clinical trials

There is a paucity of clinical trials in thyroid cancer (Table 48.4).

Areas of research

- Identification of:
  - Genetic and molecular pathways of pathogenesis
  - Molecular markers of prognosis
- Development of targeted therapies for advanced disease

Recommended reading

Almeida MQ, Hoff AO (2012) Recent advances in the molecular pathogenesis and targeted therapies of medullary thyroid carcinoma. *Curr Opin Oncol* 24(3):229–234.

American Thyroid Association Guidelines Task Force; Kloos RT, Eng C et al. (2009) Medullary thyroid cancer: management guidelines of the American Thyroid Association. *Thyroid* 19(6):565–612.

Brierley JD (2011) Update on external beam radiation therapy in thyroid cancer. *J Clin Endocrinol Metab* 96(8):2289–2295.

Cooper DS et al. for the American Thyroid Association (ATA) Guidelines Taskforce on Thyroid Nodules and Differentiated Thyroid Cancer (2009) Revised American Thyroid Association management guidelines for patients with thyroid nodules and differentiated thyroid cancer. *Thyroid* 19:1167–1214.

Ferris R, Goldenberg D, Haymart MR et al. (2012) American Thyroid Association Consensus Review of the Anatomy, Terminology and Rationale for Lateral Neck Dissection in Differentiated Thyroid Cancer. *Thyroid* [Epub ahead of print].

Harris PJ, Bible KC (2011) Emerging therapeutics for advanced thyroid malignancies: rationale and targeted approaches. *Expert Opin Investig Drugs* 20(10):1357–1375.

Harris PJ, Bible KC (2011) Emerging therapeutics for advanced thyroid malignancies: rationale and targeted approaches. *Expert Opin Investig Drugs* 20(10):1357–1375.

Hay ID, Thompson GB, Grant CS et al. (2002). Papillary thyroid carcinoma managed at the Mayo Clinic during six decades (1940-1999): temporal trends in initial therapy and long-term outcome in 2444 consecutively treated patients. *World J Surg* 26(8):879–885.

Jonklaas J, Sarlis NJ, Litofsky D et al. (2006) Outcomes of patients with differentiated thyroid carcinoma following initial therapy. *Thyroid* 16(12):1229–1242.

Lee N, Tuttle M (2006) The role of external beam radiotherapy in the treatment of papillary thyroid cancer. *Endocr Relat Cancer* 13(4):971–977.

Lee SL (2012) Radioactive iodine therapy. *Curr Opin Endocrinol Diabetes Obes* 19(5):420–428.

McLeod SN, Sawka AM, Cooper DS (2013) Controversies in primary treatment of low-risk papillary thyroid cancer. *Lancet* 381:1046–1057.

Nikiforova MN, Nikiforov YE (2009) Molecular diagnostics and predictors in thyroid cancer. *Thyroid* 19(12):1351–1361.

NCCN Treatment guidelines in Oncology: Thyroid Carcinoma Version 3.2012 NCCN.org

Pacini F, Castagna MG, Brilli L, Pentheroudakis G; ESMO Guidelines Working Group (2010) Thyroid cancer: ESMO Clinical Practice Guidelines for diagnosis, treatment and follow-up. *Ann Oncol* 21(Suppl 5):v214–219.

Smallridge R, Ain K, Asa SL et al. (2012) American Thyroid Association Guidelines for Management of Patients with Anaplastic Thyroid Cancer. *Thyroid* 22(11):1104–1139.

Sacks W, Fung CH, Chang JT, Waxman A, Braunstein GD (2010) The effectiveness of radioactive iodine for treatment of low-risk thyroid cancer: a systematic analysis of the peer-reviewed literature from 1966 to April 2008. *Thyroid* 20(11):1235–1245

Sawka AM, Brierley JD, Tsang RW et al. (2008) An updated systematic review and commentary examining the effectiveness of radioactive iodine remnant ablation in well-differentiated thyroid cancer." *Endocrinol Metab Clin North Am* 37(2):457–480.

Schvartz C, Bonnetain F, Dabakuyo S et al. (2012) Impact on overall survival of radioactive iodine in low-risk differentiated thyroid cancer patients. *J Clin Endocrinol Metab* 97(5):1526–1535.

Steward D (2012) Update in utility of secondary node dissection for papillary thyroid cancer. *J Clin Endocrinol Metab* 97(10):3393–3398

Tennvall J, Lundell G, Wahlberg P et al. (2002) Anaplastic thyroid carcinoma: three protocols combining doxorubicin, hyperfractionated radiotherapy and surgery. *Br J Cancer* 86(12):1848–1853.

49 Adrenal tumours

Minerva Angélica Romero Arenas[1], Mouhammed Amir Habra[2] and Nancy D. Perrier[1]

[1]Department of Surgical Oncology, Section of Surgical Endocrinology, The University of Texas M. D. Anderson Cancer Center, Houston, TX, USA
[2]Department of Endocrine Neoplasia and Hormonal Disorders, The University of Texas M. D. Anderson Cancer Center, Houston, TX, USA

Summary	Key facts

Introduction	• Majority of adrenal masses are benign:
	  ▪ Found in 4% of patients undergoing abdominal imaging
	  ▪ Found in 9% of autopsies
	• Incidence of adrenocortical carcinoma (ACC) is 1–2 cases per million
	  ▪ Affects more women; bimodal age distribution
	• Phaeochromocytoma affects young adults, both genders equally
	• Metastases to the adrenal are more common:
	  ▪ Adrenal lesion will be metastatic in 30–50% of patients with a history of cancer

Presentation	• Symptoms are based on excess hormone secretion, if any
	• Cushing syndrome (CS) is the most common endocrinopathy:
	  ▪ Characteristic physical findings: moon facies, dorsocervical fat pads, purple striae
	  ▪ History: diagnosis of hypertension and diabetes mellitus
	  ▪ Non-specific symptoms: weight gain, fatigue, weakness and headaches.
	• Non-functional tumours can occasionally cause symptoms of mass effect, such as pain and abdominal fullness
	• Adrenal incidentalomas (AIs) are increasingly diagnosed

Scenario	• Treatment for ACC:
	  ▪ When resectable, open adrenalectomy offers maximum survival benefit
	  ▪ Mitotane is the most commonly used medical adjunctive therapy
	  ▪ No established survival benefit from mitotane, chemotherapy or radiation
	• Phaeochromocytoma mandates alpha-adrenergic blockade prior to operation
	• Adrenal metastectomy appeared to benefit selected patients in retrospective series

Trials	• Owing to the rarity of adrenal malignancies, few phase III trials have been carried out
	• FIRM-ACT: mitotane + etoposide + doxorubicin + cisplatin (EDP-M) versus streptozocin + mitotane:
	  ▪ No difference in overall survival (OS)
	  ▪ Progression-free survival was better with EDP-M
	• GALACCTIC: recently completed trial of OSI-906, an insulin-like growth factor-1 receptor (IGF1R) inhibitor:
	  ▪ The lack of significant benefit led to early study termination
	• ADIUVO: prospective evaluation of mitotane in low-risk patients:
	  ▪ Underway

UICC Manual of Clinical Oncology, Ninth Edition. Edited by Brian O'Sullivan, James D. Brierley, Anil K. D'Cruz, Martin F. Fey, Raphael Pollock, Jan B. Vermorken and Shao Hui Huang. © 2015 UICC. Published 2015 by John Wiley & Sons, Ltd.

Introduction

Adrenal tumours have various patterns of presentation depending on their endocrine functionality and oncological potential. Evaluation of the patient with an adrenal tumour requires a thorough understanding of adrenal physiology and proper application of imaging and biochemical testing to guide therapeutic recommendations, which may include surgical intervention. Diagnostic evaluation of the adrenal mass must answer two questions:

1. Is the lesion functional, i.e. does it secrete hormones?
2. Do the radiographic characteristics appear benign or malignant?

Although rare, primary adrenal malignancy dictates a different therapeutic approach from that for benign disease, particularly from a surgical standpoint.

The incidence and characteristics of the different types of adrenal lesion are given in Table 49.1.

Adrenal anatomy

An adult adrenal gland weighs 4–5 g and is rubbery in consistency. It is composed of two embryologically distinct structures: the outer cortex and inner medulla. The thin cortex, of mesodermal origin, synthesizes steroid hormones. Its bright yellow hue easily demarcates the adrenal gland from the surrounding retroperitoneal adipose tissue during surgery. The maroon inner medulla, formed from chromaffin cells from the neural crest, synthesizes neuroendocrine hormones involved with the sympathetic system. The anatomical and physiological differences in the adrenal structures result in distinct endocrinopathies and symptoms in the diseased state.

Table 49.1 Incidence of various types of adrenal lesions

Type	Characteristics and incidence
Adrenocortical carcinoma	Incidence: 1–2 cases per million worldwide May be functional or non functional
Phaeochromocytoma	Incidence: 2–8 per million persons annually Primary tumour of the adrenal medulla: • Rare, usually benign tumours • Secrete catecholamines
Metastatic disease	Common 30–50% of adrenal lesions are metastatic in patients with a history of cancer
Adenoma	May secrete hormones: cortisol, aldosterone, androgens Most common is cortisol

Functional diseases of the adrenal cortex

The adrenal cortex has three discrete functional layers, each responsible for the production of a steroid hormone. The most superficial layer, the zona glomerulosa (ZG), produces mineralocorticoids, the zona fasciculata (ZF) produces glucocorticoids, and the zona reticularis (ZR) produces androgens. The hypersecreted hormone determines the clinical manifestations of functional adrenocortical lesions (Table 49.2).

Aetiology and physiology

Aetiology and physiology: Functional diseases of the adrenal cortex	Description

Cushing syndrome (hypercortisolism)	• Most common aetiology is exogenous intake of steroids
	• Excess endogenous production of cortisol:
	  ▪ Pituitary disease (70%)
	  ▪ Primary adrenal lesions (15%)[a]
	  ▪ Ectopic adrenocorticotrophic hormone (ACTH) (15%)[b]
	• ZF secretes 10–20 mg of cortisol daily; can increase to 50–70 mg in times of stress:
	  ▪ Owing to the diurnal rhythm of ACTH secretion, plasma cortisol levels peak in the early morning and reach a nadir in the late afternoon
	• Hypothalamic–pituitary–adrenal axis (HPAA):
	  ▪ Corticotropin-releasing factor (CRF) from the hypothalamus stimulates pituitary secretion of ACTH, which then stimulates cortisol secretion by the adrenals
	  ▪ Cortisol provides negative feedback to the pituitary and hypothalamus, inhibiting the synthesis of both CRF and ACTH

Conn syndrome (hyperaldosteronism)	• First described in 1955 in a patient with hypertension and hypokalaemia from an adrenal adenoma • Major causes: a unilateral aldosteronoma and bilateral adrenal hyperplasia (BAH) • Rare causes: unilateral adrenal hyperplasia, familial hyperaldosteronism, aldosterone-secreting ovarian tumours and ACC (approximately 2% produce aldosterone) • Aldosterone is produced in the ZG in small amounts (100–150 µg/day)

Aetiology and physiology: Functional diseases of the adrenal cortex	Description

	• Plays a major role in the regulation of electrolyte excretion and fluid balance, and blood pressure:
	  ▪ Released from the juxtaglomerular cells of the macula densa in response to decreased volume (pressure) or sodium concentration
	  ▪ Targets type I receptors in the distal renal tubules to increase sodium reabsorption and potassium secretion
	  ▪ Also promotes secretion of hydrogen ions
	• Renin–angiotensin system (RAS):
	  ▪ Renin hydrolyses angiotensinogen to angiotensin I in the liver
	  ▪ Angiotensin-converting enzyme (ACE) in the lung will then cleave angiotensin I to angiotensin II, a potent vasoconstrictor and trophic hormone to the ZG
	  ▪ Aldosterone is released in response to angiotensin II

Virilizing syndromes (hyperandrogenism)	• Prevalence is estimated at 8% of the population in the USA:
	  ▪ Approximately 50% appear in childhood
	  ▪ After puberty adrenogenital syndrome is more frequently recognized in females
	• Adrenal glands produce:
	  ▪ 80% of dehydroepiandrosterone (DHEA)
	  ▪ All DHEA-sulphate (DHEAS)[c]
	  ▪ 50% of androstenedione and 25% of circulating testosterone
	  ▪ Adrenal androgen secretion is dependent on ACTH secreted by the anterior pituitary

Adrenocortical carcinoma	• Incidence: 1–2 per million persons worldwide
	• Bimodal age distribution: peaks in children <5 years of age and in the fifth and sixth decades of life
	  ▪ Children in Southern Brazil reported to have a 10-fold higher-than-normal incidence
	  ▪ Women are affected slightly more often than men (58.6% vs 41.4%)
	• 0.2% of cancer-related deaths
	• Aetiology is unknown:
	  ▪ Recent studies have noted chromosomal abnormalities and altered growth factor production
	  ▪ Genetic syndromes have been associated with ACC:
	    ○ TP53, menin and the APC
	    ○ Beckwith–Wiedemann syndrome and Carney complex
	  ▪ A few ACC cases are associated with adrenal hyperplasia, leading to the theory that hyperplasia is a predisposing factor for ACC, but no evidence for progression from hyperplasia to adenoma or carcinoma
	  ▪ Epidemiological studies suggesting an increased risk of ACC in men who smoke cigarettes and women who use oral contraceptives are viewed with caution

[a]Cortisol hypersecretion from adrenal tumours is most often due to a benign adenoma, although it can occur in patients with ACC, and rare forms of BAH, including primary pigmented nodular adrenal dysplasia and ACTH-independent macronodular adrenal hyperplasia.
[b]Ectopic ACTH-production is usually a paraneoplastic process commonly seen in patients with neuroendocrine-derived tumours of the lung, thymus, gastrointestinal tract or pancreas.
[c]Because DHEAS is not secreted by the ovaries, it is used as a marker of adrenal androgen secretion in females.

Table 49.2 Clinical manifestations of adrenocortical hormone excess

Manifestation	Cortisol	Androgen	Oestrogen	Aldosterone
Hypertension	✓	–	–	✓
Glucose intolerance	✓	–	–	–
Hirsutism	–	✓	–	–
Hallmarks or manifestations specific to hormone	Truncal obesity Buffalo hump Moon facies Abdominal purple striae Easy bruising Osteoporosis Psychiatric changes Thin skin*	Male pattern baldness Voice changes Breast atrophy Libido change Oligomenorrhoea or amenorrhoea Increased muscle mass	Gynaecomastia Mastodynia Testicular atrophy Decreased libido	Hypokalaemia Polyuria Weakness Mild hypernatraemia Metabolic alkalosis

*Not all these signs and symptoms are present in all cases, and may be absent or subtle in subclinical disease.

Presentation and natural history

Presentation and natural history: Functional diseases of the adrenal cortex	Description

Cushing syndrome (hypercortisolism)	• Most common feature is weight gain:
	  ▪ Some patients may offset this through diet and exercise
	  ▪ Others may have weight loss especially in association with malignant tumours (approximately 20% of patients with ectopic CS, and occasionally in ACC)
	• Hyperglycaemia, body fat redistribution, altered immune function
	• Additional physical manifestations are listed in Table 49.2
	• Cortisol may affect bone resorption, cardiovascular system, digestive tract and renal function[a]

Conn syndrome (hyperaldosteronism)	• Symptoms are non-specific and usually mild: ▪ Headache, muscle weakness, fatigue, polydipsia, polyuria and/or nocturia • Increased retention of water and sodium by the kidneys, expanding the extracellular fluid compartment and eventually resulting in higher intravascular volume, increased cardiac output and elevation of blood pressure • Hypokalaemia is usually associated with aldosterone-producing adenomas while many cases of BAH may be normokalaemic
Virilizing syndromes (hyperandrogenism)	• Virilizing tumours producing primarily androgens are striking • Females may experience a deepening of the voice, acne, thickening and darkening of facial hair, assumption of a male hair distribution, clitoral hypertrophy, menstrual cessation and breast atrophy • May go undetected initially in adult male patients • Patients should be asked about changes to libido • Androgen-secreting tumours have higher malignant rate and should raise a suspicion of ACC

Adrenocortical carcinoma	• Highly aggressive, frequently metastasize to lungs and liver
	• Often large (>5 cm), bulky and locally invasive (Fig. 49.1):
	  ▪ Yet, nearly half are localized to the adrenal gland
	• Approximately half are functional tumours:
	  ▪ Frequently associated with virilizing syndromes
	• Non-functional tumours: symptoms result from mass effect
	• Early series found nearly half of all patients were Stage IV at diagnosis; however, more recent series have shown an increasing proportion of patients with early-stage (I, II) disease

[a]The morbidity and mortality associated with CS can be in part related to the severity of abnormalities caused by excessive cortisol (opportunistic infections, venous thromboembolism, hypertension, hyperglycaemia or hypokalaemia) as well as the cause of the hormonal excess (adenoma, hyperplasia or malignancy).

Diagnostic work-up

Diagnostic work-up: Functional diseases of the adrenal cortex	Description
Cushing syndrome (hypercortisolism)	**Biochemical studies** • 24-hour urinary cortisol or midnight salivary cortisol are usually elevated in the presence of low ACTH levels (usually <15 pg/mL) • An overnight 1-mg dexamethasone suppression test can also be used as a screening test for CS in patients with adrenal tumours who have a less remarkable presentation: ▪ A morning cortisol level of 1.8 μg/dL (60 nmol/L) was found to have 100% sensitivity and 67% specificity to diagnose CS in patients with adrenal tumours • Plasma ACTH levels are also helpful to identify the aetiology as ACTH dependent or independent (suggestive of adrenal source)

Diagnostic work-up: Functional diseases of the adrenal cortex	Description
	Imaging • Abdominal computed tomography (CT) is helpful in identifying an adrenal aetiology of CS • Imaging is helpful for operative planning: establishes the laterality of the lesion (unilateral or bilateral) and the likelihood that the mass is a benign cortisol-producing adenoma (size <4 cm, smooth well-rounded borders, homogenous appearance) or suspicious for ACC (large, irregular borders, inhomogeneous lesion)

Conn syndrome (hyperaldosteronism)	**History**
	• Findings of hypertension and hypokalaemia should raise suspicion of primary hyperaldosteronism:
	  ▪ Review of medications is required to rule out hypokalaemia as a side effect of medications, especially in patients with pre-existing hypertension which may be treated with diuretics (Box 49.1)
	
	Biochemical tests
	• Complete electrolyte panel may reveal hypochloraemic metabolic alkalosis
	• A morning plasma aldosterone-to-plasma renin ratio of >30 in association with a plasma aldosterone concentration of >15 ng/dL or higher is highly suggestive of primary hyperaldosteronism
	• Confirmation of diagnosis requires aldosterone levels after high sodium intake (urinary aldosterone after either 3 days of a high-salt diet or plasma aldosterone concentration after 2 L of normal saline given over 4 hours)
	• Adrenal vein sampling (gold standard):
	  ▪ Differentiation between a unilateral adenoma and BAH is essential
	  ▪ Aldosterone levels will be increased on the affected side, if unilateral
	
	Imaging
	• Adrenal imaging (CT) helps preoperative planning and in determining risk of malignancy

Virilizing syndromes (hyperandrogenism)	**Biochemical studies**
	• Adrenal pathology is suggested by significantly elevated testosterone or DHEAS serum levels, especially if combined with elevated cortisol:
	  ▪ DHEAS values >700 ng/dL (7 µg/mL, 18 µmol/L)
	• Abnormal levels of urine 17-ketosteroid suggest a virilizing or feminizing tumour and should raise suspicion for ACC
	
	Imaging
	• CT or magnetic resonance imaging (MRI):
	  ▪ Either technique may help differentiate between benign and malignant neoplasms based on appearance, size and enhancement features

Adrenocortical carcinoma	**Biochemical studies**
	• Approximately half of ACC are hormonally active:
	  ▪ Up to 50% produce cortisol resulting in CS
	  ▪ Another 10–20% of tumours produce androgens, oestrogens or aldosterone
	• Elevation of serum DHEAS or other androgens
	
	Imaging
	• Masses of >6 cm in diameter have about a 25% likelihood of being ACC, although smaller size does not rule out malignancy
	• CT characteristics suggestive of malignancy:
	  ▪ Heterogeneity, irregular shape, irregular borders and attenuation >10 Hounsfield units (HU)
	  ▪ Thoracic and abdominal CT may identify lesions not evident on physical exam and metastatic ACC
	• Image-guided needle biopsy is often unnecessary and ordered in select cases:
	  ▪ Malignant seeding by the biopsy tract may thwart the potential of curative resection for ACC

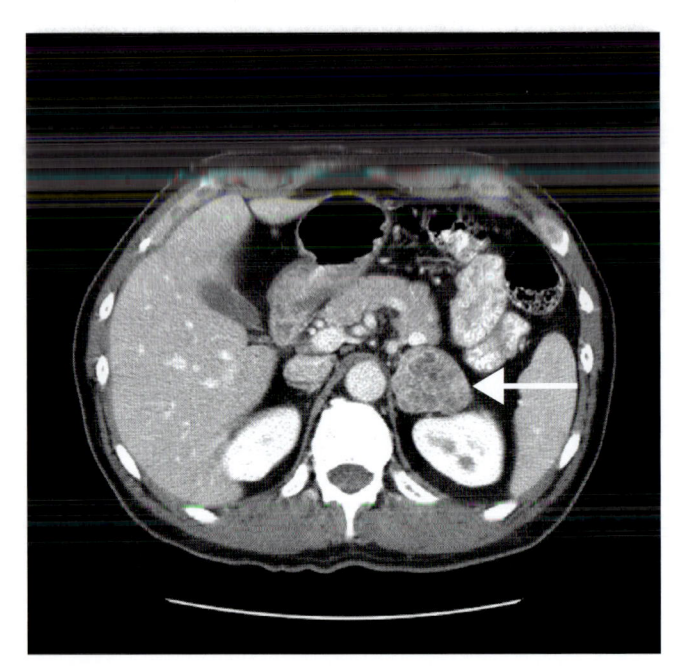

Figure 49.1 Computed tomography scan of the abdomen demonstrates adrenocortical carcinoma on the left side. Note the heterogeneous consistency of the mass and its large size. Irregular borders (not shown here) would also suggest malignancy.

Box 49.1 Drugs associated with hypokalaemia

- Diuretics: carbonic anhydrase inhibitors, loop diuretics, thiazide
- Steroid therapy
- Penicillins
- Bicarbonate
- Amphotericin B
- Gentamicin
- Beta-agonist intoxication
- Mannitol

Patients with adjacent organ invasion or fixed positive lymph nodes are considered to have Stage IV disease, as are patients with distant metastatic disease. More recent proposals recommend staging those patients with locally invasive tumours as Stage III, reserving the Stage IV category for patients with distant metastatic disease. This modification to the traditional staging system would more accurately reflect the natural history of the disease, as well as the correct application of surgical and medical therapy, and is in agreement with cancer-staging systems used for other solid tumours.

Staging and prognostic grouping

Adrenocortical carcinoma

UICC TNM staging

The UICC staging system for ACC was last updated in 2010 and is the same as the most recent (seventh edition) American Joint Committee on Cancer (AJCC) staging system (Table 49.3).

Table 49.3 UICC TNM categories and stage grouping: Adrenal cortical carcinoma

TNM categories	
T1	≤5 cm, no extra-adrenal invasion
T2	>5 cm, no extra-adrenal invasion
T3	Local invasion
T4	Adjacent organs
N1	Regional
M1	Distant metastasis

Stage grouping			
Stage I	T1	N0	M0
Stage II	T2	N0	M0
Stage III	T1, T2	N1	M0
	T3	N0	M0
Stage IV	T3	N1	M0
	T4	Any N	M0
	Any T	Any N	M1

Sobin (2010). Reproduced with permission of John Wiley & Sons.

Prognostic factors

See Table 49.4.

Table 49.4 Prognostic factors for survival in ACC

Prognostic factors*	Tumour related	Host related	Environment related
Essential	T, N, M categories Biochemical status: • Improved survival in patients with functional tumours		Resectability
Additional	Response to mitotane	Age	
New and promising	Molecular profile: • Higher tumour grade, described by Ki-67 or mitotic rate is associated with poorer prognosis • Chromosomal aberrations associated with poor survival: gain in chromosomes 6, 7, 12 and 19; and loss in chromosomes 3, 8, 10, 16, 17 and 19 • Increasing degree of aberration is associated with shorter survival		

*Factors have been studied retrospectively.

Treatment

Treatment: Functional diseases of the adrenal cortex	Description

Cushing syndrome (hypercortisolism)	**Medical management**
	• Focuses on minimizing the symptoms of cortisol excess
	• Mitotane, metyrapone or ketoconazole.
	Surgical intervention
	• Primary production of cortisol due to hyperplasia or a neoplasm of an adrenal gland:
	  ▪ Bilateral adrenalectomy is usually required for patients with BAH; thereafter, these patients require lifelong replacement of glucocorticoid and mineralocorticoid hormones
	  ▪ Retrospective data favours bilateral adrenalectomy for patients who do not respond to medical management to improve metabolic and functional status
	  ▪ Patients with ectopic ACTH syndrome where primary tumour is unresectable and not responsive to medical therapy may also benefit
	• Referral to an endocrine surgeon with experience in the operative treatment of CS is important

Conn syndrome (hyperaldosteronism)	**Medical management**
	• Patients with BAH are best treated medically with mineralocorticoid receptor antagonists:
	  ▪ Spironolactone or eplerenone
	  ▪ Adrenalectomy is reported to help <20% BAH patients
	Surgical intervention
	• Unilateral aldosteronomas benefit from adrenalectomy:
	  ▪ Corrects hypokalaemia in nearly all
	  ▪ Cures hypertension in 30%:
	    ○ 70% whose hypertension persists usually require fewer medications
	• Adrenalectomy may be open or laparoscopic:
	  ▪ Minimally-invasive adrenalectomy should be offered for patients with adenomas:
	    ○ Lower morbidity and an equal cure rate compared to open adrenalectomy
	    ○ Anterior or posterior retroperitoneoscopic approach
	  ▪ If there is any suspicion of aldosterone-producing ACC, an open adrenalectomy should be performed

Virilizing syndromes (hyperandrogenism)	**Surgical intervention** • Adrenalectomy is the standard therapy for adrenal tumours that result in hyperandrogenism: ▪ Suspicion of ACC should prompt open (instead of laparoscopic) adrenalectomy

Adrenocortical carcinoma	**Surgical intervention**
	• Complete resection is the only potential cure for localized ACC:
	  ▪ Whenever an adrenal mass suspicious for malignancy is confined to the abdomen on imaging, adrenalectomy is warranted, and should be performed by an open technique (see later)
	  ▪ Patients who undergo a complete resection have a median survival of 43 months and a 5-year survival rate of 32–48%, compared to median survival of <1 year for those whose resection is incomplete
	• Carefully selected patients with localized recurrence of ACC or isolated metastasis may also benefit from operative intervention
	Adjuvant systemic therapy
	• No prospective data on the effectiveness of adjuvant systemic therapy, most commonly mitotane
	• Recent trials failed to demonstrate improvement in overall survival

FUNCTIONAL DISEASES OF THE ADRENAL MEDULLA

Aetiology and physiology

Aetiology and physiology: Functional diseases of the adrenal medulla	Description
Phaeochromocytoma	• Catecholamine-secreting tumours arising from the chromaffin cells of the adrenal medulla • Annual incidence of 2–8 cases per million • Found equally in men and women

(continued)

Aetiology and physiology: Functional diseases of the adrenal medulla	Description
	- Most commonly present in the third through fifth decades of life
- Approximately 10–20% of patients have a germline mutation associated with the hereditary syndromes multiple endocrine neoplasia (MEN) 2A or 2B, neurofibromatosis type 1, Von Hippel–Lindau (VHL) and familial phaeochromocytoma or paraganglioma syndrome
- Norepinephrine and epinephrine are derived from tyrosine though the intermediary dopa, a pathway in which tyrosine hydroxylase is the rate-limiting step
- Metabolites of this pathway can be converted to vanillylmandelic acid (VMA) and are detectable in urine
- Phaeochromocytoma: lesion in the adrenal gland(s)
- Paraganglioma: lesion occurs elsewhere:
- Along the para-aortic lymph nodes
- Organ of Zuckerkandl
- Bladder wall
- Along the parasympathetic chain (neck to pelvis)

Presentation and natural history

Presentation and natural history: Functional diseases of the adrenal medulla	Description
Phaeochromocytoma	- *Symptoms*:
- Hypertension, sustained or paroxysmal
- Characteristic hyperadrenergic spells:
- Palpitations, pallor, tremor, headache, diaphoresis
- May be precipitated by postural change, anxiety, medication, exercise, medical procedures or increased intra-abdominal pressure (i.e. Valsalva)
- Majority of patients with these symptoms are not hyperadrenergic and do not have phaeochromocytoma
- May also be asymptomatic
- *Signs*:
- Hypertension, especially when refractory to medical therapy:
- Evidence of end-organ damage caused by hypertension (hypertensive retinopathy, cardiomyopathy and myocardial infarction with normal coronary arteries) may be subtle yet unrecognized signs
- Rarely orthostatic hypotension
- Hyperglycaemia, diabetes mellitus, hypercalcaemia and erythrocytosis

Presentation and natural history: Functional diseases of the adrenal medulla	Description
Malignant phaeochromocytomas	- Malignancy is more commonly seen with paragangliomas
- Disease course is indolent in about half of patients and rapidly progressive in the other half
- Prognosis is therefore variable, from 20 years for indolent to 1–3 years for aggressive disease

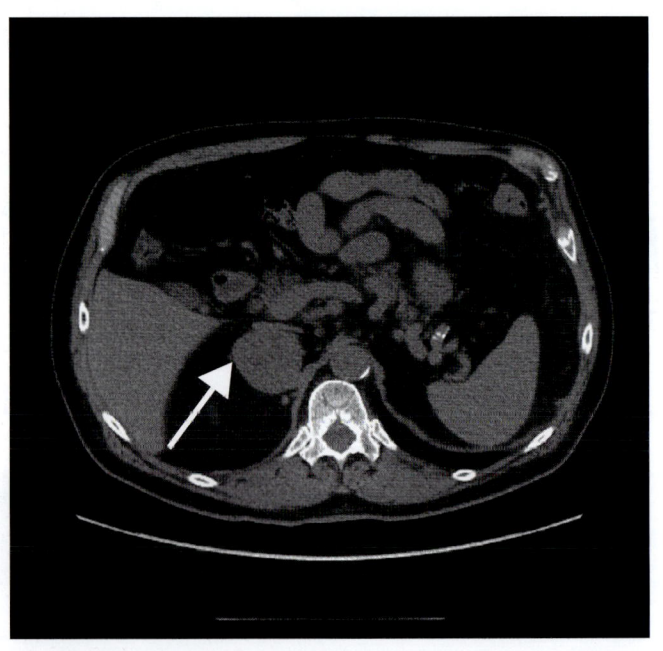

Figure 49.2 Computed tomography scan of the abdomen demonstrates a large phaeochromocytoma on the right side.

Diagnostic work-up

Diagnostic work-up: Functional diseases of the adrenal medulla	Description

Phaeochromocytoma	**Biochemical studies**
	• Plasma free-metanephrines and nor-metanephrines:
	  ▪ 24-hour urine collection to measure metanephrines and catecholamines:
	    ○ Plasma free-metanephrines are particularly helpful in high-suspicion cases and are ideal in children and other patients in whom 24-hour urine collection would be difficult or unreliable
	• Measurement of urinary VMA
	• Rarely, phaeochromocytomas may also be associated with ectopic hormonal production of ACTH, parathyroid hormone-related peptide and growth hormone-releasing hormone
	
	Imaging
	• Abdominal CT or MRI should follow biochemical confirmation:
	  ▪ Each test has a reported sensitivity of >95% and specificity of >65%
	  ▪ Mayo Clinic reported a 98% true-positive rate for either test
	  ▪ Phaeochromocytomas tend to have marked enhancement on CT after intravenous contrast agent administration and to have high signal intensity on T2-weighted MRI (adrenal mass-to-liver ratio >3) (Fig. 49.2)
	• ^{123}I meta iodobenzylguanidine scintigraphy scan indicated when cross sectional imaging reveals a:
	  ▪ Large tumour
	  ▪ Paraganglioma, which increases the risk of having additional extra-adrenal sites of disease
	  ▪ Negative study despite biochemical confirmation

Malignant phaeochromocytoma	• May be difficult to distinguish malignant from benign phaeochromocytoma • Histological evidence of malignancy can be demonstrated in approximately 10% of cases: ▪ Both benign and malignant lesions may show penetration of the tumour capsule, invasion of veins draining the gland, cellular pleomorphism, mitoses and atypical nuclei • Malignant potential is only confirmed in the presence of distant metastasis or invasion of adjacent organs during adrenalectomy • Patients with succinate dehydrogenase B mutations are more likely to have malignant disease and other neoplasms, such as renal cell carcinoma

Treatment

Treatment: Functional diseases of the adrenal medulla	Description

Phaeochromocytoma	**Medical management**
	• Alpha-adrenergic blockade:
	  ▪ Phenoxybenzamine is commonly used in the preoperative period for control of blood pressure and arrhythmias
	  ▪ Starting dose is 10 mg once or twice daily
	  ▪ Dose is then increased by 10 mg every 2–3 days as needed to achieve mild orthostatic hypotension (a dose as high as 100 mg daily may be needed)
	  ▪ If blood pressure is mildly to moderately elevated before surgery, or if long-term alpha-adrenergic blockade will be necessary (i.e. metastatic phaeochromocytoma), selective antiadrenergic drugs, such as prazosin, terazosin or doxazosin, have fewer side effects and thus may be better tolerated
	• Beta-blockers:
	  ▪ Should be administered only after establishment of effective alpha-adrenergic blockade
	• Patients are often advised to increase sodium intake in preparation for surgery to avoid major blood pressure drops that could ensue after resection of the phaeochromocytoma
	• Other pharmacological therapies include metyrosine and the calcium-channel blockers, most commonly nicardipine and diltiazem

(continued)

Treatment: Functional diseases of the adrenal medulla	Description
	Surgical intervention • Operative intervention for paraganglioma may be open or laparoscopic depending on the suspicion for malignancy • Benign-appearing lesions may be resected using a laparoscopic approach for unilateral adrenalectomy • Cortical-sparing adrenalectomy has been successfully performed for patients with bilateral phaeochromocytoma (VHL, MEN 2) to avoid the need for chronic steroid replacement therapy and lessen the risk of addisonian crisis
Malignant phaeochromocytoma	• Metastatic lesions should be resected if possible or treated with radiotherapy or cryoablation

NON-FUNCTIONAL ADRENAL DISEASE

Presentation and natural history

Presentation and natural history: Non-functional adrenal disease	Description

Adrenal incidentaloma	• Incidence:
	  ▪ Up to 4% on abdominal imaging (CT or MRI)
	  ▪ Increases with age:
	    ○ <1% at age 30 years and 7% at 70 years
	• 1 in 4000 malignant
	• Term adrenal incidentaloma is applied to:
	  ▪ Clinically inapparent (asymptomatic, non-functional) mass
	  ▪ Found during radiographic study for a non-adrenal aetiology
	  ▪ Definition excludes adrenal metastases found on imaging for cancer staging or surveillance

Myelolipoma	• Benign lesion of fat and myeloid elements

Metastatic disease	• 30–50% of adrenal lesions are metastatic in patient with history of cancer
	• Cancers frequently metastasizing to the adrenal gland:
	  ▪ Lung (35%), prostate (31%), breast (31%)
	  ▪ Melanoma, renal, uterine, colon
	• May have specific symptoms that prompt imaging, or
	• May be detected during imaging for cancer surveillance:
	  ▪ New adrenal lesions in patient with known cancer should raise suspicion for metastasis and/or recurrence
	  ▪ Imaging will often suggest primary malignancy in patients without history of cancer
	• Primary cancer may produce substances causing a paraneoplastic syndrome
	• Bilateral adrenal metastases may cause adrenal insufficiency:
	  ▪ Weight loss, skin hyperpigmentation, dizziness, hypotension, nausea, vomiting and abdominal pain

Diagnostic work-up

Diagnostic work-up: Non-functional adrenal disease	Description
Adrenal adenoma	• Work-up follows the protocol for any adrenal mass • Diagnosis is applied only in the absence of functional disease or suspicion of malignancy • On unenhanced CT, appear homogenous, attenuation value <10 HU and have smooth borders • Delayed imaging on contrast-enhanced CT will demonstrate rapid washout of contrast

Diagnostic work-up: Non-functional adrenal disease	Description
Myelolipoma	• Definite diagnosis can be rendered by CT: 　▪ Attenuation value of <0 HU because of fat content 　▪ Areas of soft tissue attenuation are also seen and correspond to the myeloid tissue 　▪ Borders are usually smooth, with no evidence of invasion 　▪ Larger lesions may be inhomogeneous since they may bleed
Metastatic disease	• Work-up differs from that of an incidental adrenal mass • If the history or imaging suggest metastatic disease, and if it will help direct the therapy for unresectable disease, fine needle aspiration biopsy may be warranted only after excluding the possibility of phaeochromocytoma • Laboratory studies may show elevation of lactate dehydrogenase level • In cases of bilateral metastases, careful assessment is mandated to establish need for steroid replacement

Treatment

Treatment: Non-functional adrenal disease	Description
Adrenal incidentaloma	• True adrenal incidentaloma has low malignant potential • Risks and benefits of operation should be carefully considered against continued surveillance • Treatment is dependent on the malignant potential, the patient's clinical risk for operation and the patient's anticipated lifespan • If suspicion for malignancy is low and the mass characteristics permit, minimally-invasive adrenalectomy may be considered • Any suspicion for ACC mandates open adrenalectomy
Myelolipoma	• No indication to operate on a patient whose diagnosis of myelolipoma is clear, lest their presenting symptoms are specifically attributable to said lesion
Metastatic disease	• Mainstay is systemic therapy for the primary disease: 　▪ Goals of care in the setting of advanced disease need to be discussed with the patient • Occasionally, highly selected patients may benefit from adrenal metastasectomy: 　▪ In retrospective series, characteristics associated with improved survival following adrenalectomy include isolated adrenal metastasis; a long period between primary tumour treatment and development of adrenal metastasis; and patients with certain types of primary cancer (melanoma, kidney, lung and pancreatic cancers) 　▪ When operation is offered, preferred approach is laparoscopic, and some surgeons advocate specifically for the posterior retroperitoneoscopic approach to further minimize the risks to the patient

Operative treatment of adrenal masses

Selecting the right approach for surgical resection of an adrenal mass requires consideration of a multitude of factors, including the size of the tumour and degree of suspicion of malignancy. Tumours of >4 cm (and more recent experience suggests tumours up to 6 cm may be resected laparoscopically) and any tumour suspected of being ACC or malignant phaeochromocytoma should be resected by open adrenalectomy. Other factors influencing the therapeutic approach include laterality of the disease, presence of multiple or extra-adrenal tumours, additional intra-abdominal disease, distant metastases, history of prior abdominal surgery, the patient's body habitus and the surgeon's experience. The operative approaches are summarized in Box 49.2.

Anatomical considerations

The adrenal glands are highly vascularized; they receive arterial blood from branches of the inferior phrenic arteries and renal artery, and directly from the aorta. Nutrient arteries form a capsular arterial plexus that sends capillaries coursing through the cortex. These capillaries then form a venous portal system that drains into the adrenal medulla. There the vessels reach confluence with the central adrenal vein. Additionally,

Box 49.2 Approaches to adrenal mass surgery

Open approach
- *Indications*:
  - Known or suspected primary adrenal malignancy
  - Large tumours (>6 cm)
- *Positioning*: supine or semilateral
- *Incision*: midline, bilateral subcostal or Makuuchi (hockey stick shape)
  - Subcostal (tumours <10 cm) or thoracoabdominal (tumours ≥10 cm) incision maximizes exposure, minimizes the chance of tumour spillage, and allows vascular control of the IVC, aorta and renal vessels if necessary
- *Left-sided adrenalectomy*:
  - Mobilization of the splenic flexure of the colon is performed along the inferior border of the pancreas
  - Medial visceral rotation of the spleen and pancreatic tail may be helpful for large tumours
  - Exposure of the renal hilum, and dissection and ligation of the adrenal vein are key steps
- *Right-sided adrenalectomy*:
  - Mobilization of the right triangular ligament of the liver allows anteromedial rotation of the liver
  - Kocher manoeuvre facilitates exposure of the right kidney and IVC
  - Right adrenal vein is very short owing to its direct drainage to the IVC, so care is taken to dissect and control it
- *Considerations*:
  - Surgeon should be prepared for en bloc resection of adjacent structures, including the liver, IVC, kidney, spleen and pancreas
  - Thoracoabdominal approach provides the broadest exposure and is useful for anticipated wide en bloc resection or extensive lymph node dissection
  - Lateral approach may be useful in obese patients and those who have undergone prior abdominal surgeries
- *Adrenalectomy for ACC*:
  - As much of the tumour as possible should be excised
  - Contralateral adrenal gland should be inspected for occult tumour
  - Prognosis is strongly influenced by completeness of resection:
    - Invasion of the IVC should not be considered metastatic disease, but rather tumour extension than mandates a more aggressive resection
    - Local invasion of other vascular structures (such as the coeliac axis, aorta or superior mesenteric artery) is clear evidence of an unresectable tumour
- *Adrenalectomy for phaeochromocytoma*:
  - Early ligation of the left adrenal vein helps limit the release of catecholamines
  - Open approach is recommended to avoid leaving residual medullary tissue

Laparoscopic approach
- Procedure of choice for benign disease
- *Contraindications*:
  - Primary adrenal malignancy
  - Large tumours
- *Benefits*:
  - Shorter convalescence (2–3 days compared to approximately 1 week following open adrenalectomy)
  - Reduced discomfort
  - Better cosmetic results
- *Anterior approach*:
  - Position: lateral decubitus position
  - Skin is prepared from the nipple to below the iliac crest and from the umbilicus to the vertebral column
  - Port placement:
    - Port is placed below the costal margin approximately 10–15 cm anterior to the anterior axillary line for insufflation
    - Once pneumoperitoneum is established, three additional trocars are placed under direct visualization with the laparoscope (two placed at the anterior and posterior axillary lines and one 5 cm posterior to the posterior axillary port)
  - Adrenal gland is dissected from the retroperitoneal fat using a harmonic scalpel; gland is mobilized entirely and the adrenal vein is ligated just prior to specimen removal:
    - Vein may be safely ligated using a vascular stapler or titanium clips placed on the proximal side of the vessel
  - Anterolateral approach makes bilateral adrenalectomy cumbersome, as the patient requires repositioning midway through the procedure

Posterior retroperitoneoscopic adrenalectomy
- Developed as an alternative minimally-invasive approach
- Indications and contraindications are the same as those for standard laparoscopy

- *Advantages*:
  - Direct approach to adrenal gland; avoid peritoneal cavity; no need to mobilize adjacent organs; avoid hostile abdomen in patients with prior abdominal operation
  - No need for repositioning in bilateral procedures
  - Patients may be discharged as early as first postoperative day
  - Retroperitoneal insufflation does not alter cardiovascular and respiratory parameters as much as peritoneal insufflation and is generally better tolerated
- *Positioning*:
  - Prone jack-knife position on a Cloward table
  - Hips and knees are flexed at 90° angles
  - All pressure points are appropriately padded
  - Abdominal wall must be allowed to hang free from the hip support
  - Anaesthesia team needs to be ready to manage adrenal-related pathologies with the patient in the prone position
  - Care must be taken to protect the endotracheal tube, eyes and face.
- Operative technique has been described in detail by Walz and Perrier (see Recommended reading)

the adrenal medulla is supplied by arteriae medullae; these penetrate directly into the substance of the medulla. Although some small veins drain from the surface of the adrenal cortex, most arterial blood flows from the capsular plexus, through the cortex and medulla, and out through the central vein.

The right adrenal vein is short and wide; it exits the gland and immediately enters the posterolateral aspect of the inferior vena cava (IVC). The left adrenal vein exits anteriorly and usually drains into the left renal vein, although it occasionally enters the IVC directly.

Perioperative considerations

Perioperative medical management

Perioperative medical management	Discussion
Hypercortisolism	- Most commonly used regimen: hydrocortisone 100 mg intravenously every 8 hours - Steroids should be considered for patients with non-functional tumours to compensate for any subclinical production - Steroids should be tapered slowly once the patient is stabilized in the postoperative phase and later discontinued after the confirmation of the recovery of the HPAA - Patients undergoing bilateral adrenalectomy will require lifelong steroid replacement

Hyperaldosteronism	- Monitoring and normalizing blood pressure and potassium levels preoperatively is essential:
	  - Spironolactone or eplerenone
	  - May be used with other antihypertensive medications

Phaeochromocytoma	- At least 2 weeks of intense preoperative medical management consisting of alpha-adrenergic blockade and volume loading:
	  - Many patients also require beta-blockade to treat the resultant tachycardia
	- Acute hypertensive crisis may occur before or during operation and should be treated with intravenous sodium nitroprusside, phentolamine or nicardipine
	- Hypotension may be controlled with phenylephrine or ephedrine
	- Anaesthesia should be induced with:
	  - Propofol, etomidate or barbiturates in combination with synthetic opioids
	  - Fentanyl, ketamine and morphine may stimulate catecholamine release and should be avoided
	  - Anaesthetic gases other than halothane and desflurane may be used

Standard preoperative precautions

For all patients, preoperative antibiotics, prophylactic measures for deep venous thrombosis, and general endotracheal anaesthesia are required. It is important to have a dedicated anaesthesia team that is comfortable with managing adrenal pathologies.

Continuing care

Postoperative hypotension may result from manipulation of the adrenal glands, inadequate alpha-adrenergic blockade and adrenocortical insufficiency. Generally, postoperative hypotension responds to initial treatment with fluids. Postoperative follow-up should include physical examination with cross-sectional imaging if indicated in light of final pathology. If the tumour was functional, biochemical monitoring should also be included.

Non-operative treatment of adrenal neoplasms

Treatment	Description
Radiotherapy	• May be used for palliation of metastases from ACC and phaeochromocytoma or paraganglioma

Mitotane	• Insecticide derivative used to treat ACC for over five decades
	• Mechanism of action: reduces corticoid biosynthesis and induces structural damage to mitochondria, leading to cell necrosis:
	  ◦ Patients have difficulty tolerating side effects:
	    ▪ Up to 80% experience nausea, vomiting, diarrhoea and/or anorexia
	    ▪ Up to 25% report neuropsychiatric symptoms such as ataxia, dysarthria, confusion, lethargy and/or somnolence
	    ▪ Skin rashes reported by <10%
	    ▪ Rarer side effects: hepatotoxicity and hypercholesterolemia
	    ▪ Side effects are usually reversible and/or reducible with decreases in dose or cessation of therapy
	  ◦ Affects both normal and abnormal adrenal tissue; thus, steroid replacement is necessary
	• Appears to have a dose-dependent effect, with higher serum levels (>14 µg/mL) correlating with improved response
	• No prospective evidence to suggest it improves survival
	• Tumour regression and improvement of endocrine symptoms in 30% of patients with unresectable or metastatic ACC
	• Because it affects both normal and abnormal adrenal tissue, steroid replacement with cortisol, and occasionally fludrocortisone, is necessary:
	  ◦ When therapy is stopped, steroid replacement should be tapered slowly

Chemotherapy	• Cisplatin-based combination chemotherapy is the most widely used regimen to treat ACC:
	  ◦ EDP-M reported to produce a 50% response rate
	  ◦ Recent study found response rate of 23% in patients with unresectable or metastatic ACC treated with EDP-M
	  ◦ No standard second-line treatment for patients who do not respond to EDP-M: these patients should be enrolled in clinical trials whenever possible
	• Very little published on chemotherapy for patients with unresectable or metastatic malignant phaeochromocytoma:
	  ◦ Cyclophosphamide + vincristine + dacarbazine: small series of 14 patients with malignant phaeochromocytoma showed a 57% response rate

Other agents	• Ketoconazole, an antifungal, suppresses androgen and corticosteroid production without inhibiting tumour growth: ◦ Can provide long-term hormonal suppression and is used for patients with CS or ACC • Metyrapone inhibits adrenal cortisol production and is helpful for patients in whom mitotane and ketoconazole fail

Controversies

Adrenocortical carcinoma

While curative intent of operation for ACC mandates an open approach, the role of adjuvant medical therapy, such as mitotane, for early-stage (I and II) ACC is subject to debate. There has been no prospective validation of survival benefit with mitotane therapy.

As noted earlier, controversy persists about whether to include adjacent invasive disease or fixed positive lymph nodes in Stage III or IV ACC. They are included in the latter in the most recent UICC and AJCC systems. However, survival for patients with advanced-stage ACC appears better than that for patients with distant metastases. Evaluation of the staging system must be ongoing as new information on the natural progression of disease is established.

The value of postoperative radiological surveillance after adrenalectomy for ACC remains unclear. However, we support radiological surveillance after adrenalectomy for ACC because patients with isolated recurrence may benefit from operation, and patients with multiple recurrence sites may benefit from systemic therapy.

Adrenal incidentalomas

Whether to treat adrenal incidentalomas has been debated due to two main driving forces:
- Increased use of cross-sectional imaging has led to an exponential increase in the incidence and prevalence of these lesions. Surveillance of patients with true incidentalomas (non-functional, benign-appearing lesions) has resulted in an extremely low incidence of malignancy
- Costs to patients and the healthcare system of continued surveillance against risk of operation for low-risk lesions.

Phase III clinical trials

See Table 49.5.

Table 49.5 Phase III clinical trials

Trial name	Results
FIRM-ACT Fassnacht et al. (2012) N Engl J Med 366(23):2189–2197	• EDP-M versus streptozocin + mitotane (Sz-M) • Disappointing response to either regimen: ▪ Progression-free survival of 5 months in the EDP-M group and 2 months in the Sz-M group. • Median overall survival did not differ significantly between the two groups

Areas of research

- *Insulin-like growth factor*:
  - Gene for insulin-like growth factor (IGF) is consistently over-expressed in ACC
  - Receptors appear to lead to downstream activation of the AKT/mTOR pathway
- OSI-906:
  - Antagonist to IGF 1
  - Recent phase I trial found the combination of an IGF-1R inhibitor (cixutumumab) with an mTOR inhibitor (temsirolimus) was well tolerated and resulted in stable disease for >6 months in 11 (42%) of 26 patients; but Phase III trial could not confirm a significant benefit from using OSI906 as a single agent in ACC
- *Tyrosine kinases*:
  - Emerging research including on epidermal growth factor and fibroblast growth factor
- *Genomic markers of ACC*:
  - Microarray-based comparative genomic hybridization analysis has helped identify chromosomal aberrations shared by ACC tumours:
    - Linked to ACC oncogenesis and may be potential targets for therapeutic intervention
  - Accumulation of gains and losses in specific regions can also be linked to survival differences, creating a genetic footprint for ACC survival and progression of disease

Acknowledgements

The authors would like to thank Ms Melissa Burkett for editorial assistance in preparation of this chapter.

Recommended reading

Abrams HL, Spiro R, Goldstein N (1950) Metastases in carcinoma: Analysis of 1000 autopsied cases. *Cancer* 3(1):74–85.

Allolio B, Fassnacht M (2006) Clinical review: adrenocortical carcinoma: clinical update. *J Clin Endocrinol Metab* 91(6):2027–2037.

Bussey KJ, Demeure MJ (2009) Genomic and expression profiling of adrenocortical carcinoma: application to diagnosis, prognosis, and treatment. *Future Oncol* 5(5):641–655.

Conn JW (1955) Primary aldosteronism, a new clinical entity *J Lab Clin Med* 45:3–17.

Fassnacht M et al. (2012) Combination chemotherapy in advanced adrenocortical carcinoma. *N Engl J Med* 366(23):2189–2197.

Figueiredo BC, Stratakis CA, Sandrini R et al. (1999) Comparative genomic hybridization analysis of adrenocortical tumors in childhood. *J Clin Endocrinol Metab* 84:1116–1121.

Lee JE, Berger DH, el-Naggar AK et al. (1995) Surgical management, DNA content, and patient survival in adrenal cortical carcinoma. *Surgery* 118(6):1090–1098.

Lee JE, Curley SA, Gagel RF, Evans DB, Hickey RC (1996) Cortical-sparing adrenalectomy for patients with bilateral pheochromocytoma. *Surgery* 120(6):1064–1070.

Lughezzani G, Sun M, Perrotte P et al. (2010) The European Network for the Study of Adrenal Tumors staging system is prognostically superior to the international union against cancer-staging system: a North American validation. *Eur J Cancer* 46(4):713–719.

Mittendorf EA, Evans DB, Lee JE, Perrier ND (2007) Pheochromocytoma: advances in genetics, diagnosis, localization, and treatment. *Hematol Oncol Clin North Am* 21(3):509–525.

Mittendorf EA, Lim SJ, Schacherer CW et al. (2008) Melanoma adrenal metastasis: natural history and surgical management. *Am J Surg* 195:363–369.

Morris LF, Harris RS, Milton DR et al. (2013) Impact and timing of bilateral adrenalectomy for refractory ACTH-dependent Cushing syndrome. *Surgery* 154(6):1174–1183; discussion 1183–1184.

Naing A, Lorusso P, Fu S et al. (2013) Insulin growth factor receptor (IGF-1R) antibody cixutumumab combined with the mTOR inhibitor temsirolimus in patients with metastatic adrenocortical carcinoma. *Br J Cancer* 108(4):826–830.

National Institute of Health (2002) *NIH State-of-the-Science Statement on management of the clinically inapparent adrenal mass ("incidentaloma")*. NIH Consens State Sci Statements 19(2):1–23.

Perrier ND, Kennamer DL, Bao R et al. (2008) Posterior retroperitoneoscopic adrenalectomy: preferred technique for removal of benign tumors and isolated metastases. *Ann Surg* 248(4):666–674.

Valli N, Catargi B, Ronci N et al. (2001) Biochemical screening for subclinical cortisol-secreting adenomas amongst adrenal incidentalomas. *Eur J Endocrinol* 144(4):401–408.

Vazquez BJ, Richards ML, Lohse CM et al. (2012) Adrenalectomy Improves Outcomes of Selected Patients with Metastatic Carcinoma. *World J Surg* 36:1400–1405.

Veerapong J, Lee JE (2012) Adrenal tumors. In: FeigBW, ChingCD, eds. (2012)*The MD Anderson Surgical Oncology Handbook*, 5th edn. Philadelphia: Lippincott, Williams & Wilkins:518–549.

Walz MK, Alesina PF, Wenger FA et al. (2006) Posterior retroperitoneoscopic adrenalectomy – results of 560 procedures in 520 patients. *Surgery* 140(6):943–948.

Zeiger MA, Thompson GB, Duh QY et al. (2009) AACE/AAES Adrenal incidentaloma guidelines. *Endocr Pract* 15(5):450–453.

50 Neuroendocrine tumours

Dermot O'Toole[1,2], **Laura H. Tang**[3], **Robert T. Jensen**[4], **Massimo Falconi**[5], **U.-F. Pape**[6] **and Dik Kwekkeboom**[7]

[1]Department of Clinical Medicine & Gastroenterology, Trinity Centre for Health Sciences, St James's Hospital & Trinity College, Dublin, Ireland
[2]Department of Neuroendocrine Tumours, St Vincent's University Hospital, Dublin, Ireland
[3]Department of Pathology, Memorial Sloan-Kettering Cancer, New York, NY, USA
[4]Cell Biology Section, Digestive Diseases Branch, National Institute of Diabetes and Digestive and Kidney Diseases (NIDDK), NIH, Bethesda, MD, USA
[5]Pancreatic Surgery Unit, Salute e Vita University-San Raffaele Hospital, Milan, Italy
[6]Division of Hepatology and Gastroenterology, Department of Internal Medicine, Campus Virchow-Klinikum, Berlin, Germany
[7]Department of Nuclear Medicine, Erasmus MC, Rotterdam, Netherlands

Summary	Key facts
Introduction	<ul><li>The World Health Organization classifies all neuroendocrine tumours as neoplasms (NEN)</li><li>Incidence is increasing and, as patients with NEN live a long time, the prevalence is high</li></ul>
Presentation	<ul><li>Presentation depends on whether or not the neoplasm is secretory and site of origin</li><li>40–60% of gastroenteropancreatic NEN are functional and 30% of small intestinal carcinoids can be associated with the carcinoid syndrome</li><li>Non-secretory neoplasms can present with symptoms of advanced malignancy or alternatively can be incidentally found</li></ul>
Scenario	<ul><li>Dependent on site of origin and whether secretory or non-secretory</li><li>Tumour grading (mitotic count and Ki-67 index) as well as tumour stage (TNM) are important predictors of outcome and deciding therapy</li><li>*Localized*:<ul><li>Surgery</li></ul></li><li>*Locally advanced*:<ul><li>Surgical resection if possible</li><li>Palliative resection if secretory</li></ul></li><li>*Metastatic*:<ul><li>Surgical resection if possible</li><li>Palliative resection if secretory</li><li>Depends on grade and site</li><li>Symptomatic therapy for functional syndromes</li></ul></li></ul>
Trials	<ul><li>Several multicentric placebo-controlled phase III trials have been conducted</li></ul>

Introduction

The most recent 2010 World Health Organization (WHO) system renders all neuroendocrine tumours as neoplasms (NEN) with a malignant potential, and the acronym NEN is recommended. Several national registries have published interesting data in this field, and although comparisons between countries are sometimes hampered by types of registries and the data recorded (e.g. capture fields used, definition of malignancy and nomenclature issues), the sheer body of recent work attests to the

UICC Manual of Clinical Oncology, Ninth Edition. Edited by Brian O'Sullivan, James D. Brierley, Anil K. D'Cruz, Martin F. Fey, Raphael Pollock, Jan B. Vermorken and Shao Hui Huang. © 2015 UICC. Published 2015 by John Wiley & Sons, Ltd.

growing interest in gastroenteropancreatic (GEP)-NEN. The incidence is increasing and as patients with NEN can live a long time, the prevalence of disease is high.

Incidence, aetiology and screening

Incidence, aetiology and screening	Description
Incidence	• Incidence of GEP-NEN is increasing across the world. ▪ Appears to be the result of both an increase in real incidence and increased detection using new imaging and endoscopic screening • Global age-adjusted incidence of 5.25 per 100,000 in 2004 • Prevalence: 29-year limited duration prevalence of 35 years per 100,000

Aetiology	• Majority of NEN are sporadic
	• Inherited predispositions:
	  ▪ Multiple endocrine neoplasia 1 (MEN 1)
	  ▪ Von Hippel–Lindau (VHL)
	  ▪ Neurofibromatosis 1 (NF 1)

Screening	• No proven role apart from in MEN 1

Pathology and natural history

The most important classification of NEN distinguishes between well-differentiated NEN and poorly differentiated neuroendocrine carcinomas (NEC). They represent different pathogenic pathways, clinical presentations, outcomes and, most importantly, require distinct therapeutic strategies.

Pathology and natural history	Description
Well-differentiated NEN	• Group of tumours which share similar phenotype • Many historically designated as carcinoid tumours (a term that is now discouraged due to its inherent connotation of a benign process) • Wide spectrum of clinical behaviour ranging from protracted disease-free survival to frequent recurrence and metastasis • WHO classification of well-differentiated NEN is based on tumour proliferative index (Table 50.1) and mitotic counts
Poorly differentiated NEC	• Highly malignant neoplasms that can occur at any anatomical site with epithelial linings • Pathologically recognized as small cell or large cell high-grade NEC: ▪ Evolving pathological and molecular studies suggest that they are more related to conventional carcinoma than to well-differentiated NEN; therefore they are listed under the adenocarcinoma chapters of the corresponding anatomical sites • WHO classification defines poorly differentiated NEC by proliferative index alone; clinical characteristics of these tumours are also important in the diagnosis of this entity (Table 50.2) • High-grade NEC collectively have a poor clinical course regardless of the anatomical site

Presentation

NEN may present with or without a specific functional syndrome due to raised circulating levels of specific hormones or peptides. Many tumours also secrete measurable substances that do not result in specific symptoms (so-called non-functional tumours). Advanced tumours may present with typical cancer-related symptoms of anorexia, weight loss and general cachexia. In well-differentiated NEN, 80% are hypervascular and demonstrate somatostatin receptors on their cell surface, which can aid in detection and staging.

- 40–60% of pancreatic NEN are associated with a specific syndrome:
  - Insulinoma > gastrinoma > others (VIPomas, GRFomas, glucagonomas, somatostatinomas)

Table 50.1 WHO classification of GEP-NEN (2010)

	Mitoses (per 10 HPF)	Ki-67 index (%)
Well-differentiated NEN (grade 1)	<2	≤2
Well-differentiated NEN (grade 2)	2–20	3–20
Poorly differentiated NEC	>20	>20

Data from Bosman et al. World Health Organization Classification of Tumours of the Digestive System, Fourth Edition. IARC, Lyon, (2010).

Table 50.2 Clinical and pathological characteristics of well-differentiated neuroendocrine tumour (WD-NET) and poorly differentiated neuroendocrine carcinoma (PD-NEC)

	WD-NET	PD-NEC
Histogenesis	Neuroendocrine cells	Surface epithelial cells
Pathology	Typical morphology + staining for chromogranin A and/or other marker: • Synaptophysin • NCAM • Leu 7 (CD57) • PGP9.5	Typical morphology (chromogranin A may be negative): • Synaptophysin • p53 (may be useful)
Tumour grade	Low Intermediate	High
Mean age	50s	60s
Neuroendocrine-associated syndromes	Carcinoid syndrome Functional NEN associated with specific hormonal/peptide-inducing symptoms (e.g. gastrinoma, insulinoma)	Paraneoplastic syndromes more commonly seen in small cell carcinoma (Cushing, hypercalcaemia)
Serum markers	Neuroendocrine/peptide hormones (chromogranin A, gastrin, insulin)	Carcinoma associated antigens (CEA, CA19.9, CA125)
Clinical imaging features	Somatostatin receptor-positive imaging (e.g. Octreoscan™ or gallium-PET-CT) in the majority FDG-PET usually negative in low-grade NEN	Somatostatin receptor-positive imaging (e.g. Octreoscan™ or gallium-PET-CT) in majority is negative FDG-PET is positive with high standard uptake value (SUV)
Combined with conventional carcinoma	No	Up to 75%
Molecular pathogenesis	Mutation of oncogene/tumour suppressor genes (*TP53*, *RB1*) uncommon Occasionally part of hereditary disease (MEN 1, VHL, tuberous sclerosis, NF1)	Similar to conventional carcinoma (mutations of common oncogene tumour suppressor genes [*TP53*, *RB1*])
Prognosis	Site specific but generally protracted clinical course	Generally rapid progression 2-year survival <25%

- Small intestinal carcinoids are frequently associated with the carcinoid syndrome (diarrhoea, flushing and/or wheezing)
- Non-functional pancreatic NEN and gastrointestinal NEN can present with advanced metastatic disease with liver metastases
- Incidentally discovered NEN (discovered on imaging for unrelated issues) include:
  - Gastric, rectal, pulmonary, duodenal NEN, but also pancreatic NEN
- Patients with advanced hepatic metastatic disease and who have long survival or are in good health should be suspected of having metastatic NEN

Diagnostic work-up

Diagnostic work-up	Description

Histological classification	• Diagnosis can be made by cytology but is best made by biopsy to allow proper classification/grading
	• Histology based on:
	  ▪ Characteristic morphology
	  ▪ Immunohistochemical staining (chromogranin, synaptophysin)

Diagnostic work-up	Description

Tumour markers	- General markers:
	  - Plasma chromogranin A (raised in 80% and may be in proportion to tumour size)
	    - False positives include antisecretory medications (e.g. proton pump inhibition), renal failure, chronic atrophic gastritis (pernicious anaemia)
	- Suspected specific hormonal syndromes:
	  - Measure specific hormone: insulin for insulinoma, gastrin for gastrinoma, urinary 5-hydroxyindoleacetic acid (5-HIAA) in carcinoid syndrome

Imaging	- Depends on tumour type and location - Contrast-enhanced techniques may also be helpful - Luminal tumours (e.g. gastric, duodenal, bronchial, colorectal) may require endoscopic evaluation and/or endoscopic ultrasound (EUS) (especially useful for T staging of small tumours and regional nodes)

Tumour stage evaluation	- For NEN with risk of advanced disease (locoregional or metastatic disease), minimal staging tests:
	  - Triphasic computed tomography (CT) of the abdomen and/or thorax, and/or magnetic resonance imaging (MRI) of the liver (diffusion-weighted imaging and/or Primivist®)
	  - Somatostatin receptor imaging (e.g. scintigraphy with ^{111}In-labelled somatostatin analogues or ^{68}Ga-labelled somatostatin analogues, positron emission tomographic [PET]-CT)
	  - ^{18}F-fluorodeoxyglucose (FDG) with PET scanning is useful for high-grade NEN and poorly differentiated NEN
	  - Intraoperative ultrasound is helpful in assessing pancreatic NEN location/extent and for all NEN to assess liver metastases location/extent

Site-specific key features of well-differentiated NEN are summarized in Tables 50.3, 50.4, 50.5, 50.6, 50.7, 50.8 and 50.9.

Table 50.3 Stomach

	Type I	Type II	Type III
Frequency (%)	70–80	6	15–20
Age (years)	63	50	55
Male-to-female ratio	1:2.5	1:1	2.8:1
Neuroendocrine cell lineage	Enterochromaffin cell like (ECL)	ECL	Multiple neuroendocrine origins
Size	0.5–1.0 cm	≤1.5 cm	Variable; One-third >2 cm
Location	Corpus	Corpus	Variable
Presentation and association	Chronic atrophic (immune or non-immune) gastritis (e.g. pernicious anaemia)	Occurs in 20–30% of MEN 1 associated with Zollinger–Ellison syndrome (ZES)	Sporadic
Laboratory tests	Achlorhydria Hypergastrinaemia Antiparietal cell antibody Anti-intrinsic factor antibody Anaemia (macrocytic)	Hyperchlorhydria Hypergastrinaemia Chromogranin A elevated *MEN 1* gene mutation	Chromogranin A (variable)
Key pathological features	Multifocal NEN Spectrum of neuroendocrine cell hyperplasia (linear, micronodular ECL proliferation) Atrophic gastritis with intestinal metaplasia Lacking or reduced parietal cell volume	Multifocal May have duodenal and/or pancreatic NEN Peptic ulcers	Solitary
Natural history	Lymph node (LN) metastasis <5% Liver metastasis <2%	LN metastasis 30% Liver metastasis 10%	LN metastasis 71% Liver metastasis 69%

Table 50.4 Duodenum

	Gastrinoma	Somatostatinoma and gangliocytic paraganglioma (GCPG)	Others non-functioning NEN
Frequency (%)	48	30–40	10–20
Age (years)	39	40s–50s	50s–60s
Male-to-female ratio	1:1	1:1	1.5:1
Neuroendocrine cell lineage	G cell	Delta-cell (somatostatinoma) Trilineage of ganglion, Schwann and pancreatic polypeptide-producing epithelial cell (GCPG)	Variable enterochromaffin cell like (ECL) cell, pancreatic polypeptide secreting cell)
Size	<1 cm	Usually <2 cm	Usually <2 cm
Location	ZES-associated NEN: 90% in first and second part of the duodenum	Ampulla or periampullary region	Most are located in the first and second part of the duodenum
Presentation and association	50% of gastrinoma found in ZES/MEN 1 Peptic ulcer disease	20% associated with NF1 Rare in MEN 1, VHL Jaundice secondary to biliary obstruction Gastrointestinal (GI) bleeding	Often asymptomatic GI bleeding
Laboratory tests	Chromogranin A Hypergastrinaemia *MEN 1* gene mutation	Chromogranin A Serum somatostatin Calcitonin *NF1* gene mutation	Chromogranin A Urinary 5-HIAA in carcinoid syndrome
Key pathological features	Occult primary is common Large periduodenal/peripancreatic Lymph node (LN) metastasis	Prominent glandular pattern mimicking adenocarcinoma Psammoma bodies Infiltrative edge GCPG exhibits mixed epithelial, Schwann and ganglion cells.	Non-specific general insular or trabecular pattern
Natural history	LN metastasis 60% Liver metastasis 5–10%	LN metastasis 30% Liver metastasis rare	LN metastasis 45% Liver metastasis 5%

Table 50.5 Small intestine (distal jejunum and ileum)

Frequency	26% of all gastrointestinal well-differentiated NEN
Age (years)	>30s, peak 60s–70s
Male-to-female ratio	1:1
Neuroendocrine cell lineage	Majority are enterochromaffin cell like (ECL) cells with serotonin production
Size	Usually <2 cm at primary site Large mesenteric nodal metastasis
Location	>70% in ileum with distal ileum most common; up to 30% multiple along small intestine
Presentation and association	Crampy abdominal pain Carcinoid syndrome (flushing, diarrhoea, valvular heart disease) in 18% of functional localized NEN, and in 95% liver metastasis
Laboratory tests	Chromogranin A 24-hour urine 5-HIAA
Key pathological features	Mucosal lesions with solid nests and peripheral granulated cell palisading Multiple tumours in 20–25% Mesentery fibrosis Mesentery nodal metastasis can be larger than primary
Natural history	Lymph node metastasis 36–39% Distant metastasis 64% (commonly liver and bone)

Table 50.6 Colorectum

	Right and transverse colon (midgut)	Left colon and rectosigmoid region (hindgut)
Frequency (%)	46	54 Prevalent in Asian/Pacific Islanders, Native Americans, African–Americans
Mean age (years)	66	56
Male-to-female ratio	1.02:1	0.66:1
Neuroendocrine cell lineage	Enterochromaffin cell like (ECL) (serotonin)	L cell (GLP), pancreatic polypeptide (PP)/peptide tyrosine tyrosine (PYY) cells
Size	4.9 cm	1–2 cm
Location	Caecum/right colon	4–20 cm above dentate line
Presentation and association	Diarrhoea Abdominal pain Similar to symptoms of adenocarcinoma May have increased risk for other GI malignancy	Incidental finding (>80%) Change in bowel habits Blood per rectum, pain, discomfort Increased risk for other GI malignancy
Laboratory tests	Chromogranin A 24-hour urine 5-HIAA	Chromogranin A Enteroglucagon and pancreatic polypeptide
Key pathological features	Mucosal lesions with solid nests with peripheral granulated cell palisading	Submucosal nodule/polyp Predominant trabecular pattern with irregular trabeculae and acini 80% express GLP, PP/PYY 80–100% express prosaposin (PSAP)
Natural history	Localized 16% Distant metastasis >40%	Localized 75–85% Distant metastasis <10%

Table 50.7 Appendix (excluding goblet cell carcinoid tumour)

Frequency	19% of all GI NEN
Age	Mean: 30 years Peak: male 20–24 years; female 15–19 years
Male-to-female ratio	1:2
Neuroendocrine cell lineage	Most are serotonin-producing enterochromaffin cell like (ECL) cells Rare glucagon-like peptide-producing L cells
Size	Mean: 0.9 mm 80% >1 cm 6% >2 cm
Location	75% at the tip
Presentation and association	Majority are incidentally seen in appendectomy associated with acute appendicitis Up to 29% association with secondary malignancy
Laboratory tests	Rarely useful (chromogranin A and 24-hour urinary 5-HIAA in rare advanced cases)
Key pathological features	Majority (87%) are low grade (grade 1) and insular type with solid nests with peripheral granulated cell palisading Tubular subtype, particularly mural lesion
Natural history	Low stage (UICC or ENET Stage T1 and T2) with complete surgical removal have 10-year disease-specific survival of 100% High stage (UICC or ENET Stage T3 and T4), including large size, mesoappendix or extra-appendiceal involvement, and positive resection margin are associated with unfavourable prognosis; and right hemicolectomy is recommended for complete staging

Table 50.0 Pancreas

Frequency	1–2% of pancreatic neoplasms
Mean age (years)	50s
Male to female ratio	1:1
NE cell lineage	Functional tumour associated with normal counterpart neuroendocrine cells Non-functional tumour is not well known
Size	Functional NEN: <2 cm Non-functional NEN: 3.6 cm (although smaller non-functional tumours are increasingly recognized incidentally due to advanced and more frequent imaging)
Location	Anywhere in the pancreas
Presentation and association	Functional NEN (29%): symptoms caused by hypersecretion of hormones (insulin, glucagon, vasoactive intestinal peptide [VIP], gastrin, somatostatin) Non-functional NEN: mass and invasion-associated symptoms; up to 50% incidentally identified without symptoms MEN 1 and VHL associated with multiple NEN Tuberous sclerosis (rare)
Laboratory tests	Chromogranin A (universal marker) Insulin, glucagon, VIP, gastrin, somatostatin in functional NEN (depending on symptoms)
Key pathological features	Diverse histological patterns: loosely cohesive, nesting, trabecular, tubuloacinar, glandular, gyriform and pseudorosette arrangement Multiple NEN commonly seen in hereditary conditions such as MEN 1 and VHL Abnormal histology of islets ranging from atypia to microadenomatosis seen in MEN 1 Co-exist with serous cystic neoplasm in VHL

Natural history	Small functional insulinomas (<1.0 cm) have a benign clinical course and rarely metastasize
	Others:
	• Lymph node metastasis ~30%
	• Distant metastasis:
	  ▪ 10–15% synchronous
	  ▪ >50% metachronous

Table 50.9 Bronchopulmonary

	Typical carcinoid	Atypical carcinoid
Frequency	2% of all lung malignancies	0.2% of all lung malignancies
	90%	10%
Age (years)	45–50	60
Male-to-female ratio	1:1	1:1
Neuroendocrine cell lineage	Diffuse idiopathic pulmonary neuroendocrine cell proliferation secondary to chronic injury leading to tumourlet (<5 mm) formation and carcinoid tumour (>5 mm)	
Size	2.1 cm	3.5 cm
Location	75% central	60% central
	Endobronchial location most common: • 75% lobar bronchi, 10% bronchus main stem • 15% periphery	
Presentation and associations	Smoking 40%	Smoking 60%
	>50% asymptomatic Dyspnoea, haemoptysis, cough and postobstructive pneumonia Carcinoid syndrome (1–3%) Cushing (<1%) Rare acromegaly, hypoglycaemia and hypercalcaemia 5% associated with MEN 1	
Laboratory tests	Chromogranin A 24-hour 5-HIAA	

Table 50.9 Bronchopulmonary (Continued)

	Typical carcinoid	Atypical carcinoid
Key pathological features	Low grade Mitosis <2 per 2 mm² (10 HPF)	Intermediate grade Mitosis <2–10 per 2 mm² (10 HPF) or punctate necrosis
	Organoid/nested pattern is most common with round or spindle cell morphology Trabecular and glandular pattern is less common	
Natural history	Lymph node (LN) metastasis 10–15% Distant metastasis 5%	LN metastasis 40–50% Distant metastasis 15%

Staging

Two similar staging systems have been proposed by the European Neuroendocrine Tumor Society (ENETS) and UICC. Poorly differentiated neuroendocrine carcinoma should be staged as for adenocarcinoma of the corresponding anatomical site.

UICC TNM staging

See Table 50.10.

Table 50.10 UICC TNM categories and stage grouping: Appendiceal and non-appendiceal gastrointestinal well-differentiated NEN

TNM categories: Appendix: Well differentiated NEN	
T1a	≤1 cm
T1b	>1–2 cm
T2	>2–4 cm; caecum
T3	>4 cm; ileum
T4	Perforates peritoneum; other organs or structures
N1	Regional
M1	Distant metastasis

Stage grouping: Appendix: Well-differentiated NEN			
Stage I	T1	N0	M0
Stage II	T2, T3	N0	M0
Stage III	T4	N0	M0
	Any T	N1	M0
Stage IV	Any T	Any N	M1

TNM categories: Non-appendiceal gastrointestinal well-differentiated NEN	
Stomach	
Tis	Mucosa <0.5 mm
T1	Mucosa 0.5 mm to 1 cm or submucosa ≤1 cm
T2	Muscularis propria or >1 cm
T3	Subserosa
T4	Perforates serosa; adjacent structures
Small intestine	
T1	Lamina propria or submucosa and ≤1 cm
T2	Muscularis propria or >1 cm
T3	Jejunal, ileal: subserosa Ampullary, duodenal: invades pancreas or retroperitoneum
T4	Perforates serosa; adjacent structures
Large intestine	
T1	Lamina propria or submucosa and ≤2 cm
T1a	<1 cm
T1b	1–2 cm
T2	Muscularis propria or >2 cm
T3	Subserosa, or pericolorectal tissue
T4	Perforates serosa; adjacent structures

Stage grouping: Non-appendiceal gastrointestinal well-differentiated NEN			
Stage I	T1	N0	M0
Stage IIA	T2	N0	M0
Stage IIB	T3	N0	M0
Stage IIIA	T4	N0	M0
Stage IIIB	Any T	N1	M0
Stage IV	Any T	Any N	M1

Treatment philosophy

Given the generally excellent prognosis of patients with well-differentiated NEN, the goal of treatment is cure with minimal morbidity. Surgical (or occasionally endoscopic) resection should be considered to provide cure where possible. Patients with functionally symptomatic tumours may require treatment to control symptoms prior to embarking on specific antioncological measures.

- Oncological principles of management in patients with GEP-NEN depend on many factors and require a multidisciplinary approach
- Treatment often requires individualization

- Surgery is the only definitive cure but is rarely possible in patients with metastatic disease, and other approaches are therefore necessary
- Antiproliferative treatment decisions depend on:
  - Origin of the primary tumour
  - Histological differentiation
  - Tumour grade (or proliferative capacity)
- There is an ever increasing need to enrol patients into clinical trials in the field of NEN

Treatment

Surgery

Surgical treatment of NEN should be individualized according to both tumour features and patients' co-morbidities. Tumour size, extent and grading are the most powerful preoperative predictors of aggressiveness and the extent of surgical resection is always correlated with these variables. In general, a standard oncological resection, as for the more common carcinomas arising from the same sites, is always recommended. Surveillance or limited resections are possible and recommended according to the size and site of the lesion, and when a malignant behaviour is ruled out; full oncological resection is favoured where the metastatic potential is intermediate to high even in the absence of overt metastases. Surgery often can be proposed in some patients with Stage IV disease and while it may not be curative, excellent palliation can result and overall good recurrence-free progression can be expected in some cases. Occasionally, a so-called debulking surgical procedure can be proposed to try to control the bulk of the tumour burden and/or symptoms that are resulting from the tumour. There is currently no evidence to support adjuvant therapy following resection of grade 1 and grade 2 NEN; in rare cases where surgery is performed for grade 3 NEN or NEC, adjuvant therapy might be considered on an individual bases. Following a good response to systemic therapy in patients with grade 1/2 NEN, then secondary surgery can be rediscussed on an individual basis.

Important considerations are:
- A standard resection should be performed in the case of positive margins after local excision
- In patients with functional symptoms due to carcinoid syndrome, perioperative intravenous somatostatin analogues should be used to prevent a carcinoid crisis
- Surgery may be the only method of controlling symptoms due to functioning tumours
- Patients with poorly differentiated or grade 3 tumours rarely benefit from surgery due to the tumour bulk and especially the tumour biology.

Surgery	Description

Resection of early tumours with curative intent	**Gastric neuroendocrine neoplasms**
	• Type 1 tumours:
	  ▪ T1 and <2 cm: endoscopic resection
	  ▪ >T1 or >2 cm: limited surgery
	• Type 3 sporadic tumours: oncological resection
	
	Duodenal neuroendocrine neoplasms
	• Tumours <1 cm (T1): endoscopic excision or surgical resection only if periampullary
	• Tumours between 1 and 2 cm (T1): endoscopic resection if feasible
	• Tumours >2 cm (>T2) or grade 3: surgical resection
	
	Colonic neuroendocrine neoplasms
	• Tumours <2 cm (T1): endoscopic polypectomy if feasible
	• Tumours >2 cm or grade 3 (or >T1): typical colectomy with lymphadenectomy
	
	Rectal neuroendocrine tumours
	• Tumours <2 cm (T1): endoscopic resection (using an endoscopic mucosal resection technique) or transanal endoscopic microsurgery (TEM)
	• Tumours >2 cm (or >T1): standard locoregional resection, including low anterior resection and abdominoperineal excision
	
	Pancreatic neoplasms
	• Tumours <2 cm:
	  ▪ Surveillance if asymptomatic (depending on patient age and other co-factors)
	  ▪ When symptomatic: pancreatic resection (classical or atypical pancreas-sparing resections)
	• Tumours >2 cm: standard pancreatectomy according to the tumour site (i.e. pancreaticoduodenectomy or distal pancreatectomy) associated with regional lymphadenectomy
	
	Jejunal and ileal tumours
	• Segmental resection with wide lymphadenectomy

Surgery	Description

	Appendiceal neuroendocrine tumours
	• Tumours <2 cm: simple appendectomy (with no poor pathological features^)
	• Tumours >2 cm (or <2 cm with poor pathological features*): right-sided hemicolectomy
	
	*Deep (>3 mm) mesoappendiceal invasion or lymphovascular invasion
	
	Bronchopulmonary neuroendocrine tumours
	• Main therapy is surgical resection
	• Dependent on the size, location and tissue type:
	    ▪ Surgical techniques of choice are lobectomy or sleeve resection
	    ▪ Pneumonectomy should be avoided except in selected cases
	• Systemic nodal dissection should be performed since lymphonodal metastases may be present in up to 25% of cases in typical carcinoids and >50% in atypical carcinoids
	• Protracted follow-up should always be performed, including in patients who have undergone radical operation

Locally-advanced non-metastatic disease	• Surgical approach with curative intent is always recommended in the presence of well-differentiated NEN (grade 1/2) • Surgery of advanced forms includes vascular resection and/or resection of nearby organs • Palliative surgery is mandatory in the presence of functional tumours with refractory syndrome

Metastatic disease	• *Curative surgery:*
	    ▪ Surgery with curative intent is limited to well-differentiated NEN (grade 1/2) regardless of the site of origin (foregut, midgut, hindgut):
	    ▪ Curative resection (R0/R1) for both midgut and hindgut tumours is associated with better survival
	        ○ Mortality and morbidity rates are 0–5% and 30%, respectively
	• *Palliative surgery:*
	    ▪ Presence of functionality is the most important factor influencing the decision for surgery
	    ▪ Debulking surgery (R2): decision to remove the majority (traditionally ≥90%) is associated with an improved quality of life, but benefit in terms of survival has not been demonstrated
	    ▪ Resection of the primary tumour may be recommended to avoid local complications such as intestinal occlusion, mesenteric retraction and haemorrhage (and allows therapy focused on a single organ, e.g. the liver)
	• *Liver transplantation:*
	    ▪ Rare selected cases
	    ▪ Requirements: absence of extrahepatic disease, previous removal of the primary tumour and the presence of a well-differentiated NEN (grade 1/2)
	    ▪ Also considered for those patients with severe endocrine syndrome refractory to all other treatments

Systemic therapy

Systemic therapy of NEN generally covers two biological aspects of the disease:
- Control of hormone hypersecretion symptoms (i.e. functionality)
- Control of proliferation.

Since some medications are effective for both situations, they are mentioned below in both scenarios.

While specific symptomatic therapy (i.e. antihormonal effects) needs to be considered in relation to the functional syndrome, medical antiproliferative treatment is considered according to NEN grading and primary tumour localization. In all cases, surgical resectability needs to be ruled out prior to the initiation of treatment. General principles of oncological treatment, such as antiemetics, prehydration and careful monitoring for toxicities are not specifically mentioned in the following sections.

Symptomatic therapy

Systemic therapy: symptomatic	Description
Carcinoid syndrome (CS)	• Somatostatin analogues (SSA) effectively control hypersecretion of serotonin and other mediators of CS: 　▪ Octreotide: 50–500 µg SC b.i.d. or t.i.d. 　▪ Octreotide long-acting release (LAR): 10–30 mg IM monthly 　▪ Lanreotide autogel: 60–120 mg deep SC monthly • Peri-interventional continuous IV infusion of SSA: initial 100 µg bolus, then 50 µg/hour (not approved but common practice (and recommended to avoid carcinoid crisis) • Somatostatin receptor–non-specific SSA: 　▪ Pasireotide 600–1200 µg SC b.i.d (not approved, under development) • Interferon-alpha (IFN-α) may also be used to control hypersecretion of serotonin and other mediators of CS: 　▪ IFN-α 2b: 3–5 MIU SC three times weekly 　▪ PEG IFN α 2b: 80–180 µg SC once weekly • Telotristate etiprate (tryptophan hydroxylase inhibitor) specifically inhibits synthesis of serotonin (under development)
Insulinoma syndrome (Whipple triad)	• Diazoxide controls insulin hypersecretion by inhibiting K_{ATP}-channels 　▪ 25–150 mg b.i.d. or t.i.d. • SSA may very effectively control insulin hypersecretion: • Everolimus may control insulin hypersecretion in refractory cases not amenable to surgical treatment: 　▪ 5–10 mg PO daily (not approved, individual approach)
Zollinger–Ellison syndrome (ZES; gastrinoma)	• Proton-pump inhibitors (PPI) very effectively control gastric acid hypersecretion of ZES: 　▪ Omeprazole: equivalent of 80 mg/day titrated according to symptoms and follow-up of acid studies and/or endoscopic findings • SSA may control hypersecretion of gastrin in cases of insufficient control by PPI
Glucagonoma syndrome	• Standard antidiabetic treatment • SSA effectively control hypersecretion of glucagon
Verner Morrison syndrome (VIPoma)	• SSA effectively control hypersecretion of VIP • Additional standard antidiarrhoeal treatment may be necessary: 　▪ Loperamide: 2–4 mg PO t.i.d. 　▪ Tinctura opii 1%: titrate according to effect 　▪ Careful fluid balance (blood bicarbonate/base excess, etc.)
Atypical carcinoid syndrome	• SSA may effectively control hypersecretion of histamine • Antihistaminic drugs may provide some additional antihistaminic symptom control

Systemic antiproliferative therapy

Systemic medical antiproliferative treatment of NEN generally needs to consider the following issues:
- Tumour grading (i.e. NEN grade 1/2 or NEC grade 3)
- Primary tumour localization (pancreatic NEN vs midgut/jejunoileal NEN vs other gastrointestinal NEN)
- Tumour velocity (kinetics) according to previous treatment (partial response/stable disease/progressive disease)
- Clinical TNM stage and hepatic and extrahepatic tumour load (Stage III or IV, hepatic tumour load <10%, <50%, >50%)
- Clinical symptoms (pain, weight loss, fatigue, insufficiently controlled functional syndromes, etc.)

In cases of cancer of unknown primary (CUP), imaging studies and/or immunohistochemistry may be considered to locate a primary to a specific region and aid the choice of treatment strategy:

- Imaging, e.g. mesenteric lymph nodes suggest a non-detected midgut primary
- Immunohistochemistry:
  - Serotonin positivity suggests an undetectable midgut primary
  - CDX-2 positivity suggests a non-pancreatic gastrointestinal primary
  - ISL-1 positivity suggests a pancreatic primary
  - TTF-1 positivity suggests a bronchopulmonary primary.

If there is no indication of the specific region of the primary, treatment options for other gastrointestinal/bronchial NEN should be considered.

In general, antiproliferative medical treatment options include:
- *Biotherapy* with peptide analogues to physiological oligo- or poly-peptides (SSA or IFN-α)

- Classical *chemotherapy* as single or combination protocols with either IV or PO administration or a combination of both
- *Molecular targeted therapy* such as the mTOR inhibitor everolimus, the multikinase inhibitor sunitinib, or the monoclonal vascular endothelial growth factor (VEGF) antibody bevacizumab.

Systemic antiproliferative therapy in pancreatic NEN

There are a number of treatment options for progressive pancreatic NEN grade 1/2; however, no evidence-based recommendations with regard to the order in which these should be applied exist. Most guidelines recommend first-line streptozotocin (STZ)-based chemotherapy, followed by either molecular targeted therapies or temozolomide-based chemotherapy (depending on availability and approval status in the respective country), peptide receptor radiotherapy (PRRT) (in cases of SSTR-2-receptor positive NEN) and ultimately (with least data available), oxaliplatinum-based chemotherapy in cases of rapidly progressing NEN in spite of low-to-intermediate proliferative index (grade 1/2).

Systemic therapy: Antiproliferative pancreatic NEN (grade 1/2)	Description

Chemotherapy (streptozotocin based)	• Combination chemotherapy of STZ with either 5-fluorouracil (5-FU) or doxorubicin (DOX) induces a partial response (PR) in 30–40% and stable disease (SD) in an additional 20–30% (data form outdated Phase III studies and some phase II trials)
	• Example regimens:
	  ■ STZ + 5-FU:
	    ○ STZ 500 mg/m² body surface area (BSA) IV over 1 hour, Days 1–5
	    ○ 5-FU 400 mg/m² BSA IV as bolus, Days 1–5
	    ○ Repeat both on Day 43
	    ○ Treat until best response or for nine cycles
	  ■ STZ + DOX:
	    ○ STZ 500 mg/m² BSA IV over 1 hour, Days 1–5
	    ○ DOX 50 mg/m² BSA IV over 1 hour, Days 1 and 22
	    ○ Repeat both on Day 43
	    ○ Treat until best response or for nine cycles
	    ○ CAVE: cumulative DOX dose: 500 mg/m²

Molecular targeted therapy (everolimus)	• Induces SD/PR in approximately 70% and prolongs progression-free survival (PFS) against placebo from 4.6 to 11.0 months (phase III study) • 10 mg daily • Treat until PD
Molecular targeted therapy (sunitinib)	• Induces SD/PR in approximately 70% and prolongs PFS against placebo from 5.5 to 14.0 months (phase III study) • 37.5 mg daily • Treat until PD
Chemotherapy (temozolomide based)	• Combination chemotherapy of temozolomide (TMZ) with capecitabine (CAP) induces PR in 40–70% and SD in an additional 20% (phase II study) • TMZ: 200 mg/m² BSA PO daily, Days 10–14 • CAP: 750 mg/m² BSA PO b.i.d., Days 1–1 • Repeat both on Day 30 • Treat until PD Not approved by authorities
Biotherapy (somatostatin analogues)	• Appear to increase PFS compared to placebo (phase III CLARINET trial: early positive results presented at ESMO 2013, not currently approved)

Chemotherapy: (oxaliplatin based)	• Combination chemotherapy of oxaliplatin (OX) with either 5-FU and leucovorin (folinic acid [FOL]) (FOLFOX) or capecitabine (CAP) may induce tumour control in 30–40% of rapidly progressing pancreatic NEN or such with high tumour load (evidence from phase II trials only)
	• FOLFOX:
	  ■ OX: 85 mg/m² BSA IV over 2 hours, Day 1
	  ■ FOL: 200 mg/m² BSA IV over 2 hours, Days 1 and 2
	  ■ 5-FU: 400 mg/m² BSA IV as bolus, Days 1 and 2
	  ■ 5-FU: 600 mg/m² BSA 22-hour infusion, Days 1 and 2
	  ■ Repeat cycle on Day 15
	  ■ Treat until PD (not approved by authorities)

(continued)

Systemic therapy: Antiproliferative pancreatic NEN (grade 1/2)	Description

	• CAPOX:
	  ■ OX: 130 mg/m² BSA IV over 2 hours, Day 1
	  ■ CAP: 1000 mg/m² BSA PO b.i.d., Days 2–15
	  ■ Repeat both on Day 21
	  ■ Treat until PD (not approved by authorities)

Molecular targeted therapy (bevacizumab)	• Bevacizumab may induce prolonged PFS as a reserve medication alone or in combination with SSA or TMZ
	• Bevacizumab in combination with SSA:
	  ■ 15 mg/kg IV over 1–2 hours, Day 1
	  ■ Repeat on Day 21
	  ■ Treat until PD (not approved by authorities)
	• Bevacizumab in combination with TMZ:
	  ■ 5 mg/kg IV over 1–2 hours, Day 1
	  ■ Repeat on Day 15
	  ■ Treat until PD (not approved by authorities)

Systemic antiproliferative therapy in midgut/jejunoileal NEN

For progressive midgut/jejunoileal NEN (SI-NEN), probably due to a different tumour biology resulting in a lower proliferative index in most cases, the treatment options differ significantly from those for pancreatic NEN. Tumour growth inhibition using molecular pathways that are either receptor mediated (SSA and IFN) or via inhibition of cellular signalling pathways (everolimus and, possibly, sunitinib) are the most effective options for controlling NEN proliferation. SI-NEN should for the large part be considered chemotherapy insensitive. However, in the very rare case of a highly proliferative and rapidly progressing SI-NEN, a chemotherapy trial with either a TMZ-based regimen or a regimen suitable for NEC grade 3 may be considered. The actual proliferative index may be re-evaluated prior to such a decision to target the high proliferative capacity and thus aggressively and urgently treat the NEN disease.

Systemic therapy: Antiproliferative midgut/jejunoileal NEN (grade 1/2)	Description
Biotherapy (somatostatin analogues)	• Increases SD from 37% to 67% and prolongs PFS from 6.0 to 14.3 months, both compared to placebo (phase III trial of sandostatin LAR vs placebo) • Octreotide LAR: 30 mg IM monthly • Lanreotide autogel: 120 mg deep SC monthly (phase III CLARINET trial: early positive results presented at ESMO 2013, not currently approved)
Molecular targeted therapy (everolimus)	• May induce tumour shrinkage in approximately 75% vs 45% and prolong PFS from 11.3 to 16.4 months, both compared to placebo (Radiant 2 phase III trial of everolimus vs placebo); this did not achieve statistical significance • 10 mg daily (not approved by authorities)

Chemotherapy (temozolomide based)	• TMZ alone or in combination with CAP (TEMCAP) may induce tumour control in up to 40% of pretreated SI-NEN
	• TMZ single therapy 100 mg/m² BSA PO daily, Days 1–5:
	  ■ Repeat on Day 29
	  ■ Escalate dose to 200 mg/m² BSA if tolerated
	  ■ Treat until PD (not approved by authorities)
	• For TEMCAP-protocol, see pancreatic NEN section

Molecular targeted therapy (sunitinib)	• May be an option for SI-NEN in the future • Currently being investigated in combination with SSA (phase III SUNLAND trial)

Systemic antiproliferative therapy in NEN from other parts of the gastrointestinal tract or from the bronchial tract

For progressive NEN grade 1/2 from other parts of the gastrointestinal tract (i.e. stomach, duodenum, rectum and CUP-NEN) and from the bronchial tract (GI- or bNEN), very limited data and no specific studies on systemic medical treatments have been published. However, by extrapolating from published studies and the other entities, the following approaches have been recommended on a common-sense basis (and according to consensus guidelines). Peptide receptor radionuclide therapy (PRRT) may be considered early in these patients due to lack of other specifically established treatment options.

Systemic therapy: Antiproliferative other gastrointestinal and bronchial NEN (grade 1/2)	Description
Biotherapy (somatostatin analogues)	• May be a future option but have not been systematically and prospectively studied • For treatment protocols, see pancreatic NEN or SI-NEN sections
Molecular targeted therapy (everolimus)	• May also be a future option and is currently under investigation for some non–pancreatic-and jejunoileal-NEN (RADIANT-IV trial) • For treatment protocols, see pancreatic NEN or SI-NEN sections
Chemotherapy (temozolomide based)	• TMZ alone or in combination with capecitabine (TEMCAP) may also induce some tumour control, but has not been systematically and prospectively studied • For treatment protocols, see pancreatic NEN or SI-NEN sections
Chemotherapy (oxaliplatin based)	• May be an individual option, particularly in rapidly progressing GI- or bNEN, but has not been systematically and prospectively studied • For treatment protocol, see pancreatic NEN section
Chemotherapy (streptozotocin based)	• May be an individual option particularly for foregut NEN (bronchial, thymic, gastric), but has not been systematically and prospectively studied • For treatment protocols, see pNEN section

Systemic antiproliferative therapy in NEC

Highly proliferative, poorly differentiated NEC grade 3 requires a systemic combination chemotherapy regimen. Currently, only first-line data using cisplatinum or carboplatinum in combination with etoposide have been studied prospectively. However, retrospective data are available for TMZ-based regimens in NEC grade 3 with a Ki-67 index between 20% and 60% and for irinotecan-based treatment in the second-line situation, as well as for oxaliplatinum-based regimens. Whether the latter is still effective after prior use of a cisplatinum- or carboplatinum-based chemotherapy has not been studied, but it may be considered on an individual base.

Systemic therapy: Antiproliferative NEC (grade 3)	Description
Chemotherapy (cisplatinum based)	• Combination chemotherapy of cisplatinum + etoposide (VP16) induces a complete response (CR)/PR in 60–70% with a time to progression (TTP) of approximately 9–11 months • Cisplatinum: 45 mg/m^2 BSA IV over 1–2 hours, Days 2 and 3 • Etoposide: 130 mg/m^2 BSA IV over 1–2 hours, Days 1–3 • Repeat both on Day 29 • Treat until PD (not approved by authorities)
Chemotherapy (oxaliplatin based)	• Combination chemotherapy of oxaliplatin (OX) with either 5-FU and leucovorin (folinic acid [FOL]) (FOLFOX) or capecitabine (CAP) may induce tumour control in 30–40% or provide a less toxic alternative to the cisplatinum + etoposide protocol • For FOLFOX protocol, see pancreatic NEN section • For CAPOX protocol, see pancreatic NEN section
Chemotherapy (temozolomide based)	• TMZ in combination with capecitabine (TEMCAP) may also induce some tumour control in NEC of non-small cell phenotype with a Ki-67 index below 60%, but has not been systematically and prospectively studied • For treatment protocol, see pancreatic NEN section

Chemotherapy (irinotecan based)	• Combination chemotherapy of irinotecan (IRI) with 5-FU and leucovorin (folinic acid [FOL]) (FOLFIRI) may induce tumour control in 30–40% as a second-line therapy
	• FOLFIRI:
	  ▪ IRI 180 mg/m^2 BSA IV over 2 hours, Day 1
	  ▪ FOL 400 mg/m^2 BSA IV over 2 hours, Day 1
	  ▪ 5-FU 400 mg/m^2 BSA IV as bolus, Day 1
	  ▪ 5-FU 1200 mg/m^2 BSA IV over 46 hours, Days 1 and 2
	  ▪ Repeat cycle on Day 15
	  ▪ Treat until PD (not approved by authorities)

Other forms of therapy
Peptide receptor radionuclide therapy

The majority of GEP-NEN express somatostatin receptors and can be treated with PRRT with radiolabelled somatostatin analogues (Fig. 50.1). The most commonly used analogues in PRRT are [^{90}Y-DOTA^0, Tyr^3]octreotide and [^{177}Lu-DOTA^0, Tyr^3]octreotate. Response and survival data with this modality are given in Table 50.11. Tumours must have high avidity on somatostatin receptor scintigraphy to be considered for PRRT. To date no Phase III data have been published.

Peptide receptor radionuclide therapy	Description
Early disease	- No role

Metastatic disease	- PRRT as therapy
	- Cumulative dose:
	  - [^{90}Y-DOTA^0, Tyr^3]-octreotide: usually 360 mCi (two to four cycles)
	  - [^{177}Lu-DOTA^0, Tyr^3]octreotate: usually 800 mCi (four cycles)
	- *Important inclusion criteria*:
	  - Inoperable/metastatic well-differentiated (grade 1/2) NEN
	  - Sufficient tumour uptake on diagnostic somatostatin receptor scintigraphy
	  - Sufficient bone marrow reserve (grade 1/2 haematological toxicity is usually accepted)
	  - Creatinine clearance of >50 mL/min
	  - Karnofsky performance score of >50
	  - Signed informed consent
	- *Side effects*:
	  - Acute:
	    - Nausea after 25% of administrations
	    - Vomiting after 10% of administrations
	    - (Abdominal) Pain after 10% of administrations
	    - Temporary hair loss in 60% of patients after [^{177}Lu-DOTA^0, Tyr^3]octreotate
	    - Grade 3/4 haematological toxicity in <15% of patients
	    - Hormonal crises in <1% of patients
	  - Long term:
	    - [^{90}Y-DOTA^0, Tyr^3]octreotide:
	      – Renal insufficiency in 1–9%
	      – Myelodysplastic syndrome (MDS) in 2%
	    - [^{177}Lu-DOTA^0, Tyr^3]octreotate:
	      – Renal insufficiency in <1%
	      – MDS in 1–2%)

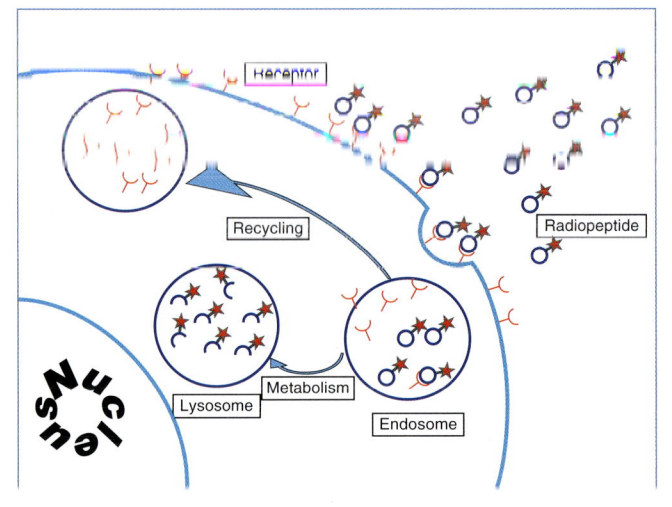

Figure 50.1 Mechanism of action of PRRT. The radiolabelled somatostatin analogues are internalized, and the breakdown products of the radiolabelled peptides are stored in lysosomes, thus enabling a long irradiation of tumour cells.

Symptoms and quality of life
- [^{177}Lu-DOTA^0, Tyr^3]octreotate: 265 Dutch patients; EORTC QLQ-C30 questionnaire:
  - Improved Global Health Score in 36% who scored suboptimally at baseline
  - Improved symptomatology in 40–70% of patients who had certain symptoms

Other studies
- Combinations of ^{90}Y- and ^{177}Lu-labelled peptides:
  - Three retrospective human studies reporting better PFS
  - No randomized trials
- Intra-arterial PRRT for liver-predominant disease:
  - Better response rates reported in several studies
  - No data on PFS
  - No randomized trials
- Chemosensitization:
  - No data
  - Randomized trial ongoing
- Neoadjuvant PRRT for pancreatic NEN:
  - Several case report but no real evidence exists
  - No randomized trials
- Adjuvant PRRT:
  - No data

Registration trials
- [^{177}Lu-DOTA^0, Tyr^3]octreotate vs high-dose somatostatin analogues in patients with metastatic NEN of midgut origin, and which are progressive under somatostatin analogue treatment:
  - Primary endpoint: PFS
  - Trial started 2012 in the European Community and the USA

Table 50.11 Tumour response and survival data with PRRT

Centre	Ligand	Patients	Objective response (%)	PFS (months)	OS (months)
Milan	[^{90}Y-DOTA^0, Tyr^3]octreotide	21	29		
Basel	[^{90}Y-DOTA^0, Tyr^3]octreotide	74	24		
Basel	[^{90}Y-DOTA^0, Tyr^3]octreotide	33	33		
Multicentre	[^{90}Y-DOTA^0, Tyr^3]octreotide	58	9	29	37
Multicentre	[^{90}Y-DOTA^0, Tyr^3]octreotide	90	4	16	27
Copenhagen	[^{90}Y-DOTA^0, Tyr^3]octreotide	53	23	29	
Warsaw	[^{90}Y-DOTA^0, Tyr^3]octreotide	58	23	17	22
Rotterdam	[^{177}Lu-DOTA^0, Tyr^3]octreotate	310	29	33	46
Gothenburg	[^{177}Lu-DOTA^0, Tyr^3]octreotate	26	38		
Lund	[^{177}Lu-DOTA^0, Tyr^3]octreotate	12	17		
Milan	[^{177}Lu-DOTA^0, Tyr^3]octreotate	42	31		

- [^{177}Lu-DOTA^0,Tyr^3]octreotate vs everolimus or sunitinib in patients with pancreatic NEN:
  - Primary endpoint: PFS
  - Trial comparing PRRT to high-dose octreotide near completion (2015) in the European Community and the USA

Transarterial embolization and chemoembolization

Transarterial chemoembolization (TACE) is based on the administration of a cytotoxic agent (streptozotocin or doxorubicin) directly into the hepatic artery followed by a transient embolization, inducing ischaemia in the metastases. Bland embolization without concomitant cytotoxics may be as effective as TACE.

- *Indications:*
  - Controls symptoms in functional tumours (e.g. carcinoid syndrome, VIPoma)
  - Antiproliferative control
- *Results:*
  - Tumour response in 1/3 of cases
  - Symptomatic response is seen in 60–95%
- *Contraindications:*
  - Portal venous thrombosis
  - Hepatic insufficiency
  - Biliary–digestive anastomosis
- *Side effects:*
  - Postembolization syndrome (abdominal pain, nausea, vomiting, fever and an increase in hepatic transaminases); frequent but usually mild
  - Severe but rare complications:
    - Liver failure, cholecystitis, gastric ulcers, liver abscess
    - Carcinoid crisis
  - In case of a large tumour burden, to limit adverse events, the liver can be treated on one side over two sessions (interval of 4–8 weeks)

Radioembolization for liver metastases in NEN

Radioembolization is based on the administration of radiolabelled (^{90}Y is most commonly used) microspheres (mostly resin or glass), which will strand in the small arteries, as a selective internal radiotherapy (SIRT) through the hepatic transarterial approach.

- *Response rates:*
  - 40–65% (median duration of therapeutic effect not reported)
- *Main contraindications:*
  - Shunt of 20% or more to the vascular bed of the lungs, and therefore a pretherapeutic scintigraphy with ^{99m}Tc-labelled microparticles (macroaggregated albumin) should be performed
- *Specific complications:*
  - Radiation-induced liver disease, hepatic abscess
  - Arterial shunting to the lung, radiation
  - Microsphere-induced gastric ulceration and bleeding
  - Acute cholecystitis or acute pancreatitis

Phase III clinical trials

For trials in NEN grade 1/2, see Table 50.12.

There are no phase III clinical trials in NEC, but one reported phase II trial for NEC grade 3:

- Moertel et al. (1990) Cancer 65(10 Suppl):2415–2418: Monocentric prospective phase II trial establishing the cis-platinum + etoposide protocol for 'anaplastic' NEC (likely large compared to NEC grade 3 of the WHO 2010 classification) (n = 45; 18 anaplastic NEC):
  - CR: 17%
  - PR: 50%
  - Median TTP: 11 months (range 2–21 months)
  - Median OS: 19 months (range 5–36 months)

Table 50.12 Phase III clinical trials in NEN (grade 1/2)

Trial name	Results

PROMID
Rinke et al. (2009) J Clin Oncol 27(28):4656–4663
	• Multicentric, placebo-controlled, phase III trial establishing the antiproliferative activity of the SSA octreotide in midgut NEN versus placebo (n = 85):
	  ▪ SD: 67% vs 37%
	  ▪ Median PFS: 14.3 vs 6.0 months; $P<0.001$
	  ▪ Median OS: not reached (>77.4 vs. 73.7 months; not statistically significant)

CLARINET Caplin et al. (2014) N Engl J Med. 371:224–233	• Multicentric, placebo-controlled, phase III trial establishing the antiproliferative activity of the SSA lanreotide in midgut and intestinal NEN versus placebo (n = 204): ▪ Median PFS: not reached vs 18 months; $P<0.0002$

RADIANT-3
Yao et al. (2011) N Engl J Med 364(6):514–523
	• Multicentric, placebo-controlled, phase III trial establishing the antiproliferative activity of everolimus in progressive pancreatic NEN versus placebo (n = 410):
	  ▪ PR + SD: 72.2% vs 25.9%
	  ▪ Median PFS: 11.4 vs 5.4 months; $P<0.001$
	  ▪ Median OS: not reached in both arms

Raymond et al. (2011) N Engl J Med 364(6):501–513	• Multicentric, placebo-controlled, phase III trial establishing the antiproliferative activity of sunitinib in progressive pancreatic NEN versus placebo (n = 171):
	  ▪ PR + SD: 72% vs 60%
	  ▪ Median PFS: 11.4 vs 5.5 months; $P<0.001$
	  ▪ Median OS: not reached in both arms

RADIANT-2
Pavel et al. (2011) Lancet 378:2005–2012
	• Multicentric, placebo-controlled, phase III trial investigating the antiproliferative activity of everolimus + concomitant SSA in progressive NEN with carcinoid syndrome versus placebo + SSA (n = 429):
	  ▪ PR + SD: 84% vs 81%
	  ▪ Median PFS: 16.4 vs 11.3 months; $P = 0.026$
	  ▪ Median OS: not reached in both arms

Moertel et al. (1992) N Engl J Med 326(8):519–523	• Multicentric, three-arm phase III trial in advanced pancreatic NEN comparing tumour response to antiproliferative treatment with STZ + DOX, STZ + 5-FU or chlorozotocin (n = 105)
	  ▪ CR+ 'any regression': 83% vs 49% vs 36%
	  ▪ Median PFS: 22 vs 13 vs 21 months
	  ▪ Median OS: 2.2 vs 1.4 vs 1.5 years; $P<0.001$
	  ▪ Comment: chlorozotocin, although more effective than STZ + 5-FU in this trial, is no longer available. This advantages has not been proven in further observational reports. Also, toxicity, particularly cardiotoxicity, has been a problem with STZ + DOX and thus, STZ + 5-FU is now the most commonly used and recommended chemotherapy regimen in pancreatic NEN

Recommended reading

Bergsma H, van Vliet EI, Teunissen JJ et al. (2012) Peptide receptor radionuclide therapy (PRRT) for GEP-NETs. Best Pract Res Clin Gastroenterol 26:867–881.

Bosman FT, Carneiro F (2010) WHO Classification of Tumours of Digestive System, 4th edn. Lyon: International Agency for Research on cancer (IARC).

Caplin M, Sundin A, Nillson O et al.; Barcelona Consensus Conference participants (2012) ENETS Consensus Guidelines for the management of patients with digestive neuroendocrine neoplasms: colorectal neuroendocrine neoplasms. Neuroendocrinology 95(2):88–97.

Delle Fave G, Kwekkeboom DJ, Van Cutsem E et al.; Barcelona Consensus Conference participants (2011) ENETS Consensus Guidelines for the management of patients with gastroduodenal neoplasms. Neuroendocrinology 95(2):74–87.

ENETS Consensus Guidelines for the Standard of Care for Patients with Digestive Neuroendocrine Tumors. Available at http://www.enets.org/guidelines_tnm_classifications.html

Falconi M, Bartsch DK, Eriksson B et al.; Barcelona Consensus Conference participants (2012) ENETS Consensus Guidelines for the management of patients with digestive neuroendocrine neoplasms of the digestive system: well-differentiated pancreatic non-functioning tumors. Neuroendocrinology 95(2):120–134.

Jensen RT, Cadiot G, Brandi ML et al.; Barcelona Consensus Conference participants (2012) ENETS Consensus Guidelines for the management of patients with digestive neuroendocrine neoplasms: functional pancreatic endocrine tumor syndromes. Neuroendocrinology 95(2):98–119.

Kianmanesh R, Ruszniewski P, Rindi G et al.; Palma de Mallorca Consensus Conference Participants (2010) ENETS consensus guidelines for the management of peritoneal carcinomatosis from neuroendocrine tumors. Neuroendocrinology 91(4):333–340.

Klöppel G, Rindi G, Perren A, Komminoth P, Klimstra DS (2010) The ENETS and AJCC/UICC TNM classifications of the neuroendocrine tumors of the gastrointestinal tract and the pancreas: a statement. Virchows Arch 456(6):595–597.

Kos-Kudła B, O'Toole D, Falconi M et al.; Palma de Mallorca Consensus Conference Participants (2010) ENETS consensus guidelines for the management of bone and lung metastases from neuroendocrine tumors. *Neuroendocrinology* 91(4):341–350.

Oberg K, Casanovas O, Castaño JP *et al.* (2013) Molecular pathogenesis of neuroendocrine tumors: implications for current and future therapeutic approaches. *Clin Cancer Res* 19(11):2842–2849.

Pape UF, Perren A, Niederle B *et al.*; Barcelona Consensus Conference participants (2012) ENETS Consensus Guidelines for the management of patients with neuroendocrine neoplasms from the jejunoileum and the appendix including goblet cell carcinomas. *Neuroendocrinology* 95(2):135–156.

Pavel M, Grossman A, Arnold R *et al.*; Palma de Mallorca Consensus Conference Participants (2010) ENETS consensus guidelines for the management of brain, cardiac and ovarian metastases from neuroendocrine tumors. *Neuroendocrinology* 91(4):326–332.

Pavel M, Baudin F, Couvelard A *et al.*; Barcelona Consensus Conference participants (2012) ENETS Consensus Guidelines for the management of patients with liver and other distant metastases from neuroendocrine neoplasms of foregut, midgut, hindgut, and unknown primary. *Neuroendocrinology* 95(2):157–176.

Pavel M, Kidd M, Modlin I (2013) Systemic therapeutic options for carcinoid. *Semin Oncol* 40(1):84–99.

Rindi G, Klöppel G, Alhman H *et al.*; all other Frascati Consensus Conference participants, European Neuroendocrine Tumor Society (ENETS) (2006) TNM staging of foregut (neuro)endocrine tumors: a consensus proposal including a grading system. *Virchows Arch* 449(4):395–401.

Rindi G, Arnold R, Bosman FT *et al.* (2010) Nomenclature and classification of neuroendocrine neoplasms of the digestive system. In: Bosman TF, Carneiro F, Hruban RH, Theise ND, eds. *WHO Classification of Tumours of the Digestive System*, 4th edn. Lyon: International Agency for Research on cancer (IARC):13.

Sundin A (2012) Radiological and nuclear medicine imaging of gastroenteropancreatic neuroendocrine tumours. *Best Pract Res Clin Gastroenterol* 26:803–818

Travis WD, Brambilla E (2004) Path Genetics Tumours of Lung Pleura Thymus Heart.

Yao JC, Hassan M, Phan A *et al.* (2008) One hundred years after "carcinoid": epidemiology of and prognostic factors for neuroendocrine tumors in 35,825 cases in the United States. *J Clin Oncol* 26(18):3063–3072.

Zappa M, Abdel-Rehim M, Hentic O, Vullierme MP, Ruszniewski P, Vilgrain V (2012) Liver-directed therapies in liver metastases from neuroendocrine tumors of the gastrointestinal tract. *Target Oncol* 7(2):107–116.

51 Skin

Basal cell carcinoma, squamous cell carcinoma and Merkel cell carcinoma

Sandro V. Porceddu[1], Michael J. Veness[2] and H. Peter Soyer[3]

[1]Princess Alexandra Hospital & School of Medicine, University of Queensland, Brisbane, Queensland, Australia
[2]Westmead Hospital and University of Sydney, Sydney, New South Wales, Australia
[3]Dermatology Research Centre, University of Queensland, School of Medicine, Translational Research Institute, Brisbane, Queensland, Australia

Category	Key facts
Introduction	• Non-melanoma skin cancer (NMSC) is the most common cancer worldwide • Mortality rates from basal cell carcinoma (BCC) and squamous cell carcinoma (SCC) are very low • Solar ultraviolet (UV) exposure is the most common cause • Prevention is aimed at education about risks of UV radiation and the need for reducing sun exposure
Presentation	• Commonly arise within sun-exposed or photodamaged areas • Four clinicopathological BCC types: nodular, superficial, morphoeic, fibroepithelial • SCC ranges from well to poorly differentiated • Merkel cell carcinomas (MCC) consist of small blue cells with hyperchromatic nuclei • Spread to regional nodes or distant sites is uncommon with BCC/SCC (≤5%), but more frequent with MCC (20–50%)
Scenario	• Surgery is the predominant treatment of choice as it provides high cure rates and histopathological information • Goal is complete removal of disease with optimal functional and cosmetic outcome • Radiotherapy (RT) is an alternative option where surgery is not an option due to medical unresectability, a technically difficult location or patient preference • High-risk patients warrant consideration of postoperative RT (PORT) • Options such as topical therapies may be considered for very superficial lesions, but may result in lower cure rates • Immunosuppression is a high-risk feature that increases the likelihood of local, regional and distant recurrence
Trials	• Paucity of phase III trials in skin cancer

Introduction

Non-melanoma skin cancer (NMSC) is the most common cancer observed worldwide. Basal cell carcinoma (BCC) is more common than squamous cell carcinoma (SCC), while Merkel cell carcinoma (MCC) is rare. They commonly occur on the head and neck region with solar radiation as the major causative agent.

Surgery is the predominant treatment modality as it provides histological information and high cure rates. With the exception of MCC and in the presence of immunosuppression, the development of regional and/or distant metastases is rare; if present, it is associated with a poorer prognosis. Patients with high-risk features warrant referral to specialist clinicians and multidisciplinary clinics.

UICC Manual of Clinical Oncology, Ninth Edition. Edited by Brian O'Sullivan, James D. Brierley, Anil K. D'Cruz, Martin F. Fey, Raphael Pollock, Jan B. Vermorken and Shao Hui Huang. © 2015 UICC. Published 2015 by John Wiley & Sons, Ltd.

Incidence, aetiology and screening

Incidence, aetiology and screening	Description

Incidence	**Basal and squamous cell carcinoma**
	• Exact global incidence is unknown as registries do not routinely report NMSC cases
	• Estimated >3.5 million cases of NMSC occurred in approximately 2.5 million individuals in the USA in 2006
	• BCC is the most common skin cancer in the world (incidence rates likely to be under-reported):
	  ▪ Increasing by 3–10% per year
	  ▪ Increases with age
	  ▪ Inversely associated with equatorial latitude
	• Australia has the highest rate of skin cancer:
	  ▪ BCC age-standardized incidence rate (ASIR): 884 per 100,000
	  ▪ SCC ASIR: 387 per 100,000
	• At younger age (<55 years), NMSC is more common in women
	• At older age, more common in men:
	  ▪ By 80 years male-to-female ratio: 2–3:1
	• Mortality rates are low:
	  ▪ Estimated age-standardized mortality rate (ASMR) for BCC: 0.12 per 100,000
	  ▪ Estimated ASMR for SCC: 0.26 per 100,000
	
	Merkel cell carcinoma
	• Increasing incidence:
	  ▪ Incidence of 0.2 per 100,000 Caucasians in the US population
	  ▪ Incidence has tripled in the last 40 years
	• More common in males
	• Incidence higher in older patients (median age 70 years)
	• Mortality rates 25–30%

Aetiology	**Basal and squamous cell carcinoma**
	• *Environmental exposure* (most common):
	  ▪ UV exposure:
	    ○ BCC: intermittent exposure
	    ○ SCC: cumulative exposure
	    ○ Lower threshold of solar exposure for malignant development to BCC
	  ▪ Ionizing radiation
	  ▪ Chemicals, e.g. arsenic
	  ▪ Infections, e.g. human papillomavirus (HPV) (SCC only)
	  ▪ Smoking (SCC only)
	• *Skin phenotype*:
	  ▪ Fair skin, red hair, freckling
	• *Genetic conditions*:
	  ▪ Xeroderma pigmentosum
	  ▪ Nevoid BCC (NBCC) syndrome (also known as Gorlin syndrome)
	• *Immunosuppression*:
	  ▪ Solid organ transplantation
	  ▪ Long-term oral corticosteroid use
	  ▪ Immunosuppressive conditions, e.g. chronic lymphocytic leukaemia, human immunodeficiency virus (HIV)
	• *Other*:
	  ▪ Previous BCC or SCC
	  ▪ Chronic ulcers, sinus tracts and scars
	  ▪ Long-standing inflammatory skin conditions, e.g. chronic discoid lupus erythematosus, lichen sclerosus and atrophicus
	  ▪ Long-term PUVA
	
	Merkel cell carcinoma
	• *Environmental*:
	  ▪ UV exposure
	• *Viral* (probable):
	  ▪ Merkel cell polyomavirus (MCV) may play a role
	• *Immunosuppression*

(continued)

Incidence, aetiology and screening	Description

Screening and prevention	- Prevention aimed at education about risks of UV radiation and need for reduction of sun exposure:
	   - Sunscreen
	   - Protective clothing/hats
	- Advise against artificial UV radiation tanning devices
	- Early detection by:
	   - Public education to seek prompt medical advice
	   - Improving diagnostic skills of clinicians
	- Diets high in antioxidant-rich foods and green leafy vegetables reduce risk of SCC in high-risk patients
	- Reduction/cessation of immunosuppressive drugs if possible
	- Retinoids used as prophylaxis against skin cancer development in solid organ transplant recipients, patients with NBCC syndrome and patients with multiple NMSC

Pathology

Pathology	Description

Basal cell carcinoma	- Common feature: aggregations of follicular germinative (basaloid) cells within a variable fibromyxoid stroma:
	   - Cells are characterized by small, oval, monomorphous nuclei and scant cytoplasm
	   - Cells at the periphery of aggregations are columnar and arranged in a palisade
	   - Clefts (retraction spaces) between aggregations of basaloid cells and adjacent stroma are characteristic when present
	- Numerous (>20) morphological subtypes with no universally accepted classification system:
	   - Transitions between patterns are commonly observed
	- Four major clinicopathological types:
	   - *Nodular*:
	      ○ Large round or oval aggregations of basaloid cells extending into the reticular dermis
	      ○ Cystic or nodulocystic variant consists of mucinous pools
	      ○ Micronodular variant is composed of smaller aggregations of basaloid cells extending into the reticular dermis
	   - *Superficial*:
	      ○ Small buds of basaloid cells extending from the epidermis and confined to the papillary dermis
	      ○ Skip lesions along the epidermis, which are actually interconnected, resulting in the inaccurate description *multifocal superficial*
	   - *Morphoeic (morpheiform)*:
	      ○ Similar histopathological features to sclerosing, fibrosing and infiltrative variants
	      ○ Fibrotic/sclerotic component sometimes predominates over the epithelial component characterized by strands and cords of basoloid cells
	      ○ Usually no peripheral palisading
	      ○ Commonly a nodular component observed in the upper part
	   - *Fibroepithelial (fibroepithelioma of Pinkus)*:
	      ○ Fenestrated by cords and columns of pink-staining epithelial cells and by abundant fibroplasia
	      ○ Blue-staining germ-like structures protrude from the epithelial columns

Squamous cell carcinoma (invasive)	- Defined as invasive when extending into the dermis
	- Differentiation ranges from well to poorly to undifferentiated:
	   - *Well differentiated*:
	      ○ Aggregations of eosinophilic keratinocytes containing nuclei with some degree of pleomorphism and mitoses
	      ○ Intercellular bridges (desmosomes), keratin pearls and apoptotic cells are common
	   - *Poorly differentiated*:
	      ○ Progressive and overlapping features with well-differentiated SCC with lack of overt keratinization
	      ○ Highly infiltrative and sometimes spindle cell morphology
	      ○ More commonly associated with stromal sclerosis, desmoplasia and neurotropism
	      ○ Immunostaining for cytokeratin can help distinguish them from melanoma and certain sarcomas
	- Related conditions:
	   - Actinic keratosis (also known as solar keratosis)

Pathology	Description

	- Proliferation of atypical keratinocytes beginning in the basal layer and confined to the epidermis
	- Several histopathological variants have been described, including pigmented, acantholytic, atrophic, bowenoid, lichenoid, hypertrophic (hyperkeratotic)
	- Basosquamous cell carcinoma:
	  - Variable definitions
	  - Mixed histopathological features of BCC and SCC or BCC with presence of keratinization

Squamous cell carcinoma (*in situ*)	- Commonly called Bowen disease - Clinical variants include pigmented (due to melanin) and verrucous - Full-thickness atypia of epidermis over a broad zone and atypical keratinocytes extend down the adnexa (in contrast to actinic keratosis) - Pleomorphic nuclei and apoptotic cells are florid - Diffuse confluent parakeratosis more common than in actinic keratosis
Keratoacanthoma (KA)	- Unknown whether it is part of the well-differentiated spectrum of SCC or a benign tumour (pseudomalignancy) - Typically a crater-like architecture with a central keratin core - Well-differentiated keratinocytes with brightly eosinophilic glassy cytoplasm - Neurotropism may be present - Fibrosis seen at the base in the regressive phase

Merkel cell carcinoma	- Normal Merkel cells are located at the dermoepidermal junction
	- Proposed neural crest origin
	- Small blue cells with hyperchromatic nuclei
	- Mitoses common; minimal cytoplasm
	- Three cellular patterns:
	  - Intermediate (most common)
	  - Small cell
	  - Trabecular
	  - Histopathological variants not prognostic
	- Commonly CK20 and CD56 positive
	- Thyroid transcription factor 1 (TTF-1) negative

Presentation and natural history

NMSC typically arises from sun-exposed or photodamaged areas such as the head, extremities and trunk. There are four common clinicopathological variants of BCC. Invasive SCC can present with a variety of appearances and grow at variable rates with doubling times ranging from weeks to months. They can either arise de novo or from pre-existing SCC *in situ* and actinic keratoses. KA typically grow rapidly over a period of weeks to months, forming a lesion with raised edges and a keratotic core, and then spontaneously regress over many months leaving a residual scar. The exact cause of these lesions is unknown. Because of their rarity, the diagnosis of MCC can often be delayed. They tend to be more aggressive tumours with a high propensity for spread in-transit, to lymph nodes and distantly.

Presentation and natural history	Description

Basal cell carcinoma	- Arise within photodamaged skin commonly on trunk and face
	- Usually amelanotic but can be pigmented, especially in Asians
	- *Nodular*:
	  - Most common subtype (50%)
	  - Commonly occurs on face (forehead, nasolabial)
	  - Rarely seen on non–hair-bearing regions
	  - Papule or nodule, pearly raised edges, telangiectasia, haemorrhagic central crust, ulceration (rodent ulcer)
	- *Superficial*:
	  - Usually occurs at a younger age compared with other subtypes

(continued)

Presentation and natural history	Description

	■ Commonly on trunk and extremities, multiple lesions
	■ Erythematous macules/plaques, shiny, scaly
	■ Growth pattern is typically horizontal with thin rolled edges
	• *Morphoeic*:
	  ■ Less common subtype
	  ■ Similar body site distribution to nodular
	  ■ Pale lesion resembling a scar with ill-defined borders
	  ■ Smooth surface with areas of ulceration, crust and telangectasia
	  ■ Aggressive local behaviour
	• *Fibroepithelial*:
	  ■ Rare
	  ■ Commonly on trunk, especially lower back
	  ■ Skin- or pink-coloured sessile plaque or pedunculated nodule

Squamous cell carcinoma (invasive)	• Usually arises within photodamaged skin • Common sites are the scalp, face, neck, forearms, dorsum of hands, shins • Present with a variety of appearances including skin-coloured, erythematous or pigmented (less common), papulonodular, plaque, papillomatous, exophytic, ulcerative, crusting • Rate of growth varies widely with doubling time ranging from many months to weeks • Can be associated with pain and neurological symptoms; suggest perineural invasion (PNI)
Squamous cell carcinoma (*in situ*)	• Commonly arise within sun-exposed areas • Scaly erythematous plaques • Arise *de novo* or within AK

Keratoacanthoma	• Mostly occur on sun-exposed areas
	• Rapidly enlarging lesion which develops into a well-circumscribed, crateriform nodule with a keratotic core and may resolve slowly over weeks to months
	• May leave scarring
	• Common variant is solitary KA
	• Other variants:
	  ■ Multiple
	  ■ Grouped
	  ■ Giant
	  ■ Centrifugum marginatum
	  ■ Subungual
	• Associated with syndromes:
	  ■ Multiple spontaneously regressing (Ferguson–Smith)
	  ■ Multiple non-regressing, generalized eruptive (Grzybowski)
	  ■ Muir–Torre syndrome
	• Associated with infections (HPV), chemical exposure, immunosuppression

Merkel cell carcinoma	• Difficult to diagnose clinically: ■ Delay in diagnosis due to rarity; under-diagnosis as benign lesion • Rapid growth (<3 months) in majority • Blue or violaceous colour • Epidermis commonly intact • Rarely arises in non–sun-exposed areas

Routes of spread

Routes of spread		Description
Basal cell carcinoma	Regional (nodal)	• <1% involvement at diagnosis or as site of relapse
	Distant	• <0.1% involvement at diagnosis or as site of distant relapse

Routes of spread		Description
Squamous cell carcinoma	Regional (nodal)	• ≤5% involvement at diagnosis or as site of relapse • Associated with high-risk primary disease • 10–15% of head and neck cases have no identifiable index lesion
	Distant	• 1–2% will develop distant relapse • Sites include bone, lung, liver and brain • Development of metastases tends to be sequential; initially regional nodes then distant sites • Isolated distant metastases are uncommon
Merkel cell carcinoma	Regional (nodal)	• 30–50% at diagnosis • 15–20% have unknown index lesion • More commonly seen with groin nodes
	Distant	• ~5% at diagnosis • 20–30% distant relapse • Metastases occur at almost any site, commonly lung

Diagnostic work-up (Table 51.1)

A clinical history and physical examination, including any change in or symptomatology of a skin lesion, is essential. Dermoscopy, performed by an appropriately trained clinician, can enhance the diagnosis of a BCC by visualizing specific dermoscopic criteria, such as arborizing vessels, typical for BCC. Stretching the skin assists with determining the variant of BCC. Biopsy techniques, such as shave, punch, incisional or excisional, may be appropriate. Biopsy should precede management of a single erythematous scaling lesion. Diagnostic imaging, such as computed axial tomography (CT) or magnetic resonance imaging (MRI) to assess regional lymph node involvement or distant spread, should be performed when suspected. The threshold for performing diagnostic imaging is lower in the presence of high-risk features, particularly for SCC, suspicion of perineural involvement (PNI), immunosuppression or MCC.

Staging and prognostic risk grouping

UICC TNM staging
See Table 51.2.

Prognostic factors
See Tables 51.3 and 51.4.
- BCC and SCC generally share the same risk factors for local and regional recurrence (see Table 51.3)
- Factors that predict for local recurrence generally tend also to predict for risk of nodal involvement/relapse
- Division into low and high risk is arbitrary as it forms part of a continuous spectrum
- Majority of recurrences (primary/nodal) occur within ≤2 years of the initial primary diagnosis
- Risk factors for MCC are slightly different from those for BCC and SCC (see Table 51.3)

Table 51.1 Key patient and tumour features to elicit in the diagnostic work-up

Patient profile	Tumour profile	Tumour extent

Age
Sex
Skin type
Sun exposure
Previous precancerous/skin cancer, scarring
Previous treatment
Smoking (for SCC)
Carcinogenic exposure
Genetic risk factors
Family history
Immunosuppression
	Type:
	• BCC:
	  ▪ Subtypes
	• SCC:
	  ▪ *In situ*
	  ▪ invasive
	• MCC
	• Other, e.g. basosquamous
	Location
	Size
	Depth and invasion into other structures
	Borders; well vs poorly defined
	Differentiation
	Rate of growth
	PNI and/or lymphovascular space invasion (LVSI)
	De novo vs recurrent
		Local:
		• Single
		• Multiple
		Spread:
		• Regional
		• Distant
		Diagnostic imaging where extensive disease is suspected

Table 51.2 UICC TNM categories and stage grouping: Carcinoma of skin of eyelid and Merkel cell carcinoma

TNM categories: Carcinoma of skin of eyelid	
T1	≤5 mm, not in tarsal plate or lid margin
T2a	>5–10 mm or tarsal plate or lid margin
T2b	>10–20 mm or full thickness eyelid
T3a	>20 mm or adjacent ocular/orbital structures, perineural
T3b	Needs enucleation, exenteration, or bone resection
T4	Not resectable due to extensive invasion
N1	Regional
M1	Distant metastasis

Stage grouping: Carcinoma of skin of eyelid			
Stage 0	Tis	N0	M0
Stage IA	T1	N0	M0
Stage IB	T2a	N0	M0
Stage IC	T2b	N0	M0
Stage II	T3a	N0	M0
Stage IIIA	T3b	N0	M0
Stage IIIB	Any T	N1	M0
Stage IIIC	T4	Any N	M0
Stage IV	Any T	Any N	M1

TNM categories: Merkel cell carcinoma		
T1		≤2 cm
T2		>2–5 cm
T3		>5 cm
T4		Deep extradermal structures (cartilage, skeletal muscle, fascia, bone)
N1		Regional
	N1a	Microscopic
	N1b	Macroscopic
N2		In-transit metastasis
M1		Distant metastasis
	M1a	Skin, subcutaneous tissues or non-regional lymph nodes
	M1b	Lung
	M1c	Other site(s)

Stage grouping: Merkel cell carcinoma			
Stage 0	Tis	N0	M0
Stage I	T1	N0	M0
Stage IA	T1	pN0	M0
Stage IB	T1	cN0	M0
Stage IIA	T2, T3	pN0	M0
Stage IIB	T2, T3	cN0	M0
Stage IIC	T4	N0	M0
Stage IIIA	Any T	N1a	M0
Stage IIIB	Any T	N1b, N2	M0
Stage IV	Any T	Any N	M1

Table 51.3 Prognostic factors for low- and high-risk BCC, SCC and MCC

Prognostic factors	Low risk	High risk
BCC and SCC		
Location/area	Area: • L <20 mm • M <10 mm • H <6 mm	Area: • L ≥20 mm • M ≥10 mm • H ≥6 mm
Tumour thickness (SCC)	<2 mm	≥6 mm
Borders	Well defined	Poorly defined
Margin status	Negative	Positive
Size and invasion of surrounding tissues	T1–2	T3–4
Sites		Lip, ear, genitalia
Perineural invasion	None or single focus, asymptomatic	Multiple, named nerve or symptomatic
Lymphovascular space invasion (LVSI)	Absent	Present
Rapidly growing	Absent	Present
SCC differentiation	Well	Poorly
SCC subtype		Basosquamous, adenoid, adenosquamous, desmoplastic
BCC subtype	Nodular, superficial	Micronodular, infiltrating, sclerosing, morphoeic
Immune status		Immunosuppressed
MCC		
Size	≤10 mm	>10 mm
Tumour thickness	≤10 mm	>10 mm
Excision margins	≤5 mm	>5 mm
LVSI	Absent	Present
Immune status		Immunosuppressed

L, trunk and extremities; M, cheeks, forehead, scalp and neck; H, mask areas of face (central face, eyelids, eyebrows, periorbital, nose lips [cutaneous and vermillion], chin, mandible, pre- and post-auricular, temple, ear), genitalia, hands and feet.

Table 51.4 Tumour-, host- and environment-related prognostic factors for skin cancer

Prognostic factors	Tumour related	Host related	Environment related
Essential	TNM Histopathological type Location Thickness PNI (clinical)	Immune suppression Recurrent disease	Surgical margins Previous RT
Additional	Tumour borders Differentiation Rate of growth LVSI PNI (incidental)	Genetic factors Gorlin syndrome Age Chronic inflammation, scars, burns	Smoking (SCC)
New and promising	SLNB Perturbed cellular pathways	Viral aetiology Highly conformal RT Chemoradiotherapy Targeted therapies Intralesional therapy	

BASAL AND SQUAMOUS CELL CARCINOMA

Treatment philosophy

Most low-risk lesions are suitable for treatment in the community by adequately trained clinicians. Complex and high-risk cases should be managed by specialized clinicians and considered for referral to a multidisciplinary clinic (Box 51.1).

Box 51.1 Situations where consideration should be given to specialist treatment/referral to a multidisciplinary clinic

- Uncertainty of diagnosis
- Any high-risk tumours
- Immunosuppression
- Difficulty in obtaining complete margins
- Tumours in complex locations (face, lip, eyes)
- Multiple primary disease
- Cosmetic considerations
- Suspected/confirmed lymph node metastases
- Distant metastases

Scenario: BCC and SCC	Treatment philosophy

Local disease	• Aim is complete surgical removal with the least functional deficit and optimal cosmetic result
	• Surgery is the preferred option as it is often curative, provides histopathological information and adequacy of excision:
	  ▪ Lesions with positive margins warrant consideration for further surgery
	  ▪ Radiotherapy (RT) should be considered when further surgery is not considered
	• Definitive RT may be used where surgery is contraindicated, impractical or not preferred
	• Patients with high-risk tumours and close margins warrant close surveillance or consideration of adjuvant RT
	• Adjuvant RT is recommended for extensive pathological (incidental) PNI or large nerve involvement
	• Topical treatments may be used in superficial low-risk lesions, but may provide lower cure rates and mask deeper extension or recurrences
	• Local disease should be treated as soon as feasible to prevent spread to regional nodes or the development of *in-transit* metastases

Regional (nodal) disease	• Remains curative
	• Often requires surgery and adjuvant RT:
	  ▪ 3-year regional control of 60–85% following surgery/PORT
	• In specific high-risk primary disease, regional nodes may be treated electively with either surgery or RT
	• *Subclinical (N0):*
	  ▪ Elective nodal treatment in BCC almost never warranted
	  ▪ Elective nodal treatment considered in high-risk primary SCC
	  ▪ Where regional disease suspected:
	    ○ Diagnostic imaging performed to assess disease extent
	    ○ Fine needle aspiration (FNA) performed to confirm diagnosis and repeated if negative
	    ○ Open lymph node biopsy may be required
	• *Clinical (N+):*
	  ▪ If regional disease confirmed with no evidence of distant metastases, operable patients should undergo a regional lymph node dissection
	  ▪ Postoperative radiotherapy recommended in the presence of any of the following:
	    ○ Multiple nodes
	    ○ Single node ≥3 cm

(continued)

Scenario: BCC and SCC	Treatment philosophy
	○ Extracapsular extension (ECE) ○ Residual disease ○ Unable involvement of important structures such as bone, nerves, and orbit ■ Immunosuppression • Use of concurrent chemotherapy in the presence of ECE remains investigational • Inoperable patients should be considered for definitive RT ± chemotherapy
Distant disease	• Incurable • Treatment is aimed at palliation: ■ Consider palliative RT to symptomatic sites and/or chemotherapy in the presence of multiple sites

Recurrent primary and/ or regional disease	• Depending on the extent and location of recurrence, treatment intent may still be curative:
	   ■ *Recurrent (relapse) local disease*:
	     ○ Consider curative re-excision and/or RT
	   ■ *Recurrent (relapse) regional disease*:
	     ○ Operable: further surgery ± RT (if no previous RT)
	     ○ Inoperable: RT (curative or palliative) or palliative chemotherapy
	• Patients warrant management by specialist clinicians and referral to a multidisciplinary clinic

Guidelines

Evidence guiding skin cancer management is predominantly based on non-randomized cohort series and low-level systematic reviews. Randomized data and meta-analyses are lacking. Recommended guidelines are:

- The National Comprehensive Cancer Network (NCCN) Clinical Practice Guidelines in Oncology Basal Cell and Squamous Cell. Available at http://www.nccn.org/professionals/physician_gls/f_guidelines.asp:
  - Skin Cancers Version 2.2012 Guidelines are predominantly based on lower-level evidence with uniform NCCN consensus that the intervention is appropriate (level 2A).
- http://www.cancer.org.au/health-professionals/clinical-guidelines/

Surgery

Type of surgery and repair/reconstruction is dependent on location, extent of disease and patient co-morbidities.

Recommended surgical margins and local control for BCC and SCC are described in Table 51.5. Table 51.6 gives the estimated local control following surgery according to T stage for BCC and SCC.

Table 51.5 Recommended surgical margins and 3-year local control for BCC and SCC

	Recommended minimal margin (mm)	3-Year local control (%)
BCC low risk	2–4	≥98
BCC high risk	5–10	90–95
SCC low risk	4–6	80–90
SCC high risk	10	60–80

Table 51.6 Estimated 5-year local control following surgery according to T stage for BCC and SCC

T stage	BCC (%)*	SCC (%)
1	95–99	95–99
2	85–90	70–85
3	70–75	60–75
4	50	<40

*Relapses can occur at 10 years.

Surgery: BCC and SCC	Description

Local disease	• Curettage and electrodesiccation
	• Excision with margin assessment:
	   ■ Secondary intention healing
	   ■ Side-to-side primary closure
	   ■ Excision with skin graft or flap repair
	• Mohs or resection with complete circumferential peripheral and deep margin assessment with frozen or permanent section

Regional disease	• *Elective resection*:
	   ■ Considered when the perceived risk of nodal involvement is ≥20%, based on high-risk features
	   ■ In the head and neck may involve some form of parotidectomy ± neck dissection (level I–III, I–IV, I–V, II–IV or II–V)
	• *Therapeutic resection*:
	   ■ Nodal basin dissection

Distant disease	• Palliative resection of symptomatic sites not amendable to palliative RT or chemotherapy

Radiotherapy

Estimated 5-year local control following radiotherapy according to T stage for BCC is given in Table 51.7.

Table 51.7 Estimated 5-year local control following RT according to T stage for BCC

T stage	BCC (%)
1	95–97
2	90–92
3	70–80
4	50–60

Beam, energy and techniques

- Superficial lesion: superficial (50–150 kV), orthovoltage (150–300 kV), electrons (typically 6–9 MeV)
- Kilovoltage, prescribe to Dmax (skin)
- Electrons: select energy for 90% isodose coverage on tumour, with appropriate skin bolus
- Consider more complex megavoltage photon beams and techniques such as 3D or intensity-modulated RT (IMRT), with appropriate skin bolus for technically difficult locations, extensive or deep tumours or those surrounded by critical structures
- Brachytherapy considered in specific scenarios in departments with appropriate expertise

Radiotherapy: BCC and SCC	Description

Local disease	• Considerations for the type of beam, energy, technique, volume, dose, fractionation and overall treatment time include:
	  ▪ Histology and risk factors (low risk vs high risk)
	  ▪ Thickness
	  ▪ Size/area
	  ▪ Location
	  ▪ Relative importance of cosmetic result
	  ▪ Surrounding organs and tissues
	  ▪ Intent (adjuvant, definitive, palliative)
	  ▪ Increased radiosensitivity, e.g. scleroderma, use of methotrexate
	  ▪ Previous RT
	  ▪ Patient preference
	• Volumes:
	  ▪ Clinical target volume (CTV) on the gross tumour volume (GTV) or high-risk tumour volume (HTV), minimum of 0.5 cm:
	    ○ Consider larger minimum CTV margin (1.0 cm) for high-risk disease and all SCC
	  ▪ Volumes and doses may need to be modified due to nearby structures
	  ▪ CTV includes back of the skull base/origin for named nerve involvement
	  ▪ Expansion from CTV to planning target volume depends on site and stability
	• Doses, time and fractionation schedule:
	  ▪ Definitive (gross disease):
	    ○ 64–66 Gy in 32–33 fractions over 6.4–6.6 weeks
	    ○ 55 Gy in 20 fractions over 4 weeks
	    ○ 45–50 Gy in 15 fractions over 3 weeks
	    ○ 35 Gy in five fractions over 5 days
	  ▪ Postoperative (clear margins):
	    ○ 60 Gy in 30 fractions over 6 weeks
	    ○ 50 Gy in 20 fractions over 4 week
	  ▪ Postoperative (positive margins):
	    ○ As per definitive therapy
	• For optimal cosmetic outcome and reduced risk of late effects, use small dose per fraction

Regional disease	• Elective or therapeutic regional irradiation may be considered as an alternative where surgery is contraindicated or not preferred
	• Doses, time and fractionation schedule:
	  ▪ *Unresected:*
	    ○ 66–70 Gy over 6.6–7 weeks
	  ▪ *Resected:*
	    ○ Head and neck with ECE: 60–66 Gy in 30–33 fractions over 6–6.6 weeks

(continued)

Radiotherapy: BCC and SCC	Description

	○ Head and neck without ECE: 56–60 Gy in 28–30 fractions over 5.6–6 weeks
	  ○ Axilla, groin with ECE: 60 Gy in 30 fractions over 6 weeks
	  ○ Axilla, groin without ECE: 54 Gy in 27 fractions over 5.4 weeks
	 - Elective:
	  ○ 50 Gy in 25 fractions over 5 weeks
	• Consider synchronous PORT to the nodal basin and primary site where nodal disease has occurred ≤12 months after resection of primary disease (no prior RT)
	• Refer to POST TROG 05.01 protocol for adjuvant RT guidelines, including volumes in high-risk head and neck skin SCC (NCT00193895, Section 7)

Systemic therapy

There are no universal standard protocols for locally-advanced, unresectable and distant disease due to limited phase II/III data.

Cytotoxic chemotherapy

Cytotoxic chemotherapy: BCC and SCC	Description
Local early disease	• BCC: - No role, including as adjuvant therapy • SCC: - Very rare - Widespread multifocal disease

Locoregional advanced disease	• BCC:
	 - No role, including as adjuvant therapy
	• SCC:
	 - May be combined with RT as potential curative treatment for unresectable disease
	 - Role of concurrent chemoradiotherapy (CCRT) for advanced local disease remains investigational
	 - Used for palliation of medically inoperable or unresectable disease
	 - Adjuvant protocol for high-risk disease:
	  ○ Concurrent cisplatin 100 mg/m^2 IV Weeks 1 and 4 + 7
	 - Protocol for unresectable disease:
	  ○ Active agents: cisplatin, 5-fluorouracil (5-FU), bleomycin, doxorubicin
	  ○ Suggested regimens:
	   – Cisplatin 100 mg/m^2 IV Day 1 + 5-FU 650 mg/m^2 continuous IV Days 1–5, repeat every 21–28 days
	   – Cisplatin 75 mg/m^2 IV Day 1 + doxorubicin 50 mg/m^2 IV, repeat every 21 days
	  ○ Response rates 15–60%
	  ○ Median duration of response 4–6 months

Distant disease	• BCC: - Undefined - Role of CCRT for nodal metastatic disease remains investigational • SCC: - Used in the palliation of symptomatic disease - Protocol for metastatic disease: as for locally advanced disease

Destructive and topical therapies

- Used for:
  - Solar keratosis
  - SCC *in situ*
  - Superficial BCC/SCC

- Treatment options:
  - Diathermy, electrodesiccation, curettage
  - Cryotherapy
  - Topical 5-FU, imiquimod, diclofenac gel, ingenol mebutate
  - Intralesional interferon
  - Photodynamic therapy (PDT)

MERKEL CELL CARCINOMA

Treatment philosophy

- Has a high rate of local, regional and distant recurrence
- Highly radiosensitive:
  - Durable in-field disease control with either adjuvant or definitive RT
  - Lower doses of RT required compared with BCC and SCC
- Adjuvant RT is considered in high-risk primary disease or nodal involvement with any of the following:
  - >1 node
  - ≥3-cm single node
  - Residual disease
  - ECE
  - In-transit disease
- RT is considered for local and/or regional disease where surgery is contraindicated or not preferred

Surgery

Surgery: MCC	Description

Local disease	- Aim is to achieve clear margins:
	  - Minimum 0.5–1.0-cm margin, but within location constraints
	  - Repair/reconstruction depends on defect and location
	- Consider sentinel lymph node biopsy (SLNB) at time of primary surgery, especially for limbs/trunk
	- Surgery alone acceptable in low-risk disease:
	  - Small lesions (<1.0 cm)
	  - Thin lesions (<1.0 cm)
	  - Adequate excision margins
	- Adjuvant RT considered for high-risk primary disease

Regional disease	- *Elective resection*:
	  - Consider nodal basin dissection for high-risk primary disease or RT
	  - Indication for adjuvant RT (as above)
	- *Therapeutic resection*:
	  - Nodal basin dissection required
	  - Indication for adjuvant RT (as above)
	  - Definitive RT if unsuitable for surgery

Distant disease	- Limited role for surgery - Excellent response for palliative RT

Radiotherapy

Beam, energy and technique principles are as for BCC and SCC. Volume principles also are as for BCC and SCC but:
- Consider wider CTV (3–4 cm) to encompass nearby dermal lymphatics
- Extremity lesions may require discontinuous RT to nodes, excluding in-transit tissues.

Radiotherapy	Description

Local disease	- *Definitive (gross disease)*:
	  - 50–54 Gy in 25–27 fractions over 5–5.4 weeks, or
	  - 50–55 Gy in 20–25 fractions over 4–5 weeks, or
	  - 25–30 Gy in 5–6 fractions twice per week over 2.5–3.0 weeks
	- *Postoperative (clear or positive margins)*:
	  - 50–54 Gy in 25–27 fractions over 5–5.4 weeks, or
	  - 50–55 Gy in 20–25 fractions over 4–5 weeks
	  - Consider higher dose range for positive margins
	  - RT should not be delayed beyond 3–4 weeks

Regional (nodal) disease	- *Unresected and resected disease*:
	  - As for definitive RT for primary site
	- *Elective*:
	  - 40–50 Gy in 23–25 fractions over 4.6–5.0 weeks, or
	  - 45–50 Gy in 18–20 fractions over 4.6–5.0 weeks

Metastatic disease	- RT to symptomatic sites:
	  - 20–30 Gy in 5–10 fractions over 1–2 weeks
	  - 6–10 Gy single fraction

Systemic therapy

Cytotoxic chemotherapy: MCC	Description
Local early disease	- No role
Locoregional advanced disease	- Undefined, remains investigational - As adjuvant therapy, also undefined

Metastatic disease	- Chemotherapy:
	  - Platinum and etoposide, similar to small cell lung cancer protocols
	  - Duration of response is often short (3–4 months)

Post-treatment assessment and follow-up

Post surgery

Postoperative surgical wound care follow-up is individualized and aimed at assessing the rate of healing, monitoring for the development of infection, haematoma and dehiscence, and ensuring viability of the graft/flap.

Post radiotherapy

The frequency of follow-up in the immediate post-RT period for either definitive or adjuvant treatment depends on dose, volume, location and patient factors.

Side effects of radiotherapy are:

- *Acute* (typically resolve in 4–6 weeks):
  - Typical:
    - Skin reaction (ranging from erythema, dry to moist desquamation)
    - Pain
    - Loss of hair
    - Lethargy
    - Head and neck region: mucositis, dry mouth, change in taste
  - Postoperative
    - May result in wound or graft/flap breakdown
- *Late*:
  - Typical:
    - Hyperpigmentation (3–6 months) followed by hypopigmentation (years)
    - Alopecia
    - Skin and subcutaneous atrophy
    - Telangectasia
    - Loss of sweat glands
    - Fibrosis, scarring
    - Oedema
  - Uncommon:
    - Non-healing ulcer
    - Osteoradionecrosis
  - Rare:
    - Radiation-induced cancer
    - Named nerve palsy
  - Risk of other late effects relate to location of tumour and surrounding structures
  - Postoperative:
    - Risk of late effects greater with surgery and RT than with RT alone.

Follow-up

- 30–50% risk of developing a new lesion within 3–5 years of NMSC diagnosis
- Ongoing follow-up and education about sun protection and self-examination
- Low threshold for biopsy of a new lesion
- Frequency of follow-up depends on risk status (Table 51.8)

Special consideration: Immunosuppression (see also Chapter 59.3)

- Solid organ transplant recipients and patients with conditions associated with prolonged immunosuppression are at greater risk of developing NMSC, especially SCC, compared with the normal population:

Table 51.8 Frequency of follow-up

BCC	Low risk	Every 6–12 months for Years 1–5
	High risk	Every 4–6 months for Years 1–2 years Every 6–12 after year 2
SCC	Low risk	Every 3–6 months for Years 1–2 Every 6–12 months for Year 3–5 Every 12 months after Year 5
	High risk	Every 1–3 months for Year 1 Every 3–4 months for Year 2 Every 4–6 months for Years 3–5 Every 6–12 months after Year 5
MCC		As per high-risk SCC

  - Prolonged duration and increasing dosage of immunosuppressive therapy increases the risk
- 5-year cumulative incidence of developing NMSC appears higher in cardiac (31%) compared with renal (25%) or liver (8%) transplant recipients, presumably due to the higher doses of immunosuppressive therapy
- Tumours are often more aggressive with higher rates of local recurrence, regional spread and distant metastases
- Management of these patients is complex and is best with multidisciplinary specialist care
- These patients warrant long-term close surveillance
- Reducing the immunosuppression can improve prognosis
- Retinoid chemoprophylaxis reduces the development of SCC in renal transplant recipients:
  - Cessation of retinoid chemoprophylaxis results in the loss of skin cancer suppression
  - Because of the need for long-term therapy, it is recommended that retinoids be instituted only when SCC are causing significant morbidity

Controversies

Solariums

Solariums emit UVA and UVB radiation, which are both known causes of skin cancer. There is strong evidence of an association between artificial tanning and the development of SCC, with the risk doubling compared with non-users. The evidence for BCC is inconclusive.

Vitamin D deficiency

Vitamin D is involved in maintaining musculoskeletal health and reducing the risk of bone fracture. Vitamin D forms in the skin as a result of UVB exposure. Concerns have been raised about sun protection campaigns leading to vitamin D deficiency. Further studies are required to determine the amount of UV exposure required to produce adequate amounts of vitamin D. Those at high risk of skin cancers, such as the immunosuppressed, should continue to minimize sun exposure and have their vitamin D levels monitored.

Perineural invasion

PNI is broadly divided into pathological (incidental) or clinical.

Clinical PNI implies that the patient is symptomatic and normally involves large/named nerves, more commonly occurs in the head and neck, is of SCC histopathology and is seen on radiography (MRI). It is associated with increased risk of recurrence. The extent of nerve resection required and optimal adjuvant RT dose and volumes remain unknown.

Pathological PNI is asymptomatic and an incidental finding usually involving small calibre nerves. It can be confined within the tumour or extend beyond its margins. There is no standardized grading of degree of PNI. It is unknown whether incidental PNI is a precursor to clinical PNI. The prognostic significance of incidental PNI remains uncertain and the need for adjuvant RT remains controversial. However, where there is extensive incidental PNI, it is generally considered as high risk.

Adjuvant chemoradiotherapy in high-risk SCC

Adjuvant chemoradiotherapy has been shown to be superior to adjuvant RT alone in high-risk mucosal head and neck cancer. There is no direct evidence that it is of benefit in cutaneous SCC, either locally advanced or where there is nodal involvement, particularly in the presence of nodal ECE. Despite the lack of evidence, it is used in this setting.

Sentinel lymph node biopsy

SLNB has been shown to be of benefit in selected melanoma patients. Its use in cutaneous SCC is not considered routine and its role remains controversial.

Merkel cell carcinoma

There are no randomized controlled studies comparing surgery with RT in the management of:
- Primary disease: early and advanced
- Subclinical nodal disease
- Clinically positive nodal disease.

The role of chemotherapy in the definitive and adjuvant setting remains undefined. Many patients are elderly and intolerant to systemic therapy.

The role of MCV in the aetiology and management of MCC is also undefined.

Phase III clinical trials/meta-analyses

There is a paucity of landmark phase III clinical trials, prospective trials and meta-analyses in skin cancer (Table 51.9).

Table 51.9 Phase III clinical trials/meta-analyses

Trial reference	Results
Tang et al. (2012) 366:2180–2188	• Vismodegib, a systemic inhibitor of the hedgehog signalling pathway, reduces the BCC tumour burden and blocks growth of new tumours in patients with Gorlin syndrome • Treatment was discontinued in 54% of patients due to adverse events
Brewster et al. (2007) J Clin Oncol 25:1974–1978	• Adjuvant 13-cis-retinoic acid + interferon-alpha does not prevent tumour recurrence and second primary tumours of skin SCC among patients with aggressive skin SCC
Marcil, Stern (2000) Arch Dermatol 136:1524–1530	• 3-year cumulative risk of developing a subsequent skin cancer (BCC or SCC) is increased by 10-fold compared with the incidence of first tumours in a comparable general population
Lewis et al. (2006) Arch Dermatol 142:693–700	• Patients not receiving adjuvant radiotherapy for MCC were 3.7 and 2.9 times more likely to develop local and regional recurrence respectively, if treated with surgery alone
Lebwohl et al. (2012) N Engl J Med 366:1010–1019	• Randomized double-blind studies demonstrated that ingenol mebutate gel is effective for field treatment of actinic keratosis

Areas of research

- Role of adjuvant chemoradiotherapy in high-risk cutaneous SCC (TROG 05.01 [NCT00193895])
- Definitive chemoradiotherapy for unresectable/medically inoperable SCC
- Development of targeted therapies for advanced disease:
  - Inhibitors of the hedgehog signalling pathway in BCC
  - Signalling pathway and epidermal growth factor receptor in SCC
  - Intratumourally injected DNAzyme in BCC
- MCC:
  - Efficacy of chemoradiotherapy in PET Stage II and III MCC of the skin (NCT01013779)

Recommended reading

(2008) *Basal Cell Carcinoma, Squamous Cell Carcinoma (and Related Lesions) – A Guide to Clinical Management in Australia*. Sydney: Cancer Council Australia and Australian Cancer Network.

Bath FJ, Bong J, Perkins W, Williams HC (2003) Interventions for basal cell carcinoma of the skin. *Cochrane Database Syst Rev* 2:CD003412.

Bavinck JN, Tieben LM, Van Der Woude FJ et al. (1995) Prevention of skin cancer and reduction of keratotic skin lesions during acitretin therapy in renal transplant recipients: a double-blind, placebo-controlled study. *J Clin Oncol* 13(8):1933–1938.

Brantsch KD, Meisner C, Schönfisch B et al. (2008) Analysis of risk factors determining prognosis of cutaneous squamous-cell carcinoma: a prospective study. *Lancet Oncol* 9:713–720.

Cho E-A, Moloney FJ, Cai H et al. (2013) Safety and tolerability of an intratumorally injected DNAzyme, Dz13, in patients with nodular basal-cell carcinoma: a phase 1 first-in-human trial (DISCOVER). *Lancet* 381:1835–1843.

Clayman GL, Lee JJ, Holsinger FC et al. (2005) Mortality risk from squamous cell skin cancer. *J Clin Oncol* 23:759–765.

Grant WB, Garland CF, Gorham ED (2007) An estimate of cancer mortality rate reductions in Europe and the US with 1,000 IU of oral vitamin D per day. *Cancer Res* 174:225–234.

International Agency for Cancer Research (2007) The association of use of sunbeds with cutaneous malignant melanoma and other skin cancers: A systematic review. *Int J Cancer* 120(5):1116–1122.

Maubec E, Petrow P, Scheer-Senyarich I et al. (2011) Phase II study of cetuximab as first-line single-drug therapy in patients with unresectable squamous cell carcinoma of the skin. *J Clin Oncol* 29(25):3419–3426.

Pellitteri PK, Takes RP, Lewis JS Jr et al. (2012) Merkel cell carcinoma of the head and neck. *Head Neck* 34:1346–1354.

Poulsen MG, Rischin D, Porter I et al. (2003) High-risk Merkel cell carcinoma of the skin treated with synchronous carboplatin/etoposide and radiation: A Trans-Tasman Radiation Oncology Group study-TROG 96:07. *J Clin Oncol* 21(23):4371–4376.

Rogers HW, Weinstock MA, Harris AR et al. (2010) Incidence estimate of nonmelanoma skin cancer in the United States, in 2006. *Arch Dermatol* 146:283–287.

Ross AS, Schmults CD (2006) Sentinel lymph node biopsy in cutaneous squamous cell carcinoma: a systematic review of the English literature. *Dermatol Surg* 32:1309–1321.

Rubin AI, Chen EH, Ratner D (2005) Basal-cell carcinoma. *N Engl J Med* 353:2262–2269.

Rowe DE, Carroll RJ, Day CL Jr (1992) Prognostic factors for local recurrence, metastasis, and survival rates in squamous cell carcinoma of the skin, ear, and lip. Implications for treatment modality selection. *J Am Acad Dermatol* 26:976–990.

Soyer HP, Rigel DS, Wurm EM (2012) Actinic keratosis, basal cell carcinoma and squamous cell carcinoma. In: Bolognia JL, Jorizzo L, Schaffer JV, eds. *Dermatology*, 3rd edn. London: Elsevier: 1773–1794.

Veness MJ, Palme CE, Morgan GJ (2006) High-risk cutaneous squamous cell carcinoma of the head and neck: results from 266 treated patients with metastatic lymph node disease. *Cancer* 106:2389–2396.

Veness MJ, Porceddu S, Palme CE, Morgan BJ (2007) Cutaneous head and neck squamous cell carcinoma metastatic to parotid and cervical lymph nodes. *Head Neck* 29(7):621–631.

Veness MJ, Richards S et al. (2012) Radiotherapy. Chapter 139. In: Bolognia JL, Jorizzo L, Schaffer JV, eds. *Dermatology*, 3rd edn. London: Elsevier:2291–2301.

Von Hoff DD, LoRusso PM, Rudin CM et al. (2009) Inhibition of the hedgehog pathway in advanced basal-cell carcinoma. *N Engl J Med* 361:1164–1172.

52 Melanoma

Kim Margolin[1], Brian O'Sullivan[2] and Raphael Pollock[3]

[1]Division of Oncology, Pigmented Lesion and Melanoma Program, Stanford University, Stanford, CA, USA
[2]Department of Radiation Oncology, The Princess Margaret Cancer Centre, University of Toronto, Toronto, ON, Canada
[3]Department of Surgery, The James NCICCC/Ohio State University, Columbus, OH, USA

Summary	Key facts
Introduction	<ul><li>Incidence is rising steeply, while the mortality rate is rising less rapidly</li><li>Sun exposure behaviours and genetic factors do not fully account for the risks of melanoma</li><li>Efforts at early detection need to be optimized</li><li>No prevention strategies have been identified other than ultraviolet protection</li></ul>
Presentation	<ul><li>Change in the appearance of an existing mole or appearance of a new or atypical mole is the most common factor triggering a skin evaluation</li><li>Rarely, melanoma presents with palpable lymphadenopathy without a history or simultaneous occurrence of a primary melanoma</li></ul>
Scenario	<ul><li>*Stage I–II*:<ul><li>Excision/wide excision of primary with adequate resection margin</li><li>Sentinel lymph node (SLN) biopsy in melanoma with a tumour thickness of >0.75–1 mm and/or ulceration is necessary for accurate staging</li></ul></li><li>*Stage III*:<ul><li>cN0: wide resection of primary + sentinel nodal biopsy:<ul><li>Complete lymph node dissection for sentinel node-positive and/or elective lymph node dissection</li></ul></li><li>cN+: therapeutic lymph node dissection:<ul><li>Postoperative radiotherapy (RT) to nodal basin in selected patients based on location, size and number of involved nodes, or bulky lymph node metastases, or presence of extracapsular extension (ECE)</li></ul></li><li>Interferon for selected cases with tumour thickness of >1 mm</li></ul></li><li>*Stage IV (metastatic disease)*:<ul><li>Limited disease<ul><li>Resectable: surgical resection ± systemic therapy</li><li>Unresectable: radiotherapy ± systemic therapy</li></ul></li><li>Disseminated:<ul><li>Systemic therapy</li><li>Palliative radiotherapy/surgery for symptom relief</li><li>Best supportive care (BSC)</li></ul></li></ul></li></ul>

(continued)

UICC Manual of Clinical Oncology, Ninth Edition. Edited by Brian O'Sullivan, James D. Brierley, Anil K. D'Cruz, Martin F. Fey, Raphael Pollock, Jan B. Vermorken and Shao Hui Huang. © 2015 UICC. Published 2015 by John Wiley & Sons, Ltd.

Summary	Key facts
Trials	- Multicentre randomized trial of 2-cm vs 4-cm resection margins; Gillgren et al. (2011) Lancet 378:1635:
- 2 cm margins are adequate
- Multicenter Selective Lymphadenectomy Trial (MSLT-I) of sentinel node biopsy versus nodal observation; Morton et al. (2006 and 2010) N Engl J Med 355:1307–1317 and 370(7):599–609:
- Although overall survival (OS) was similar between the groups, sentinel node biopsy-based management prolongs disease-free survival (DFS) for all patients and prolongs distant control and cause-specific survival for patients with nodal metastases from intermediate-thickness melanomas
- Meta-analysis of interferon-alpha (IFN-α) for high-risk melanoma; Mocellin et al. (2010) J Natl Cancer Inst 102:493–501:
- In patients with high-risk cutaneous melanoma, IFN-α adjuvant treatment significantly improved both DFS and OS
- Ipilimumab (Ipi) versus Ipi + a melanoma peptide vaccine versus vaccine alone; Hodi et al. (2010) N Engl J Med 363(8):711–723:
- Ipi improved survival in patients with metastatic melanoma
- BRIM-3 trial: dacarbazine versus vemurafenib in melanoma with BRAF V600E mutation; Chapman et al. (2011) N Engl J Med 364(26):2507–2516:
- Improved survival with vemurafenib

Incidence, aetiology and screening

Malignancies of the skin are common, affecting over 225 million people worldwide per year, but the vast majority are non-melanoma cancers (see Chapter 51) that have little potential for regional or distant spread and rarely cause the death of the patient (Table 52.1).

While solar ultraviolet A and B (UVA and UVB)-induced DNA damage is paramount in the oncogenesis of all four types of skin cancer (melanoma, squamous, basal and Merkel), the contribution of host genetics and other environmental causes appears to differ between these types. For melanoma in particular, germline or acquired alterations of the expression and function of genes that control the cell cycle, apoptosis and metabolic pathways have all been identified in some scenarios and may provide therapeutic targets not only for advanced disease, but also as further investigation opens opportunities for prevention strategies by identifying subjects at high risk.

Table 52.1 Incidence and mortality for the four types of skin cancer

Histology	Yearly incidence (thousands)		Yearly deaths	
	USA	Global	USA	Global
Melanoma	80	230	9500	Approx 10% of new cases
Squamous	700		2500	
Basal	2800		Rare	
Merkel	1.5		500	

Incidence, aetiology and screening	Description
Incidence	- Worldwide is rising rapidly, due at least in part to changes in sun exposure behaviour:
- Includes tanning salon use, often by teenagers and young adults for cosmetic reasons as well as providing an addictive sense of well-being (use of recreational drugs and tobacco are also higher in regular tanning-bed users)
- Particularly prevalent and rising in incidence in countries like Australia, where the majority of the population has fair skin that tans poorly and the climate is sunny, providing high exposures to the damaging UVA and B frequencies of sunlight
- Mortality from melanoma is not rising as rapidly as incidence:
- Probably in large part due to early detection and prompt management:
○ Vast majority of patients are diagnosed and treated in the early stages and have a favourable outcome
- While improvements in survival after metastatic disease have also been achieved over the past few years, these impact only a relatively small number of patients and are unlikely to account for the overall trends

Incidence, aetiology and screening	Description

	- Age of onset:
	  - Melanoma is a disease of relatively young adults, but the risk does not diminish with age and it can occur across the entire spectrum of ages:
	    - Risk factors, sites of origin, tumour characteristics and overall prognosis vary across the age spectrum.
	    - In infants, most likely to arise from a congenital nevus
	    - Infants have been described who were born with metastatic melanoma as a result of transplacental dissemination from maternal metastatic melanoma
	- Although the overall incidence of melanoma is very low in Asians, Native Americans, African–Americans and other dark-skinned populations, different histopathological and genetic types and locations of melanoma predominate in populations of more darkly-pigmented races

Aetiology	- Complex interactions of solar exposure with skin type, genetic polymorphisms for genes affecting pigmentation and mole numbers, UV damage repair, and cell cycle proteins and other factors contributing to melanomagenesis are under active investigation
	- *Genetic*:
	  - Familial melanoma syndromes are rare but have been informative in demonstrating the importance of genes controlling cell cycle progression and DNA repair in melanomagenesis:
	    - Most common (<2% of cutaneous melanomas worldwide) is a loss-of-function mutation of the cyclin kinase inhibitor CDKN2A, encoded by the *p16* or *p14^{ARF}* genes on chromosome 9, or less commonly an activating mutation of the cyclin kinase CDK4
	    - Interactions of these proteins with p53 and retinoblastoma protein (Rb) to control proliferation and apoptosis are altered in the presence of germline mutations, and the latter can also contribute to sporadic melanomagenesis when acquired as somatic mutations
	  - Predisposition also reported with other germline cancer syndromes such as Cowden (loss of function of PTEN) and several genetic syndromes characterized by abnormal DNA repair, such as *BRCA 2* and xeroderma pigmentosum
	- *Environmental*:
	  - Rising incidence of melanoma, particularly in age and gender groups that can be correlated with specific UV exposure behaviours (middle-aged men and young adult women), and a less steep rise in the death rate from melanoma are evidence of the role of environmental factors, since genetic risks, while subject to evolutionary selection, are less likely to change over short periods of observation
	  - Sun exposure is recognized but not well understood, because patterns of exposure, genetic factors and other environmental factors also play a role:
	    - Sporadic, early acute sun damage, such as seasonal childhood sunburns in fair-skinned Caucasians, contribute the greatest risk from the sun
	    - Chronic exposure, while associated with the risk of squamous and basal cancers (and the rarer non-melanoma skin tumour, Merkel cell carcinoma), is probably a risk factor
	  - Regular tanning bed use, often for cosmetic purposes but also associated with other potentially pleasurable and addictive behaviours such as cigarette smoking and use of recreational drugs, has recently been documented as a risk factor

Screening and prevention	- *Primary screening*:
	  - Population-based screening is fraught with many limitations, including the high incidence of false positives and negatives in unselected populations and the expense, risks and questionable cost–benefit relationship of screening
	  - Given the dramatically different outcomes of melanoma diagnosed early and managed effectively with surgery versus the still suboptimal therapies for advanced disease, melanoma should be the 'poster child' for effective screening and early intervention:
	    - Recent German demonstration project suggested that screening measures can reduce mortality; these strategies are being applied to other populations in order to validate the German data and identify other factors that may mitigate or alter the approach needed in other settings

(continued)

Incidence, aetiology and screening	Description

	• Melanoma chemoprevention is a very important goal that has been elusive, reflecting the extremely complex nature of this malignancy as well as the need to 'customize' interventions to the major contributing risk factors.
	   ■ Educational efforts directed at sun behaviours, recognition of early lesions and general principles of good skin care, starting with young children and their parents:
	     ○ These measures must remain in place even if additional chemopreventive measures are introduced into the melanoma risk-reducing lifestyle
	   ■ Anti-tanning bed measures (behavioural modification and legislation), directed particularly at the highest users, young Caucasians with light skin, who are also at higher risk for later melanoma development
	   ■ Use of risk-modifying dietary or medicinal substances, e.g. lipid-lowering statins, epigallocatechin (found in Asian green tea) and vitamin D supplementation (may have modest cancer-preventive effects; readily obtained from sources *other* than sun exposure) has not been adequately demonstrated to modify risk of melanoma

Pathology

The diagnosis of melanoma can be challenging, particularly in equivocal lesions that lack clear-cut features pathognomonic of malignancy. This is particularly true in children and adolescents, who may have a range of lesions termed 'atypical Spitzoid lesions', not all of which have the natural history of malignant melanoma. The reader is referred to more specialized literature for current information on this category.

Molecular characterization of melanoma has recently demonstrated great value for diagnostic and therapeutic decision-making, although many of the therapeutic options remain investigational despite the identification of likely molecular targets. Half of cutaneous melanomas harbour an activating mutation of the gene encoding BRAF, a critical member of the MAP kinase pathway. Activating mutations of the *NRAS* oncogene occur with similar frequency across all the subsets of melanoma detailed below and are nearly always mutually exclusive of *BRAF* mutations. Other molecular changes may occur in cells carrying activated 'driver' oncogenes (e.g. loss-of-function mutations of the negative regulator PTEN that controls the highly complex downstream PI3K pathway) which, while not yet diagnostic, may provide therapeutic targets.

Pathology and molecular characteristics	Description
Superficial spreading melanoma (SSM)	• Most common category of melanoma, occurring in all cutaneous sites with a slightly higher frequency in men than women and a tendency to occur in areas exposed to intermittent high-intensity sun: ■ Women have a higher incidence on the skin of the extremities, while men have an increased incidence on the trunk and back, possibly related to attire and likely also genetic factors • Intermediate behaviour, starting with a radial growth phase that has minimal metastatic potential but evolving to a vertical growth phase with increased aggressiveness • Presence of a *BRAF* mutation at amino acid 600 (most commonly an activating mutation of valine to glutamic acid or, less frequently, valine to lysine) in about 50% of cases
Nodular melanoma	• Rarely occurs *de novo* • May be mistaken for benign or other proliferative skin lesions of much less concern, because it is often non-pigmented (amelanotic) and features a vertical growth phase that is not preceded by a radial growth phase • Most common site of origin in both genders is the trunk, and more common in younger individuals • *BRAF* mutations are common
Lentigo maligna	• Typically found on the face of older individuals and has a very indolent behaviour, although with metastatic potential • Often less pigmented and may be easily confused with non-malignant solar damage occurring in a similar setting • May have a component of melanoma *in situ* and often a wide area of involvement and location on the cosmetically-sensitive face; its management requires an experienced team of plastic and oncological surgeons: • *BRAF* mutations are rare

Pathology and molecular characteristics	Description

Acral lentiginous	• Occurs on the distal extremities (acral)
	• Varies in its aggressiveness but is often diagnosed after a delay due to misdiagnosis as an inflammatory or post-traumatic lesion:
	  ▪ Subungual form can easily be confused with benign or post-traumatic changes in the nail or nailbed:
	    ○ Pigmented lesions, which also feature a prominent nodular phase at diagnosis, may be very aggressive and not uncommonly feature distant metastases at the time of diagnosis
	• *BRAF* mutations are less common (10–15%) than in other cutaneous sites
	• *c-Kit* mutations may be found in 10–15%

Mucosal melanoma	• Together with acral melanomas, this subtype is the one most frequently occurring in pigmented races who rarely develop cutaneous melanoma
	• Can arise on the mucous membranes of the nasal cavity and paranasal sinuses, oral cavity and pharynx, vagina and lower gastrointestinal tract
	• Diagnosis is often difficult, because presentations vary widely but often feature bleeding and/or symptoms of the mass effect such as nasal obstruction
	• Pathological features are not unique and staging is not straightforward; stage-based prognostic indicators are harder to define than for cutaneous melanoma.
	• Mucosal melanomas of upper aero-digestive tract are aggressive tumours with ominous outcomes, and T1 and T2 are omitted from the T classification as are stages I and II (i.e. only stage III and IV are defined)
	• Molecular characteristics have been reported for fewer mucosal melanomas than cutaneous melanomas:
	  ▪ *BRAF* mutation is rare
	  ▪ Suggested to have the highest incidence of c-Kit over-expression, particularly by mutation, which confers potential sensitivity to molecularly-targeted therapies

Uveal melanoma	• Unique, rare and somewhat distinct group of melanomas • Most common primary intraocular malignancy in adults, managed almost exclusively by experienced ophthalmologists in specialized centres (see Chapter 54)

Natural history and presentation

Melanoma should be considered a highly aggressive malignancy characterized by the propensity to widespread metastasis via both lymphatic and haematogenous routes. No body site appears to be protected, and melanoma is the malignancy with the highest incidence of metastases to the brain as well as to unusual sites rarely involved by other tumours, such as the heart and the small intestine. Cutaneous melanoma also metastasizes readily to other skin and nodal distributions generally and at a distance from the site of origin. Spontaneous haemorrhage also characterizes this highly-vascular tumour and is not uncommonly the immediate cause of death, particularly when due to uncontrolled central nervous system (CNS) metastasis.

- Patients often come to medical attention after becoming aware of changes in a mole (most commonly increase in size, changes in the shape or colour, development of bleeding or pruritus) or a new mole
- Women most often present with primary lesions on the arms and legs
- Men more often develop primary melanoma on the back and trunk:
  ▪ Older men with chronic sun exposure have a higher propensity to melanoma of the face and scalp
- Rarely, the patient has already developed palpable adenopathy in the draining lymph node basin
- Diagnosis is often delayed in patients with less common sites of primary melanoma such as mucosal or acral melanoma, which are often neglected for long periods or initially misdiagnosed

Natural history and presentation	Description
Presentation	Locoregional: • Patients or their partners likely notice changes in a pre-existing nevus or a new, unusual nevus (including the 'ugly duck' sign: a mole of concern just does not look like the others) • Small percentage have overt spread to regional nodes or even distant metastases at the time of diagnosis, due either to delayed primary diagnosis and treatment or to a particularly aggressive tumour

(continued)

Natural history and presentation	Description
	• Melanoma of unknown primary site is diagnosed in about 10% of patients who present with clinically-evident adenopathy and are found on biopsy to have melanoma in the node: 　▪ This presentation of Stage III disease has been reported to have a similar or even slightly better prognosis than Stage III melanoma with a known primary, possibly due to the development of an effective immune response that ablated the primary tumour *Metastatic:* • Rarely found at the time of initial diagnosis and management of cutaneous melanoma • Historically heralded a grim, nearly always fatal outcome: 　▪ Recent developments in immunotherapy have changed the outcome for a small proportion of patients 　▪ Rapidly expanding developments in both tumour immunology and molecularly targeted therapy are improving the prognosis • Yield of initial staging with scans and laboratory assessments is limited, since most patients present with early-stage disease: 　▪ Nevertheless, accurate initial staging is extremely valuable, since the discovery of possible metastatic disease may have major implications for surgical and medical management
Routes of spread	*Local:* • Most cutaneous melanomas start growing radially in the epidermis, and in their radial phase, melanomas have little to no propensity to invade or spread • Once a melanoma has developed a vertical growth phase, however, its invasiveness is established, and dissemination can then occur via both lymphatic and vascular channels • Although theoretically possible for a primary melanoma to grow to a large size and become deeply invasive into local structures without metastasizing, this is exceedingly rare, and most patients seek attention at the point when their primary melanoma is readily manageable surgically *Regional:* • First site of spread for most melanomas is the regional lymph node bed • Haematogenous spread without evidence of lymph node involvement occurs on occasion • Melanoma in-transit refers to the occurrence of cutaneous metastases in the region between the primary excision site and the draining lymph nodes: 　▪ Most commonly seen in the lower limb and may be difficult to impossible to control with surgery, radiotherapy or systemic therapy 　▪ Regional strategies that include isolation of the tumour circulation and delivery of high doses of cytotoxic chemotherapy or biological therapies may be useful in controlling this extremely challenging problem 　▪ While melanoma in-transit often remains a locoregional problem for long durations, patients who do not succumb to its complications almost always go on to develop distant metastatic disease *Metastatic:* • Among all solid tumours, melanoma has the greatest propensity to spread far and wide, in a seemingly 'predictably unpredictable' fashion: 　▪ Sites that are almost never involved with other solid tumour metastases, such as the small intestine and the heart, can also be affected, leading to complications such as haemorrhage and pain that may raise diagnostic as well as therapeutic challenges

Diagnostic work-up

Diagnostic work-up	Description
Visual examination and dermoscopy	• Visual exam and dermoscopy of a concerning mole as well as complete skin exam and, if possible, mole mapping with photographic documentation (also important in surveillance and screening for development of new melanomas and other skin cancers) 　▪ Suspicious lesions are characterized by **A**symmetry, **B**order irregularities, **C**olour heterogeneity, **D**iameter, **E**volving (the 'ABCDE rule')

Diagnostic work-up	Description

Biopsy	• Diagnosis should be made by excisional biopsy of the full thickness of the tumour with a small peripheral margin:
	  ▪ Recommendations for excisional biopsy are based on principles of surgery and pathological evaluation, which demand that the lesion be fully excised whenever possible in order to preserve its architecture, optimize the accuracy of pathological evaluation (including margin assessment) and avoid transection of the tumour whenever possible
	• Incisional biopsy is usually confined to large or cosmetically-difficult lesions in order to confirm the diagnosis and plan the definitive excision and margins, if malignant
	• Melanoma *in situ* should be excised with negative margins but does not require wide margins or lymph node evaluation
	• Invasive melanoma should be excised in an effort to achieve clear resection margins without disturbing the local anatomy
	• Compromise in resection margins may be indicated to avoid complex or cosmetically/medically unfavourable outcomes
	• Tumours with a Breslow depth of at least 0.75–1 mm or with one or more risk factors, such as ulceration, mitoses of >1/mm^2 or perineural or lymphovascular invasion, are appropriate for surgical staging with sentinel lymph node (SLN) biopsy:
	  ▪ Using lymphoscintigraphic detection of lymph node drainage patterns followed by lymphazurin dye tracing for detection within the draining basin of the sentinel node

Imaging	• Computed tomography (CT):
	  ▪ Commonly used for evaluation of potential metastatic sites in the lungs, lymph nodes, bone and liver:
	    ○ Particularly useful for the detection of purely lytic lesions not apparent on radionuclide bone scan
	    ○ Better sensitivity and similar specificity for detection of abdominal metastases compared to ultrasound
	  ▪ Indicated for high-risk melanoma with a positive SLN
	• Magnetic resonance imaging (MRI):
	  ▪ Recommended for Stage IV, optional for Stage III and not indicated for Stage I–II
	  ▪ Useful to differentiate between benign versus metastatic lesions in the liver
	  ▪ Superior for the delineation of vascular involvement and identifying signal in bone marrow
	  ▪ More sensitive than CT for detection of metastatic disease in the brain, spinal cord and leptomeninges
	• ^{18}FDG-PET (positron emission tomography) scanning is more accurate than CT or MRI alone in the diagnosis of metastases since melanoma is highly FDG avid:
	  ▪ Should complement conventional CT or MRI in the staging work-up of patients with solitary or oligo-metastases amenable to surgical resection
	  ▪ Substantial frequency of both false-negative and false-positive ^{18}FDG-PET scans should be kept in mind in order to avoid under-, over- or mis-treating melanoma

Tumour markers	• No circulating markers have proven valuable in any stage of melanoma, although many approaches, ranging from detection of circulating whole tumour cells by flow cytometry to polymerase chain reaction-based assays for tumour- or mutation-specific nucleic acids, have been studied • Pathological examination can be aided by immunohistochemical stains for melanoma-associated differentiation antigens such as HMB-45 (gp100) and MART-1/Melan-A, and the less-specific S-100 protein • Mutational analysis, while sensitive and of major value for therapeutic decisions in advanced disease, is not very specific, since moles and other malignancies can have some of the same mutations (e.g. *BRAF* V600E, *NRAS*, c-*KIT*): ▪ Superficial spreading and nodular melanomas present a much higher frequency of *BRAF* and *NRAS* mutations than other melanoma types • In advanced melanoma, the serum lactate dehydrogenase (LDH) level has prognostic impact and is used to upstage patients with metastatic disease to the highest-risk M stage (M1c) due to its association with an unfavourable prognosis independent of other factors

Staging and prognostic grouping

While earlier staging systems were developed based on factors known to be prognostic and widely available at the time, rapid changes in the field have led to the need for near constant revision of the staging system, and current efforts are underway to incorporate principles of molecular biology as well as a growing understanding of tumour–host biology.

Ideally, future staging systems will also include not only prognostic information, but also predictive factors that apply to the interaction of tumour and host with therapeutic interventions.

An example from outside of melanoma is illustrated by the biomarker HER2neu, which possesses independent (unfavourable) prognostic value in breast cancer (see Chapter 21). Incorporation of such valuable and biologically-rational information into future staging systems (which will also raise the questions of access to therapy and resource allocation) will be a necessary but challenging task for the staging committees.

UICC TNM staging

See Table 52.2.

Table 52.2 UICC TNM categories and stage grouping: Skin malignant melanoma and mucosal melanoma of the upper aerodigestive tract

TNM categories: Skin malignant melanoma	
pT1a	≤1 mm, <1 mitosis/mm², no ulceration
pT1b	≤1 mm, ≥1 mitosis/mm², or ulceration
pT2a	>1–2 mm, no ulceration
pT2b	>1–2 mm, ulceration
pT3a	>2–4 mm, no ulceration
pT3b	>2–4 mm, ulceration
pT4a	>4 mm, no ulceration
pT4b	>4 mm, ulceration
N1	1 node
N1a	Microscopic
N1b	Macroscopic
N2	2–3 nodes or satellites/in-transit without nodes
N2a	2–3 nodes microscopic
N2b	2–3 nodes microscopic
N2c	Satellite(s) or in-transit without nodes
N3	≥4 nodes; matted; satellite(s) or in-transit without nodes
M1	Distant metastasis
M1a	Skin, subcutaneous tissues, lymph node(s) beyond the regional
M1b	Lung
M1c	Other sites; any site with elevated LDH

Stage grouping: Skin malignant melanoma			
Stage 0	pTis	N0	M0
Stage I	pT1	N0	M0
Stage IA	pT1a	N0	M0
Stage IB	pT1b	N0	M0
	pT2a	N0	M0
Stage IIA	pT2b	N0	M0
	pT3a	N0	M0
Stage IIB	pT3b	N0	M0
	pT4a	N0	M0
Stage IIC	pT4b	N0	M0
Stage IIIA	pT1a–4a	N1a, 2a	M0
Stage IIIB	pT1a–4a	N1b, 2b, 2c	M0
	pT1b–4b	N1a, 2a, 2c	M0
Stage IIIC	pT1b–4b	N1b, 2b, 2c	M0
	Any pT	N3	M0
Stage IV	Any pT	Any N	M1

TNM categories: Mucosal melanoma of the upper aerodigestive tract	
Melanoma: Upper aerodigestive	
T3	Epithelium/submucosa (mucosal disease)
T4a	Deep soft tissue, cartilage, bone, or overlying skin
T4b	Brain, dura, skull base, lower cranial nerves, masticator space, carotid artery, prevertebral space, mediastinal structures

Stage grouping: Mucosal melanoma of the upper aerodigestive tract			
Stage III	T3	N0	M0
Stage IVA	T4a	N0	M0
	T3, T4a	N1	M0
Stage IVB	T4b	Any N	M0
Stage IVC	Any T	Any N	M1

Note: Mucosal melanomas are aggressive tumours, therefore T1 and T2 are omitted as are stages I and II (i.e. only stage III and IV are defined)

Prognostic risk factors

The prognosis for patients with melanoma is primarily determined by the thickness of the primary tumour, ulceration, mitotic rate, and presence and extent of metastatic disease (Table 52.3). New concepts for assessing outcomes, including molecular and immunological, host, tumour and environmental factors will be increasingly incorporated into the databases used to define TNM stage and develop stage and prognostic groupings.

In addition to those factors that have emerged in multivariate analysis as having sufficient prognostic impact to be used in staging, other characteristics of the tumour and host may impact the outcomes of one or more stage groups and can be used to refine the prognostic grouping as well as in the design of new therapeutic trials. Rapid progress in tumour biology is

Table 52.3 Prognostic factors for melanoma

Prognostic factors	Tumour related	Host related	Environment related
Essential	Tumour thickness Mitotic rate Ulceration Extent of metastatic disease	Lymphocyte infiltrate Regression	Medications, especially immunosuppressives
Additional	Lymphovascular Perineural	Site of primary, family history Personal medical history, especially immunodeficiency Gender (female more favourable) Age (younger age more favourable)	Sun exposure history Tanning bed use
New and promising	Molecular: mutational, gene expression, proteomics, miRNA	Immunogenetics Other characteristics of host immune response	

Note: *BRAF* mutation, an iconic biomarker in melanoma, is predictive for response to RAF kinase inhibitors, but it remains uncertain whether it is a prognostic biomarker in itself; therefore, it is not included.

Data from Dummer *et al*, (2012) *Ann Oncol* 23 (suppl 7): vii86–vii91. NCCN Clinical Practice Guidelines in Oncolog. Melanoma v.3.2014 http://www.nccn.org/professionals/physician_gls/pdf/melanoma.pdf

expected to introduce new paradigms in the development of cancer staging and stage grouping.

Treatment philosophy

The mainstay of therapy for melanoma is prompt identification of a suspicious lesion and its surgical excision. In view of the historically profound resistance of melanoma to systemic therapies and even radiotherapy (RT), surgical management, even of disseminated disease, has played a larger role than for other metastatic cancers. Patients with solitary or oligo-metastatic melanoma can survive many years after resection of one or more metastatic lesions.

RT may play a part in enhancing regional control of high-risk sites following surgery, and is also used for palliation of symptoms from unresectable metastatic disease.

Systemic therapies have been notoriously inactive for melanoma, with minimal control by cytotoxic agents and infrequent durable responses achieved with immunotherapy. Adjuvant systemic therapy has also failed to show substantial benefit. Recent identification of molecular targets or 'drivers' of melanoma has led to the development of drugs that inhibit these pathways; these drugs are being tested in the adjuvant setting for advanced melanoma. However, responses to single agents and even combination inhibitors in this class have been of relatively limited duration, due to the high propensity of melanoma to acquire new alterations that confer resistance. Advances in immunotherapy have also provided new optimism in the treatment of metastatic melanoma, particularly with the advent of immune checkpoint-blocking agents that appear to reverse immunosuppression in the tumour microenvironment and unleash an existing immune response to tumour antigens not only in melanoma but in many other malignancies. Increasingly evident is the need for combination and complex strategies that will restore the balance of immune control from 'evasion' back to 'elimination' as effectively as has been achieved in other settings, such as allogeneic bone marrow transplantation for haematological malignancies.

Scenario	Treatment philosophy

Local disease	• Lentigo maligna:
	  ▪ Moh's micrographic surgery is a valid option to minimize disfiguration due to its less aggressive nature
	  ▪ Primary radiotherapy in selected cases (usually elderly)
	• Invasive melanoma should be excised in an effort to achieve clear resection margins:
	  ▪ Wide local excision with adequate resection margins
	  ▪ Avoid disturbing the local anatomy, since re-excision for definitive margins will often include local tumour bed injection of lymphoscintigraphic and dye tracers to guide the sentinel node biopsy that is done at the time of definitive wide local excision; both should be performed soon after the initial diagnostic biopsy by an experienced surgeon/surgical oncologist
	• Adjuvant RT to the primary site is indicated to reduce risk of local recurrence in specific settings (see Box 52.1)
	• Primary RT alone is rarely used but can be considered for patients unsuitable for or refusing surgery

(continued)

Scenario	Treatment philosophy

Regional disease	- SLN biopsy in melanoma with a tumour thickness of >1 mm and/or ulceration is necessary for precise staging:
	  - If positive, a complete lymphadenectomy of regional lymph nodes should be performed, although there is no proven survival benefit
	- Complete lymph node dissection for patients with a positive SLN is commonly recommended
	- Therapeutic lymph node dissection for clinically-palpable lymphadenopathy:
	  - Management follows the same surgical principles as for the SLN
	  - Generally consists of an attempt to surgically clear all palpable and readily-accessible nodes in the nodal bed
	- Complications of lymphadenectomy depend on the experience and skill of the surgeon as well as the site and underlying condition of the patient. Even under optimum conditions, lymphoedema is common following axillary and inguinal lymphadenectomy, and bacterial infection complicates a high percentage, especially in inguinal surgeries.
	- Adjuvant RT to the site of involved nodes and adjacent nodal regions following surgical excision of involved nodes has been shown to improve regional control and is indicated in specific settings (see Box 52.1)
	- Palliative RT for unresectable nodal, satellite or in-transit disease

Metastatic disease	- Limited disease
	  - Resectable: surgical resection ± systemic therapy
	  - Unresectable: radiotherapy ± systemic therapy
	- Disseminated:
	  - Systemic therapy
	  - Palliative radiotherapy/surgery for symptom relief
	  - Best supportive care (BSC)
	
	Treatment indications:
	Radiotherapy
	- Can be considered for:
	  - Brain metastases
	  - Other potentially symptomatic soft tissue and/or bone metastases
	Surgery
	Considered for single metastases in parenchymal organs, including the CNS following imaging studies to exclude further metastases
	Systemic therapy
	- *Immunotherapy*: first-line treatment of choice:
	  - Interleukin-2 (originally known as 'T-cell growth factor'):
	    - Requires high doses which are associated with multiorgan toxicities due to cytokine cascade-induced capillary leak syndrome
	    - Autoimmune events are rare, generally limited to hypothyroidism
	    - Responses occur within weeks
	    - Provides remissions in 15–20% of patients, half of which are durable
	  - Ipilimumab, inhibitor of CTLA-4:B7.1 complex-induced negative signalling in T cells
	    - Acute side effects are immune-related colitis, hypophysitis, hepatitis, dermatitis
	    - Responses are slow to develop and may be observed after initial tumour growth
	    - Provides remissions in about 15% of patients and prolonged stable disease in 10%, thus benefiting about 25% of patients long term
	- *Molecularly-targeted agents*:
	  - Targeting the mutated, activated BRAF with the oral kinase inhibitors vemurafenib or dabrafenib provides remissions in about 50% of patients, with another 25–30% of patients experiencing minor tumour regression
	  - Complete response is rare, and median response duration only 6 months
	  - Combination strategies have shown an increased frequency and duration of response
	  - 'Vertical' combined-pathway inhibition using drugs that block sequential enzymes in the same pathway (MAPK, using the BRAF inhibitor dabrafenib and the MEK inhibitor trametinib) is under investigation
	  - 'Horizontal' blockade using drugs that block enzymes in parallel pathways to prevent or overcome resistance is also under investigation
	  - Generally, single or combination targeted agents are used in patients who fail to achieve durable remission with immunotherapy, or those who present with aggressive, high-volume, symptomatic metastatic disease that is unlikely to be controlled with immunotherapy, or those with contraindications to immunotherapy such as autoimmune syndromes

Scenario	Treatment philosophy

Recurrent disease	• Patients with metastatic melanoma rarely have more than one chance to achieve durable complete remission with standard therapies
	• Second-line therapy should always consider enrolment on an available clinical trial
	• Alternatives include cytotoxic chemotherapy approved for use in melanoma but without proven survival benefit, particularly in second-line systemic therapy
	• *Isolated local recurrence*:
	  ▪ At the site of the original surgical scar or one in-transit lesion: re-excision ± adjuvant RT
	  ▪ More than one in-transit lesion: immunotherapy, systemic chemotherapy or regional chemotherapy with isolated limb perfusion
	• *Lymph node recurrence*:
	  ▪ Therapeutic lymph node dissection ± adjuvant RT
	• *Distant recurrence*:
	  ▪ Treated in the same way as for Stage IV melanoma (i.e. M1 disease)

Follow-up	• Physical examination is the most important element of melanoma follow-up
	• Laboratory tests may be valuable for assessing the general health of the patient, but do not provide sensitive or specific markers of melanoma recurrence
	• A substantial fraction of melanoma recurrences as well as new primary lesions are found by the patient or a family member
	• Cutaneous and nodal recurrences often occur without or precede the appearance of visceral metastases
	• Modalities used for detection of visceral metastases have been inadequately studied:
	  ▪ CT scans may detect early, asymptomatic metastases with surgical implications, but impact on overall survival is unknown
	  ▪ ^{18}FDG-PET-CT provides greater sensitivity but adds vast expense and also raises many additional questions
	  ▪ False positives and negatives are common with both modalities
	• Symptom-driven assessment with laboratory and imaging tests is encouraged until further data emerge regarding the best way to follow and screen melanoma survivors

---

Box 52.1 Indications for radiotherapy

Adjuvant radiotherapy

- Primary site: indicated to reduce risk of local recurrence in the following settings:
  - Desmoplastic melanoma
  - Compromised margins where surgical revision is not possible
  - >4-mm thickness, especially if ulcerated or with satellite nodules
  - Neurotropism
  - In-transit or satellite lesions on wide local re-excision
  - Recurrent local disease (relative indication)
  - Adjacent to a radiotherapy field for lymph node recurrence less than 1 year following original primary treatment (relative indication)
- Involved nodes and adjacent nodal regions: indicated in selected patients with the following pathological findings after surgical excision:
  - Multiple or bulky lymph node metastases
  - Gross nodal extracapsular extension
  - Parotid: ≥1 involved node, any size of involvement
  - Cervical: ≥2 involved nodes and/or ≥3 cm of tumour within a node
  - Axillary: ≥2 involved nodes and/or ≥4 cm of tumour within a node
  - Inguinal: ≥3 involved nodes and/or ≥4 cm of tumour within a node
  - Recurrent nodal disease
  - Patients with positive SLN but for whom complete nodal dissection is not planned

Primary radiotherapy

- As an alternative to surgery for patients unsuitable or refusing surgery; including for functional and cosmetic considerations (e.g. elderly patients with lentigo maligna)

Radiotherapy in the palliative setting

- Unresectable nodal, satellite or in-transit disease
- Oligometastases
- Brain metastasis
- Bone metastasis
- Other typical symptom relief settings (e.g. bleeding, spinal cord compression, pain, superior vena cava syndrome, etc.)

Treatment

Surgery

Surgery	Description
Lentigo maligna	• The only subtype often managed with Moh's micrographic surgery because of the need to minimize disfiguration and its less aggressive behaviour than other cutaneous melanomas
Early disease	• Wide excision of primary with adequate resection margin ± SLN ± adjuvant RT • Recommended clinically adequate margins are: • In-situ disease: 0.5–1.0-cm resection margin • Tumour thickness of ≤1.0 mm: 1.0-cm resection margin • Tumour thickness of 1.0–2.0 mm: 1.0–2.0-cm resection margin • Tumour thickness of >2 mm: 2-cm resection margin • Modifications may be needed for preservation of function in acral and facial melanomas • SLN biopsy in melanoma with a tumour thickness of >1 mm and/or ulceration is necessary for accurate staging

Advanced without distant metastasis	• Wide excision of primary with adequate resection margin + SLN
	• Complete lymph node dissection for sentinel node-positive and/or elective lymph node dissection
	• Therapeutic lymph node dissection for macroscopic nodal involvement
	• Adequacy of regional lymph node dissection includes:
	  ▪ An anatomically complete dissection of the involved nodal basin
	  ▪ In the groin, consider elective iliac and obturator lymph node dissection if clinically positive superficial nodes or three or more superficial nodes are positive
	  ▪ Iliac and obturator lymph node dissection indicated if CT pelvis is positive or if Cloquet's node is positive
	  ▪ For primary melanomas of the head and neck with clinically or microscopically positive lymph nodes in the parotid gland, a parotidectomy and appropriate neck dissection of the draining nodal basins is recommended

Metastatic disease	• Palliation of symptoms • Curative intent in the case of single or very limited resectable metastases: ▪ Surgery of visceral metastases may be appropriate for selected cases with good performance status and isolated tumour manifestations; in principle, the goal is R0 resections in these patients

Radiotherapy

Radiotherapy	Description

Early disease	• Rarely used as the primary treatment in malignant melanoma
	• Can be considered for:
	  ▪ Lentigo maligna: 12–50-kV X-rays (so-called 'soft X-rays'), as an alternative to surgery for cosmetic consideration if the resection area is too extensive and most often in elderly patients:
	    ○ Suggested doses: 100–120 Gy (12 kV) or 42–54 Gy (20–50 kV) at 3–4-day intervals for seven to nine fractions as these superficial X-rays only affect the epidermis and upper dermis
	  ▪ Patients unsuitable or refusing surgery:
	    ○ Suggested radiation doses are 50–55 Gy in 20 fractions or 60–70 Gy in 30–35 fractions

Locally-advanced non-metastatic disease	• Adjuvant RT to the site of involved nodes and adjacent nodal regions following surgical excision of involved nodes remains controversial: ▪ Results of the only rigorous randomized trial using current methods of RT and follow-up supported a role for RT to improve regional control, but without a survival benefit and at the cost of toxicity • Postoperative RT is considered in selected cases (see Boxes 52.1 and 52.2)

Locally-advanced and metastatic disease	• RT for metastatic melanoma remains useful as a palliative modality, without playing a role in curative therapy:
	  ▪ May be considered especially for symptomatic brain or painful bone metastases
	• Typical dose: 20 Gy in five fractions, 30 Gy in ten fractions, 40 Gy in 15 fractions, 24 Gy in three fractions over 3 weeks (on Days 0, 7 and 21)
	• Brain metastases:
	  ▪ Whole-brain radiation therapy may provide some relief of symptoms:
	    ○ Typical dose: 20 Gy in five fractions and 30 Gy in ten fractions
	  ▪ Stereotactic RT, which delivers a high dose of RT focused on a very small target, can also be used for each individual metastatic brain lesion

Box 52.2 Adjuvant radiotherapy dose/volume design

Typical RT doses
- Conventional fractionation: 50–60 Gy in 25–30 fractions over 5 weeks:
  - Smaller or conventional fraction size regimens may mitigate late toxicity
- Hypofractionation: 48 Gy in 20 fractions over 4 weeks TROG 02.01. [Burmeister (2012) *Lancet Oncol* 13(6):589–597] or 30 Gy in five fractions over 2.5 weeks (two fractions per week) (MD Anderson regimen):
  - Toxicity may offset disease control with hypofractionation regimens (larger fraction size)

Typical RT volume
- *Primary disease*:
  - Wider clinical target volume (CTV) margin is recommended
  - High-dose CTV margin: 5 mm from original gross tumour where it can be defined by presurgical photograph or surgical clips and surgeon's description
  - Elective CTV margin: 2 cm from the original site of gross disease where this can be defined:
  - Based on the Scandinavian surgical margin trial: demonstrated that the potential zone of microscopic tumour infestation is within 2 cm from gross tumours of >2 mm thickness
- *Nodal disease*:
  - High-dose CTV should encompass the original site of gross disease, e.g. dissected lymph node field, with the adjacent echelons at risk of harbouring microscopic disease receiving an elective dose to address potential microscopic disease
  - Primary site may be included if nodal recurrence has occurred within 1 year, especially if it is adjacent to or overlying the regional nodal target volume
  - Lymphadenectomy scar should be included in the elective microscopic volume
- *Specific considerations*:
  - *Parotid neck*: ipsilateral RT is recommended to:
    - Parotid bed
    - Level I, II, III, IV and V neck nodes
    - Lymphadenectomy surgical scars (and primary site when included) to have full bolus to give tumour dose on skin
    - Primary site may also be included in the treatment volume if it is:
      – Stage III
      – Abutting or overlying RT node fields
      – Excised <1 year before nodal recurrence
  - *Axilla/supraclavicular*: ipsilateral RT is recommended to:
    - Axillary level I, II and III nodes
    - Supraclavicular fossa in continuity (5-cm margin on proximal operative clips)
    - Skin dose to surgical scars and any encompassed primary site
  - *Inguinal/iliac*: ipsilateral RT is recommended to:
    - Femoral and inguinal and external iliac nodes (or 5-cm margin on cephalic clipped surgical bed)
    - Surgical scars with full skin dose using tissue-equivalent materials ('bolus')
  - Primary site with 3-cm normal tissue margin may also be considered for inclusion in the treatment volume if primary site is:
    - Within 5 cm of the required field
    - Excised <1 year prior to nodal metastases

Systemic therapy

Systemic therapy	Description
Early	- None
Advanced non-metastatic disease	- None

Metastatic disease	- *High-dose interleukin-2 (IL-2)*:
	  - Administered in the intensive care unit or a similar facility at a hospital with an experienced team of physicians and nurses:
	    - Dose and schedule: 600,000 IU/kg IV over 15 minutes, infused every 8 hours up to 14 doses over a 5-day period; repeat after a rest period of 9 days
	    - Doses are withheld for severe hypotension, volume overload or organ toxicity using algorithms and guidelines

(continued)

Systemic therapy	Description

	- All patients receive adjunctive antipyretics, antibiotics, and inflammatory agents, antacids and antiemetics
	- Additional symptom management provided as indicated
	- Post-IL-2 therapy assessment and management until stable condition:
	  ○ Assessment of tumour status at about 4 and 8 weeks after completion of the two-cycle course of therapy, with retreatment planned for responders or those with stable disease who tolerated IL-2 well
	- *Ipilimumab*:
	  ■ Exclude patients with autoimmune disease or on steroid therapy
	  ■ Dose and schedule: 3 mg/kg IV every 3 weeks for four doses
	  ■ Immune-related toxicities during therapy:
	    ○ May require dose delay or withholding to allow resolution
	    ○ Prednisone 1 mg/kg for persistent or severe reactions; 2 mg/kg for very severe reactions and short-term use
	    ○ Additional immunosuppressants such as antitumour necrosis factor (anti-TNF) antibodies, mycophenolate mofetil or tacrolimus may be needed
	    ○ Immune-related diarrhoea, particularly with other signs and symptoms of severe colitis, should generally be evaluated endoscopically to seek and treat other causes and to assess the extent and severity of drug-related changes
	  ■ Assessments start at 3–4 weeks after last dose of ipilimumab:
	    ○ Delayed response may occur even after initial progression and/or new lesions appearing, so changing therapy after ipilimumab is discouraged unless there is definite evidence of progression, including worsening symptoms requiring another intervention
	- *Vemurafenib or combination of dabrafenib + trametinib*:
	  ■ Recommended as second-line therapy for patients who do not achieve durable benefit from initial immunotherapy
	  ■ Patients with bulky disease, significant symptoms or rapid progression and evidence of *BRAF* mutation should generally start treatment with the molecularly-targeted therapy, which is generally continuous until progression or intolerance
	  ■ Potential benefit of intermittent dosing is under investigation
	  ■ Toxicities include rash, sun sensitivity, fatigue, gastrointestinal disturbances such as diarrhoea and nausea, and joint pain and swelling:
	    ○ Combination of dabrafenib + trametinib causes high fevers and sometimes a systemic inflammatory response syndrome; patients who newly develop this syndrome should be assessed for possible infection

Controversies

Lymph nodes

Management of regional nodal disease remains an area of important controversy and investigation, due to the relatively low incidence of nodal involvement at diagnosis and the expense and morbidity associated with nodal biopsy and potential lymph node dissection. Non-invasive techniques to detect nodal involvement, most commonly using special ultrasound detection methods, are under intense investigation, represented by the MSLT-2 trial which has randomized patients with a positive sentinel node between the traditional complete lymph node dissection and serial follow-up ultrasounds of the nodal basin.

Adjuvant therapy

The initial wave of enthusiasm regarding the benefits of adjuvant IFN-α was based in large part on significant improvements of both relapse-free and overall survival during the period of observation and follow-up. Subsequent trials showed more modest benefit, and longer follow-up also demonstrated that the initial impact of therapy appears to wane over time. Thus, for patients followed over 10 years, there remains only a modest relapse-free benefit, mostly during the period of active treatment, and almost all of the initial survival benefit is lost. Despite data from meta-analyses showing a small aggregated improvement in survival with adjuvant IFN-α, it has a very poor therapeutic index. To date, no other form of adjuvant immunotherapy has shown a greater advantage, and more aggressive approaches like multi-agent chemotherapy and immunomodulatory cytokines have also been overly toxic and insufficiently active.

Phase III clinical trials

See Table 52.4.

Table 52.4 Phase III clinical trials

Trial name	Results
Local disease	
Gillgren et al. (2011) Lancet 378:1635	• Randomized multicentre trial of 2-cm versus 4-cm surgical excision margins for primary cutaneous melanoma >2 mm (n = 936; clinical Stage IIIa–c) • 5-year survival was 65% in both groups • Conclusion: 2-cm margins are adequate

MSLT-1 Morton et al. (2006) N Engl J Med 355:1307–1317	• Randomized trial of sentinel node biopsy versus nodal observation in intermediate-thickness (1.2–3.5 mm) cutaneous melanoma (n = 1269)
	• Overall survival was equal between the groups:
	  ▪ Relapse-free survival favoured the sentinel node biopsy group, who generally went on to complete lymph node biopsy
	  ▪ Incidence of sentinel node positivity was 16%, similar to the incidence of nodal relapse in patients randomized to observation
	  ▪ More nodes were involved in patients relapsing from observation than in those who underwent complete lymph node dissection after a positive sentinel node
	• Sentinel lymph node biopsy is generally recommended for patients who do not participate in a clinical trial:
	  ▪ Although the primary endpoint of overall survival was not impacted by sentinel node biopsy in MSLT-1, the benefit for the patient subset with positive nodes has been used as a strong argument for recommending it as standard surgical practice
	  ▪ MSLT-2 trial is addressing the role of complete lymph node dissection by randomizing patients between complete lymph node dissection and serial ultrasounds of the draining lymph node bed
	  ▪ Prognostic impact of the sentinel node, together with the benefit of early surgery for patients who turn out to have one or more positive nodes, is also important in designing prospective trials, particularly of systemic adjuvant therapy

TROG 02.01 Burmeister et el. (2012) Lancet Oncol 13(6):589–597	• Randomized trial of adjuvant RT versus observation alone following therapeutic lymphadenectomy for patients with macroscopic nodal involvement (n = 250)
	• At a median follow-up of 40 months, there was a significant decrease in the rate of nodal relapse among patients randomized to RT
	• No difference in the overall relapse rate, which included local plus distant relapses
	• No survival benefit from RT:
	  ▪ Non-significant difference in overall survival favouring the non-radiated patients
	  ▪ RT did not increase the wound complications of infection or seroma formation, but was associated with severe dermatitis in 15% of patients
	• Nodal radiation is currently recommended only for patients at extreme risk of local relapse

Adjuvant systemic	
EORTC 18991 Eggermont et al. (2012) J Clin Oncol 30(31):3810–3818	• Randomized trial of adjuvant therapy with pegylated (PEG)-IFN-α 2b for 5 years (or until relapse) versus observation in Stage III melanoma post lymphadenectomy (n = 1256) • At a median follow-up of 7.6 years, relapse-free survival favoured the IFN-treated patients (hazard ratio 0.87) • Survival was not affected by treatment • Toxicities were substantial, reflected in a reduction in health-related quality of life measures and a high rate of treatment discontinuation among the patients on IFN • Subset analysis demonstrated survival benefits for patients with ulcerated primary melanoma and/or microscopically-involved sentinel node(s) • A follow-up study specifically in patients with an ulcerated primary is underway

Kirkwood et al.; Eastern Cooperative Oncology Group (2004) Clin Cancer Res 10(5):1670–1677	• Long-term data for adjuvant high-dose therapy from four completed randomized trials of the Eastern Cooperative Oncology Group were pooled, with median follow-up intervals ranging from 2.1 to 12.6 years:
	  ▪ Previously reported data favouring relapse-free survival among patients randomized to high-dose IFN were confirmed, although the magnitude of the benefit had diminished from the time of initial reporting of E1684 and E1690
	  ▪ Overall survival, which had been reported to favour the high-dose interferon group in E1684 but not in E1690, was no longer significant in pooled analysis of the high-dose IFN-treated patients compared with untreated patients
	  ▪ Prognostic factors confirmed in these series included ulceration of the primary, age >49 years and delayed nodal recurrence
	• Subsequent meta-analyses have shown a very modest survival benefit for IFN at the risk of significant toxicities, and the expert opinion remains divided regarding the use of adjuvant IFN for patients with resected melanoma at risk of recurrence

(continued)

Table 52.4 (Continued)

Trial name	Results
Lian et al. (2013) Clin Cancer Res 19(16):4488–4498	• Phase II randomized trial comparing adjuvant high-dose IFN-α 2b versus adjuvant chemotherapy (temozolomide + cisplatin) versus observation for Stage II or III resected mucosal melanoma (n = 189 Chinese patients) • At 27 months' median follow-up, the chemotherapy group had the longest relapse-free and overall survivals, followed by the IFN group • Statistical power of these results was limited by the randomized phase II design and the challenge of accruing sufficient eligible patients • Generalizability of these data to non-Chinese patient populations with mucosal melanoma remains to be determined
Advanced disease and metastatic disease	
Hodi et al. (2010) N Engl J Med 363(8):711–723	• Patients with advanced melanoma treated with one prior systemic therapy were randomized in a 1:3:1 ratio to receive ipilimumab, ipilimumab + melanoma peptide vaccine, or vaccine alone (n = 676) • Ipilimumab alone or with peptide improved median survival and hazard ratio for survival compared with peptide alone • Survival plateau in the ipilimumab treatment groups suggested that this form of immunotherapy has the potential for long-term control of advanced melanoma • Subsequent experience has shown that patients relapsing after initial control with ipilimumab can be safely retreated and may re-respond to therapy
Robert et al. (2011) N Engl J Med 364(26):2517–2526	• Patients with advanced melanoma who had received no prior systemic therapy were randomized to dacarbazine or ipilimumab + dacarbazine, using a regimen that featured a higher ipilimumab dose than in the above study and included maintenance ipilimumab (n = 502) • Median survival, hazard ratio for overall survival and landmark survivals at 1, 2 and 3 years all favoured the ipilimumab-containing regimen, which also resulted in a survival plateau • Toxicities of combination therapy were greater than those of ipilimumab alone, particularly hepatotoxicity • Current practice and approved dosing of ipilimumab is 3 mg/kg IV every 3 weeks for four doses, with the option to retreat patients who achieve benefit for at least 3 months • Toxicity patterns and likelihood of response are at least as favourable upon retreatment, possibly because the patients are a more select group who had initial benefit and did not experience toxicities at the level precluding retreatment
BRIM-3 trial Chapman et al. (2011) N Engl J Med 364(26):2507–2516	• Patients with advanced melanoma carrying mutation *BRAF V600E* were randomized to receive dacarbazine or vemurafenib, an inhibitor of the serine-threonine kinase activity of constitutively activated BRAF (n = 675) • After an interim analysis demonstrating a significant survival benefit for vemurafenib, cross-over was recommended for patients randomized to dacarbazine • Final analysis demonstrated objective responses in 48% of the vemurafenib group versus 5% of the dacarbazine group (hazard ratio for overall survival significantly favoured vemurafenib) • Median duration of response to vemurafenib was 6 months, and patients often experienced rapid disease progression, although occasional patients had disparate responses such as progression at one or more sites despite control at others • Toxicities included fatigue, diarrhoea, increased sun sensitivity, proliferative squamous lesions of the skin, arthralgias, fever and laboratory abnormalities, including elevated hepatic enzymes

Areas of research

The best therapy for a patient with malignancy is participation in a clinical trial. Clinical trials are critical for the advancement of the field and the achievement of success in individual cases as well as for present and future cancer patients.

Recent strides in both immunotherapy and molecularly targeted therapy for melanoma have led the way to new hope for therapeutic success against melanoma. Nevertheless, the disease continues to be lethal for a substantial fraction of patients, and understanding of the necessary and sufficient steps for this lethal potential remains inadequate. Clearly, this 'smart' tumour has the ability to evade or escape control, due to factors that are likely to reflect tumour plasticity based on both tumour and host biology, impacted further by selective evolutionary pressure from the environment, including therapeutic interventions.

While the principles and practice of surgical and radiotherapeutic management are unlikely to change rapidly in the foreseeable future, the rapid emergence of new discoveries in tumour biology and in drug development is expected to result in new and better therapies over the next several years. These will include well-designed combinations and/or sequences of targeted agents, customized to both the tumour biology and the host. Examples of agents and strategies currently under investigation include a variety of new pathway inhibitors, including several enzymes in the pathway downstream from the tumour suppressor PTEN; cyclins that interact with Rb and p53; and modulation of the determinants of gene expression such as histone deacetylase inhibitors and demethylating agents. In the immunotherapy arena, proteins that block the interaction of cell-signalling receptors in immune effector cells with their ligands on tumour or other cells appear likely to dramatically improve patient outcomes and are currently being incorporated into numerous investigational strategies. The rapidly-growing field of adoptive T-cell therapy, using a variety of methods to select or engineer the optimal antigen-specificity and signalling cascade, is also likely to provide further therapeutic success in the relatively near future. Finally, the field is just beginning to see some advances in understanding the biology and origin of brain metastasis, a complication of particularly high frequency in melanoma that is almost always lethal. It is probable that better systemic therapies will soon reduce the incidence of brain metastasis and that additional therapeutic discoveries will reduce their threat, resulting in a substantial overall benefit to patients with melanoma.

Recommended reading

Belum VR, Fischer A, Choi JN et al. (2013) Dermatological adverse events from BRAF inhibitors: a growing problem. *Curr Oncol Rep* 15:249–259.

Burmeister BH, Henderson MA, Ainsle J et al. (2012) Adjuvant radiotherapy versus observation alone for patients at risk of lymph-node field relapse after therapeutic lymphadenectomy for melanoma: a randomised trial. *Lancet Oncol* 13(6):589–597.

Dudley ME, Yang JC, Sherry R et al. (2008) Adoptive cell therapy for patients with metastatic melanoma: evaluation of intensive myeloablative chemoradiation preparative regimens. *J Clin Oncol* 26:5233–5239.

Dummer R, Hauschild A, Guggenheim M, Keilholz U, Pentheroudakis G; ESMO Guidelines Working Group (2012) Cutaneous melanoma: ESMO Clinical Practice Guidelines for diagnosis, treatment and follow up. *Ann Oncol* 23(Suppl 7):vii86–91.

Flaherty KT, Infante JR, Daud A et al. (2012) Combined BRAF and MEK inhibition in melanoma with BRAF V600 mutations. *N Engl J Med* 367:1694–1703.

Flaherty KT, Robert C, Hersey P et al. (2012) Improved survival with MEK inhibition in BRAF-mutated melanoma. *N Engl J Med* 367:107–114.

Gillgren P, Drzewiecki KT, Niin M et al. (2011) 2-cm versus 4-cm surgical excision margins for primary cutaneous melanoma thicker than 2 mm: a randomized, multicentre trial. *Lancet* 378:1635–1643.

Hamid O, Robert C, Daud A et al. (2013) Safety and tumor responses with lambrolizumab (anti-PD-1) in melanoma. *N Engl J Med* 369:134–144.

Katalinic A, Waldmann A, Weinstock MA et al. (2012) Does skin cancer screening save lives?: an observational study comparing trends in melanoma mortality in regions with and without screening. *Cancer* 118:5395–5402.

Kaufman HL, Kirkwood JM, Hodi FS et al. (2013) The Society for Immunotherapy of Cancer consensus statement on tumour immunotherapy for the treatment of cutaneous melanoma. *Nat Rev Clin Oncol* 10(10):588–598.

Liew DN, Kano H, Kondziolka D et al. (2011) Outcome predictors of Gamma Knife surgery for melanoma brain metastases. Clinical article. *J Neurosurg* 114:769–779.

Menzies AM, Haydu LE, Visintin L et al. (2012) Distinguishing clinicopathologic features of patients with V600E and V600K BRAF mutant metastatic melanoma. *Clin Cancer Res* 18:3242–3249.

Mocellin S, Pasquali S, Rossi CR et al. (2010) Interferon alpha adjuvant therapy in patients with high-risk melanoma: a systematic review and meta-analysis. *J Natl Cancer Inst* 102:493–501.

NCCN. Clinical Practice Guidelines in Oncology. Melanoma v.3.2014. Available at http://www.nccn.org/professionals/physician_gls/pdf/melanoma.pdf

Rosenberg SA, Yang JC, Sherry RM et al. (2011) Durable complete responses in heavily pretreated patients with metastatic melanoma using T-cell transfer immunotherapy. *Clin Cancer Res* 17:4550–4557.

Topalian SL, Hodi FS, Brahmer JR et al. (2012) Safety, activity, and immune correlates of anti-PD-1 antibody in cancer. *N Engl J Med* 366:2443–2454.

Weber JS, Dummer R, de Pril V et al. (2013) Patterns of onset and resolution of immune-related adverse events of special interest with ipilimumab: detailed safety analysis from a phase 3 trial in patients with advanced melanoma. *Cancer* 119:1675–1682.

Wolchok JD, Kluger H, Callahan MK et al. (2013) Nivolumab plus ipilimumab in advanced melanoma. *N Engl J Med* 369:122–133.

Zhang M, Qureshi AA, Geller AC et al. (2012) Use of tanning beds and incidence of skin cancer. *J Clin Oncol* 30:1588–1593.

53 Central nervous system

Caroline Chung[1], Do-Hyun Nam[2] and Roger Stupp[3]

[1]Department of Radiation Oncology, The Princess Margaret Cancer Centre, University of Toronto, Toronto, ON, Canada
[2]Department of Neurosurgery, Samsung Medical Center, Sungkyunkwan University School of Medicine, Gangnamgu, Seoul, Republic of Korea
[3]Department of Oncology and Cancer Center, University Hospital Zurich, Zurich, Switzerland

Summary	Key facts
Introduction	- Sixth most common cancer globally: - Incidence has significantly increased since the year 2000, especially in developed countries, possibly due to improved imaging and the ageing population - Aetiology: prior cranial radiation - Histology: >60% of primary central nervous system (CNS) malignant tumours are glioblastomas

Presentation	- Dependent on tumour location and CNS function:
	  - Generalized fatigue
	  - Increased intracranial pressure: headaches, nausea/vomiting
	  - Seizures
	- Symptoms specific to tumour location:
	  - Cognitive deficits
	  - Personality changes
	  - Decreased memory
	  - Dysphasia/aphasia
	  - Focal motor deficits
	  - Sensory deficits

Scenario	- *Gliomas:*
	  - Resection followed by radiotherapy in combination with temozolomide is standard therapy for glioblastomas
	- *Meningioma:*
	  - Grade I:
	    - Gross total resection
	    - Consider radiotherapy for incompletely resected or recurrent tumour
	  - Grade II:
	    - Gross total resection
	    - Radiotherapy for incompletely resected tumour
	  - Grade III:
	    - Maximal surgical resection followed by radiotherapy
	- *CNS lymphoma:*
	  - Methotrexate-based chemotherapy with or without consolidative radiotherapy
	  - If elderly patient, consider palliative radiotherapy alone

UICC Manual of Clinical Oncology, Ninth Edition. Edited by Brian O'Sullivan, James D. Brierley, Anil K. D'Cruz, Martin F. Fey, Raphael Pollock, Jan B. Vermorken and Shao Hui Huang. © 2015 UICC. Published 2015 by John Wiley & Sons, Ltd.

Summary	Key facts
	- *Medulloblastoma and primitive neuroectodermal tumour:* - Maximal safe resection followed by radiotherapy (craniospinal with boost to the primary tumour site) - *Brain metastases:* - Surgical resection for larger tumours causing mass effect, histological confirmation or single metastasis - Whole-brain radiotherapy (WBRT) for multiple brain metastases (typically >4 metastases) or leptomeningeal disease - Radiosurgery for limited number (typically 1–4) brain metastases with or without WBRT or for salvage treatment following prior WBRT

Trials	- EORTC-NCIC; Stupp *et al.* (2009) *Lancet Oncol* 10(5):459–466:
	  - Phase III randomized trial of radiotherapy with concomitant and adjuvant temozolomide versus radiotherapy alone on survival in glioblastoma
	  - Addition of concurrent and adjuvant temozolomide to radiotherapy improves overall survival
	- EORTC 22845; van den Bent *et al.* (2005) 366:985–990:
	  - Phase III randomized trial of early versus delayed radiotherapy for low-grade astrocytoma and oligodendroglioma in adults
	  - Early radiotherapy improves progression-free survival but not overall survival for patients with low-grade glioma
	- RTOG 9802; Shaw *et al.* (2012) *J Clin Oncol* 30(25):3065–3070:
	  - Phase III randomized trial of radiotherapy plus procarbazine + lomustine + vincristine (PCV) versus radiotherapy alone for supratentorial adult low-grade glioma
	  - Addition of PCV to radiotherapy for low-grade glioma improves progression-free survival
	  - Subsequent abstract publication (Mehta *et al.* (2014) *Int J Radiat Oncol Biol Phys* 90(1):S37–S38) showed a substantial survival benefit
	- EORTC 26951; van den Bent *et al.* (2013) *J Clin Oncol* 31(3):344–350:
	  - Phase III randomized trials of radiation alone vs radiation with adjuvant procarbazine + lomustine + vincristine (PCV) chemotherapy for anaplastic oligodendroglial tumours
	  - Addition of PCV after radiation for anaplastic oligodendroglial tumours improves progression-free and overall survival
	- G-PCNSL-SG-1; Thiel *et al.* (2010) *Lancet Oncol* 11(11):1036–1047:
	  - Phase III randomized non-inferiority trial of high-dose methotrexate with or without WBRT for primary CNS lymphoma
	  - WBRT after high-dose methotrexate improves progression-free survival but not overall survival for patients with primary CNS lymphoma
	- Patchell *et al.* (1998) *JAMA* 280(17):1485–1489:
	  - Randomized trial of postoperative radiotherapy in the treatment of single metastases to the brain
	  - Addition of postoperative WBRT for patients with a single brain metastasis improves survival

Introduction

Tumours affecting the central nervous system (CNS) are commonly metastases of extracranial origin, while primary tumours of the CNS account for only 3–5% of all malignancies in adults (in children up to 25%). The most common primary tumours in adults are meningiomas, a usually benign and slow growing tumour arising from the meninges. Glioblastoma accounts for >50% of all gliomas which occur at all ages, but with an increasing incidence in the elderly (peak in the seventh decade of life). In younger patients, low-grade glioma and anaplastic astrocytoma account for approximately 10% of CNS tumours.

Primary brain tumours are grouped according to the World Health Organization (WHO) classification based on the cell of origin, and the histological aggressiveness from grade 1 to grade 4. However, molecular features are becoming an integral part of the classification of brain tumours, and are important markers for prognostication and treatment selection (see Fig. 53.2). The management of most brain tumours is multidisciplinary, involving neurosurgery, radiation oncology and neuro-oncology.

Clinical presentation

The clinical presentation of CNS tumours varies widely, depending largely on the location and function of the affected zone, but also on the rapidity of the tumour growth and the presence or absence of perilesional oedema. The most common presenting symptoms can be categorized into three clinical scenarios that may present in parallel: raised intracranial pressure, seizures or specific neurological deficits progressing over several days to weeks. Increased intracranial pressure may induce headaches, nausea, vomiting, ataxia, confusion and a decreasing level of consciousness (Table 53.1). Cortical tumours commonly present with generalized seizures or partial seizure equivalents. Focal neurological deficits reflect

Table 53.1 Clinical presentation of brain tumours associated with brain location

General	Fatigue Seizures
Focal neurological deficits	Cognitive deficits Personality changes Decreased memory Dysphasia/aphasia Focal motor deficits Sensory deficits Visual or auditory disturbance Imbalance/dizziness
Increased intracranial pressure	Headaches Nausea/vomiting Confusion Decreased level of consciousness

the region of the CNS affected by the tumour and the associated peritumoural oedema. Patients may present with motor and/or sensory deficits, cognitive and behavioural changes, speech disturbances and visual deficits. These focal deficits can present over weeks to months.

Imaging features (Table 53.2)

The imaging modality of choice to evaluate intracranial tumours is magnetic resonance imaging (MRI), which typically includes a gadolinium-enhanced T1-weighted sequence to evaluate the enhancing tumour, and a non-contrast, T2-weighted sequence to evaluate the extent of non-enhancing tumour and peritumoural oedema. Additional MR acquisitions such as diffusion-weighted imaging (DWI) can be useful to differentiate active tumour versus ischaemia or necrosis, but there is no definitive diagnostic imaging test and

Table 53.2 Imaging features of brain tumours

	T1 Gad	T2 weighted
Glioma		Fluid-attenuated inversion recovery (FLAIR) T2-weighted images best show the infiltrating tumour margin
	High grade: gadolinium-enhancement with central necrosis, although absence of enhancement does not definitely exclude high grade	*High grade*: hyperintense area associated with peritumoral oedema ± low-grade component of tumour
	Low grade: no gadolinium enhancement	*Low grade*: hyperintense area, often demonstrating mass effect
Meningioma	Intense gadolinium enhancement with a sharp tumour border	Generally isointense with grey matter Histological subtypes can vary: • Angioblastic → hyperintense • Fibroblastic → hypointense
CNS lymphoma	Homogeneously gadolinium-enhancing mass	Homogeneous hypointense mass with surrounding vasogenic oedema
Medulloblastoma/primitive neuroectodermal tumour (PNET)	Heterogeneous gadolinium enhancement, commonly with leptomeningeal seeding	Hyperintense mass ± cystic components and low signal calcifications
Germ cell tumour	*Germinoma*: well-demarcated homogeneously gadolinium-enhancing mass in the pineal region, often multicystic *Teratoma*: well-demarcated heterogeneously gadolinium-enhancing mass in the pineal region, often multicystic	*Germinoma*: slightly hyperintense mass on the pineal region *Teratoma*: heterogeneous masses with calcifications (hypointense) and fatty deposits (hyperintense)
Brain metastases (secondary)	Typically well-demarcated gadolinium-enhancing mass with variable patterns: punctate, homogeneous or ring-enhancing due to central necrosis	Typically hyperintense lesion with surrounding peritumoural oedema that is often out of proportion to the tumour size
	Note: If haemorrhage is present, the T1-weighted sequence prior to gadolinium injection will be hyperintense	Note: If haemorrhage is present, there may be areas of hypointensity

histological confirmation is recommended prior to the initiation of therapy in most cases. Similarly, MR spectroscopy has shown promise in helping to distinguish active tumour from infection in the pretreatment setting, and from post-therapeutic alterations in the blood–brain barrier (BBB) due to surgery or radiation (e.g. pseudoprogression or radiation necrosis) in the post-treatment setting.

Principles of management

Ideally, all cases should be reviewed at a multidisciplinary tumour board by a multidisciplinary team composed of neurosurgery, otolaryngology (skull base tumours), radiation oncology, neuro-oncology, neuropathology and neuroradiology for a recommendation on management.

Surgery

For most brain tumours, maximal safe complete resection should be attempted if feasible. While metastases tend to be well demarcated and encapsulated, an infiltrative, diffuse and ill-delineated growth pattern is characteristic for primary brain tumours, which limits the ability to achieve a complete resection. The ability to achieve a gross total resection can depend on a number factors: tumour location (involvement of eloquent areas), surgeon experience and availability of additional image guidance (e.g. cortical mapping, intraoperative imaging, fluorescence).

Radiotherapy

External beam radiotherapy is typically recommended adjuvantly for higher-grade tumours following surgical resection, whereas radiotherapy is often reserved for treatment of recurrent or progressive lower-grade tumours. The radiation treatment volume, dose and duration depend on the tumour location, patient's clinical presentation and prognostic factors. Generally, aggressive CNS tumours are treated up to a total dose of approximately 60 Gy delivered in 1.8–2.0 Gy fractions once daily on week days. With modern radiotherapy techniques (e.g. intensity-modulated radiotherapy [IMRT]), MRI and computed tomography (CT) images are used for delineation of the target volumes and organs at risk in order to guide the generation of the treatment plan.

Chemotherapy

The brain is protected by the BBB, and although this may be disrupted within a malignant tumour, it will still protect infiltrative tumour parts from many therapeutic agents. Alkylating agents like nitrosourea (e.g. lomustine [CCNU], carmustine [BCNU], nimustine [ACNU], fotemustine) and temozolomide (TMZ) readily cross the BBB and are the most commonly used chemotherapy agents against brain tumours. Other agents that penetrate the BBB are platinum derivatives, high-dose methotrexate if administered in high doses (>2500 mg/m^2), camptothecins (irinotecan and topotecan) and etoposide.

Corticosteroids

Corticosteroids are frequently used to relieve neurological symptoms from CNS tumours and peritumoural oedema. The most commonly used agent is dexamethasone. When patients present acutely with significant symptoms, a loading dose of dexamethasone 10 mg intravenous (IV) may be administered, followed with either oral or IV maintenance doses of up to 16 mg daily. For alert patients who are able to swallow and who have no gastrointestinal issues, there is no advantage in IV administration. Once symptoms are addressed and the tumour is being treated (with surgery, radiation and/or chemotherapy), the dexamethasone dose should be rapidly tapered by 2–4 mg every 2–5 days, as tolerated. Common toxicities associated with corticosteroids include hyperglycaemia, gastrointestinal (GI) irritation (heartburn, gastritis, GI bleed), insomnia, weight gain, peripheral oedema and myopathy. In order to address the common toxicities, a GI protectant medication (proton pump inhibitor and/or H1-blocking agent) is recommended concurrently with the start of corticosteroids, and patients with known diabetes are recommended to monitor glucose more closely while taking corticosteroids.

Antiepileptics

Prophylactic administration of antiepileptic agents in patients without a prior history of seizures is not recommended; however, patients with CNS tumours often present with an inaugural epileptic seizure and thus require antiepileptics to prevent further seizures. Nevertheless, after tumour treatment (surgery, radiation) long-term antiepileptic therapy may not be required.

Antiepileptic agents commonly cause drowsiness or fatigue, occasionally unsteady gait and nausea. Most patients do adjust to these medications to some degree over time. Some older antiepileptic agents, including phenytoin, phenobarbital and carbamazepine, can induce the hepatic p450 enzyme complex, and therefore can impact the metabolism of other medications, including many chemotherapeutic agents that are also metabolized by this pathway (e.g. irinotecan or vincristine). In these patients, the use of non–enzyme-inducing agents (e.g. valproic acid, levetracetam and other third-generation agents) are preferred. Nitrosoureas or TMZ are not metabolized by this pathway and therefore are not affected.

GLIOMA

Gliomas are primary brain tumours that arise from glial progenitor cells (Fig. 53.1).

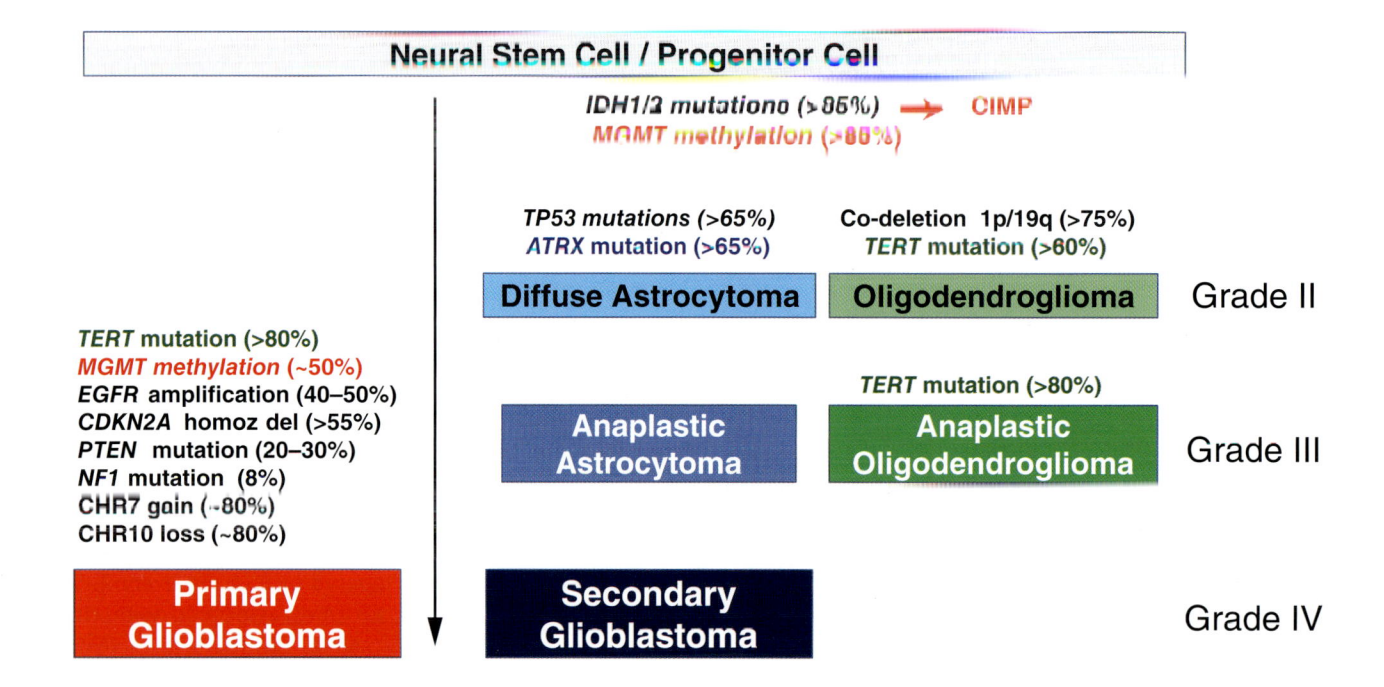

```
                    Neural Stem Cell / Progenitor Cell
                              │
                              │  IDH1/2 mutations (>85%)  →  CIMP
                              │  MGMT methylation (>80%)
                              │
                              │   TP53 mutations (>65%)     Co-deletion 1p/19q (>75%)
                              │   ATRX mutation (>65%)      TERT mutation (>60%)
                              │   ┌─────────────────┐       ┌─────────────────┐
                              │   │ Diffuse Astrocytoma │   │ Oligodendroglioma │   Grade II
                              │   └─────────────────┘       └─────────────────┘
TERT mutation (>80%)          │
MGMT methylation (~50%)       │                              TERT mutation (>80%)
EGFR amplification (40–50%)   │   ┌─────────────────┐       ┌─────────────────┐
CDKN2A homoz del (>55%)       │   │   Anaplastic    │       │   Anaplastic    │
PTEN mutation (20–30%)        │   │   Astrocytoma   │       │ Oligodendroglioma│   Grade III
NF1 mutation (8%)             │   └─────────────────┘       └─────────────────┘
CHR7 gain (~80%)              │
CHR10 loss (~80%)             ▼
  ┌─────────────┐                  ┌─────────────┐
  │   Primary   │                  │  Secondary  │                              Grade IV
  │ Glioblastoma│                  │ Glioblastoma│
  └─────────────┘                  └─────────────┘

mean age : 55 years              39 years
```

Figure 53.1 Pathogenetic/epigenetic evolution of glioma in the adult. Molecular alterations, non-exhaustive list of alterations differentiating subtypes.
Reprinted by permission from Macmillan Publishers Ltd: from Hegi, Stupp (2013), Killela et al. (2013), Bady et al. (2012), Ozawa et al. (2014), Catalogue of Somatic Mutations in Cancer [COSMIC]; http://cancer.sanger.ac.uk/cosmic/).

Pathology

Pathology: Gliomas	Description

Glioblastoma (GBM)	**WHO 2007 classification: astrocytoma grade IV**
	• *Histological features:*
	  ▪ Invasive primary glial tumour with marked cellularity, hyperchromatism and nuclear pleomorphism associated with increased vascularity and areas of necrosis
	  ▪ Primary and secondary GBM cannot be distinguished morphologically
	• *Genetic features and molecular markers:*
	  ▪ Common alterations include loss on chromosome 10q, *TP53* mutations and epidermal growth factor receptor (EGFR) over-expression
	  ▪ Isocitrate dehydrogenase (*IDH*) mutations are pathognomonic for secondary GBM (5–8% of GBM)
	  ▪ MGMT gene promoter hypermethylation is associated with improved survival (prognostic) and increased response to alkylating agent chemotherapy (e.g. TMZ) (30–45% of GBM)
	  ▪ EGFR variant III (EGFRvIII) constitutively activates the EGFR pathway and is associated with a more aggressive course:
	    ○ EGFRvIII is under investigation as a specific treatment target (e.g. kinase inhibitors, immunotoxins and peptide vaccines)

Anaplastic glioma (also referred to as grade III astrocytoma, oligoastrocytoma, oligodendroglioma)	**WHO 2007 classification: astrocytoma grade III**
	• *Genetic features and molecular markers*:
	  ▪ IDH mutations are pathognomonic for secondary high-grade gliomas and are associated with a better prognosis
	  ▪ 1p19q loss of heterozygosity in oligodendroglial tumours is associated with better prognosis and predicts for response to TMZ
	• Anaplastic oligoastrocytoma has a better prognosis than glioblastoma
	• Anaplastic astrocytoma tends to have a better prognosis than glioblastoma in younger patients; in elderly patients, the prognosis is similar for all high-grade astrocytomas

Pathology: Gliomas	Description

Low-grade gliomas	**WHO grade I**
	• *Histological subtypes*:
	  ▪ Pilocytic astrocytoma (PA)
	  ▪ Dysembryoplastic neuroepithelial tumour (DNET)
	  ▪ Pleomorphic xanthoastrocytoma (PXA)
	  ▪ Ganglioglioma
	• *Histological features*:
	  ▪ Pilocytic: often associated with neurofibromatosis type 1 (NF1)
	  ▪ *K1AA1548:BRAF* fusion in 50–70% (potential target for future therapy)
	
	WHO grade II
	• *Histological subtypes*:
	  ▪ Fibrillary astrocytoma
	  ▪ Oligodendroglioma
	  ▪ Mixed gliomas
	• *Histological features*:
	  ▪ *IDH1* mutation in 50–80% (better prognosis)
	  ▪ 1p19q loss of heterozygosity (LOH) in 50–70% with oligodendroglial component (better prognosis, more likely to respond to TMZ)

Diagnostic work-up: Imaging features

Imaging features: Gliomas	Description

Glioblastoma (GBM)	• *Contrast-enhanced T1-weighted MRI*:
	  ▪ Enhancing mass due to breakdown of the BBB with central necrosis due to rapid tumour proliferation resulting in outgrowth of vascular supply
	• *T2-weighted MRI*:
	  ▪ Hyperintensity representing both infiltrative tumour and peritumoural oedema

Anaplastic glioma (grade III astrocytoma, oligoastrocytoma, oligodendroglioma)	• *Contrast-enhanced T1-weighted MRI*:
	  ▪ Enhancing mass due to breakdown of the BBB with central necrosis due to rapid tumour proliferation resulting in outgrowth of vascular supply
	• *T2-weighted MRI*:
	  ▪ Hyperintensity representing both infiltrative tumour and peritumoural oedema

Low-grade gliomas	• *Grade I*: enhancing intra-axial mass (diffusely enhancing in paediatric and young adult patients) • *Grade II*: diffusely non-enhancing infiltrative lesions with expansion of involved brain

Staging

No TNM (tumour, node, metastases)-based staging system exists for CNS tumous.

Treatment philosophy

The standard treatment options for gliomas involve surgery, radiation and chemotherapy (Fig. 53.2).

Treatment is personalized to individual patients based on their age, clinical presentation, overall performance status, medical co-morbidities and social support, with the aim of optimizing overall survival and quality of life.

Scenario: Gliomas	Treatment philosophy
Glioblastoma (GBM)	• For patients with good prognostic factors, maximal surgical resection followed by radiotherapy with concomitant and adjuvant TMZ chemotherapy is recommended (Fig. 53.2; see Table 53.5). ▪ Key molecular and clinical prognostic factors to consider in management decisions for patients to optimize their survival and quality of life are summarized in Tables 53.3 and 53.4 • For patients with limited performance status, older age or more extensive disease (e.g. gliomatosis), the radiation and systemic therapy options are adjusted to minimize duration of therapy and toxicity of treatment (see Table 53.5)
Anaplastic glioma (grade III astrocytoma, oligoastrocytoma, oligodendroglioma)	• Recommended overall management approach for high-grade gliomas is summarized in Fig. 53.4
Low-grade gliomas	• *Grade I*: indolent, potentially curable neoplasm with complete or maximal resection and individualized post-surgical management • *Grade II*: slow-growing neoplasm that is managed with a combination of surgery, radiotherapy and chemotherapy over the course of disease with individualized approaches, considering all tumour and patient factors

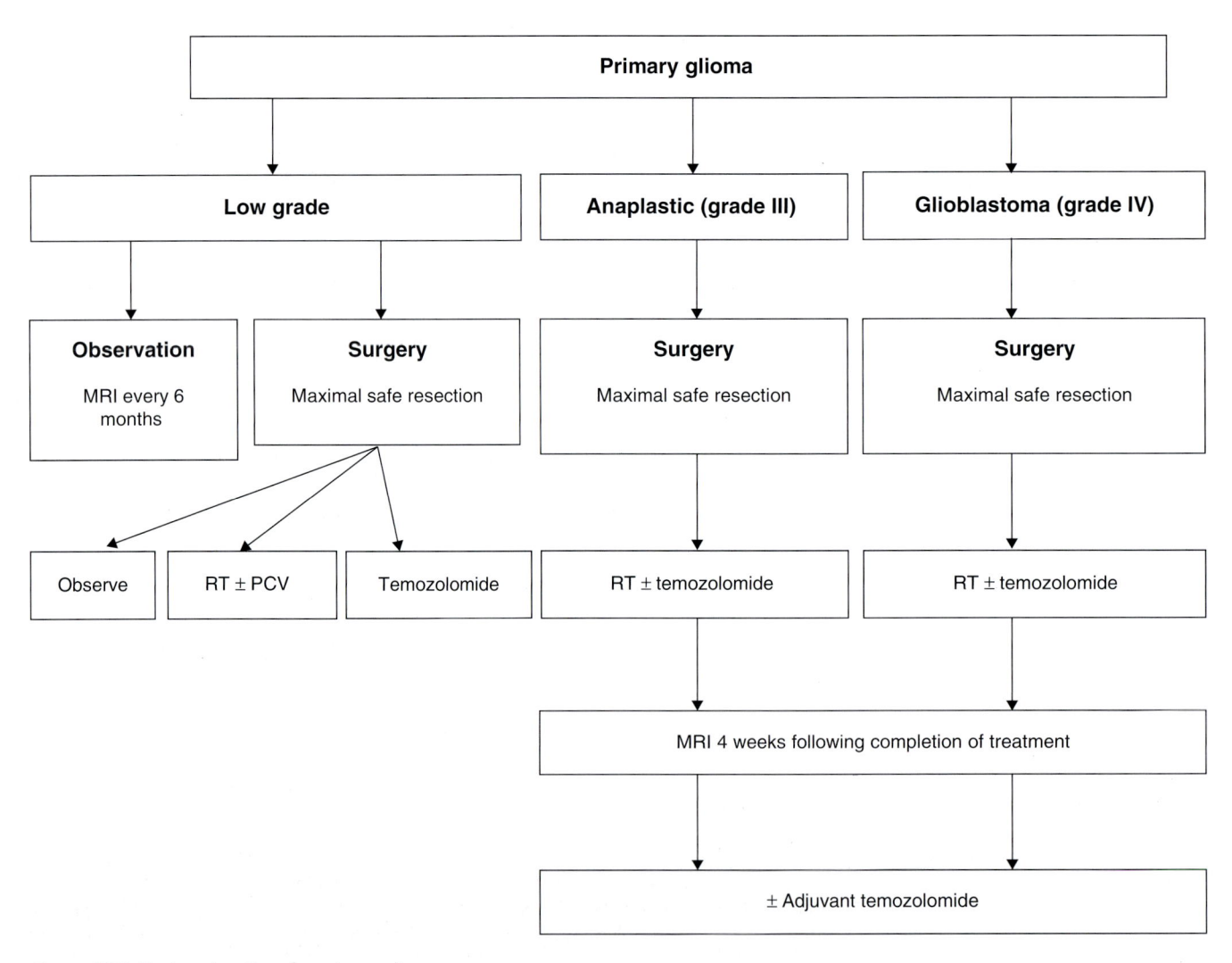

Figure 53.2 Treatment options for primary glioma.

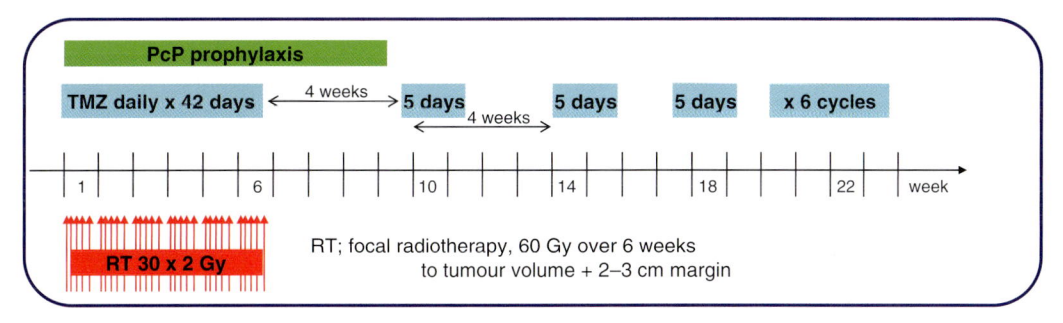

Figure 53.3 Summary of combined radiotherapy and temozolomide for glioblastoma.

Source: Reprinted from Mino et al. (2013) Central nervous system. In: Dicato MA, ed. *Side Effects of Medical Cancer Therapy*. London: Springer, with permission.

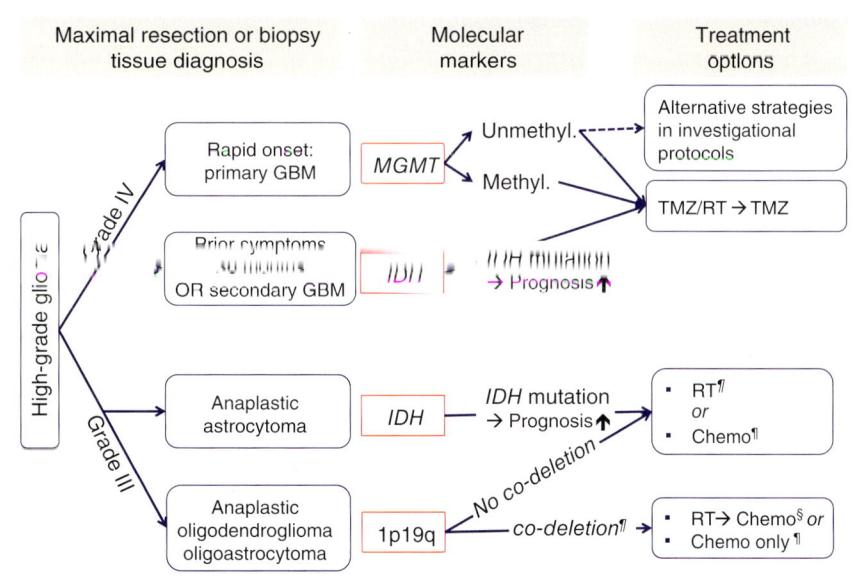

Figure 53.4 Management algorithm for high-grade gliomas.

¶RT or chemotherapy first, and at progression chemotherapy or RT, respectively (according to NOA-04).
§Subgroup analysis and long-term follow-up of RTOG and EORTC randomized studies demonstrated prolonged survival for patients treated with RT → PCV.
GBM, glioblastoma; *MGMT*, methylguanine methyltransferase gene promoter methylation status; *IDH*, isocitrate dehydrogenase gene mutation; LOH 1p/19q, loss of heterozygosity of chromosomes 1 and 19; RT, radiotherapy; Chemo, chemotherapy with either PCV or temozolomide; PCV, procarabine + lomustine (CCNU) + vincristine; TMZ, temozolomide.

Table 53.3 Prognostic factors for brain tumours

Brain tumour type	Prognostic factors	Tumour related	Host related	Treatment related
Diffuse low-grade astrocytoma (grade II)	Essential	Size of tumour (>5–6 cm) Extension across the midline IDH	Age (>40 years) Performance status	Gross total resection
	Additional	Gemistocytes (unfavourable) Oligodendrocytes (favourable) Proliferation rate (MIB-1/Ki-67) VEGF expression TP53 mutation		
	New and promising	BRAF V600E, FGFR1,		
High-grade glioma (grade III + IV)	Essential	Histological grade MGMT gene promoter methylation	Age (>50 years, >70 years) Performance status	Extent of resection Concomitant chemoradiotherapy (grade IV)
	Additional	IDH mutation ATRX or LOH 1p/19q		Radiotherapy or chemotherapy (grade III)
	New and promising	TP53, EGFR, EGFRviii, PDGFR, PTEN, FGFR1/3, TERT		
Oligodendroglioma (grade III)	Essential	Histological grade Co-deletion on chromosomes 1p/19q	Age Performance status	Extent of resection Adjuvant chemotherapy Radiotherapy
	Additional	IDH mutation		
	New and promising	TERT, CIC, FUBP1		
Meningioma	Essential	Histological grade Location (skull based vs non-skull based)	Age Performance status	Extent of resection Treatment with fractionated radiotherapy or radiosurgery
	Additional	Proliferation rate (MIB-1/Ki-67) TP53 over-expression		
	New and promising	Proportion of cells in S-phase Telomerase activity Upregulation of hTERT mRNA PDGF-BB, VEGF/SEMA3A ratio EGFR		
Medulloblastoma or PNET	Essential	Histology: high risk – PNET, anaplastic or large cell medulloblastoma CSF spread – if present, then high risk	Age Performance status	Extent of resection (≥1.5 cm³ is high risk) Treatment with fractionated radiotherapy and/or chemotherapy

Table 53.4 Prognostic factors from recursive partitioning analysis for patients treated with surgery, radiation and chemotherapy for GBM

RPA risk group	Prognostic factors	Median survival (weeks)
1 (lowest risk)	<40 years old Frontal tumour	132
2	<40 years old Tumour beyond frontal lobe	71
3	40–65 years old KPS >70 Subtotal/total resection	63
4 (highest risk)	>65 years old or 40–65 years old KPS <80 or any age with only biopsy	37

Surgery

Surgery: Gliomas	Description
Glioblastoma (GBM)	- Maximal safe resection with the aim of a gross total resection should be attempted whenever feasible - For unresectable disease, stereotactic biopsy for histological diagnosis (for molecular marker analyses) as sufficient tumour material is needed in order to extract DNA or RNA
Anaplastic glioma (grade III astrocytoma, oligoastrocytoma, oligodendroglioma)	- Maximal safe surgical resection

Low-grade gliomas	- Grade *I*:
	  - Curative complete resection when possible or maximal safe surgical resection
	  - *Post-surgical options:*
	    - Observation
	    - Radiotherapy only
	    - Chemotherapy alone (often reserved for recurrence)
	    - Decision is individualized based on various prognostic factors: age, extent of resection, volume of brain requiring radiation, involvement of eloquent brain (motor strip, internal capsule, brain stem), neurological deficit, performance status and histological/molecular features (see Table 53.3)
	- Grade *II*:
	  - Maximal safe surgical resection
	  - *Post-surgical options:*
	    - Observation
	    - Radiotherapy alone
	    - TMZ alone
	    - Decision is individualized based on various prognostic factors: age, seizures, histology (presence of worrisome features, elevated proliferative indices, presence or absence of oligo component), enhancement on MRI, performance status, tumour bulk, neurological deficit, involvement of eloquent brain, presence/absence of co-deletion of 1p19q

Salvage treatment	- Salvage treatments are individualized based on the clinical presentation and prognostic factors, including patient age, performance status and ability to obtain effective further resection

Radiotherapy

Radiotherapy: Gliomas	Description

Glioblastoma (GBM) (Table 53.5)	- For patients up to the age of 70 years with adequate general health and function (Karnofsky performance status [KPS] ≥70), the following dose prescriptions are recommended (IRCU 62):
	  - Target volume contours:
	    - Gross tumour volume (GTV): enhancing tumour and surgical cavity (but excluding the surgical approach changes in brain that were previously uninvolved with tumour)
	    - Clinical target volume (CTV): 1.5 cm (that will encompass the majority of the surrounding T2 hyperintensity)
	    - Planning target volume (PTV): 0.5 cm (depending on set-up error at the institution)
	  - If the tumour is a secondary GBM with a dominant non-enhancing component, the following treatment volumes are recommended:
	    - GTV: surgical cavity (exclude surgical approach) + tumour on T2-weighted imaging (usually FLAIR)
	    - CTV: 1 cm
	    - PTV: 0.5 cm (depending on set-up error at the institution)
	  - Dose prescription:
	    - Approximately 60 Gy is prescribed over approximately 6 weeks (commonly 2 Gy/fraction × 30 fractions or 1.8 Gy/fraction × 33 fractions), typically delivered with concurrent TMZ chemotherapy
	    - If the tumour is particularly large such that excessive brain will receive high-dose radiotherapy, dose may be reduced to respect normal tissue tolerances (e.g. a total dose of 54 Gy delivered in 1.8 Gy/fraction × 30 fractions)

(continued)

Radiotherapy: Gliomas	Description
	• For elderly patients and patients with low performance status, accelerated hypofractionated irradiation schemes are often proposed: (e.g. 40 Gy in 15 fractions delivered over 3 weeks, 3.4 Gy × 10 fractions over 2 weeks) • Small randomized trials have demonstrated similar outcome and hypofractionated regimens with concomitant TMZ chemotherapy are being investigated in a randomized clinical trial • In patients with poor performance status, whole-brain radiotherapy (WBRT) to a dose of 30 Gy in ten fractions delivered over 2 weeks may be offered for palliation: ▪ In some cases, it may be more appropriate to omit radiotherapy to focus on supportive care and optimization of quality of life
Anaplastic glioma (grade III astrocytoma, oligoastrocytoma, oligodendroglioma)	• Adjuvant radiotherapy up to 60 Gy, with the same approach for target volume (GTV/CTV/PTV) delineation as for GBM

Low-grade gliomas (typically only grade II)	• GTV: surgical cavity (excluding surgical approach) + FLAIR abnormality
	• CTV: grade I 0.5 cm; grade II 1.0 cm
	• PTV: grade I 0.3–0.5 cm; grade II 0.5 cm (depends on institutional set-up error with immobilization ± image guidance)
	• Dose: 50 Gy in 25 fractions or 54 Gy in 30 fractions:
	   ▪ Alternative dose prescription for patients aged >65–70 years or those with compromised performance status:
	      ○ Partial brain: 40 Gy in 15 fractions to same GTV, CTV, PTV as described above
	      ○ Whole brain: 20 Gy in five fractions or 30 Gy in ten fractions

Table 53.5 Summary of radiotherapy and systemic therapy for GBM

Patient population	Radiotherapy	Systemic therapy
Age <70 years and KPS >70	60 Gy in 30 fractions (2 Gy/fraction) or 33 fractions (1.8 Gy/fraction) over 6 weeks (five fractions/week)	Temozolomide 75 mg/m^2 PO daily, 7 days/week over 6 weeks during radiotherapy
Age >70 years and good KPS	40 Gy in 15 fractions (2.66 Gy/fraction) over 3 weeks (five fractions/week) or 34 Gy in ten fractions (3.4 Gy/fraction) over 2 weeks (five fractions/week)	Uncertain benefit of adding temozolomide with hypofractionated radiation (ongoing randomized study)
Poor KPS Leptomeningeal or multifocal disease	30 Gy in ten fractions to the whole brain (3.0 Gy/fraction) over 2 weeks (five fractions/week)	None

Systemic therapy

Systemic therapy: Gliomas	Description

Glioblastoma (GBM) (Table 53.5)	• Temozolomide (TMZ) is an oral, alkylating agent
	• For patients <70 years old with a KPS of >70, the current standard treatment involves TMZ 75 mg/m^2 daily, which is administered 7 days a week concurrently with 6 weeks of radiation (60 Gy in 30 fractions delivered 5 days a week) followed by adjuvant TMZ 150–200 mg/m^2 daily in a 5-day/28-day schedule for 6–12 cycles after the completion of radiotherapy:
	   ▪ Landmark phase III randomized controlled trial conducted by the European Organization for the Research and Treatment of Cancer (EORTC) and the National Cancer Institute of Canada demonstrated that this combined regimen resulted in significant prolongation of survival (hazard ratio 0.63)
	• During treatment, monitoring as follows:
	   ▪ Weekly complete blood counts (CBC) during daily concurrent TMZ and radiotherapy
	   ▪ Monthly CBC during monthly adjuvant TMZ
	      ○ Usually well tolerated, but may induce mild-to-moderate nausea and vomiting and myelosuppression:
	   ▪ Main toxicity is profound lymphocytopenia and thrombocytopenia, occurring late in the treatment cycle after 21–28 days
	   ▪ Prophylaxis for thrush, herpes and pneumocystis should be considered, especially in patients with absolute lymphocyte counts of <500 μL

Systemic therapy: Gliomas	Description

Anaplastic glioma (grade III astrocytoma, oligoastrocytoma, oligodendroglioma)	• Added value of concomitant and/or adjuvant TMZ has not been evaluated prospectively
	• Clinical trials have suggested improved survival with (neo)adjuvant PCV chemotherapy (procarbazine + lomustine [CCNU] + vincristine) in patients with newly diagnosed anaplastic oligoastrocytoma and oligodendroglioma with co-deletion of 1p/19q
	• Patients may be considered for upfront chemotherapy rather than radiotherapy:
	  ■ A recent trial with short follow-up of 4.5 years has shown similar time to failure following initial chemotherapy or radiation:
	    ○ No observed difference in efficacy between PCV or TMZ chemotherapy

Low-grade gliomas	• *Grade I*:
	  ■ Chemotherapy most often given at recurrence following radiotherapy in adults
	  ■ Typical agents:
	    ○ TMZ in 5-day/28-day cycle, 150–200 mg/m^2
	    ○ Vincristine + carboplatin (associated with 65% progression-free rate [PFS] at 3 years)
	    ○ Weekly vinblastine (used at salvage with a 50% response rate)
	• *Grade II*:
	  ■ Recent data support the use of TMZ (5-day/28-day cycle, 150–200 mg/m^2) either as an upfront post-surgical approach (particularly in cases with co-deletion of 1p19q) or for recurrence following radiotherapy

Recurrent glioma

Salvage treatment: Gliomas	Description
Repeat surgery	• Can provide rapid palliation of symptoms by debulking tumour and decompressing the brain • Can provide histological confirmation of the clinical and radiological suspicion
Salvage radiotherapy	• Offered at the time of progression after initial surgery and chemotherapy • Repeat irradiation may be considered for highly selected patients: ■ Good performance status and focal disease recurrence after a durable period of tumour control following initial radiation treatment • Various dose and fractionation schedules using both fractionated IMRT and radiosurgery have been evaluated, but no standard salvage radiotherapy regimen has been established

Salvage systemic therapy	• More commonly utilized at the time of tumour recurrence following prior radiotherapy with or without TMZ
	• Salvage regimens include:
	  ■ TMZ rechallenge:
	    ○ 150–200 mg/m^2 for 5 days every 28 days
	    ○ 75 mg/m^2 daily
	  ■ Nitrosureas + carmustine (BCNU) + lomustine (CCNU), nimustine (ACNU) + fotemustine
	  ■ Studies have shown that combination therapy results in added toxicity with no significant benefit over single-agent treatment
	  ■ Bevacizumab (monoclonal antibody to vascular endothelial growth factor [VEGF]):
	    ■ Approved by the US Food and Drug Administration (FDA) for GBM recurrence and progression after initial therapy based on the results of a phase II trial showing significantly better 6-month PFS of 50.3% with salvage bevacizumab and irinotecan versus 42.6% with irinotecan alone
	    ■ Definitive studies demonstrating an improvement in overall survival are still lacking
	    ■ Normalizes vascular permeability, thus reduces steroid requirement and leads to a decrease of the enhancing tumour volume without reduction of tumour size or destruction of tumour cells; this radiological phenomenon (pseudoresponse; see below) presumably accounts for the high response rates observed with bevacizumab without improvement in overall survival

Assessment of treatment response

A phenomenon called pseudoprogression, a self-limiting reaction to therapy that radiologically and clinically mimics tumour progression, is frequently observed weeks to months after initial radiotherapy. It may occur in up to 30–50% of patients with GBM treated with concurrent radiation and TMZ, and is more frequent in patients with MGMT methylated tumours. Although MR spectroscopy or positron emission tomography (PET) scan may occasionally help distinguish pseudoprogression from true tumour progression, there is currently no gold standard imaging test for this differentiation. Clinically, patients who have symptoms as well as these radiological changes are more likely to have true tumour progression over pseudoprogression. Therefore, in patients who are clinically well, a differential diagnosis of pseudoprogression should always be considered when radiological progression is observed following treatment, before embarking on salvage treatment with repeat surgery or second-line chemotherapy.

Follow-up

- *High-grade gliomas (glioblastoma and anaplastic gliomas):*
  - Clinical assessment every 3–4 months with MRI
- *Low-grade gliomas:*
  - Clinical assessment and MRI brain post treatment:
    - Every 3–4 months for Year 1
    - 6 monthly for Years 2–5
    - Once yearly for Years 5–10

MENINGIOMA

Pathology

Pathology: Meningioma	Description
Meningothelial, fibroblastic, transitional, angiomatous, microcystic, secretory, lymphoplasmacytic metaplastic, psammomatous (90% of cases)	- WHO grade I - Do not fulfil criteria for grade II or III

Chordoid, clear cell (7%)	- WHO grade II (atypical)
	- Four or more mitotic cells per 10 HPF and/or three or more of the following in an otherwise grade I tumour:
	  - Increased cellularity
	  - Small cells
	  - Necrosis
	  - Prominent nucleoli
	  - Sheeting
	  - Brain invasion

Papillary, rhabdoid (3%)	- WHO grade III (anaplastic or malignant) - 20 or more mitoses per 10 HPF and/or obviously malignant cytological characteristics such that tumour cells resemble carcinoma, sarcoma or melanoma

Table 53.6 Simpson grading for resection of meningioma

Grade	Definition
1	Gross total resection with excision of involved dura, sinus and bone
2	Gross total resection with coagulation of dural attachments
3	Macroscopic resection without resection or coagulation of dural attachment
4	Subtotal resection
5	Biopsy

The most common genetic alteration is loss of the *NF2* gene on chromosome 22q, which encodes a tumour suppressor protein known as merlin (or schwannomin).

Prognostic factors (see Table 53.3) are:
- Age: older age associated with worse prognosis
- Histological grade
- Simpson resection grade (Table 53.6).

Diagnostic work-up

- Typical radiological features:
  - Contrast-enhanced T1-weighted MRI: diffusely enhancing mass arising from the meninges
  - T2-weighted MRI: iso- or hypo-intense mass arising from the meninges

Treatment philosophy

Scenario: Meningioma	Treatment philosophy

WHO grade I	- *Surgery*: complete surgical resection if feasible, or maximal safe surgical resection:
	  - Simpson grading classifies tumours following surgery based on extent of resection (see Table 53.6)
	- *Postoperative management*: following partial resection with gross residual disease (Simpson grade 4), radiotherapy can be considered immediately after surgery or may be delayed until tumour progression
	- *Unresectable or recurrent/progressive grade I meningioma:*
	  - For symptomatic meningioma that cannot be surgically resected (e.g. cavernous sinus, optic nerve), radiotherapy is recommended
	  - For recurrent meningiomas, radiotherapy with or without additional surgical resection is usually recommended

Scenario: Meningioma	Treatment philosophy

WHO grade II	• *Surgery*: complete surgical resection if feasible, or maximal safe surgical resection
	• *Postoperative management*:
	  ▪ *Gross total resection*: observation is reasonable as the rate of recurrence at 10 years is about 50%
	  ▪ *Gross residual or recurrent tumour*: radiotherapy is recommended

WHO grade III	• *Surgery*: complete surgical resection if feasible, or maximal safe surgical resection • *Postoperative management*: radiotherapy is recommended in all cases

Treatment

Radiosurgery

- *Indications*:
  - Maximal tumour diameter of 3 cm
  - Initial treatment for skull base meningiomas
  - Treatment of small residual/recurrent grade I meningiomas
  - Treatment of recurrent grade II/III meningiomas after prior fractionated radiation
- *Immobilization*: radiosurgery frame or relocatable stereotactic frame with image guidance
- *Imaging*: CT and MRI T1 gadolinium, T2
- *Target volumes and dose*:
  - GTV: T1-gadolinium enhancing tumour
  - CTV: none
  - PTV: none (unless institutional measurements suggest margin for set-up error)
  - Dose: 12–16 Gy based on location and aggressiveness of tumour

Fractionated radiotherapy

- *Indications*:
  - All tumours with a maximal dimension of >3 cm
  - All tumours with a prior partial resection
  - All grade II and III tumours
- *Immobilization*: thermoplastic frame or stereotactic relocatable frame
- *Imaging*:
  - Preoperative imaging (CT, MRI) to identify initial tumour location
  - Planning CT and planning MRI (T1 gad, T2)
- *Target volumes and dose*:
  - GTV: surgical cavity and enhancing tumour, excluding surgical approach
  - CTV:
    - 0 cm for grade I meningiomas with no prior surgery
    - 0.5 cm for grade I meningiomas with prior surgery, all grade II/III tumours
  - PTV: 0.5 cm (depends on institutional set-up variability)
  - Dose:
    - Grade I meningioma 50 Gy in 25 fractions or 54 Gy in 30 fractions
    - Atypical or malignant meningioma 60 Gy in 30 fractions ± optional boost to GTV with 0.3-cm PTV margin of additional 10 Gy in five fractions (i.e. total dose of 70 Gy in 35 fractions)

Systemic therapy

There are no chemotherapeutic or targeted agents known to be effective for any grade of meningioma. Initial promising reports for the use of interferon, progesterone (i.e. mifepristone [RU486]), hydroxyurea and other agents have not been confirmed in trials. Novel treatments are needed.

Follow-up

- *Grade I*: clinical assessment and MRI:
  - At 6 months
  - Then 12 monthly until Year 5
  - Then once every 2 years
- *Grade II/III* (atypical/malignant): clinical assessment and MRI:
  - 6 monthly until Year 5
  - Then once yearly

CNS LYMPHOMA

CNS lymphoma accounts for <1% of intracranial tumours and <1% of non-Hodgkin lymphomas. It generally occurs in patients in their sixth and seventh decades, but can be seen at all ages. The incidence is higher in immunocompromised patients.

Pathology

- Most cases are diffuse large B-cell non-Hodgkin lymphomas
- Prognosis is poor regardless of histology:
  - Main prognostic factors are age and performance status

Diagnostic work-up

- *Typical radiological features*:
  - Contrast-enhanced T1-weighted MRI: single or multiple deep, diffusely enhancing masses, often with a serpentiginous or white matter tract pattern of spread
- *Biopsy*:
  - Efforts should be made to biopsy before steroids are given
  - If steroids need to be started to control mass effect, the biopsy should be done within 12 hours of starting steroids

- *Staging investigations* should include:
  - Brain MRI (or CT if MRI is not available)
  - CT chest, abdomen and pelvis
  - Ophthalmological examination
  - Bone marrow biopsy
  - Cerebrospinal fluid (CSF) examination

Treatment philosophy (immunocompetent patients)

Chemotherapy is the treatment of first choice at initial diagnosis of primary CNS lymphoma. The main role for surgery is in histological confirmation (i.e. biopsy only).
- *Younger patients with good performance status*: upfront chemotherapy, followed by radiotherapy for consolidation unless there is a complete response
- *Older patients with good performance status*: upfront chemotherapy, then observation, reserving short-course radiotherapy for recurrence
- *Older, less well patients (generally age 70+ years)*: upfront short-course radiotherapy with possible palliative chemotherapy at recurrence, although salvage rate post-radiotherapy recurrence is <20%

Treatment

Radiotherapy
Randomized trial data suggest that inclusion of WBRT improves progression-free survival but does not necessarily improve overall survival. A recent trial demonstrated promising results of improved long-term disease control with minimal toxicity with the addition of rituximab to methotrexate + procarbazine + vincristine followed by consolidative reduced-dose WBRT and cytarabine. Overall, however, the efficacy of WBRT to improve PFS needs to be weighed against the increased neurotoxicity in long-term survivors.
- *Target volumes:*
  - GTV: whole brain
  - CTV: none
  - PTV: 1 cm beyond cranial bone
- Dose:
  - Younger patient following response to chemotherapy: 40 Gy in 20 fractions
  - Younger patient progressing on chemotherapy: 50 Gy in 25 fractions
  - Younger patient who cannot continue chemotherapy due to toxicity: 50 Gy in 25 fractions
  - Older patient as primary treatment or for recurrence: 20 Gy in five fractions
  - Patient with ocular involvement: to a total dose of 35–40 Gy in 1.5–2-Gy fractions should be delivered to bilateral orbits

Systemic therapy
Intermediate-to-high dose methotrexate (MTX), typically in the range of 3–4 g/m^2, in a multiagent chemotherapy regimen seems to be associated with the best results. Table 53.7 summarizes the chemotherapy regimens evaluated for initial therapy of primary CNS lymphoma.

Follow-up
- Clinic visit and MRI brain every 3–4 months

MEDULLOBLASTOMA AND PRIMITIVE NEUROECTODERMAL TUMOUR

Medulloblastoma and PNET account for <2% of intracranial malignancies in adults, but occur more frequently in children. Medulloblastomas are more common than PNET and present in the posterior fossa. In general, the prognosis for PNET is worse than that for medulloblastoma. Medulloblastomas are associated with Gorlin and Turcot syndrome, usually as the first manifestation of either syndrome.

Pathology

Medulloblastomas and PNET are WHO grade IV tumours.
Histologically, these are highly cellular neoplasms composed of cells with small-to-medium sized, hyperchromatic nuclei and little cytoplasm. They have high mitotic rates, tumour necrosis and cellular apoptosis with nuclear pyknosis, fragmentation or karyorrhexis. Homer Wright ('neuroblastic') rosettes are seen in approximately 40% of cases.
- *Molecular/genetic features:*
  - Positive prognostic marker:
    - Expression of nuclear beta-catenin (15–20% of medulloblastomas) is associated with activation of the WNT signalling pathway (potential therapeutic target), loss of chromosome 6 and TRK-C expression
  - Negative prognostic markers:
    - Chromosome 1q gain, *MYCN* amplification, C-ERBB2 over-expression and *TP53* mutation/expression, *MYCC* gene amplification (10% medulloblastomas, usually anaplastic)
- *Prognostic features* (see Table 53.3):
  - Extent of locally residual tumour post surgery
  - Presence or absence of CSF spread

Diagnostic work-up

- *Typical imaging features*:
  - Contrast-enhanced T1-weighted MRI: hypointense lesion with heterogeneous enhancement

Table 53.7 Chemotherapy regimens evaluated for initial therapy of primary CNS lymphoma

Initial chemotherapy	Radiotherapy	Additional chemotherapy
Methotrexate (MTX) 4 g/m^2 IV over 4 hours on Day 1 of a 14-day cycle, × 6 Ifosfamide 1.5 g/m^2 IV over 3 hours on Days 3–5 of a 14-day cycle × 6	45 Gy in 30 fractions	Cytarabine (ara-C) 3 g/m^2 IV over 3 hours on Days 1–2 of a 21 day cycle × 4
MTX 3.5 g/m^2 IV over 2 hours on Day 1 of a 14-day cycle with leucovorin rescue Vincristine 1.4 mg/m^2 (max 2.8 mg) IV on Day 1 of a 14-day cycle Procarbazine 100 mg/m^2 PO on Days 1–7 for cycles 1, 3 and 5, starting 24 hours after MTX infusion	45 Gy (40–50 Gy in 1.8–2-Gy fractions)	Ara-C 3 g/m^2 IV over 3 hours on Days 1–2 × 2 cycles, 1 month apart

- *Staging investigations*:
  - MRI brain and spine should ideally be acquired preoperatively
  - Lumbar puncture should be done no sooner than 14 days postoperatively (CSF contamination during surgery)

Treatment philosophy

Maximal surgical resection of the primary tumour is attempted to avoid the development of hydrocephalus followed by adjuvant craniospinal radiotherapy with or without chemotherapy.

Treatment

Surgery
- Maximal safe resection of the primary tumour will address the issue of hydrocephalus in order to avoid the need for a CSF shunt
- Postoperative brain MRI is recommended within 24–48 hours of surgery to best assess extent of locally residual disease and extent of resection

Radiotherapy
- *Craniospinal fields:*
  - Lateral opposed fields to cover all intracranial contents and cervical cord:
    - Gantry rotation of the lateral brain/cervical cord fields should be matched to the superior border of the spinal field
  - Direct posterior field to cover the whole spine down to the S2–S3 junction in order to treat the entire thecal sac with a margin
  - Extended source-to-skin distance (SSD) or a junctioned third field at the inferior border of the primary spinal field may be necessary
- *Dose*:
  - Low/average risk: 36 Gy in 20 fractions without chemotherapy
  - High risk: 39.6 Gy in 22 fractions with neoadjuvant or adjuvant chemotherapy
- *Boost to primary tumour:*
  - GTV: surgical cavity plus residual tumour
  - CTV: 1 cm
  - PTV: 5 mm
  - Dose: boost to 55.8 Gy in 31 fractions to primary site, 54 Gy in 30 fractions to metastatic gross areas of disease (both for intracranial and spinal regions)

Systemic therapy

- Chemotherapy is recommended as part of initial management of adults with high-risk medulloblastoma or PNET:
  - Repeat cycles of a combination of active agents like cisplatin or ifosfamide + carboplatin + etoposide (ICE regimen) or cyclophosphamide are commonly used
- At recurrence, a variety of chemotherapy regimens may be considered, although no standard of care exists in this situation and all are non-curative:
  - Simple oral approaches such as TMZ, CCNU, procarbazine, cyclophosphamide
  - More intensive regimens are cisplatin based

Follow-up

- Years 1–2: clinical assessment every 4–6 months with MRI brain ± spine, if prior gross spinal disease was present
- Years 3–5: clinical assessment with MRI every 6 months
- Years 5–10: clinical assessment with MRI once yearly
- Beyond 10 years: clinical assessment with MRI every 2 years

BRAIN METASTASES

The incidence of brain metastases is rising with longer survival and better extracranial disease control in patients with metastatic cancer.

Pathology

Most common primary cancers, in order, are lung, breast, melanoma, renal, colorectal and others.

A number of prognostic indices have been developed for patients with brain metastases. Many of these indices share common prognostic factors, as summarized in Table 53.8.

Diagnostic work-up: imaging features

- Contrast-enhanced T1-weighted MRI: single or multiple enhancing, typically round tumours
- T2-weighted MRI: hypointense tumour with surrounding vasogenic oedema

Treatment philosophy

- *Surgery* is indicated for:
  - Mass effect: large tumour, moderate tumour with excessive oedema resulting in symptomatic mass effect, posterior fossa mass
  - Histological confirmation
  - Single metastasis or solitary metastasis
- *Radiosurgery* is indicated for:
  - As a boost for one to four brain metastases at presentation in patients with good performance status and minimal or controlled extracranial disease
  - Salvage radiosurgery following WBRT
- *WBRT* is indicated for:
  - Multiple (≥4) brain metastases at initial presentation or recurrence following prior radiosurgery
  - Leptomeningeal disease
  - Histology: small cell lung cancer, lymphoma
  - Postoperative
- *Chemotherapy* is indicated in chemosensitive disease (histologies known to respond [e.g. small cell lung cancer], patients not having received prior chemotherapy):
  - Asymptomatic brain metastases may respond similarly to systemic therapy as do visceral metastases

Radiotherapy

- *Radiosurgery planning*:
  - GTV: enhancing tumour on contrast-enhanced T1-weighted MR images
  - CTV: 0 cm
  - PTV: 0 cm (unless institutional set-error in stereotactic immobilization suggests adding a PTV margin)
  - Dose prescription (typically to the 50% isodose for Gamma Knife and 80% isodose for linear accelerator-based treatment).
    - Tumour volume 4–10 cm^3: 21–24 Gy
    - 10–20 cm^3: 18 Gy
    - >20 cm^3: 15 Gy
- *Radiotherapy planning*:
  - Fields: lateral parallel opposed fields to encompass the whole brain
  - Dose prescription:
    - 20 Gy in five fractions
    - 30 Gy in ten fractions
    - 37.5 Gy in 15 fractions

Follow-up

- Clinical assessment and MR brain every 3–4 months, if indicated

Controversies

Bevacizumab for glioblastoma

Two randomized clinical trials, Radiation Therapy Oncology Group (RTOG) and AVAglio (Roche sponsored), have investigated whether or not adding bevacizumab to standard

Table 53.8 Prognostic indices for brain metastases

Prognostic index	Age	KPS	Extracranial disease status	Primary tumour control	Volume of largest met	Number of mets
RPA classification	✓		✓	✓		
Golden Grading System	✓	✓	✓			
Basic Score for Brain Metastases (BS-BM)		✓	✓	✓		
Score Index for Radiosurgery (SIR)	✓	✓		✓	✓	✓
Graded Prognostic Assessment (GPA)*	✓	✓	✓			✓

*Disease-specific GPA (DS-GPA) = GPA with tumour histology incorporated.

therapy (TMZ/RT → TMZ) improves patient outcomes. Both demonstrated improvement in PFS but failed to show an improvement in overall survival. The current standard care following resection remains radiotherapy in combination with TMZ without bevacizumab.

WBRT for one to four brain metastases

Prior studies have raised concern about the neurocognitive toxicities of standard WBRT for patients with brain metastases. Motivated by these concerns, recent and ongoing studies have focused on the neurocognitive outcomes of brain metastases treatment, including the benefit of hippocampal-sparing WBRT techniques.

Two large randomized trials have aimed to address the benefit and toxicity of upfront WBRT in patients with a new diagnosis of one to four brain metastases. Recognizing that patients with brain metastases may die from progression of their extracranial disease, both studies utilized a primary endpoint of neurocognitive function, which may significantly impact quality of life and may reflect intracranial control. The first study N0574 randomized patients with one to three brain metastases to either radiosurgery alone or radiosurgery with WBRT. This study recently met target accrual and results will be presented at ASCO 2015. The second study, N107C, randomized patients with one to four brain metastases following surgical resection of one metastases to either radiosurgery alone to the surgical cavity and unresected metastases or WBRT alone. This study is still actively open to accrual.

Systemic therapy

The BBB protecting the brain against toxic agents remains a major challenge in the treatment of brain tumours. Many agents will not reach the tumour cells in sufficient concentration, in particular in the infiltrative and non-enhancing parts of the tumour.

Phase III clinical trials

See Table 53.9.

Recent advances and future directions

Surgical advances

The use of advanced intraoperative imaging, neuronavigation tools and tissue fluorescence with 5-aminolevolinic acid (5-ALA) to guide surgical resection are increasing the capability to achieve more extensive tumour resections while maintaining functional outcome in patients. In low-to-intermediate-grade gliomas, the more tumour removed, the better the outcome (a difference that can be measured in years, not just weeks or months). Also, maximum safe resection without leaving neurological deficits has been recently advocated even in higher grade glioma. To achieve the goal of maximum safe cytoreduction of the tumour, advanced surgical techniques such as intraoperative imaging, neurophysiological mapping during awake surgery, tumour resection under the guidance

Table 53.9 Phase III clinical trials

Trial name	Results
High-grade gliomas	
EORTC-NCIC Stupp et al. (2009) Lancet Oncol 10(5):459–466	• Phase III trial of radiotherapy with concomitant and adjuvant TMZ vs radiotherapy alone in glioblastoma • Overall survival (OS) at 2 years was 27.2% with TMZ vs 10.9% without TMZ
AVAglio Chinot et al. (2014) N Engl J Med 370(8):709–722 RTOG 0825; Gilbert et al. (2014) N Engl J Med 370(8):699–708	• Randomized trial of bevacizumab • First line use of bevacizumab in combination with radiation and TMZ prolonged progression free survival (PFS), but did not improve OS
RTOG 0525 Gilbert et al. (2013) J Clin Oncol 31(32):4085–491	• Phase III trial comparing conventional adjuvant TMZ with dose-intensive TMZ in patients with newly diagnosed glioblastoma • OS was similar between dose-intensive adjuvant TMZ (75–100 mg/m² × 21 days) every 4 weeks (median survival 14.9 months) and standard adjuvant TMZ (150–200 mg/m² × 5 days) every 4 weeks (median survival 16.6 months) • Greater grade ≥3 toxicity in the dose-intensive treatment arm with greater lymphopenia and fatigue
Low-grade gliomas	
EORTC 22845 van den Bent et al. (2005) Lancet 366:985–990	• Phase III randomized trial of early postoperative radiotherapy vs observation until progression for low-grade glioma • 5-year PFS 55% with radiotherapy vs 35% without • Similar OS of 7.4 year with radiotherapy vs 7.2 years without

Table 53.9 (Continued)

Trial name	Results
EORTC 22033-26033/CE.5 Shaw et al. (2002) J Clin Oncol 20(9):2267–2276	• Phase III randomized trial of postoperative radiotherapy vs TMZ for high risk supratentorial low grade gliomas • No difference in PFS or OS between radiotherapy and TMZ • NCCTG Phase III randomized trial of standard post-operative radiotherapy (50.4 Gy) versus high dose radiotherapy (64.8 Gy) for low grade glioma • No difference in PFS or OS but higher rates of neurotoxicity in the high-dose arm (Grade 3–5 neurotoxicity: 5% versus 2.5% at 2 years)
RTOG 98-02 Shaw et al. (2012) J Clin Oncol 30(25): 3065–3070	• Phase III randomized trial of radiotherapy with adjuvant PCV (procarbazine + lomustine + vincristine) vs radiotherapy alone • With median follow-up of 5.9 years, the 5-year PFS was 63% with PCV vs 46% without
CNS lymphomas	
(G-PCNSL-SG-1) Thiel et al. (2010) Lancet Oncol 11(11):1036–1047	• Phase III non-inferiority trial of high-dose methotrexate with or without WBRT for primary CNS lymphoma • Median OS was similar for patients who received high-dose methotrexate with or without WBRT (45 Gy in 30 daily fractions, 1.5 Gy/day) but patients who received WBRT had longer PFS
Brain metastases	
Patchell et al. (1998) JAMA 280(17):1485–1489	• Randomized trial of surgery in the treatment of single metastases to the brain • Surgical resection with WBRT resulted in better OS than WBRT alone
RTOG 95-08 Andrews et al. (2004) Lancet 363: 1665–1672	• Phase III trial of WBRT with or without stereotactic radiosurgery boost for patients with one to three brain metastases • Addition of radiosurgery boost to WBRT improved local control and was associated with better functional status compared to WBRT alone • Radiosurgery boost resulted in better OS only for patients with a single brain metastasis
Aoyama et al. (2006) JAMA 295(21):2483–2491	• Stereotactic radiosurgery (SRS) + WBRT therapy vs SRS alone for the treatment of brain metastases • Patients had better intracranial control with combined SRS + WBRT compared with SRS alone • Both treatments resulted in similar OS

of neuronavigation systems and tumour removal using fluorescence dye have reached routine clinical practice.

Navigation-guided surgery

Presurgical planning and image re-registration during surgery can aid optimal surgical resection. In addition, functional imaging incorporated into this navigation system, which also facilitates maximal safe resection. However, neuronavigation based on preoperative acquired images is limited by the lack of accuracy due to intraoperative brain shift. To compensate for this, intraoperative imaging such as intraoperative MRI or intraoperative CT can improve image guidance and correct the brain shift during surgery. However, this is time-consuming and cost intensive.

Awake surgery

Awake surgery with real-time functional electrostimulation mapping can facilitate safe resection without neurological deficits and maximize the extent of resection in the surgery of gliomas. Awake surgery can be performed using 'asleep–awake–asleep' protocols. In the first stage, cortical mapping should be done to detect the eloquent areas using a bipolar electrode with a 5-mm space between the tips (Nimbus, Newmedic, Hemodia) and delivering a biphasic current. After completion of cortical mapping, the glioma can be removed by alternating resection and subcortical stimulation. To optimize the tumour removal with preservation of function, all resections are pursued until eloquent structures are encountered around the surgical cavity. As a result, awake surgery with intraoperative mapping allows a significant increase of the extent of resection, and thus of overall survival.

Fluorescence-guided surgery

Although the role of the extent of resection is being increasingly emphasized, gross total resection is often hindered by the challenging differentiation between tumour and the surrounding oedematous brain using standard white light microscopy. To overcome this shortcoming, preoperative administration of 5-ALA can be helpful to define the resection margin of the tumour from the surrounding parenchyma. 5-ALA is a natural precursor of protoporphyrin IX in the haem biosynthesis pathway. It is a non-fluorescent prodrug that leads to intracellular accumulation of fluorescent porphyrins in malignant gliomas, but only slight or no accumulation in normal brain. Several studies demonstrating the clinical value of total and subtotal extent of resection have developed new surgical technique using tissue fluorescence (5-ALA). In particular, the ALA study, which was a surgical trial on a well-defined collection of patients with restricted entry criteria (resectable tumours, KPS 70–100, age 18–75 years), showed better control of progression in the complete resection group with 5-ALA than in the incomplete surgical group. With the aid of an appropriately fitted microscope, fluorescence-guided surgery with 5-ALA enables the surgeon to better define the tumour bulk of malignant gliomas.

Systemic therapy advances

Numerous novel agents have been investigated in newly diagnosed and recurrent glioma. Approaches targeting EGFR, integrins or vascular endothelial growth factor(receptor) (VEGF[R]) have failed to improve outcome. Ongoing trials are investigating novel targeted agents often in combination with cytotoxic chemotherapy or other signaling pathway inhibitors. These include agents that are targeting the metabolic pathways in IDH mutated tumours.

A novel treatment modality exploiting physical forces aimed at disrupting the cell membrane and organelle assembly during mitosis using alternating electrical fields is currently undergoing phase III testing.

Radiotherapy advances

Advances in radiotherapy planning and delivery with greater incorporation of image guidance in terms of delineating the target volume and normal tissue structures (e.g. use of fused MRI and CT images) as well as for treatment set-up and delivery (e.g. online cone-beam CT guidance) have improved conformal radiation treatment. The greater sparing of normal tissues with more conformal radiation delivery using techniques such as IMRT has increased the potential for re-irradiation in highly selected cases, even in CNS tumours.

Advances in imaging with incorporation of multiparametric MRI (diffusion-weighted imaging, perfusion imaging, hypoxia imaging, spectroscopy) or molecular imaging with PET have potential to further advance radiotherapy. For example, these modalities could be utilized to identify subregions of tumour that may benefit from dose escalation (e.g. hypoxic regions or metabolically more active regions). Ongoing research to improve the interpretation of conventional and advanced imaging data, including studies that provide pathological correlation, are essential steps to allowing these advances to translate to the clinical setting.

Areas of research

- Targeted therapies
- Immune therapies
- Investigation of radiological characterization of treatment response:
  - Pseudoprogression
  - Pseudoresponse
- Genomics and epigenomics: functional and chemical genomic approach to discover the driver gene
- Detection of biomarkers for better treatment selection
- Detecting/treating and preventing treatment toxicity:
  - Radionecrosis
  - Neurocognitive outcomes
  - Quality of life

Recommended readings

Brandes AA, Franceschi E, Tosoni A et al. (2008) MGMT promoter methylation status can predict the incidence and outcome of pseudoprogression after concomitant radiochemotherapy in newly diagnosed glioblastoma patients. J Clin Oncol 26(13):2192–2197.

Brandsma D, van den Bent MJ (2009) Pseudoprogression and pseudoresponse in the treatment of gliomas. Curr Opin Neurol 22(6):633–638.

Cairncross G, Wang M, Shaw E et al. (2013) Phase III Trial of Chemoradiotherapy for Anaplastic Oligodendroglioma: Long-Term Results of RTOG 9402. J Clin Oncol 31(3):337–343.

Friedman HS, Prados MD, Wen PY et al. (2009) Bevacizumab alone and in combination with irinotecan in recurrent glioblastoma. J Clin Oncol 27(28): 4733–4740.

Parsons DW, Jones S, Zhang X et al. (2008) An integrated genomic analysis of human glioblastoma multiforme. Science 321:1807–1812.

Stupp R, Hegi ME, Mason WP et al. (2009) Effects of radiotherapy with concomitant and adjuvant temozolomide versus radiotherapy alone on survival in glioblastoma in a randomised phase III study: 5-year analysis of the EORTC-NCIC trial. Lancet Oncol 10(5):459–466.

Taal W, Brandsma D, de Bruin HG et al. (2008) Incidence of early pseudo-progression in a cohort of malignant glioma patients treated with chemoirradiation with temozolomide. Cancer 113(2):405–410.

van den Bent MJ, Brandes AA, Taphoorn MJ et al. (2013) Adjuvant procarbazine, lomustine, and vincristine chemotherapy in newly diagnosed anaplastic oligodendroglioma. Long-term follow-up of EORTC Brain Tumor Group Study 26951. J Clin Oncol 31(3):344–350.

Wick W, Hartmann C, Engel C et al. (2009) NOA-04 randomized phase III trial of sequential radiochemotherapy of anaplastic glioma with procarbazine, lomustine, and vincristine or temozolomide. J Clin Oncol 27(35):5874–5880.

54 Eye

Choroidal melanoma, retinoblastoma, ocular adnexal lymphoma and eyelid cancers

Paul T. Finger

The Ocular Tumor Services: The New York Eye Cancer Center; New York University School of Medicine; The New York Eye and Ear Infirmary of Mount Sinai and The Manhattan Eye, Ear and Throat Hospital, New York, NY, USA

Summary	Key facts

Introduction	• *Uveal melanoma* (UM): most common primary intraocular malignancy in adults:
	  ▪ Can arise in the iris, ciliary body or choroid:
	    ○ When in the choroid, it is called *choroidal melanoma*
	• *Retinoblastoma* (Rb): most common primary intraocular cancer of childhood causally associated with a genetic mutation or hereditary factors
	• *Ocular adnexal lymphoma* (OAL): most common orbital malignancy in adults:
	  ▪ Most are extranodal marginal zone lymphoma (ENMZL) or mucosa-associated lymphoid type (MALT) and can be associated with systemic lymphoma
	• *Basal cell carcinoma* (BCC): most common eyelid malignancy:
	  ▪ Squamous cell, sebaceous cell and malignant melanoma also occur on the eyelid

Presentation	• *Uveal melanoma*: typically unilateral, solid, pigmented and asymptomatic:
	  ▪ Clinically diagnosed by a combination of indirect ophthalmoscopy, ultrasound imaging and complex photographic techniques (fundus autofluorescence, optical coherence tomography and angiography)
	• *Retinoblastoma*: typically presents in the first 3 years of life:
	  ▪ Early stages present as leukocoria (white pupil reflex) or strabismus
	  ▪ Indirect ophthalmoscopy reveals solitary or multiple masses in the retina (one or both eyes)
	  ▪ Ultrasound imaging demonstrates intratumoural calcifications
	  ▪ Cranial magnetic resonance imaging (MRI) is used to rule out extraocular extension and 'trilateral' disease (pinealoblastoma)
	• *Ocular adnexal lymphoma*: presents in the conjunctiva, lacrimal gland and orbit:
	  ▪ When externally visible, appear as 'salmon-coloured patches'
	• *Basal cell carcinoma*: typically found on the lower eyelid, and are commonly nodular with intrinsic vascularity:
	  ▪ Can induce eyelash loss and eyelid distortion

Scenario	• *Uveal melanoma*: ophthalmic plaque radiation therapy (brachytherapy) is the most widely used eye and vision-sparing treatment
	  ▪ Indications for enucleation (removal of the eye) include tumours too large for radiation, those with extraocular extension and blind, painful eyes
	  ▪ Metastatic UM is associated with poor survival
	• *Retinoblastoma* (depending on stage): treated with enucleation or eye-sparing combinations of chemotherapy, laser photocoagulation, cryotherapy or radiation:
	  ▪ Late detection with extraocular extension is more common in less developed countries and is associated with metastasis and death
	  ▪ Patients whose eye(s) is (are) staged with high-risk features and those with treatable systemic metastasis require intravenous chemotherapy
	  ▪ Orbital extension may also require radiation therapy

UICC Manual of Clinical Oncology, Ninth Edition. Edited by Brian O'Sullivan, James D. Brierley, Anil K. D'Cruz, Martin F. Fey, Raphael Pollock, Jan B. Vermorken and Shao Hui Huang. © 2015 UICC. Published 2015 by John Wiley & Sons, Ltd.

Summary	Key facts

	• *Ocular adnexal lymphoma*: typically treated with tumour biopsy followed by orbital external beam radiation therapy (EBRT):
	  ▪ Biologicals and chemotherapy have been less effective for local control
	• Eyelid tumours are treated with complete tumour excision using controlled microscopic margins:
	  ▪ Unlike eyelid sebaceous carcinoma and melanoma, squamous and basal cell carcinomas rarely metastasize

Trials	• Immunotherapy and monoclonal antibody therapy for metastatic melanoma • Antivascular endothelial growth factor (VEGF) treatment for radiation retinopathy • Chemotherapy, autologous stem cell transplant and/or radiation therapy in treating young patients with metastatic retinoblastoma

UVEAL MELANOMA

Introduction

UM (Fig. 54.1) is the most common primary intraocular malignant tumour in adults. It arises most frequently in the choroid, less frequently in the ciliary body and least often in the iris. This tumour can simultaneously involve one or more such uveal structures. UM often invades the underlying sclera, but rarely extends to the orbit (extrascleral extension), and typically metastasizes haematogenously to visceral organs. The liver is the most common initial metastatic site (>95%) and is commonly used for surveillance. However, when metastasis is detected, 75% of patients have multiorgan involvement. Whole-body positron emission tomography (PET)-computed tomography (CT) imaging has been particularly useful in identifying and staging multiorgan metastatic disease. Synchronous non-ocular primary cancers have been found in 3.3% at the time of UM diagnosis.

Incidence and aetiology

Incidence and aetiology	Description
Incidence	• In North America: 6–8 per million per year • More commonly affects those of older age; mean 60 years • Rarely affects children, 1.1% of cases (<20 years old) • Typically affects Caucasians > Hispanics > Asians and rarely those of African descent
Aetiology	• Genetic predisposition • Ultraviolet light exposure • Less pigmented irides (blue more commonly than brown) • Can arise from pre-existing uveal nevus or *de novo* • Association with dysplastic nevus syndrome, ocular melanosis and the Nevus of Ota

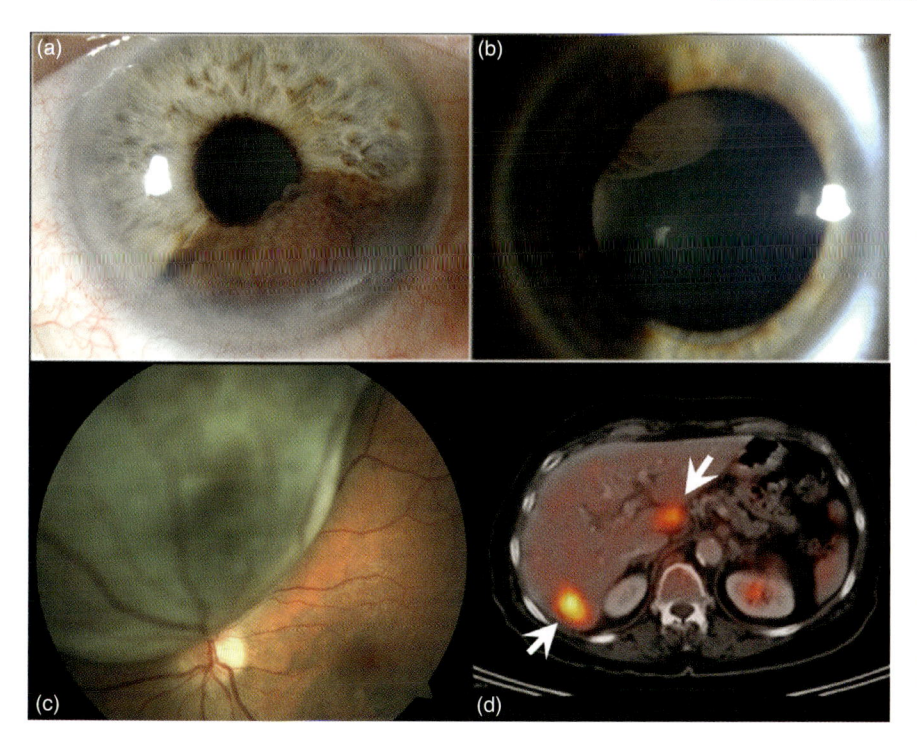

Figure 54.1 Uveal melanoma. (a) Slit-lamp photograph shows an anterior uveal melanoma (T2N0M0) of the inferior quadrants of the iris. Note the pigmented mass with intrinsic vascularity, distortion of the adjacent pupil and pigment dispersion onto the other quadrants of iris stroma. (b) Slit-lamp photograph shows a ciliary body melanoma (T4bN0M0) on dilated examination. Note the pigmented mass originating in the superior nasal ciliary body. There is anterior displacement of the iris. (c) Fundus photograph shows a posterior pigmented uveal 'choroidal' melanoma in the superior nasal quadrant, touching and obscuring a portion of the optic disc. (d) Axial PET-CT reveals two positron-avid hepatic melanoma metastases (arrows).

Pathology

- Marked variation in cytological composition ranges from spindle A cells, plump spindle B cells, epithelioid cells or mixed cell types
- A multicentre international study revealed most iris melanomas to be spindle cell type (54%)

Presentation

- Most uveal melanomas are asymptomatic
- Blurred or distorted vision (typically due to associated exudative retinal detachment)
- Flashing lights or floaters in vision
- Sector loss of peripheral vision
- For iris melanoma:
  - Irregularly-shaped pupil
  - Change in iris colour
  - Eye pain or ipsilateral headache (due to secondary glaucoma)

Diagnostic work-up

- Medium and large sized choroidal melanomas can be diagnosed through clinical exam (no biopsy) in 99.6% of cases
  - Clinical exam for posterior tumours includes:
  - Dilated indirect ophthalmoscopy
  - Ultrasound imaging (A- and B-scan)
  - Fundus photography
  - Angiography (fluorescein and indocyanine green)
  - Optical coherence tomography (OCT)
  - Fundus autofluorescence imaging (FAF)
- Clinical exam for anterior tumours also includes:
  - Ultrasound biomicroscopy (UBM)
  - Slit-lamp examination with photography
  - Gonioscopy with photography
  - Transillumination of the globe
- Magnetic resonance imaging (MRI), CT and PET-CT imaging are rarely used to establish a diagnosis, but can help in select cases

Specific features	Description

Posterior uveal melanoma	• On dilated ophthalmoscopy, most common diagnostic features:
	  ▪ Dr Finger's mnemonic device: **MOST**, choroidal **M**elanoma = **O**range pigment lipofuscin + **S**ubretinal fluid + **T**hickness >2 mm:
	     ○ Pigmented (can be variably pigmented or amelanotic)
	     ○ Orange pigment (lipofuscin) on tumour surface, best seen on FAF
	     ○ Subretinal fluid (range from small dependent fluid to large serous retinal detachment, best seen on OCT)
	     ○ Raised lesion (thickness >2 mm can help differentiate it from a choroidal nevus, best measured on ultrasound imaging)
	• B-scan ultrasound:
	  ▪ Dome or mushroom-shaped solid tumour; less often irregular, peaked or diffuse shape
	  ▪ Serous 'shifting' exudative retinal detachment
	  ▪ Vascularity can be seen on dynamic examination as 'twinkling' (within larger-sized tumours)
	• A-scan ultrasound:
	  ▪ Low-to-moderate reflectivity within the tumour
	• Angiography:
	  ▪ Tumour vascular pattern (tumour vessels and/or microaneurysms)
	  ▪ Focal hyperfluorescence with increasing intensity over timed study

Anterior uveal melanoma	• Slit-lamp examination diagnostic features:
	  ▪ Typically brown tumour
	  ▪ Location in inferior quadrants
	  ▪ Intrinsic tumour vascularity (best seen in lightly pigmented tumours)
	  ▪ Involves >3 clock hours of the iris
	  ▪ >1 mm in thickness
	  ▪ Corectopia (abnormal shaped pupil)
	  ▪ Ectropion uveae (iris pigment epithelium pulled onto iris stroma)
	  ▪ Unilateral glaucoma (look for pigment dispersion and/or angle invasion)
	  ▪ Sector cataract
	  ▪ Can rarely involve 360° of the iris (diffuse type) or invade all or most of the ciliary body (look for ring melanoma)
	  ▪ Sentinel vessels (enlarged vessels on the sclera):
	     ○ Typically anterior and a sign of an underlying malignancy
	• High-frequency ultrasound or UBM features:
	  ▪ Club or irregular shaped
	  ▪ Angle blunting (52%)
	  ▪ Other: iris root disinsertion, invasion of the supraciliary space and/or the underlying iris pigment epithelium

Staging and prognostic grouping

UICC TNM staging
See Table 54.1.

Table 54.1 UICC TNM categories and stage grouping: Conjunctiva carcinoma, malignant melanoma of conjunctiva, uveal malignant melanoma, sarcoma of orbit and lacrimal gland carcinoma

TNM categories: Conjunctiva carcinoma	
T1	≤5 mm
T2	>5 mm
T3	Adjacent structures
T4	Orbit and beyond
N1	Regional

Stage grouping: Conjunctiva carcinoma
No stage grouping is currently recommended

TNM categories: Malignant melanoma of conjunctiva	
T1	Bulbar conjunctiva
pT1	Bulbar conjunctiva (Melanoma in situ)
pT1a	≤0.5 mm, substantia propria
pT1b	>0.5–1.5 mm, and >1.55 mm substantia propria
pT1c	>1.5 mm, substania propria
T2	Non-bulbar conjunctiva
T3	Eyelid, globe, orbit, sinuses,
pT2	Palpebral, forniceal, caruncular conjunctiva
pT2a	≤0.5 mm, substantia propria
pT2b	>0.5–1.5 mm, and >1.55 mm substantia propria
pT2c	>1.5 mm, substantia propria
pT3	Eye, eyelid, nasolacrimal system
T4	CNS pT4 CNS

Stage grouping: Malignant melanoma of conjunctiva
No stage grouping is currently recommended

Note: Clinical staging using involved quadrants to define T categories. Quadrants are defined by clock hour, starting at the limbus (e.g., 6, 9, 12, 3) extending from the central cornea, to and beyond the eyelid margins. This will bisect the caruncle.

TNM categories: Uveal malignant melanoma	
Iris malignant melanoma	
T1	Limited to iris
T1a	≤3 clock hours
T1b	>3 clock hours
T1c	Glaucoma
T2	Into ciliary body/choroid
T2a	With glaucoma
T3	Scleral extension
T3a	With glaucoma
T4	Extraocular extension
T4a	≤5 mm
T4b	>5 mm

Ciliary body and choroid malignant melanoma	
T1	Category 1
T1a	Without ciliary body involvement and extraocular extension
T1b	With ciliary body involvement
T1c	Without ciliary body involvement but extraocular extension ≤5 mm
T1d	With ciliary body involvement and extraocular extension ≤5 mm
T2	Category 2
T2a	Without ciliary body involvement and extraocular extension
T2b	With ciliary body involvement
T2c	Without ciliary body involvement but extraocular extension ≤5 mm
T2d	With ciliary body involvement and extraocular extension ≤5 mm
T3	Category 3
T3a	Without ciliary body involvement and extraocular extension
T3b	With ciliary body involvement
T3c	Without ciliary body involvement but extraocular extension ≤5 mm
T3d	With ciliary body involvement and extraocular extension ≤5 mm
T4	Category 4
T4a	Without ciliary body involvement and extraocular extension
T4b	With ciliary body involvement
T4c	Without ciliary body involvement but extraocular extension ≤5 mm
T4d	With ciliary body involvement and extraocular extension ≤5 mm
T4e	Any tumour size with extraocular extension >5 mm

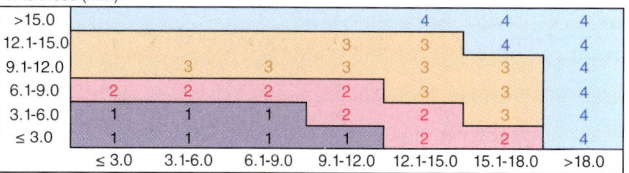

Thickness (mm)	≤ 3.0	3.1–6.0	6.1–9.0	9.1–12.0	12.1–15.0	15.1–18.0	>18.0
>15.0					4	4	4
12.1–15.0				3	3	4	4
9.1–12.0		3	3	3	3	3	4
6.1–9.0	2	2	2	2	3	3	4
3.1–6.0	1	1	1	2	2	3	4
≤ 3.0	1	1	1	1	2	2	4

Largest basal diameter (mm)

Classification for ciliary body and choroid uveal melanoma based on thickness and diameter.

(continued)

Stage grouping: Uvea malignant melanoma			
Stage I	T1a	N0	M0
Stage IIA	T1b–d, T2a	N0	M0
Stage IIB	T2b, T3a	N0	M0
Stage IIIA	T2c–d	N0	M0
	T3b–c	N0	M0
	T4a	N0	M0
Stage IIIB	T3d	N0	M0
	T4b–c	N0	M0
Stage IIIC	T4d–e	N0	M0
Stage IV	Any T	N1	M0
	Any T	Any N	M1

TNM categories: Lacrimal gland carcinoma	
T1	≤2.0 cm, limited to gland
T2	>2.0–4 cm, limited to gland
T3	>4 cm, extraglandular extension into orbital soft tissue, including optic nerve or globe
T4	Invades adjacent structures
T4a	Periosteum
T4b	Orbit bone
T4c	Adjacent structures
N1	Regional

Stage grouping: Lacrimal gland carcinoma

No staging currently recommended

TNM categories: Sarcoma of orbit	
T1	≤15 mm
T2	>15 mm
T3	Invades orbital tissues/bony walls
T4	Invades globe periorbital structures or CNS
N1	Regional

Stage grouping: Sarcoma of orbit

No stage grouping is currently recommended

Prognostic factors

See Table 54.2.

The 7th Edition AJCC–UICC Ophthalmic Oncology Task Force researchers found that the 10-year survival rates by stage among 7585 UM patients were:
- T1: 90%
- T2: 78%
- T3: 58%
- T4: 40%.

Treatment philosophy

UM treatment (radiation, enucleation) is locally curative in most cases. The 3 main goals are:
- Prevention of metastatic death
- Retention of vision
- Retention of the cosmetic use of the globe.

At the time of diagnosis, systemic metastases are rarely found (about 2%). Therefore, local treatment is employed to destroy the primary cancer, followed by periodic surveillance for pretreatment subclinical disease. In cases where systemic metastasis is discovered at the time of diagnosis (mostly T4 staged tumours), local treatment can be offered as palliative therapy to prolong functional vision, for eye retention and to prevent secondary glaucoma.

Table 54.2 Prognostic factors for survival for uveal melanoma

Prognostic factors	Tumour related	Host related	Environment related
Essential	Largest tumour diameter (typically width) Higher UICC T stage (associated with worse survival)	Advanced age	
Additional	Extrascleral 'extraocular' extension Location (iris tumours are typically smaller at diagnosis, while ciliary body tumours are less visible and typically larger at diagnosis) Histopathological cell type (spindle cell more favourable than epithelioid) Mitotic activity Microvasculature patterns		
New and promising	PET-CT standardized uptake value (SUV): higher SUV associated with worse prognosis Monosomy 3, abnormalities of chromosomes 6 and 8* Genetic expression profiling (class 1 more favourable than 1A and 2)		Immunotherapy

*Test has been independently confirmed at multiple centres.

Scenario	Treatment philosophy
Suspicious choroidal nevi and small choroidal melanoma	• As treatments for posterior choroidal melanomas risk vision loss, many eye cancer specialists will offer patients 'observation as treatment', looking for change or growth • Growth or change within 6 months of observation can indicate that tumour growth or associated retinal detachments will eventually affect vision, making treatment risk more acceptable • Observation of small melanomas should only be undertaken after informed consent • Though the Collaborative Ocular Melanoma Study (COMS) demonstrated that 3% of COMS small tumours metastasized, there exists no statistical quantification of the risk of observation as treatment

Large uveal melanoma (≥10 mm thickness or ≥16 mm width)	• COMS Large Tumor Trial found no advantage to 20-Gy pre-enucleation radiation therapy (PERT) for large melanomas
	• Most of these eyes are no longer enucleated
	• Eye-sparing treatments:
	  ▪ Select cases can be treated with larger plaques than those used in the COMS
	  ▪ Proton beam irradiation
	  ▪ Both plaque and proton beam for larger tumours are associated with increased ocular morbidity and lower rates of local control
	  ▪ Higher secondary enucleation rates compared to follow-up after treatment of T1, T2 or T3 tumours
	  ▪ Metastatic rate: 40–45% at 10 years (COMS)

Iris and iridociliary melanoma	• Small iris tumours (<5 mm in largest diameter):
	  ▪ Most can be observed for change prior to treatment due to a low incidence of metastasis:
	    ○ Multicentre international study reported 10.7% metastasis for biopsy-proven iris melanoma
	  ▪ Transcorneal Finger Iridectomy Technique (FIT) small incision biopsy found to be safe and effective
	• Surgical iridectomy and iridocyclectomy (less common):
	  ▪ These intraocular procedures can cause haemorrhage, infection, cataract, permanent glare (enlarged 'keyhole' pupil)
	  ▪ Yields more tissue for histopathology and immunohistochemical analysis
	• Plaque brachytherapy (more common):
	  ▪ Fewer surgical risks (not an intraocular procedure)
	  ▪ Causes radiation cataract
	  ▪ No radiation maculopathy or optic neuropathy reported
	  ▪ Iris-sparing retains function, eliminates keyhole pupil, reduces glare and photophobia

Uveal melanoma with systemic or regional metastasis at diagnosis	• 1–4% of patients (depending on tumour T stage, typically T4) • No known cure for metastatic uveal melanoma: ▪ After diagnosis of metastasis, the COMS metastatic death rate was 80% at 1 year and 92% at 2 years • Long-term survival (>5 years) after diagnosis of metastasis is uncommon • Early detection of metastasis allows for intervention and end of life planning • Systemic therapy includes: hepatic interventions, immunotherapy and chemotherapy to prolong survival • Local treatment may be used as palliative therapy to prevent vision loss or a blind painful eye

Treatment

Treatment	Description
Plaque brachytherapy	• Radionuclides: palladium-103 (^{103}Pd), iodine-125 (^{125}I), ruthenium-106 (^{106}Ru) • Radioactive seeds are affixed into a gold carrier which is sewn onto the eye (sclera) over the tumour for 5–7 days • Typical tumour apex dose 70–85 Gy (^{125}I and ^{103}Pd) to >100 Gy (^{106}Ru) • Local control rate: 85–97% • Eye retention rate: 74–96%
Proton beam irradiation	• Tantalum rings are sewn to the sclera as reference points • External source of radiation enters the front of the eye and is directed towards the tumour • Head is immobilized and the eye monitored for movement • Typically in four to five daily sessions; typical dose 60 Gy • Local control rate: 81–97% • Eye retention rate: 75–94%
Enucleation	• Typically not used for T1 to T3-sized tumours • Best employed for T4e, blind or blind painful eyes, where radiation is not possible and at patient request

Post-treatment assessment

- *Local tumour control:*
  - Following radiation, the tumour residua is monitored by periodic ophthalmic examinations and ultrasound imaging
  - Recurrence is treated by transpupillary thermotherapy (TTT), repeat irradiation or enucleation
  - Local recurrence is associated with an increased risk for metastatic disease
  - Following enucleation, the orbit is periodically inspected and palpated for recurrence
- *Metastasis:*
  - Most common sites: liver (95%), lung (24%) and bone (16%)
  - Patients monitored periodically with:
    - Abdominal hepatic imaging (MRI, CT, ultrasound)
    - Chest X-ray
    - Whole-body PET-CT in high-risk patients to evaluate suspected metastasis and to assess viability of the primary UM
    - Liver function studies have a high specificity (92.3%), but low sensitivity (14.7%)
- *Ocular radiation side effects:*
  - Radiation maculopathy
  - Radiation optic neuropathy
  - Radiation cataract
  - Neovascular glaucoma
  - Dry eye

CONTROVERSIES

Secondary radiation retinopathy

Radiation-related macular degeneration (radiation maculopathy) is the most common cause of permanent vision loss following radiotherapy. Separate studies (two centres) have found that laser ablation of the choroid and retina immediately posterior to the tumour decreases circulation within the tumour and delays the incidence of radiation maculopathy. This was likely the first evidence that tumour-generated vascular endothelial growth factor (VEGF) could be reduced with laser treatment.

Efficacy of intravitreal anti-VEGF

Multiple centres have shown that intravitreal anti-VEGF agents (e.g. bevacizumab, ranibizumab) can induce regression of radiation-induced macular oedema. However, controversy over the efficacy of intravitreal anti-VEGF agents likely relates to the effect of macular radiation dose and to the frequency and timing of subsequent anti-VEGF treatment. For example, radiation-related retinal oedema (as well as iris neovascularization) is noted to be more sensitive to anti-VEGF treatment if given in the early stages of the disease and at regular, continuous intervals (typically every 1–3 months). Treatment is typically continuous, ceased for loss of functional vision or patient preference.

Exudative retinal detachment

Choroidal melanomas naturally leak serous fluid, causing the overlying and adjacent retina to detach. When the retinal detachment involves the macula it affects vision. Exudative retinal detachment is the second most common cause of UM-related vision loss (after radiation retinopathy) and longstanding detachment of the macula results in permanent loss of retinal function. There is no broadly applicable treatment.

Resolution of exudative retinal detachment typically takes an average of 6 months (despite radiation therapy). Laser devascularization of the tumour and anti-VEGF treatment may help speed fluid reabsorption (depending upon the size of the retinal detachment and the location of the tumour).

Biomarkers

Biomarkers to evaluate prognosis for metastatic UM have been proposed but are not universally accepted. Examples are:
- Gene expression profiling
- PET-CT SUV
- Chromosome alterations (chromosome 3, 6p and 8q).

RETINOBLASTOMA

Introduction

Retinoblastoma (Rb) is the most common primary intraocular cancer of childhood (Fig. 54.2) (3% of all childhood malignancies). It can affect one or both eyes. When both are affected, it is more likely to be heritable. However, only about 10% will present with a family history of Rb. The most common early presentation is leukocoria or white pupil. It can also present as strabismus or with neovascular glaucoma. In less developed countries, it can present as a massive fungating mass. It can spread through the choroid, into the orbit or through the optic nerve. Metastasis involves the brain, bones and viscera. Survival drops dramatically in patients with local extraocular and metastatic disease. Early detection and prompt treatment is critical for patient prognosis. In the developing world, Rb is most commonly fatal. However, with early detection and treatment, the majority of children in North America and Europe (>98%) survive Rb.

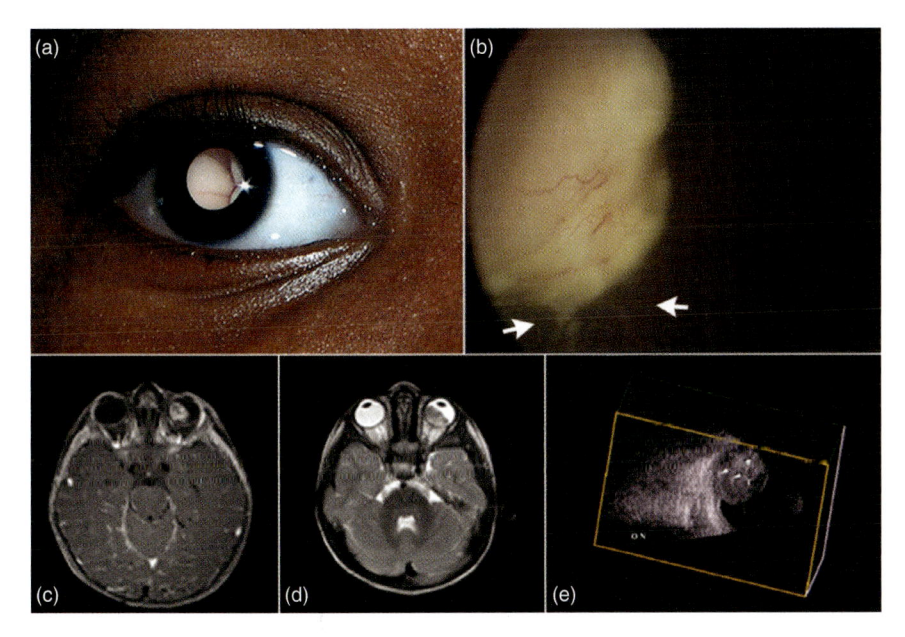

Figure 54.2 Retinoblastoma. (a) External photograph demonstrating leukocoria (white pupil) in a child with (T4N0M0) retinoblastoma. Leukocoria is the most common presenting sign of retinoblastoma. (b) Fundus photograph reveals a solitary off-white retinoblastoma with vitreal seeding (arrows). (c) MRI (axial) T1-weighted image of a retinoblastoma tumour in the left eye. The tumour is hyperintense relative to the vitreous. (d) MRI (axial) T2-weighted image of a retinoblastoma tumour in the left eye. The tumour is hypointense relative to the vitreous. (e) Three-dimensional reconstruction B-scan ultrasound image of a retinoblastoma. Note the high reflective components (arrows) corresponding to calcifications within the tumour. ON, optic nerve

Incidence, aetiology and screening

Incidence, aetiology and screening	Description
Incidence	• Worldwide, about 9000 cases each year • In the USA, 350 cases each year • Seventh most common paediatric cancer in the USA • Affects 1 in every 11,000–30,000 live births, depending on country • Average age of diagnosis: 12 (bilateral) to 24 (unilateral) months • No racial or gender predilection
Aetiology	• Deletions or mutation of *RB1* on the q14 band of chromosome 13 • 40% of cases have the germinal form of the disease (autosomal dominant inheritance, mutation of the *RB1* gene) and 10% have an antecedent family history • Patients with heritable Rb have an increased non-ocular cancer risk • 60% of Rb cases are the non-germinal form, which is non-inheritable: ■ Typically unilateral (one eye affected) • Associated with pinealoblastoma, a primitive neuroectodermal tumour (PNET)
Screening	• Standard of care for family history of Rb is evolving to molecular diagnosis to identify infants at risk in each family: ■ Most cannot afford this, even in the USA • Screening programmes for less developed countries • *In utero* detection of Rb

Pathology

- Deep blue cells with little cytoplasm
- Flexner–Wintersteiner and Homer–Wright rosettes
- Other features: calcification, staining of blood vessels and necrosis with islands of Rb

Presentation

- Most common in the developed world:
  - Leukocoria (over 50%)
  - Strabismus (exotropia or esotropia)
- Most common in the developing world:
  - Painful and red eye
  - Change in iris colour (due to neovascular glaucoma, haemorrhage of anterior chamber, tumour seeding)
  - Orbital, sinus and intracranial extension
  - Failure to thrive

Diagnostic Work-up

- Correctly diagnosed through clinical exam in >95% of cases (without a biopsy)
- Examination under general anaesthesia involves slit-lamp exam, dilated ophthalmoscopy, digital fundus photography and ultrasound imaging (A- and B-scan):
  - Fluorescein angiography is primarily used to evaluate recurrent disease
- CT imaging:
  - Can detect intraocular calcification as well as extraocular and intracranial extension
- MRI:
  - Preferred due to no risk of radiation-induced secondary malignancy (particularly for children with the heritable form)
  - More difficult to access and more expensive.

- Brain and orbits.
  - On T1-weighted images, Rb tumours have low intensity and can be difficult to distinguish from vitreous, but on T2-weighted images they demonstrate very low intensity compared to vitreous
  - T2 images: calcium is more pronounced
- Evaluation for optic nerve or extraocular extension
- Evaluation of the pineal region for PNET, also called trilateral Rb
- X-ray: when ultrasound and MRI are not available, may be the only technique that can identify intraocular calcification (particularly in patients with opaque media)
- Molecular diagnosis:
  - Standard of care for family history of Rb is evolving to molecular diagnosis to identify infants at risk in each family
  - Genetic analysis can help to differentiate Rb from other conditions (in hereditary Rb only)
- Tumour biopsy:
  - Opening the eye is contraindicated due to risk of extraocular tumour extension
  - Easily performed in cases presenting with orbital extraocular extension

Specific features

- On dilated ophthalmoscopy:
  - Exophytic, endophytic or mixed growth patterns
  - Can be solitary or multifocal in one or both eyes
  - Unilateral 75%; bilateral 25%
  - Location: retina and vitreous
  - Can involve the optic disc
  - Retinal detachment
  - Vitreous or anterior chamber seeding – 'snowballs' of tumour cells
- On B-scan ultrasound:
  - High internal reflectivity, calcifications with orbital shadowing
  - Presence of retinal detachment, extrascleral or intraneural tumour extension and/or vitreous seeding

Staging and prognostic grouping

UICC TNM staging

See Table 54.3.

Table 54.3 UICC TNM stage grouping and summary: Retinoblastoma

TNM categories				
T1	No more than two-thirds of eye volume, no vitreous/subretinal seeding		pT1	Tumor confined to eye with no optic nerve or choroidal invasion
	T1a	No tumor in either eye is >3 mm in size, and >1.5 mm from the optic nerve/fovea		
	T1b	At least 1 tumor is >3 mm or <1.5 mm to optic nerve/fovea		
	T1c	At least 1 tumor is >3 mm or <1.5 mm to optic nerve/fovea, retinal detachment/subretinal fluid beyond 5 mm from tumour base		
T2	Tumors no more than two-third volume of eye with vitreous or subretinal seeding with retinal detachment		pT2	Minimal optic nerve and/or choroidal invasion
	T2a	Focal vitreous and/or subretinal seeding	pT2a	Superficial invasion optic nerve
	T2b	Massive vitreous and/or subretinal seeding	pT2b	Superficial invasion optic nerve, focal choroidal invasion
T3	Severe intraocular disease		pT3	Significant invasion optic nerve and/or choroidal invasion
	T3a	Tumor fills more than two-thirds of eye	pT3a	Invasion of optic of the eye nerve past lamina cribrosa but not to surgical resection line or massive choroidal invasion
	T3b	One or more tumor-related intraocular complications	pT3b	Invasion of optic nerve past lamina cribrosa (not to surgical resection line, massive choroidal invasion)
T4	Extraocular tumour		pT4	Invasion of optic nerve to resection line or extraocular extension
	T4a	Invasion of optic nerve	pT4a	Invasion of optic nerve to resection line, no extraocular extension
	T4b	Invading into the orbit	pT4b	Invasion of optic nerve to resection line, extraocular extension
	T4c	Intracranial, not past chiasm		
	T4d	Intracranial, past chiasm		
N1	Regional lymph node involvement		pN1	Regional lymph node involvement
M1	Distant metastasis		pM1	Distant metastasis
			pM1a	Single metastasis to sites other than CNS
			pM1b	Multiple metastasis to sites other than CNS
			pM1c	CNS metastasis
			pM1d	Discrete mass(es) without Leptomeningeal and/or CSF involvement
			pM1e	Leptomeningeal and/or CSF involvement
Stage grouping				
No stage grouping is at present recommended.				

Prognostic factors

See Table 54.4.

Table 54.4 Prognostic factors for survival for retinoblastoma

Prognostic factors	Tumour related	Host related	Environment related
Essential	Massive = > or equal to 3-mm' uveal invasion Extrascleral tumour extension Optic nerve invasion Anterior chamber extension Higher UICC T stage	Immunosuppression (i.e. AIDS) Germline mutation *RB1* allele	Access to care
Additional	Multidrug resistance gene(s) Heritability		Cyclosporine therapy Experienced multidisciplinary team (local control)
New and promising			Screening programmes for less developed countries Telepathology for evaluation of enucleated eyes *In utero* detection of Rb

Treatment philosophy

Rb treatment can be divided into two scenarios. The first is found in countries with well-developed and readily accessible medical systems. Here, most cases are diagnosed early, while the Rb is contained within the eye(s), and treatment is typically curative. This is not the case in less developed countries where children often present with massive extraocular extension and metastases. Here, the primary goal is palliation and pain control. Rb typically metastasizes to the bone marrow, skeletal system and viscera. World-wide mortality from Rb is reported to be 70%. In contrast, if diagnosed and treated while the Rb is contained within the eye, >95% can be cured. within the eye, >95% of patients can be cured.

Treatment

Treatment	Description
Enucleation	• Only method that removes the primary tumour • Used prior to adjuvant therapy for very large tumours, those with extrascleral extension or intraneural tumour invasion, massive choroidal, vitreous, subretinal or anterior chamber tumour seeding • Method of choice if the tumour relapses after all eye-sparing treatments are exhausted
Plaque brachytherapy	• Rb is radiation sensitive • Primary brachytherapy for smaller, anterior, solitary Rb • Used for salvage in cases of residual or recurrent tumours • Radionuclides: ^{125}I, ^{103}Pd, ^{106}Ru • Radioactive plaque is sewn onto the eye (sclera) over the tumour • Typical tumour apex dose 40–45 Gy delivered over 2–5 days
Laser therapy	• Photocoagulation with infrared 810 nm (TTT) or argon laser 532 nm • Used after chemotherapy-induced tumour reduction for small (≤2.5–3.0 mm) individual or multifocal tumours • Compared to TTT, argon laser is more focal (associated with less laser scar enlargement over time)
Intravenous chemotherapy	• For presumed microscopic metastasis in high-risk Rb patients with massive choroidal invasion, extrascleral or intraneural tumour extension • For treatment of metastatic disease • Agents include vincristine, cyclophosphamide, carboplatin, cisplatinum and etoposide • Systemic chemotherapy is toxic for bone marrow; may cause infertility and secondary non-ocular malignancies
External beam radiation	• Rarely used due to side effects of radiation: secondary malignancy, disturbs growth of orbital bones and teeth • Used for ocular salvage cases of chemotherapy failure and tumour recurrence in the only eye • For treatment of orbital tumour invasion (after enucleation) • For intracranial, sinus Rb • For metastatic Rb
Cryotherapy	• Less commonly used, but can be helpful for small anterior tumours

(continued)

Treatment	Description
Intra-arterial chemotherapy	• Investigational treatment • Requires interventional radiology specialist • Chemotherapy is injected directly into the ophthalmic artery under radiographic fluoroscopy • Goal is to improve local control and minimize systemic chemotherapy side effects • Agents: typically melphalan and topotecan • Average of three sessions per eye, at 4-week intervals • Vitreal and anterior chamber tumour seeding and haemorrhage are predictive factors for the treatment failure • Residual Rb can be treated with laser, cryotherapy or plaque brachytherapy • Risks include thromboemboli in the optic nerve, down-staging due to lack of histopathology, risk of untreated occult metastases and fluoroscopic radiation exposure

Post-treatment assessment

- *Systemic examination:*
  - Metastatic sites:
    - Regional: preauricular and cervical lymph nodes
    - Distant: liver, other visceral organs, bone marrow, skeletal system
  - Paediatric patients should be monitored by a paediatric oncologist
  - Physical examination and blood tests (especially those treated with chemotherapy or radiation therapy)
  - Survivors of the hereditary form of Rb have a genetic predisposition to develop additional non-ocular cancers:
    - Estimated risk is 1%/year that a survivor with germinal retinoblastoma will develop a second cancer (i.e. 50% chance at age 50 years)
- *Follow-up examinations:*
  - Exam under anaesthesia (EUA) evolving to office-based ophthalmic exam to evaluate for:
    - Development of recurrent or subsequent Rb in the same or other eye
    - Development of chorioretinal toxicity after chemotherapy
    - Development of radiation retinopathy and optic neuropathy
  - Electroretinogram (ERG) is used to indirectly measure visual acuity before and after intra-arterial chemotherapy
  - Typical EUA schedule:
    - Every 4 months until age 3 years, then
    - Every 6 months until age 5 years
    - Outpatient examinations every year thereafter
  - After being disease-free for 44 months, it is unlikely that a patient with unilateral Rb will develop new disease in the fellow eye
  - However, patients can still develop new tumours
  - Those with only a family history of Rb (but without the disease) need to be screened at least until age 28 months
  - Entire nuclear family should be screened for Rb

Controversies

- Benefit of IV chemotherapy after enucleation for prevention of distant metastasis
- Treatment of Rb with vitreous or anterior chamber seeding with intra-arterial and/or intravitreal chemotherapy
- Long-term complications after intra-arterial chemotherapy (e.g. vascular)
- Long-term radiation-related oncogenic risk associated with fluoroscopy during intra-arterial chemotherapy on patients with heritable Rb

OCULAR ADNEXAL LYMPHOMA

Introduction

The most common orbital malignancy, ocular adnexal lymphoma (OAL) (Fig. 54.3), can originate in the conjunctiva, eyelids, lacrimal gland and orbit. There is a wide spectrum of

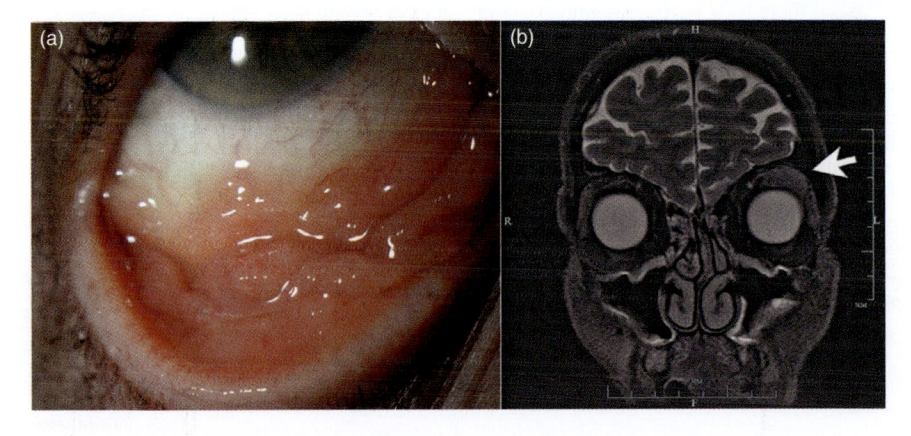

Figure 54.3 Ocular adnexal lymphoma (OAL). (a) Slit-lamp photograph shows salmon patch OAL in the inferior fornix (T1bN0M0), pathologically-proven to be an extranodal marginal zone lymphoma (ENMZL). (b) MRI (coronal) T2-weighted image of an OAL tumour in the superotemporal left orbit (T2N0M0) (arrow). Note that the tumour is hypointense relative to the vitreous and hyperintense relative to the orbital fat. Like most OAL, this tumour conforms to rather than invades or infiltrates the eye or orbital bones.

subtypes, with the most common considered to be low grade (extranodal marginal zone B-cell non-Hodgkin lymphoma [ENMZL] MALT-type).

Incidence and aetiology

Incidence and aetiology	Description

Incidence	- Incidence poorly documented
	- Increasing with the use of immunosuppression
	- More commonly affects those in sixth to seventh decades of life
	- More prevalent in Asia and Europe than in North America
	- Lymphomas comprise 55% of all malignant orbital tumours
	- Most common subtypes:
	  - ENMZL of the MALT-type (up to 80%)
	  - Follicular lymphoma
	- Less common subtypes:
	  - Diffuse large B-cell lymphoma
	  - Mantle cell lymphoma
	  - Follicular
	  - T cell
	  - Hodgkin
	  - Plasmacytoma
	- Rare subtypes:
	  - Burkitt lymphoma
	  - Peripheral T-cell lymphoma
	  - Mycosis fungoides
	  - Extranodal NK/T-cell lymphoma
	  - Anaplastic large cell lymphoma

Aetiology	- Clonal proliferation of B or T lymphocytes - Most OAL are non-Hodgkin type (NHL) of the B-cell type - Most are primary tumours; however, up to 30% are found in the setting of disseminated lymphoma - May be a result of antigenic inflammation or autoimmune disorders - May be associated with microbial pathogens (*Helicobacter pylori, Chlamydia pneumonia, Chlamydia psittaci*)

Pathology

- Spectrum ranges from benign reactive lymphoid hyperplasia to malignant lymphoma
- Biopsy should yield a sufficient specimen for pathological staging and subtyping on the basis of morphology and immunophenotype
- Genotypes: trisomy 3 and 18;t(14; 18), and A20 deletion on chromosome 6
- Flow cytometry with fresh tissue (as possible)
- Suspected lymph node or extranodal involvement should be histopathologically confirmed
- Assessment of tumour cell growth factor (Ki-67, MIB-1)

Presentation

- Most frequent site of origin is the orbit, followed by the conjunctiva, lacrimal gland and eyelid
- Unilateral (most cases)
- Conjunctival involvement:
  - Salmon patch lesion
  - Follicular conjunctivitis
  - Can present as conjunctivitis and be masked by topical steroid therapy
- Orbital / lacrimal gland involvement:
  - Orbital/eyelid oedema
  - Palpable mass
  - Proptosis
  - Diplopia
  - Can cause papilloedema and decreased vision
  - Rare bone erosion (high-grade B-cell tumours)
- Eyelid involvement:
  - Eyelid swelling (oedema)
  - Ptosis

Natural history

- MALT and low-grade follicular lymphoma are considered low grade and relatively indolent
- Diffuse large B-cell and mantle cell lymphoma are considered high grade and more aggressive

Diagnostic work-up

- Slit-lamp examination of all conjunctival surfaces with eversion of the upper and lower eyelids as well as photographic documentation
- Hertel exophthalmometry
- Visual field testing
- Colour vision
- Ocular motility evaluation
- CT typically reveals a homogeneous tumour that moulds to the globe and does not affect the orbital bones
- MRI (T1-weighted images dark tumour compared to orbital fat)
- Imaging of orbits/brain/sinuses utilizing axial and coronal sections to determine tumour location and extension
- Orbital ultrasound

Systemic examination

- Referral to haematologist–oncologist for staging of disease
- Most common sites of metastasis are other extranodal tissues
- Preauricular, submandibular and cervical lymph node palpation

- Whole-body (scalp to toe) PET-CT is preferable; if not available, CT imaging of the neck, chest, abdomen and pelvis
- Routine blood studies
- Serum protein electrophoresis
- Serum lactate dehydrogenase (LDH)
- Serum β2-microglobulin
- Bone marrow biopsy

Table 54.5 AJCC staging: Ocular adnexal lymphoma

Primary Tumor (T)	
TX	Lymphoma extent not specified
T0	No evidence of lymphoma
T1	Lymphoma involving the conjunctiva alone without orbital involvement
T1a	Bulbar conjunctiva only
T1b	Palpebral conjunctiva +/- fornix +/- caruncle
T1c	Extensive conjunctival involvement
T2	Lymphoma with orbital involvement +/- any conjunctival involvement
T2a	Anterior orbital involvement (+/- conjunctival involvement)
T2b	Anterior orbital involvement (+/- conjunctival involvement + lacrimal involvement)
T2c	Posterior orbital involvement (+/- conjunctival involvement +/- anterior involvement and +/- any extraocular muscle involvement)
T2d	Nasolacrimal drainage system involvement (+/- conjunctival involvement but not including nasopharynx)
T3	Lymphoma with pre-septal eyelid involvement (defined above) +/- orbital involvement +/- any conjunctival involvement
T4	Orbital adnexal lymphoma extending beyond orbit to adjacent structures such as bone and brain
T4a	Involvement of nasopharynx
T4b	Osseous involvement (including periosteum)
T4c	Involvement of maxillofacial, ethmoidal and/or frontal sinuses
T4d	Intracranial spread
Regional LYMPH Nodes (N)	
NX	Regional lymph nodes cannot be assessed
N0	No evidence of lymph node involvement
N1	Involvement of ipsilateral regional lymph nodes*
N2	Involvement of contra lateral or bilateral regional lymph nodes*
N3	Involvement of peripheral lymph nodes not draining ocular adnexal region
N4	Involvement of central lymph nodes
*The regional lymph nodes included preauricular (parotid), submandibular, and cervical	
Distant Metastasis (M)	
M0	No evidence of involvement of other extranodal sites (no pathologic M0; use clinical M to complete stage group)
M1a	Noncontiguous involvement of tissues or organs external to the ocular adnexa (e.g., parotid glands, submandibular gland, lung, liver, spleen, kidney, breast, etc.)
M1b	Lymphomatous involvement of the bone marrow
M1c	Both M1a and M1b involvement

No stage grouping is currently recommended.

Source: Edge *et al.* (2010) Reproduced with permission of Springer.

Staging and prognostic grouping

AJCC staging
See Table 54.5.

Prognostic factors
See Table 54.6.

Treatment philosophy

The goal of OAL treatment is local cure and surveillance for or treatment of systemic disease. However, in those with advanced disseminated disease, palliative therapy may be needed. Palliative therapy can reduce proptosis, diplopia and exposure keratopathy, and prolong functional vision.

Table 54.6 Prognostic factors for survival for ocular adnexal lymphoma

Prognostic factors	Tumour related	Host related	Environment related
Essential	Lymphoma type (ENMZL more favourable prognosis)	Advanced age	
	Primary site other than conjunctiva (eyelids, lacrimal gland, orbit)		
	Lymph node involvement		
	Advanced disease stage		
Additional	Elevated Ki-67	Presence of B symptoms	
	Cell-cycle markers, e.g. for chronic lymphocytic leukaemia (CLL) subtype: *TP53* and fluorescence *in situ* hybridization (FISH) prognostic profile	Elevated serum LDH	
		Elevated β2-microglobulin	
		Immunocompromised (e.g. HIV)	
	Immunohistochemical and gene expression profile subtyping, e.g. for diffuse large cell B lymphoma		
New and promising	Molecular genetics and gene expression profiling (for certain subtypes)		Improved local control associated with less systemic recurrence
			Immunotherapy

Treatment

Treatment	Description
Observation	• ENMZL (or MALT) conjunctival tumours are less aggressive and associated with low morbidity • Once a pathological diagnosis is established, most patients can be observed during systemic work-up
Surgical resection	• Small tumours are typically removed for pathological analysis • Larger tumours undergo partial resection for pathological analysis • Negative surgical margins typically are not feasible
External beam radiation	• OAL are typically radiation sensitive (with some variation depending on cell type) • EBRT is the gold standard for local disease • 30 Gy (range 20–40 Gy) in 180–200-cGy daily fractions • Very high EBRT local control rates suggest utilizing the lower end of the acceptable dose range for ENMZL disease • Patient must be monitored post-treatment for radiation side effects (dry eye, cataract, radiation retinopathy, optic neuropathy)
Intravenous chemotherapy	• Combined chemotherapy regimens (cyclophosphamide + doxorubicin + vincristine + prednisone [CHOP]) used for more aggressive subtypes such as diffuse large B-cell or mantle cell lymphoma • Moderately high local control rates seen • Less commonly used due to systemic side effects
Immunotherapy	• Monoclonal antibody rituximab • Approved for relapsed or refractory low-grade B-cell NHL and follicular lymphoma • Typically given in cycles of 4-weekly infusions • Not established to replace EBRT for local ophthalmic treatment • Favourable toxicity profile (compared to CHOP) • Unknown local control and systemic efficacy
Antibiotic therapy	• In those with confirmed microbial infection, a trial with doxycycline 100 mg PO b.i.d. for 3 weeks can result in a complete or partial resolution
Radioimmunotherapy	• Yttrium-90 ibritumomab tiuxetan (beta-brachytherapy) • Experimental treatment to maximize radiation dose to tumour cells while minimizing dose to critical organs (bone marrow) • Given in two injections 7 days apart • Early results suggest a response rate similar to that for EBRT • Main side effect is pancytopenia

Post-treatment assessment

- *Local tumour control:*
  - Comprehensive ophthalmic examination:
    - Pupillary, ocular motor and adnexal/nodal palpation
  - Slit-lamp biomicroscopy with photography (as needed) and indirect ophthalmoscopy
  - Visual fields, colour vision and Hertel exophthalmometry
  - Periodic CT or MRI of orbits/sinuses/head
- *Metastasis:*
  - Systemic examination with a haematologist–oncologist
  - Patients monitored periodically with:
    - Physical examination
    - CT abdomen, chest and pelvis
    - Whole-body PET-CT
    - Blood tests (CBC, LDH)
- *Radiation side effects:*
  - Radiation maculopathy
  - Radiation optic neuropathy
  - Radiation cataract
  - Neovascular glaucoma
  - Dry eye

Controversies

OAL represents a spectrum of lymphoid malignancies, ranging from the more common and less aggressive ENMZL MALT-type to those more resistant to treatment and likely to be associated with systemic disease. In each case, the approach should be to establish a pathological diagnosis and perform systemic staging. This will allow for adjustments in EBRT dose or systemic

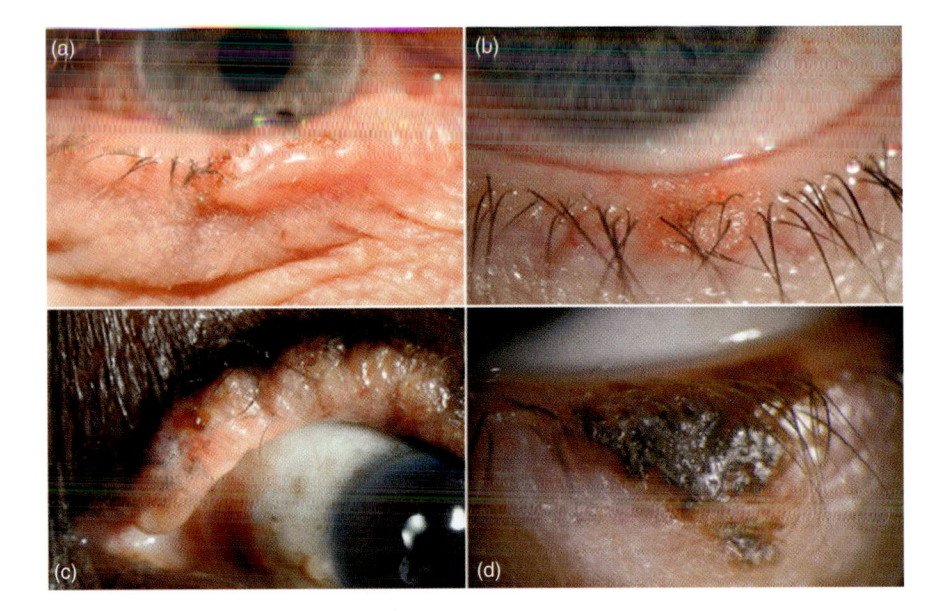

Figure 54.4 Eyelid cancers. (a) Slit-lamp photograph reveals a basal cell carcinoma (BCC) of the lower lid displaying telangiectactic vessels and a central crater (T2aN0M0). Note the minimal induration with some loss of hair follicles. (b) Slit-lamp photograph shows a squamous cell carcinoma of the lower lid (T2aN0M0). This tumour is relatively flat and indurated compared to the basal cell carcinoma. (c) Slit-lamp photograph of a sebaceous carcinoma of the upper eyelid (T2bN0M0). Here there is extensive eyelash loss and misdirection. The tumour diffusely invades the eyelid stroma. (d) Slit-lamp photograph of an eyelid melanoma. It did not affect the eyelashes; however, it does extend onto the lid margin (T2bN0M0). Note the diagnostic incisional biopsy site.
Source: Schwarcz (2013). Reproduced with permission of Wolters Kluwer Health.

therapy. However, most evidence suggests that EBRT offers the best rates of local control. Newer biological therapies and radioimmunotherapy (rituximab and beta-brachytherapy) are still considered investigational. Follow-up evaluations should be influenced by the methods of primary treatment. For example, after EBRT, patients must be periodically assessed for ophthalmic radiation side effects. Multidisciplinary care is crucial to optimize outcomes for patients with OAL.

EYELID CANCERS

Introduction

The most common type of eyelid cancer is basal cell carcinoma (BCC) (90%). Other less common eyelid cancers include squamous cell carcinoma (SCC), sebaceous cell carcinoma and malignant melanoma (Fig. 54.4). Most eyelid cancers can be removed with surgery. However, if left untreated, eyelid tumours can grow around the eye and into the orbit, sinuses and brain, as well as metastasize.

Incidence and aetiology

Incidence and aetiology	Description
Incidence	• BCC: 90% • Malignant melanoma, SCC, sebaceous cell carcinoma, miscellaneous: 10%
Aetiology	• Ultraviolet light exposure • Fair skin • Outdoor occupations • Aetiology of sebaceous cell carcinoma is unknown

Pathology

It is important to note that descriptions of eyelid cancers are given, and description of primary conjunctival cancers with eyelid involvement (especially for SCC, which is more common on the conjunctiva and less commonly affects the eyelid) is not included.

Pathology	Description
Basal cell carcinoma	• Typically firm, indurated pink nodular tumour (can present as pigmented or without a nodule) • Central crater with nodular margins • Typically occurs in sixth to eighth decades of life • Typically slow growing with no discomfort • Usually affects lower eyelid (>50%); but can develop on the medial canthus or upper eyelid; rarely the lateral canthus • Can induce ectropion (eversion of the eyelid) • Morpheaform (or sclerosing) BCC variant with flat, diffuse edges (indistinct margins) • Can invade orbit and sinuses • Rare metastasis
Squamous cell carcinoma (SCC) of the eyelid	• Spectrum from premalignant actinic keratosis to invasive SCC • Appearance can range from hypervascular flat lesion to thickened tumour • Typical reddish colour • Can be surrounded by inflammation (induration) • With or without exfoliation on the surface • Can invade orbit and sinuses • Can be found associated with conjunctival SCC: ▪ All conjunctival surfaces should be inspected, including eversion of upper and lower eyelids • Metastasis seen with very large tumours and in the immunosupressed

Pathology	Description
Malignant melanoma of the eyelid	• Pigmented or variably pigmented lesion • Can change size or colour, or bleed • Can be found associated with conjunctival melanoma: ▪ All conjunctival surfaces should be inspected, including eversion of upper and lower eyelids • Metastatic rates similar to those for cutaneous melanoma
Sebaceous cell carcinoma of the eyelid	• From sebaceous glands in the tarsus, eyelash margin, eyebrow or within smaller pilosebaceous units that cover the eyelid and caruncle • Average age is sixth decade of life • More common in upper eyelid • Can present as non-responsive blepharitis or chronic, recurrent chalazion • Eyelash loss • Spread along conjunctival surface • Can be aggressive with orbital extension and lymphatic based systemic metastasis • Metastatic rate up to 27% (dependent on the size, location and degree of infiltration) • Can be associated with Muir–Torre syndrome: a hereditary condition prone to cancers of the colon, breast, genitourinary tract and skin (including sebaceous tumours)

Presentation

- Growth on or in the eyelid
- Red, brown or black
- Loss of eyelashes
- Chronic conjunctivitis or chronic chalazion
- Can distort eyelid position
- Massive orbital extension can lead to displacement of the eye, proptosis and optic nerve compression

Diagnostic work-up

- Slit-lamp examination with photographic documentation
- Assessment of optic nerve and ocular motor function
- If orbital extension is suspected, CT or MRI is needed to examine the posterior extent and for extension into the sinuses
- Palpation of regional lymph nodes: preauricular, parotid, infra-auricular (cervical, submandibular and supraclavicular) chains
- Incisional or excisional biopsy can determine if an eyelid tumour is malignant
- Radiographic imaging of the cervical lymph node chains may lead to PET-CT or sentinel node biopsy

Staging and prognostic grouping

AJCC staging and prognostic grouping
See Table 54.7.

Prognostic factors
See Table 54.8.

Treatment philosophy

The primary goal is cure with relative sparing of unaffected eyelid tissues. Depending on the tumour type, this can be accomplished by excision with negative margins (nodular BCC, smaller SCC, sebaceous cell tumours and melanomas). Larger margins are used for sebaceous carcinoma and melanoma. Alternatively, cryotherapy or radiation therapy has been used as primary treatment or to extend treatment margins.

Table 54.7 AJCC staging and prognostic grouping: Carcinoma of the eyelid

Primary Tumor (T)	
TX	Primary tumor cannot be assessed
T0	No evidence of primary tumor
Tis	Carcinoma in *situ*
T1	Tumor 5 mm or less in greatest dimension. Not invading the tarsal plate or eyelid margin.
T2a	Tumor more than 5 mm, but not more than 10 mm in greatest dimension. Or, any tumor that invades the tarsal plate or eyelid margin.
T2b	Tumor more than 10mm, but not more than 20 mm in greatest dimension. Or, involves full thickness eyelid.
T3a	Tumor more than 20 mm in greatest dimension. Or, any tumor that invades adjacent ocular, or orbital structures. Any T with perineural tumor invasion.
T3b	Tumor complete resection requires enucleation, exenteration or bone resection.
T4	Tumor is not resectable due to extensive invasion of ocular, orbital, craniofacial structures or brain.

Regional LYMPH Nodes (N)	
NX	Regional lymph nodes cannot be assessed.
N0	No regional lymph node metastasis, based upon clinical evaluation or imaging. No regional lymph node metastasis, based upon lymph node biopsy.
N1	Regional lymph node metastasis.

Distant Metastasis (M)	
M0	No distant metastasis (no pathologic M0; use clinical M to complete stage group)
M1	Distant metastasis

Anatomic Stage • Prognostic Groups

Clinical

GROUP	T	N	M
☐ 0	Tis	N0	M0
☐ I A	T1	N0	M0
☐ I B	T2a	N0	M0
☐ I C	T2b	N0	M0
☐ II	T3a	N0	M0
☐ III A	T3b	N0	M0
☐ III B	Any T	N1	M0
☐ III C	T4	Any N	M0
☐ IV	Any T	Any N	M1

☐ Stage unknown

Pathologic

GROUP	T	N	M
☐ 0	Tis	N0	M0
☐ I A	T1	N0	M0
☐ I B	T2a	N0	M0
☐ I C	T2b	N0	M0
☐ II	T3a	N0	M0
☐ III A	T3b	N0	M0
☐ III B	Any T	N1	M0
☐ III C	T4	Any N	M0
☐ IV	Any T	Any N	M1

☐ Stage unknown

Edge *et al.* (2010) Reproduced with permission of Springer.

Treatment

Treatment	Description
Surgical resection	• Tumour excision with negative margins using frozen section control or same with Moh's technique • Eyelid reconstruction • Small tumours are usually removed by pentagonal wedge resection • Medium-sized tumours often require reconstruction with transpositional flaps (Tenzel, Mustarde, glabellar) • Large tumour resections are typically reconstructed with Hughes, Hewes or Cutler–Beard techniques
Cryotherapy	• For treatment of select typically smaller tumours after biopsy, to extended margins and for patients who cannot undergo surgery
External beam radiation	• Used primarily for morpheaform (diffuse-type) BCC, as an adjuvant to surgery in cases with limited orbital extension, and after radical neck dissection • Extensive or recurrent disease and those unresponsive to all other therapies may require exenteration with subsequent orbital EBRT

Post-treatment assessment

- *Local tumour control:*
  - Following treatment, the eyelid is inspected (with eversion of the eyelids) and palpated for recurrence
  - Periodic comparative photography is helpful to detect recurrence

Table 54.8 Prognostic factors for survival for eyelid cancers

Prognostic factors	Tumour related	Host related	Environment related
Essential	Location (worse prognosis if tumour involves the orbit or sinus)	Immunosuppression Perauricular and/or cervical lymph node involvement Systemic metastatic disease at presentation	
Additional	BCC: nodular better than morpheaform type Sebaceous and melanoma tumours have a worse prognosis than BCC or SCC		
New and promising	Improvements in local control have been associated with less systemic recurrence Universally accepted AJCC staging		

- *Metastasis:*
  - Regional lymph nodes are palpated
  - Periodic CT or MRI of the brain and orbits for cases of orbital/sinus extension
  - Patients with sebaceous cell carcinoma and melanoma should be monitored periodically for systemic disease (CT, MRI, PET-CT) as directed per medical oncology

Phase III clinical trials

There is a general lack of new, ongoing phase III clinical trials for eye cancers.

Uveal melanoma

The Collaborative Ocular Melanoma Study (COMS) was the first large, prospective, standardized, multicentre study for patients with choroidal melanoma. Treatments investigated included observation, plaque brachytherapy and enucleation. Though limited to select posterior choroidal melanomas, the results of this landmark study shaped the way we manage UM, and continues to play a role in patient education and informed consent.

- Small Choroidal Melanoma Study (observation for growth): 21% of small tumours grew and 3% metastasized
- Medium-sized Choroidal Melanoma Study (1317 patients enrolled): no survival advantage between plaque and enucleation for survival at up to 12 years' follow-up
- Large-sized Choroidal Melanoma Study (1003 patients enrolled): no survival advantage associated with 20-Gy pre-enucleation EBRT at up to 10 years' follow-up
- Medium and large choroidal melanomas: in multivariate analysis, both advanced patient age and larger basal tumour diameter were the most important risk factors for metastasis
- Accuracy of clinical diagnosis was 99.6%
- Mean patient age was 60 years

Areas of research

- Genetic and molecular pathways of pathogenesis
- Biomarkers for prognosis
- Development of therapies to prevent the development of metastatic disease
- Treatment of metastatic UM:
  - With no known cure, there are multiple phase III trials, most recently with a focus on immunotherapy and monoclonal antibodies such as ipilimumab, nivolumab, PD-1, MEK inhibitors and Allovectin-7
- Treatment of metastatic Rb:
  - Phase III study is evaluating the effect of combination chemotherapy, autologous stem cell transplant and/or radiation therapy in patients with extraocular Rb
- *Early* detection of Rb:
  - Early detection programmes using flash from cameras to screen for leukocoria
  - Intrauterine ultrasonography for high-risk pregnancies
- Radiation retinopathy:
  - Anti-VEGF therapy has been shown in small case series and phase I/II trials to suppress retinopathy associated with radiation, but to date there has been no prospective randomized trial to validate its benefit
- Rb screening programmes for less developed countries
- Immunotherapy and radioimmunotherapy for treatment of OAL
- Understanding of genetic alterations that cause development of OAL
- Effect of microbial infection on OAL development and progression
- EyeCancerBIG (http://eyecancerbig.com) ocular tumour registry programmes active for uveal melanoma, retinoblastoma, conjunctival melanoma, ocular adnexal lymphoma, lacrimal gland carcinoma and eye lid carcinoma.

Recommended reading

American Brachytherapy Society - Ophthalmic Oncology Task Force (2014) The American Brachytherapy Society consensus guidelines for plaque brachytherapy of uveal melanoma and retinoblastoma. *Brachytherapy* 13:1–14.

Chiu-Tsao ST, Astrahan MA, Finger PT et al. (2012) Dosimetry of 125I and 103Pd COMS eye plaques for intraocular tumors: Report of Task Group 129 by the AAPM and ABS. *Med Phys* 39:6161–6184.

Collaborative Ocular Melanoma Study Group (2006) The COMS randomized trial of iodine 125 brachytherapy for choroidal melanoma: V. Twelve-year mortality rates and prognostic factors: COMS report No. 28. *Arch Ophthalmol* 124:1684–1693.

Coupland SE, Krause L, Delecluse HJ et al. (1998) Lymphoproliferative lesions of the ocular adnexa. Analysis of 112 cases. *Ophthalmology* 105:1430–1441.

Coupland SE, Hummel M, Stein H (2002) Ocular adnexal lymphomas: Five case presentations and a review of the literature. *Surv Ophthalmol* 47:470–490.

Dimaras H, Kimani K, Dimba EA et al. (2012) Retinoblastoma. *Lancet* 379:1436–1446.

Finger PT (1997) Radiation therapy for choroidal melanoma. *Surv Ophthalmol* 42:215–232.

Finger PT (2009) Radiation therapy for orbital tumors: Concepts, current use and ophthalmic side effects. *Surv Ophthalmol* 54:545–568.

Finger PT, Chin K (2007) Anti-vascular endothelial growth factor bevacizumab (Avastin) for radiation retinopathy. *Arch Ophthalmol* 125:751–756.

Finger PT, Harbour JW, Karcioglu ZA (2002) Risk factors for metastasis in retinoblastoma. *Surv Ophthalmol* 47:1–16.

Finger PT, Chin KJ, Duvall G; Palladium-103 for Choroidal Melanoma Study Group (2009) Palladium-103 ophthalmic plaque radiation therapy for choroidal melanoma: 400 treated patients. *Ophthalmology* 116:790–796.

Finger PT (2014) Intraocular melanoma. In: DeVita VT Jr, Lawrence TS, Rosenberg SA, eds. Cancer. Principles & Practice of Oncology, 10th edn. Philadelphia, PA: Wolters Kluwer Health/Lippincott Williams & Wilkins Publishers; 1770–1779.

Freton A, Chin KJ, Raut R, Tena LB, Kivelä T, Finger PT (2012) Initial PET/CT staging for choroidal melanoma: AJCC correlation and second nonocular primaries in 333 patients. Eur J Ophthalmol 22:236–243.

Graue G, Finger PT, Maher E et al. (2013) Ocular adnexal lymphoma staging and treatment: American Joint Committee on Cancer versus Ann Arbor. Eur J Ophthalmol 23:344–355.

Kivela T, Kujala E (2013) Prognostication in eye cancer: the latest tumor, node, metastasis classification and beyond. Eye 27:243–252.

Khan S, Finger PT, Yu GP et al. (2012) Clinical and pathologic characteristics of biopsy-proven iris melanoma: a multicenter international study. Arch Ophthalmol 130:57–64.

Margo CE, Waltz K (1993) Basal cell carcinoma of the eyelid and periocular skin. Surv Ophthalmol 38:169–192.

Moshfeghi DM et al. (2000) Enucleation. Surv Ophthalmol 44:277–301.

Murphree AL (2005) Intraocular retinoblastoma: the case for new group classification. Ophthalmol Clin North Am 200:41–53.

Rasmussen PK, Coupland SE, Finger PT et al. (2014) Ocular adnexal follicular lymphoma: a multicenter international study. JAMA Ophthalmol 132:851–858.

Rosenberg C, Finger PT (2008) Cutaneous malignant melanoma metastatic to the eye, lids and orbit. Surv Ophthalmol 53:187–202.

Schwarcz RM, Coupland SE, Finger PT (2013) Cancer of the Orbit and Adnexa. Am J Clin Oncol 36:197–205.

Semenova E, Finger PT (2013) Palladium-103 radiation therapy for small choroidal melanoma. Ophthalmology 120:2353–2357.

Semenova E, Finger PT (2014) Palladium-103 plaque radiation therapy for American Joint Committee on Cancer T3- and T4-staged choroidal melanomas. JAMA Ophthalmol 132:205–213.

The AJCC-UICC Ophthalmic Oncology Task Force (2009) Ophthalmic sites. In: EdgeSE, Byrd DR, CarducciMA, ComptonCA, eds. AJCC Cancer Staging Manual, 7th edn. New York, NY: Springer:521–590.

The AJCC Ophthalmic Oncology Task Force (2015) International Validation of the American Joint Committee on Cancer's 7th Edition Classification of Uveal Melanoma. JAMA Ophthalmol. 2015;133(4):376-383.

Wilson MW, Czechonska G, Finger PT, Rausen A, Hooper ME, Haik BG (2001) Chemotherapy for eye cancer. Surv Ophthalmol 45:416–444.

55 Bone (osteosarcoma)

Elizabeth J. Davis[1], Geoffrey Siegel[2], Mary Feng[3], J. Sybil Biermann[4] and Rashmi Chugh[1]

[1]Division of Hematology/Oncology, Department of Internal Medicine, University of Michigan, Ann Arbor, MI, USA
[2]Department of Orthopaedic Surgery, Wayne State University School of Medicine, Oakwood Heritage Hospital, Taylor, MI, USA
[3]Department of Radiation Oncology, University of Michigan, Ann Arbor, MI, USA
[4]Department of Orthopaedic Surgery, University of Michigan, Ann Arbor, MI, USA

Summary	Key facts
Introduction	- Osteosarcoma is the most common primary malignant bone tumour (about 45% of all bone tumours) - Bimodal age distribution: adolescence and sixth decade - Risk factors: retinoblastoma, Li–Fraumeni, Rothmund–Thomson syndrome, multiple hereditary exostosis, radiation exposure, Paget disease
Presentation	- Often presents as a firm, painful mass, adjacent to bone - Most common sites are the distal femur, proximal tibia and proximal humerus - Most are intramedullary tumours, but some are surface lesions - Initial evaluation includes history, physical exam, blood work (complete blood count, comprehensive metabolic panel, lactate dehydrogenase, alkaline phosphatase), plain film of primary site, CT/MRI of primary site and CT chest
Scenario	- *Local disease and low-grade disease:* initial treatment is wide local excision - *High-grade disease:* chemotherapy followed by surgery and additional chemotherapy - *Metastatic disease:* chemotherapy followed by evaluation for surgical resection of primary site and metastatectomy with adjuvant chemotherapy - Limited role for radiation

Trials	- Eilber *et al.* (1987) *J Clin Oncol* 5:21–26:
	   - Established role for adjuvant chemotherapy in patients with localized high-grade osteosarcoma
	- POG 8651; Goorin *et al.* (2003) *J Clin Oncol* 21(8):1574–1580:
	   - Survival was similarly improved by either pre- or post-surgical chemotherapy
	   - Established a benchmark outcome for future studies
	- ISG/OS-1; Ferarri *et al.* (2012) *J Clin Oncol* 30(12):2113–2118:
	   - Ifosfamide should only be considered in patients who have a poor histological response to methotrexate + cisplatin + doxorubicin
	- OS 06/OS-91, Daw *et al.* (2006) *Cancer* 106(2):403–412:
	   - Established role of cisplatin given improvement in overall survival
	- Goorin *et al.* (2002) *J Clin Oncol* 20(2):426–433:
	   - Combination of etoposide + high-dose ifosfamide is effective induction chemotherapy for patients with metastatic osteosarcoma

UICC Manual of Clinical Oncology, Ninth Edition. Edited by Brian O'Sullivan, James D. Brierley, Anil K. D'Cruz, Martin F. Fey, Raphael Pollock, Jan B. Vermorken and Shao Hui Huang. © 2015 UICC. Published 2015 by John Wiley & Sons, Ltd.

Introduction

Primary malignant bone tumours are very rare, whereas metastases to bone from a variety of primary sites are fairly common. *Osteosarcoma* is the most common malignancy originating within the bone and is the focus of this chapter. It is composed of osteoid and may have an intramedullary (most common), bone surface or extraskeletal location. The most common variant is conventional osteosarcoma, which is a high-grade tumour that is often located at the distal femur, proximal tibia or proximal humerus.

Incidence and aetiology

Incidence and aetiology	Description

Incidence	- Bone tumours are rare cancers
	- 3–5% of childhood and 1% of adult cancers
	- Osteosarcoma is the most common type:
	  - Incidence has a bimodal distribution with peaks in the young and in the elderly:
	    - Earlier incidence peak in adolescent girls than in boys, likely linked to earlier growth spurt
	  - In those aged <24 years: men 4.3 per 1,000,000 and women 3.4 per 1,000,000
	  - In those aged 25–59 years: men 1.9 per 1,000,000 and women 1.4 per 1,000,000
	  - In those aged >60 years: men 4 per 1,000,000 and women 3.1 per 1,000,000
	- Male predominance of osteosarcoma at younger ages:
	  - <24 years old: 1.43:1
	  - 25–59 years old: 1.28:1
	  - >60 years old: 1:1

Aetiology	- Association between rapid bone growth/turnover and development of osteosarcoma
	- Most have complex, unbalanced karyotypes:
	  - Highest frequency of loss of heterozygosity (LOH) is for chromosomes 3q, 13q, 17p and 18q
	- Risk factors:
	  - *Hereditary*: Li–Fraumeni, retinoblastoma, Rothmund–Thomson syndrome, multiple hereditary exostosis
	  - *Non-hereditary*: prior radiation exposure, Paget disease, polyostotic fibrous dysplasia

Screening	- No role for screening in osteosarcoma

Data Source: *Int. J. Cancer:* 125, 229–234 (2009).

Pathology

Pathology	Description
Conventional, intramedullary	- 75–85% of all osteosarcomas - Most are high grade - Characterized by dominant matrix in the tumour: bone (osteoblastic), cartilage (chondroblastic) or fibrous tissue (fibroblastic) - Spindled-polyhedral tumour cells - Pleomorphic and hyperchromatic nuclei
Parosteal, surface	- <5% of osteosarcomas - Usually on the distal posterior femur - Characterized by parallel bone trabeculae with bone spicules that are thicker at the base of the lesion - Intertrabecular spaces contain fibrous tissue - Most are associated with the outer fibrous layer of the periosteum
Periosteal, surface	- Less common than parosteal osteosarcoma - Matrix is mostly cartilaginous. - Often arises between the cortex and cambium layer of the periosteum

Other	- *Telangiectatic*:
	  - Composed of multiple blood-filled sinusoids with little tissue
	  - Resemble an aneurysmal bone cyst at low power
	  - Nuclear pleomorphism and high mitotic rate are more apparent at high power

Pathology	Description
	<ul><li>Extracellular matrix is often sparse</li><li>Often contain foci of osteoclast-like giant cells</li></ul><ul><li>Small cell:<ul><li>Rare type of osteosarcoma (1–2%)</li><li>Small cells with round, hyperchromatic nuclei and little nuclear pleomorphism</li><li>Occasional spindling of tumour cells and production of osteoid</li><li>Controversy about this subtype given its overlap with Ewing tumours: can have the t11; 22 translocation or positive membrane staining for CD99</li></ul></li><li>Epithelioid:<ul><li>Poorly differentiated tumour cells, making distinction between sarcoma and carcinoma difficult</li><li>Tumour cells are often round or polyhedral with round or ovoid enlarged nuclei, and may contain one or more prominent nucleoli</li></ul></li><li>Osteoblastoma like:<ul><li>Resemble osteoblastoma producing microtrabecular bone lined by osteoblasts</li><li>Characterized by tumour and aneuploid mitotic activity interfacing with normal bone</li></ul></li><li>Chrondroblastoma like:<ul><li>Characterized by osteoid or bone formation, atypical mitotic activity and infiltration of adjacent intertrabecular spaces</li></ul></li></ul>

Presentation and natural history

Osteosarcoma often presents as a firm, tender mass adjacent to underlying bone. Bones of the knee and proximal humerus are most commonly affected and pain may be worse at night. Overlying erythema or evidence of increased vascularity may be present. Loss of range of motion or function of a limb may occur.

Presentation and natural history		Description
Presentation	Local	<ul><li>Painful, firm mass</li><li>Possible limitations on range of motion or use of limb</li></ul>
	Metastatic	<ul><li>Lungs are most common site for metastases</li><li>Often asymptomatic</li><li>Metastases are present in 10–20% of patients at diagnosis</li></ul>
Routes of spread	Local	<ul><li>Tumour may extend locally and into surrounding structures</li></ul>
	Metastatic	<ul><li>Most commonly spread to lung</li><li>Bone is second most common site</li><li>Skip metastases via the medullary canal also occur</li><li>Lymphatic spread is rare</li><li>Metastases often occur within 2 years of initial diagnosis</li></ul>

Diagnostic work up

- Plain films, magnetic resonance imaging (MRI) ± computed tomography (CT) of the primary site
- Chest CT
- Biopsy of primary site for diagnosis and staging:
  - Biopsy placement is critical to maintain option of limb-sparing surgery
  - Core needle biopsy:
    - Safe direct path to tumour mass is possible from skin
    - Lower cost and morbidity
  - Open (surgical) biopsy:
    - Short longitudinal incision in line with projected surgical approach for resection
    - Meticulous haemostasis
    - Avoid contamination between muscle compartments or of neurovascular structures
- Lactate dehydrogenase (LDH), alkaline phosphatase
- No tumour markers

Staging and prognostic grouping

The Enneking system for the surgical staging of bone and soft tissue tumours is based on grade, site and metastasis. It uses histological, radiological and clinical criteria. Grade 1 is low grade and grade 2 is high grade. Site is represented by T: T1 is intracompartmental and T2 is extracompartmental. M0 represents absence of metastatic disease and M1 represents presence of metastases.

Table 55.1 UICC TNM categories and stage grouping: Bone

TNM categories	
T1	≤8 cm
T2	>8 cm
T3	Discontinuous tumours in primary site
N1	Regional
M1a	Lung
M1b	Other sites
	Low grade
	High grade

Stage grouping				
Stage IA	T1	N0	M0	Low grade
Stage IB	T2–3	N0	M0	Low grade
Stage IIA	T1	N0	M0	High grade
Stage IIB	T2	N0	M0	High grade
Stage III	T3	N0	M0	High grade
Stage IVA	Any T	N0	M1a	Any grade
Stage IVB	Any T	N1	Any M	Any grade
	Any T	Any N	M1b	Any grade

Note: Use N0 for NX
For T1 and T2, use low grade if no grade is stated

UICC TNM staging

The UICC staging system is based on grade, tumour, node and metastases (Table 55.1). Grade 1 or 2 is low grade while grade 3 or 4 is high grade. T1 is <8 cm, T2 is >8 cm and T3 is a tumour that has spread to another site within the same bone. N0 represents no nodal involvement; N1 indicates nodal involvement. M0 indicates no metastases; M1a represents lung metastases only and M1b represents other sites of metastases.

Prognostic factors

The significance of various factors in the prognosis of osteosarcoma remains somewhat controversial given the heterogeneity of data. Most studies agree that poor response to neoadjuvant chemotherapy, positive margin resection, presence of and location of metastases at diagnosis, and elevated enzyme markers (LDH, alkaline phosphatase) are poor prognostic factors (Table 55.2). A large tumour is also considered a poor prognostic factor; however, a standard size has not been established (10 cm has been repeatedly used as a cut-off in multiple studies). The significance of age as a prognostic factor has been debated, with two large retrospective studies reporting <14 and >40 years old as poor prognostic factors; however, a large, international retrospective study failed to confirm this. Treatment type (i.e. amputation, combination therapy with chemotherapy, radiation and surgery) has been associated with poor prognosis; however, there are likely confounding factors as patients with larger tumours or more extensive disease are more likely to receive these therapies.

Treatment philosophy

Conventional osteosarcoma

The goal of treatment for conventional osteosarcoma depends on the stage at diagnosis; however, even metastatic disease, if there are limited lung metastases, can be treated with curative intent. For non-metastatic, high-grade osteosarcoma, treatment should include neoadjuvant chemotherapy, wide local excision and adjuvant chemotherapy. The goal of neoadjuvant chemotherapy is to treat occult metastatic disease and assess necrosis induced by treatment to determine an adjuvant regimen. Low-grade disease may be treated with wide local excision alone. The 5-year overall survival (OS) has improved in the last few decades and is estimated at 50–70%. About 80–90% of these patients are candidates for limb salvage surgery. Surgery is the only curative treatment.

In metastatic disease, survival rates are more dismal (10–40%) and vary based on location and resectability of metastases. Metastatic osteosarcoma should be treated with chemotherapy and may be followed by surgery depending on the location, number and size of metastases. If surgery is performed, adjuvant chemotherapy should be administered. Radiation

Table 55.2 Prognostic factors for osteosarcoma

Prognostic factors	Tumour related	Host related	Environment related
Essential	Location, size, extent of disease Tumour response to neoadjuvant chemotherapy	Age	Residual disease after resection
Additional	LDH Alkaline phosphatase	Gender Performance status	Management by a multidisciplinary sarcoma team Local recurrence
New and promising	Biomarkers		

therapy may be useful in the metastatic setting, especially if the tumour remains unresectable after neoadjuvant chemotherapy, in which case it is given with palliative intent for local disease control.

Patients with osteosarcoma have a high rate of relapse; around 30% in patients with localized disease and 80% in those with metastatic disease. Treatment can include surgical resection, chemotherapy or radiation therapy depending on site and extent of relapsed disease.

Parosteal osteosarcoma

The prognosis for parosteal osteosarcoma is better than that for the high-grade variants of osteosarcoma, and treatment for this disease is surgical. Preoperative MRI and CT allow for precise surgical planning with the goal of negative margins. Because parosteal osteosarcoma selectively involves the bone surface, more limited resections are sometimes possible with better limb function preservation than is possible with the high-grade variants. Patients should be followed postoperatively as early detection may result in limb-sparing options for recurrence. Local recurrence or distant relapse tends to occur later than with the high-grade variants, and there is a transformation rate of about 25% into high-grade osteosarcoma.

Periosteal osteosarcoma

The prognosis of periosteal osteosarcoma is similar to that of parosteal osteosarcoma, and treatment for this disease is primarily surgical. Long-term OS after surgical resection is around 80%. No benefit has been demonstrated for adjuvant chemotherapy. Patients should be followed for local recurrence or metastatic disease.

Scenario	Treatment philosophy
Local disease	- *Low-grade osteosarcoma*: wide local excision - *High-grade osteosarcoma*: chemotherapy followed by wide local excision and adjuvant chemotherapy
Metastatic disease	- Metastatectomy if possible, chemotherapy and/or radiation
Recurrent disease	- Chemotherapy or resection

Follow-up	- History, physical exam, chest X-ray and imaging of the primary site:
	  - Every 3 months for Years 1 and 2
	  - Every 4 months in Year 3
	  - Every 6 months in Years 4 and 5
	- Blood work as clinically indicated

Treatment

Surgery

Surgery	Description

Early disease	- Wide resection
	- Negative margins:
	  - Intraoperative frozen sections may be helpful in confirming negative margin resections
	- Surgical dissection ideally proceeds *en bloc* through normal tissue so as not to seed tumour cells into the surgical field:
	  - Must include unviolated cuff of healthy tissue
	  - Biopsy tract/scar must be resected with tumour specimen *en bloc*
	- No role for lymph node dissection
	- Coordinate pathological evaluation of specimen to achieve analysis of margins and treatment effect in patients treated with neoadjuvant chemotherapy
	- No reconstruction needed for 'expendable' bones (e.g. fibula, wing of ilium)
	- Skeletal reconstruction options:
	  - Allograft:
	    - Allows near-anatomical muscle/tendon reattachment site
	    - No immediate structural support; requires period of non-weight bearing
	    - Potential non-union, especially in smokers

(continued)

Surgery	Description

	• Endoprostheses:
	  ◦ May be used alone or as composite with allograft
	  ◦ Allows immediate structural support
	  ◦ Durable surface for joint restorations
	  ◦ Longevity of implants is limiting factor
	• Implants currently available for skeletally immature patients, which allows for expansion for anticipated limb growth

Advanced non-metastatic disease	• Wide resection • Negative margins • Limb-sparing surgery when possible • Amputation if neurovascular involvement precludes limb salvage or if amputation will confer better functional outcome • No difference in long-term survival between amputation and limb salvage, but local recurrence rate higher with limb salvage
Metastatic	• Role for surgery only if isolated lung metastases amenable to complete resection

Radiotherapy

Radiotherapy	Description
Early disease	• Typically not part of initial curative treatment of resection ± chemotherapy depending on tumour grade
Advanced non-metastatic disease	• Typically not part of initial curative treatment of resection ± chemotherapy depending on tumour grade • If a resection is not possible, or if resection margins are positive, radiotherapy can provide local control, particularly if doses of >55 Gy in standard fractionation (1.8–2 Gy/day) or equivalent in larger doses per fraction, are given

Metastatic disease	• For small metastases, consideration should be given for stereotactic body radiotherapy (SBRT) since sarcomas are less radiosensitive than other tumour types:
	  ▪ Doses of 50–60 Gy in three to five fractions are common for lung, liver and bone metastases
	  ▪ Lower doses are used near the spinal cord to maintain safety
	  ▪ May provide better local control and faster pain relief for bone metastases compared with standard fractionated radiotherapy of 1–10 treatments for a total of 8–30 Gy

Systemic therapy

Systemic therapy	Description

Early disease	• Chemotherapy is indicated prior to wide local excision in high-grade osteosarcoma.
	• Adjuvant chemotherapy should be given after surgery:
	  ▪ If histological response to neoadjuvant therapy was poor (<90% necrosis), changing chemotherapeutic agents can be considered
	• Neoadjuvant therapy is given for two cycles followed by four cycles of adjuvant chemotherapy
	• If only adjuvant therapy is given, six cycles are administered
	• Cisplatin + doxorubicin are the mainstays of therapy:
	  ▪ Cisplatin 100–120 mg/m² IV + doxorubicin 60–75 mg/m² IV over 48-hour continuous infusion every 3 weeks
	  ▪ Cisplatin often discontinued after four cycles of therapy or if evidence of neurotoxicity
	  ▪ Typically given with granulocyte-colony stimulating factor (G-CSF) support
	• Role of methotrexate is controversial given nephrotoxicity and lack of survival benefit:
	  ▪ Cisplatin + doxorubicin + methotrexate (MAP):
	    ◦ Cisplatin 50–60 mg/m²/day IV × 2 days (Days 1 and 2) + doxorubicin 30–37.5 mg/m²/day IV over 2 days (Days 1 and 2) + methotrexate 8–12 g/m² × one dose (cap of 20 g/dose) IV on Days 22 and 29 (with hydration, alkalinization and leucovorin rescue) of a 35-day cycle (Table 55.3)

Systemic therapy	Description

	• Role of ifosfamide in first-line treatment remains controversial:
	  ▪ 2–3 g/m²/day
	  ▪ No improvement in event-free or overall survival when added to MAP and compared to MAP alone
	  ▪ Can be considered when poor histological response to neoadjuvant therapy; although preliminary data from a recent multicentre phase III study demonstrated no improvement in outcome with the addition of ifosfamide and etoposide to post-operative treatment
	  ▪ Consider use of G-CSF

Advanced non-metastatic disease	• Same as for early disease

Metastatic disease	• Ifosfamide 3.5 g/m²/day + etoposide 100 mg/m²/day for 5 days every 3 weeks:
	  ▪ G-CSF on Day 6
	• Ifosfamide 1.8 g/m²/day + etoposide 100 mg/m²/day + carboplatin 400 mg/m²/day on Days 1–5 every 3 weeks:
	  ▪ G-CSF on Day 6
	• Cisplatin, doxorubicin or methotrexate as for localized disease

Table 55.3 Schedule for methotrexate, doxorubicin and cisplatin (MAP) perioperatively

WEEK	1	2	3	4	5	6	7	8	9	10	11	12	13	14	15	16	17	18	19	20	21	22	23	24	25	26	27	28	29
TREATMENT	AP				M	M	AP			M	M	SURGERY		AP		M	M	AP		M	M	A		M	M	A		M	M

Adapted from EURAMOS-1 protocol as cited by Janeway, Grier (2010), with permission from Elsevier.

Controversies

Use of methotrexate

The role of methotrexate remains controversial. Studies have demonstrated conflicting results about survival benefit, and expertise for administration is required. The optimal dose is also debated. Bacci et al. found that patients given high-dose methotrexate had a trend toward higher OS rates at 5 years compared to those given moderate doses (58% vs 42%; $P = 0.07$). Their subsequent study found the complete remission rate at surgery to be related to methotrexate level. A study by the European Osteosarcoma Intergroup compared outcomes of patients who received doxorubicin + cisplatin versus doxorubicin + cisplatin + methotrexate. Overall survival was similar in the two groups, but event-free survival was improved in the group that did not receive methotrexate. However, the methotrexate group received lower total doses of doxorubicin + cisplatin, which could account for the difference.

Use of ifosfamide

Initial studies using low-dose ifosfamide (4.5–9 g/m²/cycle) did not demonstrate an improvement in patient prognosis. In 2008, the results of Intergroup-0133, a phase III, randomized, prospective trial investigating the addition of ifosfamide (9 g/m²) to chemotherapy, reported no improvement in event-free or overall survival. However, a subsequent Japanese phase II study that investigated adding high-dose ifosfamide (16 g/m²) to the treatment regimen for patients who had a poor histological response to neoadjuvant chemotherapy reported improved prognosis. Patients did have notable haematological toxicities, often limiting their ability to receive the full course of intended treatment. A recent phase III Italian Sarcoma Group trial examined the addition of ifosfamide to methotrexate + cisplatin + doxorubicin (MAP). There was no improvement in the good responder rate and haematological toxicity was increased. There was no benefit in event-free or overall survival at 5 years. The role of ifosfamide in local disease remains unclear and requires further study to determine how to optimize the dose while minimizing therapy-related toxicities.

Use of muramyl tripeptide phophatidyl-ethanolamine (MTP-PE)

MTP-PE is a component of the cell wall of Bacille Calmette-Guerin (BCG). It is encapsulated in liposomes and acts as an immune stimulator. The Children's Oncology Group conducted a phase III randomized trial examining the addition of MTP-PE to chemotherapy in the adjuvant setting. There was

Table 55.4 Phase III clinical trials

Trial name	Results
Local disease	
Eilber et al. (1987) J Clin Oncol 5:21–26	• Established role for adjuvant chemotherapy in patients with localized high-grade osteosarcoma
POG 8651 Goorin et al. (2003) J Clin Oncol 21(8):1574–1580	• Established that survival was similarly improved by either pre- or post-surgical chemotherapy • Established a benchmark outcome for future studies
ISG/OS-1 Ferarri et al. (2012) J Clin Oncol 30(12):2113–2118.	• Adding ifosfamide to methotrexate + cisplatin + doxorubicin (MAP) from the preoperative phase does not improve the good responder rate and increases haematological toxicity • Ifosfamide should only be considered in patients who have a poor histological response to MAP
Adjuvant systemic treatment	
Link et al. (1986) N Engl J Med 314(25):1600–1606	• 2-year relapse-free survival was significantly higher in patients with osteosarcoma of the extremity receiving adjuvant chemotherapy versus those on observation
Lewis et al. (2007) J Natl Cancer Inst 99(2):112–128	• Dose intensification of cisplatin + doxorubicin resulted in increased dose received and a statistically significant increase in good histological response rate, but not in increased progression-free or overall survival
Meyers et al. (2008) J Clin Oncol 26 (4):633–638	• Adding ifosfamide to MAP did not enhance event-free or overall survival for patients with osteosarcoma • Adding MTP to the same regimen resulted in a statistically significant improvement in OS and a trend toward better event-free survival
Advanced disease and metastatic disease	
OS-86/OS-91 Daw et al. (2006) Cancer 106(2):403–412	• Compared ifosfamide + cisplatin + doxorubicin + high-dose methotrexate to the same agents at similar doses, but with substitution of cisplatin with carboplatin • Established role of cisplatin given improvement in OS
Bacci et al. (2003) Ann Oncol 14(7):1126–1134	• Confirmed the prognosis of patients with metastatic osteosarcoma of the extremity remains poor, despite the use of aggressive treatment with combination chemotherapy and surgery
Goorin et al. (2002) J Clin Oncol 20(2):426–433	• Combination of etoposide + high-dose ifosfamide is effective induction chemotherapy for patients with metastatic osteosarcoma

a statistically significant improvement in overall survival at 6 years (78% vs 70%; $P = 0.03$) in patients receiving MTP-PE versus those who did not, and a trend towards improvement in event-free survival (68% vs 61%; $P = 0.08$). When patients with metastatic disease were examined in isolation, the trends toward improvement in overall and event-free survival persisted but were not statistically significant. Based on these data, MTP-PE was not approved by the FDA for use in the USA. It is available in Europe, but use of this agent is still widely debated.

Phase III clinical trials

See Table 55.4.

Areas of research

- Assessing whether changing chemotherapeutic agents after a poor histological response can improve outcomes
- Determining whether the addition of interferon-alpha as maintenance therapy improves outcomes
- Identifying pathways required for osteosarcoma cell proliferation and survival, and development of targeted therapies

Recommended reading

Anninga JK, Gelderblom H, Fiocco M et al. (2011) Chemotherapeutic adjuvant treatment for osteosarcoma: where do we stand? *Eur J Cancer* 47:2431–2445.

Bacci G, Picci P, Ruggieri P et al. (1990) Primary chemotherapy and delayed surgery (neoadjuvant chemotherapy for osteosarcoma of the extremities. *Cancer* 65:2539–2553.

Bakhshi S, Radhakrishnan V (2010) Prognostic markers in osteosarcoma. *Expert Rev Anticancer Ther* 10(2):271–287.

Bernthal NM, Federman N, Eilber FR et al. (2012) Long-term results (>25 years) of a randomized, prospective clinical trial evaluating chemotherapy in patients with high-grade, operable osteosarcoma. *Cancer* 118:5888–5893.

Bielack SS, Kempf-Bielack B, Branscheid D et al. (2009) Second and subsequent recurrences of osteosarcoma: presentation, treatment, and outcomes of 249 consecutive cooperative osteosarcoma study group patients. *J Clin Oncol* 27:557–565.

Bramwell VHC, Burgers M, Sneath R *et al*. (1992) A comparison of two short intensive adjuvant chemotherapy regimens in operable osteosarcoma of limbs in children and young adults: The first study of the European Osteosarcoma Intergroup. *J Clin Oncol* 10:1579–1591.

Briccoli A, Rocca M, Salone M, Guzzardella GA, Balladelli A, Bacci G (2010) High grade osteosarcoma of the extremities metastatic to the lung: long-term results in 323 patients treated combining surgery and chemotherapy, 1985-2005. *Surg Oncol* 19:193–199.

DeLaney TF, Park L, Goldberg SI *et al*. (2005) Radiotherapy for local control of osteosarcoma. *Int J Radiat Oncol Biol Phys* 61(2):492–498.

Iwamoto Y, Kazurhiro T, Isu K *et al*. (2009) Multiinstitutional phase II study of neoadjuvant chemotherapy for osteosarcoma (NECO study) in Japan: NECO-93J and NECO-95J. *J Orthopaed Sci* 14:397–404.

Janeway KA, Grier HE (2010) Sequelae of osteosarcoma medical therapy: a review of rare acute toxicities and late effects. *Lancet Oncol* 11(7):670–678.

Klein MJ, Siegal GP (2006) Osteosarcoma anatomic and histologic variants. *Am J Clin Pathol* 125:555–581.

Meyers PA, Schwartz CL, Krailo MD *et al*. (2008) Osteosarcoma: The additional of muramyl tripeptide to chemotherapy improves overall survival- a report from the children's oncology group. *J Clin Oncol* 26(4):633–638.

Mirabello L, Troisi RJ, Savage SA (2009) International osteosarcoma incidence patterns in children and adolescents, middle ages and elderly persons. *Int J Cancer* 125:229–234.

NCCN Treatment guidelines in oncology: Bone Cancer Version 2.2013 NCCN.org.

Mankin HJ, Mankin CJ, Simon MA (1996) The hazards of the biopsy revisited. *J Bone Joint Surg* 78(5):656–663.

Marina N, Smeland S, Bielack SS *et al*. (2014) MAPIE vs MAP as postoperative chemotherapy in patients with a poor response to preoperative chemotherapy for newly-diagnosed osteosarcoma: results form EURAMOS-1. CTOS abstract 032.

Ritter J, Bielack SS (2010) Osteosarcoma. *Ann Oncol* 21(Suppl 7):vii320–vii325.

Yasko AW (2009) Surgical management of primary osteosarcoma. *Cancer Treat Res* 152:125–145.

56 Soft tissue

Colleen Dickie[1], Abha Gupta[2], Raphael Pollock[3] and Brian O'Sullivan[1]

[1]Department of Radiation Oncology, The Princess Margaret Cancer Centre, University of Toronto, Toronto, ON, Canada
[2]Department of Medical Oncology, The Princess Margaret Cancer Centre, University of Toronto, Toronto, ON, Canada
[3]Department of Surgery, The James NCICCC/Ohio State University, Columbus, OH, USA

Summary	Key facts
Introduction	<ul><li>Soft tissue sarcoma is a rare malignancy derived from mesenchymal tissue</li><li>Comprises approximately 1% of adult cancers in the USA:<ul><li>11,000 new cases annually</li></ul></li><li>Soft tissue masses deep to the investing fascia with a history of growth should be considered sarcoma until proven otherwise</li></ul>
Presentation	<ul><li>Median age of onset is 50–55 years</li><li>Approximately 50% originate in the extremities, 40% in the trunk and retroperitoneum, and 10% in the head and neck:<ul><li>In general, superficial extremity lesions and those in the head and neck region are smaller due to earlier detection</li><li>Some sites can escape detection for significant lengths of time (e.g. the retroperitoneum, abdominal and intrathoracic cavity, and those originating deep to fascia)</li></ul></li><li>Characterized by wide heterogeneity in anatomical site, pathological subtype and clinical behaviour:<ul><li>Over 50 histological subtypes, the most common being the liposarcoma and undifferentiated pleomorphic sarcoma subtypes</li><li>Primary gastrointestinal stromal tumours (GIST) are uncommon (approximately 14% of all sarcomas), most frequently involving the gastrointestinal tract</li></ul></li><li>Any superficial or deep abnormality with a history of radiation exposure requires careful examination</li><li>Most common site of metastasis is the lungs:<ul><li>Tumours arising in the abdominal cavity/retroperitoneum more commonly metastasize to the liver and peritoneum</li></ul></li></ul>
Scenario	<ul><li>Should be managed by a multidisciplinary team with expertise in sarcoma</li><li>Treatment approach is surgery with or without local radiation therapy for extremity, torso, head and neck, and retroperitoneal tumours:<ul><li>Low-grade, superficial, small tumours (<5 cm): cure with surgery alone</li><li>High-grade and/or large tumours: commonly require a combined-modality approach including neoadjuvant or adjuvant radiotherapy with function-preserving surgery</li><li>Role of chemotherapy remains controversial and in general is restricted to established chemoresponsive subtypes and high-risk cases</li><li>Surgery alone is the current standard for retroperitoneal sarcoma; the role of adjuvant radiotherapy is being investigated</li></ul></li><li>Surgery is the mainstay of treatment for GIST (complete resection is possible for approximately 85% of primary tumours):<ul><li>Imatinib should be considered for tumours which are large, mitotically active or arising from small bowel</li></ul></li><li>Overall 5-year survival remains at 50–60% for all stages and sites combined</li></ul>

UICC Manual of Clinical Oncology, Ninth Edition. Edited by Brian O'Sullivan, James D. Brierley, Anil K. D'Cruz, Martin F. Fey, Raphael Pollock, Jan B. Vermorken and Shao Hui Huang. © 2015 UICC. Published 2015 by John Wiley & Sons, Ltd.

Summary	Key facts

Trials	• Rosenberg et al. (1982) *Ann Surg* 196:305–314:
	  ▪ Limb-sparing surgery + radiation therapy led to no difference in survival compared to amputation alone
	• Yang et al. (1998). *J Clin Oncol* 16:197–203.
	  ▪ Significant decrease in local recurrence with adjuvant postoperative radiation therapy for high- and low-grade lesions versus surgery alone, but no difference in overall survival
	• O'Sullivan et al. (2002) *Lancet* 359:2235–2241:
	  ▪ Higher wound complication rate, lower fibrosis rate at 2 years and no difference in 5-year survival rate for preoperative versus postoperative radiation therapy
	• Pisters et al. (1996) *J Clin Oncol* 14:859–868:
	  ▪ Addition of brachytherapy for high-grade lesions significantly improved local control after complete resection, with no significant difference in outcome for superficial trunk and extremity tumours versus surgery alone
	• Dematteo et al. (2009) *Lancet* 373:1097–1104:
	  ▪ Adjuvant imatinib mesylate after resection of localized, primary GIST significantly improved recurrence-free survival compared with placebo

Incidence, aetiology and screening

Soft tissue sarcomas (STS) are a heterogeneous group of rare malignant tumours derived from mesenchymal tissue. Several risk factors have been identified for STS but no clearly defined aetiological factor exists for most STS. General screening in high-risk patients using imaging or laboratory tests is not supported by clinical evidence.

Incidence, aetiology and screening	Description
Incidence	• Comprise just under 1% of adult cancers in the USA: ▪ 11,410 new cases were predicted for 2013, of which 6290 male and 5120 female • Global incidence is difficult to report due to the low prevalence of this disease

Aetiology	• Median age at onset is 50–55 years
	• *Genetic predisposition*:
	  ▪ Li-Fraumeni syndrome: associated with *TP53* mutation
	  ▪ Von Recklinghausen disease: neurofibromatosis
	  ▪ Retinoblastoma
	  ▪ Gardner syndrome/familial adenomatous polyposis
	  ▪ Carney triad
	  ▪ Werner syndrome
	  ▪ Gorlin syndrome
	  ▪ Tuberous sclerosis
	  ▪ Basal cell nevus syndrome
	• *Industrial chemicals*:
	  ▪ Manufacturing thorotrast
	  ▪ Vinyl chloride and arsenic: hepatic angiosarcomas
	  ▪ Phenoxyherbicides
	  ▪ Chlorophenols
	  ▪ Dioxins
	  ▪ Phenoxyacetic acids
	  ▪ Certain herbicides
	• *Past medical history*:
	  ▪ Lymphoedema associated with lymphangiosarcoma
	  ▪ Prior radiotherapy
	  ▪ Viral infections, including human herpesvirus 8 (HHV-8) and human immunodeficiency virus (HIV)

Screening	• General screening has limited use in STS given its rarity • Lesions deep to the superficial fascia require investigation, especially with a history of growth • Any superficial or deep lesion of skin or soft tissue in patients with a history of prior radiation increases risk • Patients with predisposing genetic factors require detailed clinical evaluation

Pathology

There are many STS subtypes with varying biological behaviours. Malignant fibrous histiocytoma has been the most common pathological subtype for the past two decades (40%); however, more recently this entity has been reclassified as part of a heterogeneous group termed undifferentiated pleomorphic sarcoma. Liposarcoma is the second most common STS (25%).

Pathology	Description
Fibroblastic/myofibroblastic	• Fibromatoses: superficial and deep (benign) • Fibrosarcoma • Myxofibrosarcoma, low grade • Low-grade fibromyxoid sarcoma • Sclerosing epithelioid fibrosarcoma

Fibrohistiocytic tumours (or other synonyms)	• Undifferentiated pleomorphic sarcoma (formerly malignant fibrous histiocytoma):
	  ▪ Pleomorphic
	  ▪ Giant cell
	  ▪ Myxoid/high-grade myxofibrosarcoma
	  ▪ Inflammatory forms

Adipocytic tumours	• Atypical lipoma
	• Liposarcoma:
	  ▪ Well differentiated
	  ▪ Dedifferentiated
	  ▪ Myxoid/round cell
	  ▪ Pleomorphic

Smooth muscle sarcomas	• Leiomyosarcoma • Epithelioid leiomyosarcoma
Skeletal muscle	• Rhabdomyosarcoma (embryonal, alveolar and pleomorphic forms)
Vascular	• Epithelioid haemangioendothelioma • Angiosarcoma, deep • Lymphangiosarcoma • Kaposi sarcoma
Perivascular	• Malignant glomangiosarcoma • Malignant haemangiopericytoma
Neural tumours and tumours of the peripheral nerves	• Malignant peripheral nerve sheath tumour (MPNST, neurofibrosarcoma) • Primitive neuroectodermal tumour (PNET)
Chondro osseous tumours	• Extraskeletal chondrosarcoma (mesenchymal and other variants) • Extraskeletal osteosarcoma
Paraganglionic	• Malignant paraganglioma
Tumours of uncertain differentiation	• Synovial sarcoma • Epithelioid sarcoma • Alveolar soft part sarcoma • Clear cell sarcoma of soft tissue • Extraskeletal myxoid chondrosarcoma • PNET/extraskeletal Ewing tumour • Desmoplastic small round cell tumour • Extrarenal rhabdoid tumour • Undifferentiated sarcoma; sarcoma, not otherwise specified (NOS)

Presentation and natural history

- Typical signs and symptoms of STS vary depending upon the location, size, depth and pathological characteristics of the primary tumour:
  - Most frequently observed symptom of extremity and superficial torso STS is a painless mass that gradually increases in size over a period of time.
  - Some STS may be asymptomatic and when growth is unimpeded are large at presentation (e.g. retroperitoneal liposarcoma)
  - Early-stage STS may not cause signs or symptoms (painless mass) until growth into surrounding tissues or organs
  - Pain on presentation suggests origin from or invasion of neurovascular structures
- Interval between onset of symptoms and diagnosis is shorter for extremity and head and neck STS than for abdominal or retroperitoneal tumours due their easier detection
- Superficial lesions and those that develop in the head and neck region are usually smaller than those in the retroperitoneum and those originating deep to fascia
- The natural history of certain pathological subtypes is inconsistent with the general behaviour of STS and will be described separately (i.e. cutaneous/superficial angiosarcoma).
- In general, the major route of spread is local extension. Regional lymphatic spread is less common and distant metastases are present in approximately 10% of cases at initial diagnosis.

Presentation and natural history	Description
STS of extremity, trunk or head and neck	**Extremity and superficial torso** • Usually present as a painless mass • Erythema and warmth may be present • Large, slow-growing lesions may restrict joint movement • Larger tumours may ulcerate skin and/or invade adjacent muscle compartments and bone, leading to fracture in rare cases • Lesions are usually controlled at the local site and death results from lung metastases, usually within 2–3 years of the initial diagnosis in those at risk **Head and neck** • In addition to a mass, additional symptoms include nasal obstruction, cranial nerve dysfunction and proptosis • Associated mass effect may occur in more restrictive head and neck locations and may result in pain, odynophagia, pharyngeal obstruction and/or airway compromise • Local control is lower in head and neck lesions than in the extremity presumably related to anatomic constraints due to the wish to minimize functional and aesthetic consequences in the head and neck

Retroperitoneal or intra-abdominal STS	• Represent 10–15% of STS:
	  ▪ Liposarcoma (30–60%) and leiomyosarcoma (20–30%) are the most common histologies
	• Symptoms often develop late and are non-specific (e.g. abdominal pain)
	• Low-grade tumours may grow at a slow rate without symptoms and may be large at presentation
	• Anorexia and subacute intestinal obstruction with subsequent weight loss may occur with large tumours
	• Nausea and vomiting may appear
	• Growth rate is a determinant of clinical response
	• Have a greater propensity to recur locally than at a distant site many years after initial treatment:
	  ▪ Rate of local relapse of these often biologically indolent tumours is 40–50%

Gastrointestinal stromal tumours (GIST)	• May arise anywhere in the gastrointestinal tract but occur most commonly in the stomach or small intestine • Prognostic factors include site (stomach is best), size, mitotic index and mutation status • Metastasize to peritoneum and liver

Desmoid tumours (aggressive fibromatoses)	• Benign locally aggressive tumours defined by over-expression of beta-catenin
	• Originate in the deep muscular aponeuroses, scar tissue and tendons
	• Women are affected twice as commonly as men
	• Usually occur in the third and fourth decades of life, but may occur in children
	• Categorized as extra-abdominal (70%), intra-abdominal (10%) and those in the abdominal wall (20%):
	  ▪ Intra-abdominal forms are associated with Gardner syndrome
	• Unpredictable natural history:
	  ▪ Growth arrest or even regression without intervention in some
	  ▪ Capable of local infiltration and destruction, hence the name 'aggressive fibromatoses'
	  ▪ Local recurrence following resection alone is quite common

Non-pleomorphic rhabdomyosarcoma	• Fifth most common cancer in childhood • Classified into embryonal, botryoid, alveolar and pleomorphic subtypes • Prognostic factors include: translocation positivity for alveolar subtype, age >10 years, lymph node or distant metastases and site of primary • Rarely, these tumours may develop synchronous or metachronous metastases in one or both breasts • May exhibit lymph node and CNS relapse

Angiosarcoma	• Superficial angiosarcoma often occurs in the dermal tissues of the head and neck, typically on the scalp (approximately 50%) or facial skin:
	  ▪ Radial growth pattern within the dermis of the scalp and facial tissues frequently results in satellite lesions:
	    ○ Involvement of the eyelid and periorbital tissues is particularly troublesome due to risk to optic anatomy of this location
	  ▪ May present on the chest wall of women who have had prior radiotherapy for breast cancer or a *de novo* disease in the breast
	  ▪ Rarely forms in the heart, where it is one of the commonest tumours at this site

(Continued)

Presentation and natural history		Description
		• Commonly present as purple, bruise-like lesions in elderly Caucasian men, with rare occurrence in patients of African origin
• Macules frequently become nodular, may coalesce into flat masses of substantial size and may ulcerate
• Frank bleeding may be an ongoing problem
• Lymph node involvement occurs unpredictably, but with higher rates than for other soft tissue sarcomas
• Apparent multifocal nature
Liposarcoma		• Second most commonly encountered subtype of STS
• Myxoid/round cell liposarcoma (MLS):
▪ Most common variant associated with *FUS-CHOP* t(12;16)(q13;p11) translocation
▪ Unusual/unpredictable pattern of recurrence in soft tissues
▪ May present multifocally or recur at two or more anatomically separate soft tissue sites (more frequently in the retroperitoneum and mediastinum)
▪ Oligometastases and widespread vertebral bone metastases without initial lung metastases may occur and may not be revealed by scintigraphy
▪ More favourable survival independent of other prognostic factors such as grade, size and depth
Synovial sarcoma		• Exhibit a characteristic chromosomal translocation t(X; 18) (p11; q11) in 100% of biphasic and 96% of monophasic synovial sarcomas
• Affect young adults
• Typically occur in the para-articular areas of the tendon sheaths and joints:
▪ 50% present in the lower limbs, especially the knee
▪ 50% originate in the upper limbs
▪ Rarely arise from synovial tissue
• Calcification may be apparent
• Risk of lymph node metastases has been reported
Routes of spread	Local	• Longitudinal spread within the muscle groups of origin, typically an extremity
• Invasion of contiguous structures and muscle may occur as growth progresses
• May encase major neurovascular structures
• *Extremity STS*: barriers to tumour spread such as bone and major facial planes limit axial spread beyond the originating compartments
• *Non-extremity STS*: similar patterns of spread; therefore, recognizing and accounting for facial planes in surgical and/or radiotherapy target volumes is required
	Regional	• Lymph node metastasis is uncommon:
▪ Increased risk reported for epithelioid sarcoma, clear cell sarcoma, angiosarcoma and rhabdomyosarcoma
▪ Traditionally associated with an adverse prognosis
▪ Isolated lymph node metastasis is potentially curable with prognosis similar to Stage III overall
	Metastatic	• 10% present with overt distant metastasis
• Most common site is pulmonary
• Spread to bone may follow lung metastasis, but may be the first site of spread for MLS
• MLS may also develop isolated soft tissue metastases
• For retroperitoneal and intra-abdominal visceral sarcomas, the liver is more commonly the first site of metastasis

Diagnostic work-up

Abundant literature exists in biomarker assessment of soft tissue sarcoma. Thus far, important diagnostic information has emerged rather than predictive markers that can be targeted. In addition, no circulating markers are yet available for clinical use in soft tissue sarcoma.

Diagnostic work-up	Description
Work-up	- Complete history and physical exam
- Prebiopsy imaging:
- Adequate cross-sectional imaging: computed tomography (CT) ± magnetic resonance imaging (MRI) of a suspicious primary lesion
- Plain radiograph optional
- Biopsy and pathology assessment:
- Carefully planned along future resection axis to avoid compromising curative resection
- Core needle or incisional biopsy (with minimal dissection)
- Fine needle aspiration may be acceptable in institutions with sarcoma expertise
- Should establish grade and histological subtype
- The anatomic site of biopsy intrusion should ordinarily be addressed either by inclusion in the radiation therapy treatment volume or in the surgical resection
- Chest CT to assess for distant metastases:
- Chest CT or chest X-ray for low-grade T1 lesions for metastatic assessment
- CT abdomen/pelvis for abdominal/retroperitoneal lesions:
- Usual to perform an intravenous pyelogram at baseline CT scan or a differential renal isotope scan to appreciate the function of the kidney contralateral to the side involved by the disease for abdominal/retroperitoneal lesions
- Creatinine clearance test for abdominal/retroperitoneal lesions
- Some unique clinical situations/exceptions:
- *Myxoid/round cell liposarcoma:*
○ Consider total spine MRI for provocation for spine metastases not evident on bone scanning
○ Consider CT abdomen for risk of retroperitoneal disease at presentation in addition to CT chest to exclude mediastinal disease
- *Alveolar soft part sarcoma, malignant peripheral nerve sheath tumour, rhabdomyosarcoma and angiosarcoma:*
○ Consider central nervous system (CNS) imaging due to higher risk of brain metastases in these tumours compared to other soft tissue sarcomas
- *Angiosarcoma:*
○ Apparent multifocal nature of this disease obscures accurate definition of margins for surgery and radiation therapy, and is very challenging
○ Meticulous clinical examination of the skin is the only real means of identifying any areas of multifocal involvement
- *Non-pleomorphic rhabdomyosarcoma:*
○ Initial evaluation is similar to STS but should also include bone marrow examination and bone scan, and may include cerebrospinal fluid (CSF) examination for parameningeal sites
○ Parameningeal sites (middle ear, nasopharynx, paranasal sinuses, infratemporal and pterygopalatine fossae and parapharyngeal region) may relapse in the leptomeninges
○ Consider sentinel node examination for extremity lesions
- *Desmoid tumours* (benign and locally aggressive):
○ Tissue confirmation is needed to rule out malignant disease
○ MRI has importance in determining infiltration into other organs, size of lesion and response to therapy
Tumour markers	- Common diagnostic markers:
- *PAX3–FOXO1* or *PAX7–FOXO1* from t(2; 13) or t(1; 13) chromosomal translocations in the alveolar subtype of non-pleomorphic rhabdomyosarcoma
- *FUS–DD1T3* (*TLS–CHOP*) or *EWSR1–DD1T3* (*EWSR1–CHOP*) from t(12; 16) or t(12; 22) in myxoid/round cell liposarcoma
- *MDM2* amplification in atypical lipomatous tumour/well-differentiated and dedifferentiated liposarcoma
- *ASPL–TFE3* from der(17)t(X; 17) in alveolar soft part sarcoma
- *EWSR1–AFT1* or *EWSR1–CREB1* from t(12; 22) or t(2; 22) in clear cell sarcoma
- *COLIA1–PDGFB* from t(17; 22) in dermatofibrosarcoma protuberans
- *SS18–SSX1*, *SSX2* and *SSX4* from t(X; 18) in synovial sarcoma
- Selected targets with FDA approved agents (target, drug and tumour type)
- KIT or PDG–FR A and B with imatinib in GIST
- VEGFR 1, 2 and 3 or PDGFR A and B or FGFR 1 and 3 or KIT or FMS with pazopanib in soft tissue sarcomas, except well-differentiated/dedifferentiated liposarcomas
- VEGFR 1, 2 and 3 or KIT or TIE-2 or PDGFR B or FGFR 1 or RET or RAF with regorafenib in GIST
- VEGR or VEGFR 1 or PDGFR A and B or FLT3 or KDR or KIT or RET with sunitinib in GIST

Table 56.1 UICC TNM categories and stage grouping: Soft tissue sarcoma

TNM categories with tumour grade	
T1	≤5 cm
T1a	Superficial
T1b	Deep
T2	>5 cm
T2a	Superficial
T2b	Deep
N1	Regional
Grade	Grade 1 (G1)
	Grade 2 (G2)
	Grade 3 (G3)
M1	Distant metastasis

Stage grouping				
Stage IA	T1a, T1b	N0	M0	G1
Stage IB	T2a, T2b	N0	M0	G1
Stage IIA	T1a, T1b	N0	M0	G2, G3
Stage IIB	T2a, T2b	N0	M0	G2
Stage III	T2a, T2b	N0	M0	G3
	Any T	N1	M0	Any G
Stage IV	Any T	Any N	M1	Any G

Note: Use low grade for GX; use N0 for NX.

UICC TNM staging

The TNM classification system is probably used most widely and incorporates the established prognostic hallmarks of grade, size and depth (Table 56.1). Another classification system is the Surgical Staging System of the Musculoskeletal Tumor Society, which accounts for grade, local extent/anatomical boundaries, and presence or absence of metastasis, but does not consider size of the primary tumour.

Prognostic factors

Additional important prognostic factors beyond tumour size, depth and histological grade include anatomical site, presentation status (primary vs recurrent) and surgical margins (Table 56.2). Mitotic index, tumour size and tumour location are valuable prognostic factors for GIST.

Expected survival of STS at 5 years is approximately 60%, with the majority of patients achieving local control (apart from certain sites, e.g. the retroperitoneum). The benchmark for local control in extremity sarcomas is 90%.

Staging and prognostic grouping

Clinical staging and diagnosis depends upon patient history and physical examination, imaging and laboratory tests. Tumour grade is important in STS and contributes to the stage grouping along with the designations for size, depth and presence of distant metastases. This approach represents a historic approach in this site. It is anticipated that future editions of UICC TNM may position grade within a Prognostic Grouping schema, instead of in the anatomic Stage Groups, for soft tissue sarcoma, a formalisation that is emerging for other cancers to permit inclusion of non-anatomic factors in the TNM.

Table 56.2 Prognostic factors for soft tissue sarcomas

Prognostic factors	Tumour related	Host related	Environment related
Essential	Anatomical site Histological type Size of tumour: • < or >5 cm in general • ≤2, 2–≤5, 5–≤10 and >10 cm for GIST Depth of invasion Grade (well to poorly differentiated) M category Mitotic rate for GIST (<5 mitoses and ≥5 mitoses/50 HPF)		
Additional	Presence of *c-Kit* mutation for GIST Mutational site in *c-Kit* or *PDGFRA* gene for GIST EWS–FL11 fusion transcript for Ewing sarcoma SYT–SSX fusion transcript for synovial sarcoma FOXO1 translocation for alveolar rhabdomyosarcoma Surgical resection margins Presentation status (primary vs recurrence)	Neurofibromatosis (NF1) Radiation-induced sarcomas Age	Quality of surgery and radiotherapy
New and promising	TP53 Ki-67 Tumour hypoxia		

Treatment philosophy

STS should be managed in a multidisciplinary setting with expertise in sarcoma.

Surgery is the main curative treatment modality for STS with the goal of achieving negative margins. There are rare exceptions to the use of surgery in STS:
- Rhabdomyosarcomas are generally very sensitive to both radiotherapy and chemotherapy and surgical intervention is reserved for selected sites
- Angiosarcomas of the face and scalp often present overwhelming surgical challenges due to the improbability of achieving useful margins in advanced lesions.

A combination of RT and surgery is the usual option for these cases and chemotherapy may also be given.

Radiation therapy (RT) may be used either pre- or post-operatively to reduce the risk of local failure for deep, high-grade or large (>5 cm) tumours. If fascial boundaries are compromised intraoperatively or margins are close or involved, re-excision and/or adjuvant RT should be considered.

Although every effort should be made to attempt resection, certain cases may require definitive RT owing to a combination of medical co-morbidity and/or unresectability, or to achieve palliation when surgery is deemed inappropriate. RT is usually administered by external beam photons (EBRT) or by brachytherapy either pre- or post-operatively. RT permits less extensive operations and has generally been shown to improve local control without affecting survival when combined with surgery.

The role of adjuvant chemotherapy remains unproven in most STS subtypes. An integral role for chemotherapy is reserved for certain high-risk cases and/or chemosensitive tumours, e.g. extraosseous Ewing sarcoma and rhabdomyosarcoma.

The National Comprehensive Cancer Network (NCCN) guidelines for management of adult STS address the following disease subtypes and settings:
- STS of extremity, trunk or head and neck
- Intra-abdominal or retroperitoneal STS
- GIST
- Desmoid tumours (aggressive fibromatoses)
- Rhabdomyosarcoma

Scenario	Treatment philosophy

Localized disease	• Surgical excision is the primary treatment of STS:
	  ▪ Function/structural preservation is achievable in most patients
	  ▪ Inappropriate surgical violation of fascia should be avoided since tumours can ordinarily be considered to involve either the deep or the superficial compartment but rarely both; transgression across compartments results in tumour contamination of previously uninvolved areas
	• If the deep compartment is involved, or has been contaminated (as may be the case in an unplanned excision or misguided biopsy), re-excision, RT or a combination of the two may be required
	• In general, adjuvant RT is recommended for:
	  ▪ Deep tumours since adequate wide excision is often not possible
	  ▪ Close (<2 cm) or positive surgical margins
	  ▪ Tumours of >5 cm if higher grade and anatomical constraints to resection exist
	• Multiagent chemotherapy is mandatory in non-pleomorphic rhabdomyosarcoma:
	  ▪ May be considered in:
	    ○ Liposarcoma (usually myxoid) or synovial sarcoma which generally show significant responses to chemotherapy
	    ○ High-risk cases of locally-advanced, unresectable disease, for the purpose of cytoreduction to facilitate surgical resection
	• MLS:
	  ▪ Radiosensitive and chemosensitive, and consequently have very favourable local control following adjuvant radiotherapy
	• GIST:
	  ▪ Complete R0 surgical excision is also required for GIST at all sites
	  ▪ Imatinib may be given neoadjuvantly to achieve cytoreduction to assist a complete resection (as above), or in the adjuvant setting for patients with high-risk tumours (based on large size, non-gastric site and high mitotic index)

Regional disease	• Certain histologies are associated with a higher propensity for lymph node metastases, including epithelioid sarcoma, clear cell sarcoma, angiosarcoma and rhabdomyosarcoma • Isolated lymph node (LN) metastasis has the same prognosis as Stage III disease in the seventh edition of TNM (rather than Stage IV as in prior editions) • However, treatment of the LN disease is required in all situations with surgery and/or RT if the patient is considered for curative management • Aggressive approaches including regional LN dissection for both synchronous or metachronous nodal disease may result in prolonged control

(Continued)

Scenario	Treatment philosophy
	• Adjuvant RT is generally advised where there is a high risk of recurrence within the surgically dissected tissues due to extracapsular nodal spread or for very large and/or multiple nodes: ▪ Should target the LN pathway and include the next echelon of apparently uninvolved nodal tissues

Metastatic disease	• Doxorubicin-based systemic chemotherapy remains the first-line treatment for patients with metastatic disease:
	   ▪ With the exception of rhabdomyosarcoma where multiagent chemotherapy is offered
	• Other drugs including pazopanib, gemcitabine, ifosfamide or trabectedin may be considered
	• *Metastatic GIST*: imatinib remains first-line therapy
	• In selected cases, pulmonary metastasectomy can prolong the disease-free period
	• Stereotactic RT delivered in a single high-dose fraction or a small number of fractions may provide equivalent local control and overall survival (OS) for pulmonary metastases in a less invasive fashion:
	   ▪ Optimal benefit seen for patients presenting with one to three oligometastases peripherally located with no evidence of disease elsewhere
	• Treatment of metastatic bone disease is usually palliative, except in rare myxoid liposarcoma cases:
	   ▪ RT is indicated for management of symptoms of bone metastases and in cases with large malignant lesions adjacent to critical structures
	• Surgery has an important role in the relief of obstruction or for mechanical problems, including fracture:
	   ▪ Rarely, debulking surgery in the chest, abdomen or elsewhere may prevent morbidity from intestinal obstruction, ureteral obstruction compressive syndromes and respiratory embarrassment
	• Soft tissue metastasis, when treated effectively, may be associated with long disease-free survival (DFS), especially in selected cases of myxoid liposarcoma

Locally recurrent disease	• 10–25% of STS will recur locally depending on site of original disease (in retroperitoneum may reach 40–50%)
	• Salvage treatment should be carefully considered as selected patients may enjoy long disease-free outcomes following the appropriate intervention:
	   ▪ Consider the dual goals of tumour control and normal tissue protection
	• In patients with STS not previously treated with RT or chemotherapy, combined modality therapy should be used if they can be administered safely
	• Treatment of previously irradiated lesions requires greater individualization:
	   ▪ Brachytherapy combined with a wide local excision may be used
	   ▪ IMRT delivered preoperatively probably has an advantage in the treatment of previously irradiated lesions due to the smaller doses and volumes involved
	• Local recurrence with concurrent metastases following a short disease-free interval is generally best managed with palliative approaches

Follow-up	• At 4–6 weeks following primary treatment (surgery or surgery + RT)
	• Every 3–4 months for Years 1 and 2
	• Every 6 months for Years 3–5
	• Annually thereafter
	• Procedures at each visit:
	   ▪ Complete history and physical exam
	   ▪ Chest imaging (plain radiograph or CT chest)
	   ▪ CT or MRI of the abdomen and pelvis (if retroperitoneal primary or GIST)
	   ▪ Consider baseline and periodic imaging of primary site based on estimated risk of locoregional recurrence
	   ▪ Evaluation for rehabilitation (occupational and physical therapy): continue until maximal function is achieved
	• *GIST*:
	   ▪ Consider triphasic CT of the abdomen and pelvis (with intravenous and oral contrast) or MRI every 3–6 months for 3–5 years, then annually
	   ▪ Consider endoscopic surveillance every 6–12 months for tumours with low-risk features on endoscopic ultrasound

Treatment

In general, surgical techniques that preserve function are the current standard of care.

Surgery	Description

Early-stage disease	- *Role:*
	  - Main management of STS at most sites (retroperitoneal, extremity, GIST)
	  - May be used alone for the treatment of low-grade tumours or localized superficial small STS (<5 cm) provided the fascial boundaries are not compromised intraoperatively and surgical margins are wide
	  - If surgical excision margins are involved by tumour or close (<2 cm), re-excision or adjuvant/neoadjuvant RT should be strongly considered
	  - Quality of the excision margin should also be considered:
	    - Barriers to tumour spread such as the periosteum, muscular fascia, epineurium and vascular adventitia may allow for smaller margins
	- Sarcoma operations should be carefully planned to avoid an unplanned resection or 'surgical error' that compromises fascial containment of disease
	- Goal is to resect the entire lesion with an adequate margin of normal tissue to reduce the risk of microscopic residual disease

Advanced non-metastatic disease	- Combined modality approach is usually considered for high-grade, large primary lesions (>5 cm) that includes function-preserving surgery + RT
	- For lesions ≥10 cm, conservative resection where possible ± RT may be considered with high rates of local control expected
	- In the extremity, amputation may be required if multicompartmental involvement and/or neurovascular encasement (approximately 5% of extremity lesions)
	- *Recurrent lesions without prior RT:*
	  - Combined modality approach should be considered including function-preserving surgery, chemotherapy and RT
	- *Recurrent lesions with a history of RT:*
	  - Function-preserving surgery may still be an option combined with brachytherapy or highly conformal EBRT

Metastatic disease	- Pulmonary metastasectomy has the potential to offer prolonged remission in selected cases:
	  - Adverse features for pulmonary metastasectomy generally include:
	    - More than four metastatic lesions
	    - Incomplete resection
	    - Disease-free interval <12 months
	- May have a role in relieving obstruction (e.g. intestinal, ureteral, intrathoracic, etc.) and stabilizing mechanical problems such as fracture may be repeated as needed
	- Palliative amputation may restore the ambulatory status of a patient in extreme pain/dysfunction

Radiotherapy

Radiotherapy	Description

Early-stage disease	- *Role:*
	  - Pre- or post-operative radiotherapy for deep tumours or tumours of >5 cm is usually required
	  - Adjuvant treatment for marginal or positive surgical resections
	  - Brachytherapy is an option in selected cases
	- *General principles:*
	  - STS generally respect barriers to tumour spread, such as bone, interosseous membrane and major fascial planes, and this concept should be exploited in tissue/function-preserving radiotherapy planning, especially for extremity lesions
	  - In the event of an 'unplanned' surgical resection with positive margins, the RT target volume needs to generously include all disturbed muscle compartments in addition to other tissues considered to be directly involved
	  - Suspicious peritumoural changes, frequently referred to as 'oedema', may harbour microscopic disease; oedema is usually most obvious in the craniocaudal dimension and is ordinarily encompassed in the RT target volume

(Continued)

Radiotherapy	Description
	<ul><li>For RT target volume definition, CT simulation imaging should be performed:<ul><li>MR image fusion may enhance target delineation</li></ul></li><li>Radiotherapy target coverage is typically based on the experience of extremity STS; for other sites (e.g. head and neck) these need to be adjusted for feasibility</li><li>Gross disease (gross tumour volume [GTV]) is defined by physical examination and imaging</li><li>RT error margin (planning target volume [PTV]) that accounts for patient and set-up uncertainties should be 0.5–1.0 cm surrounding the clinical target volume (CTV), and is determined by individual institutional protocols/procedures</li></ul><ul><li>*Preoperative RT* (generally for extremity lesions):<ul><li>50 Gy in 2-Gy fractions is ordinarily used and target volumes include the GTV, CTV and PTV</li><li>Preoperative CTV:<ul><li>Includes all areas at risk of subclinical spread defined by the distance from the GTV or oedema, or surgically disturbed tissue by initial biopsy or attempted excision</li><li>RT coverage should approximate a 3–4-cm margin in the longitudinal dimensions and a 1.5-cm margin in the radial dimension, limited to but including any anatomical barrier to tumour spread (e.g. bone or fascia)</li></ul></li></ul></li><li>*Postoperative RT* (generally for extremity lesions):<ul><li>66 Gy is ordinarily used or potentially 60 Gy in margin-clear, low-grade cases</li><li>Postoperative GTV (tumour bed) should identify the original site of the tumour</li><li>Strategy:<ul><li>Generally, a low-risk volume encompassing all sites or microscopic involvement is treated to 50 Gy in 25 fractions (or an equivalent dose fractionation regimen)</li><li>Tumour bed is treated to a 'boost' dose of 60–66 Gy</li><li>This strategy may be achieved by the traditional 'shrinking field' technique or by simultaneous integrated boost (54–56 Gy in 30–33 fractions for the microscopic volume) using IMRT</li></ul></li><li>Low-risk 'microscopic' volume is usually larger than the preoperative scenario:<ul><li>Discussion with the surgeon and review of surgical and pathology reports will facilitate the decision about whether or not a seroma, lymphocele or haematoma should be included</li></ul></li></ul></li><li>*Retroperitoneal RT:*<ul><li>Preoperatively, the CTV includes the GTV + a 2-cm margin in the longitudinal dimensions and a 0.5–2.0-cm margin in the radial dimension limited to but including any anatomical barrier to tumour spread and critical anatomy, e.g. if the tumour is approximating an intact liver, 0.5 cm of the liver is included</li><li>2-cm margins are usually used posteriorly to include fatty tissues and vessels</li><li>Ipsilateral kidney may need to be sacrificed provided the contralateral kidney has acceptable function (see Diagnostic work-up section):<ul><li>In such a case, dose to the uninvolved opposite kidney should be kept as low as reasonably achievable</li></ul></li><li>*Postoperatively*, target definition is problematic and difficult to administer because of normal tissue tolerances (e.g. bowel, liver in right-sided lesions) and often severely compounded by bowel loop fixation</li><li>Intraoperative radiotherapy (IORT) may be employed in specialized centres but reports have almost always combined it with EBRT (usually preoperatively)<ul><li>Prospective assessment shows favourable toxicity profiles when combined with preoperative RT although IORT toxicity reporting is usually confounded by retrospective series that combined EBRT and IORT</li></ul></li></ul></li><li>Brachytherapy allows for treatment delivery in the perioperative period over a shorter time course than EBRT:<ul><li>Can be used alone or in combination with EBRT, particularly when one modality may result in a higher than normal probability of complication</li><li>Various methods are used including low-dose rate (LDR), fractionated high-dose rate (HDR) and intraoperative HDR</li><li>Evidence supporting brachytherapy use is limited to small case series, and comparisons are difficult due to non-standardization of target volumes, dose prescription points and delivered dose</li><li>No robust large series evaluating HDR brachytherapy exist</li><li>Concern remains over reduced local control in proximally located tumours</li><li>The American Brachytherapy Society recommends:<ul><li>Its use after complete resection of intermediate- or high-grade lesions with negative margins</li><li>To be avoided as sole modality treatment when (1) CTV is not fully encompassable, (2) critical organ proximity precludes delivery of meaningful dose, (3) skin involvement</li></ul></li></ul></li></ul>
Advanced non-metastatic disease	<ul><li>For unresectable residual gross disease, 70 Gy in 2-Gy fractions or equivalent dose fractionation may be used depending on tissue tolerance</li></ul>
Metastatic disease	<ul><li>Palliative treatment may be used in primary or metastatic foci</li><li>Selected small volume pulmonary metastases may undergo metastasectomy or stereotactic RT</li></ul>

Systemic therapy

Systemic therapy	Description
Early-stage disease	• In patients with localized, resectable sarcoma, the role of adjuvant chemotherapy is limited • Multiagent chemotherapy is necessary for patients with non-pleomorphic rhabdomyosarcoma and extraosseous Ewing sarcoma regardless of disease stage

Advanced non-metastatic disease	• For locally advanced, non-metastatic scenarios, chemotherapy may offer cytoreduction to facilitate surgical resection
	• Protocols include:
	  ▪ Doxorubicin 60–75 mg/m² IV every 3 weeks, or
	  ▪ Doxorubicin 60–75 mg/m² IV + ifosfamide (5–9 g/m²) every 3 weeks

Metastatic	• Chemotherapy may be offered to prolong life
	• Protocols include:
	  ▪ Doxorubicin (schedule as above)
	  ▪ Pazopanib 800 mg PO b.i.d.
	  ▪ Gemcitabine 1000 mg/m² IV Days 1, 8 and 15, every 4 weeks
	  ▪ Gemcitabine 900 mg/m² on Days 1 and 8 + docetaxel 100 mg/m² on Day 8, every 3 weeks
	  ▪ Trabectedin 1.5 mg/m² (24-hour infusion), every 3 weeks

Targeted therapy

GIST represents the first solid tumour to exhibit a consistent favourable response to molecular *c-Kit* targeted therapy.

Additional considerations

Desmoid tumours
- For asymptomatic or non-progressive disease, watchful waiting may be most appropriate
- Surgery alone, RT alone, a combination of surgery + RT, and systemic therapy alone are all reasonable options:
  - There are no data to suggest that one approach is better than another
  - Many centres are moving away from ablative operations due to the high rate of local recurrence and potential morbidities
- Enlarging or symptomatic tumours may require systemic therapy, including non-steroidal anti-inflammatory drugs (NSAIDs), hormonal therapy (e.g. tamoxifen, toremifene), methotrexate and vinblastine/vinorelbine, low-dose interferon, doxorubicin-based regimens or tyrosine kinase inhibitors (TKIs) (e.g. imatinib, sorafenib)

Angiosarcoma
- Surgical resection is challenging due to its wide infiltrative nature
- RT is commonly offered using wide margins
- Taxane-based chemotherapy or oral TKIs are available for patients with locally-advanced or metastatic disease

Rhabdomyosarcoma
- Standard paediatric regimens include vincristine + actinomycin + cyclophosphamide
- Surgery and/or radiotherapy are ordinarily used for local control
- Treatment of adult patients or young patients with metastatic disease can also include vincristine + doxorubicin + cyclophosphamide alternating with ifosfamide + etoposide

Controversies

- There remains uncertainty about whether RT should be administered pre- or post-operatively:
  - Different toxicity profiles govern the decision-making in individual cases
- Need for a postoperative boost following positive surgical margin resection with preoperative radiotherapy is controversial
- The volume required in post-operative external beam radiotherapy has been studied in a completed randomised trial addressing volume reduction (VORTEX NCT00423618)
- Role of radiotherapy in retroperitoneal sarcoma remains unproven: various strategies (preoperative, postoperative and intraoperative) are used; an ongoing EORTC study is addressing the role of preoperative radiotherapy compared to surgery alone (STRASS NCT01344018 trial)
- Role of brachytherapy remains uncertain:
  - Apart from one underpowered randomized trial, evidence supporting its use is limited to small case series
  - Control rates seem lower than with EBRT/IMRT
- Routine use of systemic chemotherapy in adult STS remains an ongoing area of controversy
- Isolated limb perfusion (ILP) with and without extracorporeal bypass is used in specialized centres:
  - Techniques are complex with significant late treatment-related toxicities reported
  - Randomized trials comparing this approach with conventional adjuvant RT are needed for patients who might benefit (e.g. borderline resectable cases)
- Hyperthermia trials have been undertaken but this approach has not yet been adopted widely
- Role of intensity modulated radiotherapy (IMRT) has been reported for two completed Phase 2 trials addressing protection of normal tissue and target volume reduction while maintaining high local control in extremity soft tissue sarcoma (NCT00589121 and NCT00188175)

Phase III clinical trials

See Table 56.3.

Table 56.3 Phase III clinical trials

Trial reference	Results
Local control	
Rosenberg et al. (1983) Cancer 52(3):424–434	• 43 cases of high-grade extremity sarcoma were randomized to amputation or to limb-preservation surgery + RT • No difference in survival with surgery + RT: 5-year OS 83% vs 88% ($P = 0.99$)
O'Sullivan et al. (2002) Lancet 359:2235–2241	• 190 cases of extremity sarcoma were randomized to pre- or post-operative RT • Wound complication rate in the preoperative arm was 35% vs 17% in the postoperative arm • 2-year fibrosis rates were 31.5% (preoperative) vs 48.2% ($P = 0.07$) • No difference in 5-year local recurrence rate or OS
Pisters et al. (1996) J Clin Oncol 14:859–868	• Intraoperative randomization of 164 patients after complete excision of superficial trunk or extremity tumours to brachytherapy or observation • 5-year local control rate: 82% (RT arm) vs 69% ($P = 0.04$) • 5-year disease-specific survival rate: 84% vs 81% ($P = 0.65$) • No significant difference in low-grade tumours
Sindelar et al. (1993) Arch Surg 128(4):402–410	• Single-institution randomized controlled trial comparing postoperative EBRT with IORT and EBRT • 40% vs 80% local recurrence rate ($P <0.001$) in favour of adding IORT • Significantly higher radiation enteritis and neuropathy in IORT arm with no significant difference in median survival (45 vs 52 months)
Yang et al. (1998) Clin Oncol 16(1):197–203	• To assess the impact of postoperative EBRT and limb-sparing surgical resection vs surgery alone • With a median follow-up of 9.6 years, a significant decrease in local recurrence was seen with postoperative RT for high- and low-grade lesions • No difference in OS
Adjuvant systemic, advanced disease and metastatic disease	
Dematteo et al. (2009) Lancet 373:1097–1104	• Trial investigating whether adjuvant imatinib treatment would improve recurrence-free survival compared with placebo after resection of localized GIST • Interim analysis showed imatinib significantly improved recurrence-free survival compared with placebo (8% in the imatinib group vs 20% in the placebo group had tumour recurrence or had died)
PALETTE van der Graaf et al. (2012) Lancet 379:1879–1886	• Patients with advanced STS received pazopanib (n = 246) or placebo (n = 123) • Median PFS was 4.6 months for pazopanib (CI 3.7–4.8) vs 1.6 months for placebo (CI 0.9–1.8) • New treatment option for patients with metastatic non-adipocytic soft tissue sarcoma after failure of standard chemotherapy
Demetri et al. (1997) J Clin Oncol 31(19):2485–2492	• 702 patients were randomized to receive maintenance therapy with placebo vs ridaforolimus after routine therapy • Small improvement in PFS in treated patients • Ridaforolimus induced a mean 1.3% decrease in target lesion size vs a 10.3% increase with placebo ($P <0.001$) • Median OS with ridaforolimus was 90.6 weeks vs 85.3 weeks with placebo (HR 0.93; 95% CI 0.78–1.12; $P = 0.46$) • Toxicities were seen with ridaforolimus treatment

Areas of research

- Radiotherapy volume and dose reduction trials
- Avoidance of radiotherapy in selected cases of local disease
- Role of preoperative RT versus surgery alone in retroperitoneal sarcoma (STRASS NCT01344018 trial)
- Role of maintenance therapy with mTOR inhibitors or other agents
- Role of combining targeted therapies with standard cytotoxic chemotherapy
- Evaluation of technical radiotherapy delivery including IMRT, Stereotactic RT, and hadron treatments (protons and heavy ion) in radiotherapy volume optimization for the combined modality treatment of soft tissue sarcoma

Recommended reading

Dematteo RP, Ballman KV, Antonescu CR et al. (2009) Adjuvant imatinib mesylate after resection of localised, primary gastrointestinal stromal tumour: a randomised, double-blind, placebo-controlled trial. Lancet 373:1097–1104.

Demetri GD, Chawla SP, Ray-Coquard I et al. (1997) Results of an international randomized phase III trial of the mammalian target of rapamycin inhibitor ridaforolimus versus placebo to control metastatic sarcomas in patients after benefit from prior chemotherapy. J Clin Oncol 31(19):2485–2492.

O'Sullivan B, Davis AM, Turcotte R et al. (2002) Preoperative versus postoperative radiotherapy in soft-tissue sarcoma of the limbs: a randomised trial. Lancet 359:2235–2241.

Pisters PW, Harrison LB, Leung DH, Woodruff JM, Casper ES, Brennan MF (1996) Long-term results of a prospective randomized trial of adjuvant brachytherapy in soft tissue sarcoma. J Clin Oncol 14(3):859–868.

Rosenberg SA, Tepper J, Glatstein E et al. (1983) Prospective randomized evaluation of adjuvant chemotherapy in adults with soft tissue sarcomas of the extremities. Cancer 52(3):424–434.

Sarcoma Meta-analysis Collaboration (1997) Adjuvant chemotherapy for localised resectable soft-tissue sarcoma of adults: meta-analysis of individual data. Lancet 350:1647–1654.

Sindelar WF, Kinsella IJ, Chen PW et al. (1993) Intraoperative radiotherapy in retroperitoneal sarcomas. Final results of a prospective, randomized, clinical trial. Arch Surg 128(4):402–410.

van der Graaf WT, Blay JY, Chawla SP et al. (2012) Pazopanib for metastatic soft-tissue sarcoma (PALETTE): a randomised, double-blind, placebo-controlled phase 3 trial. Lancet 379:1879–1886.

Yang JC, Chang AE, Baker AR et al. (1998) Randomized prospective study of the benefit of adjuvant radiation therapy in the treatment of soft tissue sarcomas of the extremity. J Clin Oncol 16(1):197–203.

57 Paediatric tumours

Hatel Moonat[1], Anna R. Franklin[1], Andrea Hayes-Jordan[2], Mary Frances McAleer[3] and Winston W. Huh[1]

[1]Division of Pediatrics, The University of Texas, M. D. Anderson Cancer Center, Houston, TX, USA
[2]Department of Surgery, The University of Texas, M. D. Anderson Cancer Center, Houston, TX, USA
[3]Department of Radiation Oncology, The University of Texas, M. D. Anderson Cancer Center, Houston, TX, USA

Introduction

Childhood cancers are rare and represent only 1% of all new cancer diagnoses (Fig. 57.1). The overall worldwide incidence rate varies between 50 and 200 million, with a higher incidence rate noted in developed countries (but with decreased mortality rates). Although overall mortality rates have consistently declined in the past 40 years (down by 66%), cancer still ranks as the second most common disease-related cause of death in children.

LEUKAEMIA

Incidence, aetiology and screening

Acute lymphoblastic leukaemia (ALL) is the most common malignancy of childhood, while chronic leukaemias are rare. In children under 5 years of age, 80% of leukaemia cases are ALL, 15% acute myeloid leukaemia (AML) and only 2–3% chronic myeloid leukaemia (CML). In adolescents aged 15–19 years, the distribution changes to 50% ALL, 35% AML and 10% CML. The immunophenotype of ALL in children is predominantly pre-B cell (85%), with T-cell (15%) and mature B-cell (<5%) being less common.

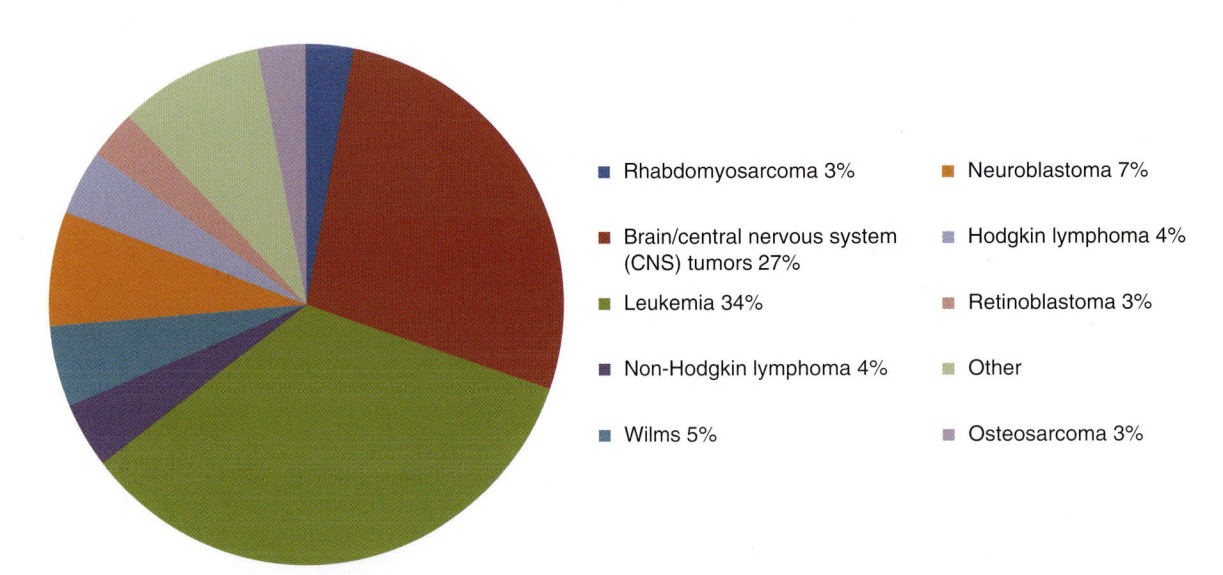

Figure 57.1 Distribution of childhood cancer according to the American Cancer Society Cancer Facts & Figures 2012. Data from http://www.cancer.org/research/cancerfactsstatistics/cancerfactsfigures2012/index

- Rhabdomyosarcoma 3%
- Brain/central nervous system (CNS) tumors 27%
- Leukemia 34%
- Non-Hodgkin lymphoma 4%
- Wilms 5%
- Neuroblastoma 7%
- Hodgkin lymphoma 4%
- Retinoblastoma 3%
- Other
- Osteosarcoma 3%

UICC Manual of Clinical Oncology, Ninth Edition. Edited by Brian O'Sullivan, James D. Brierley, Anil K. D'Cruz, Martin F. Fey, Raphael Pollock, Jan B. Vermorken and Shao Hui Huang. © 2015 UICC. Published 2015 by John Wiley & Sons, Ltd.

Paediatric tumours

Incidence, aetiology and screening: Leukaemia	Description

Incidence	- Most common paediatric cancer
	- Annual incidence:
	  - ALL: 80–90 cases per million at 2–3 years; 10 cases per million by 20 years
	  - AML: 5–10 cases per million in first 20 years of life
	- Survival rate:
	  - ALL 5-year survival rate of 88% for age <15 years and 61% for age 15–19 years
	  - AML 5-year survival rate of 60% for age <15 years and 47% for age 15–19 years
	- Peak age:
	  - ALL: 2–5 years
	  - AML: infancy and adolescence
	- ALL: slight male predominance
	- AML: equal sex ratio
	- In the USA, Caucasians have a two-fold greater risk of developing ALL compared to African–Americans, possibly related to difference in susceptibility and/or environmental exposures
	- T-cell ALL: more common in adolescent boys and African–Americans

Aetiology	- Unknown - Acquired risk factors: exposure to ionizing radiation, cytotoxic chemotherapy agents, benzenes - Congenital conditions: neurofibromatosis, Down syndrome (particularly megakaryocytic AML subtype), Wiskott–Aldrich syndrome, Kostmann syndrome, Shwachmann–Diamond syndrome, Diamond–Blackfan anaemia, ataxia telangiectasia, Li–Fraumeni syndrome, Bloom syndrome, Fanconi anaemia - Increased incidence of ALL in siblings of patients with ALL; additional increased risk in twins
Screening	- No role in healthy children - Those with an underlying disorder that carries an increased risk: follow closely with interval physical examinations and complete blood count (CBC) with differential

Presentation

- Direct result of bone marrow, liver, spleen, lymph node invasion
- Common clinical features:
  - Fevers (61%), fatigue (50%), pallor (40%)
  - Neutropenia causing fevers, infection, buccal mucosa ulceration
  - Anaemia causing tachycardia, dyspnoea, congestive heart failure (in severe cases)
  - Thrombocytopenia causing petechiae, easy bruising, bleeding from mucous membranes
  - AML M3, acute promyelocytic leukaemia (APL): can present as a serious bleeding diathesis
  - ALL with central nervous system (CNS) involvement at diagnosis: <5% of cases (even fewer in AML)
  - Other sites of leukaemic infiltration: testes, tonsils, adenoids, anterior mediastinum (often in T-cell ALL), gastrointestinal tract, bone/joint, renal (more common in T-cell ALL or mature B-cell ALL), skin, pericardium, pleura
  - Sanctuary sites for lymphoblasts: CNS, testes

Diagnostic work-up

Diagnostic work-up: Leukaemia	Description
Work-up	- Initial laboratory work-up: CBC/differential, peripheral blood smear, electrolytes, liver/kidney function, immunoglobulin levels, coagulation studies, infectious disease evaluation (including varicella, cytomegalovirus, herpes simplex virus, hepatitis antibody titres) - Bone marrow aspiration/biopsy and lumbar puncture to evaluate for presence of leukaemic blasts - Chest radiograph (CXR) to evaluate for mediastinal mass (often in T-cell leukaemia) - Baseline electrocardiogram (ECG) and echocardiogram
Tumour markers	- Cytochemical stains, immunohistochemistry, flow cytometry and cytogenetics determine specific subtype of leukaemia - Pre-B-ALL: positive for TdT, CD10, CD19, CD22 and CD20 - AML is myeloperoxidase positive and immunophenotype varies with subtype

Prognostic factors

Age and initial white blood cell count (WBC) at diagnosis are strong prognostic factors used to determine treatment (Table 57.1). Early treatment response also greatly influences outcome. Treatment response is determined morphologically and via flow cytometry or polymerase chain reaction (PCR) to quantify presence of minimal residual disease (MRD) 4–12 weeks post therapy. MRD of >0.01% at the end of induction significantly increases the risk of relapse

Cytogenetic changes in paediatric leukaemia are either structural or numerical alterations, with the most common structural changes being chromosomal translocations. Cytogenetics and molecular alterations are prognostic in both ALL and AML, and are used to determine treatment intensity (Table 57.2).

In 2000–2004 5-year survival rates were 87.5% for ALL and 59.9% for AML (for patients aged <15 years), with an expected increase to 90.6% for ALL and 64.8% for AML in 2005–2009 (based on a linear trend from previous estimates). For adolescents aged from 15 to 19 years, survival rates were much lower in 2000–2004: 61.1% for ALL and 47.2% for AML. Infant ALL, seen in patients aged <1 year, is uncommon and carries a very poor prognosis.

Table 57.1 Prognostic factors in pre–B-cell ALL that affect treatment intensity

	Low risk	High risk
Age (years)	1–9	<1, >10
WBC (per mm3)	<50,000	≥50,000
CNS disease	Negative	Positive
Response	Rapid	Slow

Treatment philosophy

Acute lymphoblastic leukaemia

Risk stratification determines treatment intensity in order to optimize the balance between efficacy and treatment-related toxicity. Adolescents and young adults have improved outcomes when treated according to paediatric versus adult treatment regimens. Treatment is typically divided into four phases: induction, CNS prevention, consolidation and maintenance. The intensive phases last 6–8 months and maintenance lasts 2–3 years.

Table 57.2 Prognostic impact of cytogenetic and molecular changes in paediatric acute leukaemia

Leukaemia	Prognostic impact	Cytogenetic and molecular change
ALL	Favourable	t(12; 21) ETV6-RUNX1 Hyperdiploidy (>53 chromosomes) Trisomies of chromosomes 4 and 10 NOTCH mutations (T-cell ALL)
	Unfavourable	t(9; 22) BCR-ABL1 (Philadelphia chromosome) Philadelphia chromosome–like acute lymphoblastic leukemia (Ph-like ALL) Translocations of 11q23 (MLL) Hypodiploidy (<44 chromosomes) Intrachromosomal amplification of chromosome 21 (iAMP21) 1KZF1 gene alteration (encodes IKAROS) JAK mutations CRLF2 overexpression
AML	Favourable	Core binding factor leukaemias: • t(8; 21), ETO-AML1 • Inversion 16, MYH11-CBF • t(15; 17), PML-RAR NPM (nucleophosmin) CEBPα (CCAAT/enhancer binding protein α)
	Intermediate	Normal karyotype
	Unfavourable	Monosomy 5 Monosomy 7 Deletion 5q Translocations of 11q23 (MLL) Complex cytogenetics (>3 distinct cytogenetic abnormalities) FLT3-ITD (FMS-like tyrosine kinase 3; internal tandem duplication) WT1 (Wilms tumour 1)

Treatment phase: ALL	Description
Induction	- *Goal*: rapid induction of remission
- Risk stratification based on age and WBC at diagnosis:
- *Standard risk*: three-drug regimen:
- Vincristine + asparaginase + corticosteroids
- *High risk*: four-drug regimen:
- Addition of an anthracycline (either doxorubicin or daunorubicin) to standard-risk three-drug regimen
- Includes intrathecal chemotherapy
- Corticosteroids: dexamethasone confers superior event-free survival (EFS) versus prednisone, but has increased toxicity
Consolidation	- *Goal*: CNS prophylaxis
- CNS is a sanctuary site for lymphoblasts
- Treatment consists of weekly intrathecal chemotherapy as well as systemic chemotherapy with agents that penetrate the blood–brain barrier:
- Intrathecal methotrexate is most commonly used, but some regimens use triple intrathecal chemotherapy (methotrexate + cytarabine + hydrocortisone)
Interim maintenance	- *Goal*: decrease intensity treatment prior to re-intensification
- Varies based on risk stratification
- High-risk ALL patients who received high-dose methotrexate (5000 mg/m^2/dose) and leucovorin rescue during interim maintenance had better results compared to those who received escalating low-dose methotrexate
Delayed intensification	- *Goal*: repeat intensive chemotherapy in a setting of minimal disease burden
- Vincristine + asparaginase + anthracycline + corticosteroids
Maintenance	- *Goal*: minimize risk of recurrence
- Daily oral 6-mercaptopurine
- Weekly oral methotrexate
- Varied schedules of vincristine and steroid pulses
- Intensive chemotherapy continues for 2 years for girls and 3 years for boys
Special considerations	- CNS irradiation is rarely used (reserved for patients with CNS disease at diagnosis and high-risk T-cell ALL)
- Tyrosine kinase inhibitors (TKIs) added for Philadelphia-positive ALL:
- Imatinib (*BCR-ABL1* TKI) following induction showed improved 3-year EFS (80% vs 35% in historical controls)
- Longer follow-up needed to compare its impact with that of sibling donor haematopoetic stem cell transplant (HSCT)
- Nelarabine in newly diagnosed T-cell ALL is under evaluation
- Down syndrome patients have increased treatment-related mortality
Relapsed ALL	- Site and timing of relapse are the two most influential prognostic factors
- *Site of relapse*:
- Isolated bone marrow relapse
- Combined bone marrow and extramedullary relapse
- Isolated extramedullary relapse
- *Timing of relapse:*
- Early: <18 months from diagnosis
- Intermediate: 18–36 months from diagnosis
- Late: >36 months from diagnosis
- Treatment primarily consists of systemic and intrathecal chemotherapy
- CNS radiation is required for any CNS relapse
- Stem cell transplantation is reserved for high-risk patients

Acute myeloblastic leukaemia

Treatment for AML focuses on achieving initial remission with induction therapy, followed by consolidation therapy to maintain and prolong remission. Increased intensity has been shown to improve outcome in AML, but has been limited by treatment-related toxicity. CNS-directed therapy with intrathecal chemotherapy is included.

Treatment phase: AML	Description

Induction	- One to two courses of high cumulative doses of anthracycline + cytarabine
	- Etoposide or 6-thioguanine often included
	- APL induction: all *trans*-retinoic acid (ATRA) combined with chemotherapy leads to remission in 90–95% of cases
	- AML with Down syndrome:
	  - Increased treatment-related mortality with conventional AML therapy
	  - Patients <4 years of age have higher remission and overall survival rates with less intensive treatment due to increased sensitivity to cytarabine

Consolidation	- Two to five courses of non–cross-resistant drug combinations - HSCT in first complete remission (CR1) can be used as consolidation therapy for high-risk patients
Relapse	- Duration of CR1 is prognostic with improved outcomes if >1 year - Bone marrow is the most common site of relapse - Chemotherapy regimens include antimetabolites and anthracyclines - Intrathecal chemotherapy included - Allogeneic SCT recommended in second complete remission

Chronic myeloblastic leukaemia

- Divided into the chronic phase (CP), accelerated phase (AP) and blast crisis (BC):
  - CP lasts about 3 years
  - AP is more aggressive and defined as <20% blasts
  - BC is similar to acute leukaemia with >20% blasts
- Ionizing radiation is a known environmental risk factor
- Philadelphia chromosome (Ph+) results in a BCR-ABL fusion protein that leads to a constitutively activated tyrosine kinase (TK) that makes cells resistant to apoptosis
- TKI therapy with either imatinib or dasatinib is first-line for newly diagnosed CML in paediatric patients
- HSCT is the preferred treatment for those who progress past the CP, who are unable to achieve a complete cytogenetic response or who have persistent Ph+ at 12 months

Lymphoma

Paediatric lymphomas are divided into Hodgkin and non-Hodgkin lymphoma (NHL). The four major subtypes of NHL in children are lymphoblastic lymphoma (LBL), diffuse large B-cell lymphoma (DLBCL), anaplastic large cell lymphoma (ALCL) and Burkitt lymphoma (small, non-cleaved cell). Most paediatric B-cell lymphomas are high grade with a rapid growth rate.

Non-Hodgkin lymphoma

Incidence, aetiology and screening: NHL	Description

Incidence	- Slightly more common worldwide compared to Hodgkin lymphoma
	- Global incidence
	  - ASR per million for women 0.7
	  - ASR per million for men 1.3
	- Annual incidence:
	  - Approximately 45% of paediatric lymphomas
	  - 800 new cases diagnosed annually in the USA
	- Male predominance
	- More common in Caucasians versus African–Americans

Incidence, aetiology and screening: NHL	Description

Aetiology	- Most cases are sporadic
	- Congenital or acquired immunodeficiencies: Wiskott–Aldrich syndrome, ataxia telangiectasia, common variable immunodeficiency, human immunodeficiency virus, human T-lymphotropic virus, post transplant
	- Epstein–Barr virus (EBV):
	  - Seen in almost all endemic cases of Burkitt lymphoma but rare in sporadic form (which is more common in North America and Europe)
	  - Involved in Hodgkin lymphoma

Screening	- Patients with underlying predisposing conditions should be followed closely for early signs/symptoms of lymphoma:
	  - Serial history
	  - Physical exams
	  - Laboratory studies and imaging when history and physical exam are concerning

Presentation

- Extranodal sites of involvement are common
- *Lymphoblastic lymphoma*:
  - Can have bulky lymphadenopathy
  - Frequent emergency presentations include a large anterior mediastinal mass or tonsillar enlargement causing airway obstruction, superior vena cava (SVC) syndrome and pleural/pericardial effusions
- *Diffuse large B-cell lymphoma*:
  - Typically involves diffuse nodes and soft tissue sites
- *Sporadic Burkitt*:
  - Most often presents with abdominal symptoms, including abdominal pain (intussusception), distension, nausea, vomiting and gastrointestinal bleeding
  - Can involve head and neck:
    - Endemic form commonly as jaw or orbital masses
- Bone marrow and CNS disease occasionally seen in LBL and Burkitt lymphoma
- Tumour lysis syndrome is frequent and severe in first few days of treatment of Burkitt lymphoma

Diagnostic work-up

Diagnostic work-up: NHL	Description

Work-up	- Excisional lymph node biopsy
	- Routine blood work including EBV status and CXR is essential
	- CT neck, chest, abdomen and pelvis
	- Positron emission tomography (PET) fused with computed tomography (CT) is useful for diagnosis and to evaluate treatment response
	- Bone marrow aspiration/biopsy and lumbar puncture
	- For patients with large mediastinal masses or SVC syndrome, minimally invasive diagnostic procedures should be used due to the high general anaesthesia risk:
	  - Fine needle aspiration or core biopsy of lymph node
	  - Bone marrow aspiration
	  - Evaluation of a malignant effusion or ascites
	- Ultrasound can be used to evaluate suspicious intra-abdominal masses, especially when resources are limited

Tumour markers	- *Lymphoblastic lymphoma*: same cell of origin as T-cell ALL in 85–90% of cases and has translocations in the T-cell receptor genes
	- *Anaplastic large cell lymphoma*:
	  - Can be B, T or null phenotype
	  - CD30 (Ki-1) receptor positivity is characteristic
	  - Typically has the fusion product of the translocation between nucleolar phosphoprotein gene (*NPM*) and anaplastic lymphoma kinase (*ALK*)
	- *Burkitt tumour cells*:
	  - Positive for late-stage B-cell phenotype with surface IgM expression (CD19, CD20, CD22, CD10, BCL6 cell surface markers)
	  - Commonly has the translocation t(8; 14)(q24; q32), fusing *c-MYC* with the immunoglobulin heavy chain gene that then leads to overexpression of c-MYC

Staging and prognostic factors

Staging
One of the most common staging systems used is the St Jude/Murphy staging system (Table 57.3).

Prognostic factors
Poor prognostic factors include DLBCL in females, *c-MYC* rearrangements, primary mediastinal B-cell lymphoma and lactate dehydrogenase (LDH) of >500 U/L.

Estimated 5-year survival rates for paediatric NHL range from 70% to >95%, depending on stage and histology.

Treatment philosophy
Treatment for NHL entails using combination chemotherapy with intensity depending on specific subtype and stage.

Table 57.3 St Jude/Murphy staging system for paediatric NHL

Stage	Description
I	Single site (excluding abdomen or mediastinum)
II	Single extranodal site with regional nodes Two or more nodal sites, same side of diaphragm Two extranodal sites, same side of diaphragm Primary gastrointestinal (GI), complete resection
III	Two extranodal sites, both sides of diaphragm Two or more nodal sites, both sides of diaphragm Primary thoracic Primary GI, unresectable Paraspinal, epidural
IV	CNS and/or bone marrow (<25%)

Data source: Murphy (1989). Reproduced with permission of Springer.

Treatment: NHL	Description

Systemic chemotherapy	• *Lymphoblastic leukaemia*:
	  ▪ Good survival with ALL-based therapy, including CNS prophylaxis with intrathecal chemotherapy
	  ▪ Shown to be as effective as prophylactic cranial irradiation
	• *Diffuse large B-cell lymphoma*:
	  ▪ Best results with regimens for Burkitt lymphoma including CNS prophylaxis
	• *Anaplastic large cell lymphoma*:
	  ▪ Optimum treatment is less clear
	  ▪ Targeted agents combined with standard chemotherapy are currently being trialled in newly diagnosed patients
	• *Burkitt lymphoma*:
	  ▪ Localized: can be completely resected surgically with minimal chemotherapy
	  ▪ Advanced stage: needs aggressive combination chemotherapy with CNS prophylaxis

Radiotherapy	• Typically not used electively except in acute emergencies refractory to initial chemotherapy (i.e. superior mediastinal syndrome)

Recurrence	• Optimizing upfront treatment to prevent relapse is crucial since relapsed high-grade B-cell NHL carries a very poor prognosis
	• Primary focus of treatment for relapse:
	  ▪ Induce remission with chemotherapy followed by consolidation with SCT:
	    ◦ Choice of autologous versus allogeneic SCT depends on timing and balancing benefit with toxicity
	    ◦ Autologous SCT can be as effective as allogeneic in relapsed paediatric NHL, except for LBL where allogeneic SCT is more effective
	• *Anaplastic large cell lymphoma*:
	  ▪ Vinblastine or *cis*-retinoic acid with/without interferon-alpha can be used as salvage therapy in certain cases
	  ▪ Brentuximab vedotin and ALK inhibitors are being evaluated

Hodgkin lymphoma

The diagnosis of Hodgkin lymphoma in children is similar to that in adults (see Chapter 34).

Therapy in paediatrics and young adults is based on risk status and degree of early response to treatment. Favourable low risk features include localized disease with no constitutional (B) symptoms (unexplained fevers, unintentional weight loss, night sweats) or bulky disease. Unfavourable high-risk features include B symptoms, bulky disease, extranodal involvement or advanced stage. Treatment typically includes multiagent chemotherapy (including anthracyclines, alkylating agents and bleomycin), with or without consolidative involved field radiation therapy (IFRT). Risk of

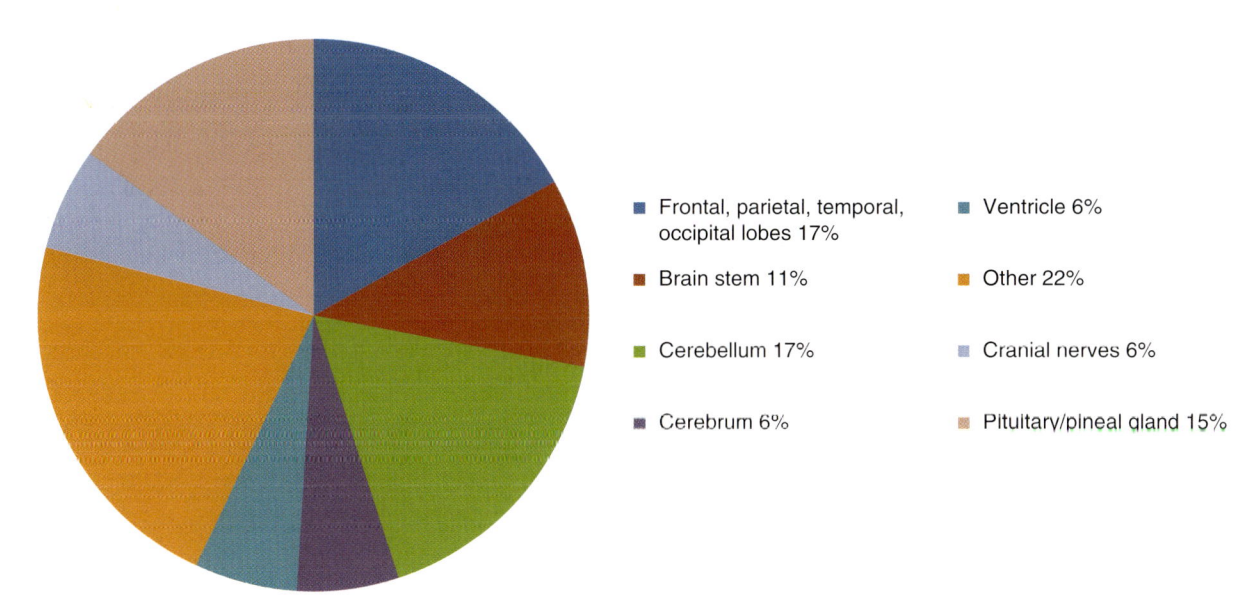

Figure 57.2 Distribution of brain tumours in children/adolescents aged 0-19 years based on location. Data from http://www.cbtrus.org

- Frontal, parietal, temporal, occipital lobes 17%
- Brain stem 11%
- Cerebellum 17%
- Cerebrum 6%
- Ventricle 6%
- Other 22%
- Cranial nerves 6%
- Pituitary/pineal gland 15%

gonadal toxicity in boys and increased risk of breast cancer in girls should be taken into consideration during treatment planning. With high EFS rates, the goal of current treatment regimens is to decrease intensity to minimize treatment-related toxicity (such as secondary malignancies and cardiotoxicity) while maintaining survival rates. Favourable low-risk disease with an early response or complete remission can be treated with fewer rounds of chemotherapy with or without IFRT. Intermediate- and high-risk groups may need both treatment modalities.

Brain tumours

Brain tumours are the second most common paediatric malignancy and the most common paediatric solid tumour (Figs 57.2 and 57.3). Infratentorial tumours are more common than supratentorial tumours in paediatric patients. Pilocytic astrocytomas are the most common CNS tumour in children and are typically slow growing, while medulloblastomas are the most common malignant brain tumour and are described in greater detail following a general description of brain tumours.

Incidence, aetiology and screening

Incidence, aetiology and screening: Brain tumours	Description
Incidence	• Annual incidence (2004–2008): 4.84 per 100,000 children aged 0–19 years (includes malignant and non-malignant primary CNS tumours) • Slightly higher incidence in males versus females • Higher incidence in Caucasians versus African–Americans

Aetiology	• Majority of paediatric CNS tumours are sporadic, unknown cause
	• Variety of chromosomal abnormalities noted (only few are recurrent and characteristic)
	• Two factors known to increase risk of developing childhood primary CNS tumour:
	  ▪ Prior radiation exposure to CNS
	  ▪ Certain genetic syndromes: neurofibromatosis types 1 and 2 (NF1 and 2), familial cancer predisposition syndrome, Li–Fraumeni syndrome, tuberous sclerosis, Von Hippel–Lindau syndrome, Gorlin syndrome, Turcot syndrome

Screening	• Routine screening for healthy children is not recommended • Those with predisposing risk factors should be followed closely for developing signs/symptoms

(a)

- Pilocytic astrocytoma 18%
- Embryonal (including medulloblastoma) 15%
- Malignant gliomas NOS 14%
- Ependymoma 6%
- Craniopharyngioma 4%
- Germ cell tumour 4%
- Other 29%

(b)

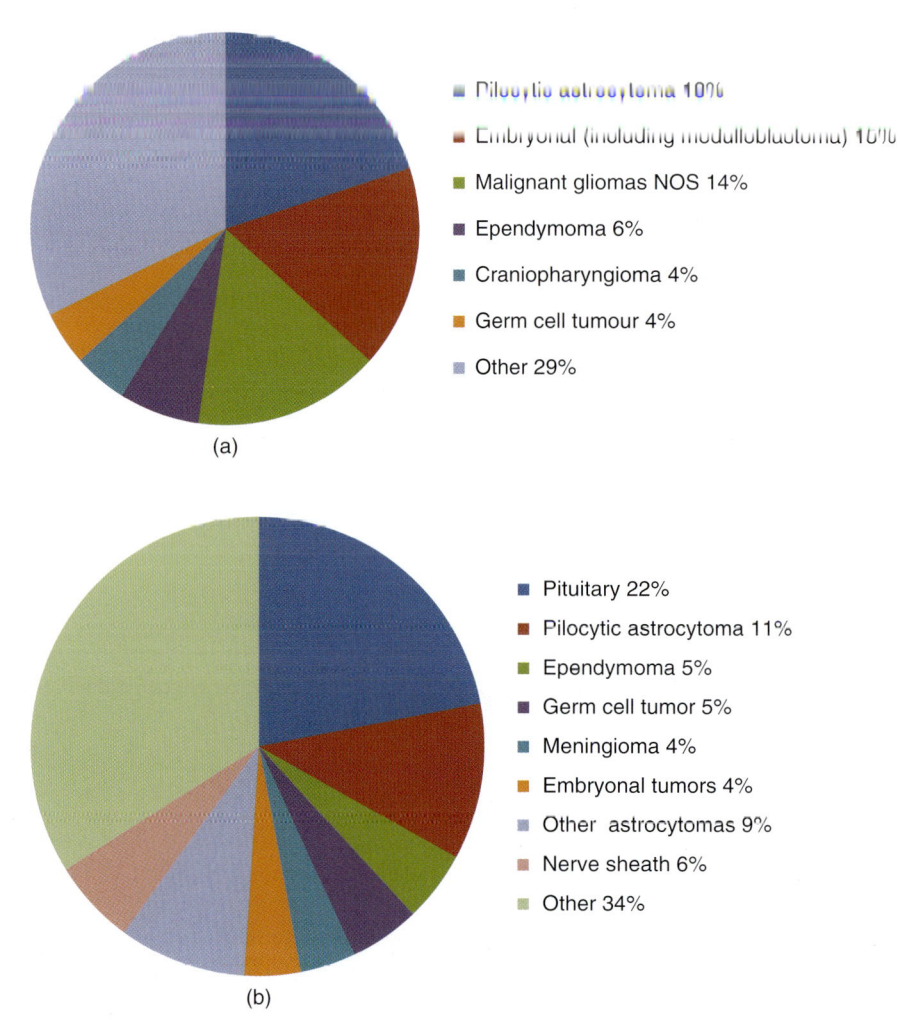

- Pituitary 22%
- Pilocytic astrocytoma 11%
- Ependymoma 5%
- Germ cell tumor 5%
- Meningioma 4%
- Embryonal tumors 4%
- Other astrocytomas 9%
- Nerve sheath 6%
- Other 34%

Figure 57.3 Distribution of paediatric brain tumours based on histology. (a) Age 0–14 years; (b) 15–19 years.
Data from http://www.cbtrus.org

Presentation

- Presenting symptoms can be:
  - Increased or obstructed intracranial pressure (ICP), or
  - Compression/infiltration of CNS
- Symptoms at presentation correlate with tumour location and growth:
  - Frontal lobe: personality changes, seizures, headaches, memory changes
  - Temporal lobe: seizures or altered speech
  - Suprasellar: endocrinopathies or vision changes
  - Thalamic: motor and sensory deficits
  - Midline tumours: can cause obstructive hydrocephalus as a result of direct invasion of the third or fourth ventricles
  - Pineal tumours: can cause vision changes (Parinaud syndrome)
  - Cerebellum: associated with nystagmus, ataxia, increased intracranial pressure
  - Brainstem: affect cranial nerves and basic life support
  - Spinal tumours: weakness, sensory disturbances, altered bowel/bladder function

Diagnostic work-up

- Symptoms indicative of increased intracranial pressure (ICP) require emergent CT scan without contrast
- Definitive imaging: high-quality magnetic resonance imaging (MRI) with and without gadolinium contrast and including the spine

Staging and prognostic factors

No uniform staging system exists for brain tumours.

Location of the tumour, presence of residual tumour and age of the child are important prognostic factors that influence the type of treatment used.

Treatment philosophy

Treatment can include a combination of surgery, radiation and chemotherapy, depending on tumour type. Initial supportive care interventions can include a ventriculostomy and/or ventriculoperitoneal shunt for acute hydrocephalus, dexamethasone or mannitol for cerebral oedema, and anticonvulsants for seizure prophylaxis.

Treatment: Brain tumours	Description
Surgical resection	• Surgical resection is the treatment of choice if anatomically feasible
Radiotherapy	• For unresectable lesions and as adjuvant therapy for residual tumours or completely resected malignant tumours • For lesions with a tendency to develop neuraxis metastases
Systemic chemotherapy	• Plays a role in certain high-risk patients, e.g. those with primitive neuroectodermal tumour (PNET), atypical teratoid/rhabdoid tumour (AT/RT) and high-grade gliomas • Used in patients under age 3 years in whom it is preferable to delay initiation of radiation due to neurocognitive effects

Medulloblastoma

Embryonal tumours are the largest group of malignant brain tumours in paediatrics and can occur anywhere in the CNS. Those located in the posterior fossa are commonly medulloblastomas, while those in the pineal region are pineoblastomas. Supratentorial PNET are another biologically distinct entity that carries a poorer prognosis compared to other PNET. Medulloblastomas are the most common subtype of malignant brain tumour in children.

Incidence and aetiology

Incidence and aetiology: Medulloblastoma	Description
Incidence	• Most common malignant brain tumour in paediatrics: ▪ Annual incidence in the USA: 400 cases • Typically present in patients under age 15 years • Slight male predominance

Aetiology	• Associated syndromes: Gorlin syndrome, Turcot syndrome, Li-Fraumeni syndrome
	• Clinical risk groups (high risk):
	  ▪ Presence of metastasis
	  ▪ Presence of residual tumour after resection (≥ 1.5 cm^2)
	  ▪ Presence of anaplasia
	  ▪ Age ≤ 3 years

Diagnostic work-up and classification

In addition to brain imaging, MRI of the spine and CSF sampling with a lumbar puncture are required. Although metastases outside the CNS are rare, they can occur in the bone, bone marrow and liver.

Risk stratification is based on age, evidence of metastatic disease, extent of surgical resection, and presence or absence of diffuse anaplasia histologically. Standard-risk patients are older than 3 years, with localized disease, a gross total resection (maximum 1.5 cm^2 of residual disease on MRI) and absence of anaplasia. All others are high risk. The World Health Organization (WHO) classifies medulloblastoma into five pathological subtypes: classic, anaplastic, large cell, nodular desmoplastic and with extensive nodularity. However, a growing body of literature from gene expression analyses has classified medulloblastoma into four distinct molecular subtypes, which are strongly associated with patient age and metastatic status (Table 57.4).

Table 57.4 Molecular subtypes of medulloblastoma

WNT	Sonic Hedgehog (SHH)	Group 3	Group 4
10% of medulloblastomas Involves monosomy of chromosome 6 and/or mutations of the beta-catenin gene (*CTNNB1*) 50% of tumours have mutations in the *DDX3X* helicase gene Excellent prognosis: • Long-term survival >90% • Almost exclusively of *classic* histology • Occurs in older children (>3 years of age)	25–30% of medulloblastomas In infants and adults, 50% of medulloblastomas are SHH type Not all tumours with this subtype can be identified by mutations of known SHH pathway genes (*PTCH1* and *SUFU* gene mutations) 30–40% have deletions in chromosome 9q 50% of SHH subtypes are *nodular desmoplastic* Intermediate prognosis	More common in males Worst outcome in paediatric and adult patients *MYC* amplification often found and carries worst prognosis of all subtypes, with higher rate of metastasis and poor outcome even with localized disease	70% have isochromosome 17q In females, 80% of tumours have loss of chromosome X Intermediate prognosis

Treatment philosophy

Surgery with gross total resection is the goal, followed by adjuvant chemotherapy, radiation therapy and maintenance chemotherapy.

Treatment: Medulloblastoma	Description

Radiotherapy	- *Standard-risk* medulloblastoma:
	  - Treatment includes craniospinal radiation with focal tumour bed boost and adjuvant chemotherapy:
	    - Use of chemotherapy has allowed craniospinal radiation to be given at lower dose of 23.4 Gy (compared to 36 Gy historically)
	  - 5-year survival rates are still >80% after gross total resection
	- *High-risk* medulloblastoma:
	  - Patients aged >3 years receive full-dose craniospinal radiation at 36 Gy and chemotherapy intensification
	  - 5-year survival rate: 70%

Systemic chemotherapy	- Typical agents: vincristine, etoposide, alkylating agents, platinum - High-risk patients aged <3 years receive upfront chemotherapy to delay and potentially even avoid radiation (with acceptable cure rates), and also can receive high-dose therapy with stem cell rescue
Recurrence	- Relapsed cases after standard treatment have poor prognosis - No standard salvage regimen
Follow-up	- Surveillance imaging: routine MRI brain and spine - Monitoring for late effects, including endocrinopathies, growth delay, neuropsychiatric effects, second malignancies such as meningiomas

NEUROBLASTOMA

Neuroblastoma (NB), a small round blue cell neoplasm, is the most common extracranial malignant solid tumour of childhood. It arises from neural crest cells that fail to differentiate normally, and is seen along tissues of the sympathetic nervous system, paraspinal ganglia and adrenal medulla.

Incidence, aetiology and screening

Incidence, aetiology and screening: Neuroblastoma	Description
Incidence	- Most common malignancy in infancy - Most common extracranial solid tumour in children - Annual incidence: 10.5 per million in children under age 15 years - Median age at diagnosis: 17–22 months: - Majority of cases are diagnosed by age 5 years - Slight male predilection - No significant difference between races

Aetiology	- Familial forms (1% of cases):
	  - Germline mutations in *ALK* oncogene may play a key role
	  - Associated with other neural crest disorders: NF1, Hirschsprung disease, congenital hypoventilation disorder

Screening	- Routine screening of infants aged <12 months has been attempted previously to identify asymptomatic tumours - This however doubled the incidence and identified tumours with a good prognosis (therefore not impacting survival)

Presentation

- Depends on tumour location, size, extent of invasion, effects of catecholamine secretion from primary tumour
- Site:
  - Typically in abdomen (65% of cases):
    - Half of these are located in the adrenal medulla
  - Other sites: chest, neck and pelvis
  - Infants can present with cervical and thoracic primary sites
  - Unknown primary site in 1% of patients
- At diagnosis:
  - Localized or regional disease in 50% of cases
  - Regional lymph node spread in 35% of cases
- Symptoms range from none to constitutional, enlarging mass, pain, abdominal distension, lymphadenopathy, respiratory distress due to compression or hepatomegaly, constipation, difficulty urinating
- Localized cervical disease can present as Horner syndrome
- Epidural or intradural extension can present with neurological deficits
- Dissemination via haematogenous or lymphatic routes involves bone marrow, liver and bone
- Classical signs of tumour dissemination:
  - Proptosis and periorbital ecchymoses (raccoon eyes)
  - Blue or obstructed intracranial pressure blueberry muffin syndrome)
- Paraneoplastic syndromes: can include extensive diarrhoea from vasoactive peptide or opsoclonus–myoclonus (rapid eye movement, myoclonus and ataxia)

Diagnostic work-up

- Baseline blood work: CBC, serum electrolytes, liver function, ferritin (typically elevated), LDH, neurone-specific enolase, and urine or serum catecholamines (specifically homovanillic [HVA] and vanillylmandelic acid [VMA])
- Initial imaging: CT scan of suspected location
- MRI useful when concern for spinal extension
- Bilateral bone marrow aspiration/biopsy to evaluate marrow involvement
- Metaiodobenzylguanidine (MIBG):
  - Norepinephrine analogue specifically concentrated in sympathetic nervous tissue
  - Radioactively-labelled MIBG allows for NB staging and evaluation of treatment response
  - PET scan for MIBG negative tumours
- Technetium bone scan if suspicion of cortical bone disease, especially in setting of negative MIBG scan
- Diagnosis confirmed by NB cells on tumour pathology or bone marrow sample, in setting of increased urine or serum catecholamines (or their metabolites)
- Core needle biopsy in setting of unresectable tumour or in those patients undergoing induction chemotherapy:
  - Not done for tumours that appear resectable on evaluation

Staging and prognostic factors
Staging

The International Neuroblastoma Staging System (INSS) is based on extent of tumour resection, assessment of lymph nodes and presence of metastatic disease. It has provided an initial framework to stage patients worldwide, although there has been some inconsistency between international collaborative groups. Based on age, histopathology, N-MYC gene amplification, DNA ploidy, stage and allelic deletions of chromosomes 1p and 11q, patients are categorized as being of low, intermediate or high risk of relapse.

The International Neuroblastoma Risk Group (INRG) classification system was recently developed to allow more universal pretreatment risk stratification and easier comparison of results between international clinical trials (Table 57.5). Patients are classified according to the following clinically relevant and statistically significant prognostic factors: patient age, extent of disease prior to surgery, tumour histology and grade of differentiation, N-MYC amplification status, chromosome 11q aberration and DNA ploidy. They are then stratified as very low, low, intermediate and high risk, which determines the treatment algorithm for them. Staging using the INRG system is based on tumour imaging and categorized as either locoregional (L1 and L2) or metastatic disease (M and MS). Locoregional disease is

Table 57.5 International Neuroblastoma Risk Group (INRG) staging system and corresponding International Neuroblastoma Staging System (INSS) stage

Stage	Description	Corresponding INSS stage
L1	Local disease No image-defined risk factors (IDRFs) (i.e. organ involvement, extension into blood vessels)	Stage 1
L2	Presence of IDRFs	Stages 2 and 3
M	Spread to distant organs (including distant lymph nodes)	Stage 4
MS	Spread to distant organs (skin, liver, and/or bone marrow) Limited to patients aged <18 months	Stage 4S

Adapted from http://www.cancer.gov/cancertopics/pdq/treatment/neuroblastoma/HealthProfessional/page3#Reference3.22.

determined from either the presence or absence of anatomical surgical risk factors identified on imaging studies. INRG stage assignment is currently being evaluated prospectively on all patients.

Survival rates are >90% for low- and intermediate-risk patients, while for high-risk patients it remains suboptimal at 40% (50–60% relapse rate). Infants with NB fare better than older children with NB.

Prognostic factors

Common genetic aberrations include whole chromosome gains causing hyperploidy and segmental chromosomal gains or losses. Hyperploidy is associated with a favourable prognosis while segmental changes have worse outcomes.

- Gain of chromosome 17q (most common genetic abnormality; 80% of cases): good prognosis
- Unbalanced translocation of chromosome 17q with either 1p or 11q: poor prognosis
- Regional deletion of chromosome 1p36 (70% of cases): associated with more aggressive disease
- N-MYC amplification, defined as ten or more gene copies per nucleus: associated with aggressive disease.
  - Seen in 25% of cases at chromosome 2p24, of which 30–40% are Stage 3 and 4 disease
- Deletions of chromosome 11q (15–22% of cases):
  - Specifically with 3p deletion and without N-MYC amplification is noted for aggressive disease

Treatment philosophy

Treatment modalities include surgical resection, chemotherapy, high-dose therapy with stem cell rescue, immunotherapy and radiotherapy, with algorithm dependent on a patient's risk stratification. Current trials are investigating additional variables that can be used in the intermediate-risk group to further refine risk assessment and reduce treatment.

Scenario: Neuroblastoma	Treatment philosophy

Low risk	- Includes:
	  - Stage 1
	  - Stage 2a/2b without N-MYC amplification
	  - Stage 4S (with favourable histology, without N-MYC amplification, DNA index of >1)
	- Surgery alone is sufficient (even for microscopic and gross residual disease
	- *Expectant observation*:
	  - Infants aged <6 months with solid adrenal masses of <3.1 cm (or cystic mass <5 cm) and no metastatic disease
	  - Follow with serial urine HVA/VMA and abdominal ultrasound
	  - For infants with tumours that show continued growth, surgical resection is preferred
	  - Asymptomatic 4S patients can be observed following initial biopsy if tumour has favourable features

Intermediate risk	- Includes:
	  - Patients aged 0–12 months with Stage 3 without N-MYC amplification
	  - Patients aged >12 months with Stage 3 without N-MYC amplification and favourable histology
	  - Infants with Stage 4 without N-MYC amplification
	  - Patients aged 1–1.5 years with Stage 4 without N-MYC amplification, and with favourable histology and DNA index of >1
	  - Symptomatic 4S patients with unfavourable tumour features
	- Biopsy confirmation is necessary prior to treatment
	- Chemotherapy and surgical resection are the treatment backbone:
	  - Goal of induction is to reduce tumour burden rapidly
	  - Common agents: cyclophosphamide, doxorubicin, cisplatin (or carboplatin), etoposide
	  - Followed by optimal surgical resection, even if response to chemotherapy is not robust

High risk	- Includes:
	  - Patients aged >1.5 years with Stage 4
	  - Any patient with N-MYC amplified tumours
	  - Patients aged >1.5 years with Stage 3 tumours and unfavourable histology
	  - Patients aged 1–1.5 years with Stage 4 disease with unfavourable histology or DNA index of 1
	- Treatment is challenging due to the poor long-term survival even for chemoresponsive tumours
	- Four stages of therapy:
	  - *Induction*:
	    - Current first-line agents: combinations of cisplatin, doxorubicin, vincristine, cyclophosphamide and etoposide
	  - *Local control*: tumour resection during or after induction

Scenario: Neuroblastoma	Treatment philosophy

	- *Consolidation*:
	  ○ Myeloablative consolidation therapy
	  ○ Different combination regimens:
	    – Carboplatin + etoposide + melphalan versus busulfan + melphalan
	    – Autologous haematopoietic stem cell rescue
	  ○ Radiation during consolidation decreases risk of local recurrence
	- *Maintenance*:
	  ○ Eliminates minimal residual disease
	  ○ High-risk patients receive 6 months of oral 13-*cis*-retinoic acid
	  ○ Immunotherapy with anti-GD2 antibody

Recurrence	- Local relapse of low and intermediate risk:
	  - Further standard treatment:
	    ○ A second surgery
	    ○ With or without moderately intensive chemotherapy
	- Local relapse of high risk:
	  - No current effective regimen with long-term benefit
	  - Targeted agents are being evaluated in ongoing trials

Treatment: Neuroblastoma	Description
Surgical resection	- *Goal*: to obtain complete resection safely: - Extent of resection correlates with risk of local recurrence
Systemic chemotherapy	- Role when patients are symptomatic owing to local tumour invasion - In intermediate- and high-risk, and recurrent disease - High-dose therapy with autologous stem cell rescue for high-risk disease
Radiotherapy	- Limited to advanced disease with unfavourable biology - External beam radiation helps with palliation, especially for metastases (e.g. bone)
Targeted agents	- Under development: - ALK, MIBG, aurora kinase A, mTOR inhibitors, TrkB inhibitors, immunotherapy (anti-GD2 antibody, ch14.18 and T cells), angiogenesis inhibitors, *N-MYC* targets, gastrin-releasing peptide (GRP) receptors, retinoids, cytokines

Osteosarcoma

Osteosarcoma is the most common malignant bone tumour of childhood and constitutes 3% of cases of childhood cancers.

Incidence, aetiology and screening

The most common genetic alterations associated with osteosarcoma have been mutations involving the *TP53* and *Rb1* genes. Patients with germline *Rb1* mutations have an approximately 500-fold increased risk of developing osteosarcoma, while those with *TP53* alterations have a 15-fold increased risk compared to the general population. Aneuploidy has also been described. Patients with Rothmund–Thomson syndrome and Bloom syndrome have defects in DNA mismatch repair, but the association with the development of osteosarcoma is unclear.

Incidence, aetiology and screening: Osteosarcoma	Description

Incidence	- Most common malignant bone tumour of childhood:
	  - Annual incidence 4.8 cases per million
	- Peak age:
	  - 12 years for females
	  - 16 years for males
	- Osteoblastic subtype is most common, followed by chondroblastic subtype
	- Slight male predominance

Aetiology	- Prior exposure to radiation - Germline retinoblastoma gene mutations (*Rb1*) - Syndromes associated with osteosarcoma include Li–Fraumeni, Rothmund–Thomson and Bloom - Associated with Paget disease of bone
Screening	- Routine screening for healthy children is not recommended

Pathology

Osteoblastic osteosarcoma is the most common histological subtype followed by chondroblastic and fibroblastic subtypes. The presence of malignant osteoid is a required feature for the diagnosis of osteosarcoma. Telangiectatic and small cell subtypes are rare. Parosteal and periosteal osteosarcoma are variants arising from the bone surface and have a more favourable prognosis.

Presentation

- Most common presentation: pain, swelling, warmth and erythema (especially for extremity tumours)
- Other: neurological signs due to nerve compression for sacral or vertebral column tumours
- Most common primary tumour sites are distal femur, proximal tibia and proximal humerus
- Most common site of metastases: lung (61% at diagnosis) and bone (16%)

Diagnostic work-up

- Plain film radiograph for extremity tumours:
  - Osteolytic lesion with soft tissue component
  - Malignant osteoid
  - Periosteal elevation (Codman triangle)
- CT scan or MRI of primary tumour site
- Whole-body bone scan
- CT chest

Staging and prognostic factors

Pretreatment staging criteria are based on the extent of disease. High-risk patients are those with unresectable tumours or presenting with metastases.

Poor clinical prognostic factors include incomplete resection or unresectable disease, presence of metastasis and poor histological response to neoadjuvant chemotherapy.

Current 10-year survival estimates are 70% for patients with standard-risk disease, while for metastatic disease the survival rate is 25%.

Treatment philosophy

Treatment is multimodal, utilizing primarily chemotherapy and surgery. For patients with extremity tumours, neoadjuvant chemotherapy is typically followed by surgical resection of the primary tumour. Adjuvant chemotherapy is influenced by the histological response of the tumour to neoadjuvant chemotherapy. A recent collaboration between the North American and European groups has attempted to study a standardized approach to therapy as well as to evaluate some new agents.

Treatment: Osteosarcoma	Description
Surgical resection	- For the majority of patients with extremity tumours, limb salvage surgery with endoprosthetic placement is the preferred procedure - Amputation is generally reserved for tumour sites where it is difficult to achieve local resection (e.g. ankle) or sites of local recurrence, or for palliation of pain - Rotationplasty is an acceptable option but is not commonly done in North America - Surgical resection of pulmonary metastasis is recommended - Long-term issues include implant failure/breakage, pathological fracture and leg length discrepancy
Systemic chemotherapy	- Neoadjuvant chemotherapy - Adjuvant chemotherapy is dependent upon histological response to neoadjuvant chemotherapy: - No international standard for patients with a poor initial histological response - Doxorubicin, cisplatin, methotrexate and ifosfamide are considered the most active agents - Early results show no additional benefit of adding adjuvant etoposide + ifosfamide to standard chemotherapy in high-risk patients - Addition of interferon as a maintenance drug did not improve outcome for those patients with a good histological response to neoadjuvant chemotherapy
Radiotherapy	- Considered a radiation-resistant tumour - Radiotherapy can be used for patients with unresectable primary tumours (pelvic site) and for sites of metastasis - Samarium (^{153}Sm-EDTMP), a beta-emitting radiopharmaceutical, has been used for relapsed/refractory osteosarcoma
Relapse	- Approximately 30% of patients experience recurrence: - Pulmonary recurrence is the most common - Negative prognostic factors include early recurrence and the inability to achieve second clinical remission status - High-dose ifosfamide (14 g/m^2 per course) and gemcitabine/docetaxel have been used - Agents that are being evaluated include zoledronate, liposomal muramyl tripeptide phosphatidylethanolamine (L-MTP-PE), RANKL antibody and anti-GD2 antibody

Rhabdomyosarcoma

Rhabdomyosarcoma (RMS) is a small round blue cell tumour that arises from mesenchymal cells that would normally develop into skeletal muscle. It is the most common soft tissue sarcoma of childhood and constitutes 3% of childhood cancers. The two predominant subtypes are embryonal (ERMS) and alveolar (ARMS). ERMS constitutes up to 70% of all RMS cases, and ARMS 20–25%. Rarer subtypes are botryoid and pleomorphic (mainly in adults).

Incidence, aetiology and screening

Incidence, aetiology and screening: Rhabdomyosarcoma	Description
Incidence	• Most common soft tissue sarcoma in children: ▪ Annual incidence: 4.5 cases per million • Mean age at diagnosis: 6–8 years • Slight male prevalence
Aetiology	• Most cases are sporadic • Higher predisposition in certain genetic syndromes: Li–Fraumeni, Beckwith–Wiedemann, NF1 • Genetic conditions with germline RAS/MAPK pathway mutations also have a higher incidence
Screening	• No role for routine screening in healthy children • Those with an underlying predisposing condition should be followed closely for any signs/symptoms

Genetics

Mutations specifically seen with ERMS include those involving the *RAS* and *FGFR4* genes, and loss of heterozygosity (LOH) of 11p15. Approximately 80% of ARMS have the characteristic translocation between the *FKHR/FOXO1* transcription factor gene (on chromosome 13) and either *PAX3* transcription factor gene (on chromosome 2) or *PAX7* gene (on chromosome 1). Mutations of *N-MYC*, *ALK* and *MET* are also seen in ARMS. Over-expression of insulin growth factor 2 (IGF-2) is common to both subtypes.

Presentation

- Presenting symptoms depend on tumour location and correspond to interference of surrounding tissues and structures by tumour growth
- Most common sites:
  - Head and neck (40%)
  - Genitourinary (GU) (20%)
  - Extremities
  - ERMS is more likely to present in head, neck and GU system
  - ARMS is more common in trunk and extremities
- Abdominal and pelvic sites are less common
- Typically presents as a painful mass (often mistaken for injury)
- *Head and neck manifestations*: diplopia, exophthalmos, headache, congestion, nasal discharge, cranial nerve palsy, obstruction, dysphagia, hearing or vision loss
- *GU manifestations*:
  - Urinary tract obstruction or constipation
  - Botryoid subtype commonly seen in the GU tract of young infants
- *Abdominal or pelvic manifestations*:
  - Abdominal pain, ascites, haematuria (in addition to abdominal mass)
- 15% of cases present with distant metastases to lung, bone marrow, bone and/or lymph nodes

Diagnostic work-up

- Radiographic imaging of primary site
- CT chest
- Total body bone scan
- Bone marrow biopsy
- Lumbar puncture (only for parameningeal RMS)

Staging and prognostic factors

Staging and risk stratification is based on the results of clinical trials from the Intergroup Rhabdomyosarcoma Study Group (IRSG) as well as other international collaborative groups. For example, in North America the Pretreatment Stage and Clinical Group systems are often used. The Pretreatment Staging system is based on primary tumour location (favourable versus unfavourable), size, invasiveness, presence of metastases and extent of lymph node involvement. Clinical Group classification is a surgical–pathology system based on extent of disease after initial surgical biopsy or resection. Based on the Pretreatment Staging and Clinical Group Classification, patients are further classified as being low, intermediate or high risk for treatment failure.

Low-risk RMS typically includes non-metastatic RMS of embryonal histology in favourable sites such as the orbit, vagina and paratesticular sites. The intermediate-risk group typically includes non-metastatic ARMS, parameningeal tumours or extremity tumours.

Overall survival for RMS is 70–75%. The 5 year EFS for low-, intermediate- and high-risk disease is 95%, 65% and 15%, respectively. Factors associated with a worse prognosis are: extremes of age (<1 or >10 years), alveolar histology, unfavourable primary tumour site (including the extremities, perineum, urinary bladder and prostate, cranial parameningeal sites, trunk and retroperitoneum) and metastatic disease. Factors with favourable outcomes include tumour size of <5 cm in greatest tumour diameter, favourable sites (including orbit, non-parameningeal head and neck, GU tract excluding the kidney, bladder and prostate), complete surgical resection, embryonal histology and no regional lymph nodes involved. Patients with metastatic disease, age <1 year, sites involving bone and bone marrow, and with three or more metastatic sites have a poor prognosis.

Treatment philosophy

Therapy is multimodal with chemotherapy, surgery and radiation, and depends on risk stratification.

Treatment: Rhadomyosarcoma	Description

Systemic chemotherapy	• Backbone of treatment
	• Regimens:
	  ▪ North America:
	    ○ Standard: three-drug regimen with vincristine + dactinomycin + cyclophosphamide (VAC)
	    ○ Regimens with ifosfamide + etoposide + topotecan did not show improved outcomes compared to VAC
	  ▪ Europe:
	    ○ Regimens are more adaptive based on clinical response
	    ○ Include anthracyclines and ifosfamide
	  ▪ *Low risk*:
	    ○ Shortened duration of therapy and decreased cumulative doses of cyclophosphamide are currently under investigation in North America
	  ▪ *Intermediate risk*:
	    ○ VAC alternating with vincristine + irinotecan is being evaluated
	  ▪ *High risk*:
	    ○ Interval compression with vincristine + doxorubicin + cyclophosphamide alternating with ifosfamide + etoposide may be of benefit (under investigation)
	• Maintenance chemotherapy: may play a role in certain RMS cases and is being evaluated in Europe
	• Myeloablative chemotherapy followed by stem cell rescue in metastatic RMS does not yield superior results over conventional therapy

Surgical resection	• Resection of primary tumour with negative margins:
	  ▪ Preferred local control
	  ▪ Influenced by surrounding structures
	• Delayed excision of an initially unresectable tumour may be more beneficial after initial tumour shrinkage occurs with chemotherapy (with or without radiation)
	• For paratesticular primary site, ipsilateral retroperitoneal lymph node sampling is recommended in patients ≥10 years of age and being treated using Children's Oncology Group (COG) protocols
	• For extremity tumours, sentinel node biopsy is recommended

Radiotherapy	• Typically used in:
	  ▪ Unresectable tumours
	  ▪ All patients with ARMS being treated using COG protocols
	  ▪ Adjuvant therapy for incomplete resections
	• Treated volumes are determined by tumour extent at diagnosis and prior to surgical resection or chemotherapy (a 2-cm margin is typically used)
	• Usually over 5–6 weeks (1.8 Gy once daily)
	• Dosing is dependent upon primary site, extent of disease, surgical margin status and lymph node involvement

Recurrence	• Complete surgical resection if possible • Radiation therapy to sites not previously irradiated • Surgical resection + radiation therapy offers best chance for long-term survival • No consensus on optimal salvage chemotherapy regimen

Wilms tumour

Wilms tumour (WT), also known as nephroblastoma, arises from primitive metanephric blastemal cells.

Incidence, aetiology and screening

Incidence, aetiology and screening: WT	Description

Incidence	- Most common malignant renal tumour of childhood
	- Annual incidence: 8 per million
	- Peak age: 2–3 years
	- No gender preference
	- Unfavourable histology is more common in:
	  - Older children (peak incidence at 5 years)
	  - African–Americans

Aetiology	- Familial: 5% of cases - Syndromes associated with WT and *WT1* gene: WAGR syndrome (WT, aniridia, genitourinary abnormalities, mental delays), Denys–Drash syndrome, Beckwith–Wiedemann syndrome, Bloom syndrome
Screening	- Routine radiographs until age 5 years are recommended for those with a predisposing syndrome

Pathology and genetics

The *WT1* gene on chromosome 11p13 is a transcription regulator that influences metanephric stem cell differentiation. A mutation in the *WT1* gene is seen in approximately 20% of cases. Other genetic mutations that have been reported include deletions in *WTX* and *CTNNB1*, and missense mutations in the *TP53* gene. Approximately 70% of WT have loss of heterozygosity or loss of imprinting on 11p15, which have been associated with increased IGF-2 expression.

The two histopathological types are favourable and unfavourable. The unfavourable histology includes anaplastic tumours that can be focal or diffuse in presentation.

Presentation

- Most common presentation: asymptomatic abdominal mass, often discovered by parent while bathing child
- Other: malaise, pain, microscopic or gross haematuria, hypertension
- Occasional subcapsular haemorrhage within tumour: leads to rapidly enlarging abdominal mass, anaemia, hypertension, pain, fever
- Intravenous tumour extension with thrombus extension to inferior vena cava (IVC)
- Most common site of metastases: lung (12% at diagnosis)
- Patients with WAGR have increased risk of bilateral WT

Diagnostic work-up

- CBC, urinalysis, chemistry panel, renal function
- Initial renal ultrasound can determine whether mass is intra- or extra-renal, and cystic versus solid
- CT abdomen/pelvis: preferred imaging modality
  - Evaluates tumour extension into renal vein or IVC
  - Evaluates contralateral kidney
- CT chest: initial staging

Staging and prognostic factors

Selection of therapy and prognosis is based on tumour stage; therefore, accurate staging with careful lymph node sampling is crucial (Table 57.6). Histological subtype also greatly impacts survival. Newer clinical and genetic risk factors to better identify patients at risk for recurrence include patient age at diagnosis, tumour weight, histological response to treatment, and allelic status of chromosomes 1p and 16q in resected tumours. Intravascular extension, if fully resected, does not affect outcome.

Most WT patients are cured with current multimodal therapy (OS rates > 90%).

Table 57.6 National Wilms Tumor Study Group staging system

Stage	Description
I	Limited to kidney with no renal vessel involvement Completely excised with negative margins Intact renal capsule surface (tumour not ruptured before or during removal)
II	Tumour extends beyond kidney Completely excised with negative margins Regional extension of tumour (renal capsule ruptured, biopsied or invaded; tumour spillage confined to flank without peritoneal involvement) Vessels outside kidney infiltrated or free-floating tumour thrombus
III	Residual tumour in the abdomen (non-haematogenous) with one or more of the following: - Lymph nodes - Tumour spillage beyond the flank - Peritoneal implants - Adherent tumour thrombus - Incomplete excision
IV	Distant haematogenous metastases (lung, liver, brain, distant lymph node)
V	Bilateral renal involvement (stage each side based on extent of local disease)

Adapted from National Wilms Tumor Study Group Staging System. (www.nwtsg.org/index.html)

Treatment philosophy

Treatment is multimodal, including surgery, chemotherapy and, in some cases, radiation therapy. The National Wilms Tumour Study Group (NWTS) and International Society of Pediatric Oncology (SIOP) have historically guided treatment recommendations. Several COG protocols have been developed based on risk classification to cover the spectrum of WT, with unfavourable histology and certain genetic aberrations requiring more intensive therapy.

Treatment: WT	Description

Surgical resection	• Resection is done cautiously:
	  ▪ Tumour spillage increases risk of recurrence and upstages patients, committing them to postoperative radiation therapy and more intensive chemotherapy
	  ▪ Through transverse or midline abdominal incision
	• Presence of IVC or right atrium thrombus should favour biopsy rather than resection
	• *NWTS:* recommends upfront nephrectomy to assess tumour stage and histology so under- or over-treatment avoided (nephron-sparing surgery and partial nephrectomy are *not* recommended)
	• *SIOP:* recommends upfront chemotherapy prior to nephrectomy
	• In North America, surgery alone is definitive treatment for non-metastatic, favourable histology tumours in:
	  ▪ Children <2 years and
	  ▪ Tumour (and kidney) weight <550 g
	• Treatment for bilateral WT:
	  ▪ Spare renal function
	  ▪ Neoadjuvant chemotherapy followed by bilateral partial nephrectomies
	  ▪ No upfront biopsy necessary

Systemic chemotherapy	• Preoperatively plays a role in:
	  ▪ Solitary kidney with WT
	  ▪ Bilateral WT
	  ▪ Horseshoe kidney
	  ▪ Hepatic vena cava extension
	  ▪ Extensive pulmonary metastases causing respiratory distress
	• Can shrink initially unresectable large tumours to more manageable size, allowing for later complete resection
	• Vincristine + dactinomycin: backbone of chemotherapy
	• Doxorubicin + cyclophosphamide + etoposide added for higher risk

Radiotherapy	• Plays a role in select cases:
	  ▪ Stage II with anaplasia (focal or diffuse)
	  ▪ Stage III patients without LOH
	  ▪ High-risk patients with favourable histology (Stage III with LOH or Stage IV metastatic disease)
	  ▪ Stage IV with pulmonary metastases with LOH
	  ▪ Stage IV with no LOH but pulmonary metastases that fail to respond rapidly to initial adjuvant chemotherapy
	• Patients with pulmonary nodules removed:
	  ▪ 12 Gy whole-lung radiation + chemotherapy
	  ▪ Controversy regarding benefit of whole-lung radiation in patients with lung metastases identified only on CT imaging

Relapse	• 15% with favourable histology will have recurrence
	• 50% recurrence rate in those with anaplastic histology
	• Typically within 2 years of diagnosis, often in lung
	• Survival after relapse:
	  ▪ Favourable histology: approximately 60%
	  ▪ Anaplastic histology: very poor
	  ▪ LOH at 16q: higher relapse and mortality rate compared to those without LOH (therefore more chemotherapy is recommended)
	• Regimen: ifosfamide + carboplatin + etoposide + cyclophosphamide
	• Roles of surgery and radiation in this setting are not defined

Recommended reading

Bollard CM, Lim MS, Gross TG; COG Non-Hodgkin Lymphoma Committee (2013) Children's Oncology Group 2013 Blueprint for research: Non-Hodgkin lymphoma. *Pediatr Blood Cancer* 60:979–984.

Colon N, Chung D (2011) Neuroblastoma. *Adv Pediatr* 58: 297–311.

Creutzig U, van den Heuvel-Eibrink MM, Gibson B et al. (2012) Diagnosis and management of acute myeloid leukemia in children and adolescents: Recommendations from an International Expert Panel. *Blood* 120:3187–3205.

Davenport KP, Blanco FC, Sandler AD (2012) Pediatric malignancies. *Surg Clin North Am* 92:745–767.

Davidoff A (2012) Wilms tumor. *Adv Pediatr* 59(1):247–267.

Fleming A, Chi S (2012) Brain tumors in children. *Curr Probl Pediatr Adol Health Care* 42:80–103.

Gore L, Trippett T (2010) Emerging non-transplant-based strategies in treating pediatric non-Hodgkin's lymphoma. *Curr Hematol Malign Rep* 5:177–184.

Gross TG, Hale GA, He W et al. (2010) Hematopoietic stem cell transplantation for refractory or recurrent non-Hodgkin lymphoma in children and adolescents. *Biol Blood Marrow Transplant* 16(2):223–230.

Hara J (2012) Development of treatment strategies for advanced neuroblastoma. *Int J Clin Oncol* 17:196–203.

Lanzkowsky P (2011) Non-Hodgkin's lymphoma. In: Lanzkowsky P, ed. *Manual of Pediatric Hematology and Oncology*, 5th edn. Academic Press, Elsevier Inc:624.

Leary S, Olson J (2012) The molecular classification of medulloblastoma: Driving the next generation clinical trials. *Curr Opin Pediatr* 24(1):33–39.

Longhi A, Errani C, De Paolis M, Mercuri M, Bacci G (2006) Primary bone osteosarcoma in the pediatric age: State of the art. *Cancer Treat Rev* 32:423–436.

Maloney KW, Giller R, Hunger SP (2012) Recent advances in the understanding and treatment of pediatric malignancies. *Adv Pediatr* 9:329–358.

Molyneux EM, Rochford R, Griffin B et al. (2012) Burkitt's lymphoma. *Lancet* 379:1234–1344.

Ora I, Eggert A (2011) Progress in treatment and risk stratification of neuroblastoma: Impact on future clinical and basic research. *Semin Cancer Biol* 21:217–228.

Park JR, Eggert A, Caron H (2010) Neuroblastoma: Biology, prognosis, and treatment. *Hematol Oncol Clin North Am* 24:65–86.

Pui CH, Carroll WL, Meshinchi S, Arceci RJ (2011) Biology, risk stratification, and therapy of pediatric acute leukemias: An update. *J Clin Oncol* 29(5):551–565.

Ray A, Huh W (2012) Current state-of-the-art systemic therapy for pediatric soft tissue sarcomas. *Curr Oncol Rep* 14:311–319.

Whelan JS, Jinks RC, McTiernan A et al. (2012) Survival from high-grade localized extremity osteosarcoma: combined results and prognostic factors from three European Osteosarcoma Intergroup randomized clinical trials. *Ann Oncol* 23:1607–1616.

Zage PE, Louis CU, Cohn SL (2012) New aspects of neuroblastoma treatment: ASPHO 2011 Symposium review. *Pediatr Blood Cancer* 58:1099–1105.

58 Cancer of unknown primary (non-head and neck)

George Pentheroudakis and Nicholas Pavlidis

Department of Medical Oncology, Medical School, University of Ioannina, Ioannina, Greece

Summary	Key facts

Introduction	- 5–15 new cases/100,000 population annually, 2–4% of cancers
	- Histologically, four major types.
	  - Adenocarcinoma of good-to-moderate differentiation (50%)
	  - Poorly differentiated adenocarcinoma (30%)
	  - Squamous carcinoma (15%)
	  - Undifferentiated neoplasm (5%)
	- Median age at diagnosis: 65 years
	- Male-to-female ratio: 1.5:1
	- Generally associated with known carcinogens

Presentation	- Histologically verified cancer in the absence of primary site after a standardized diagnostic work-up - High volume visceral metastases or locoregional disease in head and neck, axilla, groin - CT of chest, abdomen, pelvis is mandatory: - Further investigations according to symptoms, signs and laboratory work-up - Histopathological work-up consisting of H&E and immunohistochemistry is crucial; may be supplemented by multigene expression profiling tests
Scenario	- Favourable CUP subsets (20%) consist of locoregional disease, managed with a combination of resection, radiotherapy and/or chemotherapy - Poor risk CUP subsets (80%) consist of systemic visceral metastases, managed with palliative chemotherapy in patients with good performance status - Median survival <12 months in poor risk and variable (15–36 months) in favourable CUP
Trials	- Paucity of phase III trials in CUP

Introduction

Cancer of unknown primary (CUP) is a heterogeneous group of rare metastatic malignancies that are refractory to standard chemotherapy and of short survival in the majority of cases. In general, both diagnostic and therapeutic approaches for these patients constitute a challenge for the practising oncologist and the healthcare system. Clinical and translational research is a poorly met need worldwide. For optimal diagnosis and treatment, CUP multidisciplinary teams should be established in major referral hospitals, while evidence-based guidelines are of paramount importance for the optimal management of these patients.

Head and neck CUP is covered in Chapter 46 and this chapter concerns CUP at other sites.

Incidence and aetiology

Recent data from the Swedish Family Cancer Database suggest that the cause of death in CUP patients frequently matches the cancer diagnosed in a family member, implying that the

UICC Manual of Clinical Oncology, Ninth Edition. Edited by Brian O'Sullivan, James D. Brierley, Anil K. D'Cruz, Martin F. Fey, Raphael Pollock, Jan B. Vermorken and Shao Hui Huang. © 2015 UICC. Published 2015 by John Wiley & Sons, Ltd.

metastasis had probably undergone a phenotypic change of the primary cancer.

The most common sites harbouring the primary tumour in autopsy studies were the lung and pancreas, followed by other gastrointestinal, respiratory and urogenital sites. Hence, while there are no known risk factors, abstention from diets, habits and environmental factors with known carcinogenic potential (smoking, excessive alcohol consumption, fat-rich diet poor in fruit and vegetable, obesity, ionizing radiation exposure) is advised.

An increased risk of subsequent cancers in CUP patients has been reported in both Swedish and Swiss cancer databases, ranging from a standardized incidence ratio of 1.4 to 1.69. Significant excess risks were observed for cancer of the prostate, oral cavity and pharynx, as well as of the skin.

Incidence and aetiology	Description

Incidence	• 5–15 new cases per 100,000 population annually (2–4% of cancers)
	• Annual age-adjusted incidence per 100,000 population.
	   ▪ USA: 7–12
	   ▪ Australia 18–19 cases
	   ▪ The Netherlands 5.3–6.7
	• Fourth most frequent cause of cancer death
	• Median age at presentation: 65 years

Aetiology	• No known risk factors • Generally associated with known carcinogens

Pathology

Histologically, CUP is classified into four major types. The most common type is adenocarcinoma of good-to-moderate differentiation (50%), followed by poorly or undifferentiated adenocarcinomas (30%), squamous cell carcinoma (15%) and undifferentiated neoplasms (5%). Modern immunohistochemical algorithms permit the categorization of poorly differentiated CUP into carcinomas, neuroendocrine tumours, lymphomas, germ cell tumours, melanomas and sarcomas.

CUP is not very well defined with a discrete classification within the International Classification of Disease (ICD) nomenclature (ICD C77–C80).

Presentation and natural history

CUP patients carry a unique natural history. CUP is characterized by:
- Early dissemination (50% of CUP patients present with multiple sites of metastases)
- Short history of symptoms/signs related to the metastatic lesions
- Aggressive behaviour
- Unpredictable metastatic pattern.

There is a different incidence of metastatic sites between known and unknown primary tumours, e.g. hidden pancreatic cancer presenting as CUP has a 4–5-fold higher incidence of presenting with bone and lung involvement as compared to known primary pancreatic tumours. In CUP there is also a high rate of unusual secondary deposits in the scalp, skin, heart and soft tissues.

Diagnostic work-up

CUP is diagnosed when a thorough medical history and careful physical examination along with an extensive work-up consisting of full blood count, biochemistry tests, urinalysis, stool occult blood testing, specific immunohistochemistry, imaging technology (computed tomography [CT] of the thorax, abdomen and pelvis; mammography; positron emission tomography [PET] in selected cases), fail to detect the primary site.

The work-up focuses on the patient and the tumour. The patient work-up should encompass assessment of performance status, co morbidities, physical symptoms and signs, as well as the presence or absence of family and social support. The tumour work-up is oriented towards assessing the tumour profile, defining the extent and location of metastases, in addition to looking for the primary tumour.

Light microscopic examination using routine staining with haematoxylin and eosin (H&E) or other appropriate stains characterizes cell morphology and tumour differentiation. Immunohistochemical investigations using a series of antibodies against several structural tissue components (Table 58.1) contribute to identifying the tumour origin in metastatic adenocarcinomas or poorly differentiated carcinomas (Fig. 58.1).

The detection of chromosomal abnormalities can be helpful in selected cases, such as in germ cell CUP (detection of an isochromosome of the short arm of chromosome 12 [i12p]), in peripheral neuroectodermal tumours or in Ewing sarcomas (translocation t[11, 22]). Complementary DNA (cDNA) or oligonucleotide microarrays and tissue protein microarrays are powerful tools that molecularly assign CUP to primary site groups. These technologies have been made available in the form of customized platforms in CLIA-approved laboratories worldwide. Available tests are reported to have an accuracy

Table 58.1 Pathological evaluation of CUP

Step 1: Detection of broad types of cancer	
Carcinoma	Pan-cytokeratin, EMA
Lymphoma	CLA, (CD45RB) (±) EMA
Sarcoma	Vimentin, desmin, S-100, alpha-smooth muscle actin, myoD1, CD34, c-Kit, CD99
Melanoma	S-100, HMB45, Melan-A
Step 2: Detection of broad types of carcinoma	
Adenocarcinoma	Light microscopy, PAS, CK7, CK20
Squamous cell carcinoma	CK5/6, p63
Neuroendocrine carcinoma	Chromogranin, synaptophysin, PG9.5, CD56
Germ cell carcinoma	PLAP, OCT4, AFP, hCG
Step 3: Detection of adenocarcinoma origin	
Breast cancer	ER, GCDFP-15, mammaglobulin, CK7+/CK20–
Ovarian cancer	CA125, mesothelin, WT1, ER, CK7+/CK20–
Endometrial cancer	CK7+/CK20–, CA125, ER (PgR?)
Prostate cancer	PSA, PAP, CK7–/CK20–
Colon cancer	CDX2, CEA, CK7–/CK20+
Pancreatic cancer	CK7+/CK20±, CA125, mesothelin
Liver cancer	Hepar-1, AFP, polyclonal CEA, CD10, CD13
Lung cancer	TTF1, CK7+/CK20–
Kidney cancer	CD10, CK7–/CK20–
Thyroid cancer	TTF1, thyroglobulin

of 75–90% for correctly classifying solid tumours of a known primary in blinded validation sets and represent 6–30 tumour types. Molecular testing for tissue-of-origin identification has the potential to become an important tool in supporting a suspected diagnosis and excluding diagnoses included in the tissue-of-origin differential. However, an important consideration for these tests is to determine if patients derive benefit from their application in terms of clinical outcomes and cost; these benefits remain to be proven.

Radiology is the mainstay of tumour extent assessment as well as the main tool to screen for the primary tumour. Contrast-enhanced CT of the chest, abdomen and pelvis is sensitive at identifying metastatic sites, though its sensitivity to detect the primary site is only 30–35%. Magnetic resonance imaging (MRI) is very useful for identifying an occult hidden primary tumour in the breast. Mammography is used to detect breast primary sites in women with isolated axillary lymph node involvement by an adenocarcinoma; however, its sensitivity is

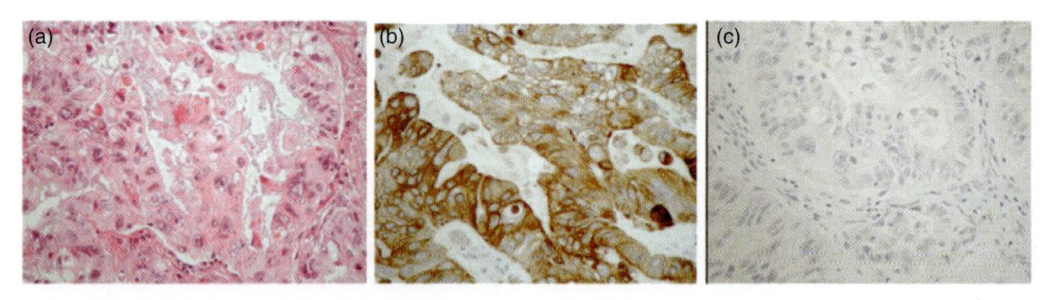

Figure 58.1 (a) Metastatic CUP adenocarcinoma (H&E × 200), suspected as of colonic origin from (b) CK20+ (CK20, DAB×200) and (c) CK7– (CK7, DAB × 200).

Source: Batistatou (2013). Reproduced with permission of Journal of OncoPathology.

not as high as that of breast MRI. The ^{111}In-Octreoscan is useful in detecting neuroendocrine CUP tumours expressing enhanced somatostatin receptors. Fluorodeoxyglucose (FDG)-PET/CT has proven to be useful in CUP patients with cervical lymphadenopathy for the detection of the primary site. In a recent meta-analysis, in a total sample size of 433 patients, the overall primary tumour detection rate, pooled sensitivity and specificity of FDG-PET/CT were 37%, 84% and 84%, respectively. FDG-PET/CT is recommended for CUP patients presenting with cervical lymphadenopathy with no primary tumour identified on ENT pan-endoscopy, providing the patient belongs to a favourable CUP subset and radical treatment is contemplated.

Endoscopic investigations should be limited to CUP patients with particular symptoms or signs, e.g. bronchoscopy in patients with haemoptysis or cough and negative imaging studies, or colonoscopy in patients with constipation, diarrhoea or overt blood loss. The sensitivity of extensive endoscopic evaluation in the absence of clinical or laboratory findings is extremely low.

Measurement of serum tumour markers has no diagnostic, prognostic or predictive value in CUP patients, as most epithelial serum tumour markers (CEA, CA15-3, CA19-9, CA125) show non-specific over-expression, with 70% of patients expressing more than two markers in their serum. However, some serum markers could be helpful in certain clinicopathological subsets, e.g. alpha-fetoprotein (AFP) or beta-human chorionic gonadotropin (β-hCG) in poorly differentiated carcinomas with midline distribution, prostate-specific antigen (PSA) in men with osteoblastic metastases, CA125 in primary peritoneal adenocarcinoma or CA15-3 in women with isolated axillary nodal adenocarcinoma.

Diagnostic work-up	Description
Patient assessment	• Physical examination including rectum/pelvis • History • Performance status • Co-morbidity • Family history • Social support
Tumour profile pathological assessment	• H&E light microscopy • Immunohistochemistry (see Table 58.1)

Tumour profile molecular assessment	• Available tests with 75–90% accuracy, but unknown impact on tailoring therapy and improving patient outcome:
	  ▪ Pathwork Tissue of Origin (Pathwork Diagnostics, Redwood City, CA, USA)
	  ▪ Theros Cancer-TYPE ID (BioTheranostics, San Diego, CA, USA)
	  ▪ MiRview Mets test (Rosetta Genomics, Philadelphia, PA, USA)

Tumour extent (radiology/endoscopy)	• CT chest, abdomen, pelvis • Mammography or breast MRI in women with isolated axillary lymphadenopathy • ^{111}In-Octreoscan in neuroendocrine CUP • PET/CT in head and neck CUP or when radical treatment is contemplated • Endoscopy guided by symptoms, signs or laboratory abnormalities
Serum tumour markers	▪ Avoid except for: ▪ AFP, β-hCG in midline CUP ▪ PSA in men with osteoblastic metastases ▪ CA125 in women with peritoneal carcinomatosis ▪ CA15-3 in women with isolated axillary adenopathy

Clinicopathological subsets and prognostic factors

Clinicopathological subsets

CUP is a heterogeneous group of diseases classified as favourable, or specific or good prognosis subsets, and unfavourable, or non-specific or poor prognosis subsets. This classification is based on age, sex, histopathology, clinical presentation and organ or tissue involvement. It offers substantial help to the practising oncologist for diagnostic and therapeutic management, and provides valuable prognostic information (Table 58.2). Patients with unfavourable CUP (80% of CUP patients) have a poor outcome despite the administration of cytotoxic chemotherapy, dependent on disease volume and patient performance status. Patients with favourable CUP (20% of CUP patients) are managed with multimodal therapy similar to that for the equivalent metastatic tumours of known primary, and frequently enjoy long-term disease control.

Table 58.2 Clinicopathological CUP subsets

Favourable	Unfavourable
Women with serous papillary adenocarcinoma of the peritoneal cavity	Adenocarcinoma metastatic to the liver or other organ
Women with adenocarcinoma involving only axillary lymph nodes	Malignant ascites from a non-papillary adenocarcinoma
Poorly differentiated carcinoma with midline distribution	Multiple cerebral metastases from adenocarcinoma or squamous cell carcinoma
Squamous cell carcinoma involving cervical lymph nodes	Multiple lung or pleural metastases from adenocarcinoma
Neuroendocrine carcinoma of unknown primary	Multiple metastatic bone disease from an adenocarcinoma without PSA expression
Adenocarcinoma with a colon cancer profile (CDX2, CK20+ and CK7−)	Squamous cell carcinoma of the abdominal cavity
Men with blastic bone metastases and PSA-positive serum or tumour	
Patients with limited disease	
Melanoma of unknown primary with localized nodal disease	

Favourable subsets

Women with serous papillary adenocarcinoma of the peritoneal cavity

This subset accounts for 7–20% of all pelvic or peritoneal serous papillary cancers. It seems to affect women who are 3–7 years older than those with ovarian carcinoma, with a median age of 55–65 years. The clinical manifestation of this disease is similar to that for patients with Stage III or IV ovarian cancer: abdominal pain and distension, ascites and palpable masses, constipation with intestinal obstruction. The disease is predominantly located on the peritoneal, mesenteric, omental and ovarian surfaces as well as in pelvic and retroperitoneal nodes. Visceral organs are involved in <15% of the cases. Serum CA125 is a useful tumour marker since it is elevated in up to 90% of patients.

Women with isolated axillary nodal metastases from adenocarcinoma

This CUP subset affects women with a mean age of 52 years, who are most commonly postmenopausal. They present with axillary lymphadenopathy of either N1 (48%) or N2–3 disease (52%). The detection of an occult primary tumour in the breast can be achieved by MRI or following mastectomy in 60–70% of cases. Ductal adenocarcinomas are the most common histology (83%). Oestrogen and progesterone receptors are expressed in around 40%, while HER2 is over-expressed in 30%.

Poorly differentiated carcinoma with midline distribution

This is a predominantly male disease with a median age of presentation of 56 years. It presents with nodal involvement of a midline distribution affecting mainly mediastinal, retroperitoneal or supraclavicular lymph nodes, occasionally with a few peripheral node, lung or pleural metastatic lesions. Elevated AFP and β-hCG levels are found in <20% of cases. Histologically, these cases are characterized as poorly differentiated or undifferentiated carcinomas.

Squamous cell carcinoma involving cervical lymph nodes

This subset represents 5% of all CUP patients. Middle-aged or elderly, mainly male, patients with a strong history of tobacco and alcohol abuse are affected. For a detailed discussion, see Chapter 46.

Neuroendocrine carcinomas of unknown primary

CUP neuroendocrine tumours are diagnosed as low-grade or high-grade malignancies. High-grade neuroendocrine tumours represent almost 80% of all cases. Poorly differentiated CUP tumours present with disseminated disease and grow rapidly. Low-grade tumours are mainly located in the liver and manifest with symptoms associated with secretion of vasoactive peptides.

Adenocarcinoma with a colon cancer profile

This recently described CUP subset refers to patients who present with predominantly liver and peritoneal metastases, and less commonly with lung, pleural, bony or ovarian deposits. Histology is compatible with adenocarcinoma staining for CK20, CDX2 and CEA, despite normal colonoscopy.

Men with blastic metastases and elevated serum PSA

This rare CUP subset consists of male patients with osteoblastic metastases from adenocarcinoma and positive immunohistochemical PSA expression or elevated serum PSA levels.

Patients with limited disease

Patients within this subset present with a single lesion in several sites, i.e. lymph nodes, skin, liver, bone, lung, brain or adrenal gland or isolated inguinal lymphadenopathy.

Unfavourable subsets

The unfavourable group accounts for 80% of all CUP patients. The most common subset in this group is that of metastatic

Table 58.3 Prognostic schemes for survival in CUP

Author	n	Multivariate	Results
Abbruzzese	657	Male sex	
		Adenocarcinoma histological type	
		Number of metastatic sites	
		Liver metastases	
Van der Gaast	79	Poor performance status Serum alkaline phosphatase	Good prognosis: • Performance status WHO 0 and alkaline phosphatase <1.25 × normal • Median survival >4 years Intermediate prognosis: • WHO 0–≤1 or alkaline phosphatase ≥1.25 × normal • Median survival 10 months Poor prognosis: • WHO ≥1 and alkaline phosphatase ≥1.25 × normal • Median survival 4 months
Culine Petrakis	150 311	Performance status 1 Elevated LDH levels Clinicopathological subgroup Poor performance status Leucocytosis	Good risk: median overall survival (OS) 11.7 months Poor risk: median OS 3.9 months I-SCOOP score with: • Low risk: median OS 36 months • Intermediate risk: median OS 11–14 months • High risk: median OS 5–8 months

liver disease. Other organs involved are the lymph nodes (35%), lungs (31%), bones (28%) and brain (15%). The most frequent histological malignancy is adenocarcinoma (60–80%) followed by undifferentiated carcinoma (20%). These patients present with miscellaneous symptoms and signs related to the underlying metastatic organ.

Prognostic factors

Several prognostic factors have been reported for patients diagnosed with CUP, though no consensus exists, probably due to the heterogeneity of the patient cohorts studied and of the disease itself. In multivariate analyses, significant adverse prognostic indicators related to histology, clinical picture or serum markers have been identified. However, these prognostic algorithms have not been validated in independent series, have not been confirmed and do not seem to add substantially to the prognostic information provided by the classification into clinicopathological subsets. A prognostic classification is sorely needed, especially for patients with unfavourable, visceral CUP.

Culine et al. published a compact and easy to use prognostic scheme that used performance status, presence of liver metastases and baseline lactate dehydrogenase (LDH) in order to assign CUP patients to a good or a poor prognosis group. Although validated, the scheme failed to incorporate the importance of CUP clinicopathological subsets. Recently, a prognostic classification incorporating clinicopathological subset, leucocytosis and performance status from a cohort of 311 CUP patients was published, though validation in an independent cohort is lacking.

Prognostic schemes in CUP are summarized in Table 58.3.

Treatment philosophy

When defining treatment intent, the physician should consider tumour and patient characteristics. In principle, favourable CUP subset patients occasionally enjoy long-term disease control, while those within unfavourable CUP subsets seldom survive >1 year from diagnosis. Accordingly, treatment should be more aggressive in the former and palliative in the latter. However, these general considerations should be modulated by patient performance status and co-morbidities, patient preferences and individual characteristics of each unique clinical scenario.

Guidelines

Widely used guidelines on the management of CUP patients are being produced and are regularly updated by the European Society of Medical Oncology (ESMO; http://www.esmo.org/Guidelines-Practice/Clinical-Practice-Guidelines/Cancers-of-unknown-primary-site) and the National Comprehensive Cancer Centre Network (NCCN; http://www.nccn.org/professionals/physician_gls/f_guidelines.asp#occult).

Scenario	Treatment philosophy
Women with serous peritoneal carcinomatosis	- Efforts at complete or major surgical cytoreduction (debulking) with a vertical midline incision from the xiphoid to the pubis are indicated - Surgical debulking is supplemented by administration of intravenous cytotoxic chemotherapy with cisplatin or carboplatin + paclitaxel for 6–9 cycles - In the presence of high-volume 'frozen' peritoneal implants, a strategy of chemotherapy initiation followed by interval debulking may be chosen - Approximately 50% survive >2 years from diagnosis (median overall survival [OS] 18–32 months), with cure seen in 10–20%
Women with isolated axillary nodal metastases from adenocarcinoma	- Axillary nodal surgical clearance supplemented by either mastectomy or external beam radiotherapy (EBRT) of the breast according to standard techniques is supplemented by administration of adjuvant cytotoxic chemotherapy for 4–8 cycles - Breast cancer-type regimens such as CMF, FEC, CAF, TAC, EC followed by taxane are recommended - Trastuzumab and tamoxifen or aromatase inhibitors should be administered as per standard indications in the presence of tumour HER2 over-expression/amplification and oestrogen receptor (ER)/progesterone receptor (PR) expression, respectively - Prognosis is similar to that for patients with node-positive breast cancer, with 5-year survival rates of 50–70%
Poorly differentiated carcinoma with midline distribution	- Platinum-based combination chemotherapy in fit patients (cisplatin + etoposide ± bleomycin, cisplatin + taxane, cisplatin + gemcitabine). - Outcome is unpredictable, since it is likely that this subset is heterogeneous, encompassing undifferentiated mediastinal tumours, lung cancer, lymphomas, melanomas or neuroendocrine tumours: - Median survival is 14–18 months, with <20% of patients enjoying long-term disease control beyond 2 years
Squamous cervical lymph nodes	- Head and neck radiotherapy ± neck dissection ± concurrent cisplatin chemotherapy (see Chapter 46 for details) - 5-year OS by N category: N1 60.8%, all N2: 51.1%, N2a 63.6%, N2b 42.5%, N2c 37.5% and N3 26.3% (see Chapter 46)

Neuroendocrine carcinomas of unknown primary High-grade neuroendocrine CUP	- Low-grade disease:
	    - Long-acting octreotide analogue (Sandostatin) is recommended, supplemented by sunitinib or everolimus upon disease progression
	- High-grade disease:
	    - Usually managed with small cell lung cancer-type regimens, such as cisplatin or carboplatin + etoposide
	    - Prognosis is rather poor, with a median OS of 12–20 months

Adenocarcinoma with a colon cancer profile	- Though the level of evidence is low, a trial of colon cancer type-chemotherapy combinations (fluoropyrimidine + oxaliplatin or irinotecan) with bevacizumab where appropriate is recommended - Median OS is 15–20 months, which is far superior to that for typical CUP patients with visceral metastases
PSA + blastic bone metastases	- Trial of androgen-deprivation therapy (luteinizing hormone-releasing hormone [LHRH] analogue ± antiandrogens) is warranted - Median OS is 10–20 months
Limited disease	- Surgical excision or EBRT

Unfavourable, visceral CUP	- Intent of antineoplastic therapy is symptom palliation, preservation of quality of life and if possible, survival prolongation:
	    - Best supportive care, and
	    - Palliative cytotoxic chemotherapy tailored to patient fitness and co-morbidities
	- Empiric chemotherapy regimens usually combine a platinum agent with either taxane, gemcitabine, vinca alkaloid or fluoropyrimidine
	- Assigning a CUP tissue of origin by means of multigene expression profiling and treating the patient with multiagent chemotherapy and biologicals for the respective primary tumour is a strategy that is gaining acceptance:
	    - Not known whether this improves outcome compared to empirical type, primary agnostic chemotherapy
	- Median survival is <12 months

Table 58.4 Chemotherapy regimens used in patients with CUP

Regimen	Dosage
Carboplatin	AUC 5 every 3 weeks
Paclitaxel	175 mg/m² every 3 weeks
Cisplatin	60–75 mg/m² every 3 weeks
Gemcitabine	1000 mg/m² on Days 1 and 8, every 3 weeks
Cisplatin	75 mg/m² every 3 weeks
Etoposide	100 mg/m² on Days 1–3, every 3 weeks
Irinotecan	160 mg/m², every 3 weeks
Oxaliplatin	80 mg/m², every 3 weeks
Irinotecan	100 mg/m² every 3 weeks
Gemcitabine	1000 mg/m² every 3 weeks
Oxaliplatin	85–130 mg/m² every 3 weeks
Capecitabine (oral)	2000 mg/m² on Days 1–14, every 3 weeks
FOLFOX	200/400/2400/85 mg/m² every 2 weeks
Bevacizumab	5 mg/KBW every 2 weeks
FOLFIRI	200/400/2400/180 mg/m² every 2 weeks
Bevacizumab	5 mg/KBW every 2 weeks

The various chemotherapy regimens commonly used in patients with CUP clinicopathological subsets are summarized in Table 58.4.

Supportive/palliative care

Supportive and palliative care is an integral part of CUP patient management, particularly in those with unfavourable CUP.

Control of pain, biliary, renal or intestinal obstruction, dyspnoea, agitation or other tumour-related disorders as well as psychosocial support are pivotal for the preservation of patient decency and quality of life. They should be instituted early and by a multidisciplinary team with relevant expertise.

Post-treatment assessment

Assessment of response to therapy, general condition of the patient and follow-up are performed according to general standards for patients with metastatic cancer. Follow-up is based on physical examination, imaging studies and appropriately selected blood tests every 2–4 months.

For favourable CUP subset patients, the same tumour markers employed for the initial work-up can be used in the follow-up phase.

As CUP is a heterogeneous mix of clinical entities, follow-up strategies are individualized according to characteristics of the patient and the tumour.

Controversies

The main controversy in the area of CUP lies in the nature of the disease. Is there a unique molecular biology that distinguishes CUP from other typical metastatic solid tumours of known primary?

Research has highlighted that there is active angiogenesis in 50–80% of cases, over-expression of several oncogenes in 10–30% of cases (TP53, HER2, EGFR, MET, MMP), activated intracellular signalling axes (AKT, MAPK, c-MYC) in 20–35% of cases, and rarely activating point mutations in either oncogenes or tumour suppressor genes (KiSS, TP53, MET, EGFR, HER2). Circulating tumour cells exist in 50% of cases in rather low numbers and no differences exist in the global microRNA profile between CUP metastases and metastases from known primary tumours.

The accumulating evidence has so far failed to identify a CUP-specific biological signature, although translational research is now focusing on the subgroup of unfavourable, visceral CUP which seems to be the biologically 'genuine' CUP subset. The debate is important because if CUP possesses no distinct signature, the therapeutic strategy should aim towards identification of the primary and administration of primary-tailored chemotherapy with biologicals. If, on the other hand, a CUP signature exists, then therapy should be aimed at the modulation of key pro-metastatic biomolecules of the signature.

Two phase III trials (GEFCAPI04, CUP02) are currently accruing CUP patients for randomization to either empirical chemotherapy or to assignment of a primary via gene expression profiling and administration of primary-tailored chemotherapy. The aim is to examine whether biological identification of the primary in CUP followed by primary-specific antineoplastic therapy will improve patient survival.

Recommended reading

Abbruzzese JL, Abbruzzese MC, Lenzi R et al. (1995) Analysis of a diagnostic strategy for patients with suspected tumors of unknown origin. J Clin Oncol 13:2094–2103.

Culine S, Kramar A, Saghatchian M et al. (2002) Development and validation of a prognostic model to predict the length of survival in patients with carcinomas of an unknown primary site. J Clin Oncol 20:4679–4683.

Golfinopoulos V, Pentheroudakis G, Salanti G, Nearchou AD, Ioannidis JP, Pavlidis N. (2009) Comparative survival with diverse chemotherapy regimens for cancer of unknown primary site: multiple-treatments meta-analysis. Cancer Treat Rev 35:570–573.

Greco FA, Spigel DR, Yardley DA et al. (2010) Molecular profiling in unknown primary cancer: accuracy of tissue of origin prediction. Oncologist 15:500–506.

Kamposioras K, Pentheroudakis G, Pavlidis N (2013) Exploring the biology of cancer of unknown primary: breakthroughs and drawbacks. Eur J Clin Invest 43(5):491–500.

Oien KA (2009) Pathologic evaluation of unknown primary cancer. Semin Oncol 36:8–37.

Pavlidis N, Briasoulis E, Hainsworth J et al. (2003) Diagnostic and therapeutic management of cancer of an unknown primary. Eur J Cancer 39:1990–2005.

Pentheroudakis G, Briasoulis E, Pavlidis N. (2007) Cancer of unknown primary site: missing primary or missing biology? Oncologist 12:418–425.

Pentheroudakis G, Golfinopoulos V, Pavlidis N (2007) Switching benchmarks in cancer of unknown primary: from autopsy to microarray. Eur J Cancer 43:2026–2036.

Pentheroudakis G, Spector Y, Krikelis D et al. (2013) Global microRNA profiling in favorable prognosis subgroups of cancer of unknown primary (CUP) demonstrates no significant expression differences with metastases of matched known primary tumors. Clin Exp Metastasis 30(4):431–439.

Petrakis D, Pentheroudakis G, Voulgaris E, Pavlidis N (2013) Prognostication in cancer of unknown primary (CUP): Development of a prognostic algorithm in 311 cases and review of the literature. Cancer Treat Rev [Epub ahead of print].

Varadhachary GR, Raber MN, Matamorous A et al. (2008) Carcinoma of unknown primary with colon-cancer profile: changing paradigm and emerging definitions. Lancet Oncol 9:596–599.

59.1 HIV-related neoplasms

Jean-Philippe Spano[1–3], Dominique Costagliola[2,3], Sylvain Choquet[4], Fabrice Bonnet[5,6], Armelle Lavolé[7,8] and Laurent Quéro[9,10]

[1]Département d'Oncologie Médicale, Hôpital Pitié-Salpêtrière-Charles Foix, APHP, Paris, France
[2]Sorbonne Universités, UPMC University of Paris, IUC, Paris, France
[3]INSERM, Institut Pierre Louis d'Epidémiologie et de Santé Publique, Paris, France
[4]Département d'Hématologie Clinique, Hôpital Pitié-Salpêtrière-Charles Foix, APHP, Paris, France
[5]Service de Médecine Interne et Maladies Infectieuses, Hôpital Saint-André, CHU de Bordeaux, Bordeaux, France
[6]INSERM, ISPED, University of Bordeaux, Bordeaux, France
[7]Service de Pneumologie, Hôpital Tenon, APHP, France
[8]Université Pierre et Marie Curie, Paris, France
[9]Service de Cancérologie-Radiothérapie, Hôpital Saint Louis, APHP, Paris, France
[10]INSERM, Université Paris Denis Diderot, Paris, France

Introduction	• Two broad categories of malignancy exist within the HIV-infected population (people living with HIV/AIDS [PLWHA]): 　▪ AIDS-defining malignancies (ADMs): Kaposi sarcoma (KS), non–Hodgkin lymphoma (NHL) and cervical cancer 　▪ Non-ADMs: Hodgkin lymphoma, anal carcinoma, lung carcinoma and hepatocellular carcinoma are the most common • Certain risk factors such as tobacco and oncogenic viruses have been demonstrated to be independent of immunosuppression or CD4 count nadir <500/mm³ and/or a high HIV viral load • Most of these cancers (AIDS or non-AIDS) are associated with co-infection by another pathogenic agent other than HIV, e.g.: 　▪ Virus-induced cancer (human herpesvirus 8 [HHV-8] and Kaposi sarcoma) 　▪ Human papillomavirus (HPV) and cancer of the cervix and anal cancer (and certain skin and head and neck carcinomas) 　▪ Hepatitis C and V viruses and hepatocellular carcinomas 　▪ Epstein–Barr virus (EBV) and Hodgkin lymphoma 　▪ *Helicobacter pylori* and stomach cancer
Presentation	• Most of these cancers and especially the non–AIDS-related cancers harbour common characteristics compared to cancers in the general population: 　▪ Younger age at diagnosis 　▪ Advanced stage at diagnosis 　▪ Poor outcome 　▪ Higher risk of recurrence 　▪ Risk of interactions between antineoplastic and antiretroviral agents 　▪ Lower survival • Risk of development of a malignancy is significantly lower if the CD4 cell count is maintained >500 cells/mm³
Scenario	• No specific guidelines for therapy • Guidelines for the management of each cancer as in non–HIV-infected patients should be used and adapted as required
Trials	• Paucity of trials: 　▪ HIV infection is an exclusion criterion for the majority of clinical trials 　▪ Trials that have been carried out have mostly been for haematological malignancies

UICC Manual of Clinical Oncology, Ninth Edition. Edited by Brian O'Sullivan, James D. Brierley, Anil K. D'Cruz, Martin F. Fey, Raphael Pollock, Jan B. Vermorken and Shao Hui Huang. © 2015 UICC. Published 2015 by John Wiley & Sons, Ltd.

Introduction

Cancer is frequent in HIV-infected individuals, and in Europe is responsible for approximately one-third of deaths in this population. Initially, three cancers known to be virus associated were identified in the list of AIDS-defining conditions because of their association with immunodeficiency: Kaposi sarcoma (associated with HHV-8), non-Hodgkin lymphoma (associated with EBV in most cases) and cervical cancer (associated with HPV). However, non-AIDS-defining malignancies (ADMs) are also more frequent in HIV-infected individuals compared to the general population by a factor of two to three. The most frequent are Hodgkin lymphoma (associated with EBV), lung, anal (associated with HPV) and liver (associated with HBV or HCV) cancers.

For discussion of the general management of specific malignancies, see the relevant site-specific chapters.

Incidence, aetiology and screening

Incidence, aetiology and screening	Description

Incidence	• *Kaposi sarcoma (KS):*
	  ▪ Western countries: about 1 in 1000 HIV-infected patients/year
	  ▪ Standardized incidence ratio (SIR) for combination antiretroviral therapy (cART)-treated patients:
	    ○ US cohort study: 3640
	    ○ Swiss cohort study: 25.3
	• *Non-Hodgkin lymphoma:*
	  ▪ Systemic NHL:
	    ○ 463 per 100,000 person-years in non-treated HIV-infected patients
	    ○ 205 per 100,000 person-years in cART-treated patients
	  ▪ Primary brain lymphoma:
	    ○ 57 per 100,000 person-years in non-treated HIV-infected patients
	    ○ 24 per 100,000 person-years in cART-treated patients
	  ▪ Despite long-term use of antiretroviral therapy, NHL remains the leading cause of AIDS death in PLWHA in developed countries:
	    ○ 24% of AIDS-related causes of death and 7% of overall causes of death in one nationwide study
	• *Cervical cancer:*
	  ▪ In the USA, 10 times higher in HIV-infected population than in non-infected population: 1.3 per 1000 person-years
	  ▪ Among HIV-infected women, no significant change in incidence was observed between 1998 and 2003 in the USA
	• *Hodgkin lymphoma:*
	  ▪ Slightly increased in HIV patients
	  ▪ Increases with immune status:
	    ○ CD4 0–49/mm^3: 20.7 per 100,000 per year (SIR compared to immunocompetent patients 5.3)
	    ○ CD4 50–99/mm^3: 32.4 per 100,000 per year (8.2)
	    ○ CD4 100–149/mm^3: 44.7 per 100,000 per year (12)
	    ○ CD4 150–199/mm^3: 53.7 per 100,000 per year (14.5)
	    ○ CD4 ≥200/mm^3: 47.2 per 100,000 per year (12.6)
	• *Anal cancer:*
	  ▪ Incidence of this rare tumour has been increasing in the USA over the past 35 years:
	    ○ Between 1975–1984 and 1995–2004, from 0.79 to 1.24 per 100,000 in men and from 1.04 to 1.47 per 100,000 in women
	    ○ During 1980–2005, the National Cancer Institute (NCI) reported that increasing incidence in the USA was related to the HIV epidemic in men
	    ○ One-third of men with anal cancer were HIV-infected and the majority of them were men who have sex with men
	    ○ In contrast, only 1% of women with anal cancer were HIV infected
	    ○ Among the HIV-infected population, primarily a disease of younger men with median age of 42–49 years
	• *Lung cancer:*
	  ▪ Most common non-ADM:
	    ○ In PLWHA: 79 per 100,000 person-years
	  ▪ Leading cause of non-ADM mortality:
	    ○ Accounted for 38% of non-ADM deaths and 8.5% of overall causes of death in a nationwide study
	• *Hepatocellular carcinoma:*
	  ▪ Despite the introduction of cART, a dramatically increased prevalence was observed during the period 1996–2009 in HIV–HCV co-infected patients

Incidence, aetiology and screening	Description
Relative risk	- *ADMs:*
- HIV infection increases the risk of developing NHL by 15–22 fold
- HIV-infected women are at higher risk for persistent HPV infection, cervical intraepithelial neoplasms and invasive cervical cancer
- Non-*ADMs* have different relative risks compared with the general population according to cancer type:
- Highest for anal cancer and Hodgkin lymphoma:
- Risk of developing anal cancer is 32 times higher in HIV-infected men and 52 times higher in HIV-infected men who have sex with men
- Risk of developing anal cancer in HIV-infected women is 24 times higher than in the general population
- Risk of invasive anal cancer was increased not only in the pre-HAART era (before 1996) but also in the HAART era: in one study rates increased from 11 per 100,000 person-years in the pre-HAART era to 55 per 100,000 in the HAART era, and continues to increase
- More moderate increased risk for lung cancer:
- HIV infection increases the risk of developing lung cancer by 2.6-fold
- Relative risk for liver cancer depends on the frequency of HCV co-infection
- Relative risks for breast and prostate cancer, two hormone-dependent cancers, is less than for the general population (0.6 for both):
- Low breast cancer risk with HIV is specifically linked to CXCR4-using variants of HIV: these variants bind to and signal through a receptor commonly expressed on hyperplastic and neoplastic breast duct cells
Aetiology	- *Infection:*
- HHV-8 infection is associated with a higher risk of KS
- HCV infection is associated with a higher risk of NHL
- Cervical cancer is associated with persistent oncogenic HPV infection in 90% of cases:
- Common high-risk HPV types are HPV 16 and 18
- Rare high risk HPV types are HPV 31, 33, 35, 42, 52 and 58
- EBV is implicated in nearly 100% of cases of Hodgkin lymphoma but only 30% of burkitt lymphoma
- HPV infection seems to be associated with most anal cancer:
- A meta-analysis reported that HPV infection prevalence in anal cancer was about 80%
- In HIV-infected patients, HPV 16 and 18 remain the most prevalent types
- Higher proportion of multiple HPV type infections among HIV-infected patients has been reported (HPV 18, HPV 51 or HPV 68), probably as a result of immunosuppression
- Chronic HCV infection and HBV infection is more common in HIV-infected patients than in non–HIV-infected patients:
- HIV and HCV share common routes of transmission, resulting in about 30% of PLWHA being co-infected with HCV; nearly 300,000 people in the USA are co-infected with HIV and HCV
- Lung cancer is the only frequent cancer in HIV-infected patients not known to be associated with viral infection
- *Immunodeficiency:*
- ADMs (KS, NHL [including cerebral] and cervical cancer) are closely associated with immunodeficiency
- Level of immunodeficiency is a risk factor for certain cancers, even when accounting for tobacco exposure for lung cancer or for HBV or HCV status for liver cancer
- Hodgkin lymphoma, lung and liver cancers also have a higher risk in organ transplant recipients who are immunosuppressed
- Relative risk in PLWHA with current CD4 >500/mm^3 remains high for KS, anal cancer, Hodgkin lymphoma and NHL
- For ADM, also important to account for viral load and cART, as these are independent risk factors
- Lower risk of cancers in treated patients with recovered immunity (evidenced by a CD4 cell count >500/mm^3) excepting anal cancer:
- However, after accounting for immunodeficiency and adjusting for viral load, combination antiretroviral therapy (cART) is still protective, except in anal cancer, an effect mediated neither by the impact of treatment on viral load control nor on CD4 cell counts
- Premature ageing may be associated with HIV infection since age-related co-morbidities, including non-ADMs, occur at younger ages (10–20 years younger) in patients infected with HIV compared to non-infected individuals:
- However, this is debated because the differences in median age at diagnosis are modest and mostly not significant after adjusting for the difference in age distribution between patients with AIDS and the general population

(continued)

Incidence, aetiology and screening	Description
	Kaposi sarcoma • HHV-8 infection • HIV via MIP-1 and HIV TAT protein • Low CD4 count or immunodeficiency • HIV replication: 　▪ HIV viral load >4 log10 copies/mL is associated with an increased risk of KS 　▪ Use of cART is associated with a significantly decreased risk of KS **Non-Hodgkin lymphoma** • HCV infection • EBV, HHV-8 and cytomegalovirus (CMV) induce B-cell expansion in those with impaired T-cell surveillance, resulting in lymphoproliferative disorders • Age • Low CD4 count (except for Burkitt lymphoma) • HIV replication: 　▪ HIV viral load >4 log10 copies/mL is associated with an increased risk of NHL • Use of cART is associated with a significantly decreased risk of NHL **Cervical cancer** • HPV infection • HIV infection, immunosuppression • Cigarette smoking • Multiple sexual partners, younger age at first intercourse, other sexually transmitted infections such as herpes simplex virus 2 (HSV 2) **Hodgkin lymphoma** • EBV positive serology • In contrast to NHL, decrease of CD4 count is inversely correlated to disease development • Use of cART slightly decreases incidence • CD4 count >200/mm^3 **Anal cancer** • HPV infection • Those with immunosuppression after organ transplantation, HIV infection or previous cervical HPV-related disease are at increased risk • Low CD4 cell counts and its duration in HIV-infected patients: 　▪ For anal cancer patients with CD4 cell counts >500/mm^3 for at least 2 years, the relative risk was 67.5 when the CD4 nadir was <200/mm^3 for >2 years and 24.5 when the nadir was >200/mm^3 for 2 years • Risk of anal cancer in PLWHA is higher in the cART era compared to the pre-cART era: 　▪ May relate to duration of immunodeficiency and not viral load (assessed by CD4 cell count) 　▪ Immune suppression appears to affect earlier stages of intraepithelial neoplasia related to HPV and progression of anal intraepithelial neoplasia towards invasive cancer is not easily reversible • Several studies have shown that cigarette smoking is an important risk factor, especially in combination with HIV or HPV infection • Multiple sexual partners, receptive anal intercourse **Lung cancer** • Increased risk among people living with HIV/AIDS is in part attributed to heavy smoking compared with non–HIV-infected individuals: 　▪ Several studies have suggested that HIV infection is associated with the risk of lung cancer even after adjusting for cigarette smoking • Risk of HIV-associated lung cancer is not closely linked to a low CD4+ cell count or to an increased HIV viral load **Hepatocellular carcinoma** • Important causes of cirrhosis and hepatocellular carcinoma (chronic HCV infection, HBV infection and alcoholic liver disease) are more common in HIV-infected patients than in non–HIV-infected patients: 　▪ Due to shared risk factors, both cirrhosis and hepatocellular carcinoma have emerged as leading causes of death among HIV-infected patients in developed countries, with 10–18% of observed deaths mainly as a consequence of HCV co-infection

Incidence, aetiology and screening	Description

Screening and prevention	• HIV-infected patients should participate in the screening and prevention programmes available to the general population
	• cART is potentially of greatest benefit in preventing the risk of cancer in HIV-infected patients when it is able to restore and/or maintain CD4 count >500/mm^3; this is facilitated by the earlier diagnosis and treatment of HIV infection
	Non-Hodgkin lymphoma
	• B-cell stimulatory cytokines and markers of immune activation such as interleukin (IL)-6, IL-10, soluble CD23, soluble CD27, soluble CD30 and C-reactive protein (CRP) are elevated several years before the diagnosis of systemic AIDS-NHL, but their clinical value has not yet been assessed
	Cervical cancer
	• Screening with cervical cytology (Pap test):
	  ▪ Screening programmes for early detection and treatment of precancerous cervical lesions should be evaluated as the HIV-infected population ages and lives longer
	• Primary prevention strategies such as vaccination should be considered to reduce HPV infection
	• Among HIV-infected women:
	  ▪ Pap smear should be obtained twice during the first year after diagnosis of HIV infection and annually thereafter if the results are normal
	  ▪ If herpes simplex virus (HSV) co-infection, previous conization or severe immunosuppression (CD4 <200/mm^3) : two Pap smears annually with colposcopy
	  ▪ HPV vaccination recommended
	  ▪ HPV test: several studies are ongoing for high-risk women; recommended for atypical squamous cells of undetermined significance (ASC-US) Pap test
	Anal cancer
	• Anal cancer is emerging as an important cause of mortality among people with a longer duration of HIV infection
	• Value of screening programmes for anal cancer in adult high-risk populations is controversial
	• No guidelines for anal cancer screening in people with HIV infection
	• For people at high risk for anal intraepithelial neoplasia (AIN), some experts recommend screening with anal cytology testing (Pap tests) and digital anal examination:
	  ▪ If digital rectal examination reveals a macroscopic lesion or the anal Pap test reveals any abnormalities, high-resolution anoscopy (HRA) is recommended
	  ▪ Anal cytology has a high sensitivity (95%) for detection of dysplasia but a low specificity (50%)
	• A randomized controlled trial showed that quadrivalent HPV vaccine reduced by 75% the rates of grade 2 or 3 AIN related to infection with HPV 6, 11, 16 or 18 among men who have sex with men
	• The Food and Drug Administration (FDA) has approved Gardasil® HPV vaccine for the prevention of AIN caused by HPV infection
	• Smoking cessation significantly reduces the risk of developing anal cancer
	• Condoms could provide some protection, but they do not fully protect against HPV
	Lung cancer
	• Screening with low-dose helical computed tomography (CT) of the chest based on the National Lung Screening Trial data is not recommended but could be considered:
	  ▪ Cost-effectiveness of this intervention is unknown
	• Screening must not be viewed as an alternative to smoking cessation
	Hepatocellular carcinoma
	• HBV and HCV testing in all HIV-infected patients is essential
	• Alpha-fetoprotein and abdominal ultrasonography monitoring is recommended for patients with cirrhosis and HIV–HCV co-infection
	• HBV vaccination is strongly recommended for all HIV-infected patients without chronic hepatitis B or immunity to HBV
	• HAV vaccination is recommended for all hepatitis A antibody-negative patients who have chronic liver disease, who are men who have sex with men or who are injection drug users
	• Patients with chronic hepatitis B disease should be advised to avoid alcohol consumption
	• Among HIV-infected patients with HCV co-infection, early antiviral therapy is recommended

AIDS-DEFINING MALIGNANCIES

Kaposi sarcoma

Concurrent with the long-term use of antiretroviral therapy, KS has substantially declined in incidence and prevalence. In addition, the natural history has changed in that its behaviour is less aggressive. Thus there has been a decrease in mortality and morbidity. The most common presentation is cutaneous lesions although visceral KS is not uncommon.

Pathology

AIDS-Kaposi sarcoma is characterized by proliferation of spindle cells that seem to originate from endothelial and mesenchymal cells.

Presentation

- High variability in the cutaneous lesion
- May be brown or wine coloured
- Sometimes painful
- May be associated lymphoedema with possible extracutaneous extent, especially in patients uncontrolled by cART or without any antiretroviral treatment
- Locations:
  - Cutaneous; any site but most frequent are:
    - Extremities
    - Trunk
    - Face
  - Mucous membranes such as the oral cavity can be involved
  - Visceral localizations: any organ but most common are:
    - Gastrointestinal tract
    - Lung
- Visceral KS is responsible for numerous symptoms and/or complications:
  - Bleeding (digestive tract)
  - Abdominal or chest pain
- Shortness of breath, cough or haemoptysis (pulmonary lesions)
- Fever
- Clinical course is more aggressive in:
  - PLWHA not undergoing cART and/or with no control of HIV replication
  - Patients with severe immunosuppression

Diagnostic work-up

- Complete physical examination
- Biopsy of accessible lesions like those in skin; may be more difficult for visceral lesions
- Computed tomography (CT) scan should be performed if there are known or suspected visceral lesions
- Gastrointestinal endoscopy for intestinal symptoms
- Bronchoscopy if abnormal chest radiograph or pulmonary symptoms

Prognostic grouping and factors

Prognostic grouping

The advent of HAART has altered the presentation and evolution of AIDS-KS. However, AIDS-related KS is still staged according to the AIDS Clinical Trials Group Classification system or 'TIS'. Patients are categorized into good or poor risk depending on tumour burden, CD4 cell count and the presence of visceral lesions (Table 59.1.1)

Prognostic factors

- Immune status
- CD4 cell count
- Age
- Occurrence of the tumour after AIDS onset
- Visceral localizations
- Presence of co-morbidities

Treatment philosophy

Therapeutic strategies depend on numerous factors: cutaneous or extracutaneous lesions, HIV viral load, CD4 cell count and co-morbidities. Strategies can be local or systemic.

- In HAART-naïve patients, antiretroviral treatment should be started without delay
- In pretreated patients, antiretroviral treatment should be reassessed:
  - Protease inhibitor or non-nucleoside reverse transcriptase inhibitors have demonstrated similar activities
  - Risk of immune reconstitution inflammatory syndrome (IRIS) when the immune system recovers

Table 59.1.1 TIS classification of Kaposi sarcoma associated with HIV infection

Good risk (all of the following)	Poor risk (any of the following)
Tumour (T): confined to skin and/or lymph nodes and/or minimal oral disease	Tumour (T): tumour-associated oedema ulceration, extensive oral KS, gastrointestinal KS, KS in other non-nodal viscera
Immune status (I): CD4 cells ≥200/μL	Immune status (I): CD4 cells <200/μL
Systemic: no history of opportunistic infection	Systemic: history of opportunistic infection and/or thrush
Illness (S): no 'B' symptoms, Karnofsky performance status (KPS) ≥70	Illness (S): 'B' symptoms present, KPS <70, other HIV-related illness (neurological disease, lymphoma)

Treatment

Treatment: KS	Description

Local treatment	• For cutaneous lesions, symptomatic control and/or cosmesis:
	  ▪ Surgical excisions
	  ▪ Radiotherapy
	  ▪ Cryotherapy
	  ▪ Local chemotherapy (intralesional: bleomycin, vinblastine)
	  ▪ Laser treatment
	  ▪ Photodynamic treatment

Systemic treatment	• *Cytotoxic chemotherapy:*
	  ▪ For patients with an aggressive presentation, significant progressive disease, life-threatening disease, symptomatic visceral involvement or multiple cutaneous lesions (>20)
	  ▪ Main active drugs are anthracyclines, especially liposomal anthracyclines, bleomycin and taxanes
	  ▪ Liposomal anthracyclines such as liposomal daunorubicin (40 mg/m^2 every 2 weeks) or pegylated liposomal doxorubicin (20 mg/m^2 every 3 weeks) have shown significantly more effectiveness with concomitant HAART treatment compared with the ABV regimen (adriamycin + bleomycin + vincristine)
	  ▪ Taxanes, such as paclitaxel or docetaxel, both have a cytotoxic effect on KS cells but also can inhibit angiogenesis:
	    ○ Paclitaxel: 135–175 mg/m^2 every 3 weeks or 100 mg/m^2 every 2 weeks.
	    ○ Paclitaxel is approved in the USA for the treatment of KS in patients with KS resistant to anthracyclines
	  ▪ Concern for potential interaction via the P450 cytochrome (CYP3A4) and in particular with the concomitant use of protease inhibitor and certain non-nucleoside reverse transcriptase inhibitors.
	    ○ Caution is necessary and treatment modifications are necessary
	• *Immunotherapy:*
	  ▪ Interferon-alpha has been approved for KS:
	    ○ More effective in patients with a CD4 cell count of >200/μL and asymptomatic HIV infection
	    ○ Can be recommended in patients with good HIV replication control, under HAART and with moderate cutaneous localizations
	    ○ Can have numerous side effects such as fever, fatigue, chills, 'flu' syndrome, neutropenia, thrombopenia
	• *Molecular targeted therapies:*
	  ▪ Role of several signalling pathways involved in KS oncogenesis has led to clinical trials with molecular targeted therapies, although none has been approved for treatment:
	    ○ Angiogenesis inhibitors
	    ○ Several tyrosine kinase inhibitors
	    ○ mTOR inhibitors, etc.

Non-Hodgkin lymphoma (see also Chapter 32)

Despite long-term use of antiretroviral therapy, NHL remains the leading cause of AIDS death in PLWHA in developed countries.

Pathology

Pathologically, AIDS-NHL is almost exclusively B-cell lymphoma of aggressive type.

The World Health Organization (WHO) classifies AIDS-NHL into three categories (Box 59.1.1):
- Lymphomas also occurring in immunocompetent patients
- Lymphomas occurring more specifically in HIV-positive patients
- Lymphomas occurring in other immunodeficiency states.

> **Box 59.1.1** WHO classification of lymphoid malignancies associated with HIV infection
>
> - Lymphomas also occurring in immunocompetent patients:
>   ▪ Burkitt
>   ▪ Diffuse large B-cell lymphomas:
>   ○ Centroblastic
>   ○ Immunoblastic (including primary central nervous system [CNS] lymphomas)
>   ▪ Extranodal mucosa-associated lymphoid tissue (MALT) lymphoma
>   ▪ Peripheral T-cell lymphoma
>   ▪ Classical Hodgkin lymphoma
>   ▪ NK-cell lymphoma
> - Lymphoma occurring more specifically in HIV-positive patients:
>   ▪ Primary effusion lymphoma
>   ▪ Plasmablastic lymphoma: lymphoma arising in HHV 8 associated multicentric Castelman Disease
> - Lymphoma occurring in other immunodeficiency states:
>   ▪ Polymorphic B-cell lymphoma (post-transplant lymphoproliferative disorder [PTLD]-like)

Presentation

The clinical course of NHL is more aggressive in PLWHA and patients present with a more advanced stage than non-infected individuals.

- Unexplained weight loss
- Fatigue/lack of energy
- Recurring fevers
- Night sweats, usually with fever
- Rashes
- Swollen lymph node
- Frequent extranodal sites involved in PLWHA:
  - Bone marrow
  - Liver
  - Meninges and CNS
  - Gastrointestinal tract
- Unusual but characteristic extranodal sites involved in people living with HIV/AIDS:
  - Anus
  - Heart
  - Mouth
  - Muscles
- Abnormalities on blood tests:
  - Anaemia
  - Thrombopenia
  - Leucopenia
- Neurological deficits suggest primary brain lymphomas
- Primary effusion lymphoma is associated with HHV-8 and presents as a pleural, pericardiac and/or peritoneal inflammatory effusion without nodes.

Diagnostic work-up

- Diagnosis should be biopsy-proven:
  - Enough tissue is needed to allow assessment of cells and architecture
  - Specimens may require flow cytometry, cytogenetics and microbiology studies in addition to routine microscopic pathology.
- CT and ^{18}FDG-positron emission tomography (PET) are recommended
- Lumbar puncture is necessary:
- If lumbar puncture shows lymphoma cells or in case of neurological symptoms, magnetic resonance imaging (MRI) of the brain is mandatory
  - MRI with gadolinium contrast is the best imaging modality to differentiate primary brain lymphoma (PBL) from other causes of brain mass

Staging and prognostic factors

For the Ann Arbor staging, see Chapter 32.

International prognostic index (IPI)

- Age (<60 years vs >60 years)
- Performance status (ECOG 0 or 1 versus >1)
- Tumour staging according to the Ann Arbor classification (Stage I or II vs Stage III or IV)
- Serum lactate dehydrogenase (LDH) (normal range vs elevated)
- Extranodal site involvement (0 or 1 vs >1)

Patients with a score of ≥2 have a <50% chance of relapse-free and overall survival at 5 years.

Prognostic factors

- CD4 lymphocytes count <100 cells/mm^3
- AIDS stage
- Control of HIV replication through antiretroviral therapy (good prognosis)

Treatment philosophy

In addition to specific antitumor treatment, the management of HIV/AIDS patients undergoing chemotherapy should include:

- In naïve patients, antiretroviral treatment should be started without delay
- In both HAART-naïve and pretreated patients, the antiretroviral combination should consider:
  - Risk of pharmacokinetic interactions between antiretrovirals and chemotherapy
  - Risk of cumulative toxicities (bone marrow, liver, kidney, peripheral nerves)
  - Previous history of antiretroviral sequences and of resistance mutations
  - HBV serological status
- Goal of antiretroviral therapy is the control of HIV RNA replication below 50 copies as associated with an increased survival
- Irrespective of the CD4 count, systematic prophylaxis against toxoplasmosis and pneumocystosis with cotrimoxazole is necessary:
  - Cotrimoxazole prophylaxis should be maintained throughout anticancer treatment and stopped after treatment if CD4 lymphocyte count is >200/mm^3 and 15% for at least 6 months
- Systematic prophylaxis of herpes infection with valacyclovir should be started before chemotherapy
- Monitoring of cytomegalovirus (CMV) DNA: if >1000 copies/mL, CMV retinitis should be evaluated and valganciclovir prophylaxis should be implemented (valacyclovir prophylaxis can be stopped)

Once these recommendations are in place, HIV patients with NHL should be treated according to guidelines developed for patients without HIV infection.

Specific treatment

Scenario	Specific treatment
Systemic NHL	- Addition of rituximab (anti-CD20 chimeric monoclonal antibody) to CHOP has been demonstrated to be superior to CHOP alone in the treatment of diffuse large B-cell lymphoma (DLBCL) in non-HIV infected patients: - However, no benefit to the addition of rituximab to CHOP in patients with a CD4 count of <50/mm^3 because of the increased risk of lethal bacterial infections

Scenario	Specific treatment
	▪ Most oncologist favour the use of rituximab with standard chemotherapy in patients with a CD4 count of >50/mm³ ▪ In patients with a CD4 count of <50/mm³, treatment should be adapted according to the risk of infection • Methotrexate may be used in patients with testicular or neurological involvement
Burkitt	• Patients with good performance status and controlled HIV infection may benefit from intensive chemotherapy such as that used in the non-HIV population (COPADM, CODOX-M/IVAC): ▪ Should include prophylactic intrathecal CNS • In patient in fragile condition, adapted chemotherapy like Short-course-EPOCH-R or R-CHOP-Méthotrexate can be proposed • Thanks to these adapted treatments, prognosis of Burkitt lymphoma is similar to high grade DLBCL but still inferior to immunocompetent Burkitt lymphoma
Primary brain lymphoma	• Reversal of advanced immunosuppression is the main goal • In addition to starting or modifying antiretroviral treatment to improve virological and immunological response, two to four cycles of methotrexate + aracytine (+ prednisone during the first days in case of cerebral oedema) may be sufficient to control disease: ▪ In patients already well controlled for HIV infection, six cycles of methotrexate + aracytine may be appropriate • Radiotherapy alone (35–40 Gy in 1.75–2-Gy fractions) is reserved for second-line treatment
NHL relapse	• Patients with well-controlled HIV infection should be treated along the same lines as non-HIV infected patients • Patients should be considered for autologous stem cell transplantation if appropriate since the prognosis is no different from that for non-HIV infected patients

Cervical cancer (see also Chapter 35)

Natural history and pathology
- Cervical carcinoma has its origins at the squamocolumnar junction
- Most cases are preceded by intraepithelial precursor lesions
- Two main types: squamous cell carcinoma and adenocarcinoma:
  - Squamous cell lesions which most often begin from the exocervix (80–90%): cervical intraepithelial neoplasia (CIN 1–3)
  - Lesions from the mucus-producing gland cells of the endocervix (15%): *in situ* adenocarcinoma, invasive adenocarcinoma
- Adenosquamous carcinomas or mixed carcinomas have features of both squamous cell carcinomas and adenocarcinomas

Presentation
- Vaginal bleeding
- Post-intercourse vaginal bleeding
- Vaginal discharge
- Pain during sexual intercourse

Diagnostic work-up
- Histopathological diagnosis: colposcopy with directed biopsy
- Local tumour staging is based on physical examination and MRI
- Distant tumour staging is based on CT
- Increasing evidence that FDG-PET-CT has a role in the primary evaluation of cervical carcinoma, in particular for evaluating lymph node status and distant metastatic disease

Staging
See Chapter 35.

Treatment
- See Chapter 35 for standard therapy
- *Specific features for HIV-infected women*:
  - Among patients undergoing chemotherapy, the antiretroviral combination should consider:
    - Pharmacokinetic interactions between antiretrovirals and chemotherapy
    - Potential interactions between antiretrovirals and radiotherapy are not known
  - Retrospective studies have reported poor outcome after radiotherapy in HIV-infected women with poor treatment compliance due to skin, gastrointestinal and genitourinary toxicities

NON–AIDS-RELATED MALIGNANCIES

Hodgkin lymphoma (see also Chapter 32)

Pathology
- Two commonest forms of Hodgkin lymphoma are:
  - Mixed cellularity
  - Lymphocyte depleted
- Less frequently: nodular sclerosis
- Association with EBV in nearly 100% of cases:
  - LMP1+
  - EBER+

Presentation
- *General symptoms:*
  - Weight loss (≥10%)
  - Fever (≥ 38°C)
  - Sweats
  - Pruritus
- *Tumoural syndrome:*
  - Nodes
  - Compressive symptoms like pericarditis, oedema, thrombophlebitis
- *Biological abnormalities:*
  - Anaemia
  - Hypereosinophilia
  - Hypoalbuminaemia
  - Inflammation

Diagnostic work-up
- Diagnosis is made by biopsy
- Extension screening comports:
  - CT neck, thorax, abdomen and pelvis
  - PET scan
- Bone marrow biopsy

Staging and prognostic factors
For Ann Arbor staging, see Chapter 32.
Prognostic factors
- Male gender
- ≥45 years old
- Albuminaemia <40 g/L
- Haemoglobin <10.5 g/dL
- White blood cells ≥15,000/mm^3
- Lymphocytes <600 /mm^3

Treatment
Treatment should whenever possible be the same as that given to immunocompetent patients. Neither overall survival nor event-free survival is decreased in HIV patients.

In addition to specific antitumour treatment, the management of HIV/AIDS patients undergoing chemotherapy should include:
- Start or modification of antiretroviral treatment adapted to prevent pharmacokinetic interactions between antiretrovirals and chemotherapy
- Control of HIV RNA replication
- Systematic prophylaxis for toxoplasmosis and pneumocystosis infections with cotrimoxazole:
  - Prophylaxis should be maintained throughout anticancer treatment and stopped after treatment if CD4 lymphocytes count is >200/mm^3
- Systematic prophylaxis of herpes infection with valacyclovir
- Monitoring of CMV DNA: if >1000 copies/mL, CMV retinitis should be evaluated and valganciclovir prophylaxis implemented (valacyclovir prophylaxis can be stopped)
- *Specific treatment*:
  - In refractory/relapsing patients, autologous stem cell transplantation may be considered

Anal carcinoma (see also Chapter 26.2)

Pathology and natural history
Squamous cell carcinoma is the most common histological subtype in HIV-infected patients.

As in cervical cancer, anal cancer is thought to be preceded by preneoplastic lesions of varying severity: anal intraepithelial neoplasia (AIN I, II or III).

Presentation
- Bleeding from the anus
- Pain in the area around the anus
- Tumour or ulceration near the anus
- Itching from the anus
- Discharge from the anus
- Change in bowel habits

Diagnostic work-up
- Histopathological diagnosis: anoscopy with directed biopsy
- Local tumour staging is based on digital rectal examination, endoanal/endorectal ultrasound and MRI
- Distant tumour staging is based on CT

Staging and prognostic factors
For staging, see Chapter 26.2.
Prognostic factors
- Tumour size
- Lymph node involvement

Treatment
The treatment of anal cancer is not dependent on HIV status.
- Standard treatment for local anal cancer is radiotherapy with concurrent 5-fluorouracil (5-FU) and mitomycin C (see Chapter 26.2)
- Several retrospective studies have reported overall 5-year survival of 62–67% in HIV-infected patients treated with combined chemoradiotherapy, which is comparable to the rate for non–HIV-infected patients
- Some studies have reported high local recurrence rates (30 – 60%) and low sphincter preservation after chemoradiotherapy in HIV-infected patients in comparison with non–HIV-infected patients (25–30%)
- Several studies have reported that HIV-infected patients have lower treatment tolerance with higher rates of severe acute skin, gastrointestinal and haematological toxicities during chemoradiotherapy, resulting in prolonged overall treatment time compared with non–HIV-infected patients:
  - Completion of chemoradiotherapy as scheduled is an important factor for tumour control and duration of radiotherapy could in part explain the low local control observed in HIV-infected patients
  - Modern radiotherapy techniques such as intensity-modulated radiotherapy (IMRT) could reduce severe skin and digestive toxicity because surrounding normal tissues such

as the small bowel, genitalia and iliac bone marrow can potentially be spared
- Close multidisciplinary monitoring by a radiation oncologist and an infectious disease specialist is recommended to adapt antiretroviral therapy and manage acute side effects during chemoradiotherapy

Lung cancer (see also Chapter 20)

Pathology
- Non-small cell lung cancer (NSCLC) represents 86–94% of cases with adenocarcinoma and is the most common histological type (30–52%)
- Squamous cell cancer is the second most common histological type (19–36%)

Presentation
- Diagnosed a decade or more earlier in PLWHA:
    - Mean age 46 years
- Respiratory complaints: cough, chest pain, haemoptysis, dyspnoea
- Unexplained weight loss
- Fatigue

Diagnostic work-up
- Obtaining adequate tissue material for histological diagnosis and molecular testing is important
- CT including brain and 18-FDG-PET is recommended
- As many as 70–90% of HIV-infected lung cancer patients are diagnosed with locally or metastatic carcinoma

Staging and prognostic factors
For staging, see Chapter 20.
Prognostic factors
- Performance status (ECOG 0 or 1 vs 2–4)
- Tumour staging
- Use of HAART (associated with increased survival)
- CD4 lymphocyte count >200 cells/mm^3 at diagnosis (associated with increased survival in one study)
- NSCLC patients with HIV have a poorer prognosis than patients without evidence of HIV

Treatment
- In the absence of scientific evidence to support otherwise, it is generally recommended to treat PLWHA with lung cancer similarly to non-infected patients (see Chapter 20)
- Surgery is the treatment of choice for localized NSCLC
- For metastatic NSCLC, the treatment strategy must take into account histology, molecular pathology, age, performance status and co-morbidities
- Platinum-based combination chemotherapy is recommended:
    - Possible potentiation of toxic effects of lung chemotherapy as several frequently employed agents (taxanes, vinca alkaloids, etoposide, erlotinib and gefitinib) are metabolized by cytochrome P450 enzymes and some antiretroviral agents, especially protease inhibitors, inhibit these enzymes

There is a need for prospective clinical trials in PLWHA with lung cancer to improve the understanding of lung cancer pathogenesis and to optimize patient care. Several clinical trials are in progress to address questions in cancer biology, screening and treatment of this disease

Hepatocellular carcinoma (see also Chapter 22)

Pathology
- Hepatocellular carcinoma
- Fibrolamellar carcinoma

Presentation
- Usually presents with symptoms of advancing cirrhosis and liver failure.
    - Jaundice
    - Pruritus
    - Ascites
    - Peripheral oedema
    - Confusion
    - Flapping tremor
    - Abdominal pain
    - Splenomegaly
    - Hepatomegaly
    - Spider naevi
    - Periumbilical collateral veins
    - Haemathemesis
    - Melaena
    - Anaemia

Diagnostic work-up
- Triple-phase, contrast-enhanced studies (dynamic CT or MRI):
    - Presence of arterial uptake followed by washout in a single dynamic study is highly specific (95–100%) for a liver tumour of 1–3 cm in diameter
- Tumour biopsy if the diagnosis is not established by dynamic imaging

Staging and prognostic factors
For staging, see Chapter 22.
Prognostic factors
- Tumour size
- Number of nodules
- Presence of vascular invasion
- Extrahepatic spread
- Performance status
- Child–Pugh score

Treatment

No consensual guideline for managing hepatocellular carcinoma in HIV-infected population is available.

- Like non–HIV-infected patients, PLWHA with early-stage disease without cirrhosis are usually treated with surgical resection
- For PLWHA with early-stage disease and established cirrhosis, orthotopic liver transplantation (OLT) is controversial:
  - HIV-infected patients should be carefully selected before OLT because of the complexity of the post-treatment management, particularly in patients with HCV co-infection
  - OLT is feasible in HIV-infected patients:
    - In a recent meta-analysis, 1-year mortality in HIV-infected patients was 16%, which was similar to the rate in non–HIV-infected liver transplant recipients (17%)
- In patients who are not eligible for surgery or OLT because of co morbidities or liver dysfunction, local ablative therapies can be used:
  - Percutaneous ethanol injection
  - Radiofrequency ablation
  - Cryoablation
  - Stereotactic body radiation therapy
  - Transcatheter arterial chemoembolization (TACE) can be considered in patients with unresectable disease and well-compensated cirrhosis
- Sorafenib is a multikinase inhibitor that has antiangiogenic, pro-apoptotic and raf-kinase inhibitory properties:
  - Approved in patients with unresectable hepatocellular carcinoma but it has not been evaluated in HIV-infected patients

Recommended readings

Biggar RJ, Jaffe ES, Goedert JJ, Chaturvedi A, Pfeiffer R, Engels EA (2006) Hodgkin lymphoma and immunodeficiency in persons with HIV/AIDS. *Blood* 108(12):3786–3791.

Bohlius J, Schmidlin K, Costagliola D et al. (2009) Incidence and risk factors of HIV-related non-Hodgkin's lymphoma in the era of combination antiretroviral therapy: a European multicohort study. *Antivir Ther* 14(8):1065–1074.

Boué F, Gabarre J, Gisselbrecht C, et al. Phase II trial of CHOP plus rituximab in patients with HIV-associated non-Hodgkin's lymphoma. *J Clin Oncol*. 2006; 24:4123-4128.

Clifford GM, Polesel J, Rickenbach M, et al. Cancer risk in the Swiss HIV Cohort Study: associations with immunodeficiency, smoking, and highly active antiretroviral therapy. *J Natl Cancer Inst*. 2005; 97:425-32.

Crum-Cianflone NF, Hullsiek KH, Marconi VC et al. (2010) Anal cancers among HIV-infected persons: HAART is not slowing rising incidence. *AIDS* 24:535–543.

Di Lorenzo G, Konstantinopoulos PA, Pantanowitz L et al. (2007) Management of AIDS-related Kaposi's sarcoma. *Lancet Oncol* 8:167–176.

Engels EA, Pfeifer RM, Goedert J et al. (2006) Trends in cancer risk among people with AIDS in the United States 1980–2002. *AIDS* 20:1645–1654.

Fraunholz I, Weiss C, Eberlein K, Haberl A, Rodel C (2010) Concurrent chemoradiotherapy with 5-fluorouracil and mitomycin C for invasive anal carcinoma in human immunodeficiency virus-positive patients receiving highly active antiretroviral therapy. *Int J Radiat Oncol Biol Phys* 76:1425–1432.

Gichangi P, Bwayo J, Estambale B et al. (2006) HIV impact on acute morbidity and pelvic tumor control following radiotherapy for cervical cancer. *Gynecol Oncol* 100:405–411

Guiguet M, Boué F, Cadranel J, Lang JM, Rosenthal E, Costagliola D, on behalf of the Clinical Epidemiology Group of the FHDH-ANRS CO4 cohort (2009) Effect of immunodeficiency, HIV viral load, and antiretroviral therapy on the risk of individual malignancies (FHDH-ANRS CO4): a prospective cohort study. *Lancet Oncol* 10:1152–1159.

Ioannou GN, Bryson CL, Weiss NS, Miller R, Scott JD, Boyko EJ (2013) The prevalence of cirrhosis and hepatocellular carcinoma in patients with human immunodeficiency virus infection. *Hepatology* 57:249–257.

Kaplan LD, Lee JY, Ambinder RF, et al. Rituximab does not improve clinical outcome in a randomized phase 3 trial of CHOP with or without rituximab in patients with HIV-associated non-Hodgkin lymphoma: AIDS-Malignancies Consortium Trial 010. *Blood*. 2005; 106:1538-43

Krown SE, Metroka C, Wernz JC (1989) Kaposi's Sarcoma in the acquired immune deficiency syndrome: a proposal for uniform evaluation, response, and staging criteria. AIDS Clinical Trials Group Oncology Committee. *J Clin Oncol*. 7: 1201-1207

Levine AM, Noy A, Lee JY et al. (2013) Pegylated liposomal doxorubicin, rituximab, cyclophosphamide, vincristine, and prednisone in AIDS-related lymphoma: AIDS Malignancy Consortium Study 047. *J Clin Oncol* 31:58–64.

Montoto S, Shaw K, Okosun J et al. (2012) HIV status does not influence outcome in patients with classical Hodgkin lymphoma treated with chemotherapy using doxorubicin, bleomycin, vinblastine, and dacarbazine in the highly active antiretroviral therapy era. *J Clin Oncol* 30(33):4111–4116.

Palefsky JM, Giuliano AR, Goldstone S et al. (2011) HPV vaccine against anal HPV infection and anal intraepithelial neoplasia. *N Engl J Med* 365:1576–1585.

Rodrigo JA, Hicks LK, Cheung MC, et al. HIV-Associated Burkitt Lymphoma: Good Efficacy and Tolerance of Intensive Chemotherapy Including CODOX-M/IVAC with or without Rituximab in the HAART Era. *Adv Hematol*. 2012;2012:735392.

Roussillon C, Henard S, Hardel L et al. (2010) Cause de décès des patients infectés par le VIH en France en 2010 : Etude ANRS EN20 Mortalité. *BEH* 46-47:541–545.

Shcherba M, Shuter J, Haigentz M (2013) Current questions in HIV-associated lung cancer. *Curr Opin Oncol* 25(5):511–517.

Shrivastava SK, Engineer R, Rajadhyaksha S, et al. (2005) HIV infection and invasive cervical cancers, treatment with radiation therapy: toxicity and outcome. *Radiother Oncol*, 74, 31-5.

Silverberg MJ, Chao C, Leyden WA et al. (2011) HIV Infection, immunodeficiency, viral replication, and the risk of cancer. *Cancer Epidemiol Biomarkers Prev* 20:2551–2559.

Simonds HM, Wright JD, Du Toit N, Neugut AI, Jacobson JS (2012) Completion of and early response to chemoradiation among human immunodeficiency virus (HIV)-positive and HIV-negative patients with locally advanced cervical carcinoma in South Africa. *Cancer* 118:2971–2979.

Spano JP, Costagliola D, Katlama C, Mounier N, Oksenhendler E, Khayat D (2008) AIDS-related malignancies: state of the art and therapeutic challenges. *J Clin Oncol* 26:4834–4842.

Wyen C, Jensen B, Hentrich M et al. (2012) Treatment of AIDS-related lymphomas: rituximab is beneficial even in severely immunosuppressed patients. *AIDS* 26:457–464.

Xicoy B, Ribera JM, Miralles P, et al. Results of treatment with doxorubicin, bleomycin, vinblastine and dacarbazine and highly active antiretroviral therapy in advanced stage, human immunodeficiency virus-related Hodgkin's lymphoma. *Haematologica*. 2007;92(2):191-8.

59.2 Post-transplantation lymphoproliferative disease

Jean-Philippe Spano[1-3], Sylvain Choquet[4], Fabrice Bonnet[5,6], Armelle Lavolé[7,8] and Laurent Quéro[9,10]

[1]Département d'Oncologie Médicale, Hôpital Pitié-Salpêtrière-Charles Foix, APHP, Paris, France
[2]Sorbonne Universités, UPMC University of Paris, IUC, Paris, France
[3]INSERM, Institut Pierre Louis d'Epidémiologie et de Santé Publique, Paris, France
[4]Département d'Hématologie Clinique, Hôpital Pitié-Salpêtrière-Charles Foix, APHP, Paris, France
[5]Service de Médecine Interne et Maladies Infectieuses, Hôpital Saint-André, CHU de Bordeaux, Bordeaux, France
[6]INSERM, ISPED, University of Bordeaux, Bordeaux, France
[7]Service de Pneumologie, Hôpital Tenon, APHP, France
[8]Université Pierre et Marie Curie, Paris, France
[9]Service de Cancérologie-Radiothérapie, Hôpital Saint Louis, APHP, Paris, France
[10]INSERM, Université Paris Denis Diderot, Paris, France

Introduction

Post-transplantation lymphoproliferative disease (PTLD) represents the most frequent cancer following transplantation. It is a specific entity defined by the World Health Organization (WHO). Epstein–Barr virus (EBV) is not the only causative factor but high viral load is a predictive factor for the development of PTLD and should be treated. New treatments have resulted in prolonged overall survivals (>6 years), which are quite similar to those for immunocompetent patients with NHL.

Incidence, aetiology and screening

Incidence, aetiology and screening	Description

Incidence	• Most frequent cancer after transplantation:
	  ▪ 194 per 100,000 per year (173 per 100,000 per year for bronchopulmonary cancer)
	  ▪ Increased risk of 7.54 compared to the general population
	• Risk depends on the transplanted organ:
	  ▪ 1–5% after kidney or liver transplantation
	  ▪ 3–8% after heart or lung transplantation
	  ▪ >10% after gut transplantation
	  ▪ <1% for matched allogeneic stem cell transplantation
	  ▪ 2% at 2 years for cord blood transplantation
	• Increases with time from transplantation: 15% at 13 years for heart
	• Depends on age:
	  ▪ 1.74–3.28% at 5 years until 34 years old
	  ▪ 0.36–2.22% after age 50 years
	  ▪ 10.1% in children with a kidney transplant versus 1.2% for adults
	  ▪ 6.7% at 1 year in children with a liver transplant versus 1.4%

UICC Manual of Clinical Oncology, Ninth Edition. Edited by Brian O'Sullivan, James D. Brierley, Anil K. D'Cruz, Martin F. Fey, Raphael Pollock, Jan B. Vermorken and Shao Hui Huang. © 2015 UICC. Published 2015 by John Wiley & Sons, Ltd.

Incidence, aetiology and screening	Description
Aetiology	- By definition transplantation and immunosuppression
- Main risk factor is an EBV-negative status for the patient but positive for the graft, leading to a very high risk of EBV primary infection and subsequent PTLD
- Other risk factors are:
- Young age
- Gut transplantation
- Use of anti-T-lymphocyte sera (OKT3) and other antilymphocyte sera
- Total-body irradiation
- Use of azathioprine
Screening	- EBV viral load is the best predictive test of PTLD and should be treated: reduced immunosuppression ± rituximab
- Treatment is necessary if:
- High viral load (>10^5 copies/mL) in an EBV-positive patient
- Positive viral load in an EBV negative patient (= primary infection)
- Monoclonal gammopathy has been described in the past as a predictive factor of PTLD, but this has not been confirmed

Pathology

- Early lesions:
  - Plasmacytic hyperplasia
  - Infectious mononucleosis-like PTLD
- Polymorphic PTLD
- Monomorphic PTLD:
  - *B-cell neoplasms:*
    - Diffuse large B-cell lymphoma
    - Burkitt lymphoma
    - Plasma cell myeloma
    - Plasmacytoma-like lesion
    - Other
  - *T-cell neoplasms:*
    - Peripheral T-cell lymphoma, not otherwise specified
    - Hepatosplenic T-cell lymphoma
    - Other
- Classical Hodgkin lymphoma-type PTLD
- Indolent small B-cell lymphoma and mantle cell lymphoma are not considered as PTLD
- Association with EBV in nearly 50% of cases, more frequently in the first year:
  - *LMP1* +
  - *EBER* +

Presentation

- *General symptoms:*
  - Weight loss (≥10%)
  - Fever (≥38 °C)
  - Sweats
  - Pruritus
  - Tumoural syndrome
  - Nodes
  - Compressive symptoms like pericarditis, oedema, thrombophlebitis
  - Digestive bleeding
  - Bronchus obstruction, dyspnoea
- *Biological abnormalities:*
  - Anaemia
  - Hypereosinophilia
  - Hypoalbuminaemia
  - Inflammation
  - Cholestasis

Diagnostic work-up

- CT scan of the neck, thorax, abdomen and pelvis
- PET scan
- EBV viral load
- Bone marrow biopsy

Staging and prognostic factors

- Ann Arbor staging
- Consensus on:
  - General status (ECOG)
  - Cerebral localization (10% of PTLD)
- Uncertain:
  - LDH
  - EBV negative
- Extranodal localization

Treatment

- Management needs a close collaboration between transplant units and oncologist

- Decrease of immunosuppression is necessary and must be decided by the transplant team
- Careful screening for graft rejection
- *Specific treatment*
  - First step (graft resection is no longer an option):
    - Decrease the immunosuppression
    - If possible, wait 3–4 weeks until restaging
    - Decrease of immunosuppression alone can cure 5% of PTLD
  - Second step:
    - Four injections of rituximab 375 mg/m^2 at weekly intervals
  - Third step depends on the screening 4 weeks after rituximab:
    - Complete response (around 30% of cases): add four injections of rituximab
    - In other cases: R-CHOP every 21 days × 4
    - In case of partial response, some recommend further rituximab before using chemotherapy
    - If progression during rituximab, treat directly with R-CHOP
    - If T-cell PTLP: CHOP after decrease of immunosuppression
    - If the central nervous system (CNS) is involved there is no consensus on management:
      - High-dose methotrexate may be necessary (if renal function is sufficient).
      - Other considerations are high-dose cytarabine, radiotherapy and rituximab
    - Relapse/refractory PTLD: anti-EBV T lymphocytes have been used but are being assessed further
    - Radiotherapy and surgery should be considered in Stage I PTLD

Recommended reading

Engels EA, Pfeiffer RM, Fraumeni JF Jr et al. (2011) Spectrum of cancer risk among US solid organ transplant recipients. *JAMA* 306(17):1891–1901.

Hall EC, Pfeiffer RM, Segev DL, Engels EA (2013) Cumulative incidence of cancer after solid organ transplantation. *Cancer* 119(12):2300–2308.

Trappe R, Oertel S, Leblond V, et al. (2012) Sequential treatment with rituximab followed by CHOP chemotherapy in adult B-cell post-transplant lymphoproliferative disorder (PTLD): the prospective international multicentre phase 2 PTLD-1 trial. *Lancet Oncol.* 13(2): 196-206

59.3 Cancer following solid organ transplant

Jerome M. Laurence

Department of Transplantation Surgery, University of Toronto, Multi-Organ Transplant Service, University Health Network, Toronto, ON, Canada

Introduction

After infection and cardiovascular disease, malignancy is the next most common cause of death in solid organ transplant recipients. Occult malignancy may have been present in the recipient prior to transplantation or transmitted from the donor. The process of donor and recipient selection generally attempts to minimize this risk. Far more commonly, cancer develops *de novo* in the recipient some time after transplantation, with the risk increasing progressively as a function of time after transplantation. Overall, the risk of malignancy in transplant recipients is 200–300% that of age- and sex-matched controls. This increase in risk is mostly dependent upon the organ transplanted and the associated nature, intensity and duration of the immunosuppressive regimen. The magnitude of the increase in cancer risk varies by cancer type and site. The greatest increase is observed in cancers associated with oncogenic viral infections. The prognosis for each cancer is substantially inferior for transplant recipients than for patients who are not transplant recipients. This is probably due to the more advanced stage at presentation and the detrimental effect of immunosuppression on host responses to cancer.

Incidence, aetiology and screening

Incidence, aetiology and screening	Description
Incidence	<ul><li>Across all sites the relative risk (RR) of cancer compared to the non-transplanted population is:<ul><li>2–3 for kidney transplant recipients</li><li>2–2.5 for liver transplant recipients</li><li>2.5–3 for heart transplant recipients</li><li>3.5–4.5 for lung transplant recipients</li><li>This broadly parallels the intensity of the immunosuppressive regimen associated with the organ</li></ul></li><li>There is great variation in the relative risk of cancer associated with transplantation depending on the site of the primary:<ul><li>Greatest increase is observed in cases linked to a viral aetiology:<ul><li>Kaposi sarcoma: human herpesvirus 8 (HHV-8), 50-fold increased risk</li><li>Non-melanoma skin cancer (NMSC) and lip cancer: human papillomavirus (HPV), ten-fold increased risk</li><li>Post-transplantation lymphoproliferative disease (PTLD): Epstein–Barr virus (EBV), eight-fold increased risk</li><li>Squamous cancers of the anogenital region: HPV, four-fold increased risk</li></ul></li><li>Little or no increase in the risk of developing breast or prostate cancer observed in transplant recipients</li></ul></li><li>Most common malignancy is NMSC</li></ul>
Aetiology	<ul><li>Immunosuppression:<ul><li>Duration and intensity is probably more significant than the agents used</li></ul></li><li>Oncogenic viral infection (usually latent in recipient prior to transplantation, but occasionally transmitted from donor, e.g. EBV)</li><li>Rejection episodes are a risk factor for subsequent development of malignancy</li></ul>

UICC Manual of Clinical Oncology, Ninth Edition. Edited by Brian O'Sullivan, James D. Brierley, Anil K. D'Cruz, Martin F. Fey, Raphael Pollock, Jan B. Vermorken and Shao Hui Huang. © 2015 UICC. Published 2015 by John Wiley & Sons, Ltd.

Incidence, aetiology and screening	Description

Screening and prevention	• Screening recommendations are the same as for the general population except for:
	  ▪ NMSC:
	    ○ Sun protection and avoidance recommended
	    ○ Regular skin surveillance by an experienced dermatologist
	  ▪ Bowel cancer:
	    ○ Annual faecal occult blood testing (FOBT) and flexible sigmoidoscopy every 5 years (American Society of Transplant Surgeons)
	    ○ Annual immunological FOBT with colonoscopy for all positive results (European Best Practice Guidelines)
	  ▪ Cervix:
	    ○ Annual cytological screening (enhanced from every second year)
	  ▪ Renal cancer:
	    ○ Role of renal ultrasound in kidney transplant recipients (interval and cost-effectiveness) is not resolved

Pathology

- Site-specific

Presentation and diagnostic work-up

- Depends on the site involved and stage of the disease

Staging and prognostic factors

Staging is organ specific.
Prognostic factors
- Disease stage
- Extent of end-organ dysfunction in transplant recipients may preclude certain therapies e.g.:
  - Abdominal surgery in patients with recurrent portal hypertension
  - Certain chemotherapy regimens in patients with renal dysfunction after kidney transplantation
- Ability to reduce or alter immunosuppression:
  - Non-life sustaining transplants (renal, pancreas) can be removed to allow immunosuppression to be ceased
  - If graft function is stable without signs of rejection, then immunosuppression can be reduced
  - Change from calcineurin inhibitor to mammalian target of rapamycin inhibitors (mTOR) inhibitor

Treatment

- Management of solid organ malignancy requires an interdisciplinary approach involving the relevant medical, surgical and radiation oncology teams in collaboration with the transplant service
- A change in the immunosuppressive regimen (change in agent or reduction in intensity) may be beneficial to prognosis
- Monitoring of graft function is essential:
  - Where graft is not life-sustaining and cessation of immunosuppression may have a substantial impact on prognosis (advanced PTLD resistant to other treatment), graft removal can be considered
- *Specific treatment*:
  - Local resection if feasible for early-stage disease is preferred
  - mTORs have been shown to have clinically significant anticancer effects, particularly in NMSC, Kaposi sarcoma and renal cell cancer

Recommended reading

Alberú J, Pascoe MD, Campistol JM et al. (2011) Lower malignancy rates in renal allograft recipients converted to sirolimus-based, calcineurin inhibitor-free immunotherapy: 24-Month results from the CONVERT trial. *Transplantation* 92:303–310.

Chapman JR, Webster AC, Wong G (2013) Cancer in the Transplant Recipient. *Cold Spring Harb Perspect Med* 3(7).

Euvrard S, Morelon E, Rostaing L et al. (2012) Sirolimus and secondary skin-cancer prevention in kidney transplantation. *N Engl J Med* 367:329–339.

PG Expert Group on Renal Transplantation (2002) European best practice guidelines for renal transplantation. Section IV: Long-term management of the transplant recipient. IV.6.3. Cancer risk after renal transplantation. Solid organ cancers: Prevention and treatment. *Nephrol Dial Transplant* 17(32):34–36.

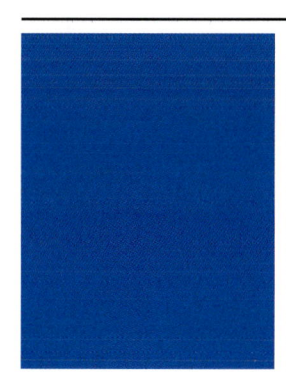

Index

Page numbers in *italics* denote figures, those in **bold** denote tables.

A

abiraterone acetate, prostate cancer **339**
ABVD regimen 136, **396**
AC220 436
acetaminophen **170**
acinic cell carcinoma **575**
Ackerman tumour **526**
acral lentiginous melanoma **692**
acromegaly 610, **612–13**
ACTH-secreting tumours **611**
    diagnosis 615–16, *616*
    treatment **621–2**
actin **601**
activated partial thromboplastin time (APTT) 151
activities of daily living (ADL) 140, 194, **195**
acute lymphoblastic leukaemia (ALL) 437–41
    classification 437
    controversies 441
    diagnostic work-up 438, **438**
    differential diagnosis 438
    paediatric 768, 770, **771**
    pathogenesis and aetiology 437
    post-treatment assessment 441
    presentation 437–8
    prognostic factors 439
    research priorities 441
    treatment 439–41, **439**
        adolescents and young adults 440–1
        allogeneic stem cell transplantation 440
        minimal residual disease 441
        monoclonal antibodies 440
        older patients 441
        Philadelphia chromosome-positive form 440
acute myeloblastic leukaemia (AML) 772, **772**
acute myeloid leukaemia (AML) 430–6
    aetiology 431
    classification 431
    controversies 436
    diagnostic work-up 432, **432**
    differential diagnosis 432
    pathogenesis 430
    post-treatment assessment 436
    presentation 431–2
    prognostic factors 433, *433*, **433**
    research priorities 436
    treatment 433–6, *434*, **434–5**
        older patients 435–6
        targeted therapy 436
    tumour markers **432**
acute promyelocytic leukaemia (APL) 436–7
adenocarcinoma
    cervix **455**
    oesophagus **282**, 291–5
        clinical trials **295**
        controversies 295
        treatment **292–4**
        treatment principles 291, **291–2**
    pancreas **272**
    salivary gland **575**
    vulva **496**
adenoid cystic carcinoma **574**
    sinonasal **588**
adenoma **92**
    adrenal **642**
    pituitary **611**, 614, 616
        treatment **623**
    salivary gland **574**
adenosquamous carcinoma
    mouth **527**
    pancreas **272**
adjustment reactions 166
adjuvant therapy 102–3, **126**, 127
    see also specific therapies
adrenal anatomy 642
adrenal disease
    functional
        cortex 642, **643**
        medulla 647–50, **647–50**
    non-functional **650–1**
adrenal insufficiency 150
adrenal tumours 641–55
    aetiology and physiology **642–3**
    clinical trials **655**
    controversies 654
    diagnostic work-up 644–6, **644–5**, *646*
    presentation and natural history **644**
    prognostic factors **646**
    research priorities 655
    staging 646, **646**
    treatment 647
        non-operative **654**
        surgery 651–3, **653**
    see also specific types
adrenocortical carcinoma 642, **643**, 654
    diagnostic work-up **645**, *646*
    presentation and natural history **644**
    prognostic factors **646**
    staging 646, **646**
    treatment **647**
adrenocorticotrophic hormone *see* ACTH
adriamycin
    ABVD regimen 136, **396**
    ALL **439**
    cardiotoxicity **201**
    myeloma **419**
    PIAF regimen **258**
    salivary gland tumours **584**
Adult Comorbidity Index-27 100
adult T-cell leukaemia/lymphoma
    pathology and natural history **404**
    treatment **412–13**
AE1 **89**
AE3 **89**
afatinib **125**
    lung cancer 213, **217**
aflibercept **125**
    colorectal cancer **323**
alcian blue **88**
alcohol
    as cancer risk factor 7–8
    use by cancer survivors 188
alemtuzumab, CLL **410**, **428**, **447**
ALK inhibitors 217
ALK gene mutations 217
ALL *see* acute lymphoblastic leukaemia
allogeneic stem cell transplantation
    ALL 440
    CML 444
all-or-none outcomes 15, **15**
α-fetoprotein (AFP) 31
    germ cell tumours **51**
    testicular cancer **51**, **371**
American Society of Anesthesiologists (ASA) score 140
American Society of Clinical Oncology (ASCO) 53, 186, 229
amidotrizoate **178**
amitriptyline 166
AML *see* acute myeloid leukaemia
amprenavir, drug interactions **143**
amputation 197–9, **198**
anaemia
    and fatigue 156
    older patients 143
    pregnancy 138
    transfusion therapy 153
anal cancer 327–32
    clinical trials 331–2, **331–2**
    diagnostic work-up 328–9
    HIV-related **798**, **800**, **801**, 806–7

UICC Manual of Clinical Oncology, Ninth Edition. Edited by Brian O'Sullivan, James D. Brierley, Anil K. D'Cruz, Martin F. Fey, Raphael Pollock, Jan B. Vermorken and Shao Hui Huang. © 2015 UICC. Published 2015 by John Wiley & Sons, Ltd.

anal cancer (*continued*)
    HPV-related 328, 798, **800**
    imaging 77
    incidence and aetiology **328**
    palliative care 331
    pathology and molecular biology 328
    prognostic factors 329, **329**
    screening **328**
    staging 329, **329**
    survivorship 331
    treatment 330–1
        chemoradiotherapy 330–1
        principles 329, **329**
        surgery 331
analgesia *see* pain treatment
anal intraepithelial neoplasia 328
analytical epidemiology 3, 4–5
    observational studies 4–5
anaplastic cell carcinoma of pancreas **272**
anaplastic glioma 710, **712**
    treatment **715, 716, 717**
anaplastic large-cell lymphoma
    biomarkers **773**
    pathology and natural history **403**
    treatment **412**
anaplastic lymphoma kinase protein (ALK1) **601**
anaplastic thyroid cancer 635–7, **635–7**
angiangiogenic therapy in lung cancer 216–17, **217**
angiogenesis 112
angioimmunoblastic T-cell lymphoma
    pathology and natural history **404**
    treatment **412**
angiosarcoma 757–8, 765
Ann Arbor staging system
    Hodgkin lymphoma 394–5, **395**
    non-Hodgkin lymphoma 405, *406*
anogenital cancer, risk factors **8**
anonymization of data 58–9
anorexia 177–9
anthracyclines 130
    nasopharyngeal cancer **520**
    patient co-morbidities **132**
    see also individual drugs
anticancer drugs *see* chemotherapy
anticholinergics **178**
anticonvulsants
    neuropathic pain 164
    pain treatment 171
antidepressants
    fatigue 156
    neuropathic pain 164
    pain treatment 171
    tricyclics 164, 166
anti-EGFR agents *see* EGFR inhibitors
anti-emetics 161, **176, 178**
    see also specific drugs
antiepileptics in CNS tumours 709
anti-HER2 agents 236
antisecretory agents **178**
antispasmodics **178**
anti-VEGF agents 127
    intravitreal 732
anxiety 166
appendix, neuroendocrine tumours
    of **661**
appetite stimulants 156
aprepitant, drug interactions **143**
ARCON trial 113
Aristolochia 10
asbestos 9
ascites, malignant 152
aspirin **170**
ASPL–TFE3 **759**

asthenia 179
astrocytoma **714**
atazanavir, drug interactions **143**
axitinib **125**
    renal cell carcinoma **365**

B
balanitis xerotica **385**
Barcelona Clinical Liver Cancer (BCLC) staging
    system 251
Barrett's oesophagus **292**
basal cell carcinoma
    incidence and aetiology **675**
    pathology **676**
    presentation and natural history **677–8**
    routes of spread **678**
    treatment
        guidelines **682**
        principles 681, **681–2**
        radiotherapy 683, **683, 684**
        surgery 682, **682**
        systemic therapy **684**
    vulva **496**
base excision repair 110
B-cell lymphoma
    pathology and presentation **400–3**
    treatment **409–12**
Bcl-2 **545**
BEACOPP regimen **396**
bendamustine
    CLL **447**
    non-Hodgkin lymphoma **411**
benzodiazepines 167
bereavement support 182
Bethesda classification **456**
bevacizumab **125**
    cervical cancer 464
    CNS tumours **717**, 722–3
    colorectal cancer 323
    CUP **795**
    lung cancer 214, **215**, 216
    neuroendocrine tumours **668**
    renal cell carcinoma **365**
bicalutamide **338, 339**
biliary cancers 263–9
    biomarkers **266**
    clinical trials **269**
    controversies 269
    diagnostic work-up **266**
    imaging 75, **75**
    incidence and aetiology **265**
    location *264*
    natural history 265, **265**
    pathology 265, *265*, **265**
    presentation 265
    prognostic factors **267**
    research priorities 269
    screening **265**
    staging 265–6, **266**
    treatment **267–8**
Binet staging system **445**
Biobanking and Biomolecular Resources Research
    Infrastructure 56
biochemical markers *see* biomarkers
bioinformatics 57–8
biological prognostic factors 27
biology guided adaptive radiotherapy
    (BiGART) 122
biomarkers 28
    biliary cancers **266**
    colorectal cancer **51**, 316
    fallopian tube cancer **492**
    gastric cancer **300**

head and neck cancers, unknown primary **601**
laryngeal cancer **545**
lymphoma **773**
nasopharyngeal cancer **515**
neuroendocrine tumours **659**
ovarian cancer **481**
pancreatic cancer **274**
response assessment 50, **51**
salivary gland tumours 579, **579**
soft tissue tumours **759**
terminology 28
testicular cancer **371**
thyroid cancers **51, 629**
see also individual biomarkers
BioMedBridges 56
biopsy 104
    testicular **371**
    see also fine needle aspiration (FNA)
bioreductive drugs 113
Biospecimen Reporting for Improved Study Quality
    (BRISQ) 27
bisphosphonates 149, 173
    breast cancer 236
bladder cancer 343–53
    biomarkers **51**
    clinical trials **351–2**
    continuing care 351
    controversies 351
    diagnostic work-up **344–5**
    imaging 81
    incidence and aetiology **343–4**
    pathology 344
    post-treatment assessment **350**
    presentation and natural history **344**
    prognostic factors **345–7**
    research priorities 353
    risk factors **8**
    staging **345**
    treatment **348–50**
        principles 347, **347–8**
        radiotherapy **349**
        surgery **348**
        systemic therapy **349–50**
bladder tumour antigen **51**
bland embolization **257**
bleeding 179–80
bleomycin
    ABVD regimen 136, **396**
    germ cell tumours **489**
    Hodgkin lymphoma **396**
    nasopharyngeal cancer **520**
    salivary gland tumours **584**
blood transfusions 153
body cavity fluids, cytopathological analysis 93
bone marrow
    aspirates 94
    clot analysis 94
bone metastases 65
    older patients 143
    pregnancy 138
    treatment 173
bone pain 172–3
bone scintigraphy 65
    lung cancer **208**
bone tumours (osteosarcoma) 745–53
    clinical trials **752**
    controversies 751–2
    imaging 78
    incidence and aetiology **746**
    paediatric 781–2, **781, 782**
    pathology **746–7**
    presentation and natural history 747, **747**
    prognostic factors 748

Index

research priorities 752
staging 748, **748**
standardized response criteria **48**
treatment **749–51**
  principles 748–9, **749**
  radiotherapy **750**
  surgery **749–50**
  systemic therapy **750–1**
bortezomib **125**, 132
  myeloma **419**, **420**, **421**
  patient co-morbidities **132**
bosutinib **443**
bowel obstruction 177, **178**
Bowen disease **385**
bowenoid papulosis **385**
brachytherapy 121, **121**
  head and neck cancers **509**
  oral cancers **536–7**
  retinoblastoma **735**
  uveal melanoma **731**
BRAF mutation 316
brain metastases 146, 721–2
  prognostic factors **722**
brain tumours *see* central nervous system tumours
BRCA mutations 10, 237
breaking bad news **181**
breast cancer 221–40
  adjuvant therapy **236**
  biomarkers **51**, 236
  BRCA gene mutations 10, 237
  breast reconstruction post-mastectomy **238**
  clinical trials **239–40**
  controversies 236
  diagnostic work-up 135, 225–7, **226**
    axillary lymph node staging 225–6
    exclusion of metastases 227
    fitness for treatment 227
    imaging 225
    tissue diagnosis 225
  hereditary 237
  imaging 72, *72*, **72**
  incidence and aetiology 222, **222**
  locoregional recurrence 237–8
  men 236–7
  natural history **224–5**
  older patients **141**
  over-treatment 236
  pathology 223, **223–4**
  post-treatment assessment 235–6
  pregnancy 134–6, 237
  prognostic factors 228–9, **228**
  research priorities 240
  risk factors 238
  screening 222, **222**
  staging 135, **227**
  treatment 135–6, 229–35
    guidelines 229
    local therapy 229–32, **229–32**
    principles 229
    systemic therapy 233–5, **233–5**
Breast Health Global Initiative (BHGI) **190**
brentuximab vedotin **412**, 413
BRIDGE project 59
brief fatigue inventory (BFI) 140
Brief Pain Inventory 169
bronchopulmonary neuroendocrine tumours **662–3**
  systemic therapy 668–9, **669**
buccal mucosa
  imaging **70**
  tumours of **535**
  see also oral cancers
buparlisib **125**

buprenorphine **171**
bupropion 156, 166
Burkitt lymphoma
  biomarkers **773**
  paediatric 773
  pathology and natural history **402**
  treatment **411**
Buschke-Lowenstein, verrucous **385**
buspirone **167**

C

C225 *see* cetuximab
CA15-3 **51**
CA19-9 **51**, 266, 274, 300
CA27.29 **51**
CA72-4 **300**
CA125 100, **300**, **481**, **492**
cabazitaxel **339**
cabozantinib **125**
cachexia **177–9**
CAM5.2 **89**, **600**
cancer Biomedical Informatics Grid (caBIG) 56
Cancer Care Ontario 55
CancerCommons 59
cancer control programmes 24, 25, **25**
Cancer Data 56
cancer fatigue 155–7
  palliative care **179**
  rehabilitation **195–6**
  screening and assessment 155–6
  in survivors **186**
  treatment 156–7
cancer informatics *see* informatics
Cancer of the Liver Italian Program (CLIP) 251, **251**
cancer registries 56
cancer of unknown primary (CUP) 788–96
  clinicopathological subsets 791–2, **792**
  controversies 795
  diagnostic work-up 789–91, **791**
  favourable subsets 792
  head and neck *see* head and neck cancers, unknown primary
  incidence and aetiology 788–9, **789**
  palliative care 795
  pathology 789, *790*, **790**
  presentation and natural history 789
  prognostic factors 793, **793**
  treatment 793–5, **794**, **795**
  unfavourable subsets 792–3
capecitabine
  anal cancer **330**
  biliary cancers **268**
  colorectal cancer 317, 321, **322**
  CUP **795**
  gastric cancer **304**
  neuroendocrine tumours **667**, **669**
  pancreatic cancer **276**, **277**
capsaicin **164**
carbamazepine **164**
  drug interactions **143**
carboplatin
  bladder cancer **350**
  cervical cancer **464**
  CNS tumours **717**
  CUP **795**
  Hodgkin lymphoma **396**
  lung cancer **218**
  nasopharyngeal cancer **520**
  oesophageal cancer **289**, **290**
  ovarian cancer **488**
  salivary gland tumours **584**
  uterine cancer **475**

carcinoembryonic antigen *see* CEA
carcinoid syndrome **666**
  atypical **666**
  see also neuroendocrine tumours
carcinoma **92**
  adrenocortical *see* adrenocortical carcinoma
  pituitary **611**, **614**
    treatment **623–4**
carcinoma cuniculatum **526**
carcinoma in situ *91*, **92**
carcinoma of unknown primary (CUP) 597
  head and neck 597–608
carcinosarcoma of salivary gland **575**
caregivers, data access 59
carfilzomib **419**, **421**
carmustine
  CNS tumours **717**
  pituitary tumours **624**
case-control studies 5, **15**
cause-specific survival 40, **41**
CD3 **89**
CD4 **432**
CD11b **432**
CD11C **432**
CD13 **432**
CD14 **432**
CD15 **89**, **432**
CD16 **432**
CD20 **89**
CD30 89, 601, 773
CD31 **89**
CD33 **432**
CD34 **89**, **432**, **601**
CD36 **432**
CD38 **432**
CD41 **432**
CD42 **432**
CD43 **601**
CD56 **89**
CD61 **432**
CD64 **432**
CD65 **432**
CD68 **89**
CD99 **601**
CD133 **432**
CD163 **89**
CDX2 **601**
CEA **51**, **89**, **100**, **300**, **629**
CEBPA^{dm} mutation **433**
celecoxib **170**
cell radiosensitizers 113
cell survival curve 110–11, *111*
Centers for Disease Control and Prevention (CDC) 4
centralized databases 55–6
central nervous system tumours 706–25
  brain metastases 146, 721–2, **722**
  clinical trials **723**, **724**
  controversies 722–3
  future studies 723–5
  glioma *see* glioma
  imaging 65–7, *66*, *67*, 708–9, **708**
    response assessment 66, **67**
  lymphoma **708**, 719–20
  medulloblastoma *see* medulloblastoma
  meningioma *see* meningioma
  older patients **142**
  paediatric 775–8, *775*, **776**, **777**, **778**
  presentation 707–8, **708**
  prognostic factors **714**
  research priorities 725
  treatment 709
    antiepileptics 709

central nervous system tumours (*continued*)
  radiotherapy 709, **715–16**
  steroids 709
  surgery 709, **715**
  systemic therapy 709, **716–17**
cephalosporins 138
cervical cancer 449–66
  anatomy and physiology 450, *450*
  Bethesda classification **456**
  clinical trials **465**
  diagnosis 136, 457–8, **458**
  epidemiology 136
  follow-up 464
  HIV-related 464–5, **798, 800, 801**, 805
  HPV-related **451**, 452–3, **454, 455**, 456–7, 798, **800, 801**
  imaging 79, *80*
  incidence and aetiology **451**
  mortality *453*
  pathology **454–5**
  pregnant women 136, 465
  presentation and natural history 456–7, **457**
  prevention 452–3
  prognostic factors **460**
  risk factors **8**
  screening **451–2**, 452
  staging 136, 458, **459**
  treatment 461–4
    principles **460–1**
    radiotherapy 463, **463**
    surgery **461–2**
    systemic therapy and chemoradiation 464
cetuximab **125**
  colorectal cancer **125**, 323
  oral cancers **538**
C-factor 38
Charlson Score 100
chemoembolization 671
chemoradiotherapy (CRT) 108, 116–17
  anal cancer 330–1
  cervical cancer 464
  colorectal cancer 314
  oesophageal cancer 290–1
  oral cancers **537**
chemoreceptor trigger zone **176**
chemotherapy 124–33
  CNS tumours 709
  cytotoxic 124
  hormone therapy 124–5
  immune therapy 126
  molecularly targeted *see* targeted therapy
  older patients 140, 142, **142**
  oral cancers **537**
  pain induced by 163, 172
  pregnancy **135**
  see also systemic therapy; and individual drugs and cancers
Child-Pugh classification 251, **251**
children *see* paediatric tumours
chlorambucil
  CLL **447**
  non-Hodgkin lymphoma **411**
chlorpromazine **176, 178**
CHOEP regimen **396**
cholangiocarcinoma *see* biliary cancers
CHOP regimen 128, **412, 739**
chromogranin **89, 601**, 659
chronic lymphatic leukaemia (CLL) 444–7
  diagnostic work-up 445, **445**
  differential diagnosis 445
  epidemiology 444
  pathogenesis 444
  presentation 444–5

prognostic factors 445, **445**
staging 445, **445**
treatment 446–7, *446*, **447**
chronic myeloblastic leukaemia (CML) 772
chronic myeloid leukaemia (CML) 441–4
  diagnostic work up 442
  pathogenesis 441–2
  presentation 442, **442**
  research priorities 444
  risk calculation 443
  treatment 442–4
    allogeneic stem cell transplantation 444
    tyrosine kinase inhibitors 442–4, **443**
cisplatin 110, 116
  adrenal tumours **654**
  anal cancer 330
  biliary cancers **268**
  bladder cancer **350**
  bone tumours 750, **751**
  cervical cancer 464
  CUP (cancer of unknown primary) **795**
  germ cell tumours **489**
  head and neck cancers 509, 606
  lung cancer 214, **218**
  nasopharyngeal cancer 520
  neuroendocrine tumours 669
  oesophageal cancer 289
  oral cancers **538**
  ovarian cancer **488**
  patient co-morbidities **132**
  penile cancer **389**
  testicular cancer 381
  uterine cancer 475
citalopram 156, 166
CK5/6 **89, 601**
CK7/20 **89, 601**
c-KIT **579**
clarithromycin 138
  drug interactions **143**
classification of cancers 23
  clinical 35, 36–7, **36**
  see also staging
clinical decision-making 43
  support systems 60, *60*
clinical endpoints 40
clinical informatics 57–8
clinical practice guidelines (CPGs) 12–22, **14**
  components of 16–22, **17–18**
  content 12–13
  CPG development group 16
  development 19–22, **20, 21**
  external review 21–2
  levels of evidence 13–16, **14, 15**
  protocol development 16–17
  quality appraisal 20, **20**
  recommendations 21, **21**
  topic selection 16
  updating 22
clinical research informatics 55–6
clinical standards 13, **14**
clinical target volume 118–19
Clinical Trial Processor 59
clinical trials 5
  adrenal tumours **655**
  anal cancer 331–2, **331–2**
  biliary cancers **269**
  bladder cancer **351–2**
  bone tumours 752
  breast cancer **239–40**
  cervical cancer **465**
  CNS tumours **723, 724**
  colorectal cancer **325**
  disclosure of data 58

gastric cancer **305–6**
head and neck cancers, unknown primary **607**
Hodgkin lymphoma **398**
interim analysis 42
laryngeal cancer **556–7**
liver cancer **260–1**
lung cancer **219**
myeloma **425**
nasopharyngeal cancer **521–2**
neuroendocrine tumours 671, **672**
oral cancers **540**
oropharyngeal cancer **569**
ovarian cancer **490**
pancreatic cancer **278**
pituitary tumours **624**
prostate cancer **341**
RCTs *see* randomized controlled trials
renal cell carcinoma **366**
salivary gland tumours **585**
sample size estimation 42
skin cancer
  melanoma **703–4**
  NMSC **687**
soft tissue tumours **766**
targeted therapy **476**
testicular cancer **382–3**
thyroid cancers **639**
uveal melanoma **743**
vs. real world learning 60–1, *61*, **61**
vulval cancer **501**
CLL *see* chronic lymphatic leukaemia
clonogenic cells *see* colony-forming cells
Clonorchis sinensis **8**
^{11}C-methionine-PET 66
CML *see* chronic myeloid leukaemia
cMPO **432**
CNS *see* central nervous system
codeine 163, **171**
CODOX-M regimen **396**
cognitive behavioural therapy 167
cognitive impairment
  cancer-related 187
  rehabilitation 199–200
cohort studies 5, **15**
  inception cohort 26
  prognostic factors 25–6
  time-zero 26
COL1A1-PDGFB **759**
colonoscopy 103–4
colony-forming cells 110
  repopulation 112
colony-stimulating factors 129, 149
colorectal cancer 308–26
  biomarkers **51**, 316
  clinical trials **325**
  controversies 325
  diagnostic work-up 313–15, **313**
  follow-up and surveillance 324
  hereditary 309–10
  imaging 76–7, *77*
  incidence and aetiology 309–10, **309**
  older patients **141**
  palliative care 325
  pathology and molecular biology 313, **313**
  prevention 310–11
  prognostic factors 316–17, **317**
  quality of life 324
  research priorities 326
  risk factors 309
  screening **309**, 311–12
  staging 314, **316**
  survivorship 325
  treatment

principles 317–19, **318–19**
radiotherapy **319**, 323–4
surgery 102, **319–20**
systemic therapy 321–3, **322–3**
unresectable cancer 320–1
colorectal neuroendocrine tumours **661**
colposcopic examination 457, **458**
common leukocyte antigen (CLA) **601**
communication 165
companion diagnostic markers 28
competing risk 40–1, **41**
computed tomography (CT) 63, **63**
CNS tumours 66
cone-beam 122
contrast-enhanced 63
lung cancer **208**
MRI **65**
multidetector 63
response assessment 43
computer-assisted intervention 54–5
cone-beam CT 122
cone biopsy 457–8
3D conformal radiotherapy (3D-CRT) 120
confounding 4–5
conivaptan 150
connective tissue, histochemical stains **88**
Conn syndrome see hyperaldosteronism
constipation 159–61
assessment 160, **160**
palliative care 176, *177*, **177**
treatment 160–1, **161**
contrast-enhanced CT 63
contrast enhanced MRI of CNS tumours 65–6, *66*
Cooperative Oncology Group (ECOG) Performance Status Scale 194
corticosteroids see steroids
cost-effectiveness of cancer drugs 132
Cox proportional hazards regression model 41
CPGs see clinical practice guidelines
cranial nerve blocks 172
crizotinib 217
cryoablation **361**
cryotherapy **742**
CT see computed tomography
CTCAE 57
cumulative risk 5
CUP see cancer of unknown primary
curative therapy
radiotherapy 117–18
supportive care 155–67
surgery 101–3
see also individual cancers
Cushing disease/syndrome see hypercortisolism
cyclin D1 **545**
cyclophosphamide
CHOP regimen 128, **412**, **739**
Hodgkin lymphoma **396**
myeloma **419**
non-Hodgkin lymphoma **411**
salivary gland tumours 584
CYP3A4 induction/inhibition **143**
cytarabine
CNS tumours **721**
Hodgkin lymphoma **396**
cytokeratins **601**
cytokines
melanoma **701–2**
renal cell carcinoma 365
side effects 153
cytopathology 91–3, *91*, **92**
methods and specimen types 92–3, *93*
screening, reporting and quality control 92
specimen collection 92

cytotoxic chemotherapy 124
colorectal cancer 321–3, **322–3**
see also individual drugs

D
dabrafenib 698
dacarbazine
ABVD regimen 136, **396**
Hodgkin lymphoma **396**
DAHANCA 5 study 113
DART initiative 55
dasatinib
CML **443**
data
anonymization 58–9
collection protocols 56
confidentiality 58
disclosure 58
infrastructure 55–6
interoperability 57, **57**
patient- and caregiver-managed 59
see also informatics
databases 56–7
centralized 55–6
federated 56
non-relational (NoSQLs) 56–7
Data governance Committee 50
data warehouses 57
DaVinci system 107
decision support 60, *60*
dehydration 156
delirium 179
demeclocycline 150
denileukin difitox **412**
Denoix, Pierre 34
depression 156
psychosocial care 166
treatment see antidepressants
descriptive epidemiology 3–4, **4**
desmin **601**
desmoid tumours **757**, 765
determinant of disease 3, **4**
dexamethasone **176**, **178**
Hodgkin lymphoma **396**
myeloma **419**, **421**
DHAP regimen **396**
diagnosis 104
see also individual cancers
diagnostic markers see biomarkers
diarrhoea 157–9
assessment **158**
exudative 157
nutritional treatment 158, **158**
osmotic 157
palliative care 176–7
patient education **159**
treatment 157–9, **159**
diclofenac **170**
DICOM standard 59
diet 156
as cancer risk factor 8–9
survivors 187
see also nutritional treatment
differential thyroid cancer 631–5
controversies 634–5
treatment 632–4
principles 631, **631**, **632**
radioactive iodine 633–4, **634**
radiotherapy 632–3
surgery **632**
systemic therapy 633
TSH suppression 633, 635

diffuse large B-cell lymphoma
paediatric 773
pathology and natural history **400**
treatment **409**
diltiazem, drug interactions **143**
dimenhydrinate **178**
diphenhydramine **176**
disclosure of data 58
disease extent 28, 29
disease-free survival 40
disease type 28
distant control 40
distant metastasis-free survival 40
distribution of disease 3, **4**
DNA
damage/repair 109–10
sequencing 95
structure 110
docetaxel
head and neck cancers 509
lung cancer **214**, **215**
oral cancers **538**
ovarian cancer **488**
prostate cancer **339**
dolasetron 153
domperidone 138, **176**
dose interval 128–9
dose-response curves in radiotherapy 110–11, *111*
dose-volume histogram 119
doxorubicin
bone tumours **750**, **751**
CHOP regimen 128, **412**, **739**
Hodgkin lymphoma **396**
salivary gland tumours 584
uterine cancer **475**
dronabinol 156
drug dose 128–9
drug-drug interactions 143, **143**
drug toxicity 41–2, 130
ductal carcinoma of breast **223**
local therapy **230**
duloxetine 166
duodenal neuroendocrine tumours **660**
dysgerminomas **482**
dysphagia 197
dysplasia **92**
dyspnoea 179

E
EBER **601**
echocardiography 130
effect size 40–1
effusions, malignant 151–2
EGFR 109, 117, **545**, **579**
EGFR inhibitors 216–17, **217**
colorectal cancer 323
oral cancers **538**
EGFR gene mutation 216, 316
electrolyte depletion 156
electrolyte replacement therapy **159**
electronic medical records 54
elotuzumab **421**
EMA **89**, **600**
emergencies 145–54
adrenal insufficiency 150
brain metastases 146
cytokine use 153
hypercalcaemia 149
malignant effusions 151–2
neutropenic fever 147–9
pain-related 173
refractory nausea and vomiting 152–3
SIADH 149–50

emergencies (continued)
  spinal cord compression 146–7
  superior vena cava syndrome 145–6, **146**
  thrombosis and hypercoagulability 150–1
  transfusion use 153
  tumour lysis syndrome 150
end of life care 182–3
  see also palliative care
endobronchial ultrasound 208
endobronchial ultrasound-guided fine needle aspiration (EBUS-FNA) 93, 208
endocrine disorders, and fatigue 156
endodermal sinus tumours **482**
endometrial cancer
  imaging 79–80
  older patients **141**
energy conservation 157
enteropathy-associated T-cell lymphoma
  pathology and natural history **404**
  treatment **413**
environment-related prognostic factors 32, **32**
enzalutamide **339**
epidemiology 3–11
  analytical 3, 4–5
  descriptive 3–4, **4**
  experimental 5
  global burden 5–7, **6**
  prevention 10–11
  risk factors 7–10, **7**
epidermal growth factor receptor see EGFR
epidural/intrathecal neurolysis 172
epirubicin
  oesophageal cancer **290**
  salivary gland tumours **584**
epithelial growth factor receptor see EGFR
epithelial markers **89**
EPOCH regimen **396**
Epstein-Barr virus 8
ERG **89**
erlotinib
  lung cancer 213, **215**, **217**
erythroid markers **432**
erythromycin, drug interactions **143**
erythroplasia of Queyrat **385**
escitalopram 166
ESHAP regimen **396**
esthesio-neuroblastoma (ENB) **588**
ethics
  end of life care 182
  palliative care 181
etoposide
  CUP **795**
  germ cell tumours **489**
  Hodgkin lymphoma **396**
  lung cancer 218
  testicular cancer **381**
European Organization for Research and Treatment of Cancer (EORTC) 169
European Union, Biobanking and Biomolecular Resources Research Infrastructure 56
euthanasia 182
everolimus
  neuroendocrine tumours **667**, **668**, **669**
  renal cell carcinoma **365**
EWSR1–AFT1 **759**
EWSR1–CREB1 **759**
EWSR1–DDIT3 **759**
exercise 157, 187
experimental epidemiology 5
exposure misclassification 5
external beam radiation
  eyelid cancers **742**
  ocular adnexal lymphoma **739**
  retinoblastoma **735**

external review of CPGs 21–2
extramedullary plasmacytoma **418**
extranodal marginal zone lymphoma, MALT type
  pathology and natural history **401**
  treatment **410**
extranodal NK/T-cell lymphoma, nasal type
  pathology and natural history **405**
  treatment **413**
exudative diarrhoea 157
eyelid cancers 740–3, *740*
  diagnostic work-up 741
  incidence and aetiology **740**
  pathology 740, **740–1**
  post-treatment assessment 742–3
  presentation 741
  prognostic factors **742**
  staging **741**, **742**
  treatment **742**
  principles 741
eye tumours see specific types

F
faecal impaction *177*
  see also constipation
fallopian tube cancer 491–4
  diagnostic work-up 492, **492**
  incidence and aetiology **491**
  pathology and natural history 491
  presentation 492
  prognostic factors **493**
  staging 492, **492**
  treatment 493–4
    principles 493, **493**
    radiotherapy 493
    surgery **493**
    systemic therapy **494**
  see also ovarian cancer
familial adenomatous polyposis 310
familial cancer syndromes 90
famotidine 178
fatigue see cancer fatigue
FDG-PET 54, 65
  Hodgkin lymphoma 398
  response assessment 46, 50
  site-specific
    CNS tumours 66
    colorectal cancer 314
febrile neutropenia 142
federated databases 56
fentanyl 163, **171**
18F-fluoroethyl L-tyrosine-PET 66
18F-fluorothymidine-PET 66, 67
field intervention trials 3
FIGO classification
  cervical cancer 79, 458, **459**
  fallopian tube cancer 492, **492**
  ovarian cancer 483, **484**
  uterine cancer **471**
  vulval cancer **497**
fine needle aspiration (FNA) 92–3, *93*, 104
  endobronchial ultrasound-guided 93
  thyroid cancers **68**, *93*, **629**
Fite stain **88**
floor of mouth
  imaging 70
  tumours of 535
Flt3-ITD mutation **433**
fluconazole, drug interactions **143**
fludarabine
  CLL **447**
  non-Hodgkin lymphoma **411**
fluorodeoxyglucose see FDG

fluorouracil (5-fluorouracil)
  anal cancer 330
  head and neck cancers **509**
  oesophageal cancer 289, **290**
  penile cancer **389**
  PIAF regimen 258
  salivary gland tumours **584**
fluoxetine 156, 166
FNA see needle aspiration
FOLFIRI **795**
FOLFOX **795**
follicular lymphoma
  pathology and natural history **400**
  prognostic factors **407**
  treatment **409**
Fontana-Masson stain **88**
Formatted Anthology Synoptic Tick (FAST) sheet 55
fosamprenavir, drug interactions **143**
Framework Convention on Tobacco Control (FCTC) 11
French-American-British (FAB) classification **431**
FUS–DDIT3 **759**

G
G-8 geriatric screening tool **140**
gabapentin 164
Gardner syndrome 310
gastric cancer 297–307
  biomarkers **300**
  clinical trials **305–6**
  controversies 304–5
  diagnostic work-up **300**
  imaging 74–5
  incidence and aetiology **298**
  natural history 299, **299–300**
  pathology 298, **299**
  prognostic factors **301**
  risk factors **8**
  screening **298**
  staging 300, **301**
  treatment 302–4
    principles 301–2, **301–2**
    radiotherapy **303–4**
    surgery **302–3**
gastric neuroendocrine tumours **659**
  systemic therapy 668–9, **669**
gastrointestinal stromal tumours **757**
  imaging 77–8, *78*
  standardized response criteria **48**
GCDFP-15 **601**
GDP regimen **396**
gefitinib **125**
  lung cancer 213, **215**, **217**
gemcitabine
  biliary cancers **268**
  bladder cancer **350**
  CUP **795**
  Hodgkin lymphoma **396**
  lung cancer 214
  nasopharyngeal cancer **520**
gemtuzumab ozogamicin **436**
Gene Expression Omnibus 56
gene therapy 126
genetic susceptibility 10
genome-wide association study 10
genomics 53
geriatric assessment scales **140**
germ cell tumours
  biomarkers **51**
  CNS **708**
  ovary 481, **482**, **488**, **489**
germinoma **708**
gigantism **613**
gingiva 70

glioblastoma **710**, **712**
 treatment **715**, **716**, 722–3
glioma 709–18, *710*
 anaplastic *see* anaplastic glioma
 diagnostic work-up **711–12**
 follow-up 718
 imaging **708**
 pathology **710–11**
 prognostic factors **714**
 recurrent **717**
 response assessment **67**
 standardized response criteria **48**
 treatment
  principles *712–13*
  radiotherapy **715–16**
  surgery **715**
  systemic therapy **716–17**
Global Alliance for Genomics and Health 56
global burden of cancer 5–7, *6*
global identifiers 55
Global Initiative for Cancer Registry Development 4
glottic cancer **549–50**
 radiotherapy vs. surgery 554–5
 see also laryngeal cancer
glucagonoma syndrome **666**
glycophorin A **432**
glycopyrrolate **178**
Gomori-methenamine silver **88**, *89*
Gomori reticulin stain **88**
governance of patient data access 59
Gram stain **88**
granisetron 153
granulocyte-colony stimulating factor (G-CSF) 153
granulocyte-macrophage colony stimulating factor (GM-CSF) 153
granulocytic markers **432**
granulosa cell tumours **483**
Groningen Frailty Indicator **140**
gross tumour volume 118
growth hormone-secreting tumours **610**
 diagnosis 616
 presentation **612–13**
 treatment 618–19, **618–19**
gynaecological cancers *see specific sites*

H
H$_2$-receptor antagonists **178**
haematopathology, diagnostic 94–5
haloperidol **176**, **178**, 179
hard palate
 imaging **70**
 tumours of **535**
hazard ratio 41
head and neck cancers 503–11
 continuing care 510
 diagnostic work-up **505**
 follow-up 510
 HPV-related **504**, **505**, *506*
 imaging 68–71, *69*, *70*, **70**, **71**
 incidence and aetiology **504**
 natural history 504
 older patients **142**
 pathology 504
  reporting 506, **506**
 post-treatment assessment 509–10
 screening **504**
 systemic therapy 509
 treatment 507–9
  brachytherapy 509
  principles 506, *506*, **507**
  radiotherapy 508–9, **508**
 recurrence/metastasis 510
 surgery 507–8
 see also individual types
head and neck cancers, unknown primary 597–608
 biomarkers **601**
 clinical trials **607**
 controversies 606
 diagnostic work-up 598–600, **599–600**
 follow-up 606
 HPV-related **598**, **599**
 incidence and aetiology **598**
 natural history 598
 pathology 598
 presentation 598
 prognostic factors 602, **602**
 screening antibodies **600**
 staging 601, **601**
 treatment 604–6
  principles 602, *603*, **603**
  radiotherapy 604–6, **604–6**
  surgery 604
  systemic therapy 606
Healthcare Information and treatment Systems Society (HIMSS) 60
health information access 58–9
 data anonymization 58–9
 governance of 59
 privacy and disclosures 58
Helicobacter pylori 8, **8**
heparin 151
hepatitis B **8**
hepatitis C **8**
hepatoblastoma **79**
hepatocellular carcinoma
 HIV-related **798**, **800**, **801**, 807–8
 imaging 75, **75**
 standardized response criteria **47**
HER2 96, *96*, **579**
histiocytic markers **89**
histochemical stains 87–9, **88**
histology 87–90, **88**, *89*, **89**
histopathological grading of tumours *37*
HIV-related neoplasms **8**, 797–808
 anal cancer **798**, **800**, **801**, 806–7
 cervical cancer 464–5, **798**, **800**, **801**, 805
 hepatocellular carcinoma **798**, **800**, **801**, 807–8
 Hodgkin lymphoma **798**, **800**, 805–6
 HPV-associated **798**, **799**, **800**, **801**
 incidence and aetiology **798–800**
 Kaposi sarcoma *see* Kaposi sarcoma
 lung cancer **798**, **800**, **801**, 807
 non-Hodgkin lymphoma **798**, **800**, **801**, 803–5, **804–5**
 screening **801**
 see also specific tumour sites
HLA-DR **432**
HMB45 **89**
Hodgkin lymphoma 394–400
 clinical trials **398**
 controversies 397–8
 HIV-related **798**, **800**, 805–6
 HPV-associated **798**, **799**, **800**, **801**
 paediatric 774–5
 pathology and natural history **394**
 prognostic factors 395, **396**
 refractory/relapsing 399
 research priorities 399–400
 risk factors **8**
 staging 394–5, **395**
 treatment 396–7, **396**, **397**
  principles 395, **395**
 see also lymphoma
home care 182
homologous recombination 110

hook effect 615
hormonal factors in cancer risk 9
hormone therapy 124–5
 uterine cancer 475, 477
hospice care 182
hospital-based cancer registries (HBCRs) 4
host-related prognostic factors 31–2
 acquired 31–2
 host demographics 31, **31**
HPV *see* human papillomavirus
β-human chorionic gonadotropin (hCG) 31, **51**
 testicular cancer **371**
human immunodeficiency virus *see* HIV
human melanoma black-antimelanoma antibody (HMB) 45 **601**
human papillomavirus (HPV) **8**
 anal cancer **328**, **798**, **800**
 cervical cancer **451**, 452–3, **454**, **455**, 456–7, **798**, **800**, **801**
 DNA testing 457
 head and neck cancer **504**, **505**, *506*, **598**, **599**
 HIV-associated **798**, **799**, **800**, **801**
 laryngeal and hypopharyngeal cancer **543**, **545**
 oesophageal cancer **281**
 oral cancers **525**
 oropharyngeal cancer 30–1, **510**, **560**, **560–1**, 561, 562, **562**, **564**, 565, 566, 570
 penile cancer **384**, **385**, **387**, 390
 sinonasal tumours **587**
 skin cancer **675**
 solid organ transplant recipients **812**
 vaccine **328**, 452–3
 vulval cancer **496**
human T-cell lymphotropic virus type 1 **8**
hydrocodone **171**
hydrocodone/acetaminophen 163
hyoscine butylbromide **178**
hyperaldosteronism (Conn syndrome) **642–3**
 clinical manifestations **643**
 diagnostic work-up **645**
 presentation and natural history **644**
 treatment **647**
  perioperative **653**
hyperandrogenism **643**
 clinical manifestations **643**
 diagnostic work-up **645**
 presentation and natural history **644**
 treatment **647**
hyperbaric oxygen 113
hypercalcaemia 149
hypercalcitonaemia 639
hypercoagulability 150–1
hypercortisolism (Cushing disease) **611**, 615–16, *616*, **642**
 clinical manifestations **643**
 diagnostic work-up **644–5**
 presentation and natural history **644**
 treatment **647**
  perioperative **653**
hyperfibrinogenaemia 150–1
hyperoestrogenism **643**
hypokalaemia **159**
hypomagnesaemia **159**
hypopharyngeal tumours 551–2
 see also laryngeal cancer
hypophosphataemia **159**
hypoxia 112

I
ibrutinib
 CLL **447**
ibuprofen **170**
ICD-10 57
ICD-O-3 classification 23, 29

ICE regimen 396
ifosfamide
    bone tumours 751
    CNS tumours 721
    Hodgkin lymphoma 396
    nasopharyngeal cancer 520
    non-Hodgkin lymphoma 413
    penile cancer 389
    testicular cancer 381
image-guided robotic surgery 55
imaging 63–82
    functional 65
    morphological 63–5, **63–5**
    response assessment 43
    site-specific studies 65–81
        breast cancer 72, *72*, **72**
        central nervous system tumours 65–7, 66, 67, 708–9, **708**
        gastrointestinal and hepatobiliary cancers 73–8, **75**, **76**, *77*
        gynaecological cancers 79–80, *80*
        head and neck cancers 68–71, 69, 70, **70**, **71**
        lymphomas and multiple myeloma 79
        musculoskeletal tumours 78–9
        thoracic cancers 72–3, **73**, *74*
        thyroid cancers 67–8, **68**, **69**
        urogenital cancers 80–1
    see also specific modalities
imatinib
    CML (chronic myeloid leukaemia) **443**
imipenem 138
immunohistochemistry 89–90, **89**
immunosuppression, and NMSC 686
immunotherapy 126
    ocular adnexal lymphoma **739**
    renal cell carcinoma 364
IMRT (also *see* intensity-modulated radiotherapy)
inception cohort 26
incidence rate 5
incidentaloma, adrenal **650**, 654
incontinence 199
indinavir, drug interactions **143**
individualized radiotherapy treatment 121–2
indomethacin **170**
infections
    as cancer risk factor 8, **8**
    pregnancy 138
informatics 53–62
    computer-assisted intervention 54–5
    databases *see* databases
    data collection protocols 56
    data interoperability 57, **57**
    decision support and learning engines 60, *60*
    electronic medical records 54
    health information access 58–9
        data anonymization 58–9
        governance of 59
        privacy and disclosures 58
    medical and scientific objectives 57–8
    operational issues 58
    patient- and caregiver-managed data 59
    patient-centred care 54
    point-of-care technology 55
    real world learning 60–1, *61*, **61**
    research data 55–6
information bias 5
instrumental activities of daily living (IADL) 140, **195**
insulinoma syndrome **666**
intensity-modulated proton therapy (IMPT) *120*
intensity-modulated radiotherapy (IMRT), *see also* IMRT 108–9, 120–1, *120*
    rotational 121

interferon-α
    non-Hodgkin lymphoma 412
    PIAF regimen 258
interleukin-2 (IL-2)
    melanoma **701**–**2**
    renal cell carcinoma 365
International Agency for Research on Cancer (IARC) 4
International Classification of Diseases for Oncology *see* ICD-O-3 classification
International Classification of Functioning (ICF) 23
International Commission on Radiation Units and Measurements (ICRU) 118–19
International Histological Classification of Tumours 39
interpretive errors 86
interventional research 191
intraoperative consultation 85–6, *85*, *86*
intraoperative therapies 103
intraspinal analgesia 172
iodine, radioactive 633–4, **634**
ionizing radiation 10
    see also radiotherapy
ipilmumab
    melanoma **702**
irinotecan
    CUP **795**
    lung cancer 218
    nasopharyngeal cancer 520
    neuroendocrine tumours 669
    penile cancer 389
iron stain **88**, *89*
isolated tumour cells 37
itraconazole, drug interactions **143**
IVAC regimen 396

K

Kadish staging system 590
Kaplan-Meier analysis 41
Kaposi sarcoma 802–3, **802–3**
    incidence and aetiology **798**, 800
    risk factors **8**
Karnovsky score 100, 194
keratoacanthoma
    pathology **677**
    presentation and natural history **678**
ketoconazole
    adrenal tumours 654
    drug interactions **143**
ketoprofen **170**
Ki-67 100
Kinyoun stain 88
KIT **757**
KRAS mutation 316

L

lactate dehydrogenase in testicular cancer **371**
Lan-DeMets approximation 42
lapatinib **125**
laryngeal cancer 542–58
    biomarkers **545**
    clinical trials **556–7**
    controversies 554–6
        neck dissection and organ preservation treatment 555–6
        neoadjuvant/induction chemotherapy in locally advanced patients 555
        radiotherapy vs. surgery in glottic cancer 554–5
        HPV-related **543**, **545**
    diagnostic work-up 545, **545**
    follow-up and continuing care 554, **554**
    imaging 70

    incidence and aetiology **543**
    pathology 543–4
    presentation and natural history 544, **544–5**
    prevention **543**
    prognostic factors 546, **547**
    research priorities 557
    staging **546**
    treatment 548–54
        adjuvant therapy **552**
        glottic cancer **549–50**
        hypopharyngeal tumours 551–2
        neck dissection **553**
        principles 546–7, **547**, **548**
        recurrence/second primary 553–4
        supraglottic cancer 550–1
laser therapy in retinoblastoma **735**
laxatives 160–1, **177**
LCA 600
learning engines 60, *60*
lenalidomide
    CLL **447**
    myeloma **419**, **420**, **421**
    patient co-morbidities **132**
lentigo maligna **692**, **700**
leucopenia in pregnancy 138
leucovorin 131
    CNS tumours **721**
    Hodgkin lymphoma 396
    oesophageal cancer **289**, **290**
leukaemia 427–48
    diagnosis 137
    epidemiology 137
    paediatric 768–72, **769–72**
    plasma cell **418**
    pregnancy 137
    staging 137
    treatment 137
    see also specific types
levels of evidence 13–16, **14**, **15**
    clinical situations 14–16
    published study designs 14
LH/FSH-secreting tumours 611
    presentation 613
lichen sclerosis 385
lidocaine patches 164
life tables 40
limb salvage 197–9
linac-based stereotactic radiotherapy 120
liposarcoma **758**
lips
    imaging 70
    tumours of 535
lithium carbonate 150
liver cancer 241–62
    clinical trials **260–1**
    controversies 258–60
        diagnosis and staging 258
        liver resection 259
        liver transplantation 259–60
        locoregional therapy 258–9
    diagnostic work-up 247–9, **247–9**, *250*, 258
    fibrolamellar 258
    incidence and aetiology **242**, *243*
    natural history 245–6, **246**
    pathology 243–5, **244–5**
    prognostic factors 252
    research priorities 261
    risk factors **8**
    screening **242**, *243*
    staging 249–51, **250**, **251**, 258
        Barcelona Clinical Liver Cancer (BCLC) system 251

Index

Cancer of the Liver Italian Program (CLIP) 251, **251**
  Child-Pugh classification 251, **251**
  Okuda system 251, **251**
  TNM 250–1, **250**
  treatment 253–8
    ablative therapies 256, **256**
    locoregional therapy 255, **255–6**, 258–9
    principles 252–3, *252*, **253**
    radiotherapy 257, **257**
    surgery 253–5, **253**, **254**
    systemic therapy 258, **258**
    transarterial therapies 256–7, **257**
liver resection 254–5
  controversies 259
liver transplantation 255
  controversies 259–60
lobular carcinoma of breast 223
  local therapy **229**
local control 40, **41**
locoregional therapy in liver cancer 255, **255–6**, 258–9
lomustine 717
lorazepam 179
low linear energy transfer radiation 113
low molecular weight heparins (LMWH) 151
LQ cell survival model 111
lung cancer 205–20
  aetiology 206, **206**
  clinical trials 219
  controversies 219
  diagnostic work-up 207–8, **207**
  HIV-related **798**, **800**, **801**, 807
  incidence 206
  non-small cell *see* non-small cell lung cancer
  older patients **141**
  pathology 206–7, **207**
  post-treatment assessments 219, **219**
  pregnancy 137
  prognostic factors **209**, **210**
  risk factors **206**
  screening 206, **206**
  small cell *see* small cell lung cancer
  staging **208**, **209**
  treatment 210–19
    principles **210**
    radiotherapy 211–13, **212**
    surgery 210–11, **210**, **211**
    systemic therapy 213–19
lymphatic invasion 38
lymph nodes
  axillary, staging 225–6
  neck, imaging **71**
  sentinel *see* sentinel lymph nodes
lymphoblastic lymphoma
  biomarkers **773**
  paediatric 773
  pathology and natural history **405**
  treatment **413**
lymphoedema 196–7
lymphoid markers **89**
lymphoma 392–414
  biomarkers **773**
  CNS 719–20
    imaging **708**
  diagnosis 136, **393–4**
  epidemiology 136
  Hodgkin *see* Hodgkin lymphoma
  imaging 79
  incidence and aetiology **393**
  non-Hodgkin *see* non-Hodgkin lymphoma
  ocular adnexal 736–40, *736*
  older patients **141**
  paediatric 772–4, **773**, **774**
  pregnancy 136–7
  presentation 393
  screening 393
  staging 136, 774, **774**
  standardized response criteria **49**
  treatment 136–7
lymphoplasmacytic lymphoma
  pathology and natural history **401**
  treatment **411**
Lynch syndrome 310
  screening for 90
lysozyme **432**

M

McDonald response assessment guidelines **67**
McGill Pain Questionnaire 169
magnetic resonance imaging (MRI) 54, 63–4, **63**, **64**
  contrast-enhanced *see* contrast-enhanced MRI
  response assessment 43
  signal intensity **64**
  site-specific
    cervical cancer 80
    colorectal cancer 314
    lung cancer **208**
    rectal cancer 77
  vs CT **65**
maintenance therapy 129
malignant ascites 152
malignant effusions 151–2
malignant melanoma *see* melanoma
mammoglobulin **601**
mammography 72, *72*, **72**, 135
mantle cell lymphoma
  Mantle International Prognostic Index 407
  pathology and natural history **400–1**
  treatment **410**
marginal zone lymphoma, nodal type
  pathology and natural history **401**
  treatment **411**
Masson trichrome **88**
MDM2 **759**
mediastinoscopy 208
medullary thyroid cancer 637–8, **637**, **638**
medulloblastoma 720–1
  diagnostic work-up 720–1
  follow-up 721
  imaging **708**
  paediatric 777–8, **777**, **778**
  pathology 720
  prognostic factors **714**
  treatment 721, **721**
megakaryocytic markers **432**
megestrol acetate suspension 156
Melan A/Mart1 **89**, **601**
melanocytic markers **89**
melanoma 689–705
  clinical trials **703–4**
  controversies 702
  diagnosis 137
  diagnostic work-up **694–5**
  epidemiology 137
  incidence and aetiology 690, **690–1**
  natural history and presentation **693–4**, 694
  oesophagus 283
  pathology 692, **692–3**
  penis 385
  pregnancy 137
  prognostic factors 696–7, **697**
  research priorities 704–5
  screening **691–2**
  sinonasal 589
  staging 695–6, **696**
  treatment 137, 700–2
    principles 697, **697–9**
    radiotherapy 699, **700**, 701
    surgery **700**
    systemic therapy **701–2**
  uveal **693**, 727–32
  vulva **496**
melphalan **419**, **420**
Memorial Pain Assessment Card 169
men
  breast cancer 236–7
  penile cancer 384–91
  testicular cancer 368–83
meningioma 718–19
  diagnostic work-up 718
  follow-up 719
  imaging **708**
  pathology 718
  prognostic factors **714**
  treatment 718–19, **719**
Merkel cell carcinoma 687
  incidence and aetiology **675**
  pathology **677**
  presentation and natural history **678**
  routes of spread **679**
  treatment 685–6, **685**, **686**
meropenem 138
mesna **396**
metabolic evaluation of tumours 50, 52
metabolomics 53
metaplasia 92
metastases
  bone *see* bone metastases
  brain 146, 721–2, **722**
  pattern of 98–9
  systemic therapy 127–8
  TNM classification 37
metastatectomy 363
methadone 163
methotrexate
  bone tumours **750**, 751, **751**
  CNS tumours **721**
  patient co-morbidities **132**
  salivary gland tumours 584
methotrimeprazine **178**
metoclopramide 138, **176**, **178**
metronidazole 138
metyrapone **654**
micrometastases 90
microorganisms, histochemical stains **88**
microwave ablation **256**
midazolam, drug interactions **143**
mirtazapine 156, 166
mismatch repair 110
missing data 42
mitotane **654**
mitoxantrone
  prostate cancer **339**
  salivary gland tumours 584
mixed ductal-endocrine carcinoma 273
molecular epidemiology 3
molecularly targeted chemotherapy 125–6, **125**
molecular markers *see* biomarkers
molecular pathology 95–6
  DNA sequencing 95
  predictive/prognostic significance 95–6
molecular targeting agents 117
monoclonal antibodies
  ALL 440
  see also specific antibodies
monoclonal gammopathy of undetermined significance (MGUS) **418**

monocytic markers **432**
MOPP regimen **396**
morbidity, surgery-associated 99–100
morphine 163, **171**
mounting of specimens 87
MRI see magnetic resonance imaging
mucicarmine stain **88**, 89
mucin, histochemical stains 88
mucinous non-cystic carcinoma **273**
mucoepidermoid carcinoma **574**
mucosal melanoma **693**
mucositis 164–5
multidetector CT 63
multigated acquisition (MUGA) scan 130
multi-institutional data sharing 56
multimodality treatment plans, surgery 100–1
multiple myeloma **418**
  see also myeloma
muramyl tripeptide phosphatidylethanolamine 751–2
muscle markers 89
musculoskeletal tumours
  imaging 78–9
  see also bone tumours; soft tissue tumours
My Cancer Genome database 96
mycosis fungoides
  pathology and natural history **404**
  treatment **412**
myelodysplastic syndrome, standardized response criteria **49**
myeloid leukaemia
  acute 430–6
  chronic 441–4
myelolipoma **650**, 651
myeloma 415–26
  clinical trials **425**
  controversies 423–4
  diagnostic work-up 417, **417–18**
  imaging 79
  incidence and aetiology 416–17, **416**
  post-treatment assessment 422, 423
  presentation and natural history 417
  prognostic risk factors 418–19, **419**
  research priorities 424
  staging 418, **418**
  standardized response criteria **49**
  treatment 419–23, **419**, **420–2**
MyoD1 **601**
myogenin **601**

N

naproxen sodium **170**
nasal cavity tumours see sinonasal tumours
nasopharyngeal cancer 512–23
  biomarkers **515**
  clinical trials **521–2**
  controversies 520–1
  diagnostic work-up **515**
  imaging 70
  incidence and aetiology 513, **513**
  pathology 513, **513–14**
  presentation and natural history 514, **514–15**
  prognostic factors 515, **516**
  research priorities 522
  risk factors **8**
  screening 513, **513**
  staging 515, **516**
  treatment 517–20
    principles 515–16, **516–17**
    radiotherapy **518–19**
    surgery **517–18**
    systemic therapy **520**

National Comprehensive Cancer Network (NCCN) 175, 229
National Electrical Manufacturers Association (NEMA) 59
nausea and vomiting
  mechanism of 175, **176**
  nutritional treatment 162, **162**
  older patients 142–3
  palliative care 175–6, 175, **176**
  pregnancy 138
  refractory 152–3
  supportive care 161–2, **162**
nefazodone, drug interactions **143**
nelfinavir, drug interactions **143**
neoadjuvant therapy 103, **126**, 127
neoplasm 92
nephrectomy **361**
  cytoreductive 363
neuroblastoma
  imaging 79
  paediatric 778–81, **778–81**
  staging 779, **779**
  treatment 780–1, **780–1**
neuroendocrine markers 89
neuroendocrine tumours 656–73
  biomarkers **659**
  clinical trials 671, **672**
  diagnostic work-up **658–63**
  incidence and aetiology 657, **657**
  pathology and natural history 657, **657**, **658**
  presentation 657–8
  staging **663**
  treatment 664–71
    chemoembolization 671
    principles 663–4
    radioembolization 671
    radionuclide therapy 670–1, 670, **670**, **671**
    surgery 664, **664–5**
    systemic therapy 665–9, **666–9**
    transarterial chemoembolization 671
  WHO classification **657**
  see also specific sites
neurone-specific enolase **371**
neuropathic pain 164, 169, 173
neutropenia 153
neutropenic fever 147–9
NG2 homologue **432**
nilotinib **443**
nitrogen mustard **396**
NHL (also see non-Hodgkin Lymphoma)
NMP1 mutation **433**
NMP22 **51**
NMSC see skin cancer, non-melanoma
nodular melanoma **692**
nomograms 29
non-Hodgkin lymphoma 400–14
  B-cell
    pathology and presentation **400–3**
    treatment **409–12**
  HIV-related **798**, **800**, **801**, **803–5**, **804–5**
  mature B-cell/T-cell subtypes **399**
  paediatric 772–4, **773**, **774**
  prognostic factors 405–6, **406**
    International Prognostic Index 405, 407
  refractory/relapsing 413–14
  risk factors **8**
  staging 405, 406
  T-cell
    pathology and presentation **403–5**
    treatment **412–13**
  treatment, principles 407–8, 408
  see also individual types
non-relational databases (NoSQLs) 56–7

non-small cell lung cancer (NSCLC)
  imaging 72–3, **73**, 74
  treatment
    radiotherapy 211–12
    surgery 210
    systemic therapy 213–18, **214**, **215**, **217**
nortriptyline 166
novibine **289**
NRAS mutation 316
NSCLC see non-small cell lung cancer
NSE **432**
nuclear matrix protein see NMP
nutritional treatment
  constipation 160
  diarrhoea **158**
  mucositis 165
  nausea and vomiting 162, **162**

O

obesity as cancer risk factor 8, 188
obinutuzumab **447**
observational studies 4–5
  case-control studies 5
  cohort studies 5
occupational risk factors 9
octreotide **178**
ocular adnexal lymphoma 736–40, 736
  controversies 739–40
  diagnostic work-up 737–8
  incidence and aetiology **737**
  natural history 737
  post-treatment assessment 739
  presentation 737
  prognostic factors **738**
  staging **738**
  treatment **739**
    principles 738
oesophageal cancer 280–96
  adenocarcinoma **282**, 291–5
    clinical trials **295**
    controversies 295
    treatment **292–4**
    treatment principles 291, **291–2**
  diagnostic work-up **283**
  HPV-related **281**
  imaging 73–4
  incidence and aetiology 280, **281**
  pathology and natural history **281–3**
  presentation 281
  prognostic factors 284, **284**
  screening 280, **281**
  squamous cell carcinoma **281–2**, 285–91
    clinical trials **291**
    controversies 290–1
    treatment **286–90**
    treatment principles 285, **285–6**
  staging 283, **283–4**
oesophageal endoscopic ultrasound 208
oesophagectomy 290, 295
oestrogen receptor **601**
ofatumumab **447**
Okuda staging system 251, **251**
olanzepine **176**, **178**, 179
older patients 139–44
  ALL 441
  AML 435–6
  chemotherapy 140, 142, **142**
  definition 139–40
  radiotherapy 140, **141–2**
  screening tools 140
  surgery 140
  treatment principles 143–4

treatment-related issues 142–3
   anaemia 143
   bone health 143
   drug-drug interactions 143, **143**
   febrile neutropenia 142
   nausea and vomiting 142–3
oligodendroglioma **714**
oligometastasis
OncotypeDx Recurrence Score Assay(R) 236
ondansetron 138, 153, **176**, **178**
operations research 58
opioid analgesics 163, 170–1, **171**, **178**
   side effects 171
Opisthorchis viverrini **8**
oral cancers 524–41
   clinical trials **540**
   controversies 539
   diagnostic work-up **529–30**
   follow-up and continuing care 538, **538–9**
   HPV-related **525**
   incidence and aetiology 525, **525**
   palliative care 538
   pathology 526, **526–7**
   presentation and natural history 527, **527–8**
   prognostic factors 530–2, **531**
   research priorities 539–41
   screening **526**, 539
   staging **530**
   treatment 533–8
     principles 530, *532*, **533–5**
     radiotherapy 536, **536–7**
     surgery **535–6**
     systemic therapy 537, **537–8**
oral hygiene and cancer risk 10
oral rehydration therapy 158
orchiectomy **371**
organs at risk 119
organ transplantation
   cancer following 812–13, **812–13**
   liver 255, 259–60
   post-transplantation lymphoproliferative disease 809–11
oropharyngeal cancer 559–70
   clinical trials **569**
   controversies 569
   diagnostic work-up 563, **563**
   HPV-related 30–1, **510**, 560, **560–1**, 561, 562, **562**, **564**, 565, 566, 570
   imaging **70**
   incidence and aetiology 560, **561–2**
   metastatic 568
   non-metastatic
     follow-up and continuing care 568
     managment 564–7, *565*, **566**, **567**
     treatment response 567
   pathology 561, **561**
   presentation and natural history 562, **562**
   prevention **561**
   prognostic factors 563, **564**
   research priorities 570
   risk factors **8**
   staging 563, *563*, **564**
   treatment failure 568, **569**
osmotic diarrhoea 157
osteoporosis 143
osteosarcoma *see* bone tumours
outcome reporting 40–52
   clinical endpoints 40
   effect size and competing risk 40–1
   interim analysis of clinical trials 42
   missing data 42
   multiple variables 41
   quality of life 42

response assessment *see* response assessment
sample size in clinical trials 42
toxicity reporting 41–2
ovarian cancer 479–91
   clinical trials **490**
   diagnostic work-up 481, **481**
   imaging 80
   incidence and aetiology 479–80, **480**
   pathology and natural history 481–3, *482*, **482–3**
   pregnancy 137
   presentation 480
   prognostic factors 483–5, **485**
   research priorities 491
   screening **480**
   staging 483, **484**
   treatment 486–9, **489**
     principles 485, **485–6**, **488**
     recurrent disease 489, **489**
     surgery **486–7**
     systemic therapy **487–8**
   see also fallopian tube cancer
overall survival 40, 41, **41**
oxaliplatin
   CUP **795**
   neuroendocrine tumours 669
   oesophageal cancer **289**, **290**
   patient co morbidities **132**
oxycodone 163, **171**
oxygen enhancement ratio 113
oxygen, hyperbaric 113

P
p16 **601**
p63 **601**
paclitaxel
   CUP (cancer of unknown primary) **795**
   head and neck cancers 509
   lung cancer 214
   nasopharyngeal cancer **520**
   oesophageal cancer **289**, **290**
   ovarian cancer **488**
   penile cancer **389**
   salivary gland tumours 584
   testicular cancer **381**
   uterine cancer 475
paediatric tumours 768–87, *768*
   brain tumours 775–8, *775*, *776*, **777**, **778**
   leukaemia 768–72, **769–72**
   lymphoma
     Hodgkin 774–5
     non-Hodgkin 772–4, **773**, **774**
   neuroblastoma 778–81, **778–81**
   osteosarcoma 781–2, **781**, **782**
   palliative care 183
   rhabdomyosarcoma 783–4, **783**, **784**
   solid tumours, imaging 79
   Wilms tumour 785–6, **785**, **786**
Paget disease of nipple **223**
pain 162–5
   assessment 162–3, 169
   definition 168
   emergencies 173
   epidemiology 168
   measurement 169
   mucositis 164–5
   neuropathic 164, 169, 173
   pathophysiology 168–9
   in survivors 186
pain syndromes 163, 172–3
   bone pain 172–3
   post-chemotherapy 172
   see also neuropathic pain

pain treatment 163–5, 169–72
   adjuvant analgesics 171–2
   bowel obstruction **178**
   interventional approaches 172
   non-opioid analgesics 170, **170**
   opioid analgesics 163, 170–1, **171**
   pregnancy 138
   topical 164
   WHO three-step analgesic ladder 170
palliative care 174–83
   bereavement support 182
   cancer of unknown primary 795
   colorectal cancer 325
   EEMAA principles 174
   end of life 182–3
   ethics 181
   paediatric 183
   radiotherapy 118
   research 182–3
   services models *175*
   social issues 181
   spiritual 181
   surgery 105
   symptom control 175–81
     anorexia and cachexia syndrome 177–9
     bleeding 179–80
     bowel obstruction 177, **178**
     constipation 176, *177*, **177**
     delirium 179
     diarrhoea 176–7
     dyspnoea 179
     fatigue and asthenia 179
     nausea and vomiting 175–6, *175*, **176**
     psychological reactions 180–1, *180*, **181**
   systemic therapy 127
   see also supportive care
palonosetron 153
palpation 43–4
pancreatic cancer 270–9, *271*
   biomarkers **51**, **274**
   clinical trials **278**
   controversies 277
   diagnostic work-up *274*, **274**
   imaging 75–6, **76**
   incidence and aetiology **271–2**
   natural history 273, **273**
   pathology 272, **272–3**
   presentation 273
   prognostic factors 275, **275**
   research priorities 278
   screening **272**
   staging 275, **275**
   treatment **275–7**
pancreatic neuroendocrine tumours **662**
   systemic therapy 667, **667–8**
panitumumab
   colorectal cancer 323
panobinostat **421**
panomics 53, 55
Papanicolaou (Pap) test 92
papilloma, sinonasal **587**
paranasal sinus tumours *see* sinonasal tumours
parapharyngeal masses, imaging **71**
parenteral nutrition 179
paroxetine 166
partial organ irradiation 116
pathological classification of tumours 35–6
pathology 83–97
   cytopathology 91–3
   diagnostic haematopathology 94–5
   hallmarks of cancer 30
   molecular pathology 95–6
   surgical *see* surgical pathology
   terminology 92

Patient-Centered Outcomes Research network 59
patient-centred care 24, 25, **25**, *54*
patient education
　cancer survivors 192
　　constipation **161**
　　diarrhoea **159**
patient-managed data 59
patient-reported outcome (PRO) measures 27
　response assessment 52
PAX3-FKHR **759**
Pax5 **89**
PAX7-FKHR **759**
pazopanib
　renal cell carcinoma **365**
PDG-FRA/B **757**
pemetrexed
　bladder cancer **350**
　lung cancer 129, **214**, **215**, 216
penile cancer 384–91
　aetiology and incidence 384, **385**
　continuing care 390, *390*
　controversies 390
　diagnostic work-up **386**
　HPV-related 384, **385**, **387**, 390
　pathology and natural history **385**
　post-treatment assessment 390
　presentation 385
　prognostic factors 387, **387**
　research priorities 390
　screening 385
　staging 386, **386**
　systemic therapy 389, **389**
　treatment 388–9
　　principles 387, **387**
　　radiotherapy 389, *389*, **389**
　　surgery 388, *388*, **388**
pentazocine **171**
peptide receptor radionuclide therapy 670–1, *670*, **670**, **671**
percutaneous ethanol injection **256**
pericardial effusion/tamponade 151–2
perineural invasion 38
　NMSC **687**
periodic acid-Schiff (PAS)-alcian blue **88**
periodic acid-Schiff (PAS) stain **88**
perioperative risk **100**
peripheral nerve blocks **172**
peripheral neuropathy 194–5, **195**
peripheral T-cell lymphoma, not otherwise specified **403**
Perl's iron stain **88**, *89*
peroxy radicals 113
PET 50, 65
　FDG *see* FDG-PET
　site-specific studies, CNS tumours 66, *67*
PET-CT 65
　site-specific
　　lung cancer **208**
　　NSCLC *74*
Peutz-Jeghers syndrome 310
PGP 9.5 **601**
phaeochromocytoma **642**
　aetiology and physiology **647–8**
　diagnostic work-up **649**
　presentation and natural history *648*, **648**
　treatment **649–50**
　　perioperative **653**
phenobarbital, drug interactions **143**
phenytoin, drug interactions **143**
phylloides tumours **223**
physical examination for response assessment 43–4
PI3K mutation 316

PIAF regimen **258**
PICO(T) process 19
Picture Archival and Communication System (PACS) 54
piroxicam **170**
pituitary tumours 609–25
　clinical trials **624**
　diagnostic considerations 614–16, *614*, *615*
　diagnostic work-up **614**
　incidence and aetiology **610**
　pathology and natural history **610–11**
　presentation 612, **612–14**
　research priorities **624**
　screening **610**
　staging 617, **617**
　treatment 618–24
　　principles 617–18, **617**
　see also specific types
placental alkaline phosphatase **371**
planning organ at risk volume 119
planning target volume 119
plaque brachytherapy **731**, **735**
plasmablastic lymphoma
　pathology and natural history **402**
　treatment **412**
plasma cell leukaemia **418**
plasmacytoma
　extramedullary **418**
　solitary of bone **418**
pleomorphic adenoma **574**
pleomorphism **92**
pleural effusions 152
PO_2 112
point-of-care technology 55
pollution as cancer risk factor 9
pomalidomide **421**
ponatinib **443**
population-based cancer registries (PBCRs) 3–4
positron emission tomography *see* PET
POSSUM 140
postoperative surveillance **106**
post-thoracotomy syndrome 197
post-transplantation lymphoproliferative disease 809–11
　incidence and aetiology **809–10**
　screening **810**
　treatment 810–11
pralatrexate **412**
predictive markers *see* biomarkers
prednisone
　ALL **439**
　CHOP regimen 128, **412**, **739**
　melanoma **702**
　myeloma **420**
　nausea and vomiting 138
　non-Hodgkin lymphoma **396**
　prostate cancer **339**
pregabalin **164**
pregnancy 134–8
　breast cancer 134–6, 237
　cervical cancer 136, 465
　leukaemia 137
　lung cancer 137
　lymphoma 136–7
　malignant melanoma 137
　obstetric considerations **134**, **135**
　ovarian cancer 137
　soft tissue sarcoma 137–8
　supportive care 138
prevention 10–11
preventive surgery **106**

primary cutaneous CD30+ T-cell lymphoproliferative disorders
　pathology and natural history **403–4**
　treatment **412**
primary cutaneous follicle centre lymphoma
　pathology and natural history **402**
　treatment **411**
primary mediastinal (thymic) large B-cell lymphoma
　pathology and natural history **401**
　treatment **411**
primitive neuroectodermal tumour (PNET) 720–1
privacy 58
procarbazine
　CNS tumours 717, **721**
　Hodgkin lymphoma **396**
processing of specimens 87
prochlorperazine **176**, **178**
profiling 28
Prognosis Research Strategy (PROGRESS) Group 24
prognostic factors 23–4, *24*
　biological 27
　classification 29–33, **30**
　　clinical relevance-based 32–3
　　subject-based 30–2, **30**, **31**
　and combination treatment algorithms 28–9
　environment-related 32, **32**
　host-related 31–2, **31**
　purpose of analysis 24–5, **25**
　studies of
　　challenges 26–7
　　endpoints 27
　　methodological pitfalls **28**
　　population selection 25–6
　　statistical techniques 27–8, **28**
　　taxonomy 28–9
　traditional 27
　tumour-related 30–1, **30**
　uncertainties in attribution 26–7
　　co-morbidity 26–7
　　non-baseline factors 26
　　responding vs. non-responding cases 26
　see also individual cancers
prognostic groups 28
prognostic markers *see* biomarkers
progression-free survival 40, 41, **41**, 43
prolactinomas **611**
　diagnosis 614–15
　presentation **613**
　treatment **620–1**
propoxyphene **171**
prostate cancer 333–42
　clinical trials **341**
　continuing care 340–1
　d'Amico risk classification **335**
　diagnostic work-up **334**
　imaging 80–1
　incidence and aetiology **334**
　older patients **141**
　pathology and natural history 334, **334**
　post-treatment assessment 340
　presentation 334
　prognostic factors **335**
　research priorities 341
　screening **334**
　staging **335**
　standardized response criteria 48
　treatment 337–40
　　principles **336–7**
　　radiotherapy **337–8**
　　surgery **337**
　　systemic therapy **338–40**
prostate-specific antigen (PSA) 31
proteomics 53

proton beam irradiation 595
  uveal melanoma **731**
psychosocial care 165
  adjustment reactions 166
  anxiety 166
  communication 165
  depression 166
  follow-up and re-evaluation 166
  screening and assessment 165
  suicide risk 167
  treatment plan 166
psychosocial distress 187
PTEN mutation 316
public health **4**
pulmonary function tests **208**

Q
quality appraisal in CPGs 20, **20**
quality assurance
  cytopathology 92
  radiotherapy 119
quality of care 106
quality of life 42
QUANTEC program 116, 119

R
radiation biology 109, *109*
  molecular/cellular aspects 109–17
    cell survival curve 110–11, *111*
    DNA damage/repair 109–10
    dose–response relationship 110–11, *111*
    fractional sensitivity 111, *111*
    tumour and normal cell repopulation 112
  tissue reactions *see* radiation injury
  tumour microenvironment 112–13
  see also radiotherapy
radiation injury
  acute 113–14
  fractionation and tissue tolerance 115
  late 114–15
  normal tissue complication probability (NTCP) 116
  partial organ irradiation 116
  re-irradiation of previously treated tissue 115–16
radiation retinopathy 732
radioactive iodine 633–4, **634**
radioembolization
  liver cancer **257**, 259
  neuroendocrine tumours 671
radiofrequency ablation **256**
  renal cell carcinoma **361**
  stereotactic 120
radioimmunotherapy in ocular adnexal lymphoma **739**
radionuclide therapy of neuroendocrine tumours 670–1, *670*, **670**, **671**
radiosurgery in meningioma 719
radiotherapy 108–23
  adrenal tumours **654**
  biliary cancers **268**
  biological basis 109–17
  bladder cancer **349**
  bone tumours **750**
  brachytherapy 121, **121**
  cervical cancer 463, **463**
  CNS tumours 709, **715–16**, 719, 720, 721
  brain metastases 722, 723
  colorectal cancer **319**, 323–4
  combination with chemotherapy 116–17
  curative radiotherapy 117–18
  departmental organization 122–3, *122*
  dose distribution and modality 120–1, *120*
  dose per fraction 115

dose–response curves 110–11, *111*
dose–volume parameters 119
fallopian tube cancer 493
gastric cancer **303–4**
global context 108–9
growth hormone-secreting tumours 618
head and neck cancers 508–9, **508**
  unknown primary 604–6, **604–6**
ICRU concepts 118–19
individualized 121–2
liver cancer 257, **257**
low linear energy transfer 113
lung cancer 211–13, **212**
lymphoma **774**
nasopharyngeal cancer **518–19**
oesophageal cancer
  adenocarcinoma **294**
  squamous cell carcinoma 287–8
older patients 140, **141–2**
oral cancers 536, **536–7**
oropharyngeal cancer **567**
pain induced by 163
palliative 118
pancreatic cancer **276–7**
penile cancer 389, *389*, **389**
planning aims 119
pregnancy **135**
prostate cancer **337–8**
renal cell carcinoma 363
role of 117–18
salivary gland tumours 583, **583–4**
sinonasal tumours 594–5, **594**, **595**
skin cancer
  melanoma 699, **700**, 701
  NMSC 683, **683**, **684**, **685**
soft tissue tumours **764**
target volumes 118–19
therapeutic ratio *109*
thyroid cancers
  anaplastic **636**
  differential thyroid cancer **632–3**
  medullary **638**
treatment optimization 119
uterine cancer **474–5**
vulval cancer 500, **500**
see also specific modalities
Rai staging system **445**
randomized controlled trials (RCTs) 14, **15**, 60
see also clinical trials
ranitidine 178
RANO 67
rasburicase 150
R-CHOP regimen **396**
RCTs *see* randomized controlled trials
real world learning 60–1, *61*, **61**
RECIST system 44–6, **44**, 55
  best overall response 45–6
  measurable and non-measurable lesions 45
  response assessment 45
  special considerations 46
  target and non-target lesions 45
reconstructive surgery 105–6
rectal cancer *see* colorectal cancer
refractory/relapsing cancer 129–30
regional control 40
rehabilitation 194–202
  activities of daily living (ADL) 140, 194, **195**
  common diagnoses 194–201
    amputation and limb salvage 197–8
    cancer fatigue 195–6
    cognitive impairment 199–200

dysphagia 197
late treatment effects 201, **201**
lymphoedema 196–7
pelvic floor dysfunction 199
peripheral neuropathy 194–5, **195**
post-thoracotomy syndrome 197
spinal accessory nerve injury 196
spinal cord compression 200–1
re-irradiation 115–16
relative risk 5
reliability 42
renal cell carcinoma 354–67
  clinical trials **366**
  continuing care 366
  controversies 366
  diagnostic work-up 357, **357**, *358*
  imaging 80
  incidence and aetiology **355**
  pathology and natural history 355–7, **355–6**
  post-treatment assessment 365–6, **366**
  presentation 357
  prognostic factors **359**
  research priorities 366
  screening **355**
  staging **359**
  standardized response criteria **48**
  treatment 360–5
    adjuvant therapy 363
    principles 359, **360**
    radiotherapy 363
    surgery 360–3, **360–2**
    systemic therapy 363–5, **364**, **365**
  tumour thrombus 362
Reporting Recommendations for Tumor Marker Prognostic Studies (REMARK) 27
research 24, 25, **25**
  cancer survivors 190–1
  data infrastructure 55–6
  palliative care 182–3
  response assessment 43
research priorities 19
  adrenal tumours 655
  biliary cancers 269
  bladder cancer 353
  bone tumours 752
  breast cancer 240
  CNS tumours 725
  colorectal cancer 326
  eye tumours 743
  Hodgkin lymphoma 399–400
  laryngeal cancer 557
  leukaemia 436, 441, 444
  liver cancer 261
  myeloma 424
  nasopharyngeal cancer 522
  oral cancers 539–41
  oropharyngeal cancer 570
  ovarian cancer 491
  pancreatic cancer 278
  penile cancer 390
  pituitary tumours 624
  prostate cancer 341
  renal cell carcinoma 366
  salivary gland tumours 585
  sinonasal tumours 596
  skin cancer
    melanoma 704–5
    NMSC 687
  soft tissue tumours 766
  thyroid cancers 639
  uterine cancer 477
  vulval cancer 502
resectability of tumours 99–100

response assessment 42–3
  applications 43
  biomarkers 50, **51**
  definition 42–3
  imaging 43
  limitations 46, 50
  metabolic evaluation of tumours 50, 52
  patient-reported outcomes 52
  physical examination 43–4
  RECIST system 44–6, **44**
  standardized response criteria **47–9**
  see also specific tumour sites
Response Assessment in Neuro-oncology see RANO
Response Evaluation Criteria In Solid Tumors see RECIST system
response rate 43
reticulin stains **88**, 89
retinal detachment, exudative 732
retinoblastoma 732–6, 733
  controversies 736
  diagnostic work-up 733–4
  incidence and aetiology **733**
  pathology 733
  post-treatment assessment 736
  presentation 733
  prognostic factors **735**
  screening 733
  staging **734**
  treatment **735–6**
    principles 735
retromolar trigone
  imaging 70
  tumours of **535**
rhabdomyosarcoma **757**, 765
  imaging 79
  paediatric 783–4, **783**, **784**
rifabutin, drug interactions **143**
rifampin, drug interactions **143**
rifapentine, drug interactions **143**
risk factors for cancer 7–10, **7**
  alcohol 7–8
  diet 8–9
  genetic susceptibility 10
  hormonal factors 9
  infections 8, **8**
  obesity 8
  occupation 9
  pollution 9
  radiation 10
  tobacco 7
risk of malignancy index 481
ritonavir, drug interactions **143**
rituximab **125**
  CLL **447**
  Hodgkin lymphoma **396**
  non-Hodgkin lymphoma **411**
robotic surgery 107
  image-guided 55
romedepsin **412**
rotational intensity-modulated radiotherapy 121
route of administration 131

S
S-100 **89**, **600**, **601**
St Jude/Murphy staging system **774**
salivary duct carcinoma **576**
salivary gland hypoplasia 114
salivary gland tumours 571–85
  biomarkers 579, **579**
  clinical trials **585**
  controversies 584
  diagnostic work-up **577–8**
  imaging **71**
  incidence and aetiology **572**
  natural history **576–7**
  pathology 573, **573**, **574–6**
  presentation 576
  prognostic factors 578, **579**
  research priorities 585
  staging **578**
  treatment 581–4
    principles 579, 580, **580–1**
    radiotherapy 583, **583–4**
    surgery 581–3, **581–2**
    systemic therapy 584, **584**
    targeted therapy 584
  WHO classification 573
salvage therapy, lung cancer 215–16
sampling errors 86
saquinavir, drug interactions **143**
sarcoma **92**
  Kaposi see Kaposi sarcoma
  oesophagus **282**
  soft tissue 137–8
  synovial **758**
Schistosoma haematobium 8
scopolamine **178**
screening
  anal cancer **328**
  biliary cancers **265**
  breast cancer 222, **222**
  cervical cancer **451–2**, 452
  colorectal cancer **309**, 311–12
  cytopathology 92
  familial cancer syndromes 90
  fatigue 155
  gastric cancer **298**
  head and neck cancers **504**
  HIV-related neoplasms **801**
  liver cancer **242**, 243
  lung cancer 206, **206**
  lymphoma **393**
  Lynch syndrome 90
  nasopharyngeal cancer 513, **513**
  oesophageal cancer 280, **281**
  older patients **140**
  oral cancers **526**, 539
  ovarian cancer **480**
  pancreatic cancer **272**
  penile cancer **385**
  pituitary tumours **610**
  prostate cancer **334**
  psychosocial needs 165
  renal cell carcinoma **355**
  retinoblastoma **733**
  skin cancer
    melanoma **691–2**
    NMSC **676**
  soft tissue tumours **755**
  surgical aspects 103–4
  testicular cancer **369**
  thyroid cancers **627**
  uterine cancer **469**
  vulval cancer **496**
secretory diarrhoea 157
selection bias 5
selective serotonin norepinephrine reuptake inhibitors see SSNRIs
selective serotonin reuptake inhibitors see SSRIs
semantic interoperability 57, **57**
seminoma **370**
sentinel lymph nodes, TNM classification 37
Sertoli-Leydig tumours **483**
sertraline 166
sex-cord stromal tumours 481, **483**, **488**
sexual dysfunction 199

Sézary syndrome
  pathology and natural history **404**
  treatment **412**
SIADH 149–50
sialyl Tn antigens **300**
sigmoidoscopy 103
signet ring cell carcinoma **273**
single nucleotide polymorphisms 10
single photon emission computed tomography see SPECT
single-strand break repair 110
sinonasal tumours 586–96
  controversies 596
  diagnostic work-up 589
  follow-up 596
  HPV-related **587**
  imaging 71
  incidence and aetiology **587**
  pathology 587, **587–9**
  presentation 589
  prognostic factors **591**
  research priorities 596
  staging **590**
  treatment 592–5
    neck 593
    primary tumour **592**
    principles 591, **592**
    radiotherapy 594–5, **594**, **595**
    surgery 593–4
    systemic therapy 595, **595**
sinonasal undifferentiated carcinoma (SNUC) **588–9**
skin cancer, non-melanoma 674–88
  assessment and follow-up 685–6, **686**
  clinical trials **687**
  controversies 686–7
  diagnostic work-up 679, **689**
  HPV-related **675**
  immunosuppressed patients 686
  incidence and aetiology **675**
  pathology **676–7**
  perineural invasion 687
  presentation and natural history 677, **677–8**
  prognostic factors 679, **680**, **681**
  research priorities 687
  routes of spread **678–9**
  screening 676
  staging **680**
  treatment 681–5
  see also specific types
sleep, strategies for 156–7
small cell carcinoma
  oesophagus **282**
  sinonasal 589
small cell lung cancer (SCLC)
  imaging 72–3, **73**
  treatment
    radiotherapy 212–13
    surgery 211
    systemic therapy 218–19, **218**
small intestinal neuroendocrine tumours **660**
  systemic therapy 668, **668**
small lymphocytic lymphoma/chronic lymphocytic leukaemia
  pathology and natural history **400**
  treatment **410**
SnNout outcomes 15
SNOMED 39, 57
Snook reticulin stain **88**
social issues in palliative care 181
soft tissue tumours 754–67
  biomarkers **759**
  clinical trials **766**
  controversies 765

diagnostic work-up 758, **759**
imaging 78–9
incidence and aetiology 755, **755**
pathology 756, **756**
pregnancy 137–8
presentation and natural history 756, 757–8
prognostic factors 760, **760**
research priorities 766
screening **755**
staging 760, **760**
standardized response criteria **48**
treatment 763–5
  principles 761, **761–2**
  radiotherapy **764**
  surgery **763**
  systemic therapy **765**
  targeted therapy **765**
solariums, and skin cancer 686
solid tumours
  paediatric **79**
  standardized response criteria **47**
solitary plasmacytoma of bone **418**
solitary pulmonary nodules **73**
somatostatin analogues in neuroendocrine tumours 668, **669**
sorafenib
  liver cancer **258**
  renal cell carcinoma **365**
specimen handling
  cytopathology **92**
  surgical pathology 83–5, *84*
  see also surgical pathology
SPECT **65**
SPECT-CT **65**
spinal accessory nerve injury 196
spinal cord
  compression 146–7, 200–1
  stimulation 172
spindle cell carcinoma of mouth **526**
spiritual care 181
splenic B-cell marginal zone lymphoma
  pathology and natural history **402**
  treatment **411**
SpPin outcomes 15
squamous cell carcinoma
  cervix **454–5**
  incidence and aetiology **675**
  mouth **526**
  nasopharynx **514**
  oesophagus **281–2**, 285–91
    clinical trials **291**
    controversies 290–1
    treatment **286–90**
    treatment principles 285, **285–6**
  pathology **676–7**
  penis **385**
  presentation and natural history **678**
  routes of spread **679**
  sinonasal **588**
  treatment
    guidelines **682**
    principles 681, **681–2**
    radiotherapy 683, **683**, **684**
    surgery 682, **682**
    systemic therapy **684**
SS18-SSX1/SSX2/SSX4 **759**
SSNRIs 164, 166
SSRIs 164, 166
  see also individual drugs
staging 28, 29, 31, 34–9
  adrenal tumours 646, **646**
  anal cancer 329, **329**

biliary cancers 265–6, **266**
bladder cancer **345**
bone tumours (osteosarcoma) 748, **748**
breast cancer 135, **227**
cervical cancer 136, 458, **459**
CLL 445, **445**
colorectal cancer 314, **316**
eyelid cancers **741**, **742**
fallopian tube cancer 492, **492**
gastric cancer 300, **301**
head and neck cancers, unknown primary 601, **601**
Hodgkin lymphoma 394–5, **395**
laryngeal cancer **546**
leukaemia 137
liver cancer 249–51, **250**, **251**, 258
lung cancer **208**, **209**
lymphoma 136, 774, **774**
myeloma 418, **418**
nasopharyngeal cancer 515, **516**
neuroblastoma 779, **779**
neuroendocrine tumours **663**
NMSC **680**
non-Hodgkin lymphoma 405, *406*
ocular adnexal lymphoma **738**
oral cancers **530**
oropharyngeal cancer 563, *563*, **564**
ovarian cancer **482**, **484**
pancreatic cancer 275, **275**
penile cancer 386, **386**
pituitary tumours 617, **617**
post-transplantation lymphoproliferative disease 811
prostate cancer **335**
renal cell carcinoma **359**
retinoblastoma **734**
salivary gland tumours **578**
sinonasal tumours **590**
soft tissue tumours 760, **760**
surgical aspects 104–5
testicular cancer 372–3, **372–3**
TNM see TNM staging
uterine cancer **471**
uveal melanoma **729–30**
vulval cancer **497**
statistical analysis of prognostic factors 27–8, **28**
stereotactic ablative radiotherapy 120
stereotactic body radiotherapy 120
stereotactic radiosurgery in growth hormone-secreting tumours 618
steroids
  anorexia-cachexia syndrome 178
  CNS tumors 709
  pain treatment 171–2, 173
  patient co-morbidities **132**
  spinal cord compression 147
  see also individual steroids
stomach cancer see gastric cancer
streptozotocin 667, **669**
suicide risk 167
sunitinib
  neuroendocrine tumours **667–8**
  renal cell carcinoma **365**
superficial spreading melanoma **692**
superior vena cava syndrome 145–6, **146**
supportive care 155–67
  constipation 159–61, **160**, **161**
  diarrhoea 157–9, **158**, **159**
  fatigue 155–7
  nausea and vomiting 161–2, **162**
  pain 162–5
  psychosocial 165–7
  see also palliative treatment

supraglottic cancer 550–1
  see also laryngeal cancer
surgery 98–107
  adrenal tumours 651–3, **653**
  anal cancer 330
  biliary cancers **268**
  bladder cancer **348**
  bone tumours **749–50**
  cervical cancer **461–2**
  CNS tumours 709, **715**, 721
  complications 106
  curative 101–3
    adjuvant therapy 102–3
    aims 101–2
    intraoperative therapies 103
    neoadjuvant therapy 103
  fallopian tube cancer **493**
  gastric cancer **302–3**
  head and neck cancers **507–8**
    unknown primary 604
  incorporation into multimodality treatment plans 100–1
  liver cancer 253–5, **253**, **254**
  lung cancer 210–11, **210**, **211**
  nasopharyngeal cancer **517–18**
  neuroendocrine tumours 664, **664–5**
  new technologies 106–7
  non-curative 103–6
    diagnosis 104
    palliation 105
    prevention 106
    reconstruction 105–6
    screening and surveillance 103–4
    staging 104–5
  oesophageal cancer
    adenocarcinoma **292–3**
    squamous cell carcinoma **286–7**, 290
  older patients 140
  oral cancers **535–6**
  ovarian cancer **486–7**
  pain induced by 163
  pancreatic cancer **276**
  patterns of tumour spread 98–9
  penile cancer 388, *388*, **388**
  postoperative surveillance 106
  prostate cancer **337**
  quality of care 106
  renal cell carcinoma 360–3, **360–2**
  resectability and operability 99–100
    anticipated morbidity 99–100
    perioperative risk 100
    surgical margins 99
    tumour behaviour 100
  robotic 55, 107
  salivary gland tumours 581–3, **581–2**
  sinonasal tumours 593–4
  skin cancer
    melanoma **700**
    NMSC 682, **682**, **685**
  soft tissue tumours **763**
  telesurgery 107
  thyroid cancers
    anaplastic **636**
    differential thyroid cancer **632**
    medullary **638**
  uterine cancer **473**
  video-assisted 208
  vulval cancer 499, *499*, **500**
surgical pathology 83–91
  clinical information 83
  communication with clinician 90–1
  gross evaluation 87
  histological evaluation 87–90, **88**, *89*, **89**

surgical pathology (*continued*)
    intraoperative consultation 85–6, *85*, *86*
    processing and mounting 87
    reporting 90, *91*
    specimen handling 83–5, *84*
surveillance
    cancer survivors 185–6
    postoperative 106
    surgical aspects 103–4
survivorship advocacy 192–3
survivorship care 184–93
    definitions of survivorship 184–5
    elements of 185–8, **185**
        persistent/late side effects 186–7
        prevention and health promotion 187–8
        surveillance 185–6
    healthcare delivery 188–9, **188**, **189**
    low and middle income countries 190
    patient and family education 192
    professional education/training 191–2
    research priorities 190–1
Survivorship Care Plan (SCP) 189, **189**
sympathetic nerve block 172
synaptophysin **89**, **601**
syndrome of inappropriate antidiuretic hormone secretion *see* SIADH
synovial sarcoma **758**
systematic reviews **15**
Systematized Nomenclature of Medicine see SNOMED
systemic therapy **126**
    adjuvant therapy 102–3, **126**, *127*
    biliary cancers 268
    bladder cancer **349–50**
    bone tumours **750–1**
    breast cancer 233–5, **233–5**
    cancer gene therapy 126
    cervical cancer 464
    chemotherapy 124–33
        cytotoxic 124
        hormone therapy 124–5
        immune therapy 126
        molecularly targeted 125–6, **126**
        older patients 140, 142, **142**
        pregnancy **135**
    CNS tumours 709, **716–17**, 719, 720, 721, **721**
    colorectal cancer 321–3, **322–3**
    cost-effectiveness 132
    drugs, dosage and dose intervals 128–9
    duration of 129
    fallopian tube cancer **494**
    head and neck cancers 509
        unknown primary 606
    liver cancer 258, **258**
    lung cancer 213–19
    lymphoma **774**
    metastatic/disseminated cancer 127–8
    monitoring 130–1
    nasopharyngeal cancer **520**
    neoadjuvant (preoperative) therapy 103, **126**, *127*
    neuroendocrine tumours 665–9, **666–9**
    oesophageal cancer
        adenocarcinoma **294**
        squamous cell carcinoma **289–90**
    oral cancers 537, **537–8**
    pancreatic cancer **277**
    patient co-morbidities 131, **131–2**
    penile cancer 389, **389**
    pregnancy 136
    prostate cancer **338–40**
    refractory/relapsing cancer 129–30
    renal cell carcinoma 363–6, **364–6**
    route of administration 131

salivary gland tumours 584, **584**
sinonasal tumours 595, **595**
skin cancer
    melanoma **701–2**
    NMSC **684**, **685**
soft tissue tumours **765**
thyroid cancers
    anaplastic **637**
    differential thyroid cancer **633**
    medullary **638**
toxicity 41–2, 130
uterine cancer 475, **475**
vulval cancer **500**
see also individual drugs

T
tamoxifen 136
tapentadol 163
targeted therapy 125–6, **125**
    AML 436
    clinical trials **476**
    lung cancer 316–17, **317**
    renal cell carcinoma 364–5, **364**, **365**
    salivary gland tumours 584
    soft tissue tumours 765
    uterine cancer 477
taxanes
    patient co-morbidities **131–2**
    see also individual drugs
taxonomy in prognostic factor studies 23, 28–9
T-cell lymphoma
    pathology and presentation **403–5**
    treatment **412–13**
^{99m}Tc-glucoheptonate 66
^{99m}Tc-sestamibi 66
^{99m}Tc-tetrofosmin 66
technical errors 86
telesurgery 107
telithromycin, drug interactions **143**
temozolomide
    CNS tumours **716**
    neuroendocrine tumours 667–8, **669**
temsirolimus
    renal cell carcinoma 365
teratoma
    CNS, imaging **708**
    ovary **482–3**
terminology
    biomarkers 28
    pathology **92**
testicular cancer 368–83
    biomarkers **371**
    clinical trials **382–3**
    diagnostic work-up 370, **371**
    follow-up 381, **381**
    imaging 81
    incidence and aetiology 368, **369**
    natural history 370, **370**
    pathology 369, **369**, **370**
    presentation 370
    prognostic factors **372**, **373**
    screening **369**
    staging 372–3, **372–3**
    treatment 375–81
        CSIIA *376*, *377*, 378, **378**
        CSIII *377*, **379**
        principles **373–4**, *375*
        relapsed/refractory tumours 380, **380**, **381**
        TIN and CSI *375*, **375–7**
testicular intraepithelial neoplasia (TIN) **370**
thalidomide
    myeloma **419**, **420**
The Cancer Imaging Archive (TCIA) 56

therapeutic ratio *109*
thoracic cancers
    imaging 72–3, **73**, *74*
    see also specific sites
thrombocytopenia 153
thrombosis 150–1
thyroglobulin **51**, **601**
thyroid cancers 626–40
    anaplastic 635–7, **635–7**
    biomarkers **51**, **629**
    clinical trials **639**
    diagnostic work-up 628–9, *629*
    differential thyroid cancer 631–5
        controversies 634–5
        treatment 631, **631–4**
    FNA **68**, *93*, **629**
    group classification **629**
    imaging 67–8, **68**, **69**
    incidence and aetiology 626–7
    medullary 637–8, **637**, **638**
    pathology and natural history **627–8**
    presentation 628
    prognostic factors 630, **630**
    research priorities 639
    screening **627**
    staging 629, **630**
thyroidectomy 634–5
thyroid stimulating hormone 67, **68**
thyrotroph-secreting tumours **611**
    presentation **613**
    treatment **622–3**
time to progression 43
time-zero 26
tirapazamine 113
tissue fixation 83–5, *84*
TNM staging 29, 31, 105
    additional descriptors 37–8
    anatomical regions and sites 36
    clinical classification 36–7, **36**
    general rules 35–6
    histopathological grading 37
    history 34–5
    isolated tumour cells 37
    operational descriptors 38
    residual tumour 38
    sentinel lymph nodes 37
    stage group 38
    see also individual cancers
tobacco
    as cancer risk factor 7
    use by cancer survivors 188
tolvaptan 150
tongue
    imaging **70**
    tumours of **535**
tositumomab tiuxetan, non-Hodgkin lymphoma **409**
TP53 **545**
traditional prognostic factors 27
tramadol 163
transarterial chemoembolization (TACE)
    with drug-eluting beads 257
    liver cancer 256–7, **256**, **257**
    neuroendocrine tumours 671
transbronchial needle aspiration (TBNA) 208
transcriptomics 53
translational bioinformatics 55–6, 58
treatment algorithms 29
treatment outcome *see* outcome reporting
treatment scenario 24
tricyclic antidepressants 164, 166
TTF-1 **601**
tumour behaviour 100
tumour blood markers 31

tumour lysis syndrome 150, 773
tumour markers see biomarkers
tumour microenvironment 112–13
tumour profile 29, 30–1, **30**
tumour-related prognostic factors 30–1, **30**
tumour spread see metastases
tyrosinase **89**
tyrosine kinase inhibitors
   CML 442–4, **443**
   resistance 444

U

UICC 29–30, **30**, 34, 35
   see also TNM system
ultrasound **63**, 64–5
   lung cancer 208
   response assessment 43
   thyroid cancers 68, **68**
unfractionated heparins 151
Union for International Cancer Control see UICC
urine cytology 93
urogenital cancers see specific sites
urothelial cancers see bladder cancer
USA
   Health Insurance Portability and Accountability Act (HIPAA) 59
   National Cancer Informatics Program 56
   National Cancer Institute 4
   National Center for Biomedical Oncology 57
uterine cancer 467–78
   controversies 477
   diagnostic work-up **470**
   incidence and aetiology **468–9**
   pathology **469**
   presentation and natural history 469–70, **470**
   prognostic risk factors 470–1, **471**
   research priorities 477
   screening **469**
   staging **471**
   treatment 473–5, 477
      hormonal therapy 475, 477
      principles 471–3, **472–3**
      radiotherapy **474–5**
      surgery **473**
      systemic therapy 475, **475**
      targeted therapy 477

uveal melanoma **693**, 727–32, *727*
   clinical trials 743
   controversies 732
   diagnostic work up 728
   incidence and aetiology **727**
   pathology 728
   post-treatment assessment 732
   presentation 728, **728**
   prognostic factors 730, **730**
   staging **729–30**
   treatment **731**
      principles 730, **731**

V

validity 43
van Gleson stain **88**
vascular endothelial growth factor see VEGF
vascular markers **89**
VEGF 545, **579**
VEGFR **757**
VEGR **757**
venlafaxine 166
venous invasion 38
venous thromboembolism 151
verapamil, drug interactions **143**
Verner Morrison syndrome **666**
VES-13 **140**
video-assisted thoracic surgery 208
vimentin **601**
vinblastine
   ABVD regimen 136, **396**
   CNS tumours 717
   Hodgkin lymphoma 396
vincristine
   CHOP regimen 128, **412**, **739**
   CNS tumours 717, **721**
   Hodgkin lymphoma 396
   patient co-morbidities **131–2**
vinflunine **350**
vinorelbine
   lung cancer **214**
   nasopharyngeal cancer **520**
   salivary gland tumours 584
VIPoma **666**
virilizing syndromes see hyperandrogenism
visual assessment 44

vitamin D deficiency 686–7
volumetric-modulated radiotherapy 120, *120*
von Kossa calcium stain **88**
voriconazole, drug interactions **143**
vorinostat **412**
vulval cancer 495–502
   clinical trials 501
   controversies 501
   diagnostic work-up **497**
   HPV-related 496
   incidence and aetiology 496, **496**
   natural history and presentation 496, **496–7**
   pathology **496**
   prognostic factors 497–8, **498**
   research priorities 502
   screening **496**
   staging **497**
   treatment 499–500
      principles 498, **498–9**
      radiotherapy 500, **500**
      surgery 499, **499**, **500**
      systemic therapy **500**

W

weight loss 156
Whipple triad **666**
Wilms tumour 785–6, **785**, **786**
   imaging **79**
women
   breast cancer 221–40
   cervical cancer 449–66
   fallopian tube cancer 491–4
   ovarian cancer 479–91
   uterine cancer 467–78
   vulval cancer 495–502
World Health Organization (WHO) 23
   Classification of Tumors 29, 39
   International Classification of Diseases for Oncology (ICD-O) 39
   three-step analgesic ladder 170
World Wide Web (www) 57

X-rays in response assessment 43

Ziehl-Neelsen stain **88**
Zollinger-Ellison syndrome **666**